SCHOOL NURSING

A COMPREHENSIVE TEXT

FOURTH EDITION

Senior Editors

Robin Adair Shannon, DNP, RN, NCSN, FNASN
Clinical Associate Professor
College of Nursing, University of Illinois Chicago
Chicago, Illinois

Catherine F. Yonkaitis, DNP, RN, NCSN, PHNA-BC, FNASN
Clinical Associate Professor
College of Nursing, University of Illinois Chicago
Chicago, Illinois

Associate Editors

Karen J. Madura, DNP, MPH, RN, PEL-CSN, NCSN
Clinical Assistant Professor
College of Nursing, University of Illinois Chicago
Chicago, Illinois

Tracy J. Perron, PhD, RN, FNAP, CNE, CSN
Professor
School of Nursing and Health Sciences, The College of New Jersey
Ewing, New Jersey

Virginia A. Reising, DNP, RN, PEL-CSN, PHNA-BC
Associate Professor
College of Nursing, Rush University
Chicago, Illinois

Tami L. Jakubowski, DNP, CPNP-PC, CSN
Associate Professor
School of Nursing and Health Sciences, The College of New Jersey
Ewing, New Jersey

F.A. DAVIS
Philadelphia

F. A. Davis Company
1915 Arch Street
Philadelphia, PA 19103
www.fadavis.com

Printed in China

Last digit indicates print number: 10 9 8 7 6 5 4 3 2 1

Publisher: Susan Rhyner
Manager of Project and eProject Management: Catherine H. Carroll
Content Project Manager2: Shannon Hill
Design and Illustration Manager: Carolyn O'Brien

As new scientific information becomes available through basic and clinical research, recommended treatments and drug therapies undergo changes. The authors and publisher used their best efforts to make this book accurate, up to date, and in accord with accepted standards at the time of publication. The authors, editors, and publisher are not responsible for errors or omissions or for consequences from application of the book, and make no warranty, expressed or implied, in regard to the contents of the book. Any practice described in this book should be applied by the reader in accordance with professional standards of care used in regard to the unique circumstances that may apply in each situation. The reader is advised always to check product information, including but not limited to package inserts, for changes and new information regarding dose and contraindications before administering any drug or treatment, or *using* any product. Caution is especially urged when using new or infrequently ordered drugs and products.

Library of Congress Cataloging-in-Publication Data

Names: Shannon, Robin Adair, editor. | Yonkaitis, Catherine F., editor. | National Association of School Nurses (U.S.), sponsoring body.
Title: School nursing : a comprehensive text / senior editors, Robin Adair Shannon, Catherine F. Yonkaitis.
Other titles: School nursing (Selekman)
Description: Fourth edition. | Philadelphia : F.A. Davis, [2025] | Includes bibliographical references and index.
Identifiers: LCCN 2024057286 (print) | LCCN 2024057287 (ebook) | ISBN 9781719649025 (paperback) | ISBN 9781719654548 (epub) | ISBN 9781719654555 (pdf)
Subjects: MESH: School Nursing | Nursing Care | Nurse's Role | Nurse-Patient Relations
Classification: LCC RJ247 (print) | LCC RJ247 (ebook) | NLM WY 113 | DDC 371.7/12—dc23/eng/20250206
LC record available at https://lccn.loc.gov/2024057286
LC ebook record available at https://lccn.loc.gov/2024057287

Acknowledgements

We gratefully acknowledge the leadership of the National Association of School Nurses for their dedication, support, and copyright of *School Nursing: A Comprehensive Textbook.* With sincere appreciation, we acknowledge our Associate Editor Team for their hard work and scholarly stewardship of their respective chapters; this text would not have been possible without you. From the bottom of our hearts, we thank our esteemed contributing authors for the time, talent, and expertise they dedicated to this important contribution to school nursing practice and student health.

With utmost respect and affection, we thank Dr. Janice Selekman for her clear vision and tireless determination on the first two editions of this textbook–we don't know how she did it solo! We thank Janice for mentoring us as junior editors with exacting expectations, infinite patience, and good humor during the 3rd edition. In this current edition, we are humbled by Janice's faith in us to continue her legacy of striving for the highest standards in clinical scholarship in our specialty practice of school nursing.

Robin Adair Shannon & Catherine F. Yonkaitis
Senior Editors

Dedication

We dedicate this textbook to the school nurses and school health leaders who use this resource on behalf of the better health and education of students and school communities–Thank you!

Robin Adair Shannon & Catherine F. Yonkaitis
Senior Editors

Preface

Who are school nurses? What do they do? What is their history? What laws and standards of practice guide them? What issues do they deal with? And what information do they need in order to provide the most current evidence-based care to children and their families? This is where I started.

It was the National Association of School Nurses (NASN) Board that initiated the idea for a textbook that would pull together all of the multiple sources of information on pediatrics and school nursing into one volume. It was Linda Wolfe (past president of NASN) who asked me to take on the task of developing and editing a comprehensive school nursing textbook in 2000.

With a host of wonderful and knowledgeable school nurses from across the country, the first edition was "birthed" in 2005 and subsequent editions helped it to grow and develop. Its success is a testament to the authors and reviewers and all the school nurses who have excelled by using its contents. What I discovered in this journey is that school nurses are very special. They must know the evolving state of the science; and they see it all. They are truly the bridge between student health, public health, and education. School nurses address acute and chronic physical, emotional, and behavioral health. They must know federal law and local laws. They are independent practitioners and can stand up to and work with the principal, the staff, the school board, and the community. They must be adept at every skill and in working with students with a full array of health conditions. Most importantly, they are role models as advocates for children and their families.

As with any child, the time comes to "cut the apron strings" and let it fly–and so the baton has been passed to new editors and new authors to take the textbook and the specialty of school nursing to new and higher levels. Regardless of your role within the specialty of school nursing, thank you for allowing me to be part of your journey and thank you for all you do for the children.

Janice Selekman, DNSc, RN, NCSN, FNASN
Professor Emerita, University of Delaware
Editor, School Nursing: A Comprehensive Textbook, 1st, 2nd, and 3rd Editions
Wilmington, Delaware

Contributors

Kruti Acharya, MD
Associate Professor, Department of Disability and Human Development
College of Applied Health Sciences and Department of Pediatrics, College of Medicine
Chicago, IL

Jennifer Adams, EdM, MSN, RN, ACCNS-P, NCSN
School Nurse
Brandywine School District
Wilmington, DE

Edith Brous, MS, MPH, JD, RN, FAAN
Nurse Attorney
Edith Brous, Esq. PC
East Stroudsburg, PA

Vicki L. Brzoza, PhD, MBA, RN, CCRN
Assistant Professor; Program Coordinator Accelerated Bachelor of Science in Nursing Program
College of Nursing, The College of New Jersey
Ewing, NJ

Margaret W. Bultas, PhD, RN, CNE, CNL
Professor
Saint Louis University School of Nursing
St. Louis, MO

Elizabeth Clark, MSN, RN, NCSN-E, FNASN
Retired School Nurse and School Nurse Administrator
Windsor, CO

Yvonne Clarke, DNP, RN
Health Services Director
Klein ISD
Klein, TX

Laurie G. Combe, MN, RN, NCSN, FNASN
Combe Consulting
Spring, TX

Mariann F. Cosby, DNP, MPA, RN, PHN, CEN, NE-BC, LNCC, CCM, CLCP, MSCC, CSN, FAEN
Legal Nurse Consultant
MFC Consulting
Sacramento, CA

Elizabeth Crespo, Esq.
Attorney
Missoula, MT

Sarah Curtis, BSN, RN
Registered Nurse
Children's Hospital of Philadelphia
Mount Laurel, NJ

Katherine L. Dato, DNP, APRN, FNP-BC
Nurse Practitioner
Community Based Practices- Rush University Medical Center
Chicago, IL

Nicole A. DiBattista, MSN, RN, CEN
Nursing Professional Development Specialist
Children's Hospital of Philadelphia
West Chester, PA

Eden J. Donahue, DNP, RN, PHN, NCSN
Associate Professor
School of Applied Health
California State Polytechnic University, Humboldt
Arcata, CA

Cynthia Galemore, MSEd, BSN, RN, NCSN, FNASN
Independent School Health Consultant; Retired Editor, NASN School Nurse; Retired, Director of Health Services, Olathe Public Schools
Olathe, KS

Patricia Gellasch, PhD, APN-C
Adjunct Faculty
School of Nursing and Health Sciences, The College of New Jersey
Ewing, NJ

Diane Gillooly, DNP, RN-BC, APN
Clinical Assistant Professor
Rutgers School of Nursing
New Brunswick & Newark, NJ

Jenny M. Gormley, DNP, MSN, BA, RN, NCSN, FNASN
Director
Northeastern University School Health Academy
Boston, MA

Jennifer S. Graber, EdD, APRN, PMHCNS-BC
Associate Dean of Academic Affairs & Practice
School of Nursing, University of Delaware
Newark, DE

Danielle Guillory, DNP, RN
Assistant Professor
College of Nursing and Health Professions, McNeese State University
Lake Charles, LA

Sarah Hallowell, MSN, BSN, CPNP-PC
Nurse Practitioner
Children's Hospital of Philadelphia—Dermatology
Philadelphia, PA

Judy E. Harkins, DNP, RN, APRN, PPCNP-BC
Assistant Professor
School of Nursing and Health Sciences, The College of New Jersey
Ewing, NJ

Kathleen Hassey, DNP, MEd, BSN, RN, FNASN
Director
Northeastern University School Health Academy (NEUSHA)
Boston, MA

Cynthia Hiltz, MSN, RN, PHN, NCSN, FNASN
Assistant Director of Support Services over Health
Anoka Hennepin ISD#11 Schools
Andover, MN

Molly Hofmann, DNP, APRN, PCNS-BC
Director Care Coordination & System Development
UIC Division of Specialized Care for Children
Peoria, IL

Tami L. Jakubowski, DNP, CPNP-PC, CSN
Associate Professor
School of Nursing and Health Sciences, The College of New Jersey
Ewing, NJ

Beth E. Jameson, PhD, RN, CNL, FNASN
Nurse Researcher/Manager
Morristown Medical Center
Morristown, NJ

Melinda Jen, MD
Professor of Pediatrics and Dermatology
Perelman School of Medicine at the University of Pennsylvania, Children's Hospital of Philadelphia
Philadelphia, PA

Kathleen H. Johnson, DNP, RN, NCSN-E, PHNA-BC, FNASN, FAAN
Affiliate Faculty
Child, Family, and Population Health Nursing
University of Washington
Seattle, WA

Joya Kabel, PhD, RN, ACM-RN
University of Delaware
Newark, DE

Connie R. Kartoz, PhD, MSN, RN, FNP-BC
Professor
College of Nursing, The College of New Jersey
Ewing, NJ

Mary Bridget Kastl, MSN, RN, CRNP, FNP-BC
Nurse Practitioner
Children's Hospital of Philadelphia – Cystic Fibrosis Center
Philadelphia, PA

Sally Lemke, DNP, WHNP-BC
Director, Community Based Practices, Rush System for Health; Assistant Professor, Rush University College of Nursing
Chicago, IL

Megan O. Lewis, MSN, RN, CPNP-PC
Pediatric Nurse Practitioner and Program Manager of the Food Allergy Center
Children's Hospital of Philadelphia
Philadelphia, PA

Karen J. Madura, DNP, MPH, RN, PEL-CSN, NCSN
Clinical Assistant Professor
College of Nursing, University of Illinois Chicago
Chicago, IL

Elizabeth Mattey, MSN, RN, NCSN, FNASN
School Nurse Consultant and Educator
Wilmington, DE

Donna Mazyck, MS, RN, LCPC, CAE, NCC, NCSN
Executive Director, NASN (Retired 2023); Board Chair, Evermore
Fulton, MD

Ellen M. McCabe, PhD, RN, PNP-BC, NCSN, FNASN
Assistant Professor
Hunter College, Hunter-Bellevue School of Nursing
New York, NY

Rachel McClanahan, DNP, RN, NCSN, CNE
Associate Professor
School of Nursing, California State University, Fullerton
Fullerton, CA

Eileen Moss, DNP, RN, NCSN
Clinical Assistant Professor
College of Nursing, University of Illinois Chicago
Chicago, IL

Tracy J. Perron, PhD, RN, FNAP, CNE, CSN
Professor
School of Nursing and Health Sciences, The College of New Jersey
Ewing, NJ

Kathy L. Reiner, MPH, BSN, RN, AE-C, FNASN
School Nurse Specialist
Colorado Department of Education
Denver, CO

Virginia A. Reising, DNP, RN, PEL-CSN, PHNA-BC
Associate Professor
Rush University College of Nursing
Chicago, IL

Nancy Santilli, MSN, PNP, FAAN
Independent Epilepsy Clinical Expert
Sunnyvale, CA

Jennifer Saylor, PhD, APRN, ACNS-BC
Associate Dean for Faculty and Student Affairs & Associate Professor
University of Delaware
Newark, DE

Robin Adair Shannon, DNP, RN, NCSN, FNASN
Clinical Associate Professor
College of Nursing, University of Illinois Chicago
Chicago, IL

Christina Silva, RN CEN
Registered Nurse
Metuchen, NJ

Jonathan M. Spergel, MD, PHD
Professor of Pediatrics; Chief, Allergy Section; Director of Center for Pediatric Eosinophilic Disease
FARE Center of Excellence at The Children's Hospital of Philadelphia; World Allergy Organization Center of Excellence; The Children's Hospital of Philadelphia; Perelman School of Medicine at University of Pennsylvania; HUB for Clinical Collaboration
Philadelphia, PA

Kimberly J. Stanislo, DNP, APRN-CNP, LSN, CPNP-PC
Research Education & Practice Director
National Association of School Nurses
Silver Spring, MD

Andrea Tanner, PhD, RN, NCSN
Assistant Professor
Indiana University School of Nursing
Consulting Research Strategist, National Association of School Nurses
Bloomington, IN

Marciarose Winston, MSN, CRNP, CPNP-PC, AE-C
Certified Pediatric Nurse Practitioner, Certified Asthma Educator
Children's Hospital of Philadelphia Division of Pulmonary and Sleep Medicine Primary Care South Philadelphia
Philadelphia, PA

Linda C. Wolfe, EdD, BSN, RN, NCSN, FNASN
School Health Consultant
Georgetown, DE

Liza Woods, MS, LPC, ACS, CCTP
Program Director and Clinical Supervisor of the AmIOK Program
School of Nursing and Health Sciences, The College of New Jersey
Ewing, NJ

Catherine F. Yonkaitis, DNP, RN, NCSN, PHNA-BC, FNASN
Clinical Associate Professor
College of Nursing, University of Illinois Chicago
Chicago, IL

Contents

part I

The Specialty Practice of School Nursing

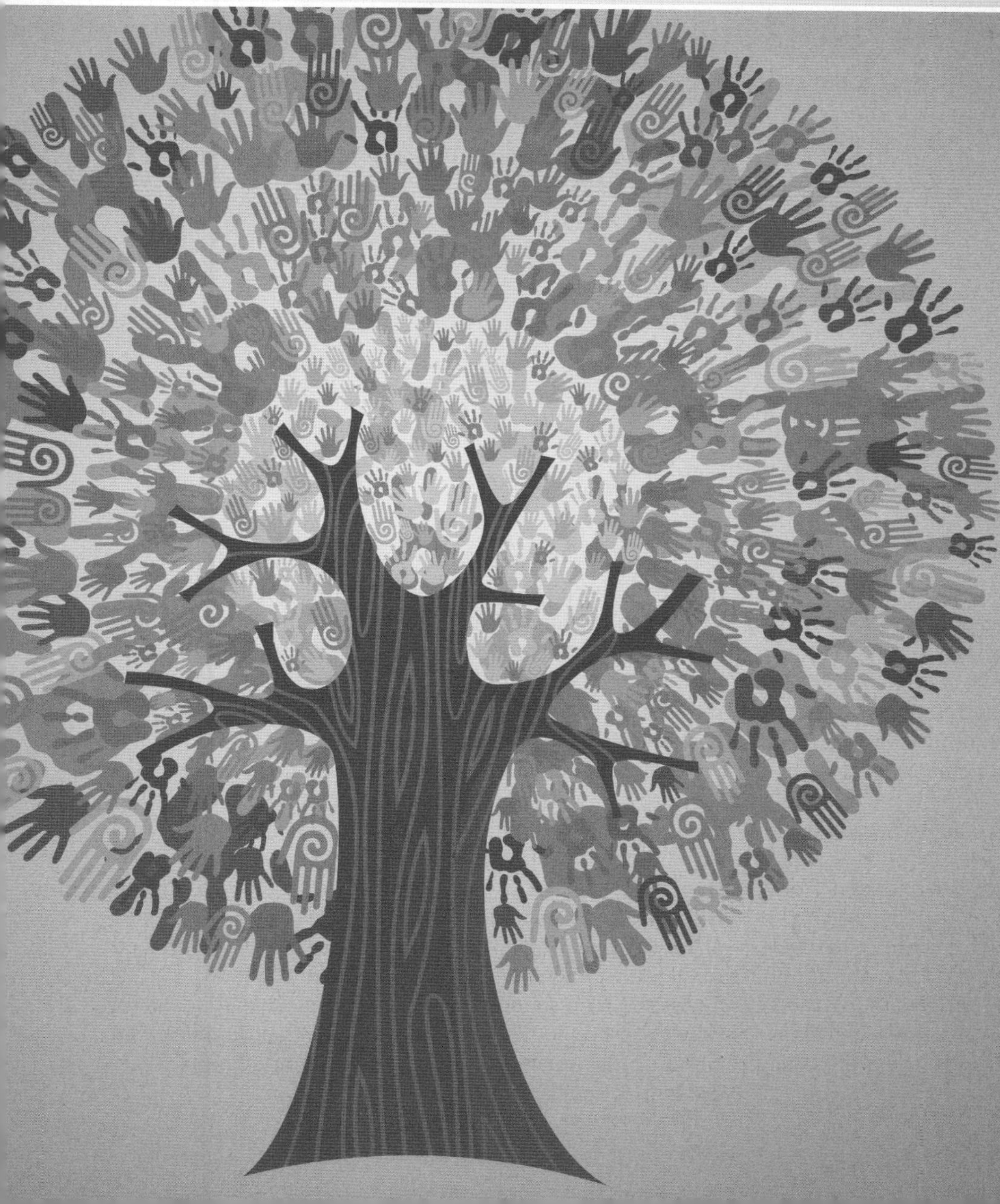

Chapter 1

Historical Perspectives of School Nursing

Linda C. Wolfe

CHAPTER OUTLINE

INTRODUCTION

School nursing is a specialty practice within the profession of nursing. Emerging from the roots of public health nursing, school nursing continues to evolve and refine practice in response to current events and changes in education, public health, medicine, and nursing. The first school nurses struggled with challenges remarkably similar to those seen today, such as high caseloads, student absenteeism, and communicable disease. With the advent of compulsory education, schools became microcosms of society. As communities changed from primarily agrarian to industrial and technological, nursing responded with changes in models of practice to meet the health needs of the school community in a changing society. The evolution of school nursing demonstrates that nurses have successfully adapted to new developments in health care and to social trends and are poised to adapt for the future.

"Those in school nursing practice today share a common bond with the visionary women who paved the way to the school door" (Zaiger, 2000, p. 12). Recurring historical themes include defining and refining the role of the school nurse, determining appropriate educational preparation and experience needed for school nursing practice, addressing the holistic needs of schoolchildren and youth, advocating for the school nurse as a valued healthcare provider within the education and health community-at-large, responding to disasters and epidemics, and expanding partnerships and collaborations. While perceptions of the role of the school nurse by educators, administrators, parents, and community leaders are the subject of ongoing dialogue, the role becomes better understood with each challenge—the most recent being the COVID pandemic. The school nurse leader continues to focus on how to best serve the needs of students, their families, and communities through high practice standards and interdisciplinary collaboration.

EMERGENCE OF SCHOOL HEALTH PROGRAMS IN EUROPE

Global History of Nursing

Early 20th-century nurse historian Agnes E. Pavey (1953) began her book with these words: "When we reflect that birth, sickness, accidental injuries and death have played an inevitable part in the life of every human being who has ever sojourned on this earth, we cannot but realize that nursing must also have had its origin with the beginning of life itself" (p. 3).

The responsibility to care for the sick and afflicted is found in ancient civilizations (e.g., Babylon, China, India, Greece), religious commandments (e.g., Christian, Hindu, Islam, Judaism), and secular entities (e.g., medieval nursing orders). As communities developed, health concerns related to communicable disease arose, especially involving waste disposal, water and food sanitation, burial of the dead, and segregating the sick (Purnell & Selekman, 2008).

Nursing has been influenced by religion, folklore, medicine, war, science, politics, and knowledge. The history of nursing in America follows, or parallels, European models and practices; however, nursing has never been exclusive to Judeo-Christian societies. Further, the profession has been and continues to be influenced by multiple cultures, such as Chinese acupuncture, the curandero of Latin Americans, and the spiritual healer of Native Americans.

European History of Nursing

The foundation of school nursing in the United States is built on the European public health nursing model. A community health approach was recorded from the earliest days of civilization (Chayer, 1931). The first reference to hospitals came in 300 A.D. when the Roman Empire "sought to place a hospital in every town under its rule" and trained both men and women as nurses (Nursing School Hub, 2022). Unfortunately, ignorance about the spread of communicable disease often led to increased deaths when injured and ill were hospitalized together. Without medication, the introduction of quarantine in 1377 was seen as the only means to control contagion (Tognotti, 2013).

Nursing during the Middle Ages was largely conducted by religious orders that provided hospital and community nursing out of a sense of Christian duty or governmental mandate (Nursing School Hub, 2022, para. 3). As such, nursing expanded through the medieval ages as nurses (nuns, monks, Christian deaconesses, and secular orders) were called on for other medical and social services (Pavey, 1953). The Poor Law of 1601 required parishes to care for its "sick poor" (Pavey, 1953), yet during the Protestant Reformation in the 1700s, there were fewer nurses as Catholic monasteries closed and their hospitals were shut down (Nursing School Hub, 2022). Then the 18th century ushered in again an emphasis on care of the sick as hospital-building proliferated in England (Pavey, 1953).

Before the 1800s, "both the quality of care and the quality of the caregiver declined" (Zaiger, 2013, p. 3). Contrary to the benevolent work of the early deaconesses in religious orders, "the secular nurse was illiterate, heavy-handed, venal, and over-worked. She divided her time between housework, laundry, scrubbing, and a pretense at nursing of the most rough and ready kind" (Dock & Stewart, 1920, p. 95).

"Before 1900, most health care was delivered in the home and community. The home was the place where babies were born, old folks died, and the injured and ill were provided care by the family" (Zaiger, 2000, p. 12). As larger segments of society moved from more isolated agrarian communities to more densely populated industrial areas, new health concerns surfaced. The outcomes of illness and injury resulted in absenteeism in both the workplace and educational settings. This concerned not only the medical community but the entire society. Efforts to address illness and the primary causes for absences fell to public health initiatives related to disease prevention (e.g., sanitation, disease treatment, and quarantine).

In 1859, modern public health nursing began with the introduction of the Visiting Nursing Association (Chayer, 1937). This movement and the work of Florence Nightingale catapulted nurses into being essential members of the health community, which soon acknowledged that "with the small number of qualified nurses available, more children in need of care could be reached by utilizing the public schools [to control communicable disease]" (p. 5).

In the late 1880s, Nightingale began to shape and elevate the practice of nursing into one with unique contributions toward patient care. Nightingale initially served and led nurses during the Crimean War (1853–1856). She was appalled by the level of high mortality and morbidity among wounded and ill soldiers for reasons that she believed were preventable. Her vision, leadership, and tenacity to improve health care had a significant influence on modern nursing. Attention to hygienic practices "reduced the death rate in the army at Scutari from 500 per thousand to 22 per thousand" (Chayer, 1931, p. 4). See Figure 1-1.

Nightingale is recognized today for significant contributions to nursing. One was her skill in data collection and statistical analysis. Her *Notes on Nursing* included volumes of data she collected and analyzed. "A master in visualizing statistics," she was the first to present data in a visual way by using pie charts and graphic reports to tell a story to bring about understanding and, ultimately, reform (Rogers, 2010). Nightingale created the framework for what is called evidence-based practice in the 21st century. Based on her findings, she initiated transformative changes in the government's approach to medicine in the army with a "new sanitary engineer system, laboratory equipment, and an army medical school" (Chayer, 1937, p. 5).

Another major contribution was her founding of the first school of nursing using the innovative approach of nurses teaching nurses. Not only was Nightingale's school

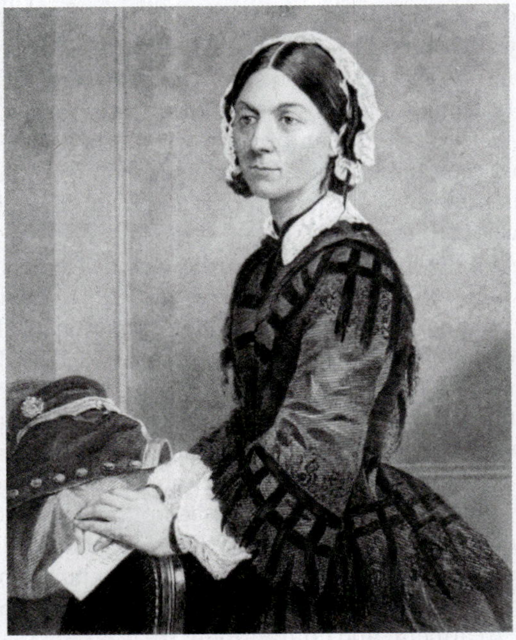

FIGURE 1-1. Florence Nightingale.

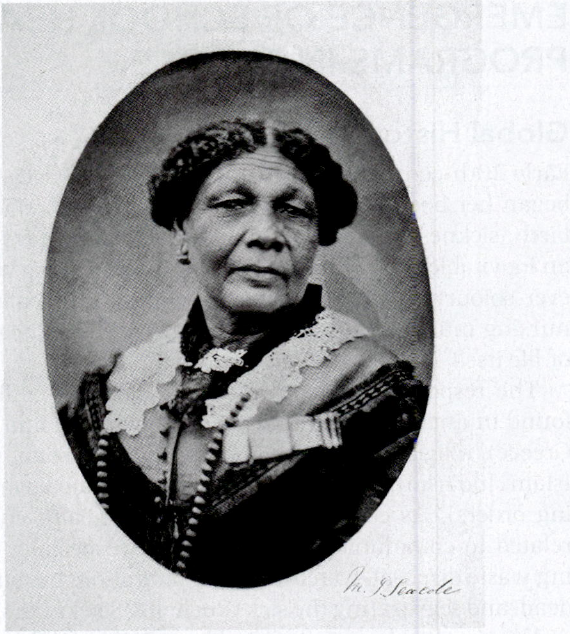

FIGURE 1-2. Mary Seacole. *(With permission from the Mary Evans Picture Library)*

solely for nursing instruction, it was also "fully endowed and therefore independent," in spite of physicians' opposition (Wold & Dagg, 1981, p. 4). Nightingale's "larger vision" was for a "health nurse" who would make home visits related to illness and health promotion (Chayer, 1937, p. 4). Intentional or not, her work set the wheels in motion for nursing to become a profession and public health nursing to emerge as a specialty. She also supported the development of the Visiting Nursing Association in Liverpool.

A contemporary of Nightingale less noted in history is Mary Seacole, who is described as a "pioneer nurse" although her informal training and social status were less recognized than Nightingale's (McDonald, 2013). Seacole, born in Kingston, Jamaica, describes herself as follows: "I am Creole and have good Scotch blood running in my veins" (Seacole, 1857, p. 1). She identified as a nurse and doctress who provided nursing services in Crimea and provided nursing services during pandemics in the Caribbean and Panama. While Nightingale led hospital reform, Seacole, a widow, was a "business-woman" who ran a lodging during the Crimean War for officers, who could pay for services. She was generous in donating medical supplies as well as volunteering and giving nursing care on the battlefield and during epidemics. She was widely known and respected. See Figure 1-2.

United States History of Nursing

The indigenous people of North and South America shared their knowledge of medicinal plants and treatments with explorers of the 16th century, who in turn introduced them to European medicine (Pavey, 1953). This included drugs such as balsam of Peru, quinine, guaiacum, sarsaparilla, and ipecac. The first recorded hospital in the Americas, the Hospital of the Immaculate Conception, was established in Mexico by explorer Hernan Cortez in the mid-16th century and staffed by a nursing brotherhood of the church (Tortorice, 2013).

Nearly 100 years later, the first hospital in the United States was founded in New Amsterdam (New York City) by the West India Company and "intended for sick soldiers and the negroes of the Company" (Pavey, 1953, p. 255). By the 1800s, hospitals across the United States housed not only those with illness, but also served as asylums for those with mental conditions, city poorhouses, penitentiaries, orphanages, and geriatric homes (Pavey, 1953). Pavey writes that "the only real nursing" took place at hospitals staffed by religious orders; secular facilities were staffed by paupers, inmates, or "undesirable" women (p. 256).

Around the same time, the current U.S. public health system grew out of a 1798 Act of Congress that established support for seamen coming out of the U.S. Marine Services (Boston University School of Public Health, 2015). Over the next two centuries, public health would develop systems to protect and support the health of those living in the United States—for example, vaccination availability (1800), government-funded research (1902), mandatory communicable disease reporting (1925), the Food and Drug Administration (1938), the Environmental Protection Agency (1970), and Homeland Security (2002).

The first recognized public health nurses, referred to as district nursing because they were assigned to a district or neighborhood, emerged in London under Nightingale's training in the mid-1800s (Morrissey, 2012). The United States was once again influenced by the English model, and the district model was established in New York City in 1877. In 1893, Lillian D. Wald established the Henry Street Settlement to provide not only health care but also social service and arts programs to the poor immigrant population on the Lower East Side of New York City. Wald became known as "one of the most influential and respected social reformers of the 20th century" (Henry Street Settlement, 2023). Wald, who was a trained nurse, became the mother of not only public health nursing in the United States, but also school nursing (see History of Nursing in Schools later in this chapter).

Early in the 20th century, public health nursing was expanded into rural areas by the American Red Cross, improving the health of children across the nation (Chayer, 1937). After the Red Cross introduced organizations in rural New York and the Kentucky Appalachians in 1896, they argued for rural nurses to be even more prepared than urban nurses because of the "lack of facilities for health work" and the "impracticality of close supervision" (p. 9). In 1912, rural nursing service was established, with 38 trained nurses providing community care, including school nursing, by 1914.

In 1920, noted Black public health nursing leader Adah Thoms urged the board of the Circle of Negro Relief (Circle) to shift from recruiting northern Black nurses to relocate to the south to educating those already living in the south (Lewenson, 2021). This led to availability of health services in rural areas that focused on Black communities. The Circle funded several demonstration projects, one of which was in Fort Valley, Georgia. Miss Hargrove, a public health nurse, provided services throughout the county, including 15 rural schools.

Stories like Thoms's are just now reaching wide audiences. Without them, nursing's history in the United States is incomplete. Missing are the significant contributions of men and women of color and male nurses. "Nurses of color have long-shaped the nursing profession and transformed health care, but their stories are underrepresented" (Uribe, 2021). The nurses of color who changed our history did so despite being denied pay or pension from the Union Army; were denied entry from nursing schools; were limited by which nursing roles they could fulfill, which patients they could serve, and which hospitals or organizations would employ them; and were excluded from organizations and sororities and so created their own.

Most historians refer to nurses as "women," but male nurses were most prevalent until the last mid-1800s (Christensen, 2017). Religious brothers and soldiers were called to care for the sick; further, the earliest school of nursing, which was in India, only accepted males (Christensen, 2017). Yet few are highlighted in recent centuries. Their unique contributions and challenges to become equal partners in the nursing workforce are less known. For example, it wasn't until 1966 that the federal government legalized the awarding of army commissions to male nurses (U.S. Army Center of Military History, 2001). It wasn't until the 21st century that a male school nurse had a seat on the National Association of School Nurses Board of Directors.

History of Nursing in Schools

France was the first country to approach improving the health of children and the community through work with school-age children. In 1833, the French government created school committees "charged with keeping the schoolhouses clean" the following year "a decree was passed that every public school should be visited by a physician who was to inspect the school grounds and make a general examination of the health of the school children" (Struthers, 1917, p. 14). Other nations, including the United States in 1907, soon followed this trend of mandatory schooling and medical oversight of the health of students in school.

In England, the mandate for compulsory elementary education began in the 1880s, yet large numbers of children failed to attend with regularity, primarily due to personal or familial illness. To address this issue, routine medical inspections by school physicians were implemented for the purpose of identifying which students needed to be excluded from school. In London and Liverpool, visiting nurses did volunteer work in schools. Miss Honnor Morton, a nurse and London School Board member, "urged the employment of nurses to follow into their homes, the children excluded from school; to see that their ailments received attention and that the children were returned to school at the earliest possible moment" (Kelly & Bradshaw, 1918, p. 3).

Amy Hughes was hired in 1892 to investigate the nutrition of schoolchildren (Wold & Dagg, 1981). Quickly her role expanded to visiting elementary schools to "treat minor ailments of the children, such as sore eyes, discharging ears, [and] festering sores" (Woodfill & Beyrer, 1991, p. 3). The board recognized the success of her program yet was unwilling to provide financial support beyond the salary of one school nurse (Wold & Dagg, 1981). Fortunately, the charitable London School Nurse Society formed to address the need. With limited contributions, the Society could only provide five nurses to cover 500 elementary schools (Zaiger, 2000). Thankfully, the positive impact on absenteeism led the London County Council to take over the school nursing program in 1904 (Pavey, 1953). In 1907, mandatory medical inspections of children in school became law in England and Wales (Struthers, 1917). Hughes's work "drew the attention of Lillian Wald, who in turn established school nursing in New York City" (Chayer, 1937, p. 14).

ESTABLISHMENT OF SCHOOL HEALTH SERVICES IN THE UNITED STATES

Lillian D. Wald

The implementation of school nursing services in the United States, although a decade behind, was strikingly similar to what occurred in Europe. Compulsory school attendance led to increased rates of communicable infections among students and, in turn, to absenteeism. In 1894, Boston was the first city to mandate medical inspection of children attending school. "Chicago followed in 1895, New York in 1897, and Philadelphia in 1898" (Struthers, 1917, p. 15).

Wald, founder of both public health nursing and school nursing in the United States, grew up in an affluent and influential family. After training for 2 years to become a nurse, she did a short study of medicine at a medical college, but her vision was to reach beyond the hospital. Her book *The House on Henry Street* (1915) documents the beginning of school nursing.

Early in Wald's career at the hospital, she created "a course of instruction in home nursing" (Wald, 1915, p. 3) for families of the patients from the Lower East Side of New York City, a poor, heavily populated side of town with many recent immigrants. During one class, Wald was asked by a young girl to go with her to visit her mother in the East Side. "A sick woman in a squalid rear tenement, so wretched and so pitiful that, in all the years since, I have not seen anything more appealing, determined me, within a half an hour to live on the East Side," wrote Wald (p. 1). She and her nurse friend Mary Brewster set about establishing what would become the Henry Street Settlement.

Wald and Brewster's goal was to bring free (or paid on a sliding scale) visiting nursing services to the Lower East Side neighborhood, where 90% of the sick resided. The nurses recognized the stigmas associated with poverty and sought to provide services in a respectful and supportive manner. Like Nightingale, Wald understood the need to document outcomes. Her 1914 records showed that Henry Street Settlement nurses cared for 3,535 patients with pneumonia with a mortality rate of 8.05%, compared with 1,612 cases in the hospitals with a mortality rate of 31.2% (Wald, 1915). Community nursing services had made a positive impact on four times as many sick people as had the hospital. The next year she was instrumental in the establishment of the first state-level position of director of the Division of Public Health Nursing.

The movement of society to the urban setting had resulted in a "demoralizing effect on public health," with little attention paid to public schools even with the compulsory attendance laws (Struthers, 1917, p. 6). In 1897 in New York City, 150 doctors were paid $30 per month to spend 1 hour a day inspecting schoolchildren. Their charge was to identify and exclude any child with contagion. However, "few received treatment," and truancy depleted many classrooms (Wald, 1915). The "policy of exclusion from school" failed to resolve the contagion, as "medical supervision of schools only meant exclusion from school for communicable or loathsome diseases, and but little attention was paid to the child after exclusion" unless the condition (smallpox, scarlet fever, or diphtheria) warranted notification to health officials or parents comprehended the need to seek remedy. The excluded child continued to play with other children, missed classroom instruction, and lost an interest in attending school.

It was Louis, a local child, who drew Wald's attention to school-age children. Because of an ongoing scalp infection, he had been unable to start school. "It needed only intelligent application of the dispensary ointments to cure the affected area and in September I had the joy of securing the boy's admittance to school for the first time in his life [at age 12]" (Wald, 1915, p. 46). "Louis set me thinking and opened my mind to many things" (p. 48).

Working with the president of the Department of Education and the Health Commissioner, Wald and colleagues convinced them to accept her offer of the services of a nurse for a one-month experiment—extracting a promise from the president that more would be hired with public funds if the experiment was successful. Thus began the One-Month Experiment.

The One-Month Experiment

Wald selected four schools (three public and one parochial) with the "greatest number of exclusions for medical causes" and an "experienced nurse, who possessed tact and initiative" (Wald, 1915, p. 51). That nurse was Lina Rogers (later known as Lina Rogers Struthers), a Canadian nurse working at the Henry Street Settlement. She became known as the first American school nurse and later started school nursing in Canada. The one-month project started on October 1, 1902.

The combined enrollment of the schools was approximately 10,000 students (Houlahan, 2018). During the month, Rogers visited each school for 1 hour each school day, working in the space available with only limited supplies and equipment (Hawkins et al., 1994; Rogers, 1905; Struthers, 1917). In Public School 12, an unused stair closet was the only available space for a dispensary, and although the nurse could not stand erect in the closet, there was sufficient room to store supplies (Struthers, 1917).

The established routine was for the physician to continue with examinations; however, students were not automatically excluded. Rather, they were sent to the nurse to confidentially treat and document the condition—for example, "disinfectant treatment of the eyes" and "collodion to ringworm" (Wald, 1915, p. 52). For those who had to be sent home, Rogers visited the home to work with the mother about obtaining the medication, applying the prescribed treatment, and ensuring good hygiene. Rogers's documentation also described conditions of the home, needs of the family, teaching, treatment, and follow-up (Struthers, 1917). The primary objective of the school nurse was to keep children in school or to have them return as soon as possible.

The results from the one-month experiment were remarkable. "At the end of a month of twenty school days (and six of these were Jewish holidays when sometimes only 30 of 2,000 attended school) the result was more than satisfactory" (Rogers, 1905, p. 767). Rogers's careful documentation showed that 893 treatments were given, 137 home visits were made, and 25 children returned to school. She was subsequently appointed by New York City Board of Health as the school nurse and "an enlightened Board of Estimate and Apportionment voted $30,000 for the employment of trained nurses, the first municipalized school nurses in the world" (Wald, 1915, pp. 52–53).

With the nurse's care, children returned to the classroom as soon as they received treatment. Rogers emphasized that "the saving of school time for the children was of the greatest importance" (1905, p. 766). Thus, the project expanded in December 1902 to add 12 nurses and then another 15 in February, with Rogers as Superintendent of School Nurses. Within 1 year, from October 1902 to September 1903, the number of children excluded for health reasons in the New York Public School system dropped from 10,567 to only 1,101. In 1903, more schools were added to the project. Ninety-eight percent of students who had been excluded for medical reasons were now in the classrooms. By 1915, New York City employed 374 school nurses.

Lina Rogers Struthers and the First Years of School Nursing

Rogers noted the policy shift from inspection and exclusion to cure and prevention with the arrival of the first school nurse (Struthers, 1917). Covering four schools with approximately 1,000 students, the nurse worked closely with mothers and teachers. Initially school nurses worked only with children excluded by the school physician. Later, inspection duties became part of the school nurse's duties. After examination, the school nurse would visit the home to explain the findings and to ensure the treatment was obtained and applied correctly. Home visits provided an opportunity to examine other children in the home, give health education, and address unsanitary conditions (through education or reporting to the Medical Officer of Health). Home visits also revealed that many children missed school for reasons other than illness, such as lack of clothing or food, childcare needed for younger siblings, child labor, and caring for sick relatives. "So the field of vision of the school nurse rapidly widened" (Struthers, 1917, pp. 22–23).

"The school nurse has become the principal's first assistant, the home health visitor, and the mother's friend and advisor, and in some communities, she is the truant officer as well" (Struthers, 1917, p. 27). The school nurse's remarkable impact on community health is perhaps best described by a public health instructor who supervised nursing students visiting schools. Data were gathered on "every available case of pediculosis, scabies, trachoma, ringworm and impetigo to be found in the Borough of Manhattan" (Baker, 1939, as reported in Houlahan, 2018, p. 207). "The response was breathtaking—because it was so meager"; only a few cases were found compared with "hundreds in every public school" just 15 years earlier (pp. 81–82).

Did You Know?

In 1917, Lina Rogers Struthers recorded effective protocols for the treatment of pediculosis.

"Saturate head and hair with equal parts kerosene and sweet oil, next day wash with solution of potassium carbonate (one teaspoonful to one quart of water) followed by soap and water. To remove 'nits' use hot vinegar" (Struthers, 1917, p. 25).

School Health Programs Expand in the United States Through the First 70 Years (1902–1975)

School nursing quickly expanded to other cities: Los Angeles and Philadelphia in 1903; Boston in 1905; Chicago in 1906; and Pueblo, Colorado, in 1909. Less is known of their beginnings. Rogers made note of an "interesting feature" in Philadelphia regarding the work of "Miss Reeve, a colored [*sic*] nurse, [who] volunteered her services for four years to the pupils in the negro section . . . [and was later] appointed to the regular staff in 1908" (Struthers, 1917, p. 33). Rogers's text does not elaborate on Reeve. More is known about Charity Collins Miles, who is credited by some as the first Black school nurse (Seltzer, 2021). Miles graduated in 1906 from Spelman College, Atlanta, and was hired as a school nurse in 1911 to serve Atlanta's segregated schools. She obtained college admission and her nursing license at a time when Black graduates were barred.

The health of children beyond urban areas was also of concern. The United States was seen as the "most healthy of all environments," but rural schoolchildren lagged behind their peers in urban settings (Barnes, 1924, p. 63). In 1908, President Theodore Roosevelt created the Country Life Commission to help farmers with "better farming, better business, and better living" (Country Life Commission, 1909, p. 11). The Commission found that the "rural population is less safeguarded by boards of health than is the urban population" (p. 48). "Easy preventable diseases hold several million-country people in the slavery of continuous ill health," (p. 13) "through poor sanitation, limited access to medical care, and lack of knowledge. They concluded that visiting nurses were needed" (p. 48). Barnes (1924) reported a subsequent 1914 study (found that children in rural areas had higher percentages of health conditions: teeth defects (48.8% compared with 33.58%), tonsils (28.14% compared with 16.42%), adenoids (23.4%

Did You Know?

The first recorded African American school nurse in the United States was Miss Reeve, who was appointed as staff in 1908 after 4 years of volunteering her services (Struthers, 1917, p. 33).

compared with 12.5%), eye defects (21% compared with 13.4%), and malnutrition (16.6% compared with 7.65%).

Expansion of school nursing services in the United States continued to follow the European approach. The Red Cross, the Frontier Nursing Service, and other privately funded organizations brought to light the needs of rural communities and the fact that municipalities were unwilling to fund school nurses. Private health organizations stepped up to fill the gap. Recommendations by the Red Cross were significant in creating the foundation of professional school nursing through a mandatory 4-month training program for nurses and a loan program for those who would work in rural areas (Chayer, 1937). By 1915, 923 school nurses worked in 26 states, primarily employed by boards of education (Kelly & Bradshaw, 1918). Just over 10 years later, in 1926, the number of nurses more than doubled to 2,087 (Tattershall, 1926, as reported in Apple, 2017, p. 137).

Guidelines for establishing rural schools emphasized the need to address and support student health. In Barnes's text *Rural School Management* (1924), she tasked teachers with health duties, such as annual vision examinations. However, she acknowledged that "in those states which employ school nurses much of the responsibility in regard to disease conditions is lifted from the teacher. Teachers will need, however, to keep in touch with school nurses and cooperate with them at all times" (p. 66). A rural school nurse served far fewer children than an urban one, but a rural community had more schools separated by significant distances. These pioneer school nurses visited "one-room schools, making their rounds by traveling the clay and dirt back roads of rural America on horseback, by buggy, and later by car" (Zaiger, 2000, p. 14). Similar to their urban colleagues, the rural school nurses focused efforts on the areas of greatest need. "Thus, the public schools became the centre of activity of the nurse [in the Midwest]" (Chayer, 1937, p. 9).

During the flu pandemic of 1918 (and beyond), public health expanded as a significant part of the medical workforce was involved in World War I. As public health continued to grow from 1925 to 1936, so did the outreach of school nursing (Chayer, 1937). The school nurse was "the most efficient means of reaching the greatest needy population" (Apple, 2017, p. 138). "In some areas, public and private agencies teamed with schools and health departments in providing school health services. By the late 1920s in Oregon and in the Territory of Hawaii, the public health concern surrounding tuberculosis gave impetus to expanding school health programming" (Zaiger, 2000, p. 14). However, in the 1930s, as school nurses' roles expanded, they became "overextended" so much so that the National Organization of Public Health Nursing's national survey, in 1934, found that nursing in schools was of the "poorest quality of any phase of public health nursing" (Wold & Dagg, 1981).

In 1937, only 50% of children ages 14 to 17 attended school; thus, the first school nurses worked with students in grades one through six or eight (Chayer, 1937). As compulsory schooling extended to high schools, school health services didn't always follow. "Too often a boy or girl goes on to college or into the business world with health handicaps that should have been discovered earlier, when preventive work could have been most effective" (Foeller, 1936, p. 617, as cited by Zaiger, 2013). The urgent need to work with young children for control of communicable diseases was not the primary concern for older students. An Oregon school nurse found that in addition to services for acute and chronic conditions, older students needed nursing care for preventive services, health promotion, health education, and mental hygiene (Zaiger, 2000).

The health of young people became increasingly important to the government in the years surrounding World Wars I and II. National Organization of Public Health Nursing held that "vitality of our democracy" was upheld by the school nurse (Axelson, 1944, as reported by Apple, 2017, p. 140). Without a healthy citizenry, the government realized that security of the United States would be compromised. Potential soldiers were turned away at enlistment sites because they were malnourished (underweight). Wesson Oil ads, circa 1936, depict a school nurse encouraging the eating of vegetables cooked in oil and the taking of a daily dose of oil to increase weight gain (L. Wolfe, personal collection).

In 1944, National Organization of Public Health Nursing saw the changing school environment and released a statement on critical services to the war effort that school nurses should provide the following services (Randle, 1944, as cited by Zaiger, 2000):

1. Advisory services to school and community leaders
2. Support and educational services to school staff on their responsibilities for student health (e.g., first aid)
3. Review, interpretation, and follow-up services from health examinations
4. Home visiting services

Practice Connection

School nurses in the 1920s were advised to maintain a nurse's handbag stocked with fountain pen, pencil, small writing pad, notebook, tincture of green soap, collodion, tincture of iodine, white precipitate ointment, absorbent cotton, gauze, narrow bandages, adhesive, toothpicks, small basin, towel, and apron. The handbag "should be large enough to hold the necessary equipment, but not so large as to be a burden" (Kelly & Bradshaw, 1918, p. 22).

Today school nurses should have a "go bag" assembled and ready to head out of the health office to attend to illness and injury in the classroom or elsewhere on the school campus. The National Association of School Nurses (NASN) Disaster Preparedness resources contains an Emergency Resources Equipment and Supplies List for Schools (NASN, 2020).

By the mid-1940s, nurses focused more heavily on health education. "Many school nurses believed themselves to be more allied with educators and education than with nurses and nursing. Some did not even consider themselves to be public health nurses" (Zaiger, 2013, p. 12). An article written by a California Public Health District Supervising Nurse examined the relationship between the school nurse and the home economics teacher (Cree, 1940): "Homemaking courses offer excellent opportunities to coordinate health education" (p. 216). Nurses contributed by "teaching special subjects, as personal and community hygiene, home hygiene and care of the sick, units on childcare, first aid or give classroom demonstrations" (p. 216). Even in the 21st century, some states denote school nurses as School Nurse Teachers, although their duties are clearly more health than education related.

As increasing numbers of school nurses were employed by boards of education, their roles and responsibilities expanded to include both public health goals and educational ones. See Figure 1-3. It follows that in the 1940s, the issue of delegation of nursing care to unlicensed assistive personnel in the schools started to appear in the literature.

An interesting depiction of the 1950s school nurse is provided in a novel by Dorothy Deming. *Hilda Baker: School Nurse* (1955), like the Cherry Ames books, was one in a series of nursing career books for young girls. Deming's depiction of nurses was credited with being "always meticulously authentic, yet ever entertaining" (p. 243). In her book on the school nurse, she introduced a competent, enthusiastic, single young woman working independently at a school under the supervision of a school physician. At the end of the year, the school nurse proudly shared her annual report showing the number of visits (by gender), percentage of students seen, length of visit, visit outcomes, repeat visits, chief complaint, and number of agency contacts.

Health education has been a cornerstone of school nurse interventions from the first days of Lina Rogers, as she educated mothers on how to apply prescribed treatment and taught children proper nose-blowing technique (Struthers, 1917). The emphasis on health education grew each decade in response to the children's health needs. School nurses soon became aware that teachers had insufficient training to provide health education and recognized an opportunity to assume the health education role (Woodfill & Beyrer, 1991). The introduction of the "Health Fairy" and the "Old Witch of Finger Nail Care" are attributed to school nurses attempting to make hygiene lessons more interesting (Brainard, 1922/1985, as cited by Zaiger, 2000). Over the first century of school nursing, health education addressed issues such as unhealthy sanitation practices in rural America in the 1920s, poor nutrition during the World Wars, communicable disease outbreaks (e.g., polio outbreak circa 1950 and increased numbers of sexually transmitted infections in the 1960s), and substance abuse in the 1970s. Many school nurse leaders envisioned their health education role evolving to school nurses leading health education and promotion in schools.

The 1960s and 1970s saw significant changes in health and education as the "Great Society and War on Poverty programs marked a new level of federal involvement" in schools and opened new funding (Allensworth et al., 1997, p. 45). In the late 1960s, Title I of the Elementary and Secondary Education Act "tripled the number of school

Did You Know?

A 1940 study in New York identified the following school nurse activities (in order of time spent): physical examinations, teaching hygiene and first aid, home visits, readmissions, vision testing, hearing testing, conferences, attendance, first aid, classroom inspection, health records, interviewing parents, weighing and measuring, related activities, guidance, classroom talks, dental examinations, cafeteria supervision, notifications, telephone conferences, sanitary inspections, tuberculosis control, gym excuses, and immunizations (*Journal of School Health*, 1940).

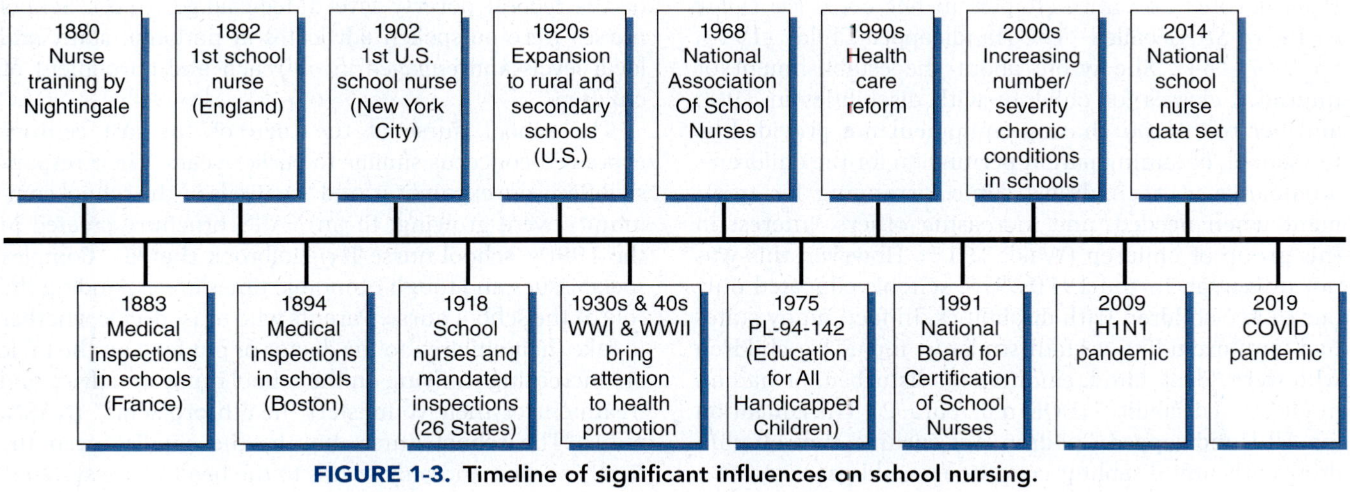

FIGURE 1-3. Timeline of significant influences on school nursing.

nurses" through funding supporting health services in schools (p. 45). Next, the implementation of the Education for All Handicapped Children Act of 1975 (Pub. L. 94-142) (see next section)—requiring schools to admit students with disabilities regardless of the amount of support services required—moved school nurses further away from health education. School nurses began to have insufficient time outside of the health office as students entered schools requiring more complex direct nursing care. It was difficult to convince education leaders of the value of health promotion; nurses were expected to focus on first aid (Woodfill & Beyrer, 1991).

During the first 70 years of school nursing, there was great variability across the United States relative to school nurse availability and services provided. Practices varied based on the school nurse's employer: public or private, boards of education or departments of health, and geography. However, the focus of school health services was consistently on early identification, treatment, and prevention of conditions that affected large cohorts of students.

An Expansion of Individualized Care (1975–2000)

School nursing roles continued to expand into the 1970s, being shaped by school administrators to fit the needs of the local school. Significant budget cuts in education were a factor too, forcing administrators to justify each school nurse position (National Nursing Coalition for School Health, 1995). In 1975, the Education for All Handicapped Children Act (Public Law 94-142 [PL94-142]) was enacted by Congress (see Chapter 7) to protect the educational rights of all students (U.S. Department of Education [DOE], n.d.). Later known as the Individuals with Disabilities Education Improvement Act (IDEA, 2004), it resulted in an increased demand for school nursing services as public schools were mandated to ensure the same educational experiences for students with or without a disability, many of which were health related or connected.

It should be noted that care for children with disabilities was not new to the role of the school nurse. Lillian Wald devoted an entire chapter in her book *The House on Henry Street* called "The Handicapped Child" (1915, pp. 117–134). She wrote about the establishment of ungraded classes for children with disabilities in 1900 and her role in purchasing equipment not provided by the school, obtaining parent permission for the children's attendance at a children's clinic, arranging for treatment when needed, and increasing others' interest in this group of children (Wald, 1915). However, this was not universal. In the 1970s, U.S. schools educated only one in five children with disabilities. In fact, many states had laws excluding certain students, including children who were "deaf, blind, emotionally disturbed, or had an intellectual disability" (DOE, n.d., para. 2). The Education for All Handicapped Children Act ensured that all children with any disabling condition would receive a free education that met their needs. Subsequent federal laws firmly established and expanded the educational rights of children and the responsibilities of the education system. Today, school nurses are members of the team for assessment and development of students' Individualized Education Program (IDEA, 2004).

Health promotion, early identification, and infection control continued to be primary goals for school nurses, but to this was added direct nursing care services for children with medical conditions requiring monitoring and nursing care during the school day. Thanks to medical advances that successfully prolonged the lives of children with severe and life-threatening conditions from infancy through school age, the number of school-age children and youth with disabilities swelled compared with previous decades. Even in locales with effective delegated service models, the school nurse's time for health education was more limited.

Many diseases treated by the first school nurses became rare in the school setting due to the success of the U.S. immunization and disease control programs (e.g., smallpox, diphtheria, measles, and tuberculosis). Yet the late 20th century continued to see conditions such as otitis media, impetigo, impaired hearing and vision, and carious teeth. The malnutrition (from underweight) of the early and mid-20th century related to the scarcity of food was replaced with overweight and obesity due to overconsumption of calorie-rich foods.

In the 1990s, national leaders considered ways to improve the health of Americans by improving the healthcare system; *healthcare reform* became prominent on political and policy agendas. It was a priority during the Clinton administration. Although an overhaul of the system was unsuccessful, one accomplishment in 1997 was a new federal law that expanded health insurance coverage to children without private or Medicaid insurance through the Children's Health Insurance Plan (CHIP; Medicaid.gov, n.d.). CHIP "provides federal matching funds to states to provide health coverage to children in families with incomes too high to qualify for Medicaid, but can't afford private insurance," minimally up to 200% (in most states) of the federal poverty level (Medicaid.gov, n.d.). School nurses were outspoken advocates at national, state, and local levels and engaged in outreach and enrollment of children.

The school nurse at the turn of the last century expressed concerns similar to earlier years. Their responsibilities were expanding, and the needs of the school community were growing. In an NASN brochure created in the 1990s, school nurse Teri Holbrook shared, "Complex social issues and tough economic times are expanding the role of the school nurse. Parents who must decide whether to take their children to the doctor or put food on the table are increasingly relying on the school nurse for advice and treatment of their youngsters' health problems" (NASN, n.d.). "The school nurse may be the child's—even the family's—first and only access to the health care system," emphasized School Nurse of the Year, Linda Salmonsen (NASN, n.d.).

> *Let's wake up! Perhaps, just perhaps, Johnny can't read or write, or add and subtract, because Johnny has health problems! Unfortunately, more children, by choice or default are relying on the schools for support related to personal, health, and developmental needs. The school nurse office or clinic, if there is one, is a safe haven for those minor ills that are sometimes related to major problems outside of school. (Feeg, 1991, p. 466)*

The 21st Century

Throughout its history and to the present day, school nursing practice has been responsive to the needs of school-age children by working collaboratively with other disciplines in order to meet their holistic (not just physical health) needs. See Figure 1-4, school nurse meeting with a parent circa 1943. Randle expressed this in 1944:

> *It is significant that each participant recognized this necessity for closer cooperation among the school, the community, and the home, and among all the professional groups concerned in the program. The field of school health is so complex that no one person or profession alone can meet its demands, if the program is to fulfil its obligations to the child. (p. 483, as cited by Zaiger, 2013, p. 13)*

This is validated today by the Centers for Disease Control and Prevention's (CDC) support of the Whole School, Whole Child, Whole Community (WSCC) model that is holistic and multidisciplinary (CDC, 2023; Lewallen et al., 2015, p. 724).

There have been changes in definitions and duties of school nurses from the earliest days, but "the changes in the responsibilities of today's [and yesteryear's] school nurses are directly related to the changes in the school setting" (Wolfe & Selekman, 2003, p. 403)—for example,

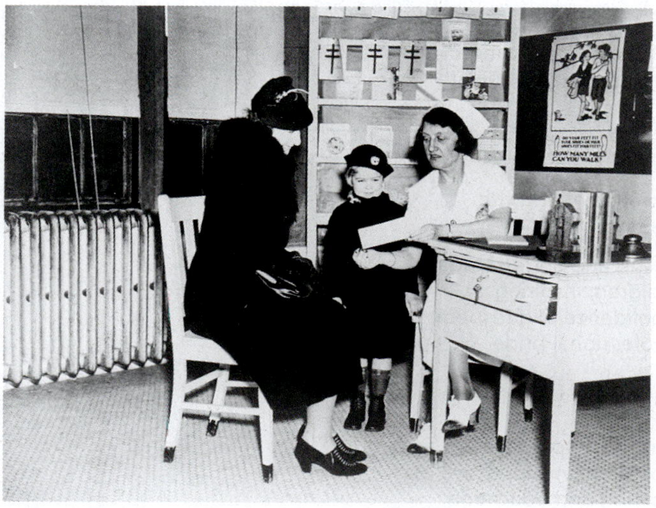

FIGURE 1-4. Parent conference. American education. Yonkers, New York, United States, ca. 1943. *(Photograph retrieved from the Library of Congress, https://www.loc.gov/item/2017877335/.)*

emergency preparedness for school violence or recent COVID testing. School nurses take it in stride and continue to focus on health promotion and disease prevention.

The classroom is a conglomeration of conditions along the health continuum. "In the same classroom, children with acute conditions such as otitis media, URIs [upper respiratory infections], and gastrointestinal upset sit alongside children with cancer, asthma, allergies, attention deficit/hyperactivity disorder, child abuse, and diabetes" (Wolfe & Selekman, 2003, p. 404). In addition, there are children with orthopedic disabilities, sensory and visual alterations, intellectual disabilities, and mental health alterations, along with children who are homeless, live in poverty. have food insecurity, live in a foster family, or cannot speak English (Wolfe & Selekman, 2003). This is the school of the 21st century, and schools continue to learn how to best recognize and support individual needs (and thus potential learning barriers) of all students.

In the first two decades of the 21st century, school nurses played a critical role in early identification and prevention of diseases that became widespread around the world, including H1N1 in 2009, Ebola in 2014, and the COVID-19 pandemic of 2019. In the case of H1N1, Mary Pappas (a private school nurse in New York City) is credited with identifying and reporting the first cases of H1N1 symptoms among U.S. students (Gaskell, 2009). More recently, most school nurses assumed roles for COVID-19 screening, quarantine, and contact tracing.

School nursing's evolution parallels public health's responses to communicable disease. Like the polio outbreak of the 1950s when vaccines and quarantines affected schools, the COVID response in schools is a good example of how external influences influence the metamorphosis of the practice. A Missouri study concluded that school nurses in the state of Missouri appeared to take their enhanced role (COVID screening, contract tracing) during the pandemic with professionalism, despite the stresses, need for information, and additional toll it took on them (Wolfe & Selekman, 2022). New responsibilities for COVID resulted in less time for direct care of students and attention to chronic disease, but increased time interacting with public health departments, community leaders, and parents. Exactly how this will change the role of the school nurse is yet to be seen, but it is likely that the future will see school nurses more involved in public health preparedness planning and more engaged with the school community.

The school nurses of the 19th and early 20th century had an active role in day-to-day education; today, school nurses are less active in classroom health education, but they still provide health promotion and are important *resident* health experts for health educators. The COVID-19 pandemic highlighted the role of school nurses as public health nurses. The early school nurses focused on health promotion and disease prevention by conducting health screenings, primary prevention such as immunizations, and health-care referrals. These activities remain important core components of current school nurses. Today's school nurse is a skilled practitioner who successfully balances the immense number of expectations from the health and education systems. The School Nursing Practice Framework (NASN, 2024) depicts this complex, demanding, and interconnected profession. See Chapter 3.

GROWING INTO A SPECIALTY PRACTICE WITHIN NURSING

Educational Preparation

Throughout the history of school nursing there have been a range of practice roles across the United States. Some of this appears to be related to geographical difference, but educational preparation is also responsible. Like Wald, Rogers advised in 1917 that school nurses should have specific training, experience, apprenticeship, and "ability, keen observation, good sense, and sound judgment" (Struthers, 1917, pp. 227–228). In the 1930s, some state boards of education began to set certification requirements, but nursing programs were deficient in addressing public and community health (Woodfill & Beyrer, 1991).

National Organization of Public Health Nursing took the national lead in the 1940s to identify core components of a school health program managed by school nurses, but it wasn't until 1948 that they called for school nursing standards (Woodfill & Beyrer, 1991). School nursing's affiliation within the National Education Association (NEA) in 1968 led newly formed school nurse associations to require members to have educational levels comparable to those of schoolteachers. In 1991, the National Board for Certification of School Nurses (NBCSN) began requiring a baccalaureate degree for all certification candidates, and in 2020 the criterion changed to a Bachelor of Science in Nursing degree (NBCSN, n.d.). See Table 1-1 for an overview.

All nurses are governed by the laws in their state, including the Nurse Practice Act which establishes the scope of practice and practice requirements for all nurses in that state. Further, educational requirements for school nurses are often mandated by the state's department of education and/or health. Currently, there is no uniformity across the United States, nor is there an accepted standard definition of school nursing, which means in some states anyone can use the title.

TABLE 1-1 School Nurse Qualifications Across the 20th Century

	1920	1956	1983	2016–Present
Credentials/Training				
Higher Education	Professional nursing training	Accredited nursing school; bachelor's degree	Bachelor's degree	Bachelor's degree in nursing from an accredited school
Nurse Licensure		Registered Nurse	Registered Nurse	Registered Nurse
School Nurse Certification		State certification	State certification	State and national certification
Specific Knowledge Areas	Surgical technique, contagious disease, dietetics, nursing ethics	20 hours in education, sociology, public health		
Characteristics				
Health	Good physical and mental health			
Communication Skills		Ability to work with parents		
Personality	Good judgment, good sense, initiative, enthusiasm	Liking and understanding children; inspiring confidence and respect; professional pride		
Personal Habits	Exquisite daintiness and neatness, prompt obedience, simplistic dress			
Other		Insights into education and community; supportive of nursing and education		

Adapted from *A handbook for school nurses*, 1918 by Kelly & Bradshaw; *The role of the nurse in the school setting: A historical perspective*, 1991 by Woodfill & Beyrer; *School health: A guide for health professionals*, 1987 by American Academy of Pediatrics; *Education, licensure, and certification of school nurses*, 2021 by National Association of School Nurses.

> **Focus on the Framework**
> **Standards of Practice**
>
> The educational requirements for school nurses have changed and evolved over the years and varies from state to state. There is also variability in the job description of school nurses. A recent study determined that 86% of school nursing responsibilities in large urban school districts align with NASN's *School Nursing Practice Framework (2024).* The Framework can be a useful guide to guide school nursing practice but must be used intentionally to develop a position description for practicing school nurses (Reising & Cygan, 2022).

A National Voice: The National Association of School Nurses

As the number of school nurses grew, they began to seek ways to enhance the specialty and to network. Before the establishment of NASN, school nurses connected with nurses through organizations such as the American Red Cross, the Visiting Nurses Association, and the American School Health Association (ASHA); nursing organizations such as the American Nurses Association (ANA); and education organizations such as the National Education Association (NEA) and the National Federation of Teachers (Zaiger, 2013). Some of these organizations, such as ASHA and the National Association of Public Health Nurses, had a section for school nurses. In 1952, the ASHA supported school nurse leaders in creating the first school nurse standards (Woodfill & Beyrer, 1991). The most recent revisions were led by NASN (2022b).

NASN was created out of a need for school nurses to have a concerted national voice. NASN historian and past president Peg Rufner (1987) wrote, "During the late 1950s and the early 1960s school nurses were not included in the professional staff structure of the public schools" (p. 2). Nor were they welcomed into nursing organizations. Fortunately, school nurse Sally Williams, with the support of the California School Nurses Organization, convinced others that a national organization was a dream whose time had come. In 1961, she met with school nurses at the national ASHA convention. Their discussions ultimately led to a vote in 1963 for "California to take the lead in forming a National Organization for Nurses employed by Boards of Education" (p. 2). After engaging state education associations in identifying school nurses, 250 school nurses representing 25 states "signed a petition in favor of organizing a school nurse organization as a department of the National Education Association" (p. 2) in 1964.

NEA embraced the formation of a steering committee, but this was not without opposition. The American Association of Physical Education and Recreation, also a department of NEA, argued against the new department, reporting that 1,800 school nurses within its ranks were opposed (p. 2). ASHA and the ANA also "campaigned against the new organization, both fearing loss of membership in their own organizations" (p. 3). Nonetheless, the NEA unanimously voted to create the Department of School Nursing (DSN) on July 4, 1968 (p. 3). See Figure 1-5. The vision "was for a national organization which would represent school nurses as an integral part of the educational community." Yet national unity was still illusive because many nurses could not meet the NEA's membership criteria to "hold degrees and be employed by Boards of Education" (p. 9). The issue somewhat resolved itself in 1975 when NEA restructured and eliminated all departments, including DSN. As a result, DSN incorporated in 1976 and changed its name to the National Association of School Nurses in 1977.

Membership in NASN has grown from 854 in 1969 (Rufner, 1987, p. 10) to over 17,000 in 2022 (NASN, 2022a). It is governed by an executive committee and board of directors, with one seat available to each U.S. state affiliate, the District of Columbia, and the Overseas School Health Nurses Association. As of 2023, all seats are filled, except for Hawaii and North Dakota (NASN, 2022a). Membership, once restricted to only school nurses employed by local boards of education, now includes public health school nurses, private school nurses, school nurse educators, school nurse researchers, state school nurse consultants, and independent school nurse consultants.

The history of NASN is closely linked with the history of school nursing in the United States. As the only organization solely representing the grassroots school nurse, NASN has a powerful voice at the federal level and empowers its members to be active in state and local decision-making. NASN's leadership for the development of national standards, professional practice position statements, and evidence-based programs continues to move the profession forward. NASN was the founder of NBCSN, which was established in 1985, incorporated in 1991, and accredited in 2008 (NBCSN, n.d.). NASN also established a successful and growing endowment fund to support school nursing education, scholarship, and innovative projects.

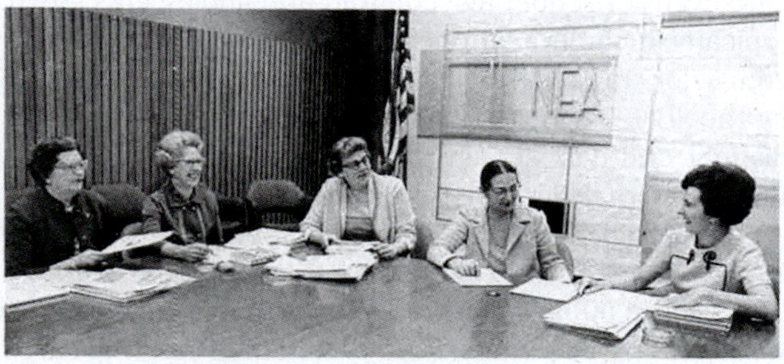

Members of DSN Organization Committee, *left to right:* Beatrice Shaffer, *corresponding secretary*, Johnstown, Pa.; Rowena McAllister, Dallas, Tex.; Sally Williams, *chairman*, Anaheim, Calif.; Ann Garber, *recording secretary-treasurer*, West Hartford, Conn.; Ruby Wheatly, Ankeny, Iowa.

FIGURE 1-5. Department of Nursing organization meeting. *(NASN archives.)*

In 2018, NASN looked back over its first 50 years. Articles outlining the accomplishments of the organization highlighted the consistent focus of school nurses on evidence-based practice, advocacy for student health, and leadership (Kiefner et al., 2018; Wolfe, 2018).

Partners and Publications

NASN has had a profound influence on the profession of school nursing, but it worked neither in isolation nor in a vacuum. Its influence and growth has been significantly augmented by other school health, education, and nursing organizations, such as the following: ASHA's bringing together school nurses under Sally Williams's leadership, NEA's establishment of DSN, ANA's establishment of a Nursing Code of Ethics and collaboration with NASN on the *School Nursing Scope and Standards of Practice*, the American School Health initiatives, and the National Association of State School Nurse Consultants (NASSNC) leadership at the state level of government to support all school nurses in the state.

State School Nurse Consultants

ASHA was also instrumental in the establishment of the NASSNC. Because state school nurse consultants (SSNCs) were not hired by local boards of education and thus were ineligible for NEA (and later NASN) membership, they served as ex officio members of state organizations but lacked a unified voice or opportunity to network. In 1975, NASSNC incorporated and opened membership to any SSNC employed by a state department of health or education. In 1981, its membership stood at 23 members (Burt, 2012) and today represents 34 states. SSNCs serve as liaisons and expert consultants to state agencies with activities such as influencing policy development, collecting and analyzing school data, providing technical assistance to schools and school nursing, and promoting quality assurance (NASSNC, 2021).

The rise of school-based health centers (SBHCs) is also closely linked with school nurses. In many states, school nurse organizations and local school nurses advocated for establishing SBHCs to meet the growing primary healthcare needs of school-age children and adolescents. SBHCs typically include a physician, nurse, social worker, and counselor. In some states, the school nurse is employed by the SBHC. "One does not replace the other. Each has a distinct and complementary function" (NASN & School-Based Health Alliance, 2021, para. 1).

The number of publications and documents increased as the school nursing profession grew. As school nursing "emerged in public health, books, manuals, and periodicals were published to address the provision of nursing care in the schools" (Zaiger, 2000, p.13). All nurses benefited from ANA's introduction of the *American Journal of Nursing* in 1900, whereas public health (and school) nurses grew with *Public Health Nursing*, the official publication of the National Organization of Public Health Nurses. ASHA's *Journal of School Health*, established in 1930 as the *School Physician's Bulletin*, continues to be a trusted resource for the entire school community (scijournal.org, n.d.). In 1981, NASN introduced the *School Nurse*, which today is the *Journal of School Nursing* (Rufner, 1987).

Professional documents served to validate the practice, maintain some uniformity in the design of school health services, and assist new locales in establishing services. The influence of these publications moved nurses *from a task orientation to an outcome orientation* that focused on the needs of the individual client and the local community.

NASN, like ASHA, was successful in obtaining grants and partnering to support publications and programs. NASN examples include Operation Uplift—Better Health for Better Learning, a drug and alcohol education program funded by NEA in 1973; PASS project, a physical assessment skills seminar program, funded by the Robert Wood Johnson Foundation in 1986; and the School Nurse Childhood Obesity Prevention Education (SCOPE) program, diabetes training funded by the CDC and the National Diabetes Education Program in 2009. The relationship with many of these foundations continues today with NASN working on several CDC grant–funded projects. Arguably one of NASN's most comprehensive projects was the development of this textbook beginning in 2006, edited by Janice Selekman, to provide a current, evidence-based resource for school nurses.

SCHOOL NURSING IN THE 21ST CENTURY

A contemporary educational researcher concluded that school nursing in the 20th century was "generally supported" with opposition "almost invariably focused on its expense" (Apple, 2017, p. 136). Many issues today are rooted in school nursing's history and influenced by finances and funding sources, educational preparation, responsibilities, workload, salaries, and ideal employers (e.g., education, health, hospital, or community systems).

Economic realities and political discourse continue today. Registered nurse availability, school budgets, and the influence of health advocates drive mandates (or lack thereof) for minimum school nurse educational preparation, school nurse responsibilities, workloads, salaries, and which students are eligible for services. Leading school health organizations continue to advocate for services that represent state-of-the-art nursing practices in promoting student health. However, without funding, legislative/local mandates, and local commitment, school nurses' struggle to maintain positions and best practices cannot be fully implemented.

"School nursing has evolved from a public-health focus to chronic conditions and medical management" (Tenenbaum, 2017, photo caption). Perhaps "evolved from" would be more accurately written as "evolved beyond."

School nurses are still focused on population health with outreach on suicide prevention, immunization updates, opioid addiction, and overdose responses. Students still come to school with stomachaches and bumped heads, and yes, the number of children with chronic physical and mental health conditions continues to grow. "[School nursing is] about kids who have trouble at home or were just released from the hospital" (para. 3) and is about kids who have no home and need help accessing services from the hospital.

NASN's position is that every student should have access to a school nurse "all day, every day" to "improve students' health, safety, and educational achievement" (NASN, 2020, para. 1). Yet staffing continues to be affected by policy and legislation, from inclusion in educational budgets to provision of health insurance for children. An increase in student enrollment or an increase in the number of students with chronic conditions does not necessarily result in an increase in school nurses for a school. School nurses continue to seek new ways and partnerships to expand services and promote health. A recent example is the expanded role of school nursing during COVID-19.

This century promises to reveal more school nursing history as researchers unveil the hidden contributions of men and women of color. The Johnson and Johnson project, *Nurses You Should Know*, has begun this important work (Uribe, 2021).

CONCLUSION

In 1920, nurses Dock and Stewart wrote, "No occupation can be intelligently followed or correctly understood unless it is, at least to some extent, illumined by the light of history interpreted from the human standpoint" (p. 1). School nursing's collective practice is built on the struggles and successes of school nurse leaders, not only seen at the national level, but also at the grassroots as new school nurses enter the practice to continue the legacy.

"Few histories of school health have documented the critical role nurses have played and their important, although contested, position today" (Apple, 2017, p. 136). The responsibilities of the school nurse "were never clearly defined," yet "nurses quickly became accepted, respected members" of the educational community while simultaneously struggling to compete with financial challenges that "limited, and continue to limit, their effectiveness in schools and communities" (p. 13). Recurring themes throughout school nursing's history show school nurses' innovative solutions and insight into how to best approach future challenges. The world has changed a great deal, but the first school nurse's core value still holds true: "The health of the child is the most vital question before any State" (Struthers, 1917, p. 257). This value was confirmed at school nursing's 100th anniversary when NASN President Wolfe spoke at the Henry Street Settlement: "At the heart of the practice are the beliefs that all children have the right to an education, and society as a whole is better off because of educating their young people" (Wolfe, 2018 p. 250). Surely the time has come for this to be fully embraced by both the health and educational communities.

School nursing history clearly is built on the dedication and determination of wise women and men who envisioned a school culture that would see education and health outcomes as one. These visionaries did not sit back and let events take the devastating toll they might have on children and the community, nor did they let circumstances destroy the profession. Rather, they responded quickly, and even proactively, to position the school nurse as a solution to the problem. The education system did not come to Lillian Wald and ask her for a solution to student absenteeism, nor did the federal government ask school nursing leaders for an approach to reducing COVID-19 infection in schools. Rather, Wald and her nursing descendants addressed the needs at hand and positioned themselves at decision-making tables. Today's school nurse is responsible for the future of the profession. From the lessons learned over the last 120+ years, competence, accessibility, partnerships, and policy will be important keys to ensuring a healthy future for both students and school nursing. It is also clear that school nurses will need to continue to advocate for themselves and their students.

Change is inevitable. The 21st century education system focuses on technology and accountability as was seen during the recent pandemic when virtual classrooms replaced in-person instruction. Health leaders focus on preventive health care as seen with recent social distancing measures to reduce infections. The school nurse continues as the bridge between health and education. Future school health teams will grow to include collaboration with medical communities and telehealth. But none of the changes depict a future in which there is no value in the school nurse who is present in a student's life to ensure that their health needs are sufficiently met in order that the student be able to fully participate in learning and meet with success.

The editors gratefully acknowledge the work of the original chapter author, Donna Zaiger.

References

Allensworth, D., Lawson, E., Nicholson, L., & Wyche, E. (Eds.). (1997). 2. Evolution of school health programs. In *Schools & health: Our nation's investment.* [Institute of Medicine Committee on Comprehensive School Health Programs in Grades K-12.] National Academies Press. https://www.ncbi.nlm.nih.gov/books/NBK232693/

American Academy of Pediatrics. (1987). *School health: A guide for health professionals.*

Apple, R. D. (2017). School health is community health: School nursing in the early twentieth century in the USA. *History of Education Review, 46*(2), 136–149.

Axelson, A. J. (1944). School nursing: What is its future? *Public Health Nursing, 36*(9), 441–442.

Baker, S. J. (1939). *Fighting for life.* Macmillan Company.

Barnes, I. G. (1924). *Rural school management.* Macmillan Company.

Boston University School of Public Health, Office of Teaching and Digital Learning. (2015). Public health in the United States. [Module, Page 8]. *History of Public Health.* https://sphweb.bumc.bu.edu/otlt/MPH-Modules/PH/PublicHealthHistory/publichealthhistory8.html

Brainard, A. M. (1922). *The evolution of public health nursing.* Garland.

Brainard, A. M. (1985). *The evolution of public health nursing.* Garland.

Burt, C. (2012). *NASSNC history 1990–2012.* https://nassnc.clubexpress.com/docs.ashx?id=985105

Centers for Disease Control and Prevention. (2023). Whole School, Whole Community, Whole Child. https://www.cdc.gov/healthyschools/wscc/index.htm

Chayer, M. E. (1931). *School nursing: A contribution to health education.* G. P. Putnam's Sons.

Chayer, M. E. (1937). *School nursing: A contribution to health education* (rev. and enlarged ed.). G. P. Putnam's Sons.

Christensen, M. (2017). Men in nursing: The early years. *Journal of Nursing Education and Practice, 7*(5), 94–103.

Country Life Commission. (1909, February 9). Report of the Country Life Commission and special message from the President of the United States transmitting the report of the Country Life Commission. https://www.fca.gov/template-fca/about/1909_Report_of_The_Country_Life_Commission.pdf

Cree, M. A. (1940). The relationship of the school nurse and the home economics teacher. *Health and Physical Education, XI*(4), 216–218, 273–274.

Deming, D. (1955). *Hilda Baker: School nurse.* Vail-Ballou Press, Inc.

Dock, L., & Stewart, I. M. (1920). *A short history of nursing: From the earliest times to the present day.* G. Putnam's Sons. http://resource.nlm.nih.gov/53730070R

Feeg, V. D. (1991). Disappearing school nurse services: Metamorphosis or endangered species? *Pediatric Nursing, 17*(5), 430, 466.

Foeller, H. (1936). The nurse in the high school. *Public Health Nursing, 28*(9), 617–619.

Gaskell, S. (2009). Mary Pappas is a true flu hero: School nurse spotted first swine flu case in New York. *New York Daily News.* http://www.nydailynews.com/new-york/mary-pappas-true-flu-hero-school-nurse-spotted-swine-flu-case-new-york-article-1.409820

Hawkins, J., Hayes, E., & Corliss, C. (1994). School nursing in America—1902–1994: A return to public health nursing. *Public Health Nurse, 11*, 416–425.

Henry Street Settlement. (2023). *Lillian Wald.* https://www.henrystreet.org/about/our-history/lillian-wald/

Houlahan, B. (2018). Origins of school nursing. *Journal of School Nursing, 34*(3), 203–210.

Individuals With Disabilities Education Improvement Act of 2004 (Public Law 108-446). https://www.gpo.gov/fdsys/pkg/PLAW-108publ446/content-detail.html

Journal of School Health. (1940, November). What the school nurse does. [Summary of paper presented by Mrs. M. T. Fay.]

Kelly, H. W., & Bradshaw, M. C. (1918). *A handbook for school nurses.* Macmillan Company.

Kiefner, J., Cogan, R., & Conway, S. (2018). Power of the past, celebrate the present, force of the future: Part 2. *NASN School Nurse, 33*(5), 299–308. https://doi.org/10.1177/1942602X18792287

Lewallen, T. C., Hunt, H., Potts-Datema, W., Zaza, S., & Giles, W. (2015). The whole school, whole community, whole child model: A new approach for improving educational attainment and healthy development for students. *Journal of School Health, 85*(11), 729–739. https://doi.org/10.1111/josh.12310

Lewenson, S. B. (2021). Rest on placement, take up preparation: The educational mission of the Circle of Negro Relief, circa 1920s. *Nursing History Review (29)*, pp. 163–178.

McDonald, L. (2013). Florence Nightingale and Mary Seacole on nursing and health care. [Debate.] *Journal of Advanced Nursing, 70*(6), 1436–1444. https://pubmed.ncbi.nlm.nih.gov/24224570/

Medicaid.gov. (n.d.). *Program history.* https://www.medicaid.gov/about-us/program-history/index.html

Morrissey, J. (2012, April 9). The history of public health nursing. *The Eagle Tribune.* https://www.eagletribune.com/news/local_news/the-history-of-public-health-nursing/article_7e21c287-599f-5103-af59-be4eb1cdf6f9.html

National Association of School Nurses. (n.d., circa 1995). *Brochure: We care for America's children.*

National Association of School Nurses. (2020). *Emergency resources, equipment and supplies list for schools.* https://higherlogicdownload.s3.amazonaws.com/NASN/8575d1b7-94ad-45ab-808ed45019cc5c08/UploadedImages/PDFs/Practice%20Topic%20Resources/Emergency_Resources_Equipment_Supplies_list_for_Schools.pdf

National Association of School Nurses. (2020). *School nurse workload: Staffing for safe care.* [Position Statement.] https://www.nasn.org/nasn-resources/professional-practice-documents/position-statements/ps-workload

National Association of School Nurses. (2021). *Education, licensure, and certification of school nurses.* (Position statement) https://www.nasn.org/nasn-resources/professional-practice-documents/position-statements/ps-education

National Association of School Nurses. (2022a). *FAQ: About NASN.* https://www.nasn.org/faq

National Association of School Nurses. (2022b). *School nursing: Scope and standards of practice* (4th ed.) Author.

National Association of School Nurses. (2024). A contemporary framework update for today's school nursing landscape: Introducing the School Nursing Practice Framework. *NASN School Nurse, 39*(3), 140–147. https://www.doi.org/10.1177/1942602X241241092

National Association of School Nurses & School-Based Health Alliance. (2021). *School nursing and school-based health centers in the United States: Working together for student success* [Joint Statement]. https://higherlogicdownload.s3.amazonaws.com/NASN/8575d1b7-94ad-45ab-808e-d45019cc5c08/UploadedImages/PDFs/Advocacy/School_Nursing_and_School-Based_Health_Centers.pdf

National Association of State School Nurse Consultants. (2021). *State school nurse consultant role.* [Position Statement.] https://nassnc.clubexpress.com/docs.ashx?id=997989

National Board for Certification of School Nurses. (n.d.). *History.* https://www.nbcsn.org/about/history/

National Nursing Coalition for School Health. (1995). School health nursing services: Exploring national issues and priorities. *Journal of School Health, 65*(9), 371–389.

Nursing School Hub. (2022). *The history of nursing.* https://www.nursingschoolhub.com/history-nursing/

Pavey, A. E. (1953). *The story of the growth of nursing: As an art, a vocation, and a profession* (4th ed.). J. B. Lippincott.

Purnell, L. D., & Selekman, J. (2008). People of Jewish heritage. In L. Purnell & B. Paulanka (Eds.), *Transcultural health care: A culturally competent approach* (pp. 278–293). F.A. Davis.

Randle, B. B. (1944). The changing school health program. *Public Health Nursing, 36*(9), 478–483.

Reising, V., & Cygan, H. (2022). School nurse job descriptions in urban districts: Alignment with the framework for 21st-century school nursing practice. *The Journal of School Nursing, 38*(4), 410–417. https://doi.org/10.1177/1059840520963621

Rogers, L. C. (1905). The nurse in the public school. *American Journal of Nursing, 5*, 764–769.

Rogers, L. C. (1908). Some phases of school nursing. *American Journal of Nursing, 8*, 966–974.

Rogers, S. (2010). Florence Nightingale, data journalist: Information has always been beautiful. *Guardian News and Media Limited.* https://www.theguardian.com/news/datablog/2010/aug/13/florence-nightingale-graphics

Rufner, P. (1987). *Visions and voices: 1969–1987* (2nd ed.). NASN.

Scijournal.org. (n.d.). *Journal of School Health* impact factor & key scientometrics. https://www.scijournal.org/impact-factor-of-j-school-health.shtml

Seacole, M. (1857). *The wonderful adventures of Mrs. Seacole.* James Blackwood.

Selekman, J. (2006). *School nursing: A comprehensive text.* F.A. Davis.

Seltzer, J. (2021, March 3). Charity Collins Miles: First black school nurse. *Nurses you should know* [Johnson & Johnson]. https://medium.com/nurses-you-should-know/charity-collins-miles-ba65c2e234a5

Struthers, L. R. (1917). *The school nurse.* G. P. Putnam's Sons.

Tattershall, L. M. (1926). Census of public health nursing in the United States. *The Public Health Nurse, 18*, 245–312.

Tennenbaum, D. (2017). News: Collaborative at UW, American Family Children's Hospital a "huge blessing" for school nurses. University of Wisconsin–Madison. https://news.wisc.edu/collaborative-at-uw-american-family-childrens-hospital-a-huge-blessing-for-school-nurses/

Tognotti, E. (2013). Lessons from the history of quarantine, from plague to influenza A. *Emerging Infectious Diseases, 19*(2), 254–259. https://pubmed.ncbi.nlm.nih.gov/23343512/

Tortorice, J. (2013, December 3). *North America's first hospital. CEUfast.com.* https://ceufast.com/blog/north-americas-first-hospital

Uribe, J. S. (2021, February). Nurses you should know: Helping change the nursing narrative. Nursing News Highlights: Nursing Leading Innovation. [Johnson & Johnson.] https://nursing.jnj.com/nursing-news-events/nurses-leading-innovation/nurses-you-should-know-helping-change-the-nursing-narrative

U.S. Army Center of Military History. (2001, January 19). Chronology. In C. M. Feller & C. J. Moore (Eds.), *Highlights in the history of the Army Nurse Corps.* [CMH Pub 85-1]. https://history.army.mil/books/anc-highlights/chrono.htm

U.S. Department of Education. (n.d.). IDEA: *A history of the Individuals with Disabilities Education Act.* https://sites.ed.gov/idea/IDEA-History#2000s-10s

Wald, L. D. (1915). *The house on Henry Street.* Henry Holt & Company.

Wold, S. J., & Dagg, N. (1981). School nursing: A passing experiment. In S. J. Wold (Ed.), *School nursing: A framework for practice* (pp. 3–19). Sunrise River Press.

Wolfe, L. C. (2018). Power of the past, celebrate the present, force of the future: Part I. *NASN School Nurse, 33*, 229–235. https://doi.org/10.1177/1942602X18779591

Wolfe, L. C., & Selekman, J. (2003). School nurses: What it was and what it is. *Pediatric Nursing, 28*(4), 403–407.

Wolfe, L. C., & Selekman, J. (2022). *COVID-19 resources for Missouri schools: Lessons learned, 2020–2021.*

Woodfill, M. M., & Beyrer, M. K. (1991). *The role of the nurse in the school setting: A historical perspective.* American School Health Association.

Zaiger, D. (2013). Historical perspectives of school nursing. In *School nursing: A comprehensive text* (2nd ed.). F.A. Davis.

Zaiger, D. S. (2000). School nursing services: The early years. *Journal of School Nursing, 16*(3), 11–19.

Chapter 2

Population Health and School Nursing Practice

Kathleen H. Johnson ▪ Catherine F. Yonkaitis

CHAPTER OUTLINE

School nursing, although its own specialty, is rooted in public health nursing. Public health and school nursing are both based in nursing, social, and public health sciences (American Nurses Association [ANA], 2022; National Association of School Nurses [NASN], 2022a). School nurses use public health concepts when they work to improve the health of individuals, families, and communities using upstream approaches and when they address social determinants of health or conduct surveillance for disease occurrence. School nursing stands on a foundation of public health nursing to practice in a manner that promotes health and provides a safe and equitable learning environment for schoolchildren (NASN, 2022b).

The birth of school nursing through the efforts of the most famous public health nurse is well documented. Lillian Wald, one of the first public health nurses, hired Lina Rogers to work as a school nurse. Nurse Rogers was charged with balancing student attendance with control of contagious illnesses in New York City (NYC) schools (Schumacher, 2002). Her work decreased absenteeism by 90% from 10,567 to 1,101 in just 1 month. As a result, the NYC Boards of Health and Education hired Nurse Rogers to continue her work, and within a few years, an additional 12 school nurses were hired to address student health. Nurse Rogers's extraordinary success was documented through her extensive collection of data, which demonstrated the link between her work and the health outcomes of her students. The impact of Nurse Rogers's work continues today as school nurses apply public health concepts to the care of children in schools to improve health and education outcomes.

CORE PUBLIC HEALTH FUNCTIONS AND CONCEPTS

School nursing uses many public health functions and concepts in the care of schoolchildren and school communities. Therefore, school nurses should be familiar with the core concepts of public health and public health nursing. Core functions of public health include (a) assessment, (b) policy development, and (c) assurance (Institute of

Medicine, 1988). These are often called the essential public health functions all public health professionals carry out.

- **Assessment** uses epidemiology and the nursing process to develop data about the health of populations. School nurses assess their communities through surveillance for health and safety issues such as playground safety assessment and infectious illness tracking.
- **Policy development** is based on the population's priorities, occurs at all levels of organizations and government, and is a form of primary prevention. School nurses influence district policy as well as state and national policy to promote the well-being of students (e.g., undesignated emergency medications).
- **Assurance** addresses compliance with laws and regulations, competence of the workforce, evaluation of efficacy of services, and research into effective strategies for care. School nurses address assurance by promoting immunization compliance, state policies on medication administration, and continuous quality improvement (QI) efforts.

Public health professionals, including public health nurses and school nurses, collaborate to deliver 10 essential public health services defined by the Centers for Disease Control and Prevention (CDC; 2020, para. 3):

1. Assess and monitor population health status, factors that influence health, and community needs and assets.
2. Investigate, diagnose, and address health problems and hazards affecting the population.
3. Communicate effectively to inform and educate people about health, factors that influence it, and how to improve it.
4. Strengthen, support, and mobilize communities and partnerships to improve health.
5. Create, champion, and implement policies, plans, and laws that affect health.
6. Utilize legal and regulatory actions designed to improve and protect the public's health.
7. Assure an effective system that enables equitable access to the individual services and care needed to be healthy.
8. Build and support a diverse and skilled public health workforce.
9. Improve and innovate public health functions through ongoing evaluation, research, and continuous quality improvement.
10. Build and maintain a strong organizational infrastructure for public health.

Figure 2-1 applies the core concept of public health to the essential public health services to show how they are connected.

Public health nursing is guided by the concepts discussed earlier; however, there are other concepts that public health nurses as well as school nurses must consider, which are

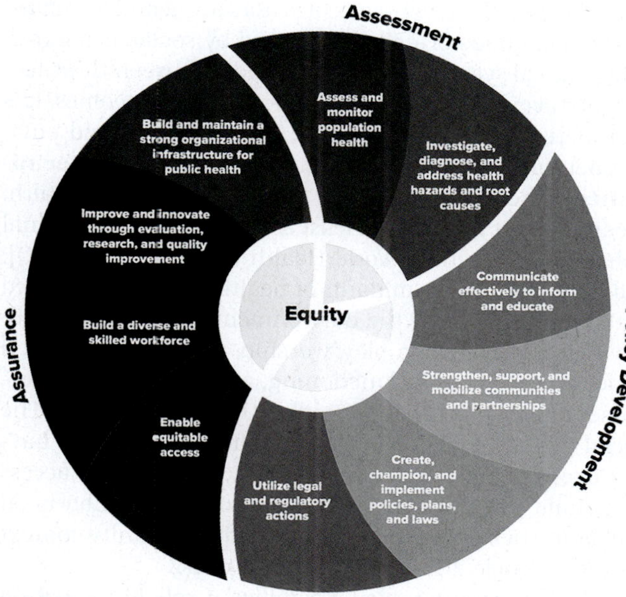

FIGURE 2-1. Core concepts of public health and 10 essential public health services. *(CDC, 2020. https://www.cdc.gov/publichealthgateway/publichealthservices/essentialhealthservices.html)*

Practice Connection

School nurses regularly collaborate with their local health department through assessment, policy development, and assurance. This was evident during the COVID-19 pandemic. School nurses in McHenry County, Illinois, worked proactively with their local health department to establish a School Nurse Task Force (SNTF). This partnership led to the creation of a toolkit to be utilized for navigating COVID-19 in the school setting.

With the pandemic in the rearview mirror, the partnership continues to meet focusing on (1) strengthening the link between public health nursing and school nursing and (2) providing the local health department with a school nursing resource to collaborate on mutually beneficial initiatives (Kunz et al., 2022).

critical to practice and incorporated into their scope and standards of practice (ANA, 2022; NASN, 2022a). These include social determinants of health, community collaboration, population health, an ecological model of health, culturally congruent practice, levels of prevention, ethics, social justice, and health equity (ANA, 2022). Each of these concepts will be discussed later in varying degrees of detail.

Social Determinants of Health

The conditions in which one lives affect health. When health outcomes differ between populations due to race, ethnicity, sex, age, disability, socioeconomic status, or geographic location, it is termed a **health disparity** (Savage et al., 2024). These nonmedical factors are generally related to the conditions of daily life shaped by social, economic, and political systems. When differences between these factors are avoidable and lead to worse health outcomes, it is considered a **health inequity.** Indeed, social and environmental conditions, often called the **social determinants of health,** account for 30% to 55% of poor health, meaning their impact is at least as significant as individual behavior or genetics (World Health Organization [WHO], n.d.). The social determinants of health (SDOH) are defined as "the conditions in the environments where people are born, live, learn, work, play, worship, and age that affect a wide range of health, functioning, and quality-of-life outcomes and risks" (Healthy People 2030, n.d., para. 1). The social determinants of health are often described as having five domains: economic stability, educational access and quality, health-care access and quality, neighborhood and built environment, and social and community context (Healthy People 2030, n.d.). See Figure 2-2.

School nurses can play a significant role in mitigating the health effects of social determinants of health at both the individual student and the population level (Bowen, 2023; Cowell, 2018). For instance, the school nurse may address individual students with asthma issues accessing health care (a SDOH) by working with families to make appointments, find transportation, or help complete paperwork for government-sponsored health insurance (Schroeder et al., 2018). They may also use a population approach to address asthma issues related to the built environment by conducting school campus surveillance for asthma triggers or advocating for school policies around air quality issues related to bus idling or poor ventilation. Through advocacy and policy implementation at school

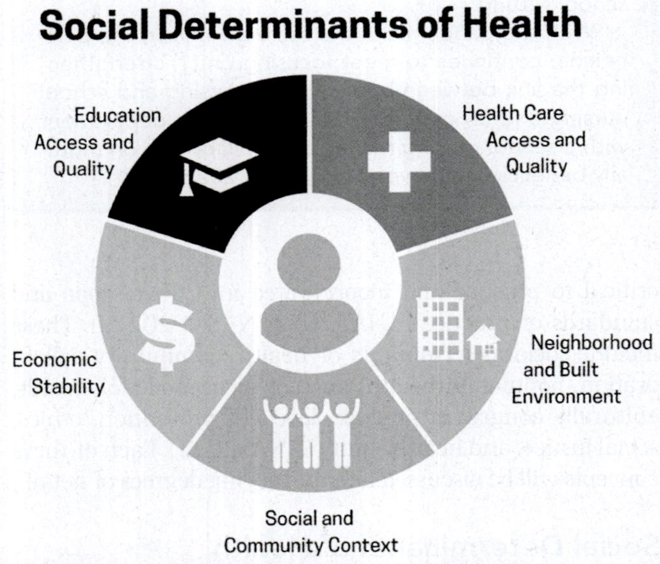

FIGURE 2-2. Social determinants of health. *(U.S. Department of Health and Human Services, Office of Disease Prevention and Health Promotion. [2023]. Social determinants of health. https://health.gov/healthypeople/priority-areas/social-determinants-health)*

and within professional organizations, school nurses have an opportunity to influence the SDOH domains of education, the built environment, and the social and community context (NASN, 2022a).

In 1980, the U.S. Department of Health and Human Services Office of Disease Prevention and Health Promotion launched the **Healthy People Initiative,** setting 10-year health and wellness goals with measurable objectives for the nation. Now in its fifth iteration, it is called Healthy People 2030. The five overarching goals for Healthy People 2030 either directly or indirectly relate to SDOH. For example, in regard to the SDOH domain of Education Access and Quality, the Healthy People 2030 (n.d.) goal is to "increase educational opportunities and help children and adolescents do well in school." Two of the 12 objectives for this goal are "increasing the proportion of children who participate in high-quality early childhood education programs" (EMC-D01) and "increasing the proportion of high school students who graduate in 4 years" (AH-08). Individuals, communities, and organizations can use these priorities to help set their own objectives toward improving the health of the populations they work with, thereby moving the national goal forward. For example, the school nurse's presence can help identify children who may benefit from public school–sponsored early childhood education through child find activities or address absenteeism, a known indicator for school attendance and high school graduation, by reducing barriers to health-care access and treatment for students and their families (Individuals With Disabilities Education Improvement Act [IDEA], 2004; NASN, 2022b; Paulson et al., 2023; U.S. Department of Education, 2019).

Community Collaboration

Communities are people "who may or may not share a sense of place and belong and who act intentionally for a common purpose" (ANA, 2022, p. 7). Community collaboration incorporates the priorities of the community and includes "full involvement" of stakeholders in decision-making "from beginning to end" addressing competing claims and conflicts of interest (ANA, 2022, p. 6). School nurses work with a variety of partners both inside and outside the school. Within the school, this could be teachers, principals, and school boards; outside the school setting, it could be extended families, faith groups, community leaders, businesses, health-care systems, and service organizations. See the Engaging Community Effectively section later in this chapter for an additional discussion of community collaboration.

Population Health

Populations are "a collection of individuals in a geographically defined area" or "group of individuals within the community" (ANA, 2022, p. 6). Examples of a population are the residents of a town or those with a specific interest or specialty. School students are considered a population. **Population health** is defined as the health outcomes and distribution of those outcomes for a group of people (ANA, 2022). That is to say that the health status and outcomes are not those of an individual but of the whole group. Population health is impacted not only by the decisions of individuals within the population but also by social determinants of health (Butterfield, 2017). The terms "population health" and "public health" are often used interchangeably. This is likely because public health initiatives and policymaking are generally focused on a population of interest. Groups or aggregates in the broader population that may share a common characteristic, such as a health condition, health behavior, risk factor, or other health threat, are called **subpopulations** (ANA, 2022). School nurses work with school populations, for example, screening during the COVID-19 epidemic or a walking club at lunchtime. They also work with subpopulations when they offer a group for students with diabetes preparing for college life or devise a medication administration policy for music students going on an overnight band trip.

Certain concepts of population health are foundational and must be understood for the public health nurse to approach care through a population-focused lens. These include systems and upstream thinking, the Health Pyramid, the Triple Aim, and population data.

Systems Thinking

Population-focused health often relies on the use of systems thinking. **Systems thinking** is a term extracted from general systems theory. Systems thinking is a means of understanding the connectedness of all systems and components within the systems that affect, influence, and define a system and system behavior (Hammond, 2010). Systems theory reminds us that a whole is greater than the sum of its parts. Therefore, the health of the community is greater than the sum of the health of its individual citizens (Rector & Stanley, 2022). Recognizing and accepting the interdependence of systems can lead to new ways of learning and sharing knowledge across disciplines. Systems thinking is a set of "synergistic analytic skills used to improve the capability of identifying and understanding systems, predicting their behaviors, and devising modifications to them in order to produce desired effects. These skills work together as a system" (Arnold & Wade, 2015, p. 675). An example of systems thinking is the dynamics of the nursing process with its interactive processes. The systems thinking approach comes naturally to school nurses who are well-schooled in the interactions of systems in the human body. What happens in one body system affects other body systems. All body systems must be considered together in planning prevention or treatment interventions. In the same way, public health nurses apply systems thinking in health promotion and disease prevention activities.

Upstream Approach

An upstream approach addresses the precursors of a problem rather than the outcome of the problem (Distelhorst et al., 2021). The upstream approach is often described using an allegory of the traditional downstream health-care approach versus what can happen if upstream thinking is applied. The story is as follows:

> *Two young men are sitting on a riverbank and suddenly notice a child being swept down the river. One of the men jumps in to bring the child to shore, and just as he does this, another child appears in the river, and the man again swims over and rescues the second child. Children continue to appear in the river, and the man uses all his strength to rescue the children who are being swept downstream. Soon the man becomes tired and wonders where his friend has gone. After saving several more children, the man's friend reappears on shore. Exhausted, the man in the river asks, "Where have you been?!" and the friend replies, "I was upstream stopping the children from falling in the river."*

Many versions of this story have been told in an effort to clearly illustrate the differences between an upstream (preventative) and a downstream (reactive) approach. Upstream thinking links directly to the preventative nature of population health impacting a population or community rather than focusing on individuals. See Figure 2-3. The Patient Protection and Affordable Care Act (2010) and other health reform initiatives have encouraged (and in some cases mandated) that those working in public health as well as all health-care providers assess health in the context of their social, emotional, and physical environment. School nurses embrace a population approach with the goal of school success for all students. They address issues related to SDOH through their work related to health-care access, their support for students with specialized health-care needs, and their advocacy for equity related to racism, poverty, and sexual minority status (Cowell, 2018).

The Health Impact Pyramid

Dr. Thomas Frieden described the many effects on an individual's health that are dependent on factors beyond medical care. He compared them to the effort required to produce change and the *degree of impact* on population health. Dr. Frieden illustrated this concept in the Health Impact Pyramid (Frieden, 2010). The tiers of the pyramid include (a) socioeconomic factors directed at future health, such as improving education and reducing

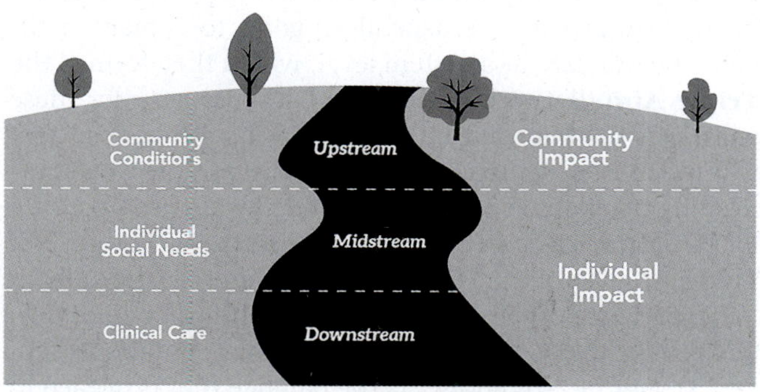

FIGURE 2-3. Upstream and downstream approaches to health. *(With permission from Brian C. Castrucci, DrPH, debeaumont.org, Bethesda, MD.)*

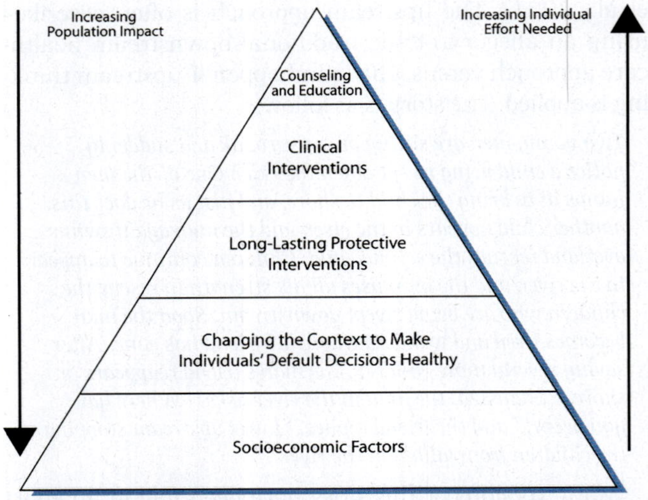

FIGURE 2-4. The Health Impact Pyramid. *(Frieden [2010]. American Public Health Association.)*

poverty; (b) contextual factors that promote healthy choices in individual decision-making, such as fluoridation of water; (c) protective interventions that prevent disease, such as promoting immunizations and preventative screenings; (d) clinical interventions, such as medical intervention to control an individual person's blood pressure or cholesterol levels; and (e) counseling and education about behaviors that reduce health risks, such as diet, smoking cessation, and exercise. See Figure 2-4. The broadest and *most impactful reach* of the five tiers occurs at the base of the pyramid—the level of improving socioeconomic factors (known also as social determinants of health)—with the *narrowest reach* in individual counseling and education at the very top of the pyramid (Frieden, 2010). This pyramid serves as a helpful reminder that school nurses' efforts might be better served in addressing issues toward the base of the pyramid rather than at the peak. There will always be a need to provide individual counseling and education; however, it should not be the school nurse's sole focus.

The Triple Aim

In 2008, the president and CEO of the Institute for Healthcare Improvement, Dr. Donald Berwick, and his colleagues introduced broad, interdependent goals to achieve high-value health care at a system level, which they termed the **Triple Aim** (Berwick et al., 2008). The impetus for these goals was the knowledge that the U.S. health-care system was the most expensive in the world but also the worst performing compared with other Western countries (Institute for Healthcare Improvement [IHI], 2023). See Figure 2-5. The three goals of the Triple Aim are to improve the individual experience of care, improve the health of populations, and reduce the per capita cost of care for populations (IHI, 2023). Figure 2-6 represents the balance that is needed to achieve the Triple Aim. Bodenheimer and Sinsky (2014) proposed adding a fourth goal to this framework, making it

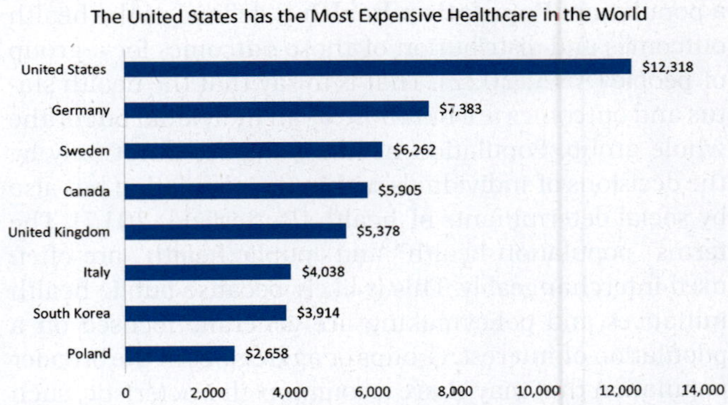

FIGURE 2-5. U.S. health-care expenditures. *(Adapted from https://cdn.statcdn.com/Infographic/images/normal/8658.jpeg)*

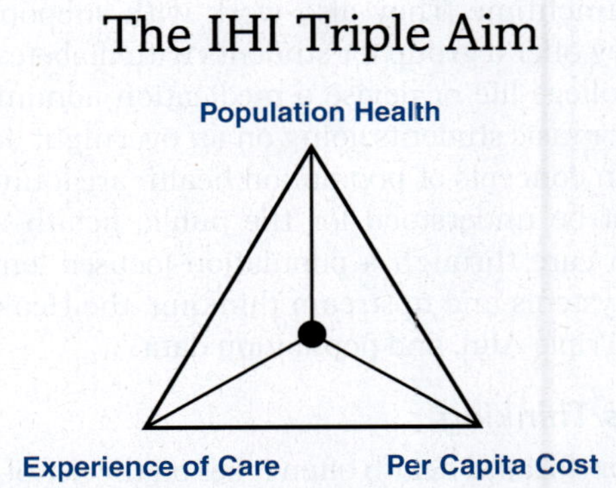

FIGURE 2-6. The Triple Aim. *(Institute for Healthcare Improvement [2023].)*

a Quadruple Aim. They suggest that the fourth goal should be to improve the lives of health-care providers. Improving the experience of providing care recognizes the impact of increasing levels of burnout and employee fatigue. More recently, further expansion to a quintuple aim has been suggested (Nundy et al., 2022). This fifth aim would add health equity to improve quality health care.

Population Health Data

Population health data is considered **big data,** a phrase that describes large, diverse amounts of data that can be studied using powerful computing software (IEEE, n.d.). Big data collection is an emerging trend in health care propelled into existence with the use of electronic medical records that collect and store multiple data points for every patient or client. The use of big data is focused on uncovering new information that can improve care. Big data pools information from patient and provider interactions to allow analysis and understanding of complex patient conditions through the sheer volume, speed, and variety of information that can be gathered and aggregated in electronic documentation systems (Wilson et al., 2017).

Population health is advanced through the aggregation of large data sets with common variables and definitions. This may include data collected by large health systems or government organizations such as the Centers for Medicare and Medicaid Services. In school nursing, population data is collected through NASN's *National School Health Dataset: Every Student Counts!* (ESC!; NASN, 2019). *Every Student Counts!* includes uniform data points and a data collection platform that allows every school in the nation to report their de-identified and aggregated data. NASN further aggregates the state-level data and reports it nationally. School nurses collect data on every student in their school—those who are well and those with chronic health conditions (e.g., through screenings, medication administration). The documentation in school nurses' records contains the most comprehensive dataset on the health of school-age children and thus lays the foundation for understanding the health needs of students and the ways that school nurses meet those needs at a population level.

Culturally Congruent Practice

Incorporating culturally sensitive practices in nursing care can improve health outcomes. The CDC's National Prevention Information Network (NPIN) defines **culture** as the "integrated patterns of human behavior that include the language, thoughts, communications, actions, customs, beliefs, values, and institutions of racial, ethnic, religious, or social groups" (NPIN, 2021, p. 1). Public health nurses integrate the "preferred cultural values, beliefs, worldview, and practices" of their clients through the application of cultural competence, sensitivity, humility, and safety (ANA, 2022, p. 11). **Cultural competence** is "a set of congruent behaviors, attitudes, and policies that come together in a system, agency, or among professionals that enables effective work in cross-cultural situations" (NPIN, 2021, p. 1). **Cultural sensitivity** describes the "ability to be open and responsive to attitudes, feelings or life circumstances" of people who practice a culture that is different from one's own whereas, **cultural humility** is a "humble and respectful attitude" that promotes lifelong learning and self-reflection on "one's own cultural biases" with the realization that we can only be experts on our own culture (ANA, 2022, p. 111).

Understanding the cultural practices of families, combined with a sense of cultural humility, builds capacity for community members' sense of safety, better communication about care, and thus more effective outcomes of care. Curtis et al. (2019) did a literature review of the importance of cultural safety to achieving health equity. They describe cultural competence as being too "narrow," and they bring attention to the "inherent power imbalance" and "othering" that may occur in merely applying cultural knowledge to care (Curtis et al., 2019, p. 13). Curtis et al. recognize that cultural competence occurs at an individual, organizational, and systems level and on a continuum from cultural safety to cultural destructiveness. Their definition of *cultural safety* therefore "encompasses a critical consciousness where healthcare professionals and healthcare organizations engage in ongoing self-reflection and self-awareness and hold themselves accountable for providing culturally safe care, as defined by the patient and their communities, and as measured through progress towards achieving health equity" (Curtis et al., 2019, p. 14). See Chapter 10 for further discussion of culturally effective school nursing care.

Did You Know?

The County Health Rankings and Roadmaps (CHR&R) program uses population-level data to quantify the impact of various factors on individual health outcomes (CHR&R, 2022). The Rankings show demographic information and provide comparisons between county, state, and national data. In addition, the CHR&R identifies successful policies and programs, details health factors, and identifies the health outcomes of Quality of Life and Length of Life. The Health Factors are broken down into four factors that influence health, and each factor is further broken down into measures of that factor. The factors include the following:

1. *Physical Environment*, which accounts for 10% of health outcomes and includes air and water quality, housing, and transit.
2. *Social and Economic Factors*, which account for 40% of health outcomes and include education, employment, income, family and social support, and community safety.
3. *Clinical Care*, which accounts for 20% of health measures such as access to care and its quality.
4. *Health Behaviors*, which account for 30% of health outcomes and include tobacco, diet and exercise, alcohol and drug use, and sexual activity.

The County Health Rankings provide aggregated data on these health factors for each U.S. county, thus providing school nurses with data specific to their school community. It also includes numerous reports on health topics and examples of effective policies and programs that could be implemented.

Levels of Prevention

The three levels of prevention are primary, secondary, and tertiary prevention (Merck Manual Consumer Version, 2022). **Primary prevention** is the prevention of disease and injury through activities such as management of immunization compliance and policy advocacy. **Secondary prevention** is the early detection of disease to minimize more acute disease or injury through surveillance for signs and symptoms of disease such as vision, hearing, and dental health screenings. **Tertiary prevention** is the management of chronic disease to prevent complications such as through medication management and coordination of care for individuals with chronic health conditions. Examples of how the levels of prevention apply to school nursing can be found in Table 2-1.

TABLE 2-1 Levels of Prevention in School Nursing

Prevention Level/Definition	Sample Strategies
Primary Prevention—Occurs before any disease or injury; includes two elements: 1. Health Promotion—Measures to promote optimal health. 2. Specific Protection—Measures to protect humans against disease or establish barriers against agents in the environment.	• Health education regarding health maintenance/enhancement (school health curriculum, health fairs) • Food and nutrition programs (serving school breakfast and lunch, weekend backpack program) • Immunizations (influenza, childhood vaccinations) • Environmental safety standards (pollution prevention—no-idling policy, maintenance of school physical plant) • Safety programs (playground safety, seatbelt campaigns, bike helmets, swimming safety)
Secondary Prevention—Occurs early in the disease process and includes two goals: 1. Early detection (diagnosis) and prompt treatment 2. Disability limitation	• Screening programs (vision and hearing, scoliosis, blood lead, body mass index, hypertension, health risk appraisal) • Case finding (following up and testing known contacts for COVID-19) • Self-detection (breast and testicular self-examination; use of smoke and home radon and/or carbon monoxide detectors • Periodic visits to health-care providers • Teaching self-care (diet, medication) • Compliance with prescribed treatment regimen (carb counting, taking prescribed medications) • Ongoing surveillance and monitoring (monthly blood pressure checks, daily blood glucose monitoring for diabetics)
Tertiary Prevention—Occurs when a defect or disability remains; the focus is on: 1. Rehabilitation 2. Supportive care for the dying and bereaved	• Rehabilitation programs • Adapted/barrier-free schools for students with physical disabilities • Inclusion of students with disabilities in general education classrooms • Support groups for bereaved students, staff, families

Adapted from CDC Colorectal Cancer Program Social Ecological Model (2015).

Ethics

All nurses are guided by the *ANA Code of Ethics* (ANA, 2015). School nurses also have the *School Nursing Code of Ethics* to guide their practice (NASN, 2021). Ethical practice includes the *precautionary principle*, which is a guide for decision-making "that, in the absence of sufficient scientific evidence," endorses "caution and avoidance of unnecessary risk" (ANA, 2022, p. 113). Ethical practice requires lifelong learning and a commitment to self-reflection and humility. There are several ethical models that can guide nurses in their practice, including "the Four Quadrant approach, the MORAL model, the DECIDE Model, the Framework for Ethical Decision-Making, and the Making Ethical Decisions—7-Step Path" (NASN, 2022a, p. 23). A collection of ethical analysis models/resources is available in online materials called OM 2-1.

Social Justice

Public health nurses define the **social justice** core concept as one that "engages in social criticism and social change," focuses on "analysis, critique, and change of social structure, policies, laws, customs, power, and privilege that disadvantage or harm vulnerable social groups through marginalization, exclusion, exploitation, and voicelessness" (ANA, 2022, p. 25). The pursuit of social justice is essential to ethical nursing practice, especially for school nurses who practice at the center of both health and education, which are critical influences on a student's future health. "School nurses have a window into the lives of children from every race, culture, religion, gender identity, economic status, and belief system," providing them with a "unique and profound opportunity" to support child health and well-being (NASN, 2022a, pp. 25–26).

Health Equity

Health equity means that every person has the ability to achieve "their full potential for health and well-being" (WHO, n.d., p. 1). It is the "absence of unfair, avoidable or remediable differences" in health whether in the form of social, demographic, geographic, or other forms of inequality (WHO, n.d., p. 1). Health equity occurs when the social determinants of health (SDOH) do not interfere with good health. Education and access to health care are key components of SDOH that school nurses have a significant opportunity to influence.

ENGAGING COMMUNITIES EFFECTIVELY

The process of working with communities includes understanding cultural influences, community engagement, models and frameworks for action in communities, and continuous evaluation of the effects of interventions on equitable health outcomes. Engaging with communities requires knowledge of models for engagement and systems theory. Previous efforts to support the health of communities often used a "top-down" or "expert" approach, which, in many cases, failed to account for the norms, values, and cultural practices of communities. Successful interventions for the health of communities require the integration of these concepts and partnerships with communities and their leaders. Working successfully with diverse communities requires lifelong learning and personal humility with self-reflection on one's strengths and biases regarding race and social justice. See Chapter 10 for a discussion of diversity, equity, and inclusion.

Community Engagement Concepts

Community engagement, which advances health equity, is "the process of working collaboratively with groups of people who are affiliated by geographic proximity, special interests, or similar situations with respect to issues affecting their well-being" (National Institutes of Health [NIH], 2011, p. xv). The CDC identifies community engagement as a key element to improve the health of communities. Effective community health improvement strategies include four concepts: (a) working together, (b) engaging the community, (c) communication, and (d) sustaining results (CDC, 2022b). The engagement process includes five steps (that align with the nursing process):

- Assess needs and resources.
- Focus on what is important.
- Choose effective policies and programs.
- Act on what is important.
- Evaluate the actions taken (CDC, 2022b).

The NIH created a free online *Principles of Community Engagement* resource highlighting the process and providing field examples for those wishing to learn more (NIH, 2011).

Coalition Building

Population-focused care requires that nurses engage with a variety of communities to support the health of the population of interest. When groups within the community are brought together, they are often called coalitions. **Coalitions** are temporary alliances formed to support shared action (Merriam-Webster, n.d.-a). Collaborative connections of groups with similar goals strengthen the potential for reaching the desired outcome. **Stakeholders** are people and groups that are "affected by a course of action" (Merriam-Webster, n.d.-b). The types of communities and organizations (stakeholders) that can be called on to support an initiative depend on the population's needs and the resources available in an individual community. Essential to working with stakeholders in those communities is the ability to effectively convey the population's needs in terms of how they align with various stakeholder interests (Johnson, 2019). An important step in organizing a coalition is to "map" stakeholders. The process of mapping stakeholders includes identifying relevant stakeholders, understanding their position on a given topic, identifying how their goals and interests align or conflict with the population's needs, developing strategies for communicating common interests, and helping the nurse find common ground for collaborative work (Johnson, 2019). Stakeholders' positions may address their level of interest in your proposal, their concern about how the topic may affect their work, and their level of influence—information that can guide the nurse in identifying points of agreement and points where negotiation may be needed. Table 2-2 describes how various stakeholders might respond to a proposal to support students with type 1 diabetes.

Messaging Effectively With Stakeholders

Ranadive (2017) describes the components of a "sticky message" that audiences pay attention to, understand, remember, believe in, care about, and act on. To make a message stick, it must be simple, unexpected, concrete, and credible; evoke an emotional response; and be accompanied by a relevant story. "When a message is Simple, people Understand it. When it is Unexpected, they Pay Attention to it. When it is Concrete, they Remember it. When it is Credible, they Believe it. When it evokes Emotion, they Care about it, and when it has a Story, they are more likely to Act" (Johnson, 2019, p. 342).

Models of Community Engagement

The Social Ecological Model of Health

The *social ecological model* is a theory-based framework that assists in identifying behavioral and organizational focal points for initiating behavioral changes to improve health in populations. The assumption on which the model is based is that health behaviors are determined through interactions of an individual with environments at different levels, and the multiple levels of influence interact across levels. Within the framework are four hierarchical levels within a social system: individual, relationship, community, and societal (CDC, 2015). The social ecological model enables recognition and understanding of factors that affect human behaviors. There are multiple levels of influence and social environments that shape behavior, and they are also shaped by behavior. See Figure 2-7.

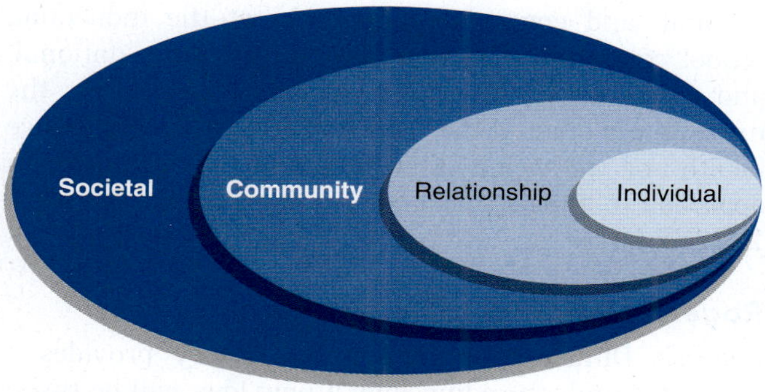

FIGURE 2-7. Social ecological model. *(CDC, 2015.)*

TABLE 2-2 Mapping Your Message: Increasing Nurse FTE* for Students With Type 1 Diabetes (T1D)

Stakeholder	Interest in Idea	Concern	Level of Influence	Position on Idea	Message Strategy
Principals	Low	Cost	High	Undeveloped	Promote interest by sharing benefits—decreased liability; parents more confident in safety; office staff more efficient
Teachers	High	Safety/ workload	Low	Supporters	Promote sharing stories of times when they were worried about T1D safety
Parents	High	Safety	Low	Supporters	Promote sharing stories of complexity of care, uncertainty about staff skill in T1D management
District Risk Management	High	Safety/ liability	High	Advocates	Promote sharing perspective on liability, safety concerns, enlist their help with administrators
Endocrinology Medical Clinic	High	Health outcomes; improved management	Low	Supporters	Request letters of support with information on potential consequences, differences noted in full- vs. part-time nurse FTE
Other Parents	Low	Cost; own child's safety	Low	Neutral	Share stories of rising numbers of students with T1D and other chronic conditions; benefits of additional nurse time for health promotion; share stories of sudden onset of some chronic conditions

FTE, Full time equivalent.
Johnson (2019), with permission.

Moving from individuals to groups, communities, and populations, public health nursing focuses on a broad view of health. Understanding how public health is administered at all three levels can be visualized using the Minnesota Intervention Wheel that defines the activities of public health professionals (Minnesota Department of Health, 2017). The Wheel identifies and defines nursing interventions at the individual/family, community, and systems levels. See Figure 2-8. School nursing practice spans from local to global to meet the needs of their school communities (NASN, 2022a). See Table 2-3.

The wide array of community stakeholders the nurse may collaborate with can be organized according to the social ecological model, including the private, organizational, and governmental entities at the individual, school community, broader community, state, national, and global levels. An ecological perspective allows the nurse to understand the "range of factors that influence health and well-being" that includes using an upstream approach to impact social determinants of health (ANA, 2022, p. 112).

Rogers's Diffusion of Innovation

Rogers's Diffusion of Innovation Theory provides a rubric for understanding how a new idea will be taken up, along with strategies for interfacing with each

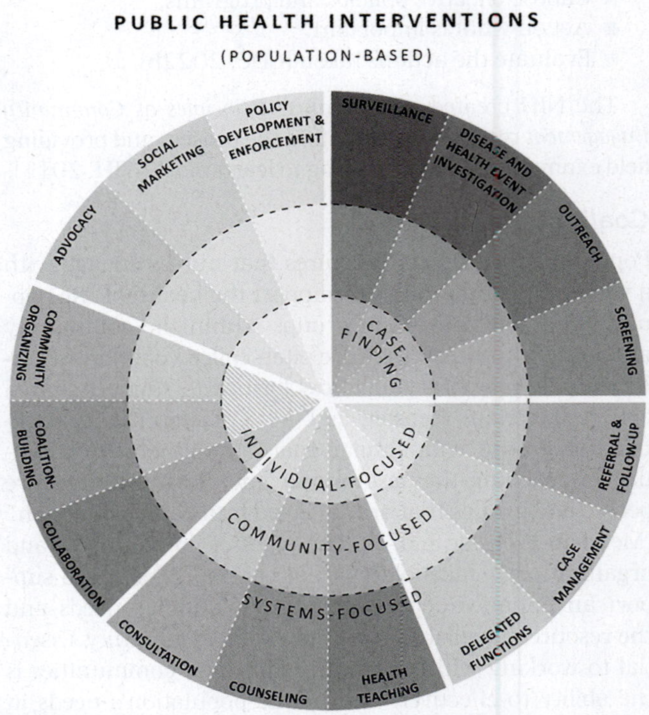

FIGURE 2-8. Minnesota wheel of public health interventions. *(Minnesota Department of Health. [2017]. Public health interventions [population-based]. https://www.health.state.mn.us/communities/practice/research/phncouncil/docs/PHInterventionsHandout.pdf)*

TABLE 2-3 Local to Global School Nursing Practice

Setting	Example
Local	Public, private, or parochial school
Regional	Regional office of education or county health department
State	State School Nurse Consultant; State Nurse Association
National	National Association of School Nurses, government agency or program (e.g., Healthy Schools Campaign, Robert Wood Johnson Foundation)
Global	International health agencies (e.g., WHO, United Nations International Children's Emergency Fund)

Adapted from National Association of School Nurses (2022a).

group—innovators, early adopters, early majority, late adopters, and laggards (CDC, 2015). The continuum spans from *innovators*, the first to try a new idea with little prompting, to *laggards*, who are generally conservative in thought, bound by tradition, and the hardest to persuade (Boston University School of Public Health, 2019). Figure 2-9 visually highlights the components of Rogers's Diffusion of Innovation.

Community-Based Participatory Research/Action

Community-Based Participatory Research/Action (CBPR/A) holds that researchers and community members "respect the strengths that each brings to the partnership, and the community participates fully in all aspects of the research process . . . to achieve social change to improve health outcomes and eliminate health disparities" (CDC, 2015, Community-Based Participatory Research section). Doornbos et al. (2015) consolidated the groundbreaking work of Israel and others in identifying nine components of CBPR/A.

> *The components are a) recognizing community as a unit of identity; b) building on strengths and resources within the community; c) facilitating collaborative, equitable involvement of all partners in all phases of the research; d) integrating knowledge and action for mutual benefit of all partners; e) promoting a co-learning and empowering process that attends to social inequalities; f) involving a cyclical and iterative process; g) addressing health from both positive and ecological perspectives; h) disseminating findings and knowledge gained to all partners; and i) involving a long-term commitment by all partners. (Doornbos et al., 2015, p. 1326)*

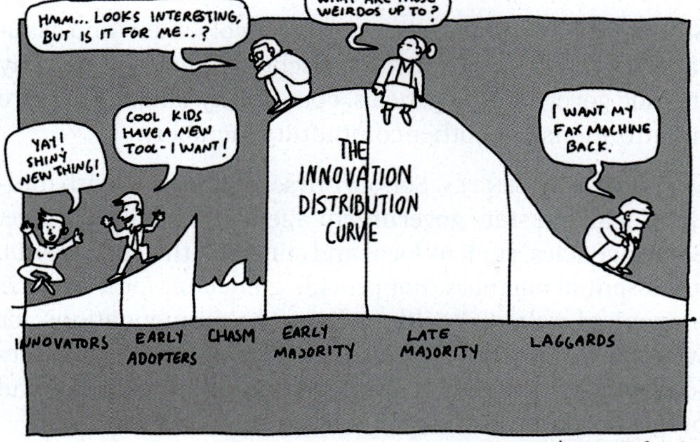

FIGURE 2-9. Rogers's Diffusion of Innovation Theory. *(With permission from Virpi Oinonen, Businessillustrator.com)*

Utilizing the principles of CBPR/Action builds trust with the community and promotes more accurate information and effective outcomes.

Translational Research

Translational research involves utilizing community participation to turn "research into practice by taking it from the bench to the bedside and into the community" and by improving the uptake of new knowledge (CDC, 2015, Translational Research section). Translational research can occur in any of the phases along the continuum of research to community. Translational research phases are framed as basic science to clinical research (T1), research that expands on current knowledge to establish relevance to patients (T2), translation into clinical practice (T3), and finally, moving the findings into the public sector through policy change (T4; CDC, 2015).

Community Collaborations by the School Nurse

Considering the number of students and staff for whom school nurses are responsible, it is imperative that school nurses collaborate with others, especially when they share common goals related to student health and education. Building collaborative partnerships takes time, commitment, and good communication. These partnerships can improve the efficiency and effectiveness of services, pool resources when budgets are tight, and allow for sharing of strategies to improve professional practice and services to students.

Collaboration With Colleagues Within the School

All students within a school population are unique with diverse academic, social, and health needs. Team members within the school community work together to ensure that these needs are met equitably. The student and family are also members of the team. School communities often have a **multidisciplinary student support team** (i.e., student assistance team, student services, or student intervention and referral team) that consists of general education teachers, special education teachers, school social workers, school psychologists, school counselors, school nurses, and school administrators. Any concern, including learning, attention, family/social issues, behavior issues, attendance issues, and health/mental health concerns, can be brought to this team.

The purpose of the student support team is to identify and assess problems, set goals, and develop a plan to provide strategies to assist the teacher in the classroom in the hopes of alleviating learning and behavior problems or barriers of individual students. Sometimes, the identified problem needs more extensive evaluation for special education services, or tiered support through the district's MTSS program. See Chapter 8. A multidisciplinary team that collaborates in school is important because educators can identify and address both subtle and sudden changes in student behavior and learning.

Parent Teacher Association or Organization. Another example of an interschool collaboration is with the Parent Teacher Association or Organization (PTA/PTO). Collaboration is one of the organization's national values: "We will work in partnership with a wide array of individuals and organizations to broaden and enhance our ability to serve and advocate for all children and families" (National PTA, n.d., PTA values). Their goal is to have parents and school leaders work closely with community organizations and businesses to engage and empower families to help all children reach their full potential.

School-Based Health Centers. School-based health centers (SBHCs) provide comprehensive care as a freestanding entity within the school setting. There are over 3,200 SBHCs in the United States, with representation in every state and Washington, DC (U.S. Department of Health and Human Services, 2022). SBHCs often are operated as a partnership between the school and a community health organization, with some offering services to the community in addition to the school. School-based health care has been described as "health care that advances health equity for children and adolescents who experience barriers to accessing care because of systemic inequities, their family income, or where they live" (School-Based Health Alliance, 2023). Over 85% of SBHCs are staffed by a nurse practitioner and about three-quarters engage a licensed social worker, counselor, or therapist to provide behavioral health (Soleimanpour et al., 2023). SBHCs operate at the intersection of health and education, and they provide a full range of age-appropriate health-care services in person or via telehealth that may include the following:

- Primary medical care
- Prevention and early intervention
- Behavioral care and health counseling
- Dental/oral health care
- Health education and promotion, including nutritional counseling
- Laboratory work and prescriptions
- Case management (NASN, 2021)

No two centers are the same; the specific services provided by SBHCs vary based on community needs and resources as determined through collaborations among the community, school district, and health-care providers.

SBHCs do not duplicate or replace school nursing services. School nurses and school-based health centers are complementary services. The school nurse facilitates access for students to use SBHC services. The school nurse is responsible for the day-to-day health of *all* students while they are in the school; only students in need of primary care and who have signed parent/guardian permission and are enrolled in the SBHC program may use the services of the SBHC. Offering comprehensive health services in schools allows children and adolescents to get back to class quickly so they can continue their education.

The SBHC and school nurse can collaborate to accomplish the following:

- Coordinate nursing and treatment care plans for clients who require follow-up care.
- Work together to collect data to study outcomes and cost-effectiveness of care.
- Develop policies and systems that ensure the quality and confidentiality of care received by students.
- Implement wellness and disease prevention programs to improve health outcomes for all school community members.

The collaboration, care coordination, and youth engagement result in improved outcomes and health literacy for students, school staff, and the community. The collaboration also contributes to positive education outcomes, including reduced absenteeism, decreased disciplinary actions and suspensions, and improved graduation rates (NASN & School-Based Health Alliance, 2021).

Community Partners

Students often have needs requiring involvement and assistance from partners outside the school building. This may include government agencies, community and health-care organizations, and other community members.

Government Agencies. School nurses collaborate with multiple local and state government agencies in daily practice. Some agencies, such as local and state health departments, are essential partners that provide guidelines for the development of school health policies, recommendations for when students need to be excluded for illness, form letters to send when there is a disease outbreak in a school, and programs on specific school-related health needs.

As mandated reporters, school nurses collaborate with Child Protective Services in cases where child abuse is suspected. State-sponsored social service agencies and mental health services often work closely with school nurses, especially for students who are in crisis, who are in foster care, or who are homeless.

Another essential government agency with which most school nurses collaborate is the department of education, as its policies often guide what happens in the schools. In addition, in many states, the **state school nurse consultant** is within the department of education. The state school nurse consultant is a valuable collaborator who can help the school nurse understand, update, and create school policy that supports student health and learning.

Police, Fire, and Emergency Medical Services. Collaboration with first responders is essential as they ensure proper response and care during emergencies. Police and fire companies can also provide fire and safety programs in the schools. The police provide security in many high schools and may offer assistance related to drug and alcohol education and policies related to violence on school property. Police can also assist in enforcing laws related to businesses that sell nicotine products or alcohol to students, ensure bike and car seat safety, and assist with programs that promote internet safety and health-promoting behaviors.

Agencies that provide emergency medical services (EMS) must work closely with schools. Emergency action plans should be discussed with EMS and first responders for students with conditions requiring their support during an emergency such as building evacuations and power outages. This might include students who are at risk for anaphylaxis or who are on portable ventilators so agencies may be prepared for emergencies involving these students.

Police, fire, and EMS are an integral part of the development, design, and training of crisis management teams in most school districts. They can collaborate with the school disaster management team to organize drills and safety training along with the local office of emergency management.

Health-care Providers and Systems. School nurses may interact with health-care providers and systems in several ways. For individual students, they may make referrals, collaborate on developing care plans, and inquire about orders or provision of care. At other times, school nurses may work with health-care professionals to provide population-level care, such as dentists and dental hygienists who provide education or mass dental screenings and preventative care at school. Collaborations with health systems can result in assistance with providing school physicals at low or no cost and donations of equipment or supplies.

Schools of Higher Education. Baccalaureate and graduate-level nursing programs collaborate with school districts as a means to provide clinical placement experiences for their students. Serving as preceptors for nursing students is an opportunity for school nurses to function as mentors and teachers and for nursing students to learn about school health. Student nurses may be required to develop a community project or capstone project related to their pediatrics or community health course. By working with the student nurses and their faculty advisors, school nurses can collaboratively initiate health-related programs such as health fairs, screening programs for mandated and nonmandated health needs, health education posters for the school, and educational programs for classroom instruction. Graduate students have the skills to assist school nurses in writing grants to fund health-related initiatives that enhance student health and have a positive impact on student academic success.

Service Organizations. Many school nurses have strong collaborative relationships with community service organizations and faith-based organizations. These organizations provide a multitude of services that support students and families in ways that lead to better health outcomes. Many of these organizations support individuals with disabilities and chronic health conditions. A prime example is the work of the Lions Club in providing free eyeglasses to eligible low-income and uninsured students. In addition, NASN partners with VSP Global to connect school nurses who are NASN members to Sight for Students gift certificates for free eye examinations and glasses for students in need (NASN, 2023).

Area Businesses. Local businesses often collaborate with local schools. Support can come in many different forms, such as volunteering, providing funds or program materials, and offering opportunities for students. They may help by posting notices of school academic events as well as school drama, music, and athletic activities to get the word out to the rest of the community. Some businesses may offer reward programs or provide discounts to teachers or students from the local area. Larger businesses may provide grants to bring speakers to school or build playgrounds. They may fund field trips for students to see plays or other events or invite classes from the school to see how their products are made or grown, such as farm-to-table visits.

CREATING COMMUNITY PROGRAMS

Public health nurses address primary and secondary health needs through health promotion and disease prevention interventions. The creation of population-focused programs to address health involves community assessment, analysis of the data, prioritization of the needs, use of models and strategies for health planning and implementation, a plan for evaluation, and purposeful engagement with the community throughout the process (Savage et al., 2024). Further discussion of health promotion programming, including several program planning models, can be found in Chapter 12.

Community/Population Assessment

Working with and within the community, the public health nurse conducts a community assessment to determine the strengths and needs of the community or population of interest. The public health nurse can conduct a community assessment in several ways, including asset mapping and windshield surveys. School nurses should understand the school community they serve by conducting an assessment before commencing health promoting interventions. Online material OM 2-2 provides a fillable community assessment tool created specifically for school community assessment. The School Health Index (SHI) assessment can also be used to assess school health and safety (CDC, 2019). When conducting a community assessment, secondary community health data resources should also be reviewed. This includes sources such as the County Health Rankings, NASN's Every Student Counts!, and health data collected at the state and local level (CHR&R, 2022; NASN, 2019).

> **Practice Connection**
>
> **School Health Index**
>
> *The School Health Index* (SHI) is a self-assessment tool used to assist in health and safety program planning and policy development for individual schools. The survey has both elementary school and middle/high school versions. It contains 11 modules, including one that examines Health Services. The survey tool is electronic, free, and anonymous.
>
> Teams can use the tool to (1) identify the strengths and weaknesses of their health programs and policies; (2) develop an action plan to improve them; and (3) involve teachers, students, parents, and community members in promoting healthy behaviors and improved health status (CDC, 2019). The SHI guides assessment to identify and prioritize actions a school can take to improve its performance in areas that received low scores on the assessment. The SHI has assisted states, districts, and schools across the nation establish policies and practices to support healthy choices and healthy lifestyles.

Health Promotion Program Planning and Implementation

The next step in the process is the planning and implementation of an intervention. The plan begins with clearly identifying the problem(s) and prioritizing which issue will be addressed first (Issel et al., 2022). The plan includes systems-focused, evidence-based solutions (Savage et al., 2024). Table 2-4 provides an overview of the steps to program planning along with suggested resources for each step.

The focus of health promotion and disease prevention programming generally focuses on one of three areas.

1. *Communication:* using various communication modalities (e.g., public service announcements, health fairs, and mass media campaigns) to increase the public/population's awareness about health behaviors
2. *Education:* providing tailored learning experiences to address health topics through courses and support groups
3. *Policy, systems, and environmental change:* to make healthy choices the easy choice for communities by changing laws and regulations (e.g., taxing unhealthy food options) or making evidence-based systems changes in organizations (e.g., adding healthy options to school vending machines; Rural Health Information Hub, 2024)

These strategies are congruent with the levels on the Health Impact Pyramid (Fig. 2-4), which highlights that the *most impactful* health promotion approaches are those that address making the healthiest decisions the default decisions (Frieden, 2010).

Evaluation of Community Interventions

As in the nursing process, evaluation is an integral component of public health interventions. Proper evaluation planning starts at the same time that the implementation plan is created. Evaluation plans should include evaluations of process, outcome, and impact (Issel et al., 2022). It is often best to consult an evaluation expert to work with the team to develop the evaluation plan and interpret and write the report. Evaluation results should be shared with the community, even when they are not what was expected (CDC, 2017). Unexpected results provide an opportunity for improvement and help identify barriers—often called moderating factors.

POLICY WORK IN COMMUNITIES

Policy work/development and implementation are vital to public health services. Public health nurses are often involved in implementing policy mandates or educating

> **Focus on the Framework**
>
> **Community/Public Health**
>
> School nurses took on many health-promoting and disease prevention roles during the COVID-19 pandemic. One intervention that gained media attention was the implementation of school-located vaccine (SLV) clinics. School-located vaccine clinics have been used in the United States since the 1850s and have helped combat smallpox, polio, and varicella (CDC, n.d.). Since the early 2000s, SLV clinics have largely focused on vaccinating school-age children against influenza improving health-care access for underserved and vulnerable populations.
>
> School nurses embraced and amplified their role in community/public health (a principle of the School Nursing Practice Framework) when they coordinated SLV clinics in their schools during COVID-19. This allowed students and staff to be vaccinated as quickly as possible (Association of Immunization Managers & NASN, 2022). Information for planners of SLV clinics can be found at https://www.cdc.gov/flu/pdf/school/SLV_information.pdf.

TABLE 2-4 Steps in Health Program Planning

The types of steps generally used in program planning are listed here, along with selected resources that may be useful at each step.

Using Evidence-Based Resources for Program Design, Implementation, and Evaluation

Step	Description	Suggested Resources
1	Identify primary health issues in your community.	• Community Health Assessment and Group Evaluation (CHANGE) • County health rankings • National Public Health Performance Standards • MAPP (Mobilizing for Action Through Planning and Partnerships)
2	Develop measurable process and outcome objectives to assess progress in addressing these health issues.	• *HP* Leading Health Indicators • HEDIS (Healthcare Effectiveness Data and Information Set) performance measures
3	Select effective interventions to help achieve these objectives.	• The Guide to Clinical Preventive Services • Health Evidence • National Guideline Clearinghouse
4	Implement selected interventions.	• Partnership for Prevention • CDCynergy
5	Evaluate selected interventions based on objectives; use this information to improve the program.	• Framework for Program Evaluation in Public Health • CDCynergy
1–5	All of the above.	• The Community Health Promotion Handbook: Action Guides to Improve Community Health • Cancer Control P.L.A.N.E.T. (Plan, Link, Act, Network With Evidence-Based Tools) • Community Toolbox • Diffusion of Effective Behavioral Interventions (DEBI)

From *Public Health Science and Nursing Practice* (Savage et al., 2024).

individuals and groups about the value and importance of behavior change needed to adhere to policies. Health policy is primarily influenced by *public concern* and *individual attitudes.* Using vaccination as an example, public concern about a measles outbreak would likely push government entities to create policy that required vaccinations whereas individual attitudes regarding the outbreak could mirror the push for increased vaccination, or if citizens desired autonomy about choosing to be vaccinated, they could push against mandated vaccination policies and advocate to make the vaccination optional. Policy work in communities is informed by the policy process, the Health in All Policies approach, and the nurse's responsibility to advocate.

Policy Process

"Policy is defined as a law, regulation, procedure, administrative action, incentive, or voluntary practice of governments and other institutions" (CDC, 2022a, p. 1). The five steps of the policy process are (1) *Problem Identification*—the identification of the root cause of the problem and writing a detailed problem statement; (2) *Policy Analysis*—working with key stakeholders to determine what policy could be most effective in addressing the problem; (3) *Strategy and Policy Development*—continued work with stakeholders to draft a policy that will address the problem; (4) *Policy Enactment*—working to have the policy officially approved and authorized; and (5) *Policy Implementation*—education of those who will be affected by the policy, creating the systems that will operationalize the policy, and identifying enforcement processes (CDC, 2022a).

Health in All Policies

Health in All Policies is a collaborative policy-making approach that engages individuals across disciplines, sectors, and institutions to consider how the policy they are making or amending can have a positive impact on health (CDC, 2016). This approach recognizes the breadth of factors that influence health, especially in areas such as transportation, education, and housing, and encourages the integration of health into policymaking. Several cities and counties have adopted this approach. The City of Boston has instituted a Health in All Policies approach within its departments. For example, they have reexamined how they can more equitably approach sidewalk repairs in areas that make fewer requests but have greater need. They have also initiated an Eviction Prevention Taskforce that is tasked with examining their eviction policies with the first assumption being that eviction represents a potential health issue (National Association of County & City Health Officials, 2019). While one might not have initially considered accessible sidewalks and fewer evictions as health-related, when viewed through a Health in All Policies lens, these small changes can affect the health of a community. Nurses can incorporate the Health in All Policies approach into their practice to improve the lives of the populations they serve.

Nurses as Policymakers

Nurses are the largest and most trusted health-care profession, and yet they generally do not impact policy (Zurmehly, 2019). Reasons why nurses don't often contribute to policymaking vary. Nurses may not have the confidence to pursue a policy change, nor do they potentiate their voices by collaborating across nursing or health professional specialties to bring policy ideas forward. Advocacy and policymaking, although included in the *Nursing: Scope and Standards* (ANA, 2022) as a responsibility of the nurse, may not have been emphasized in nursing education courses, and thus, nurses may feel unprepared to participate. However, public health nurses may be some of the best prepared to see health effects on populations. Nurses can share their concerns and start by addressing policy within the community they serve. Collaborating with professional organizations to bring policy concerns forward may also provide the support and expertise needed to advance a policy stance beyond a community setting to the local, state, or federal level.

CONCLUSION

School nursing has its roots in public health nursing. Public health theories and activities can inform community-level school nursing practice. Public health nursing core functions and competencies align well with school nursing activities and can expand understanding of population health needs. Work in communities is informed by theories and models in engaging communities, program planning, performing community assessments, creating interventions through health promotion theories and models, use of models for implementation, and assessing outcomes. Policy work is also an expectation of school nursing practice (NASN, 2022a), which is informed by an understanding of the policy process. By building skills in cultural safety, in the context of coalition building within communities, school nurses can develop strategies to work upstream to promote health and prevent illness in their school communities.

References

American Nurses Association. (2015). *Code of ethics for nurses with interpretive statements* (2nd ed.). Author.

American Nurses Association. (2022). *Public health nursing: Scope and standards of practice* (3rd ed.). Author.

Arnold, R., & Wade, J. (2015). A definition of systems thinking: A systems approach. *Procedia Computer Science, 44*, 669–678. http://doi.org/10.1177/0020731415585986

Association of Immunization Managers & National Association of School Nurses. (2022). The landscape of state and local school-located vaccination clinics. *NASN School Nurse, 37*(1), 3S–14S. https://doi.org/10.1177/1942602x211064750

Berwick, D. M., Nolan, T. W., & Whittington, J. (2008). The Triple Aim: Care, health, and cost. *Health Affairs, 27*(3), 759–769. https://doi.org/10.1377/hlthaff.27.3.759

Bodenheimer, T., & Sinsky, C. (2014). From triple to quadruple aim: Care of the patient requires care of the provider. *Annals of Family Medicine, 12*(6), 573–576. https://doi.org/10.1370/afm.1713

Boston University School of Public Health. (2019). *Behavioral change models: Diffusion of innovation theory.* http://sphweb.bumc.bu.edu/otlt/MPH-Modules/SB/BehavioralChangeTheories/BehavioralChangeTheories4.html

Bowen, F. R. (2023). Education is a social determinant of health: School nurses level the playing field. *The Journal of School Nursing, 39*(5), 10598405231191283–10598405231191344. https://doi.org/10.1177/10598405231191283

Butterfield, P. G. (2017). Thinking upstream: A 25-year retrospective and conceptual model aimed at reducing health inequities. *Advances in Nursing Science, 40*(1), 2–11. https://doi.org/10.1097/ANS.0000000000000161

Centers for Disease Control and Prevention. (n.d.). Influenza school-located vaccination (SLV): Information for planners. https://www.cdc.gov/flu/pdf/school/SLV_information.pdf

Centers for Disease Control and Prevention. (2015). Models and frameworks for the practice of community engagement. Agency for Toxic Substances and Disease Registry. https://www.atsdr.cdc.gov/communityengagement/pce_models.html

Centers for Disease Control and Prevention. (2016). Health in all policies. https://www.cdc.gov/policy/hiap/index.htm

Centers for Disease Control and Prevention. (2017). A framework for program evaluation. Office of Policy, Performance, and Evaluation. https://www.cdc.gov/evaluation/framework/index.htm

Centers for Disease Control and Prevention. (2019). *School Health Index.* cdc.gov. https://www.cdc.gov/healthyschools/shi/index.htm

Centers for Disease Control and Prevention. (2020). *Essential public health services.* www.cdc.gov/publichealthgateway/publichealthservices/essentialhealthservices.html

Centers for Disease Control and Prevention. (2022a). *CDC policy process.* Office of Policy, Performance, and Evaluation. https://www.cdc.gov/policy/analysis/process/index.html

Centers for Disease Control and Prevention. (2022b). *Tools for successful CHI efforts.* https://www.cdc.gov/chinav/tools/index.html

County Health Rankings and Roadmaps. (2022). *County health rankings model.* https://www.countyhealthrankings.org/explore-health-rankings/measures-data-sources/county-health-rankings-model

Cowell, J. M. (2018). Population health: School health services and school nursing. *The Journal of School Nursing, 34*(1), 10. https://doi.org/10.1177/1059840517748720

Curtis, E., Jones, R., Tipene-Leach, D., Walker, C., Loring, B., Paine, S. J., & Reid, P. (2019). Why cultural safety rather than cultural competency is required to achieve health equity: A literature review and recommended definition. *International Journal for Equity in Health, 18*(174). https://doi.org/10.1186/s12939-019-1082-3

Distelhorst, K., Graor, C., & Hansen, D. (2021). Upstream factors in population health. *Advances in Nursing Science, 44*(3), 210–223. https://www.doi/ 10.1097/ANS.0000000000000362

Doornbos, M. M., Ayoola, A., Topp, R., & Zandee, G. L. (2015). Conducting research with community groups. *Western Journal of Nursing Research, 37*(10), 1323–1339. https://doi.org/10.1177/0193945915573633

Frieden, T. R. (2010). A framework for public health action: The Health Impact Pyramid. *American Journal of Public Health, 100*(4), 590–595. https://doi.org/10.2105/AJPH.2009.185652

Hammond, D. (2010). *The science of synthesis: Exploring the social implications of general systems theory.* University Press of Colorado.

Healthy People 2030. (n.d.). *Social determinants of health*. U.S. Department of Health and Human Services. https://health.gov/healthypeople/priority-areas/social-determinants-health

Individuals With Disabilities Education Improvement Act of 2004 (Pub. L. 108-446). https://www.gpo.gov/fdsys/pkg/PLAW-108publ446/content-detail.html

IEEE. (n.d.) About big data. https://bigdata.ieee.org/about

Institute for Healthcare Improvement. (2023). *The IHI Triple Aim*. https://www.ihi.org/Engage/Initiatives/TripleAim/Pages/default.aspx

Institute of Medicine. (1988). *The future of public health*. The National Academies Press. https://doi.org/10.17226/1091

Issel, L. M., Wells, R., & Williams, M. (2022). *Health program planning and evaluation* (5th ed.). Jones & Bartlett Learning.

Johnson, K. (2019). Sharing your message: Every student counts. *NASN School Nurse, 34*(6), 340–344. https://doi.org/10.1177/1942602X19877566

Kunz, D. J., Manno, M. S., Ruffatti, D. M., Blohm, S. L., Wuerger, A. A., Keegan, A. J., & Karras, S. L. (2022). Collaboration between a school nurse task force and the local health department in Illinois: Development of a COVID-19 toolkit. *NASN School Nurse, 37*(1), 36–40. https://doi.org/10.1177/1942602X211015298

Merck Manual Consumer Version. (2022). *Three levels of prevention*. https://www.merckmanuals.com/home/multimedia/table/three-levels-of-prevention

Merriam-Webster. (n.d.-a). *Coalition*. https://www.merriam-webster.com/dictionary/coalition

Merriam-Webster. (n.d.-b). *Stakeholders*. https://www.merriamwebster.com/dictionary/stakeholder

Minnesota Department of Health. (2017). *Public health interventions (population-based)*. https://www.health.state.mn.us/communities/practice/research/phncouncil/docs/PHInterventionsHandout.pdf

National Association of County & City Health Officials. (2019). Health in all policies success story: Boston Public Health Commission. *NACCHO Voice*. https://www.naccho.org/uploads/downloadable-resources/BPHC-HiAP-Profile.pdf

National Association of School Nurses. (2019). *Every Student Counts!* https://www.nasn.org/research/everystudentcounts

National Association of School Nurses. (2021). *NASN code of ethics*. NASN.org. https://www.nasn.org/nasn-resources/professional-topics/codeofethics

National Association of School Nurses. (2022a). *School nursing: Scope and standards of practice* (4th ed.). Author.

National Association of School Nurses. (2022b). *Student access to school nursing services*. [Position statement.] Author.

National Association of School Nurses. (2023). *Vision care gift certificates for students*. https://higherlogicdownload.s3.amazonaws.com/NASN/8575d1b7-94ad-45ab-808e-d45019cc5c08/UploadedImages/PDFs/EyesOfHope_GiftCertificates_Flyer_-_NASN_-_2023-06.pdf

National Association of School Nurses & School-Based Health Alliance. (2021) *Joint statement: School nursing and school-based health centers in the United States*. https://higherlogicdownload.s3.amazonaws.com/NASN/8575d1b7-94ad-45ab-808e-d45019cc5c08/UploadedImages/PDFs/Advocacy/School_Nursing_and_School-Based_Health_Centers.pdf

National Institutes of Health. (2011). *Principles of community engagement (2nd ed.)*. NIH Publication No. 11-7782. Author. https://doi.org/https://www.atsdr.cdc.gov/communityengagement/pdf/PCE_Report_508_FINAL.pdf

National Prevention Information Network. (2021). *Cultural competence in health and human services*. Centers for Disease Control and Prevention. https://npin.cdc.gov/pages/cultural-competence

National PTA. (n.d.). *About PTA: Mission statement: PTA values*. https://www.pta.org/home/About-National-Parent-Teacher-Association/Mission-Values

Nundy, S., Cooper, L. A., & Mate, K. S. (2022). The Quintuple Aim for health care improvement: A new imperative to advance health equity. *Journal of the American Medical Association, 327*(6), 521–522. https://doi.org/10.1001/jama.2021.25181

Patient Protection and Affordable Care Act, Public Law No. 111-148. (2010). https://www.congress.gov/bill/111th-congress/house-bill/3590

Paulson, R. E., Plesko, C. M., Gross, D., & Bettencourt, A. F. (2023). Associations between social determinants of health, chronic absence from school, and teacher ratings of parents' engagement in early education. *The Journal of School Nursing, 39*(6),431–443. https://www.doi.org/10.1177/10598405211032958

Ranadive, A. (2017). *How to create messages that stick*. https://medium.com/@ameet/how-to-create-sticky-messages-79649c82e412

Rector, C. L., & Stanley, M. J. (2022). *Community and public health nursing: Promoting the public's health* (10th ed.). Wolters Kluwer.

Rural Health Information Hub. (2024). *Health promotion and disease prevention theories and models*. https://www.ruralhealthinfo.org/toolkits/health-promotion/1/definition

Savage, C. L., Kub, J. E., & Groves, S. L. (2024). *Public health science and nursing practice: Caring for populations*. F.A. Davis.

School-Based Health Alliance. (2023). *Social determinants of health*. https://www.sbh4all.org/what-we-do/social-determinants-of-health-sdoh/

Schroeder, K., Malone, S. K., McCabe, E., & Lipman, T. (2018). Addressing the social determinants of health: A call to action for school nurses. *The Journal of School Nursing, 34*(3), 182–191. https://doi.org/10.1177/1059840517750733

Schumacher, C. (2002). Lina Rogers: A pioneer in school nursing. *The Journal of School Nursing, 18*(5), 247–249. https://doi.org/10.1177/10598405020180050101

Soleimanpour, S., Cushing, K., Christensen, J., Ng, S., Yang, J., Saphir, M., Geierstanger, S., Even, M., & Brey, L. (2023). *Findings from the 2022 national census of school-based health centers*. School-Based Health Alliance. https://sbh4all.org/wp-content/uploads/2023/10/FINDINGS-FROM-THE-2022-NATIONAL-CENSUS-OF-SCHOOL-BASED-HEALTH-CENTERS-09.20.23.pdf

U.S. Department of Education. (2019). *Chronic absenteeism in the nation's schools*. https://www2.ed.gov/datastory/chronicabsenteeism.html

U.S. Department of Health and Human Services. (2022, Oct 3). *HSS awards nearly $25 million to expand access to school-based health services*. [Press Release.] https://www.hhs.gov/about/news/2022/05/03/hhs-awards-nearly-25-million-expand-access-school-based-health-services.html

Wilson, M. L., Weaver, C. A., Proctor, P. M., & Beene, M. S. (2017). Big data in healthcare: A wide look at a broad subject. In C. W. Delaney, C. A. Weaver, J. J. Warren, T. R. Clancy, & R. L. Simpson (Eds.), *Big data enabled nursing: Education, research and practice* (pp. 11–29). Springer.

World Health Organization. (n.d.). *Health equity*. https://www.who.int/health-topics/health-equity#tab=tab_1

Zurmehly, J. (2019). Health in policy and politics. In J. Loversidge & J. Zurmehly (Eds.), *Evidence-informed health policy: Using EBP to transform policy in nursing and healthcare* (pp. 43–61). Sigma Theta Tau International.

Chapter 3

The Specialty Practice of School Nursing

Catherine F. Yonkaitis

CHAPTER OUTLINE

School nursing in the United States developed in response to the historical and social changes of the time (see Chapter 1). As education became compulsory across the United States at the turn of the 20th century, the connection between health and education became visible as communicable diseases presented major barriers to school attendance and learning. In response, school nursing began as a public health experiment in New York City schools to determine the impact of employing a public health nurse in schools to assess students, provide interventions, and follow up with home visits to ensure continued treatment (Struthers, 1917). The experiment was successful in returning students to school, and school nursing emerged.

DEFINITION OF SCHOOL NURSING

Over the past century, the definition of school nursing evolved as the health-care needs of students and communities changed. Students' increased health-care needs also influenced the knowledge and skills needed to practice school nursing. These changes, together with wide differences among practice settings, have presented challenges to define school nursing unambiguously. See Online Materials Table OM 3-1 for the evolution of school nursing as observed through descriptions of the specialty during the past century.

The National Association of School Nurses' (NASN's) comprehensive **definition of school nursing** stresses the role of the school nurse in effecting change.

> *School nursing, a specialized practice of nursing, protects and promotes student health, facilitates normal development, and advances academic success. School nurses, grounded in evidence-based and ethical practice, are the leaders who bridge healthcare and education, provide care coordination, advocate for quality student-centered care, and collaborate to design systems that allow individuals and communities to develop their full potential.* (NASN, 2022a, p. 10)

PUBLIC HEALTH FOUNDATIONS

The connections of school nursing to public health nursing continue to be strong. Public health nursing and school nursing practice intersect within the public health system. School nursing is student-focused, and interventions to improve and protect student health help to protect the health of the entire population. The American Academy of Pediatrics (AAP) and NASN support the role of the school nurse including the school nurse's contributions to individual and population health through collaborative approaches with the school community (AAP, 2016; NASN, 2022a, 2022b, 2024a).

As school nursing evolved from its roots in public health nursing into its own specialty practice, various foundational principles, frameworks, and concepts were incorporated and created. Some of these were adopted or adapted from other disciplines, such as education, psychology, sociology, medicine, and public health, to be applicable to nursing and, subsequently, to school nursing. See Chapter 2 for more information on the school nurse's role as a public health nurse.

School Health Models

School nurses work to ensure that students are well enough to be ready to learn in the classroom. Wellness includes the dimensions of a healthy social and physical environment, health and mental health services, health and physical education, and proper nutrition. Therefore, it takes a team of school professionals working together to have an integrated school health program. This was the philosophy behind the development of the Centers for Disease Control and Prevention's (CDC) **Coordinated School Health Program Model** in 1997. The model divided the school health program into eight components: health service; counseling, psychological, and social services; health education; health promotion for staff; healthy school environment; nutrition services; physical education; and family and community involvement.

Coordinated school health programs entailed a diverse multidisciplinary team of school and community representatives, including the school nurse and parents from the school community. The components were interactive but separate, each with specific and unduplicated responsibilities, and services were designed to protect and promote the health and well-being of students and school staff. The model represented a framework that could be used across school settings with minimal additional financial and human resources.

However, in recent years several factors necessitated a reevaluation of the Coordinated Health School Program model. Social and behavioral theories and research have highlighted the role of social determinants of health in child health and well-being as well as the interactions among education, health, and health equity. The focus on health of students in the Coordinated Health School Program model did not comprehensively consider the social, psychological, emotional, cognitive, and academic development of students or connect with the educational interest of minimizing health barriers to learning and to closing achievement gaps among youth. In addition, it failed to develop synergy among the model's components; rather, the components of the coordinated health school program model operated separately and within their own knowledge domains.

These factors highlighted the need for a more collaborative model that draws from a wider range of stakeholders in school health and education. Therefore, the Coordinated School Health Program model was retired in 2007 and replaced with the Whole School, Whole Community, Whole Child model (CDC, 2023).

Did You Know?

The National Association of School Nurses (NASN) is part of the Council of Public Health Nursing Organizations (CPHNO), formerly the Quad Council of Public Health Nursing Organizations. The Council represents the education, practice, leadership, and research interests of public health nursing and publishes the *Public Health Nursing Journal* six times per year. Member organizations include the following:

- Alliance of Nurses for Healthy Environments
- American Public Health Association—Public Health Nursing Section
- Association of Community Health Nursing Educators
- Association of Public Health Nurses
- National Association of School Nurses
- Rural Nurse Organization

(CPHNO, n.d.)

Whole School, Whole Community, Whole Child Model

Responding to the need for a new model in education to focus on all factors affecting academic achievement in schools, ASCD (formerly the Association for Supervision and Curriculum Development) collaborated with the CDC to develop the **Whole School, Whole Community, Whole Child (WSCC) model** (2023). See Figure 3-1. The WSCC model added emphasis by creating a new component, *Social and Emotional Climate*, and expanding so there are two separate components connecting to the community, *Community Involvement* and *Family Engagement* (CDC, 2023). In the WSCC model, academic achievement is defined more broadly to include academic performance (grades, test scores, graduation rates), education behaviors (attendance, dropout rates, behavior problems at school), and cognitive skills and attitudes (concentration, motivation, memory, mood).

The WSCC model directs the focus of both health and education sectors on the student and includes the student as an active participant (healthy, safe, engaged, supported, and challenged) in the achievement process. The school community and the greater community have collaborative roles for coordination of policy development to support new health and education processes and practices to improve student learning and health for long-term well-being and success. The most successful approach to a

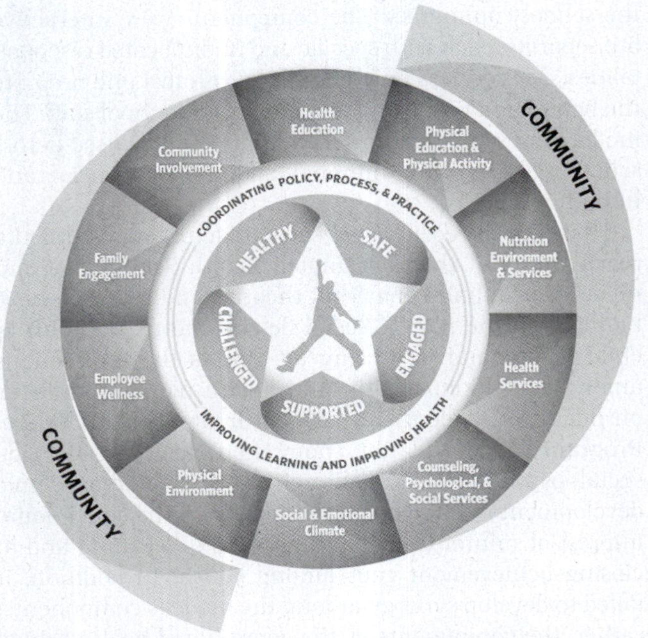

FIGURE 3-1. **Whole School, Whole Child, Whole Community Model.** *(CDC, 2023.)*

coordinated school health program follows the strategies outlined in Table 3-1.

In optimal settings, schools have pupil support services staff who specialize in each of the WSCC components: health education, nutrition services, employee wellness, school climate, physical environment, health services, counseling/psychological/social services, community involvement, family engagement, and physical education/activity. The school health services component is led by school nurses (CDC, 2023). As school health experts, school nurses are called to connect to all nine components of the WSCC model. The school nurse's role in coordinating and collaborating the WSCC approach within the school should not be underestimated.

TABLE 3-1 Strategies to Implement Coordinated School Health Programming

1. Secure and maintain administrative support and commitment.
2. Establish a school health council.
3. Identify a school health coordinator.
4. Develop a plan.
5. Implement multiple strategies through multiple components.
6. Focus on students.
7. Address priority health-enhancing and health-risk behaviors.
8. Provide professional development for staff.

U.S. Environmental Protection Agency (2023).

SCHOOL NURSING FRAMEWORKS

Wold and Dagg's Conceptual Framework for School Nursing Practice

The first conceptual framework created specifically for the specialty practice of school nursing was introduced by Wold and Dagg (1981). The following are the principles upon which this framework (Fig. 3-2) is based:

1. Students are entitled to educational opportunities that prepare them optimally to achieve their full potential as productive adults and citizens.
2. Students are entitled to optimal health.
3. The legal and moral obligation of schools is to provide a school health program that promotes and protects the health of students and the entire school community.
4. There is significant importance in collaboration with students, families, and community resources in planning, implementing, and evaluating comprehensive, coordinated school health programs.
5. The role of the appropriately credentialed school nurse in leading and coordinating the school health program is essential (Wold & Dagg, 1981).

- The principles incorporate the metaparadigm for nursing (people, environment, health, and nursing practice). The visual model describes the concepts and activities that embody school nursing. The practice of school nursing is at the center of this framework, and the surrounding concepts represent what school nurses do in practice to provide nursing care to students. Concepts in the model are overlapping and imply coordination and collaboration among disciplines and stakeholders focused on education and health.

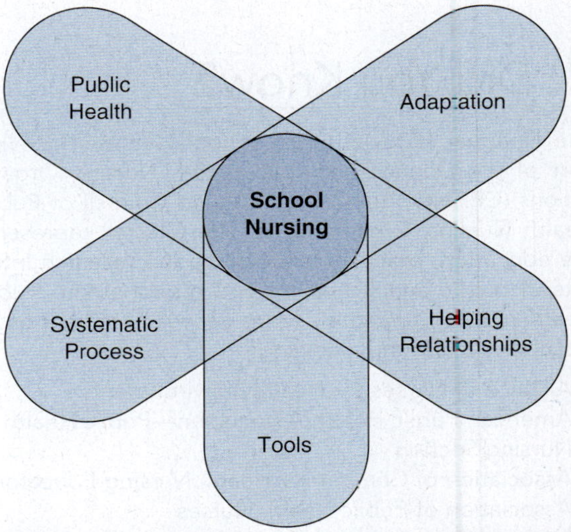

FIGURE 3-2. **Wold and Dagg's Conceptual framework for school nursing practice.** *(From Wold, S. J., & Dagg, N. V. [1981].* School nursing: A framework for practice. *Sunrise River Press.)*

School nursing does all of the following:

- Incorporates the principles of public health
- Works to enable adaptation of students to internal and external environmental changes
- Forms collaborative relationships within education, communities, and government to support effective school health programs
- Uses discipline-specific tools
- Employs systematic processes, particularly the nursing process, to achieve goals of school nursing (Wold & Dagg, 1981)

NASN's School Nursing Practice Framework

Throughout its history, school nursing has continued to develop as a nursing specialty practice with its own body of research and knowledge. As the complexity of student health and health-care needs increased, so did the depth and breadth of school nursing practice and the extent of collaborations formed to fully support student health and achievement.

To reflect these advances, *The Framework for 21st Century School Nursing Practice* (the Framework) was developed by NASN in 2016. This conceptual framework painted a picture of modern-day school nursing practice. The developers refer to the Framework as a *heuristic* framework, meaning a framework that uses general knowledge of school nursing gained through experience and applied to simple as well as complex problems in everyday practice (NASN, 2016). The elements of the Framework were explained in the context of interactions within and among components to reach the shared goal. The Framework for 21st Century School Nursing Practice was both a synthesis and an expansion of concepts from earlier models and theories. It incorporated elements from multiple frameworks from other disciplines adapted for school nursing practice. In 2024, NASN published a "refreshed" Framework to ensure it was still reflective of current practice and to clarify any questions that had been raised as the Framework was used over the prior 7 years. What resulted is a renaming into the **NASN's *School Nursing Practice Framework*** (2024a).

The *School Nursing Practice Framework* defines the specialty practice of school nursing and places students' functioning within their social environments at the center of the defining principles and concepts (NASN, 2024a). The Framework aligns with the WSCC model by using a collaborative whole child approach to student health, achievement, and well-being. The five concepts (i.e., principles) of the Framework are also in line with the metaparadigm for nursing (people, environment, health, and nursing practice) and are linked to multidisciplinary bodies of knowledge adapted for school nursing. The result is four practice principles: Community/Public Health, Leadership, Quality Improvement, and Care Coordination, all of which are rooted in the fifth principle, Standards of Practice.

The concepts within each principle of the Framework are nonhierarchical and often overlapping; they represent what school nurses do in practice to meet the health needs of students and school communities. Within each principle are school nursing practice descriptors that help describe the specialty role (NASN, 2024a). It is important to note that the practice descriptors within each principle are ever-changing and evolving as new evidence for practice develops. A pictorial image of the School Nursing Practice Framework can be seen in Figure 3-3. The depiction is meant to provide a bird's-eye view of school nursing practice with the standards of practice principle as the base and the school nurse's practice encompassing all.

Student

Students are featured at the center of the model. They are subsequently encircled and supported by three groups (NASN, 2024a). The first two, the family and the school community, are pictured in the white circle directly adjacent to the student. The third, the school nurse, is depicted in the outermost dark circle of the model as school nursing includes support of the student, family, and school community as part of their practice.

Standards of Practice

The Standards of Practice principle provides the foundation for quality practice that is evidence-based and clinically competent (NASN, 2022a). Ethically, legally, and professionally, the Standards of Practice principle underpins all the other principles of the framework. The concepts of standards of practice are discussed in detail later in this chapter.

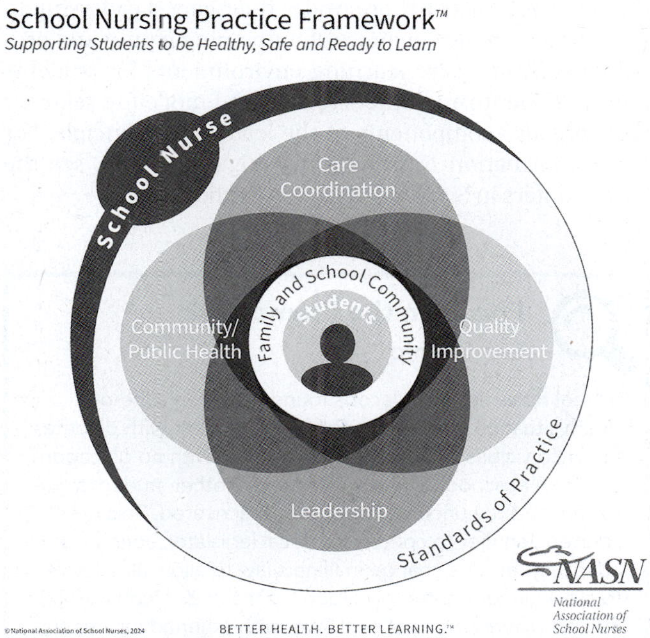

FIGURE 3-3. School Nursing Practice Framework. *(NASN, 2024a.)*

Care Coordination

The principle of *Care Coordination* is probably the most recognizable principle to the general public. It includes the direct care and school nurse–led case management school nurses provide as they bridge the health and education needs of students (NASN, 2024a). School nurses' role in chronic care management of both physical and mental health conditions includes coordination and collaboration with parents/guardians, school administrators, teachers, and support personnel, as well as community-based health-care providers. School nurses use the nursing process to assess, diagnose, plan, implement, and evaluate nursing interventions focused at both the individual and population levels. Within this principle, school nurses focus on increasing students' self-care through individual teaching in the health office or group teaching in classrooms or in the community.

Leadership

The principle of *Leadership* outlines the responsibility of school nurses to lead and supports the school nurse's ability to act as a change agent. It encourages rather than suggests all school nurses should hold formal leadership positions. Leadership can be at the school, district, local, or even national level (NASN, 2024a). School nurses lead when they develop evidence-based school policies, procedures, and programming at the school and district level, including those related to emergency and disaster preparedness. School nurses lead through advocacy for students and families as well as themselves at all levels.

The Future of Nursing 2020–2030 (National Academies of Sciences, Engineering, and Medicine, 2021) calls on all nurses to practice to the full extent of their education and training through problem-solving, effective communication, and collaboration with others and by advancing the self-care skills of those under their care. Leadership in school nursing also includes championing equity and providing safe, inclusive learning environments for students and staff. Mentoring others to lead and modeling self-care skills are also components of the leadership principle. For more information on school nursing leadership, see the four chapters in Section VII of this textbook.

> **Focus on the Framework**
> **Leadership**
>
> School nurse Jennifer Jacobs found herself in a life-or-death situation when a hypoglycemic student with diabetes fell unconscious while in the health office with no glucagon available at school. She administered another student's glucagon, and the unconscious student recovered. This event spurred Jennifer to contact her local legislator. Jennifer's advocacy led to a change in Illinois law to allow all schools to stock undesignated glucagon (Yonkaitis & Jacobs, 2022). She now works on a national level with other advocates to make stock glucagon available in other public spaces.

Quality Improvement

The principle of *Quality Improvement* is embedded in the nursing process (NASN, 2024a). This principle includes the work school nurses do when they assess, diagnose, plan, implement, and evaluate, analyzing the data they collect to improve the care they provide. Quality improvement for school nursing practice includes the collection of data to support local and state requirements and the national data set initiative. School nurses can use data to monitor population- and student-level health and academic outcomes and disseminate these outcomes through presentations and publications. Data collection by school nurses not only guides development and improvement of policies and interventions but can lead to the identification of practice questions that may benefit from additional research. These practice-related questions can be answered through academic-practice partnerships and further develop the evidence around school health and school nursing practice. See Chapter 5 for more discussion of the school nurse's role in quality improvement.

Community/Public Health

The principle of *community/public health* focuses on the role of the school nurse with school populations, the surrounding community, and the delivery of health promotion and disease prevention activities (NASN, 2024a). These include conducting health screenings, surveillance, and outreach and assessing the impact of social and environmental determinants of health. This principle captures the work school nurses do in primary, secondary, and tertiary health services, especially when they advocate for upstream solutions to address all three levels of prevention. This principle also includes concepts related to community care and community partnerships that require the nurse to interact in ways that are culturally sensitive, inclusive, and holistic. See Chapter 2 for more information on the school role as public health nurse.

The School Nursing Practice Framework has much to offer school nurses to help define and explain their practice. NASN

> **Practice Connections**
>
> **School Nurses—Coordinating Care Through a Community/School Health Partnership**
>
> School districts can partner with community health-care providers to connect low-income students to health care. Such a partnership has been operating in Columbia, South Carolina, for more than 25 years. Healthy Learners, a private nonprofit organization, works with community health-care providers and school district nurses to connect eligible students to needed services. The partnership provides dental, vision, and episodic and pediatric specialty care. Healthy Learners sets appointments, transports students during the school day, and makes reports to school nurses. The goal is to keep students in school, healthy, and ready to learn (Duff & Poole, 2016).

offers several articles and infographics that can be explored to learn more about using the Framework in daily practice. Models and frameworks provide a basis to guide school nursing practice from a systems level. However, further delineation is needed to help nurses and the public understand school nursing and delineate accountability for practice. Though all nurses practice in the same fundamental way, it is important to illustrate how nursing is practiced when in the educational setting. The specialty of school nursing is delineated first through definition and second through scope and standards.

SCOPE AND STANDARDS OF PRACTICE

It is necessary to understand all aspects of school nursing in order to appreciate the complex, ever-changing landscape of this specialty (NASN, 2022a). There are several types of standards of interest to the school nurse. Standards that exist for clients and their welfare, nursing and its practice, and the integrity of nursing as a discipline are applicable to all nurses in active practice regardless of their venue. Within school nursing, related standards may be legal standards, standards of care, nursing education standards, and learning standards. See Table 3-2.

According to NASN (2022a),

> *School nurses straddle multiple federal, state, and local statutory and regulatory frameworks. Because school nurses practice nursing in an educationally focused system, they face unique legal, policy, funding, and supervisory issues that may also have ethical dimensions. School nurses rely on the most current evidence and professional policy statements to guide the care of individual and student populations. (p. 39)*

School nurses use their knowledge of health and education laws such as the Individuals With Disabilities Education Improvement Act (IDEA; 2004), Section 504 of the Rehabilitation Act (1973), and their state's nurse practice act along with state and local laws and regulations to guide their practice. In addition to NASN's *School Nursing: Scope and Standard of Practice (2022a)*, discussed later in this chapter, school nurses consult the evidence including the literature, clinical practice guidelines, and the data they collect to determine the best interventions and approaches to use with students, families, and the school community.

The scope and standards of nursing help to provide descriptions by which others can understand the basic tenets of the specialty practice as well as provide a reliable resource on which to judge the practice (NASN, 2022a). All nurses are held to the same basic scope and standards as outlined in the ANA's *Nursing Scope and Standards of Practice* (2021). These ensure consistency not only within the profession but in the way we communicate our work to others. Standards of practice translate into standards of care by which nurses are held to account professionally, ethically, and sometimes legally.

In 1991, ANA divided the standards into two categories: Standards of Care (later retitled *Standards of Practice*) and *Standards of Professional Performance.* The *Standards of Practice* are the six steps of the nursing process. The *Standards of Professional Performance* address nursing activities and responsibilities beyond the nursing process, such as ethics, communication, and leadership. The scope was added in 2001. Although many nurses are familiar with standards and their associated competency statements, the scope of practice is often overlooked. The ***scope*** of nursing practice provides both nurses and their audience (e.g., patients, partners, community members, and interested parties) with an overview of the who, what, where, when, how, and why of nursing (ANA, 2021).

Standards are complementary to the scope. Standards articulate the roles and functions of the practice. **Standards,** or expectation statements for any kind of practice, require an understanding of the nature of the discipline under consideration for their successful development. Hence, the importance of the scope, along with a concise

TABLE 3-2 Types of Standards

Type	Description	Example
Legal Standard	Laws and statutory regulations in state or federal law	Registered Nurse Licensure (state); disposal of sharps (federal)
Standard of Care (aka Community Standard)	"What a reasonably prudent person would do under the same or similar circumstances" (Rossi-Scott & Bubert, 2013, p. 214)	Nursing: Scope and Standards of Practice: Specialty Scope and Standards of Practice
Nursing Education Standards	Regulations that address the educational preparation necessary to successfully practice nursing	National Council on the Licensure Examination for Registered Nurses (NCLEX)
School Nursing Education Standards	A body of knowledge that a nurse entering school nursing should have to practice; varies by state	Required continuing education, coursework, or certifications required by state to practice
Learning Standards	A guideline for what every student should be able to know and do at each grade level in specific subject areas such as math and language arts	State health and wellness learning standards Common Core Standards (Common Core State Standards Initiative, 2024)

and meaningful definition of nursing and school nursing. It is also crucial to consider the *Code of Ethics for Nurses with Interpretive Statements* (ANA, 2015) and the *NASN Code of Ethics* (NASN, 2022a). The NASN Code of Ethics contains nine provisions. See Table 3-3.

Standards, along with the definition of nursing, are the beginning, not the end, of a comprehensive description of nursing practice and constitute the profession's pledge of accountability to the client and the public. Standards also reflect the values and priorities of the discipline (ANA, 2021); they serve as a definitive guide for role implementation, interpretation, and evaluation, and they carry legal standing (NASN, 2022a).

There are five key concepts that apply to nursing standards, each of which helps us to understand the nature of professional practice standards. These concepts are as follows:

- Standards are authoritative statements.
- Standards apply to all practicing registered nurses.
- Standards are a declaration of expected competence and performance.
- Standards constitute "a standard of care."
- Application of standards is context and situation dependent.

School Nursing Standards

Early on, ANA recognized that certain specialties within nursing would benefit from having their own unique scope and standards. The first *Standards of School Nursing Practice* were written in 1970 and then published in 1983 by the American Nurses Association. Today, the *School Nursing: Scope and Standards of Practice* (NASN, 2022a) are published by NASN and are reviewed and revised every 5 years. All school nurses should be fully versed in the most current version of NASN's *School Nursing: Scope and Standards of Practice* and should include a copy in their personal reference library.

Did You Know?

The language of standards is intentionally broad and not intended to inform an uninitiated reader as to the specific responsibilities and expectations of nursing practice without more clarification. Nursing roles and activities may be state and/or district specific, and the uniqueness of a given position cannot be fully understood or appreciated through the use of standard statements by themselves. Therefore, standard statements optimally serve nursing practice or the recipients of nursing care when further tailored to the specifics of the role and setting by defining competencies.

Structure and Components

Similar to the ANA, NASN's *School Nursing: Scope and Standards of Practice* (2022a) begins with a thorough description of the Scope of Practice that outlines the guiding principles, characteristics, concepts and frameworks, practice settings, roles, and trends of school nursing practice.

Like ANA, the accompanying School Nursing Standards are composed of two groupings: *Standards of Practice* and *Standards of Professional Performance* (NASN, 2022a). Each standard within both groups has (1) a standard number, (2) a standard title, (3) a statement (the actual language of the standard), and (4) several competencies related to that

TABLE 3-3 National Association of School Nurses Code of Ethics

Provision 1	The nurse practices with compassion and respect for the inherent dignity, worth, and unique attributes of every person (ANA, 2015, p. 1).
Provision 2	The nurse's primary commitment is to the patient, whether an individual, family, group, community, or population (ANA, 2015, p. 5).
Provision 3	The nurse promotes, advocates for, and protects the rights, health, and safety of the patient (ANA, 2015, p. 9).
Provision 4	The nurse has authority, accountability, and responsibility for nursing practice; makes decisions; and takes action consistent with the obligation to promote health and provide optimal patient care (ANA, 2015, p. 15).
Provision 5	The nurse owes the same duties to self as to others, including the responsibility to promote health and safety, preserve wholeness of character and integrity, maintain competence, and continue personal and professional growth (ANA, 2015, p. 19).
Provision 6	The nurse, through individual and collective effort, establishes, maintains, and improves the ethical environment of the work setting and conditions of employment that are conducive to safe, quality health care (ANA, 2015, p. 23).
Provision 7	The nurse, in all roles and settings, advances the profession through research and scholarly inquiry, professional standards development, and the generation of both nursing and health policy (ANA, 2015, p. 27).
Provision 8	The nurse collaborates with other health professionals and the public to protect human rights, promote health diplomacy, and reduce health disparities (ANA, 2015, p. 31).
Provision 9	The profession of nursing, collectively through its professional organizations, must articulate nursing values, maintain the integrity of the profession, and integrate principles of social justice into nursing and health policy (ANA, 2015, p. 35).

National Association of School Nurses. (2022a). Appendix B: NASN Code of Ethics for school nurses. *School Nursing: Scope & Standards of Practice* (4th ed., pp. 131–136). Author.

standard. The Standards of School Nursing Practice comprise the six steps of the nursing process. However, there are actually eight practice standards because Standard 5, *Implementation*, has two nested standards: 5A Coordination of Care, and 5B Health Teaching and Health Promotion.

The Standards of Professional Performance for School Nursing address nursing activities and responsibilities beyond the nursing process, such as ethics, communication, and leadership. There are 12 professional performance standards that are numbered 7 through 18. Therefore, the 4th edition of *School Nursing: Scope and Standards of Practice* (NASN, 2022a) contains a total of 18 standard statements. See Table 3-4 and OM 3-2. Several adjustments were made from the 3rd edition for clarity and conciseness. Advocacy (Standard 8) was added, and Project Management (formerly Standard 18) was removed and its content interspersed throughout the other standards/competencies. Additionally, the names and definitions of several standards were refined:

- 3rd edition Standard 8. Culturally Congruent Practice → 4th edition Standard 9. Respectful and Equitable Practice
- 3rd edition Standard 13. Evidence-Based Practice & Research → 4th edition Standard 14. Scholarly Inquiry
- 3rd edition Standard 16. Resource Utilization → 4th edition Standard 17. Resource Stewardship

Figure 3-4 depicts the entire breadth of the scope and standards of school nursing practice in pictorial form,

TABLE 3-4 **School Nursing: Standards of Practice and Professional Performance**

Standards of Practice

Standard 1. Assessment
The school nurse collects pertinent data and information relative to the student, family, group, school community, or population.

Standard 2. Diagnosis
The school nurse analyzes assessment data of the student, family, group, school community, or population to describe actual or potential diagnoses.

Standard 3. Outcomes Identification
The school nurse articulates measurable expected outcomes for a plan individualized to the student, family, group, school community, or population.

Standard 4. Planning
The school nurse develops a collaborative course of action that prescribes strategies to attain expected, measurable outcomes that address the student, family, group, school community, or population.

Standard 5. Implementation
The school nurse executes an agreed upon plan/intervention for the student, family, group, school community, or population.

Standard 5A. Coordination of Care
The school nurse aligns care for the student, family, group, school community, or population.

Standard 5B. Health Teaching and Health Promotion
The school nurse employs strategies to improve the health and safety of the student, family, group, school community, or population.

Standard 6. Evaluation
The school nurse systematically appraises the progress toward attainment of student and school population goals and outcomes.

Standards of Professional Performance

Standard 7. Ethics
The school nurse integrates ethics in all aspects of practice.

Standard 8. Advocacy
The school nurse demonstrates advocacy in all roles and settings.

Standard 9. Respectful and Equitable Practice
The school nurse practices with cultural humility and inclusiveness.

Standard 10. Communication
The school nurse effectively conveys information in all areas of practice.

Standard 11. Collaboration
The school nurse collaborates with students, families, and key stakeholders.

Continued

TABLE 3-4 School Nursing: Standards of Practice and Professional Performance—cont'd

Standards of Professional Performance

Standard 12. Leadership
The school nurse leads within their professional practice setting and the profession.

Standard 13. Education
The school nurse seeks knowledge and competence that reflects current nursing practice and promotes innovative, anticipatory thinking.

Standard 14. Scholarly Inquiry
The school nurse integrates scholarship, evidence, and research findings into practice.

Standard 15. Quality of Practice
The school nurse contributes to quality nursing practice.

Standard 16. Professional Practice Evaluation
The school nurse appraises one's own and others' school nursing practice.

Standard 17. Resource Stewardship
The school nurse utilizes appropriate resources to plan, provide, and sustain evidence-based nursing services that are safe, effective, and financially responsible, and are used judiciously.

Standard 18. Environmental Health
The school nurse practices in a manner that advances environmental safety, justice, and health.

Source: National Association of School Nurses. (2022a). *School nursing: Scope and standards of practice* (pp. 57–58). Author.

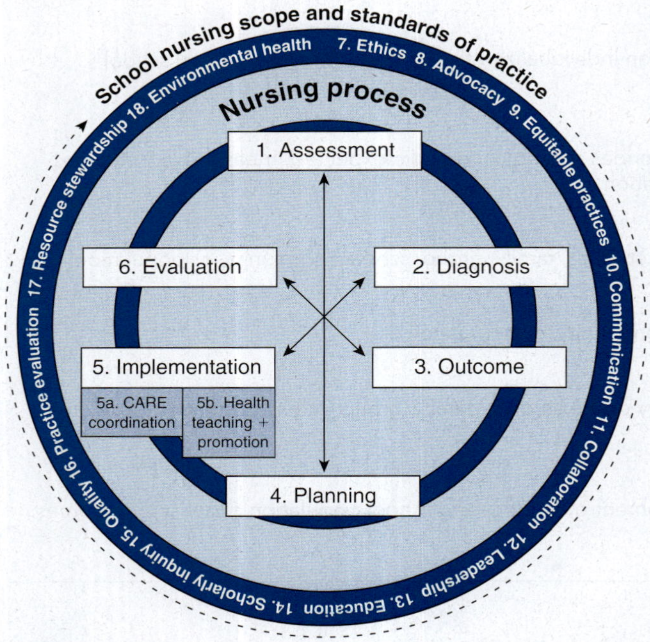

FIGURE 3-4. Scope of School Nursing Practice. *(Meza & Rau, 2021; NASN, 2022a.)*

indicating the iterative nature of the nursing process and the fact that the professional practice standards apply to all aspects of the nursing process. Together, the standards describe what competent practice should look like depending on the context and model of care in which the school nurse practices (NASN, 2022a).

Did You Know?

The competencies that augment each standard statement are grouped by expectations for basic nursing practitioners first, followed by additional competencies for the graduate-level prepared school nurse. The graduate-level prepared school nurse is defined as

a nursing leader in school nursing and health, prepared at the master's or doctoral level, who possesses specialized knowledge and skills in school nursing, public health, organization and management, health education, health promotion, administration, or other areas of study necessary to promote the health and academic success of the student and professional school nursing practice (NASN, 2022a, p. 102).

Attributes of the graduate-level prepared school nurse are the abilities to understand and work with populations, systems, and complexity and to contribute to the growth of the specialty of school nursing.

Application of the Standards to Practice

Standards are *broad, authoritative statements* framing the scope of practice of a discipline. Therefore, they need to be adapted for practical use. Standards are meant to be interpreted and applied to the contexts of practice. Strictly implementing the standards as published without critical thinking and nursing judgment can present barriers to utilization, such as the following:

- The language and competencies of the standards are purposefully broad and general; therefore, specific application to nursing duties and responsibilities can be challenging, particularly for the uninitiated.

- The standards and their accompanying competencies are best employed through the use of a graduated measurement tool, such as a Likert scale, with numerical values or word descriptors, to assess the *degree, level,* or *extent* to which a nurse meets a particular standard (Wallin & Rothman, 2020).
- Even with the published competencies in place, standards are best used as a "framework" to be further customized to individual work settings or environments by the development of district-, school-, or setting-specific competencies or objectives.
- The standards may not lend themselves to uniform application, even within a single school district. In some districts, a nurse may be able to meet the intent of some of the standards but not all of them, because of excessive pupil-to-nurse ratios, inadequate educational preparation, unique assignment or role, or the particulars of the work environment itself.

Standards of practice are a vital and essential part of practice. Standards of practice may be optimally used in the school setting in several ways, including performance evaluation/appraisal, job description development, and quality assurance/improvement.

Position (Job) Descriptions

The *School Nursing Standards* can guide the development of accurate school nurse job descriptions. Furthermore, they can assist in the revision of existing position descriptions. A *position (job) description* is a document describing the duties or functions of an individual within an organizational structure. A position description is a "what" rather than a "how to" statement of a nursing job. Job descriptions prescribe the authority, accountability, and responsibility of the individual. Role functions related to each standard can be enumerated in detail using the standards as a framework (NASN, 2023). See Chapter 31 for more information on job descriptions.

Employee Performance Evaluation/Appraisal

Standards of practice and their accompanying competencies can play an important role in the development of evaluation instruments for nurse performance appraisal or review. Indeed, competencies/objectives are almost always used in the appraisal of nursing practice. If competencies, behavioral objectives, position (job) description items, or other behavioral indicators already exist and are modeled on the standards of practice, they can be adapted for performance review as a framework for self, peer, or supervisor evaluation. In order to provide clear, actionable evaluation it is particularly helpful to incorporate qualifiers into evaluation documents, such as a Likert scale containing numerical values with words such as unsatisfactory, emerging, proficient, and exemplary (Wallin & Rothman, 2020). Congruence with the district's position (job) description is critical. A nurse hired under a position description that varies markedly from the instrument used to evaluate their performance creates a disconnect between initial expectations and what is appraised during routine evaluation.

The Connecticut State Department of Education (CTDOE) first used the NASN standards of practice to develop a school nurse self-evaluation of competencies tool, a school nurse performance evaluation tool, and other supporting documents (CTDOE, 2014). Other states have also developed their own models of evaluation based on the national standards and the *NASN School Nursing Framework*. In 2017, a suburban St. Louis district utilized the school nurse standards and the *Framework for 21st Century School Nursing Practice* to improve their school nurse evaluation process (Wallin & Rothman, 2020). Most recently, the Tennessee Department of Education (2023) created a guide for nursing supervisors and school administrators called *School Nurse Competencies and Evaluation.* See Chapter 31 for more information on performance evaluation.

Quality Improvement and Program Evaluation

The *School Nursing Practice Standards* may be used to evaluate the functions and quality of school health services programs. Outcomes Identification (Standard 3) speaks specifically to the expectation that the nurse articulate outcomes for the "student, family, group, school community, or population" (NASN, 2022a, p. 63). The language of the standard suggests that Outcomes Identification goes beyond the student and could be used as a quality improvement indicator. Additionally, Quality of Practice (Standard 15) states that nursing practice, regardless of the specialty focus, should be evaluated and that assurance of the quality and safety of care is evident.

School nurses provide direct nursing services, coordinate the delivery of other health services, provide health instruction, manage the school health program, engage in resolving issues regarding the school environment and nutrition, offer health counseling, confer and collaborate with physical education personnel, collaborate with families and community agencies, and are involved with employee health promotion (NASN, 2016). All of these activities should be evaluated, and the standards and related competencies provide a foundation for doing so.

THE PRACTICE OF SCHOOL NURSING

The school nurse's practice is highlighted by the *School Nursing Practice Framework* and the *School Nursing: Scope and Standards of Practice;* however, the specifics—the "where," "who," and "what" of school nursing—require additional elaboration. The following sections will explore these areas.

The "Where" of School Nursing

Almost all matters related to public health and public education in the United States are under the domain of the states. Education is required and free for all students until ages 16 to 18, depending on the individual state (National Center for Education Statistics, 2018). Each state has a state department of education that sets guidelines and, in some cases, curriculum for the public schools. It is headed by a state superintendent or secretary of education or a leader with a comparable title. Funding for the schools is determined by state legislatures and is usually dependent on taxes.

School Districts

States make geographical decisions to divide their territory into **school districts,** also called **local educational agencies** (LEAs), each of which is governed by a school board. Additionally, states have charter schools and private schools that may be part of the public school system or act as independent districts. The school board is either elected by the local community or appointed. It is the school board that usually sets local policies for the school district, determines curriculum, ensures that state guidelines are met, and hires a chief school officer (typically called a superintendent) to manage the schools in that district and to oversee contracts with its employees. In some districts, the school boards may play a more active role in running the schools, such as approving textbooks to be used.

Because schools are businesses within a community, the superintendent is considered the "chief education officer" or "chief executive officer" of the district. They are responsible for the distribution of designated state funds and overseeing the quality of the schools regarding both academics and built environments. Superintendents are employees of the school board and implement board policy. They meet regularly with boards to report and advise them on district policy and operational issues. They usually are not voting members of boards. The superintendent assumes a leadership role in the formation of school district policies and procedures. They also may guide research related to educational status in that district and should be knowledgeable about the science of education of children.

Each school is headed by a principal (director, headmaster) who reports to a director of schools, an assistant superintendent, or directly to the district superintendent. The school principal has the responsibility for making hiring recommendations, mentoring, and evaluating staff. They set the academic tone and work with faculty and staff to develop and maintain high educational standards. As the highest-ranking administrator in the building, the principal is responsible for the overall operation of the school according to district policies and procedures, including budget and finances, maintenance and safety of the building, student scheduling, public relations, school discipline, coordination of the instructional program, staff management, and other overall school matters. The principal's duties and responsibilities are at the discretion of the superintendent. Above all, the superintendent and principal must ensure that student instruction meets national, state, and local academic standards.

Principals also have the leadership responsibility for interacting with parents/guardians and members of the school and nearby community. This may involve working with parents through a Parent Teacher Association or Organization (PTA/PTO). In most cases, when parents/guardians have concerns, the principal will be the first person they contact. Principals may also seek financial support for school programs through local businesses, grants, and other sources, as well as find ways to meet and support community needs, through use of the school building, for example.

In most situations, the principal is also responsible for the school health program within their building. Thus, the school nurse works under the direct supervision of the principal. Often, there is another district level leader responsible for the school health program who also provides direction and possibly administrative supervision of the school nurses; this person may or may not be a nurse. Principals may not be fully aware of the scope of the school nurse role, and therefore it is incumbent on the school nurse to describe the school nurse role and to use data to explain and support the structure of the current school health program. Principals and staff depend on the expertise of the school nurse, and as a systems leader, a school nurse has great opportunity to create a school health program that truly advances health and supports education. See Chapters 30 and 31 for more about managing and supervising the school health office.

School nurses practice in a variety of settings. Most school nurses practice at the local level, assigned to one or more schools in a district (Willgerodt et al., 2023b). As highlighted earlier, the school can be public, private, charter, parochial, or a boarding school, and some students attend virtual schools or schools run by the U.S. Department of Defense. The school nurse can be assigned to a school that serves all grade levels, specific grades, special education, early childhood, or alternative schools. The responsibilities of the school nurse extend beyond the school building and can include daytime or overnight out-of-school trips, athletic events, and home visits (NASN, 2024b). During the COVID-19 pandemic, school nurses made virtual visits and devised innovative ways to educate and supervise their most vulnerable students and families (Combe, 2020).

School nursing can also entail regional, statewide, national, or global practice. Beyond the traditional school positions, school nurses can be found in school-based health centers, daycare centers, home health and temporary staffing companies, public health departments, and hospital health-care systems (NASN, 2022a). School nurses also serve at the state level as state school nurse consultants, as association presidents and board members, and as school nurse educators at colleges and universities.

School nurses also serve important roles as health educators for individual students, for staff, and in the classroom (see Chapter 4).

The "Who" of School Nursing

School Nurse Demographics

NASN periodically conducts a national survey of school nurses that includes both members and nonmembers. The School Nurse Workforce Study estimated that there are approximately 79,000 full-time equivalent school nurses with about 65,000 registered nurses/advanced practice registered nurses (RNs/APRNs) and 14,000 licensed practical nurses/licensed vocational nurses (LPNs/LVNs) in the United States (Willgerodt et al., 2023c). Only 65.7% of schools have access to a full-time nurse (RN/LPN/LVN; Willgerodt et al., 2023b). The majority of school nurses (58.2%) are assigned to work in one building; the remaining 42% are asked to cover from two to greater than six buildings. Regionally, the Northeast had the most full-time school nurses, and the West had the fewest. See Figure 3-5.

The workforce study provides additional insights into school nurse demographics. School nurses are primarily female (98.2%) and White (91.2%; Willgerodt et al., 2023b). Diversity in terms of racial and ethnic background, while troubling in nursing overall, is even more pronounced in school nursing. The lack of diversity extends into representation of gender as well.

Of additional concern is the fact that in the next few decades school nursing will likely face staffing shortage dilemmas, as almost 69% of school nurses are older than 40. Complicating things further are the low wages paid to school nurses compared with their acute care setting colleagues. Thirty-four percent of RNs working in schools earned less than $60,000/year, with 11% of those earning less than $40,000 (Willgerodt et al., 2023a).

Professional Registered Nurses Licensure

All RNs share the same basic legal requirements so that licensure and practice regulations apply equally. Most states delineate the rules of the profession through a Nurse Practice Act enacted by the legislature (see Chapter 6). The rules set by the state apply to all nursing roles in *every* setting in that state, including school health services. In some instances, several states enter into an agreement (a compact) to legally allow RNs to practice in any of the states

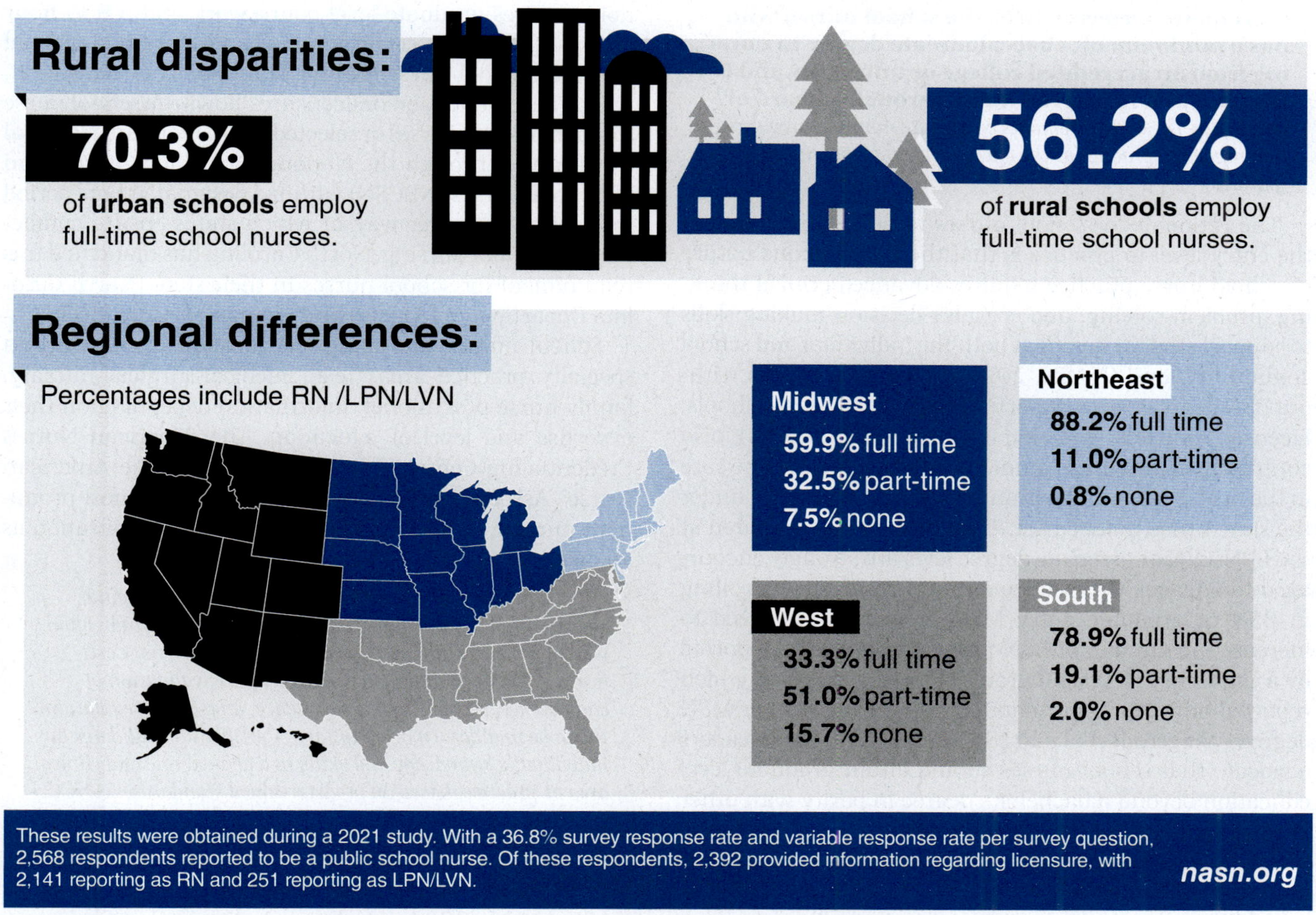

FIGURE 3-5. Distribution of Full-Time (35 hours/week) School Nursing Positions. *(Willgerodt et al., 2023b.)*

within the compact without the need to seek additional licensure. Currently, 41 states have enacted the enhanced Nurse Licensure Compact agreement, and several have legislation pending (National Council of State Boards of Nursing, 2023).

Educational Preparation for the Specialty of School Nursing

There is much diversity in the job titles and educational preparation of school nurses across the country. The American Association of Colleges of Nursing (2023) encourages nurses to seek baccalaureate or higher degree and specialty certification. All BSN programs include both community health didactic content and clinical experiences, as well as fundamentals of research, that are critical for independent practice in schools.

The American Association of Colleges of Nursing's stance supports the NASN position that the school nurse should minimally hold a Bachelor of Science in Nursing (BSN) degree to acquire the advanced skills necessary to practice autonomously and to delegate to and supervise others (NASN, 2021).

> *It is the position of the National Association of School Nurses (NASN) that every school-age child should have access to a* **registered professional school nurse (hereinafter referred to as the school nurse) who has a *minimum* of a baccalaureate degree in nursing from an accredited college or university and is licensed as a registered nurse through a board of nursing.** *These requirements constitute minimal preparation needed to practice at the entry level of school nursing. (para. 1)*

The rationale for school nurses to be BSN prepared at the entry level to practice is that the autonomous nature of school nurse practice requires advanced critical thinking, problem-solving, and complex decision-making skills to support student health at both the individual and school community level (NASN, 2021). Registered nurses without BSN degrees serve important roles as nurses in schools. Licensed practical/vocational nurses (LPNs/LVNs) also contribute to the care of students by providing routine care in the health office and within their scope of practice under the state nurse practice act. Therefore, nurses prepared at the LPN/LVN or associate degree level are strongly encouraged to advance their education and careers by enrolling in BSN or graduate entry MSN programs. The need to increase the number of BSN-prepared nurses is supported by a University of Washington school nurse survey, which reported only 63.8% of school nurses held a BSN or MSN degree (Willgerodt et al., 2018). Many school nurse leaders advocate that school nurses should attain graduate-level education beyond a bachelor's degree in parity with other professional school support personnel, such as social workers, occupational or physical therapists, and speech/language pathologists.

Additionally, continuing education, including advanced degrees and certification, is paramount to maintain nursing knowledge and skill. While important for any professional nurse, the independent nature of the school nurse's practice amplifies the need for professional development (NASN, 2022a). Understanding the demographics of school nurse educational status is important in examining the expertise of the school nurse as it relates to positive student outcomes and is consistent with the minimal level of education required for all other school professionals.

Certification/Licensure

Most state departments of education or health establish minimum criteria for nurses to practice in the school setting or to recognize school nurse expertise in the field. NASN supports state school nurse certification or licensure. Several states mandate state-specific certification or licensure beyond the registered nurse license in order to practice as a school nurse. These types of state-mandated certification or licensure often have requirements for work experience and/or continuing education; some require academic coursework. Some states require certification or licensure for school nurses that is equivalent to that of teachers, including Rhode Island and New Jersey (National Association of State Boards of Education [NASBE], n.d.). California requires 24 additional college credit hours, and West Virginia requires an RN and BSN (NASBE, n.d.). Illinois requires graduate-level coursework and a 300-hour internship for state certification as a licensed professional educator/school nurse (Illinois State Board of Education, n.d.). This certification or licensure allows the school nurse to teach health courses or selected course content. National certification through the National Board for Certification of School Nurses (NBCSN) within a designated time period from hire is another way in which states ensure competency in school nursing. North Carolina has mandated this requirement for school nurses in their state (North Carolina Department of Health and Human Services, 2022).

School nurses can obtain certification or licensure in specialty practice areas (e.g., medical-surgical nursing, family nurse practitioner, informatics) depending on their expertise and level of education. The American Nurses Credentialing Center (ANCC), an entity of the American Nurses Association Enterprise and one of the most prominent nursing certification bodies, describes certification as follows:

> *Certification is the process by which a nongovernmental agency or an association grants recognition to an individual who has met certain predetermined qualifications. Certification can be used for entry into practice, validation of competence, recognition of excellence, and/or for regulation. It can be mandatory or voluntary. Certification validates an individual's knowledge and skills in a defined role and clinical area of practice, based on predetermined standards. (ANCC, 2023, p. i)*

National Certification in School Nursing

NASN (2021, 2022a) endorses National Certification in School Nursing (NCSN). The NCSN credential is a mark of excellence in school nursing practice that reflects a commitment to competence and professionalism and demonstrates a high level of clinical practice experience, knowledge, and skills (NBCSN, 2024a). To become nationally board certified in school nursing, nurses must apply and take a certification examination through NBCSN. Qualifying criteria include the following:

- Current registered nurse license
- At least 1,000 hours of experience in school nursing (practice, leadership, teaching)
- Bachelor's degree in nursing or master's in education with concentration in school nursing or school health
- Passing score on written certification examination (NBCSN, 2022)

At the end of 2024, approximately 6,000 school nurses have earned the NCSN credential. Almost one-fourth of school nurses with national certification were from North Carolina (a state that mandates national certification), and 18% were from Massachusetts (NBCSN, 2024b). In addition, nurses working internationally can also hold the NCSN credential. School nurses who earn the NCSN credential can advocate that their school districts recognize their expertise through an annual stipend or salary increase from their school district in parity with that offered to nationally certified teaching staff.

The "What" of School Nursing

School nursing has a rich history of supporting the mission of both education and health to promote the well-being of children. Over time there have been challenges in delineating the "role expectations" of the school nurse both internally (among school nurses) and externally (among nurses, health-care providers, school administrators, educational staff, school communities, and governmental bodies). Changes and variations in school nursing service delivery models resulted in changes to role definitions, but the essence has never been lost.

From Lillian Wald at the turn of the 20th century into the 21st century, school nurses continue to support the universal goals of education and health: academic success and optimal wellness. In successful school nursing practices, these goals weave seamlessly together to create a safety net and springboard for children to grow into healthy and successful citizens—a goal that parallels the mission of NASN "to optimize student health and learning by advancing the practice of school nursing" (n.d., para 2). School nurses accomplish this goal by assisting students to improve and manage their health. See Chapter 1 for discussion of the history of school nursing.

Did You Know?

The National Board for Certification of School Nurses (NBCSN) was founded by NASN in 1986 and is now an independent, incorporated body and a member of the American Board of Nursing Specialties (NBCSN, 2024a).

Trends in student health status, school demographics, and the education and skill level of nurses all influence role definitions and task expectations of the school nurse. If, however, differences in geography, resources, institutional settings, employers, educational preparation, and tradition are erased from the equation, the question "What is the role of the school nurse?" can be easily answered: the school nurse's primary role is to advance the well-being, academic success, and lifelong achievement and health of students. This occurs as school nurses reduce or eliminate barriers to learning and health.

School Nursing: Scope and Standards of Practice (2022a) and the related competencies are well defined. School nursing practice can be affected by many factors, including student needs and school health services models that are as diverse as the students and communities they serve. The care provided by the school nurse is student-focused but refined by the external influences of the school community, the department of education or the department of public health, the theoretical model/theory on which practice is based, the boundaries of the state nurse practice act, the professional standards of school nursing, and the workload capacity of the nurse.

The AAP Council on School Health (2016) position statement on the *Role of the School Nurse in Providing School Health Services* describes the school nurse as providing both individual and population health for children and adolescents, affecting social determinants of health, providing chronic disease management, and participating in emergency preparedness, health promotion, and mental health assessment. They also highlight the role of the school nurse as a part of the team with health-care providers to participate in the coordination of care for students with specialized health-care needs.

This description coincides with NASN's current *School Nurse Workforce Study* results regarding "How school nurses spend their day," which is organized using the principles of the School Nursing Practice Framework (Willgerodt et al., 2023b). See Figure 3-6.

Forty-nine percent of the responding school nurses' day was spent in *care coordination:* assisting in acute and chronic condition management, e-mailing and creating reports, teaching and counseling, working on individual health-care plans, individualized education programs (IEPs), emergency action plans, Section 504 plans, and other activities.

Just over 24% of school nurses' time was spent in activities related to the *community/public health* principle such as compliance, vaccinations and health screenings, health promotion and prevention, and addressing social determinants of health and environmental issues.

The *leadership* and *quality improvement* principles each compose about 10% of the average workday for a school nurse. Leadership activities include advocacy, professional development, creating policies and procedures, and other

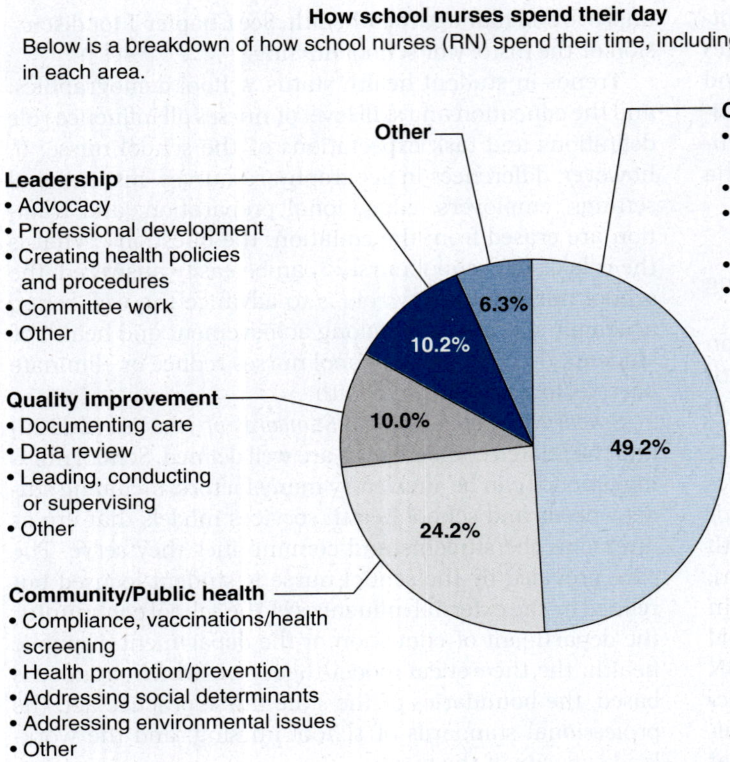

FIGURE 3-6. How School Nurses spend their day. *(Willgerodt et al., 2023c).*

committee work. Quality improvement work is described as documenting care; reviewing data; and leading, conducting, or supervising quality improvement initiatives.

FACTORS INFLUENCING SCHOOL NURSING SERVICES

Students who are not well will not learn well. In 1989, the Carnegie Corporation of New York released a landmark study on education. A key finding related to health is described in the following statement: "School systems are not responsible for meeting every need of the student, but, when the need directly affects learning, clearly the school must meet the challenge" (Adelman & Taylor, 2006, p. 121). This remains true today and was reemphasized by *The Future of Nursing 2020–2030* (National Academies of Sciences, Engineering, and Medicine, 2021).

Students With Special Health-Care Needs

The need for some level of school nursing services extends to *all* children; however, the school nursing workforce must meet the growing needs for the care coordination of students with special health-care needs (Gray et al., 2020). Children and youth need assistance at school to maintain their health. Almost 20% of children ages 0 to 17 have special health-care needs (Child and Adolescent Health Measurement Initiative, 2023). Children who attend school often require support from the school nurse related to asthma, diabetes, epilepsy, food allergies, and mental/behavioral health conditions. The number of students with physical and psychological chronic conditions continues to increase, particularly in children living in poverty (Maternal and Child Health Bureau, 2021). A national survey found that although 90% of U.S. children were judged by their caregiver to be in excellent or very good health, about 1.5% or 1 million children were reported to be in poor or fair health. These were more often American Indian/Alaska Native or non-Hispanic Black children. Poor health also was related to living in conditions of poverty. Of particular concern was the rise in emotional disorders (anxiety or depression) in children 3 to 17 years across all races/ethnicities. The school nurse addresses students' ongoing health care and safety needs that interfere with full access to the classroom. Whether from specific health conditions or the impact of social determinants of health, the needs of the students affect the amount of nursing care required in school or district.

Children with special health-care needs are protected by law and have the right to attend school. Several federal laws, including the Rehabilitation Act of 1973, the Individuals With Disabilities Education Improvement Act of 2004, and the Americans With Disabilities Act of 2008, not only allow for students to attend school but require needed nursing and health services be provided. These laws also ensure that student access issues are addressed, that transportation is provided, and that they are educated in the least restrictive environment. See Chapter 7 to learn more about federal laws that protect students with

Did You Know?

Hunger related to food insecurity is an aspect of *economic stability*—a social determinant of health and a focus of the *Health People 2030* objectives (Office of Disease Prevention and Health Promotion, n.d.). One way to address food insecurity faced by students each weekend is a backpack program. *Feeding America* (2024) has a network of over 10,000 backpack programs across the United States. These programs offer free groceries for the weekend or school break and are available through Feeding America and other nonprofit organizations. Often, the programs are coordinated through the school nurse or school social worker.

disabilities and their application to school nursing. Students with special health-care needs have the right to be evaluated by a school nurse when decisions are being made about the care to be provided at school. The school nurse is the qualified professional who contributes findings and recommendations for nursing services in special education eligibility meetings, IEP meetings, and 504 meetings. The **caseload** of students a school nurse serves with IEPs and 504 plans must be considered in terms of time needed for holding meetings with parents and the school team, developing plans of care, and providing any direct care the student may need, such as ongoing health assessment, medications, or treatments.

School employees also have health and wellness needs. **Employee wellness** is a component of the WSCC model. Therefore, depending on their job description, school nurses may be members of school wellness teams and/or lead health promotion activities for school staff to address topics such as weight management (e.g., walking clubs), stress management (e.g., yoga), personal health education (e.g., breast self-examination, blood pressure checks), and other programs. Activities may also extend to the school community (e.g., drug awareness programs or first aid instruction). Similar to working with students, all programs are culturally congruent and based on client needs. See Chapter 33 for more on promoting school staff wellness.

School Nurse Staffing

Due to the growing needs of all students, NASN's widely accepted recommendation for a school nurse-to-student ratio of 1:750 has been replaced with more comprehensive guidelines on staffing. The AAP Council on School Health (2016) has also recognized the need for all children to have access to a school nurse and revised their recommendations from a 1:750 school nurse-to-student ratio to 1:1, *one school nurse to every school*. School nurse staffing models should be based on many factors beyond ratios to include how students' health is influenced by access to care, acuity, complexity, and social determinants of health (NASN, 2020). NASN (2022b) states that "all students should have access to school nursing care by a registered, professional school nurse . . . all day, every day" (para. 1). Furthermore, NASN (2020) states that "student acuity and school community indicators should be assessed to determine appropriate staffing levels. Access to a school nurse may mean that more than one school nurse is necessary to meet the needs of the school population" (para. 1).

Factors that impact school nurse workload include funding/budgeting, laws, policies, school nurse visibility, community and parent support for school nursing services, liability, supportive administration, role confusion by the school nurse, geographical characteristics, and regional beliefs and priorities.

Variations Between States

Differences in state nurse practice acts create discrepancies in how school nurses practice across the nation. One area of discrepancy between states is what tasks a school nurse can delegate. Where delegation is permitted, school nurses may be expected to train and delegate student care to **unlicensed assistive personnel** (UAP). Sometimes school nurses are hired specifically as consultants to train these "health extenders." The UAP may be a teacher, an administrative staff member, or instructional support personnel who have primary responsibilities other than health care for students. UAP may also be employed specifically as health aides who work exclusively to provide health care to students. If the nurse practice act and the school nursing practice model of the district allow, the school nurse may be expected to train, monitor, and maintain the competency of the UAP. See Chapters 30 and 31 for further discussion of delegation.

State departments of education rules and approaches result in differences in individual practice responsibilities of the school nurse in caring for students. For example, if a student enters school without the prerequisite immunizations, the response will vary among practice settings. In many states and districts, the school nurse is responsible for ensuring compliance through referral and follow-up. Increasingly, school nurses are leading school-located vaccination clinics, especially during communicable disease outbreaks such as was the case during the COVID-19 pandemic. In yet other states/districts, the school nurse will have no or minimal accountability because the tracking is delegated by the educational administrator to a secretary. And in still another state, there may be no one to check and reinforce the requirement. See Chapter 13 for more information on disease prevention and immunizations. Education mandates may further expand the school nurse's responsibilities by assigning responsibilities for emergency care and preventative health to others by indicating that the school nurse train and supervise them (e.g., emergency medication administration).

Local Education Agencies and School Administration

School nurses are hired primarily by local education agencies (boards of education) and departments of public health and are often funded from general school or special education funds, meaning the decision to create or maintain a school nurse position may be weighed against the hiring of a teacher or purchase of educational materials (Willgerodt et al., 2018). Management goals and budget constraints differ across this diverse spectrum of environments and employers. The school or governing authority dictates the number of hours the school nurse will be onsite, the number of schools covered, the nurse-to-student ratio, and the amount of other support available to assist with nursing services (see Chapter 32).

School administrators will often determine the level of authority the school nurse has over some aspects of the environment that influence students' health status. For example, the school nurse who identifies a safety hazard on the playground may have the authority to direct a custodian to make adaptations to the playground equipment to improve its safety, or the school nurse may need to seek principal or school board approval. Schools may have a school physician or school nurse supervisor for consultation or oversight of the school health program. However, in no case can a school administrator or other individual ask or demand that the nurse breach the state's nurse practice act.

THE RELATIONSHIP BETWEEN WELLNESS AND LEARNING

U.S. policies and agencies often separate education and health, yet they are intricately linked. Research shows that educational success and health status affect one another. The evidence for the strong relationship between school nursing, good health, and readiness to learn is highlighted throughout this textbook. In the famous words of former Surgeon General of the United States Joycelyn Elders, "You can't educate a child who isn't healthy, and you can't keep a child healthy who isn't educated" (AZ Quotes, n.d.).

No step-by-step instructions or magic formulas exist for student success. Each student, setting, and challenge is unique. Optimal student wellness and learning readiness depend on access to a school nurse who can respond holistically to the needs of students as an individual. School nurses must constantly adapt to changes in student needs. One school year, let alone one school day, is never like the previous one. Success is measured by meeting established outcome goals. Through data collection and analysis, school nurses effectively identify new needs, provide new interventions, and articulate new outcomes. School nurses need to creatively assume and blend a myriad of roles on behalf of student well-being and learning.

THE FUTURE OF SCHOOL NURSING

School nursing's history lies in meeting the ever-changing needs of the school-age child. The school's responsibility to address the health needs of students and school communities is as compelling today as it was for Lillian Wald in 1902. Herein lies the future of school nursing as well. As the number of students with special health-care needs continues to increase, the need for a school nurse all day, every day in every school becomes even more imperative (NASN, 2022b).

The National Academies of Sciences, Engineering, and Medicine's *Future of Nursing 2020–2030: Charting a Path to Achieve Health Equity* (2021) highlights school nursing practice more than any other specialty in addressing health equity as a matter of social justice. The call emphasizes the critical role of community and public health nursing, specifically stating that school nurses are "the bridge between the health care and education system and other sectors as well as links to broader community health issues through the student populations they serve" (p. 2). The report also acknowledged that to enhance school nursing the nurse should be allowed to practice to the full scope of their license and that current payment structures must be improved.

School nurses increasingly play multifaceted roles in education, supporting the physical, mental, emotional, and social health of students. Nationally and internationally, school nurses can leverage *The Future of Nursing 2020–2030* (2021) and NASN's *School Nursing Practice Framework* (2024a) to synergize the power of school nursing to improve the lives of generations of students to come.

The editors gratefully acknowledge the work of the previous chapter authors, Carolyn L. Duff, Linda C. Wolfe, and Cheryl-Ann Resha.

References

Adelman, H. S., & Taylor, L. (2006). Special report on child mental health: Mental health in schools and public school. *Public Health Reports, 121*, 294–298.

American Academy of Pediatrics, Council on School Health. (2016). Role of the school nurse in providing school health services. *Pediatrics, 137*(6):e20160852. https://doi.org/10.1542/peds.2016-0852

American Association of Colleges of Nursing. (2023). The impact of education on nursing practice [Fact Sheet]. https://www.aacnnursing.org/news-data/fact-sheets/impact-of-education-on-nursing-practice

American Nurses Association. (2015). *Code of ethics for nurses with interpretive statements.* Author.

American Nurses Association. (2021). *Nursing: Scope and standards of practice* (4th ed.). Author.

American Nurses Credentialing Center. (2023). *Certification: General testing and renewal handbook.* https://www.nursingworld.org/~4a9ce2/globalassets/certification/renewals/ancc-generaltestingrenewalrequirements.pdf

AZ Quotes. (n.d.). *Joycelyn Elders.* https://www.azquotes.com/quote/715884#google_vignette

Centers for Disease Control and Prevention. (2023). Whole School, Whole Community, Whole Child (WSCC) Model. *CDC Healthy Schools.* https://www.cdc.gov/healthyschools/wscc/index.htm

Child and Adolescent Health Measurement Initiative. (2023). National performance measure/national outcome measures state comparison Map: 2020–2021. *Data Resource Center for Child and Adolescent Health*, U.S. Department of Health and Human Services, Health Resources and Services Administration (HRSA), Maternal and Child Health Bureau (MCHB). https://www.childhealthdata.org/browse/rankings

Combe, L. G. (2020). School nurses: Living the framework during COVID-19. *NASN School Nurse, 35*(4), 183–187. https://doi.org/10.1177/1942602X20929533

Common Core State Learning Standards Initiative. (2024). *Common core state standards.* https://corestandards.org/

Connecticut State Department of Education, School Nurse Competency Task Force. (2014). *Competency in school nurse practice* (2nd ed.). Author. https://portal.ct.gov/-/media/SDE/School-Nursing/Publications/Competency_in_School_Nurse_Practice.pdf

Council of Public Health Nursing Organizations. (n.d.). *About CPHNO.* https://www.cphno.org/about/

Duff, C., & Poole, C. (2016). School nurses coordinating care through a community/school health partnership. *NASN School Nurse, 31*(6), 342–346. https://doi.org/10.1177/1942602X16639379

Feeding America. (2024). *Backpack program.* https://www.feedingamerica.org/our-work/hunger-relief-programs/backpack-program

Gray, L., Klein, N., Meuret, C., Nelson, L., & Stahlnecker, L. (2020). Care coordination: A principle of 21st century school nursing practice with a focus on case management. *NASN School Nurse, 35*(4), 219–223. https://doi.org/10.1177/1942602X20928345

Illinois State Board of Education. (n.d.). *Educator licensure: PEL support personnel endorsements, school nurse–pre K–age 22.* https://www.isbe.net/Pages/PEL-School-Support-Ed-Lic.aspx

Maternal and Child Health Bureau. (2021). National survey of children's health: Data brief. *Health Resources and Services Administration.* https://mchb.hrsa.gov/sites/default/files/mchb/data-research/national-survey-childrens-health-2021-overview-fact-sheet.pdf

Meza, O., & Rau, W. (2021). *School nursing: Scope and standards of practice* [original graphic]. Lincoln Public Schools, Lincoln, NE.

National Academies of Sciences, Engineering, and Medicine. (2021). *The future of nursing 2020–2030: Charting a path to achieve health equity.* The National Academies Press. https://doi.org/10.17226/25982

National Association of School Nurses. (n.d.) *About NASN: The NASN mission.* https://www.nasn.org/about-nasn/about

National Association of School Nurses. (2016). Framework for 21st century school nursing practice. *NASN School Nurse, 31*(1), 45–53. https://doi.org/10.1177/1942602X15618644

National Association of School Nurses. (2020). *School nurse workload: Staffing for safe care* [Position Statement]. Author.

National Association of School Nurses. (2021). *Education, licensure, and certification of school nurses* [Position Statement]. Author.

National Association of School Nurses. (2022a). *School nursing: Scope and standards of practice* (4th ed.). Author.

National Association of School Nurses. (2022b). *Student access to school nursing services* [Position Statement]. Author.

National Association of School Nurses. (2023). *Supervision and evaluation of the school nurse* [Position Statement]. Author.

National Association of School Nurses. (2024a). A contemporary framework update for today's school nursing landscape: Introducing the School Nursing Practice Framework. *NASN School Nurse, 39*(3), 140–147. https://www.doi.org/10.1177/1942602X241241092

National Association of School Nurses. (2024b). *School-sponsored trips.* [Position Statement]. Author.

National Association of State Boards of Education. (n.d.). *State policy database.* https://statepolicies.nasbe.org/health/categories/health-services/school-nurse-qualifications

National Board for Certification of School Nurses. (2022). *NBCSN policies & procedures.* https://www.nbcsn.org/wp-content/uploads/2022/09/NBCSN-Policy-Manual-Revised-9-22.pdf

National Board for Certification of School Nurses. (2024a). *About NBCSN.* https://www.nbcsn.org/about/

National Board for Certification of School Nurses. (2024b). *NBCSN member search.* https://nbcsn.learningbuilder.com/Public/MemberSearch/Search

National Center for Education Statistics. (2018). *Compulsory school attendance laws, minimum and maximum age limits for required free education by state: 2017.* https://nces.ed.gov/programs/statereform/tab5_1.asp

National Council of State Boards of Nursing. (2023). *Nurse licensure compact map.* https://nursecompact.com/files/NLC_Map.pdf

North Carolina Department of Health and Human Services. (2022). *North Carolina school health program manual, Section C, School nursing practice, Chapter 1, Standards.* https://www.ncdhhs.gov/c1standardsofpractice2pdf/open#:~:text=The%20credential%20standard%20for%20school,years%20of%20date%20of%20hire

Office of Disease Prevention and Health Promotion. (n.d.). Healthy People 2030: Food Insecurity. *U.S. Department of Health and Human Services.* https://health.gov/healthypeople/priority-areas/social-determinants-health/literature-summaries/food-insecurity

Rossi-Scott, L. & Bubert, J. (2013). Leagal issues related to school nursing practice. The foundation. In J. Selekman (Ed.). School nursing: A comprehensive text. F.A. Davis.

Struthers, L. R. (1917). *The school nurse.* G. P. Putnam's Sons.

Tennessee Department of Education. (2023, August). *School nurse competencies & evaluation: A guide for nursing supervisors and school administrators.* https://www.tn.gov/content/dam/tn/education/csh/Final-School_Nurse_Evaluation_Guide.pdf

U.S. Environmental Protection Agency. (2023). *Implementing coordinated school environmental health guidelines. Healthy School Environments.* https://www.epa.gov/schools/implementing-coordinated-school-environmental-health-guidelines

Wallin, R. L., & Rothman, S. (2020). A new framework for school nurse self-reflection and evaluation. *NASN School Nurse, 35*(1), 35–42. https://doi.org/10.1177/1942602X19852295

Willgerodt, M. A., Brock, D. M., & Maughan, E. M. (2018). Public school practice in the United States. *Journal of School Nursing, 34*(3), 232–244. https://doi.org/10.1177/1059840517752456

Willgerodt, M. A., Brock, D., & Tanner, A. (2023a). Funding for public school nurses. *National School Nurse Workforce Study 2.0* [Infographic]. https://www.nasn.org/research/school-nurse-workforce

Willgerodt, M. A., Brock, D., & Tanner, A. (2023b). Public school nurses in the U.S. *National School Nurse Workforce Study 2.0* [Infographic]. https://www.nasn.org/research/school-nurse-workforce

Willgerodt, M. A. Brock, D., & Tanner, A. (2023c, June 30). School nurse workforce report. [Plenary presentation]. NASN Annual Conference, Orlando, Florida.

Wold, S. J., & Dagg N. (1981). School nursing: A passing experiment. In S. J. Wold (Ed.), *School nursing: A framework for practice* (pp. 3–19). Sunrise River Press.

Yonkaitis, C. F., & Jacobs, J. (2022). Undesignated glucagon in Illinois: An issue of access and equity. *NASN School Nurse, 37*(6), 331–336. https://doi.org/10.1177/1942602X221120820

Laws

Americans With Disabilities Amendment Act of 2008. (42 U.S.C. §§ 12101-12102). https://www.ada.gov/regs2016/adaaa.html

Individuals With Disabilities Education Improvement Act of 2004. (Pub. L. 108-446). https://www.gpo.gov/fdsys/pkg/PLAW-108publ446/content-detail.html

Rehabilitation Act of 1973. (Pub. L. 93-112). https://www.gpo.gov/fdsys/pkg/STATUTE-107/pdf/STATUTE-107-Pg718.pdf

Chapter 4

The School Nurse's Role as Health Educator

Jenny M. Gormley ▪ Kathleen Hassey

CHAPTER OUTLINE

Good teaching makes a difference. According to a research report issued by the RAND Corporation, "Teachers matter more to student achievement than any other aspect of schooling" (Opper, 2019). In the United States, the most common measures of teacher effectiveness are "structured classroom observations, teacher contributions to student achievement growth, and student perceptions of teacher effectiveness and classroom instructional climate" (Schweig, 2019, para. 2). If school nurses are going to be effective in supporting students' understanding and adoption of positive health behaviors, they need to be expert in what is taught (content) as well as how they teach students (pedagogy).

Health education has been part of the school nurse's role since the inception of school nursing. Lina Rogers Struthers, often identified as the first school nurse, wrote that "health education is the fundamental basis of all school health work" and "when the school nurse has taught the children that a healthy body and a sound mind are his greatest assets, her work will have given our educational system an inestimable force" (Struthers, 1917, pp. 11, 235). More recently, professional organizations have confirmed that health education is a key component of the school nurse's role as well as a competency for practice (American Academy of Pediatrics, 2016; Centers for Disease Control and Prevention [CDC], 2022b; National Association of School Nurses [NASN], 2022). The role of the school nurse gained significant attention during the COVID-19 pandemic, especially related to providing education and other services to school communities to reduce the spread of infection (Gormley, 2020; McIntosh et al., 2022; NASN, 2022; White House, 2022).

Effective teaching by school nurses depends on preparation, experience, evaluation, and collaboration with strong learning teams consisting of teachers and other school support personnel. Professional preparation in the specialty of school nursing is essential in order to be an effective teacher of topics relevant to school health. The school nurse must be proficient in the methods of effective teaching as well as knowledgeable on the topic presented. School nurses must also work within the educational system to promote the goals of the school, district, state, and nation.

Several states, including Massachusetts, New Jersey, and Rhode Island, refer to their school nurses as "school nurse teachers" or "school nurse educators," with some requiring specific coursework in teaching and learning for state school nurse certification. Regardless of title, every school nurse has a role in health education for students and school communities.

The purpose of this chapter is to describe the school nurse's professional role as an educator in the school setting. The objectives of this chapter are that the school nurse will be able to

- Define imperatives for health education in schools.
- Describe the context in which health education takes place in schools.
- Explain the role of the school nurse as reflected in professional nursing standards.
- Analyze how teaching components can be applied to the school nurse's role as educator.

IMPERATIVES FOR HEALTH EDUCATION

Goals from global to local initiatives, as well as federal and state standards and rules, guide programs and individuals in determining health education priorities and educator competencies. The United Nations (UN) Sustainable Development goals, the World Health Organization (WHO) Global School Health Initiative, and the U.S. *Healthy People* goals all contribute to understanding the framework in which school nurses can make a difference in promoting health for students in schools (Ross et al., 2021; UN, n.d., 2015; U.S. Department of Health and Human Services [USDHHS], n.d.b.).

Global and National Imperatives for Health Education

The *U.N. Sustainable Development Goals* (2015) set priorities to promote a healthy, sustainable world population focusing on strengthening peace, eradicating poverty, and achieving gender equality. The goals that relate most to the role of school nurse as educator include ending hunger, improving nutrition, promoting well-being, and ensuring inclusive and equitable quality education. Each goal has implications for school nurses in terms of content to be addressed when educating students and communities.

The *Global School Health Initiative* seeks to improve the health of students, school personnel, families, and other community members (Ross et al., 2021). A major goal of this initiative is to increase the number of "Health-Promoting Schools" that provide health education, health services, and health promotion programs. The *Global School Health Initiative* also aims to influence health-related behaviors, such as knowledge, skills, and attitudes through effective school nurse instruction as part of a health education collaborative team. Another component of the Global School Health Initiative is the *Global School-Based Student Health Survey*, which provides information about student health in countries around the world (CDC, 2018). The Student Health Survey includes questionnaires on major health topics, including alcohol and drug use, diet, hygiene, mental health, protective factors, sexual behavior, and violence and unintentional injury. The survey provides data for more than 90 countries. This survey mirrors the U.S. national youth survey, the *Youth Risk Behavior Survey*, which monitors six health risk behaviors that contribute to youth injury and death (CDC, 2023b). The data collected in these surveys can then be used to guide planning for educational offerings and evidence-based interventions to promote health and decrease risky behaviors.

The emphasis on equality resonates in the U.S. national health goals outlined in the *Healthy People* initiative. *Healthy People* is a collaboration between the U.S. Department of Health and Human Services and other government and professional organizations, businesses, and community members that determine goals and priorities for promoting the health of the U.S. population (USDHHS, n.d.b). *Healthy People* objectives have many implications for school health and can be used by school nurses to address the major problems faced by youth in the United States. *Healthy People 2030* includes an approach with five overarching goals that relate directly to student health and the work of school nurses:

- Attain healthy, thriving lives and well-being, free of preventable disease, disability, injury, and premature death.
- Eliminate health disparities, achieve health equity, and attain health literacy to improve the health and well-being of all.
- Create social, physical, and economic environments that promote attaining full potential for health and well-being for all.
- Promote healthy development, healthy behaviors, and well-being across all life stages.
- Engage leadership, key constituents, and the public across multiple sectors to take action and design policies that improve the health and well-being of all (USDHHS, n.d.a, Browse Objectives).

State and Local Imperatives for Health Education

Before teaching in the classroom, school nurses must be aware of existing state and local regulations that may influence the planning and delivery of health education. State guidelines range from little direction regarding what health content should be taught to specific content that clearly directs lesson planning, including health-related learning standards. When state guidelines are not present, the school health team should work together using the *National Health Education Standards* (National Consensus for School Health Education [NCSHE], 2022), described later in this chapter, and state resources while being responsive to the needs of the school community. If specific content is outlined in regulations, then public school districts need to be accountable to those regulations.

Professional Imperatives for Health Education

School nurses are committed to improving the health of students in their schools, as well as improving the health of the nation; therefore, school nurses who plan to teach need to understand and appreciate the professional standards that guide educators. Each U.S. state is mandated to provide public education for children and youth and to support that education through state funding. Because education expenses consume large portions of state budgets and much of it is tax based, there is considerable concern about providing accountability for educational expenditures. In general, it is the teachers' performance and various measures of student success that school administrators and governing bodies evaluate in determining whether taxpayer money is being well spent. Professional organizations and state and national agencies and programs assist teachers to demonstrate accountability in achieving positive student outcomes.

Two professional organizations associated with teaching in American schools are the American Federation of Teachers (AFT) and the National Education Association (NEA). The mission of AFT includes championing high-quality public education (AFT, n.d.). The purpose of the NEA, the nation's largest professional employee organization, is to "champion justice and excellence in public education" (NEA, n.d.). The NEA website provides tools and resources for educators, including best practices and expert opinions on lesson plans, classroom management, teaching strategies, and school culture. In 2021, school nurses gained representation on the NEA as New Jersey School Nurse Sheila Caldwell was named as the first Specialized Instructional Support Personnel (SISP) Fellow, working in the Education Support Professional Quality (ESPQ) department (Caldwell, 2021).

The National Board for Professional Teaching Standards (NBPTS) is an independent, nonprofit U.S. organization that seeks to identify and recognize accomplished teaching through a national certification program for educators. According to NBPTS (n.d., para. 3), highly effective teachers

- Are committed to students and their learning
- Know the subjects they teach and how to teach those subjects to students
- Are responsible for managing and monitoring student learning
- Think systematically about their practice and learn from experience
- Are members of learning communities

How does one become a highly effective teacher? For classroom teachers, teacher education preparation occurs primarily at the college level. Accountability for teacher preparation and performance rests with both the teacher preparation programs and in the performance of teachers in the classroom. Accountability approaches vary by teacher preparation program and by state, often including the *Praxis*, edTPA, NES, and/or a state-determined assessment examination (Staake, 2022). The Council for the Accreditation of Educator Preparation (n.d.) accredits teacher preparation programs to ensure quality of instruction for students learning to be teachers. This preparation and accountability are particularly important for those states that certify their nurses as teachers. However, all school nurses can benefit from keeping the NBPTS objectives in mind.

Legal Imperatives for Education

Since the late 1970s, U.S. educators have felt increased pressure to help students attain more complex outcomes. By the 1990s, every state had adopted "report cards" on how students were performing on a range of desirable school achievement goals. The federal *2001 No Child Left Behind Act* (NCLB) and subsequent acts accelerated this accountability trend.

The 2009 *Common Core State Standards* (CCSS) were developed by teachers, administrators, state leaders, governors, and state commissioners of education to bring consistency to academic standards in mathematics and English language arts/literacy across the nation (CCSS, 2017). Adoption of the Common Core State Standards by states was voluntary, although federal stimulus funding to school districts during the recession in 2009–2010 was provided to states adopting them. The CCSS have not yet yielded improvements in student achievements, and many states have rebranded the standards as state standards to reduce controversy (Goldstein, 2021).

The 2015 *Every Student Succeeds Act* (ESSA) replaced NCLB, shifting responsibility for ensuring students meet achievement thresholds and accountability for teacher effectiveness from the U.S. Department of Education to state departments of education, allowing more flexibility (U.S. Department of Education, 2020). Health and wellness measures are included in the 2015 ESSA; federal funds can now be used for health education as part of providing a well-rounded education (NASN, 2017).

TEACHING OPPORTUNITIES FOR SCHOOL NURSES

Teaching Opportunities With Students, Staff, Families, and Peers

School nurses have opportunities to teach about health daily. Learners can be any individual or group of students, staff, teachers, administrators, board members, colleagues, parents/guardians, families, and community members, as well as school nurse peer groups. Teaching can take place in the health office one-to-one, in small groups, in medium- to large-size classes, in school assemblies, in formal and informal settings, in staff and professional meetings, or through print, online, or other electronic media. The COVID-19 pandemic provided an opportunity for nurses to teach synchronously and asynchronously via platforms such as Google and Zoom to students, parents, and school communities (Marrapese et al., 2021).

The most obvious and often implemented teaching role of the school nurse occurs when educating students and their families about their health conditions and providing options for health-promoting behavior and strategies to improve health. Small-group teaching occurs when there is a special group interested in learning about a health-related topic. For example, teachers in second grade might need to learn how to work with students with allergies in their classroom. The school nurse would develop a lesson plan that addressed the teachers' ability to identify triggers, signs, and symptoms, and how to provide emergency care. Or students who are pregnant may meet with the school nurse in a small group to learn about the pros and cons of infant feeding options.

Classes in health are also obvious places where the school nurse can implement the role of educator. Other opportunities exist in government classes as a venue for talking about legal rights and responsibilities of minors in relation to health care; in math classes for learning about calculating the body mass index; in language classes for learning how to ask for health-care help when speaking to persons in another language; in English classes to learn about strategies for communicating about health concerns and studying about themes related to health in literature; in history classes to discuss the evolution of health-care concerns and the inequities faced by certain groups and what can be done to make changes for the future; in art or music classes to share strategies for relaxation and health promotion; and in science classes, which relate to almost all topics of health. The BSN-prepared nurse may be one of the few educators on campus with a science degree. Therefore, collaboration with science teachers and other faculty and coaches on topics related to anatomy, physiology and health are wonderful opportunities to highlight the expertise of the school nurse as a scientist.

Establishing the school nurse's role as educator may take time and can be accomplished in small increments. Brief messages (such as public service announcements) can be delivered together with the daily announcements. The school nurse can deliver short health messages to the entire school population via daily announcements, school newsletters or broadcasts, and school assemblies. For example, the school nurse could develop a schedule for *Myths on Monday, Tips for Tuesday, Wellness Wednesday, Thoughts on Thursday,* or *Facts on Friday* as the focus of health messages aligned with the school's health goals, *Healthy People* goals, national health observances, or current health issues of concern to the school community.

Regular, brief messages about health can be incorporated into the school community under the leadership of the school nurse so that students and staff begin to anticipate health messages. Keeping staff in the know about breaking news regarding health (whether sensationalized or legitimate) can reduce staff anxiety and remind them that the school nurse is an available, informed, expert resource. Health topics can be reinforced through a variety of venues to strengthen the message and to help educate others about the importance of the topic. This can be done in the classroom with follow-up activities provided to classroom teachers, notes home to parents, and notices in the school newsletter/website, the community newspaper, or local cable access television.

In addition to guest speaking in a class, school nurses might develop a series of classes for students or teachers with common health concerns. For example, small group learning experiences could be held for students or staff who are overweight or who have diabetes or asthma. These types of series might be held outside the regularly scheduled class sessions, as brown bag lunches, during common study hall periods, or before or after school. They may involve students, parents, staff, or a combination, depending on the topic. In most instances, parental consent must be sought before the teaching begins if the student will miss class time or stay after school.

Ideally, the expectation is that the school nurse will teach in the classroom to address health promotion strategies to improve health behaviors. In these situations, the nurse needs to develop a plan that is congruent with the mission of the school and consistent with the expectations for classroom preparation and performance of teachers in the school. At other times school nurses may be asked to share their expertise in professional meetings with other school nurses. Sharing with other school nurses is an important mechanism for promoting dialogue to improve school nursing practice and is emphasized in the school nursing *Education standard #13* (NASN, 2022). School board meetings and community meetings are another important venue for advocating for health policy change, supporting health promotion programs, and increasing understanding of the scope and responsibilities of school nursing practice. Principles for teaching and learning apply regardless of the audience and include preparing for meetings and presentations.

Teachable Moments

Using teachable moments in response to immediate concerns can readily mobilize the school community to health-care action. A teachable moment has been described as an opportunity for instruction or learning (unpredictable or planned) that produces a strong emotional response and increases perception of risk so that an individual may be motivated to change behavior (Lawson & Flocke, 2009). Starting in early

2020, the COVID-19 pandemic has been a long teachable moment for school nurses to educate school communities about signs and symptoms as well as measures to reduce virus spread, including masking, hand washing, isolation, quarantine, and vaccination (Vanderpool et al., 2020).

The news media and the Internet are constant sources of health-related content, though the reliability or thoroughness of the information the public receives may be questionable. From the COVID-19 pandemic, celebrities facing health crises, to local deaths, events have been used to capture the attention of the public and reinforce health teaching. When armed with accurate information, public and social media, community action, family discussion, and peer involvement focusing on current events can mobilize individuals to action.

Government agencies, health departments, and professional organizations such as NASN often publicize strategies that school nurses, teachers, and families can use to deal with catastrophes, epidemics, and tragedies. Federal, state, and community laws and regulations have been enacted as a result of these events, as in the case of *Megan's Law* related to sexual offenders that amended the Violent Crime Control and Law Enforcement Act of 1994 to require the release of relevant information to protect the public from sexually violent offenders.

The opportunity for addressing issues that are in the forefront for children, their parents, and the community is one that should not be overlooked. Willingness to change combined with a level of increased concern has been shown to be essential during teachable moments (Flocke et al., 2014). Taking advantage of teachable moments requires that school nurses have the skills to quickly access evidence-based materials and information. The CDC's Web sites have a wealth of materials available that can be easily accessed in response to teachable moments at school. In general, school nurses can use events (e.g., a missed period and fear of pregnancy or a publicized drowning) as teachable moments when the individual or group is attuned to the situation. These teachable moments should be integrated into a well-planned and coordinated health education program designed to address priority health concerns.

THE SCHOOL NURSE AS EDUCATOR: PROFESSIONAL STANDARDS

School nurses are committed to improving the health of students in their schools, thereby improving the health of the nation. School nurses contribute to students' learning about health in the classroom when they

1. Understand and implement educational interventions based on the standards that guide educators.
2. Speak the language of education and meet its standards for educational performance while in the school setting.
3. Collaborate with other professionals whose expertise in and commitment to education provide a foundation for understanding the educational climate in schools and who understand the role that the school nurse can play in promoting health through educational interventions.

NASN has issued standards regarding the role of the nurse as educator in the *School Nursing: Scope and Standards of Practice* (NASN, 2022). The first six standards (called the standards of school nursing practice) follow the nursing process. Embedded within the fifth standard, *Implementation*, is Standard 5B: *Health Teaching and Health Promotion.* This standard includes competencies that the nurse is expected to meet using evidence-based interventions, community resources, collaboration strategies, and systems management approaches (see Chapter 3).

The expectation is that all school nurses use health teaching to promote health with individual students and groups. Good teaching is considered a critical component of nursing practice. The *School Nursing Practice Framework* (NASN, 2024) reinforces the role of school nurse as an educator in the practice components listed in the five key principles of standards of practice, care coordination, leadership, quality improvement, and community/public health.

The question that must be addressed is, How does the school nurse become an effective teacher who can make a difference? The next section of this chapter outlines a nationally recognized approach to preparing successful teachers. This approach is used to prepare teachers in classrooms and can be useful in helping the school nurse be an active and accepted member of the school health education team.

THE DANIELSON FRAMEWORK FOR TEACHING

In *Enhancing Professional Practice: A Framework for Teaching*, Danielson (2007) describes the nature of learning and what teachers can do to promote it. She explains that constructivism, a theoretical framework that focuses on the learner's understanding of concepts, is "now acknowledged by cognitive psychologists as providing the most powerful framework for understanding how children (and adults) learn" (Danielson, 2007, p. 15).

Constructivism as a learning theory is seated in the work of Lev Vygotsky's social development theory, as well as in the work of Jean Piaget and John Dewey (Slavin, 2021). During the decades of increased accountability at the federal and state level, classroom educators increased their focus on critical thinking, problem-solving, lifelong learning, collaboration, and deeper understanding in the learning process. More attention was given to the interplay among content, the teacher, the learner, and the context.

Practice Connection

School Nursing: Standard 5B. Health Teaching and Health Promotion

The school nurse employs strategies to improve the health and a safety of students, family, group, school community, or population.

Competencies

The school nurse:

- Provides opportunities for the student and school community to identify needed health literacy, healthcare promotion, disease prevention, and self-management topics.
- Engages health promotion/health teaching considering the student and school communities' values, beliefs, health practices, developmental level, learning needs, readiness learn, language preference, spirituality, culture, and socioeconomic status.
- Uses evidence-based learning principles to communicate health promotion and disease prevention information to the student and school community.
- Engages consumer alliance and advocacy groups in health teaching and health promotion activities for students and the school community.
- Provides anticipatory guidance to students and families to promote health and prevent or reduce the risk of negative health outcomes.
- Collaborates with other school health professionals to provide appropriate and timely health promotion and health education to the student, family, and school community.
- Promotes health principles using the *Framework for 21st Century School Nursing Practice*™ and the *Whole School, Whole Community, Whole Child* model for students and the school community.
- Evaluates health information resources within the area of practice for accuracy, readability, and comprehensibility to help the school community access quality health information.
- Serves as a primary resource to the school community regarding health information and wellness.
- Evaluates evidence-based learning principles to conduct health teaching and counseling at the individual, aggregate, and population levels.
- Participates in the evaluation of health curricula and other health instructional materials and activities.
- Works in partnership with faculty, librarians, and community partners to integrate health literacy, health promotion, and illness and injury prevention into cross-curricular content.

Additional Competencies for the Graduate Level–Prepared School Nurse

In addition to the competencies of the school nurse, the graduate level–prepared school nurse:

- Assesses alignment of health education curricula within the context of national health education standards
- Identifies health education and health promotion focus based on local, state, or national data sets
- Designs health education information and programs for school community education appropriate to age, developmental level, learning needs, readiness to learn, and cultural values and beliefs of the target audience
- Evaluates effectiveness of health promotion programming using health education curriculum analysis tools (NASN, 2022, pp. 69–70)

Focus on the Framework

Community Public Health and Care Coordination

Teaching health promotion, health literacy and disease prevention in the classroom are practice components of the community/public health principle in the *Framework*. Teaching health and safety topics to faculty, staff, parents, and the larger school community are other examples of group health education. School nurses also teach individual students in the health office daily and should document learning objectives, instructional strategies, and learner outcomes in the individual student health record. This 1:1 teaching is captured in the care coordination component described as fostering developmentally appropriate independence and self-advocacy (NASN, 2024).

A constructivist approach to learning emphasizes that learning takes place when learners can make sense of the concepts for themselves. This differs based on each student's own worldview, experiences, and cognitive structures (Slavin, 2021). In other words, each person brings a unique learning style, repertoire of skills, experiences, and individual goals to the learning experience. When combined with the emotional maturity and motivation of the student, learning takes place. This means that each learner will learn what is relevant to him or her, and it may not necessarily be what other learners are learning.

For example, school nurses are often called on to teach about the pubertal changes related to growth and development. Students respond to the same learning situation in a variety of ways. Some interpret the information as too much or too scientific. Others say it clarified who they are and what is happening to them. Some students are perplexed by the whole topic, and others interpret the class to each other and their parents as a talk about sex.

The school nurse could also use constructivism to improve the potential for student learning when teaching a lesson regarding the perils of unprotected sex, for example. The lesson might include listing the top four reasons to avoid unprotected sexual activity and then having the students repeat those reasons back (knowledge). However, this does not mean that they will take the needed action to avoid unprotected sexual activity when making healthy choices (skills). To motivate behavior change, the school nurse needs to use a constructivist teaching approach that includes a safe learning environment in which students can consider the meaning of unprotected sexual activity, how it could affect their lives (dispositions), what choices they have, and what skills they need so that they truly learn the risks related to unprotected sexual activity.

Danielson's teaching framework clarifies the conditions that should be considered when planning and implementing learning experiences and how to evaluate the outcomes. School nurses can use this framework because nursing is about sharing knowledge and helping individuals, families, and communities apply that knowledge in the pursuit of health. The clarity and simplicity of the framework make it transferable to any teaching situation.

Enhancing Professional Practice: A Framework for Teaching details an evidence-based approach to help teachers meet the expected standards for student learning (Danielson, 2007; Danielson Group, n.d.a). This work was based on formal analyses of the tasks of teaching, reviews of research, analyses of state regulations for teacher licensing, and extensive pilot testing of the criteria in the author's framework. Other influences on this framework include professional teaching standards, the work of multiple educators, analyses of the concepts of teacher duties, and research on the pedagogical implications of constructivist learning (Danielson, 2007). The Danielson Group was formed in 2003 by Charlotte Danielson and a dozen other educator experts to provide consultation to states and school districts about effective teaching practices and provides learning opportunities and resources on its Web site to educators (Danielson Group, n.d.b). Danielson's *Framework for Teaching* simplifies the complexities of teaching by considering four major aspects or domains that are essential to the role of educator: (1) planning and preparation, (2) the classroom environment, (3) instruction, and (4) professional responsibilities. Each domain includes several components or activities needed for effective teaching. These domains and components provide a framework for planning, implementing, and evaluating the effectiveness of the school nurse in the role of health educator (Table 4-1). In other words, the framework addresses the what, who, when, and how of implementing the role of educator in school nursing practice.

TABLE 4-1 Danielson's Framework for Teaching Domains and Components

Domain	Components
Domain 1: Planning and Preparation	Demonstrate knowledge of content and pedagogy Demonstrate knowledge of students Set instructional goals, objectives, and outcomes Demonstrate knowledge of resources Design coherent instruction Design student assessments
Domain 2: The Classroom Environment	Develop rapport and create an environment of respect Establish a culture for learning Manage classroom procedures Manage student behavior Organize physical space
Domain 3: Instruction	Communicate with students Use questioning and discussion techniques Engage students in learning Use assessment in instruction Demonstrate flexibility and responsiveness
Domain 4: Professional Responsibilities	Reflect on teaching Maintain accurate records Communicate with families Participate in the school community Grow and develop professionally Show professionalism

Source: Republished with permission of ASCD from Danielson, C. (2007). *Enhancing professional practice: A framework for teaching* (2nd ed.); permission conveyed through Copyright Clearance Center, Inc.

Domain 1: Planning and Preparation

Demonstrate Knowledge of Content and Pedagogy

Before beginning teaching, the school nurse needs to decide what to teach and prepare for teaching. The health education curriculum approved by a local district or mandated by the state directs much of the educational content and experiences that need to be included for students. For nurses working in states that have not reached consensus on what the approved health curriculum ought to be, the school nurse can refer to the *Healthy People* objectives (USDHHS, n.d.b) as well as the *National Health Education Standards* (NHES) originally published in 1995, updated in 2007, and revised again in 2022 by experts from the following organizations: the American School Health Association, Eta Sigma Gamma, the Foundation for the Advancement of Health Education, the National Commission for Health Education Credentialing, the Society for Public Health Education, and the Society of State Leaders of Health and Physical Education (NCSHE, 2022). The overall goal of the latest edition of the NHES is to guide the development of health education curricula, instruction, and assessment for pre-K–12 students.

The eight health education standards and performance expectations are written for use by pre-K–12 teachers, local school and state directors of health education, curriculum developers, and health education teacher preparation faculty. The standards and performance expectations reflect the functional health knowledge, beliefs, and skills necessary for students to adopt and maintain healthy behaviors, achieve health literacy, and enhance health and academic outcomes.

The *National Health Education Standards* are written with performance indicators for each standard with the expectations that students will meet certain milestones by end of Grade 2, Grade 5, Grade 8, and Grade 12. The complete description can be found on their Web site. A sample (Standard #1) can be seen in Box 4-1.

BOX 4-1

National Health Education Standard #1

Standard 1: Students comprehend functional health knowledge to enhance health.

By the end of Grade 2, students will meet the following performance expectations:

1.2.1 Recognize multiple dimensions of health (e.g., physical, social, emotional, and intellectual).
1.2.2 Identify benefits of practicing health-promoting behaviors.
1.2.3 Identify potential consequences of practicing unhealthy behaviors.
1.2.4 Identify safe and unsafe situations, people, and events.
1.2.5 Identify practices and behaviors that prevent or reduce health risks (e.g., hand washing).
1.2.6 List ways to engage in healthy practices and behaviors (e.g., brushing teeth daily).
1.2.7 List ways to prevent common childhood injuries and health problems (e.g., wearing bicycle helmets and drinking water instead of sugary beverages).

By the end of Grade 5, students will meet the following performance expectations:

1.5.1 List examples of the physical, social, emotional, and intellectual dimensions of health.
1.5.2 Describe benefits of practicing health-promoting behaviors.
1.5.3 Explain potential consequences of practicing unhealthy behaviors.
1.5.4 Compare and contrast safe and unsafe situations, people, and events.
1.5.5 Describe practices and behaviors that prevent or reduce health risks (e.g., eating vegetables and fruits daily).
1.5.6 Explain ways to engage in healthy practices and behaviors (e.g., daily moderate to vigorous physical activity).
1.5.7 Explain ways to prevent common childhood injuries and health problems (e.g., recommendations for swimming safety and strategies for managing emotions).

By the end of Grade 8, students will meet the following performance expectations:

1.8.1 Describe interrelationships among physical, social, emotional, and intellectual health.
1.8.2 Analyze benefits of practicing health-promoting behaviors.
1.8.3 Analyze potential risks and consequences of practicing unhealthy behaviors.
1.8.4 Assess the risk of situations, people, and events that contribute to unhealthy behaviors and outcomes.
1.8.5 Explain why it is important to be responsible for personal health behaviors.
1.8.6 Analyze how personal practices and behaviors reduce or prevent health risks.
1.8.7 Analyze health promotion and disease prevention guidelines and recommendations for healthy behaviors from credible federal, professional, and voluntary health organizations (e.g., recommendations for rest and sleep).
1.8.8 Predict the likelihood of personal injury or illness if engaging in unhealthy behaviors.
1.8.9 Analyze the effects of family history, genetics, education level, and income on personal health status.

By the end of Grade 12, students will meet the following performance expectations:

1.12.1 Analyze interrelationships among physical, social, emotional, intellectual health, and well-being.
1.12.2 Predict how health behaviors affect the health status of self and others.
1.12.3 Compare and contrast benefits and barriers to practicing health behaviors.
1.12.4 Evaluate the effectiveness of personal practices and behaviors to reduce or prevent health risks.
1.12.5 Analyze how individual responsibility enhances personal, family, peer, school, and community health.
1.12.6 Predict how risk behaviors can affect injury, illness, or death.
1.12.7 Assess the risk of situations that can contribute to unhealthy behaviors and outcomes.
1.12.8 Analyze health promotion and disease prevention guidelines and recommendations for healthy behaviors from credible federal, professional, and voluntary health organizations (e.g., guidelines to prevent the spread of infectious diseases).
1.12.9 Analyze the likelihood of personal injury or illness if engaging in unsafe and unhealthy behaviors.
1.12.10 Evaluate how family history, genetics, education level, employment, and income can affect personal health status.

National Consensus for School Health Education. (2022). *National Health Education Standards: Model guidance for curriculum and instruction* (3rd ed.). www.schoolhealtheducation.org

The NHES place an emphasis on demonstrating skills based on the learner's ability to comprehend and analyze. The eight overall health education standards state that students will

1. Comprehend functional health knowledge to enhance health.
2. Analyze the influence of family, peers, culture, social media, technology, and other determinants on health behaviors.
3. Demonstrate health literacy by accessing valid and reliable health information, products, and services to enhance health.
4. Demonstrate effective interpersonal communication skills to enhance health.
5. Demonstrate effective decision-making skills to enhance health.
6. Demonstrate effective goal-setting skills to enhance health.
7. Demonstrate observable health and safety practices.
8. Advocate for behaviors that support personal, family, peer, school, and community health (NCSHE, 2022).

Health literacy, as a component of health education, cannot be overemphasized, as only 12% of U.S. adults have proficient health literacy skills (USDHHS, 2019). The definition of health literacy was updated in 2020 with the release of the Healthy People 2030 goals to place greater emphasis on people's ability to use health information (CDC, 2022a). The definition includes both personal and organizational health literacy:

Personal health literacy is the degree to which individuals have the ability to find, understand, and use information and services to inform health-related decisions and actions for themselves and others.

Organizational health literacy is the degree to which organizations equitably enable individuals to find, understand, and use information and services to inform health-related decisions and actions for themselves and others (CDC, 2022a, para. 1).

When teaching health lessons to parents or communicating orally with parents about their children's health concerns, school nurses can assess if instruction is delivered in a way that meets the parents' health literacy proficiency by using techniques such as "Teach-back" and "Ask Me 3." See Box 4-2. School nurses should also create written communications that have limited content and are easy to read. A team-based systematic approach to increasing health literacy that is applicable to schools can be found in the *AHRQ Health Literacy Universal Precautions Toolkit* (Brega et al., 2015). Another tool, the *Health Education Curriculum Analysis Tool* (HECAT; CDC, 2022d, can help schools evaluate their health education curricula based on the 2007 NHES Standards and CDC's *Characteristics of Effective Health Education Curricula.*

With input from teachers, administrators, staff, parents, students, community members, and school nurses, the health education curriculum should reflect the priorities for health promotion and disease prevention in the community and direct health education interventions. Topics that are relevant to the school population and community based on student needs, Youth Risk Behavior Survey data, or community concerns are often added to reflect priorities on a timely basis. The need for health education beyond the established health education curriculum may be triggered by any number of events such as students with possible anaphylaxis reactions in the school; an increase in unintended pregnancies; the prevalence of bullying or violence related to race, gender, sexual orientation, and gender identification; an increase in attempted and/or completed suicides; and/or recent morbidity or mortality from diseases or injuries.

Being an expert on the topic is important, but equally important is an understanding of teaching methodologies based on learners' developmental levels, cognitive strengths, and needs. The planning phase affords the school nurse the opportunity to consider the best way to approach the material. Because teaching in a classroom is different than teaching in the school health office or in staff meetings, school nurse preparation programs include an understanding of and opportunity to practice classroom management skills that are developmentally appropriate for the school setting. School nurses who regularly teach in a classroom must consider if they require additional education to improve their teaching skills by seeking appropriate continuing education or university-level course work.

BOX 4-2

Practical Techniques to Improve Communication with Students and Families

Teach-Back Method

- Limit content to 3–5 concepts; repeat each at least three ways.
- Provide information on one concept at a time.
- Ask questions to check for understanding.
- Avoid yes/no questions.

Ask Me 3

Ensure the student or family member can answer the following:

- What is my main problem?
- What do I need to do?
- Why is it important for me to do this?

Additional strategies include use of plain, concrete language and an interpreter if needed, avoiding medical or educational jargon, and sharing images or illustrations (Pontius, 2013).

Demonstrate Knowledge of Students

School nurses need to be prepared to work with diverse learners of all age and developmental groups. The National

Health Education Standards clearly emphasize developmentally appropriate experiences for preschool students versus students at other educational levels. Knowing who the audience is, together with the experiences, expectations, and aspirations of the individuals, is essential in the planning process to build on the learners' previous levels of knowledge and skill and to address any misconceptions or behaviors that might interfere with health-promoting activities. The school nurse should consult in advance with the classroom teacher about the class, student dynamics, and class norms or rules. It is important to be aware of any students who are English language learners or students with special learning or behavioral concerns who need differentiated instructional approaches.

Teaching parents and community members can be challenging because the school nurse must anticipate the demographics, needs, abilities, and motivation of the audience. For example, in presenting a series on adolescent development to parents and guardians of seventh-grade students, parental expectations will vary depending on their own experiences as adolescents and their parenting experiences with other teenagers. Adult learners expect to have a high degree of influence on what content is being presented and how it is being presented (Culatta, n.d.). This active participation should be encouraged in designing and implementing educational programs.

Whether the learner is a student, staff, family, and/or community member, standards of cultural competency need to be the hallmark of the planning process. The school nurse needs to consider language barriers, literacy issues, and values that influence the receptivity to the message; stereotypes or biases on the part of the school nurse also need to be considered if they could interfere with the delivery of an effective learning experience. For example, cultural expectations regarding teen dating vary widely among groups and individuals living in the same community; presenting information about "typical" adolescent behavior may not represent the norms and expectations of the learners. It is important for the nurse to be prepared to accommodate, acknowledge, and affirm the value of cultural differences in the group and the right of every person to make his or her own decisions based on a combination of informed decision making, values, and goals. See Chapter 10 for more on cultural care.

Set Instructional Goals, Objectives, and Outcomes

The goals and objectives for a lesson or class need to reflect the outcomes that are relevant for the individuals, the school, or the community. Using established goals and standards ensures that the outcomes are supported by the broader community and reflect the needs of large numbers of individuals. Health problems in a district may also direct the selection of outcomes. For instance, a recent teen death caused by illegal substance use and the increase in illegal drug transactions in the area may warrant initiation of programs to support safe and drug-free schools. The outcomes identified are not likely to be achieved in one or two classroom sessions. The school nurse needs to consider the overall outcome of the instructional process and then specifically plan the steps to achieve these measures.

Goals are the broad conditions that can be achieved over time. Specific outcomes or objectives are the measurable components of the learning process. For example, it might take several school years to demonstrate that teaching interventions resulted in increased pregnant and parenting teen graduation rates (goal). However, the *objective* of increasing the number of parenting teens who can accurately identify the school and community resources to support graduation could be measured in the short term (quarters or semesters).

When planning instruction, the school nurse should specify the learning objectives. The objectives should include who the learners are (e.g., students, parents, staff, community members) and how and when they will be able to operationalize what they have learned. Learning objectives should be SMART: *specific, measurable, achievable, realistic/relevant, and time-bound* (CDC, 2017). See Chapter 8 for more information about writing SMART objectives.

For example, a SMART objective for kindergarten students could be:

> *By the end of a hand washing lesson* (time-bound), *the kindergarten students will be able to point to three times* (measurable) *on the class schedule* (specific) *when hands should be washed* (relevant, achievable).

For high school students, a SMART goal could be:

> *Two weeks after the end of nurse-led group learning activity* (time-bound), *sophomore students will be able to report on a survey* (specific) *two actions steps* (measurable) *that they have taken to improve their sleep hygiene* (relevant, achievable).

SMART learning objectives guide teaching methods by highlighting the relationship between teaching, learning, attitudes, and action. Effective lesson plans contain factual knowledge but also consider the lived experience of the learner and how to motivate behavior change. This can be thought of as the knowledge-skills-dispositions triad (Darling-Hammond & Bransford, 2005). For example, a lesson that explores the risks related to drugs and alcohol does not prepare students with the skills to avoid such use. For learners to be competent in drug-resistance behavior, they need to know about drugs and their consequences (knowledge); to be able to recognize harmful substances and situations that put them at risk and know how to extricate themselves or ask for help when in a risky situation (skills); and for the knowledge and skills to be effective, the learners have to want to be drug free and value healthy behaviors (dispositions).

A meaningful lesson could be designed to give the students an opportunity to role-play and explore as a group how to deal with peer pressure related to underage drinking and recreational/illegal drug use.

The SMART learning objective would be:

At the end of the lesson (time-bound/achievable), *the learner will be able to demonstrate three strategies* (specific/measurable) *to avoid the use of drugs or alcohol when faced with peer pressure* (realistic).

The school nurse should start instruction by sharing the learning objectives with the group, so they understand the intent of the teaching and what is expected of them.

Objectives for effective learning must be developmentally appropriate and culturally sensitive. For instance, the school nurse would teach a lesson on good hygiene habits to kindergarteners in a way that is very different from the way it is taught to fifth graders. While the outcomes might be the same, consideration should always be given to differentiate instruction for diverse learners.

Demonstrate Knowledge of Resources

Once the school nurse has identified the health problem, understands the learners, and has determined the expected outcomes and how to measure them, the "how to" of planning begins. This entails identifying resources necessary for implementing the plan, including people, materials, and processes. **People resources** refer to identifying the best person or persons for the job. Experts in the community, peer teachers, teams of teachers, parents, students, and community members or school nurses may be the right persons to implement the lesson. The CDC's expanded coordinated school health model, called Whole School, Whole Community, Whole Child (WSCC), features a collaboration with ASCD to emphasize the whole-child approach to learning and health (CDC, 2022c). The nurse can review the WSCC model (see Chapter 2) to consider how the whole child can be addressed during teaching. In addition, it might be prudent to determine whether experts from any of the 10 WSCC component areas could support the teaching of health concepts.

Using the example of promoting safe and drug-free schools, the school nurse might invite a local law enforcement agent with the substance use task force who is an expert in drug identification, prevalence of use, and related risk behaviors to co-teach a lesson. Including a content expert in this way brings an added and realistic dimension to the lesson. Teaming with classroom teachers and others has the advantage of bringing in experts while still allowing the school nurse to maintain an active role in meeting the goals of the learning experience. Teamwork requires planning; time is needed to collaborate, coordinate, practice, and refine an integrated learning experience.

Instructional resources such as videos, games, and posters have the potential to drive a learning experience. The choice of instructional resources should support learning objectives, student outcomes, and student developmental levels, and actively engage learners to be critical thinkers. Though beneficial, some resources are expensive; therefore, the cost of materials should be feasible within instructional budgets. Using free materials creatively can be just as effective as costly branded educational products in promoting student learning.

The school nurse should use teaching materials that reflect the cultural diversity of the community, including illustrations of the community's racial, ethnic, gender, and socioeconomic diversity. Opportunities to discuss how cultural differences could affect the problem-solving and decision-making process can be incorporated into the lesson plan. Presentations on topics related to reproduction, faith, family values, drugs, tobacco and alcohol, sexuality, and risk-taking behavior all need to follow state laws on the topic and be carefully screened. A school health advisory team that includes parents, students, community members, and school staff members can evaluate resources and help the school nurse consider strategies for community buy-in before use.

Learner engagement activities (i.e., process resources) should be included to meet the learning objectives. Engagement activities consider the appropriate size of the group and the learning environment. This may mean planning in advance to move furniture, access technology, organize learners into different size groups, or teach outside of the classroom. For example, during a hand hygiene lesson, kindergartners need to practice each step of proper hand washing technique in small groups or with partners, which entails accessing sinks in the classroom or being supervised in bathroom facilities.

Design Coherent Instruction

Designing coherent instruction refers to the plan for helping the learners achieve the goal. **Coherent instruction** is a systematic and orderly process that helps learners understand the content and promotes critical thinking. The school nurse should be familiar with Bloom's taxonomy, which was developed in the 1950s and updated several times by educational researchers, to consider how to word learning objectives. See Figure 4-1. The school nurse should check with curriculum directors to learn what planning model is used in the school district. For example, educators may be expected to use a **backward design,** which calls for describing the desired results first (the student learning outcomes), then identifying the assessment methods next, and last planning the instructional activities that will align with the activities and assessment (McTighe, 2019).

A simple approach for designing instruction, regardless of the length of the lesson or the audience, is to consider **set, body,** and **closure** when planning and implementing the lesson.

Set refers to setting the stage for the learning to occur. It might start with something as simple as "Today we are going to learn three ways to prevent tooth decay." Using an impact statement might be more effective in motivating the learners for the lesson. The school nurse could display a picture of a child whose face is swollen from a dental abscess and who is in considerable pain or a picture of decayed teeth. Questions such as "How might

Did You Know?

Online Health Education Resources (Also Available in Online Materials OM4-1)

Explore the following resources for health education ideas, resources, and materials. Note that materials provided free by educational, commercial, or professional ventures should be evaluated carefully and not used solely because of availability.

- ***Adolescent and School Health*** (CDC, 2023a) provides multiple resources including data from the *Youth Risk Behavior survey* and *School Health Policies survey* and fact sheets on bullying, emergencies, healthcare disparities, school connectedness, sexual risk behaviors, social determinants of health, substance use, and other topics. https://www.cdc.gov/healthyyouth/education-materials/index.htm
- ***SHAPE America*** (Society of Health and Physical Educators, n.d.) shares a variety of skills-based learning and curriculum resources on its website in addition to resource texts. https://www.shapeamerica.org/publications/resources/default.aspx?hkey=55103b9c-7979-4a38-a483-c1669fefbc6e
- ***Kids Health in the Classroom*** (Nemours Foundation/Kids Health, n.d.) provides grade level health-related lesson plans and teaching guides that are aligned with the NHES, including discussion questions, classroom activities, handouts, videos, quizzes, and more. https://classroom.kidshealth.org/classroom/
- ***Youth Programs*** (Byrnes Health Education Center, n.d.) offers health education lesson plans, games, and activities for different grade levels on a variety of topics, including healthy eating and physical activity, dental health, and mental health. https://www.byrneshec.org/programs/youth-programs/
- ***The Health Teacher*** (n.d.) has evidence-based health curricula, "Grab & Go" projects for teaching functional health information and shaping healthy lifestyle behaviors, with a focus on adolescent health topics such as puberty, sleep, stress management, and cyberbullying. https://thehealthteacher.com

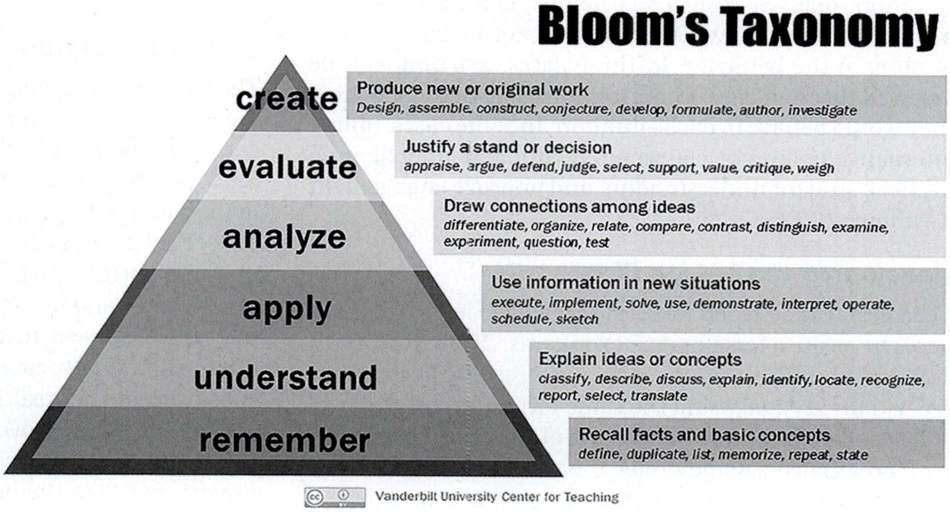

FIGURE 4-1. Bloom's taxonomy. *(From Armstrong, P. [2010]. Bloom's taxonomy. Vanderbilt University Center for Teaching. https://cft.vanderbilt.edu/guides-sub-pages/blooms-taxonomy/)*

this person be feeling?" help learners focus on what the lesson might mean to them. Impact statements, common or recent problems, analogies to other situations, and relevance to the learner's world can all be used in setting the tone for understanding the objectives of the lesson. After the students claim that they wouldn't want to experience these problems, then the school nurse can tell them that they will be learning ways (skills) to avoid this from happening to them.

Body refers to the body of the lesson. This is the knowledge, beliefs, and skills that the learner needs to have to demonstrate the new behavior. The *cognitive, affective,* and *psychomotor domains* of learning tie together the lesson so that learners can understand, practice, and incorporate the knowledge into their worldview. For instance, students might *understand* (cognitive domain/knowledge) the fact that drinking alcohol is related to impaired decision making with consequences such as motor vehicle injuries. They might also have had opportunities to *practice* (psychomotor domain/skills) refusal skills. However, if learners do not *believe* (affective domain/dispositions) they might be hurt in a drunk-driving accident then they might not put that knowledge and skill into action and still choose to drink and drive. The body of the lesson can be organized according to skills, concepts, or problems. It can be organized by moving from the simple to the complex, from the concrete to the abstract, or from the beginning to the end if there is a timeline related to the learning, or it may be an analogy to something else they know and to which they can relate.

Closure lets the learner know what they have achieved and what they are now able to do. It is the time to summarize the points of the lesson and to tie together for the learners what they have learned. No new content is introduced at this time as the lesson is pulled together into a coherent whole.

Design Student Assessments

Establishing the assessment process during the planning phase requires the school nurse to consider what behaviors will demonstrate that learning has occurred because of teaching. For example, a paper-and-pencil test or survey responses may elicit the correct answers to demonstrate knowledge on a health topic, *but it does not assess whether the student has the skills or motivation to improve health behaviors.* If the objective is that kindergarten students will demonstrate correct hand washing technique, then observing them washing their hands is a more appropriate assessment than asking students to state the steps of proper hand washing technique. Psychomotor skills are easily observable *except* in risk-taking situations (e.g., wearing a bike helmet, texting while driving, substance use) when adults are not usually present to observe the behavior. In these cases, learning can be assessed through case scenarios and asking students how they would behave in each situation. In some cases, online interactive polling or classroom technology may be used to check student understanding and improve engagement (Graham, 2023).

Developing the Lesson Plan

"The best way to teach in a well-organized, effective manner is to create a lesson plan" (Yonkaitis, 2020, p. 136). A lesson plan can be written using one of several forms. They are usually created using the same format across a school or district and are often a reflection of a school administrator's preferences. Some prefer a narrative format, others an outline format, and some a timeline. Regardless of the format, lesson plans include listing the title of the lesson, the intended audience, the goal of the lesson, the learner objectives in behavioral and measurable terms, and the measurement tools (assessment) to determine that learners met objectives. Lesson plans also include a comprehensive outline of the content, materials, teaching modalities, and the time frame for the components of instruction. Often overlooked is the teacher's own self-reflection on the lesson following the session or series of classes. Instructors should take time to reflect on what went well, what problems were encountered, and how things might be done differently the next time the lesson is taught (Rigney et al., 2019). See a sample lesson plan template in Table 4-2. (Refer to online materials OM 4-2 for an alternate fillable lesson plan template.)

Domain 2: The Classroom Environment

Develop Rapport and Create an Environment of Respect

Consensus among learning, developmental, and social theorists suggests that people learn better when they are in an environment free from fear, threat, and ridicule. Only in an environment of respect can learners feel safe to consider, try, and practice new behaviors. A culture of respect and safety can be established by developing or reviewing classroom norms and/or rules before starting the lesson (Finley, 2014).

When conducting an educational session with parents, staff, or community members, the school nurse should establish expectations at the beginning of the experience. Participants might have different educational, generational, and cultural perspectives and varying levels of comfort with the topic. In addition, some adults might dominate the discussion or challenge the teacher. The school nurse needs to be prepared for a variety of participants with a range of learning styles and personal needs. Creating an environment of respect and developing rapport with adults follows the same principles as when working with children and youth; be clear from the beginning and reinforce the guidelines during the learning experience as needed to create a civil and welcoming learning experience.

Establish a Culture of Learning

The classroom teacher is primarily responsible for establishing a culture of learning by incorporating mutual respect, caring, rapport, and cultural sensitivity (Danielson, 2007). Students should feel valued and cared for. When teaching in the classroom, supporting a culture of learning is part of the school nurse's responsibility.

An important variable to consider is who will cover the health office and be available in a health emergency when the school nurse is teaching in the classroom. The school nurse should advocate for adequate coverage or a nurse substitute in the health office while providing classroom instruction. If no coverage is available, additional planning needs to take place to make sure that (1) if the school nurse is called to the health office, another qualified adult can resume responsibility for the class; (2) the students are informed that their learning needs are important but other responsibilities may interfere with the lesson; and (3) teaching activities will be interrupted only in emergency situations. This planning contributes to the climate of learning because it lets the students know that the school nurse's instructional time with them is important.

Manage Classroom Procedures

The school nurse should consult with the classroom teacher in advance to ensure a smooth transition when teaching in the classroom (Yonkaitis, 2020). If the teacher has established norms or rules (e.g., students sitting in assigned seats, taking turns responding to questions, or raising their hands and waiting for acknowledgment before answering),

TABLE 4-2 Lesson Plan Template for Teaching Health Topics in the Classroom

General Information About Class and Teacher	
School Nurse Educator	Your name
Main Subject Area	State the broad content area (e.g., nutrition, hygiene, risk reduction, etc.)
Topic or Unit of Study	Describe the specific content area (e.g., food group choices, hand washing, substance misuse)
Classroom Teacher	Name of teacher who extended the invitation
Type of Classroom	Brief description of type of class, classroom, and number of students
Estimated Time, Time of Day, Fit in Schedule	Align with developmental level and attention span of students
Grade/Developmental Level	Grade and developmental level
Part I: Planning Student Learning	
Enduring Understanding	What overarching statement captures the essence of what is accepted knowledge about the topic? (For example, students will learn about healthy food choices using MyPlate as a visual.)
Essential Questions	What questions do you want the students to be able to answer after your lesson? (This can be written as a prompt on the board or used as a slide for projection, as well as asked of the students. It should be open-ended to stimulate interest and critical thinking, not a yes/no response question.)
State Learning Standard	Applicable State Learning Standard(s)
National Learning Standard	Applicable National Health Education Standard(s)
Title of Lesson	Title of lesson
Purpose	Brief statement of why it is important that students learn this lesson
Objectives/Learner Outcomes	State three objectives by completing this sentence: *By the end of this lesson, the students will ...*
Assessment Method(s)	What evidence will you collect that demonstrates that students have met the objectives (e.g., return demo hand washing, role-play effective strategies to resist offer to misuse medications, quiz, ticket to leave with student answering one thing learned that they can apply to their own life)?
Strategies to Assess Baseline Knowledge	How will you know what the students already know about the topic you are teaching?
Procedures and Activities	Outline your teaching plan (use bullets or brief narrative)
Strategies to Assess Readiness to Learn	How will you know if students are ready to engage with you and each other in learning, i.e., their readiness to learn?
Planning for Diverse Learners/Differentiated Instruction	Describe how you will accommodate different learning styles and abilities, such as visual/auditory learners, alternative learners, English language learners, special education students (if any), etc.
Materials and Resources	List materials, links, and evidence-based resources (e.g., from CDC, NASN, Google Scholar).
Part II: Reflection on Teaching	
Effectiveness	Were students engaged? Did they enjoy and learn content and/or skills? How do you know?
Personal Reflection	Are there specific actions you could take to improve the lesson, related to content, timing, engagement strategies for learners, etc.? What feedback did you receive from the classroom teacher?

Adapted from Yonkaitis, C. F. (2020). Lesson plan basics: Teaching in the classroom with confidence. *NASN School Nurse, 35*(3), 136–139. Copyright © 2020. https://doi.org/10.1177/1942602X19893038

then the school nurse needs to be aware of these procedures and continue with them or explain how and why the procedures might be different for the lesson. If the teacher will not be present, the school nurse needs to be familiar with the plan and be prepared for emergency procedures in case of a lockdown or evacuation.

Manage Student Behavior

The school nurse should meet with the teacher ahead of time to determine whether there are student behaviors that need to be monitored and managed. This is also a good time to establish the classroom teacher's role during the lesson. Unless this is a class period where the teacher is scheduled to be elsewhere, having an experienced teacher in the room will allow the nurse and classroom teacher to collaborate on strategies to include in follow-up about the lesson.

Typical challenging behaviors that the school nurse might encounter are student inattention, frequent interruptions, monopolizing of content, inappropriate comments, and distracting or disruptive behavior. For consistency and to promote learning, the school nurse should know and participate in the school's approach to handling this type of behavior. For example, many schools have adopted a positive behavior system, such as **Positive Behavioral Interventions and Supports (PBIS),** to encourage desirable behavior and more effectively respond to disruptive behavior (PBIS, n.d.). Behavior management techniques should be consistent with the teacher's approach. School nurses should recognize students as valuable members of the learning community, encourage them to be motivated to learn, and follow basic principles of engaging students while treating them with respect. See Chapters 7 and 28 for further discussion of student behavior management.

A well-prepared teacher will have several approaches ready to reengage distracted students. One option is to redirect the classroom activities to involve the students in more active participation through structured group work followed by a brief report. If students are talking to each other or passing notes, they can be put in separate working groups. If the activity occurs near the end of the class and there will be another session, you might ask the students to stay after class to tell them of your concern about their behavior and the need to be respectful of other students in subsequent classes.

The school nurse often teaches lesson content that has relevance to the personal lives of the students and can result in some students disrupting the class because of their concerns, embarrassment, and feelings. Topics related to sexual behavior, drugs and alcohol, bullying, and self-esteem can provoke inappropriate comments from students or other individuals. As part of the introduction to the lesson, the school nurse should emphasize that classroom discussion must be respectful of each person's comments and questions.

One strategy to help manage student behavior and maintain confidentiality is to have all questions related to the content, unless for clarification purposes, be written down on pieces of paper to be read and answered either toward the end of the class or at another time. This allows students who are uncomfortable the opportunity to ask questions in a nonthreatening manner. It also helps students who might be prone to repeated monopolizing of the classroom channel their energy by adhering to the written question approach.

Writing the questions allows the school nurse to rephrase the question with more appropriate language. The nurse might say, "There were several excellent questions about the growth of the genitals. Although some of you used terminology that you might have heard, we are going to use the correct scientific or anatomic terminology when referring to body parts."

For content that involves multiple sessions, the school nurse can leave a question box in the class and tell students that their questions will be addressed at a subsequent session. The school nurse can leave their e-mail address or use other virtual modalities such as a blog to connect with students and answer questions. If presented with student comments or behaviors that signal a danger to self or others, the school nurse should be prepared to respond following school policy and procedures.

Organize Physical Space

Depending on the objectives of the class and the methods to help students achieve those objectives, the school nurse needs to consider how the classroom is set up and how the physical space can best be organized (The Iris Center, 2021). Desks and chairs that are organized facing the front would be appropriate for a lecture or demonstration activity. Alternatively, moving the desks and chairs into dyads or triads allows students to engage in collaborative learning or practice skills. If a goal is to have student-student interaction, then the classroom needs to be set up so that all the students can see each other, either in a circle or a horseshoe formation. If students need practice skills, such as teen parents practicing feeding techniques, then the room needs to be set up so that students can realistically practice the skills and the school nurse can observe their technique to provide appropriate feedback.

Other environmental considerations include adequate ventilation in the classroom and lighting adequate for illuminating materials while avoiding direct sunlight that can cause glare and be distracting to students. Lighting consideration is also important in the use of projectors, smartboards, video monitors, or computers in the classroom to make sure that everyone can see the projection. Avoid having the room so dark that students' behavior, as well as their reactions to the material, cannot be monitored.

Domain 3: Instruction

The domain of instruction is the actual delivery of the lesson. The components of the instruction include communicating clearly, sensitively, and accurately with students; using questioning and discussion techniques; engaging students in learning; assessing learning to alter instruction; providing feedback to students; and demonstrating flexibility and responsiveness. These qualities are important with all learners, whether student, staff, or community members.

Communicate With Students

Communication in the classroom takes the form of verbal, nonverbal, visual, and auditory communication. Verbal communication requires skills in elocution, or speaking and enunciating clearly, so that students can understand. Oral presentations should be accompanied by visual cues on slides, handouts, props, or using the board in the classroom. These are especially helpful if it may be difficult for the learner to understand the teacher's spoken words.

The manner and volume of speaking is also important. Strategies such as using a microphone, conscious voice projection, and changing the tempo and volume of the voice can help maintain student interest. Silence can be a powerful and effective communication tool; it can also help learners, who have lost the pace of the lesson, refocus. The students' visual responses and body language to the presentation, including requests to repeat content, should be monitored. Encourage students to ask questions when they don't understand or need clarification.

Nonverbal communication can add to the lesson by expressing your positive regard for the students and their ability to learn. Attentive listening to their questions and concerns and asking or using their names lets students know that you value them as learners and welcome their input. The nurse might ask for a copy of the class picture composite from the teacher so that the names and faces are nearby for reference or have name cards with the students' names on them at their desks.

How the school nurse responds to an incorrect contribution from a student can also affect the instruction. Facial expressions of disbelief, distaste, or boredom convey negative messages to the learners. Neutral, smiling, or encouraging facial expressions allow the students to feel more confident as they work through trying to respond or think critically. Ask questions to engage students, and anticipate some silence that may feel uncomfortable, but allows time for students to reflect and respond.

Visual communication needs to be considered when planning and delivering a lesson. Written material needs to be clear, legible, grammatically correct, spelled correctly, and appropriate to the age, developmental level, reading skills, and culture of the learner. This supports student development of health literacy. A good rule to follow when using written or visual instructional materials is to keep it short and simple. Use key words to highlight the major concepts. When projecting written information, use no more than six lines of text with less than six words per line. Preferably, include only the key concepts and use a font that is easy to read (Courier, Times, or Arial) and large enough to be read from a distance (usually no smaller than 28 points). Contrasting colors for the font and background help highlight the text, although black background is hard to see and consumes a lot of ink if printing copies.

All learners have a preferred learning style. Some need to write notes as the speaker teaches; others are distracted by writing and just need to listen. Still others need to have the content written so that they can follow along. Most students learn well with multisensory approaches: presentation (auditory), viewing words on a slide (visual), and possibly manipulating an object (sensory; Yonkaitis, 2020). Some schools will allow students to bring their personal tablet or computer into the classroom; others provide computers or tablets to students for various learning activities, including note taking. The school nurse should know the school's policies and the classroom teachers' rules for use of electronic devices.

Use Questioning and Discussion Techniques

Giving students time to think and process information allows them to formulate questions, consider applications, and sort through any discrepancies or concerns they might have. Asking questions and promoting discussion allows learners to listen to each other's responses, opinions, and perspectives that they might not have considered themselves, thus expanding their understanding that not everyone views the same information from the same perspective (Danielson, 2007). Best practices for questioning and discussion include avoiding yes/no questions, giving time to think before expecting a response, seeking clarification ("What is an example of that?"), encouraging learners to comment on others' answers, and discouraging domination/encouraging all learners to participate.

Good questioning engages learners in exploration. Ask learners what they want to know. A good teacher engages all the learners in the discussion and focuses questions to eventually discover and explore possible solutions. The school nurse can empower students by guiding them to arrive at an acceptable answer through leading questions such as the following: What seems to work best? Does anyone want to comment on this idea? Are there any other ways of doing this? Having a handout of tips or strategies can be given as a supplement after the learners think through alternatives, consider other perspectives, and become engaged in finding solutions.

Everyone likes to feel that their contribution is valued, whether the answer to a question is right or wrong. The student who answers correctly should be given positive feedback about the contribution and how it ties into the learning activity. However, when learners provide erroneous information, give a wrong answer to a question, or go off on an irrelevant tangent, the school nurse should positively acknowledge the learner's response and help the learner consider why they provided that information. Although you do not want to reinforce incorrect information, you also do not want the person who contributed that information to feel that the learner's input is not valued. Help the learner consider why they provided that information and correct any misconceptions. Other learners can be asked if there are other options to consider. The correct answer should be confirmed, explained, and reinforced.

Another concern is the learner who wants to take over the lesson. When one learner tends to dominate the discussion, the school nurse can acknowledge the contributions and then ask others in the room to comment on their experiences or to provide another perspective. When establishing a culture for learning, the nurse can clarify the expectation that everyone will have a chance to speak and participate, and remind students of this when necessary with comments such as, "You have a lot of ideas to contribute today and I would like to hear more about it, but let's hear from others in the class and perhaps we can meet later to discuss your ideas some more." Questioning techniques and leading a discussion are at the heart of helping learners understand the application of the material to their own lives and health. Highlighting possible questions as part of the planning process can remind the school nurse to incorporate those questions at appropriate places in the lesson. In summary, discussion can be engaging and promote critical thinking when it is based on questions formulated to encourage active participation, considers a variety of perspectives, and applies the discussion to real-life situations.

Engage Students in Learning

Engaging students in learning is critical; it is the reason for teaching, and when it does not occur, the consequences of student inattention and disengagement or even disruptions become obvious (Danielson, 2007). Students need to be involved. Engagement does not mean keeping busy in the classroom or staying on task, but that learners are actively participating in and invested in the learning experience. In other words, they want to learn something that is meaningful to them. Research-based strategies for engaging students include the following (Abla & Fraumeni, 2019):

- Measuring engagement
- Focusing on relationship-building
- Seeking the right balance of structure and student autonomy
- Using technology thoughtfully
- Using effective questioning
- Connecting (instruction) with the real world

A variety of specific active learning strategies can be used to achieve this engagement. See Box 4-3. However, by themselves, audiovisual materials, physical activity, hands-on experiences, or student participation do not necessarily guarantee learning if the learner is not fully engaged in the experience. School nurses can contribute to learner engagement through both the content taught in the classroom, as described earlier, and the care provided in the health office. For instance, if students come to the health office and are hungry, feeling afraid of being bullied, pregnant, worried about a sick family member, or having difficulty breathing, they are not going to be able to be fully engaged in learning. School nurses can identify these students and help them meet their needs so that they can be ready to learn. If learner engagement is, as Danielson and others purport, the core of teaching and learning, then school nurses need to be vigilant in identifying students who are at risk for not being able to fully participate in the learning environment and in implementing interventions that effectively remove health-related obstacles to learning.

BOX 4-3

Selected Active Instructional Strategies

- Exit tickets
- Gallery walk
- Interactive technology, e.g., polling, videos, Web sites
- KWL chart (What I know, What I want to know, What I learned)
- Music and songs
- Read aloud
- Role-play/simulations/drama
- Team games
- Small-group discussion
- Sticky note graphs
- Think-pair-share
- Word wall

Source: For the Teachers (n.d.).

Use Assessment in Instruction

Formative and summative feedback is essential in the learning process. Learners need intermittent feedback so that they have a chance to determine how they are doing and what they need to do to meet the learning objectives. This kind of feedback is formative; it helps learners determine whether they are on target and what needs to be done next. Summative feedback, in contrast, occurs at the end and measures how one has done in meeting the objectives. It is often reflected in a grade or a certificate of completion. To provide feedback, it is important to assess what learners have learned in relation to the learning objectives. Are they understanding the content (knowledge), developing the needed health behaviors (skills), and integrating the health lessons into a personal belief system (dispositions) to sustain the learning over time? When the school nurse is a guest presenter in a health class, it may be challenging to assess the learners during the class time, but there still needs to be methods to assess their learning. Feedback is usually formative during the classroom learning time, providing informal feedback to students about their understanding of the concepts and the processes discussed.

The classroom teacher is most often responsible for assessing the outcome measures identified in the lesson plan and if the objectives were met. There are times, however, when the school nurse provides summative feedback. For instance, after teaching a class on first aid, babysitting care, or cardiopulmonary resuscitation (CPR), the learners might have to perform certain written, verbal, or behavioral measures to demonstrate their knowledge and skill in order to receive a certificate. If the school nurse is assigned to teach a health course that requires a grade at the end of the term, then summative feedback in the form of a grade will be necessary.

Feedback helps learners gauge their progress toward mastery, as well as indicate what areas need continued work. Some of the principles related to feedback include significance, appropriateness, comprehensiveness, constructiveness, and timeliness. All learners should get feedback, not just those who excel and not just those who are having difficulty. Learners who have worked hard to achieve need positive reinforcement for their work and guidance on ways to improve; learners who are struggling need direction.

Feedback should be geared to helping learners determine their progress toward meeting the learning objectives. For instance, when working with students to increase their physical activity, helping them see how much their endurance has improved is more appropriate than testing their understanding of pulse rates. Feedback should involve as much of the learning experience as possible. A written test that measures only vocabulary related to bones but ignores decisions about carrying books in a backpack or the intake of calcium does not let the learner appreciate the scope of what was learned or assess the true scope of the learning. Feedback also needs to be timely and constructive. Timeliness is important so that learners can relate the feedback to their current perceptions and behaviors for change to take place; it needs to be constructive to motivate learners to continue to learn (Danielson, 2007).

Demonstrate Flexibility and Responsiveness

School nurses quickly learn the importance of flexibility and responsiveness in all aspects of their role, especially that of educator. Students may speak up with inappropriate comments or sensitive personal information. Knowing how to be both sensitive to the individual student while supporting the needs of the entire class requires responsiveness and flexibility, as well as a clear understanding of school policies on working with students who are experiencing crisis. For example, imagine that the school nurse had planned to host a talk to the middle-school parent-teacher organization on pubertal changes as the first in a series on understanding adolescents. That same week it was learned that three middle-school students had been suspended because of illegal substance use. Parents come to the meeting concerned about the incidence of illegal substance use in the community, the role of the school in curbing this problem, and the need to vent their fears, concerns, and frustrations. The school nurse may need to set aside the planned lesson to respond to the needs of the audience of worried parents and concerned teachers.

Some situations may not be easily anticipated. The student who has lost a family member to a tragic death may want to talk about it in the middle of a class on another topic. Not even the school nurse is expected to do personal counseling, teach a class, and maintain confidentiality all at the same time. In an awkward or urgent moment, the school nurse can stop the lesson for a moment and instruct the students to do some reflective work such as drawing or writing on a pertinent question related to the topic for a few minutes so that the school nurse can facilitate helping the student to the appropriate source of support according to school policy.

Domain 4: Professional Responsibilities

As described previously in this chapter, the *School Nursing: Scope and Standards of Practice* and *School Nursing Practice Framework* demonstrate that school nurses are educators (NASN, 2022, 2024).

Reflect on Teaching

Evaluation of teaching and the learning that occurs is a professional imperative for any formal class or presentation. The lesson plan includes strategies to evaluate the effectiveness of the lesson. Did it meet the intended goals, and were objectives for teaching met? Were the learners able to demonstrate that outcomes were met? Were the strategies effective? Were the materials appropriate? Did the timing work? Were there questions that can be incorporated into a similar class in the future? The school nurse as educator needs to consider what worked, what did not work, and what strategies would make it more effective in the future. Although there may be a tendency to put a lesson aside until the next time, immediate reflection offers the school nurse the opportunity to consider successes and areas for improvement while the experience and feedback are still fresh (Rigney et al., 2019). See online materials OM4-3 for resources on educator reflection.

Maintain Accurate Records

Many schools require that teachers maintain and submit lesson plans, sometimes in an electronic format to a district database, so that schools can be accountable for the content taught and experiences provided. Depending on school policy, the school nurse may be held to the same standard of accountability. Even if documentation of school nurse activities as educator is not required, adequate documentation is necessary to account for time spent on health promotion activities and the outcomes.

Documentation should include copies of the materials used, including notes, handouts, electronic files, slides, and in the case of borrowed materials, their source, as well as costs involved, and a list of staff or parents who reviewed the materials. Individual teaching as part of the nurses' treatment of specific students' health needs should be documented in the individual students' health records. The accountability involved with maintaining these records can be useful to school nurses in documenting their contribution to the education of learners, time spent out of the health office, and impact on the community. It can also be used as part of a portfolio of materials for evaluation of the school nurse.

Communicate With Families

Letting families know what goes on in the classroom serves several important purposes. First, it informs them about what is taught so that they are knowledgeable about their children's education. This knowledge allows them to support and build on learning within the context of family values and expectations. It also helps families to be partners in the educational process of the school community, leading to more buy-in and support. To prepare families for different topics that might be discussed, school nurses can post information in electronic and/or paper school newsletters and Web sites and ask teachers to include information in their communications home.

Following lessons, communication with parents might include links or electronic copies for additional readings. Written tips that empower parents to feel that they are active participants in their child's education can help establish a climate in which reinforcement can take place. For instance, a brief note explaining that hand washing was taught to reduce the spread of germs can be sent home.

Many states or districts include in their regulations the provision that parents are to be notified about certain topics, to have the right to review materials, to be present during the class, or to exclude their child from the learning experience if they so desire. District policies may even dictate how to inform parents of upcoming topics that might be considered controversial, such as specific health-related topics required to be taught in certain grades, such as information on HIV. Topics considered sensitive by some include assault prevention; puberty and human sexuality; drug, alcohol, and tobacco prevention programs; and information on sexually transmitted infections (STIs), depression, and child abuse/dating violence.

As of 2023, six U.S. states require parental consent for students to participate in sex or STI/HIV education, meaning that parents have to sign permission statements for their children to participate (Guttmacher Institute, 2023). Twenty-five states and the District of Columbia require parental notification of upcoming health-related topics and 35 states and the District of Columbia allow parents to remove their children from instruction, also called *opt-out*. It is imperative that state regulations be reviewed to determine what specific content or forms need to be used when informing parents or requesting permission to teach specific content to the students in the school.

School policies about informing parents and obtaining consent need to be clearly communicated with parents or guardians on an annual basis. Some school districts include information about the health education curriculum in an annual parent/student handbook, on the district's Web site, and/or with paperwork required to be completed and signed at the start of school. If negative consent is used (when a parent who does not want their child to participate in a learning activity "opts out" of the activity), it is up to the parent to notify the school; clear guidelines need to be in place so that parents know about this option.

Schools can use a variety of communication channels to make sure that all parents receive adequate and timely notice so that they can obtain additional information and make an informed decision in advance of the learning experience. Translation of communications into languages other than English may be required and/or recommended. Communication options include electronic messaging through Web site as well as phone and e-mail blasts. For parents without access to the Internet, hard copy communication may need to go home via students' backpacks. In all cases, schools must make every effort to make sure the communication reaches the parent with sufficient time to discuss with the child and respond to the school if needed. Clear policies about parental notification should be established, in place, and communicated clearly before any controversial activities are undertaken. If they are not in place, the school nurse can advocate for their inclusion.

> **Practice Connection**
>
> **An Example of a Note Home After Hand Washing Class**
>
> Good hand washing can reduce the spread of germs and decrease the number of sick days that children experience. Today, students learned how to wash their hands before meals; before touching babies; after toileting; after coughing, sneezing, or blowing their noses; and after touching pets. They were taught to sing the *ABC alphabet song* two times in a row so that they would learn to wash for a long enough period of time.
>
> They were encouraged to have a paper towel ready before washing so that they do not have to touch the towel dispenser or faucet when in a public bathroom. Please ask your children to demonstrate this skill for you and encourage them to use it at home and when they are away from home. Thank you for your support!
>
> Signature
> Name and credentials
> Title
> School Name
> E-mail and/or Phone Contact

Participate in the School Community

School professionals can make a significant difference in the school community when they contribute beyond their day-to-day jobs (Danielson, 2007). For school nurses, this means being involved in the life of the school by way of fostering a positive environment and identifying ways to meet the goals of the school that are beyond the confines of the health office. School nurse standards related to leadership also emphasize this point (NASN, 2022). For example, a supervisor could expect a nurse who is functioning at a beginning level to participate in school events, such as an evening orientation for new students and their families, as long as this expectation aligns with the nurse's employment contract. The school nurse may identify information to help new parents and students make the transition to the school by volunteering to prepare materials and a brief motivational presentation at an open house meeting.

For the more experienced school nurse, contributions to the school or district professional community might involve assuming a leadership role in promoting school or district-wide health through student or employee fitness programs. Implementing a walk-to-school day that engages community members in making their sidewalks and neighborhoods safe and promotes students learning and practicing safe walking habits can make a substantial contribution to a healthy community and students arriving safely at school.

Grow and Develop Professionally

The NASN *Standards of Professional Performance for School Nursing* indicate a clear expectation that school nurses will continue to pursue professional development throughout their careers regardless of whether this is required by employers or state licensing boards (NASN, 2022). Professional growth in the role of school nurse can be highly rewarding on both a personal and professional level. Membership in your professional organization, attendance at professional meetings, reading evidence-based peer-reviewed journals, and getting feedback on one's performance all contribute to professional growth. National certification as a school nurse is another way to demonstrate knowledge and professional growth. Maintaining documentation of professional development activities provides evidence to licensing organizations, as well as one's employer, of efforts toward continued growth as a school nurse. See Chapter 3.

CHALLENGES IN THE ROLE OF SCHOOL NURSE AS EDUCATOR

The role of the school nurse as a health educator teaching specific lessons or classes is very dependent on role expectations and preparation of the nurse. Some states and/or districts have nurse-teachers who have been prepared beyond nursing degrees to teach schoolchildren. Most school nurses are called on to provide puberty education and intermittent education on other health-related topics, such as hand hygiene, as the need arises, which is within the scope of the registered nurse (RN). Regardless of the role expectations, the school nurse should consider key issues when implementing the educator role: time, access to students, sensitive health topics, confidentiality, expertise, and evaluation.

> **Did You Know?**
>
> The National Board for Certification of School Nurses (https://www.nbcsn.org/) has created a toolkit to help guide school nurses through the process of advocating for certification within their employment setting.

Time

Time is needed to prepare and present any lesson. Depending on the topic and type of class, this may require hours out of the nurse's day. The school nurse should clarify the expectations around teaching. Teachers' employment contracts include planning time and school nurses need to ascertain whether their contract provides the same. If not, then it is important to clarify what adjustments will be made so that the nurse will have time to prepare and teach lessons. For example, if the administration expects the health office to be open to students from the beginning to the ending bell each day, office coverage will need to be arranged to provide the nurse with uninterrupted time to plan and deliver effective lessons. Clarifying this information up front will set the tone so the nurse is seen as a professional within the school on par with other teachers.

Access to Students

Building relationships with teachers, sharing school nurse expertise and skills in health education, and finding common health goals with classroom teachers can help open the classroom doors to school nurse instruction. With the emphasis on accountability and demonstrating proficiency, some schools and teachers limit the school nurse's access to students in the classroom. One strategy to deal with this issue is to engage a coordinated school health advisory team to support the importance of the school nurse teaching students to promote health.

Sensitive Topics

Some of the topics delegated to the school nurse are those controversial topics for which classroom teachers do not have the expertise or desire to teach. Some topics might clash with family and community values, or they might provoke disruptive responses by students. Certainly, during the COVID-19 pandemic beginning in 2020, school nurses received negative and positive feedback from school communities when teaching about federal and state guidance on ways to reduce virus transmission, such as masking in school and quarantining at home when exposed. Firearm safety and human reproduction/sexuality are two other topics that can provoke concern and opposition. All potentially sensitive lessons should be planned well in advance and include as many key partners in the planning as possible. Be aware of any national, state, or local laws/policies you must follow. As indicated previously, many states mandate health education topics for students and rules for informing parents.

Teachers can help determine when best to tie the topic into the existing curriculum and can collaborate to develop strategies for transitioning to the topic. Teachers should be present during any lessons on sensitive topics so that there is additional support in the classroom. Having a second respected adult in the classroom can help maintain order, support the importance of the content to the students, and protect you and the teacher from false accusations by students regarding the nature and delivery of content.

Incorporating messages throughout all health lessons that encourage students to talk to their parents or guardians about these topics and to determine how their family values might influence their behavior now that they have been provided with this knowledge and skill are essential for linking schools and communities together. It also has the added advantage of providing health information to the parent, who can reinforce and role-model positive health behaviors. In addition to communication sent home in advance of lessons on sensitive topics, newsletter announcements and follow-up information can help to reduce the mystique of the topic and what has been discussed in class. Use of social media (e.g., Facebook, Instagram, TikTok, X [formerly Twitter]) must be used cautiously and in alignment with district communication protocols to avoid miscommunication. Communication on specific health content (e.g., reproductive health) should not be shared with students whose parents opted them out of this content. Meetings with parents in advance of topics can help them learn about the topic and provide strategies for talking about it at home and approaches to promote resiliency and reduce risk factors in youth.

Another aspect about sensitive health topics is concern about how some students may respond to topics discussed in class. As discussed previously, relating personally to any health topic is important in order to consider the value of the health behavior in relationship to the self. However, students who are emotionally fragile, who have experienced loss or adverse childhood events such as neglect or abuse, or who have family members or close friends who have experienced health concerns may be vulnerable to emotional stress when these topics are raised in class. School nurses, teachers, and guidance staff need to anticipate this possibility in advance, review the school crisis plan, and establish a mechanism for identifying students at risk and providing the appropriate support for them when sensitive issues are raised.

Confidentiality

Sensitive issues are often private issues, and respect for individual privacy needs to be preserved. The role of the school nurse as educator includes knowing the learners, being aware of resources to assist students, and creating an environment of respect and rapport that includes caring (Danielson, 2007). Inherent in teaching about health and discussing health-related topics is the importance of confidentiality. Students have a right to know that their private health information can remain private. This is sometimes challenging when students share their own and family members' health information in a classroom setting. The school nurse can help students understand the importance of respecting confidentiality and help establish guidelines, if not already in place in the classroom, about how confidentiality principles will be implemented. A school-wide discussion with staff and administrators can help develop strategies to teach and protect the rights to privacy regarding health information.

Establishing the Role of School Nurse as Health Educator

The perceptions around the role of the school nurse as an educator vary greatly. The school nurse and the school system, including teachers, parents, and administrators, may believe that "a nurse is a nurse and not a teacher." They may not recognize the contributions that a school nurse can and should make to the education and health of the school and community. Although professional standards, frameworks, and experts support the school nurse as classroom educator, research studies would provide even stronger evidence to support the role (Borawski et al., 2015; de Buhr et al., 2020); there is a need for more research on this topic. School administrators may not be aware of the educational background that some school nurses bring to the school setting, including an understanding of educational principles, supervised practice in the role of educator, and an appreciation for the components of professional teaching practice. The school nurse can learn to advocate for his or her role as an educator consistent with professional standards of practice and health goals. School nurses who lack the expertise in the role of educator should seek supervised experiences, continuing education, or course work in the foundations of education, and teaching strategies to help develop the skills and confidence to implement this role with expertise.

Evaluation of the School Nurse in the Educator Role

Evaluation of the school nurse as an educator also needs to be addressed in advance of the teaching-learning process. For instance, it is helpful to know if your teaching will be observed and evaluated by a school administrator and if the evaluation will be formative, to help you improve your performance as an educator, or summative, to determine the efficacy of this aspect of your role as a school nurse regarding this job assignment. Evaluation could affect merit considerations. In either case, the school nurse may feel threatened by this process if it has not been part of the expectation during the planning process. Anticipating the need for evaluation can help one be an active and willing participant in this institutional process of personnel evaluation and educational accountability.

An educator can evaluate the school nurse in the role of educator in terms of the nurse's strengths and needed areas for improvement regarding the components of professional practice as described by Danielson. That evaluator would need to be skilled and knowledgeable in the role of educator and the content area covered.

It is appropriate and recommended for novice school nurses to ask for a peer evaluation for their self-improvement. This would be a role for a mentor-nurse or classroom educator knowledgeable about health content to assist the novice in the planning and delivery of his or her first teaching activities. The mentor could even listen to a "practice run" of the material before it is given. Feedback can be helpful and can reinforce the school nurse's ability for the nurse's next educational experience.

CONCLUSION

The theoretical and conceptual material presented in this chapter provides the school nurse with teaching tools and strategies. No step-by-step instructions are given on how to deliver a specific lesson. The school nurse as educator considers many variables when planning, implementing, and evaluating a teaching and learning activity, most importantly the needs and characteristics of the learners that drive instruction. Equipped with evidence-based methodologies, the school nurse uses professional judgment to tailor teaching approaches to meet the needs of the learners.

Implementing the role of the school nurse as educator requires a strong conceptual base in learning theories, understanding the educational system, and understanding the community, the needs of the learners, the resources available, regulations and professional standards, and local, national, and international goals. Understanding the needs and capacity of the learners, as well as understanding one's own strengths and limitations, are essential when presenting learning opportunities to groups. Being competent as a school nurse health educator requires personal knowledge, skills, and dispositions to be able to effectively plan, implement, and evaluate the individual and overall health education programs. Effective teaching by the school nurse results in meaningful learning of students and school communities to improve health behaviors and attain, maintain, or regain one's health status in the immediate and long term.

References

Abla, C., & Fraumeni, B. R. (2019). Student engagement: Evidence-based strategies to boost academic and social-emotional results. McRel International. https://files.eric.ed.gov/fulltext/ED600576.pdf

American Academy of Pediatrics. (2016). Role of the school nurse in providing school health services. *Pediatrics, 137*(6). http://dx.doi.org/10.1542/ped.2016-0852

American Federation of Teachers (AFT). (n.d.). *Mission.* https://www.aft.org/about/mission#:~:text=The%20American%20Federation%20of%20Teachers,their%20families%20and%20our%20communities

Armstrong, P. (2010). Bloom's taxonomy. Vanderbuilt University Center for Teaching. *https://cft.vanderbilt.edu/guides-sub-pages/bloomstaxonomy/*

Borawski, E. A., Tufts, K. A., Trapl, E. S., Hayman, L. L., Yoder, L. D., & Lovegreen, L. D. (2015). Effectiveness of health education teachers and school nurses teaching sexually transmitted infections/human immunodeficiency virus prevention knowledge and skills in high school. *Journal of School Health, 85,* 189–196. http://dx.doi.org/10.1111/josh.12234

Brega, A. G., Barnard, J., Mabachi, N. M., Weiss, B. D., DeWalt, D. A., Brach, C., Cifuentes, M., Albright, K., & West, D. R. (2015). *AHRQ Health Literacy Universal Precautions Toolkit* (2nd ed.). Agency for Healthcare Research and Quality.

Byrnes Health Education Center. (n.d.). *Youth Programs.* https://www.byrneshec.org/programs/youth-programs/

Caldwell, S. (2021, September 21). *Nurse named an NEA SISP Fellow.* https://www.njea.org/nurse-named-an-nea-sisp-fellow/#:~:text=Sheila%20Caldwell%2C%20a%20school%20nurse,the%202021%2D22%20school%20year

Centers for Disease Control and Prevention. (2007). *National Health Education Standards.* https://www.cdc.gov/healthyschools/sher/standards/index.htm

Centers for Disease Control and Prevention. (2017,). *Writing SMART objectives.* https://www.cdc.gov/dhdsp/evaluation_resources/guides/writing-smart-objectives.htm

Centers for Disease Control and Prevention. (2018). Global school-based student health survey. https://www.cdc.gov/gshs/index.htm

Centers for Disease Control and Prevention. (2022a). *What is health literacy?* https://www.cdc.gov/healthliteracy/learn/index.html

Centers for Disease Control and Prevention. (2022b). *School nurses help keep students healthy.* https://www.cdc.gov/healthyschools/features/school_nurse.htm#:~:text=School%20nurses%20help%20students%20and%20families%20in%20many%20ways.&text=A%20school%20nurse%20can%20help,to%20their%20child%20at%20school

Centers for Disease Control and Prevention. (2022c). *Whole School, Whole Community, Whole Child (WSCC).* https://www.cdc.gov/healthyschools/wscc/index.htm

Centers for Disease Control and Prevention. (2022d). *Health Education Curriculum Analysis Tool (HECAT).* https://www.cdc.gov/healthyyouth/hecat/index.htm

Centers for Disease Control and Prevention. (2023a). *Adolescent and School Health.* https://www.cdc.gov/healthyyouth/index.htm

Centers for Disease Control and Prevention. (2023b). Youth risk behavior surveillance system. *Adolescent and School Health.* https://www.cdc.gov/healthyyouth/data/yrbs/index.htm

Common Core State Standards Initiative. (2017). *About the standards.* http://www.corestandards.org/about-the-standards/

Council for the Accreditation of Educator Preparation. (n.d.). *What is accreditation.* https://caepnet.org/accreditation/about-accreditation/what-is-accreditation

Culatta, R. (n.d.). *Andragogy (Malcolm Knowles).* https://www.instructionaldesign.org/theories/andragogy/

Danielson, C. (2007). *Enhancing professional practice: A framework for teaching* (2nd ed.). ASCD.

Danielson Group. (n.d.a). *The framework for teaching.* https://danielsongroup.org/framework/

Danielson Group. (n.d.b). *About us.* https://danielsongroup.org/our-story/

Darling-Hammond, L., & Bransford, J. (Eds.). (2005). *Preparing teachers for a changing world: What teachers should learn and be able to do.* Jossey-Bass.

de Buhr, E., Ewers, M., & Tannen, A. (2020). Potentials of school nursing for strengthening the health literacy of children, parents and teachers. *International Journal of Environmental Research and Public Health, 17*(7), 2577. https://doi.org/10.3390/ijerph17072577

Finley, T. (2014, August). The science behind classroom norming. *Edutopia.* https://www.edutopia.org/blog/establishing-classroom-norms-todd-finley

Flocke, S. A., Clark, E., Antognoli, E., Mason, M. J., Lawson, P. J., Smith, S., & Cohen, D. J. (2014). Teachable moments for health behavior change and intermediate patient outcomes. *Patient Education and Counseling, 96*(1), 43–49. doi.org/10.1016/j.pec.2014.03.014

For the Teachers. (n.d.). *Instructional strategies.* https://www.fortheteachers.org/instructional_strategies/

Goldstein, D. (2021, November 4). After 10 years of hopes and setbacks, what happened to the Common Core? *The New York Times*. https://www.nytimes.com/2019/12/06/us/common-core.html

Gormley, J. (2020). School nurses and the three T's of COVID: Teaching, tracing, and testing. https://neusha.org/index.php/2020/12/15/school-nurses-and-3-ts-of-covid-teaching-tracing-and-testing/

Graham, P. (2023, February 2). Engage your students with classroom polling. Cornell Center for Teaching and Learning. [Video.] YouTube. https://www.youtube.com/watch?v=V_ywS8stl-M&t=2s

Guttmacher Institute. (2023). *Sex and HIV education.* https://www.guttmacher.org/state-policy/explore/sex-and-hiv-education#:~:text=40%20states%20and%20DC%20require,sex%20education%20or%20HIV%20education

Health Teacher. (n.d.). https://thehealthteacher.com/

The Iris Center. (2021). *Classroom behavior management (part 1): Key concepts and foundational practices.* https://iris.peabody.vanderbilt.edu/module/beh1/cresource/q2/p06/#content

Lawson, P., & Flocke, S. (2009). Teachable moments for health behavior change: A concept analysis. *Patient Education and Counseling, 76*(1), 25–30. http://dx.doi.org/10.1016/j.pec.2008.11.002

Marrapese, B., Gormley, J. M., & Deschene, K. (2021). Reimagining school nursing: Lessons learned from a virtual school nurse. *NASN School Nurse, 36*(4), 218–225. doi:10.1177/1942602X21996432

McIntosh, C. E., Brelage, P. K., Thomas, C. M., Wendel, J. M., & Phelps, B. E. (2022). School nurse and COVID-19 response. *Psychology in the Schools, 60*(5), 1532-1543. https://doi.org/10.1002/pits.22708

McTighe, J. (2019). *The fundamentals of backward planning.* https://www.ascd.org/el/articles/the-fundamentals-of-backward-planning

National Association of School Nurses. (2017, March 12). *President signs "Every Student Succeeds Act" into law.* https://www.nasn.org/blogs/nasn-profile/2017/03/12/president-signs-every-student-succeeds-act-essa-into-law-school-nurses-highlighted-in-new-law

National Association of School Nurses. (2022). *School nursing: Scope and standards of practice* (4th ed.). Author.

National Association of School Nurses. (2024). A contemporary framework update for today's school nursing landscape: Introducing the School Nursing Practice Framework. *NASN School Nurse, 39*(3), 140-147. https://www.doi.org/10.1177/1942602X241241092

National Board for Professional Teaching Standards. (n.d.). *Five core propositions.* https://www.nbpts.org/certification/five-core-propostions/

National Consensus for School Health Education. (2022). *National Health Education Standards: Model guidance for curriculum and instruction* (3rd ed.). https://webnew.ped.state.nm.us/wp-content/uploads/2022/09/NHES-3rd-Edition.pdf

National Education Association. (n.d.). *Our vision, mission, and values.* https://www.nea.org/about-nea/mission-vision-values

Nemours Foundation/Kids Health. (n.d.). *Kids health in the classroom.* https://classroom.kidshealth.org/classroom/

Opper, I. M. (2019). Teachers matter: Understanding teachers' impact on student achievement. *RAND Corporation*, RR-4312. https://www.rand.org/pubs/research_reports/RR4312.html

Pontius, D. J. (2013). Health literacy. Part 1: Practical techniques for getting your message home. *NASN School Nurse, 28*(5), 246–252. doi:10.1177/1942602X13486357

Positive Behavioral Interventions & Supports (PBIS). (n.d.). *PBIS in the classroom.* https://www.pbis.org/school/pbis-in-the-classroom

Rigney, J., Ferland, T., & Dana, N. F. (2019). Understanding teacher reflectivity in contemporary times: A (re)review of the literature. *The New Educator, 15*(4), 305–326. https://doi.org/10.1080/1547688X.2019.1631923

Ross, D. A., Plummer, M. L., Montgomery, P., Kohl, K., Siegfried, N., Saewyc, E., & Baltag, V. (2021). World Health Organization recommends comprehensive school health services and provides a menu of interventions. *The Journal of Adolescent Health: Official Publication of the Society for Adolescent Medicine, 69*(2), 195–196. https://doi.org/10.1016/j.jadohealth.2021.04.036

Schweig, J. (2019). Measuring teacher effectiveness: Understanding common, uncommon, and combined methods. *Rand Corporation.* https://www.rand.org/pubs/research_reports/RR4312z4.html

Slavin, R. E. (2021). *Educational psychology: Theory and practice* (13th ed.). Pearson Education Inc.

Society of Health and Physical Educators (n.d.). *Resources and Handouts.* https://www.shapeamerica.org/publications/resources/default.aspx?hkey=55103b9c-7979-4a38-a483-c1669fefbc6e

Staake, J. (2022, Summer). *Your guide to teacher certification exams in every state.* https://www.weareteachers.com/teacher-certification-exams/

Struthers, L. R. (1917). *The school nurse: A survey of the duties and responsibilities of the nurse in the maintenance of health and physical perfection and the prevention of disease among school children.* https://play.google.com/books/reader?printsec=frontcover&output=reader&id=T4QfAAAAYAAJ&pg=GBS.PP1

United Nations. (n.d.). *Take action for the sustainable development goals.* https://www.un.org/sustainabledevelopment/sustainable-development-goals/

United Nations. (2015). Transforming our world: The 2030 agenda for sustainable development. *Department of Economic and Social Affairs.* https://sdgs.un.org/2030agenda

U.S. Department of Education. (2020). What is the Every Student Succeeds Act? *Office of Elementary & Secondary Education.* https://oese.ed.gov/families/essa/

U.S. Department of Health and Human Services. (n.d.a). *Browse objectives.* https://health.gov/healthypeople/objectives-and-data/browse-objectives

U.S. Department of Health and Human Services. (n.d.b). *Healthy People 2030 framework.* https://health.gov/healthypeople/about/healthy-people-2030-framework

U.S. Department of Health and Human Services. (2019). *Health literacy reports and publications.* https://www.hhs.gov/surgeongeneral/reports-and-publications/health-literacy/index.html

Vanderpool, R. C., Gaysynsky, A., & Sylvia Chou, W.-Y. (2020). Using a global pandemic as a teachable moment to promote vaccine literacy and build resilience to misinformation. *American Journal of Public Health, 110*(53), S284–S285. https://ajph.aphapublications.org/doi/full/10.2105/AJPH.2020.305906

Violent Crime Control and Law Enforcement Act [Megan's Law]. P. L. 104-145 (1994). https://www.congress.gov/bill/103rd-congress/house-bill/3355/text

White House. (2022, March). *National COVID-19 preparedness plan.* https://www.whitehouse.gov/wp-content/uploads/2022/03/NAT-COVID-19-PREPAREDNESS-PLAN.pdf

Yonkaitis, C. (2020). Lesson plan basics: Teaching in the classroom with confidence. *NASN School Nurse, 35*(3), 136–139. https://doi-org.proxy.cc.uic.edu/10.1177/1942602X19893038

Chapter 5

Evidence-Based School Nursing Practice

Kimberly J. Stanislo ▪ Andrea Tanner

CHAPTER OUTLINE

Optimal health and academic outcomes for school-age youth require well-designed programs of research to identify interventions that work, translation of that evidence into practice, and continuous quality improvement to maintain the highest standards of clinically competent care. For school nurses, this means using current evidence to determine and implement best practice (evidence-based practice), determining the best processes for implementation (quality improvement), and collecting and using data from these efforts to advance the profession. This chapter focuses on the interconnection between research, evidence-based practice (EBP), and continuous quality improvement (QI).

SCHOOL NURSING RESEARCH

Evidence is generated by conducting research. Before health-care providers have evidence on which to base their practice, researchers must generate that evidence through well-designed programs of research. Once researchers generate the evidence, and that evidence is translated into practice, quality improvement programs can measure how well providers execute care according to the evidence, standards, and protocols. The result is a cyclical process of building, implementing, and evaluating best practice that promotes health and emphasizes the critical role of the nurse. The goal of school nursing research is to identify practice (school nursing activities or functions) that results in optimal student health and education outcomes.

Although nursing and other scientific research literature is a foundation for practice, practice generates the research questions. Nurses in practice are essential in identifying questions in both practice and process, as they understand the issues that interfere with quality care and need more research to address them. Partnering with nurse scientists (PhD-prepared nurses), trained in formal research procedures, links these questions developed in practice with the research tools needed to answer questions when current evidence does not exist or is outdated. Partnering with nurses with practice doctorates (Doctor of Nursing Practice [DNP]), trained in EBP and the translation of research evidence into practice, links the questions developed in practice with best practices and processes based on current evidence available. This PhD-DNP partnership enables school nurse research teams to link research and practice more efficiently through scholarly inquiry.

No matter the educational degree, all school nurses can engage in scholarly inquiry. **Scholarly inquiry** is a professional activity that school nurses perform daily to identify and answer questions and solve problems. This process of inquiry is reflected in the School Nursing Practice *Framework* (Framework) within the practice principle of Quality Improvement. Nursing inquiry requires nurses to examine their practice and critically question why an approach, intervention, or procedure is utilized; question whether that practice is based on evidence or tradition; and determine whether new knowledge and practice must be developed to effectively answer the question. All school nurses are expected to be consumers of nursing research and to continually renew their knowledge of the most recent evidence for practice (National Association of School Nurses [NASN], 2022a, 2024c). Membership in professional organizations promotes this as nurse members interact with each other on topics of interest, share and explore practice questions, review journal articles, serve as participants in research to generate evidence, implement best practice, and access professional development opportunities.

Scholarly inquiry, including the integration of evidence and research findings into nursing practice, is one of the *Standards of Professional Performance for School Nursing* (NASN, 2022b). The competencies for the standard of Scholarly Inquiry (Box 5-1) speak to the role school nurses play in collaborating, generating, sharing, and using current and new knowledge.

The Research Process

Research is a systematic and rigorous process "to generate new knowledge and external evidence" that answer questions about nursing phenomena (Gallagher-Ford & Melnyk, 2022, p. 258). Answers to these questions aim to describe, explain, predict, or control phenomena. In school nursing, phenomena of interest typically involve children in the school setting and the factors that affect their health and education. The research process involves three basic components: (1) the discovery of knowledge, (2) dissemination of that knowledge to professionals and interested members of the public, and (3) the utilization of new knowledge in nursing care and policies. When undertaking nursing research, it is often helpful for the school nurse to partner with experienced researchers because

BOX 5-1

NASN Research and EBP Competencies for School Nurses

STANDARD 14. SCHOLARLY INQUIRY

Competencies

The school nurse:

- Articulates the values of research and its application relative to the practice of school nursing.
- Identifies questions in school nurse practice that may be resolved through research.
- Participates in data collection such as surveys, pilot projects, and formal studies, including the school nursing national dataset.
- Engages with the scientific literature that is foundational to school nursing practice.
- Advocates for the ethical conduct of research and translational scholarship with particular attention to the protection of the student as a vulnerable research participant.
- Investigates processes for team members to have continuous access to evidence-based practices and guidelines.
- Shares peer-reviewed research findings with colleagues to integrate knowledge into school nursing practice.
- Collaborates with researchers from outside the educational system when they seek to study student health, school nursing practices, and school communities.
- Complies with institutional, district, state, and federal policies regarding the safe conduct of research.

Additional Competencies for the Graduate-Level Prepared School Nurse

- Uses current interprofessional healthcare research findings and other evidence to expand school nurse practice.
- Connects theory and research to school nurse practice.
- Encourages other nurses to develop research skills by participating in school health research activities on a local, state, national, and global scale.
- Performs rigorous critique of evidence derived from databases to generate meaningful evidence for school nursing practice.
- Promotes a climate of collaborative research and clinical inquiry.
- Disseminates evidence-based practice outcomes and research findings through activities such as presentations, publications, consultation, and journal clubs.
- Contributes to school nursing and interprofessional knowledge through scientific inquiry to improve healthcare outcomes.
- Develops evidence-based implementation strategies to accelerate the translation of evidence into practice (e.g., toolkits).
- Develops clinical practice guidelines for school nursing practice.

Source: NASN (2022b, pp. 88–89).

the research process requires advanced skills and includes various protocols that must be followed. University schools of nursing are often looking for practice partners to build their research projects.

Regardless of the type of research being conducted, all studies use a similar scientific approach that mirrors the nursing process (Box 5-2). The research process is a way of thinking about the phenomena of interest. This process is dynamic as researchers move back and forth between the steps of constructing and implementing their projects.

Steps in the Research Process

DETERMINE THE QUESTION. The process starts by *identifying a question or problem.* As stated earlier, one of the best

BOX 5-2

Comparing Steps of Nursing Process, EBP, Continuous QI, and Research

NURSING PROCESS	EBP	CONTINUOUS QI	RESEARCH
Art and Science of Nursing	Translating research and implementing existing evidence into practice; best practice	Sustaining best practice by fixing or creating a new process specific to a local practice via existing evidence; best process	Generating new evidence via scientific method
Assessment: Collects pertinent data and information relevant to the situation	■ Ask: ■ Are we doing the best thing? ■ Ask clinical questions in PICOT format to consider	■ Ask: ■ Are we doing the best thing right and continuously? (Decide your aim) ■ (Choose your measures)	■ Ask questions: What is the best thing?
Diagnosis: Analyzes data to identify need or concern	■ Literature review to search for the best evidence	■ (Collect baseline data)	■ Literature review to help formulate question and identify gaps
Outcomes identification: Defines expected or desired outcomes	■ Appraise: Critically review all of the evidence	■ Identify outcomes to continuously monitor	■ Create a hypothesis
Planning: Develops strategies to attain the desired outcomes	■ Identify model for practice (ARCC, Hopkins, IOWA, 7-Steps of EBP) ■ Make best practice recommendations ■ Apply: Integrate the evidence with clinical expertise and client preferences and values ■ IRB or other internal review for protection of data and to meet publication requirement	■ Plan ■ Identify model for practice (PDCA, Lean, Six Sigma, FADE) ■ Identify plan to implement pilot of practice change ■ IRB or other internal review for protection of data and to meet publication requirement	■ Methodology: Study design (quantitative, qualitative, mixed), tools, Institutional Review Board (IRB)
Implementation: Carries out the strategies	■ Implement best practice recommendations	■ Do ■ Implement strategies to sustain best practice	■ Conduct research, generate new (external evidence) knowledge
Evaluation: Evaluates progress toward achieving identified outcomes	■ Assess: Evaluate the outcomes of the practice decisions or changes based on evidence ■ Measure outcomes and make recommendations for modifications (if needed) ■ Alert: Disseminate results	■ Study ■ (Outcome, process, and balance measures) Generate internal evidence ■ Act ■ (Expand and repeat; or discard) ■ Disseminate results	■ Analyze results ■ Disseminate results ■ Generalize/ transfer findings

Sources: Grys (2022); IHI (2023c); Melnyk & Fineout-Overholt (2023); NASN (2024c).

sources for research questions is practicing school nurses. Data collected in electronic health records (EHRs) or during daily practice should be examined by nurses working in the school setting to help identify research questions. Examples include "What nursing interventions can school nurses use to improve attendance rates for students experiencing chronic absenteeism?" and "Why are school nurses experiencing high levels of burnout and reporting mental distress?"

Literature Review. Once the problem is identified, then the school nurse (or research team colleagues) searches the literature to identify existing research about the topic; when, where, and how the research was conducted; and what implications the research findings had for the problem or question at hand. Publishing the synthesis of these findings and critical analysis of literature is a scholarly contribution that helps others investigating a similar topic identify a remaining gap in knowledge about the topic. Following the literature review and identification of a knowledge gap, the research team identifies the key variables that should be included in a research study, the research question(s) to guide a study, and, depending on the type of research, the *hypothesis* of the expected relationship(s) between two or more variables investigated in a study.

Methodology. Once the research question or aim is developed the research team must then decide how to best answer the question or achieve the aims. The methodology chosen depends on the type of question or aim being explored. Does the researcher seek to describe a situation or experience? If so, a qualitative method would be appropriate. For example, if the research aim is to better understand the experience of attending school as an adolescent with a mental health condition, a qualitative descriptive study might be used. Does the research want to predict and test what will happen in response to an intervention? This would require a quantitative research method. If the research aim is to predict whether chronic absenteeism is more common in certain groups, such as those who qualify for free or reduced lunch or have a chronic health condition, then a quantitative correlational methodology might be used. If the research aim is to investigate whether a specific program is effective in improving symptoms of anxiety and depression, an intervention study would be conducted. Nurse researchers have the skills to understand which methodology is most appropriate for a given question and to create a research program to effectively study the problem. The role of school nurses on the research team is essential to ensure the research question is relevant to practice and the findings are useful in the care of students. It is essential to include a practicing school nurse in research related to school health and school nursing practice.

Once the methodology is determined, tools are identified or developed to collect the data (e.g., surveys, questionnaires, or interview scripts). Tools should have a high degree of reliability (yield consistent results) and validity (measure what the tool claims to measure). Tool development is a science and specific skill that requires training. Drafting a questionnaire may seem deceptively simple. However, a bad survey design can significantly influence the validity of the results or frustrate respondents, lowering the response rate and limiting the usefulness of the study. It is better to identify and utilize an existing instrument from the literature that has good reliability and validity than to develop your own.

Research studies in schools must be approved by the district and school administrators according to protocol. Hospitals, universities, and larger school districts have *institutional review boards* (IRBs) that must review the proposal before a researcher proceeds. Some school districts use the term *research review board* (RRB). If a school district does not have an RRB, the IRB process of the partnering university should be followed. IRBs and RRBs are primarily comprised of persons with considerable research experience who follow stringent protocols to approve studies and ensure they are ethical. Most studies will require notification of parents and, in some cases, require their signed approval *(consent)*. Children must also give their oral or written *assent* to participate in research studies according to IRB guidelines. Participants must be informed about the study in a language they can understand, participation must be voluntary, and participants must be able to withdraw at any time.

Once the study is approved, the *research protocol* can be initiated, and *data collection* can begin. This may include distributing questionnaires, implementing an intervention, or accessing available data. School nurses are essential in the implementation of certain research protocols in the school setting. Following a standardized protocol is critical to ensuring uniformity and maintaining the integrity of the project. School nurses involved in implementing research protocols will receive specific training and oversight from the research team members. Data collected by school nurses must continue to maintain strict privacy standards and are typically reported back to the research team as de-identified aggregate (combined) values or through an individual de-identified coding process. The data are collected and reported to the research team, and school nurses may be involved in *data analysis*. The data analysis may include the research team members, university statisticians, or data experts from the school district. The *results* of the data analysis are reported and compared with results of similar studies. The process culminates with a discussion led by the research team regarding the implications for school nursing practice, study limitations, generalizability of findings to a broader group of people, and opportunities for future research or inquiry.

Disseminate. The last step of the research process is to share *(disseminate)* the results with stakeholders. Sharing results is a critical step in moving school nursing science forward. Research findings are disseminated to professional colleagues through two major portals: publications and presentations. The gold standard is to publish a data-based article in a peer-reviewed publication, such as *The Journal* *of School Nursing*. In this way, the study results reach the largest intended audience, and findings are available to all scholars and providers reviewing the literature. Thus, the results not only help answer the question at hand, but also add to the available literature evidence to support future school nursing research, education, and practice. Presenting the findings at professional conferences and meetings is also important to build awareness of the findings, stimulate further research, and generate ideas for translating research findings into school nursing practice. These presentations also provide school nurses with access to the latest evidence, exposure to research and its relationship to practice, and academic opportunities.

Partnerships

Partnerships between school nurses, academic or PhD-prepared researchers, and DNP-prepared school nurse experts are beneficial for conducting research that advances the science related to school health services and the health of students and school communities. Many university schools of nursing routinely use pre-K–12 schools for clinical experiences, with school nurses serving as preceptors. This relationship can be extended to include research and other scholarly endeavors through joint projects of interest to both school nurses and nursing faculty. Although school nurses may see the actual conduct of research as a daunting task, academic nurse researchers can be equally stressed by the difficulty of accessing students in schools, making an academic/practice partnership a win-win.

Complex, multisite, collaborative school health studies can require partnerships between nurse researchers, national or state professional organizations, and state school nurse consultants. Additionally, the study design, access to data, and interpretation of the data can be enhanced by partnerships of more than one discipline. Collaborative research increases resources, generalizability (to which populations the findings can apply), and validity of the evidence for determining the clinical efficacy of nursing interventions. It also promotes the value of the school nurse as a member of the education interprofessional team in practice and in the literature evidence.

In collaborative research, protocols for data ownership and reporting results must be established before the study. Ownership conveys responsibility for disseminating the findings; being responsible for its long-term storage and security; and answering any questions about the research from participants or their families, the IRB, funding agencies, or school administrators. A formal agreement includes clear authorship and presentation guidelines, data rights and access, manuscript generation and clearance, abstract and presentation policies, and publicity information. In addition to professional publications and presentations, other research dissemination activities should be considered, such as webinars, blog posts, and meetings with policy makers.

> **Practice Connection**
>
> It is essential for practicing clinicians, such as school nurses, to not only ask the questions but also share the questions with nurse researchers. If the current evidence does not answer the identified question, new research may be needed and is often informed by gaps identified in practice. The integrative review by Hoskote et al. (2022) regarding the role of school nurses in addressing adolescent mental health is an example of the importance of the link between clinical practice and research. Hoskote et al. discovered that school nurse efforts to address mental health are primarily provided at the individual level and that there is a lack of rigorous study to determine the impact of school nurse mental health interventions. This review identified gaps in knowledge that researchers could investigate alongside practicing school nurse partners.

Role of Professional Associations

The *National Association of School Nurses* (NASN) is the professional organization that represents school nurses and includes affiliate state and local level organizations. NASN advances the delivery of professional school health services through initiating, supporting, participating in, and using outcome-based research that validates school nursing practice, as detailed in *School Nursing: Scope and Standards of Practice* (NASN, 2022b). To that end, NASN supports a small grants program to fund research activities. NASN also requires educational products, including position statements, issue briefs, and clinical practice guidelines utilize EBP processes to identify and disseminate the best current evidence. Furthermore, NASN identifies national priorities for school-based research. The NASN research and evidence-based practice priorities, updated in 2024, prioritize areas where robust evidence does not exist or where additional research and translation is needed to identify the best models of practice, implementation processes, and cost effectiveness in school nursing (Box 5-3; NASN, 2024c). These priorities present areas where an academic/practice partnership would thrive. In 2022, NASN committed to promoting EBP in school nursing through the initiation of a PhD-DNP partnership model to address the research, education, and practice priorities of school nurses (Tanner & Stanislo, 2022).

EVIDENCE-BASED PRACTICE (EBP)

What is EBP?

Evidence-based practice (EBP) may be a new concept to some school nurses, as the EBP process and concept of EBP was not taught regularly in nursing programs until after 1996. Although nursing research began in 1856 and quality improvement in health care in 1966, the concept of

BOX 5-3

NASN Research and Evidence-Based Practice Priorities 2024

The National Association of School Nurses (NASN) encourages researchers and implementation scientists to invest in programs of inquiry with well-designed projects that build upon existing knowledge, meet growing evidence needs and result in improved health and well-being of students, school communities, and school nurses. A range of approaches, including 1) multisite, longitudinal, mixed methods, and intervention studies and 2) evidence-based, outcomes-driven, and replicable quality improvement projects, are essential for the advancement of school nursing knowledge and its impact on NASN's vision to keep students healthy, safe, and ready to learn. In alignment with NASN's Strategic Plan Goals, NASN champions scientific inquiry that addresses one or more of the following focus areas:

STRATEGIC PLAN GOAL	FOCUS AREA	NASN PRIORITIES INQUIRY THAT ADDRESS:
Goal 1: Engage school nurses in 21st Century Practice.	School Nurse Workforce	**School Nursing Workforce:** Advancing the understanding of the school nursing workforce factors and models of care that facilitate delivery of optimal school health services **Healthy Work Environment:** Optimizing the work environment for school nurse well-being, professional impact, workforce diversification, practice at one's full scope in alignment with the *School Nursing Practice Framework™*, and as a key member of the school health services team
Goal 2: Pursue health, education, and social equity for students through shared leadership.	Funding for School Nursing Services	**Economics of School Nursing Services:** Securing sustainable funding, understanding drivers of funding, and demonstrating cost-effectiveness of school nursing services so all students can have access to high quality school health services led by a school nurse **Health Equity and Social Determinants of Health:** Advocating for nurse-led school health services models of care that support health equity and reduce student inequities **School Violence, Disasters, and Emergency Response:** Ensuring safe learning environments for students through equitable access to school nurses and interdisciplinary team collaboration
Goal 3: Secure foundational school health evidence.	Data & School Nursing Outcomes	**Effectiveness and Outcomes of School Nursing Practice:** Building evidence of school nursing's contribution to effective school health services delivery, student learning, health, and school climate **Implementation into School Nursing Practice:** Facilitating the uptake of evidence from school nursing and related services into practice

Source: NASN (2024c).

evidence-based medicine formally began in 1990. The term was expanded to evidence-based practice in 1996 and was incorporated as an interprofessional concept between 1996 and 2009, with the development of EBP models to guide implementation (Mackey & Bassendowski, 2016).

EBP is defined as "a problem-solving approach that integrates the best evidence from research with clinical expertise and patient preferences to make decisions to improve quality, safety, and costs of healthcare as well as enhance population health outcomes" (Gallagher-Ford & Melnyk, 2022). EBP promotes evidence-based decision making to maximize patient outcomes through delivery of best practice and quality care at the lowest costs (Engle et al., 2021). As a process and problem-solving approach to implement best practices, EBP is not something a nurse does, but rather the foundation of what a nurse does (practice). As illustrated in Figure 5-1, the components of EBP integrate the following:

- **Best research and data** derived from a systematic search of current evidence *(external evidence)*, including research, EBP theories, expert panels, and critical appraisal and synthesis of the best and most relevant evidence to answer a clinical question.
- **Clinical expertise** *(internal evidence)*, which includes assessment of patient (student/population) and available resources, evidence from quality improvement or outcomes management projects, and desired patient outcomes.
- **Population/student preferences and values** that promote patient-centered care, which is a hallmark of quality healthcare by incorporating the unique

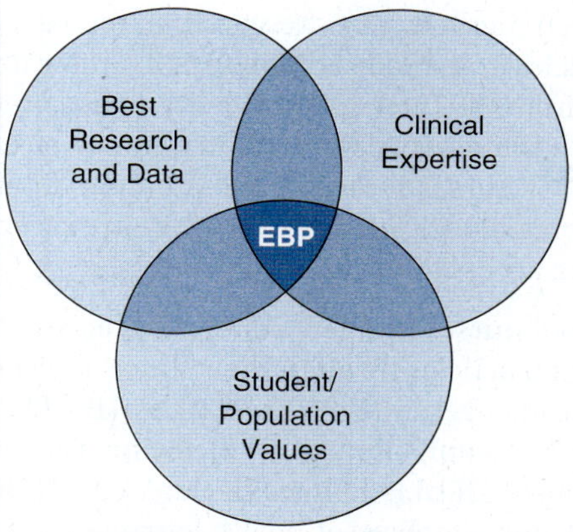

FIGURE 5-1. Evidence-based practice components.

demographics, characteristics, needs, and wants of each individual or population into the decision-making process. "Care that is respectful of and responsive to individual patient preferences, needs, and values and ensuring the patient values guide all decision" (Agency for Healthcare Research and Quality [AHRQ], 2022, para. 1). Patient/student preferences and values may include sociocultural values, demographics, quality of life beliefs, and literacy levels. This involves taking patient/student and population priorities into consideration and not just the diagnosis or identified problem to be solved.

Although EBP involves the translation and implementation of research evidence into practice, it is not the same as research utilization. **Research utilization** involves the implementation of the results from a *single* research study into practice. Evidence-based practice, on the other hand, integrates all three components of EBP (best research and data, clinical expertise, and patient values) through the synthesis of multiple studies or bodies of evidence (Melnyk & Fineout-Overholt, 2023). Quality health-care delivery depends on this translation of best evidence into practice and becomes the foundation for standards of care. School nurses may wonder why they do things a particular way in practice. EBP provides an avenue to determine best practices and promote standards of care based on evidence rather than tradition, ease, or trial and error. The steps of EBP mirror the nursing process as seen in Box 5-2.

The integration of the three components that constitute EBP can be put into action using the seven steps of EBP briefly described next and depicted in Figure 5-2 (Melnyk & Fineout-Overholt, 2023).

STEP 0: CULTIVATE A SPIRIT OF INQUIRY WITHIN AN EBP CULTURE AND ENVIRONMENT. Before school nurses can begin to ask questions about clinical practice and patient outcomes, they need to be in an environment where they feel supported to wonder and question what may be established norms. Creating an environment where clinicians can ask questions regarding patient care and challenge current practices is essential to the success of EBP efforts. Critical factors to support this environment include access to tools and resources to search and utilize evidence; administrative support for inquiry and allocation of resources to support EBP efforts; recognition of EBP efforts; job descriptions and evaluations that incorporate EBP competencies; and access to mentors to facilitate and sustain the culture of inquiry and support EBP processes. Many school nurses do not have access to structured orientations or school nurse supervisors. Nurses enter school nursing, often without the specialty knowledge to implement best practices from day one. Once school nurses become more familiar with and confident in their role, they should begin asking why certain tasks are done a certain way? How can these tasks be done better? What is the best way to do this task? Access to fellow school nurses through professional organizations, surrounding districts, or educational activities provides opportunities to wonder and gain new knowledge to support continual inquiry.

STEP 1: ASK CLINICAL QUESTIONS IN PICOT FORMAT. School nurses have many questions related to practice: What are the most effective nursing interventions for a student with asthma or with epilepsy? What is the most efficient way to

FIGURE 5-2. Evidence-based practice process. *(From Yonkaitis, C. F., & Maughan, E. D. [2018]. Finding the best evidence to support care of students with chronic conditions: CLUE #2: Acquire.* NASN School Nurse, *33(1), 23–26. https://doi.org/10.1177/1942602X17743985)*

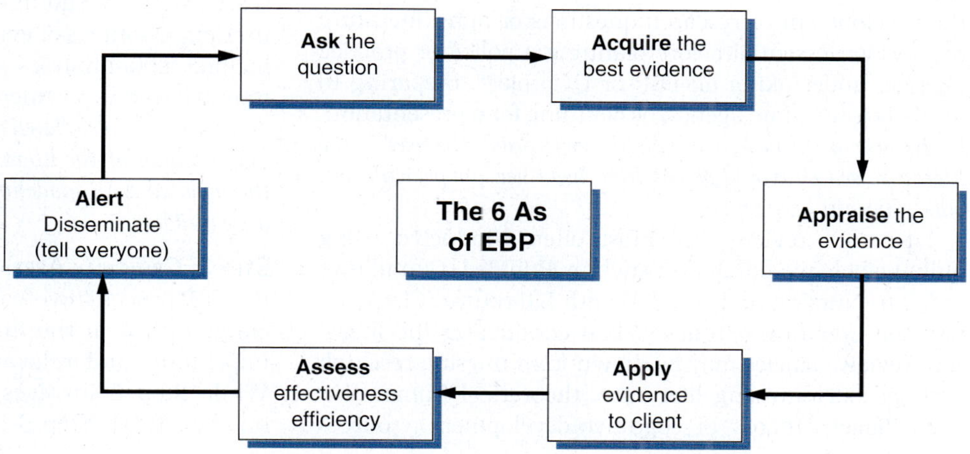

monitor immunization compliance? Which educational program will provide the desired change in health behavior or risky decision making for students? School nurses are often asked to change or reinforce policy even though it is unclear if the policy is based on evidence. This is especially challenging when the health policies are written and implemented in a nonhealth-care setting. How does the school nurse know what the evidence says? The first step is identifying the question. Formulating questions into a PICOT format facilitates the process of making evidence-based decisions. PICOT is an acronym that stands for

- P—the population of interest
- I—the intervention or area of interest
- C—the comparison intervention or group
- O—the outcome
- T—time (only used if a time constraint is appropriate for the question)

A simple example of how to write an actual question using PICOT would be: **"In ______("P"), how does ________("I") compare with ________________("C") in [increasing/decreasing] _____________ ("O")** (Melnyk & Fineout-Overholt, 2023). *For example, an elementary school suddenly has an increase in the number of students who were sent home due to head lice. The principal heard on the news that the American Academy of Pediatrics (AAP) does not support doing mass screenings for head lice or "no-nit policies" in schools (Nolt et al., 2022). The principal wants the school nurse to help develop a new policy related to head lice management. To determine whether this idea is evidence-based, the school nurse should develop a PICOT question. A PICOT question for this situation might be: In children (P), do school head lice policies without a "no-nit "exclusion guideline (I) compared with school policies with "no-nit" exclusion guidelines (C) decrease the incidence of chronic absenteeism (O)? This example will be used to illustrate how to apply each step of the EBP process (watch for italics to indicate the example).*

Step 2: Systematically Search for and Collect the Most Relevant Best Evidence. The PICOT question is a tool to guide the school nurse through the search for best evidence. The PICOT question helps the school nurse identify keywords that can be used in the literature search. Like the development of research questions or aims, literature reviews are essential before planning a policy or practice change, undertaking an EBP or QI project, preparing to testify before a state agency, or planning for a presentation. *In the case of the head lice example, keywords to be used in the literature search would be children, head lice (or pediculosis), policy, no-nits, and school.*

Literature reviews are most often conducted using online academic databases, such as PubMed, Cumulative Index to Nursing and Allied Health Literature (CINAHL), and the Cochrane Library. When conducting the literature review, articles may be drawn from nursing research and specialty nursing literature, theoretical frameworks (e.g., Piaget's theory of cognitive development), sources for research methods (e.g., research textbooks), and data-based articles from related disciplines. The literature can be retrieved from the Internet, university or hospital libraries, or through the school district library. It may be difficult for some school nurses to access these online databases and full-text journal articles; however, there are several options for gaining access to the literature:

- School nurses in a few states have access to full text journal articles through their states' registered nurse licensing agency (GoWYLD, 2022; HEALWA, n.d.).
- The National Library of Medicine provides public access to MEDLINE through PubMed. MEDLINE is an electronic database of health journals.
- Collaboration with nursing faculty, either through research collaborations or by precepting undergraduate and graduate students from local schools of nursing, can result in agreements that allow school nurses access to their university's database resources.
- Contact the librarian from the school district or local public library to find out what scientific electronic databases are available. Certain health, social science, and school research literature may be accessed through databases to which schools or communities commonly subscribe, such as EBSCO or ERIC (Education Resources Information Center). There may also be options to obtain articles through interlibrary loan systems within the state.
- Contact the author of the article to request a copy of the article. In most cases, the authors are willing to share a copy to promote the utilization of their evidence.

It is also important to investigate other sources that may not come up in an online database search, including registries of clinical practice guidelines, such as the U.S. Preventive Services Task Force (2023) or AHRQ (2023). Professional organizations, such as NASN, may provide a synthesis of evidence, including clinical practice guidelines for the care of students in schools. Government sites such as the Centers for Disease Control and Prevention (CDC) may also provide evidence that is critical for school nursing (Yonkaitis & Maughan, 2018). In the end, the literature search should result in the identification of multiple manuscripts or sources of evidence. The search results may also include meta-analyses or systematic reviews that review multiple studies pertinent to the PICOT question.

In the example related to head lice policies and school screening, a search of the literature found several articles, including the updated AAP guidelines on head lice (Nolt et al., 2022), described later.

Step 3: Critically Appraise the Evidence. The next step of the EBP process involves determining whether each article identified in the literature search is current, valid, important, and relevant to the identified population. While Step 2 involves finding relevant articles based on the PICOT, Step 3 involves evaluating the evidence presented in each article to see how strong the evidence may be in relation to the PICOT. It is important to note that much of the professional literature in nursing may not be research. In order to determine whether an article should be considered evidence, it is important to (1) access the original source (called the primary source) on the topic and (2) differentiate opinion pieces from scholarly references. Often, the type of journal will help determine whether the work is scholarly. It is important to use refereed (i.e., peer reviewed) journal articles, meaning they have been critiqued by a panel of experts before publication. This critique process, called peer review, "provides an important check and balance to ensure the manuscript is accurate and reliable and has sound conclusions" and ends with reviewers advising a journal editor "about the suitability of a manuscript for publication" (Rhudy, 2021, p. 56). Most Web sites and newsletters are not peer-reviewed and should not be used in a review of the literature.

Strength of Evidence

To help understand the concept of strength of evidence, scholars have created a pyramid that illustrates which types of evidence are considered strongest and which are weakest. See Figure 5-3. Evidence that has been synthesized into a systematic review (analyses of multiple quantitative, randomized controlled trials) is the strongest evidence (top of the pyramid), whereas case studies or texts are weaker evidence. The type of research (study design) must also be considered when assessing strength of evidence. The strongest study design is known as a randomized controlled trial (RCT). It is important to look at the study design to see how the study was conducted. Was there a comparison made between a group that received an intervention and another group that did not receive an intervention, such as an RCT?

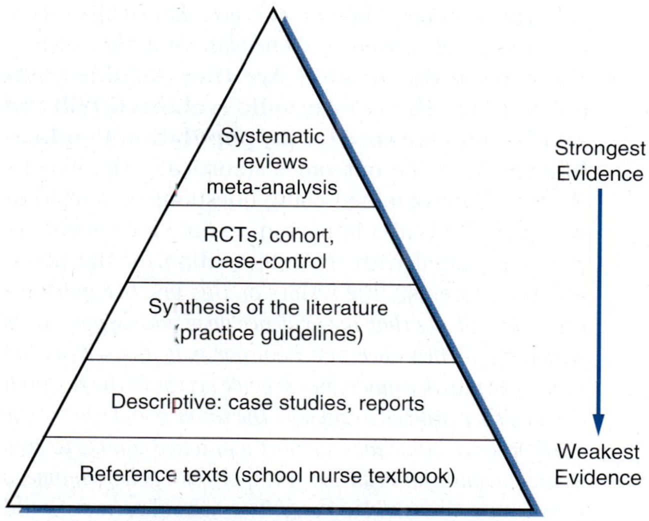

FIGURE 5-3. Pyramid of evidence.

Were efforts made to describe one group that was followed over time (cohort design)? While the goal is to look for the strongest evidence possible, sometimes that means relying on evidence that falls toward the bottom of the pyramid, such as expert opinion. School nurses must obtain and use the strongest evidence possible (Maughan & Yonkaitis, 2018).

The example article by Nolt et al. (2022) provides the AAP practice recommendations for head lice. This article would be VI level of evidence according to the pyramid (see Fig. 5-3).

Additional questions should be asked to fully evaluate the evidence, including the following:

1. **Is the evidence current?** In general, *current* refers to evidence within the past 5 years, but may include longer time frames depending on the topic and trajectory of research and research translation priorities. For example, research on a particular topic typically occurs until the evidence satisfies the question being asked. If there is consensus on the evidence, research for that topic may stop until a new question arises. This may mean the most current evidence on that topic is older than the 5-year rule. This is particularly important to remember as research in many areas stopped or slowed during the COVID-19 pandemic (National Institutes of Health [NIH], 2021). *The example article was published in 2022, so it is considered current.*
2. **What was the research question asked in the article?** Is it similar to your PICOT question? Is it asking the same type of question? This example article is not a research study, but rather practice guidelines, so there is no specific question posed in the article. Practice guidelines are a synthesis of multiple research studies and evidence to provide recommendations for practice. *The exemplar search sought articles addressing head lice that included school screening and*

Did You Know?

What is a *Primary Source* and Why is it a "Big Deal"?

When school nurses read or hear an interesting scientific fact that they might apply to their school community or nursing practice, it is important to identify where the information originated. Facts found from online sites such as Wikipedia, in a magazine or newspaper article, or even in a journal article or textbook often need to be checked for accuracy. Commonly, authors summarize information from a recent research study (the ***primary source***) to support their point. But there is a risk that this ***secondary source*** does not accurately portray the information in the primary source (think of the game of "telephone" or "whisper down the lane"). Therefore, it is important to seek out the original or ***primary*** source of the information and read the original research article to determine if the study findings are strong enough to recommend practice change (Yonkaitis & Maughan, 2018).

policy implications. The answer is yes, the example article includes school-specific recommendations in the article.

3. **What were the results? Are they reliable (reliability)? Are the results valid (validity)? Will the results help me care for my population (applicability)?** Were the outcomes statistically significant? Was the data obtained using questions or tools that were valid? It is also important to note the benefits or risks associated with the intervention for the population of interest. *The results of this practice guideline example indicate that the evidence does not support mass screening for head lice in school nor policy based on "no nits." The practice guidelines provide access to the research and evidence utilized to support the recommendations. The AAP practice guidelines support a practice change to stop mass screening for head lice in school and a policy change to remove any "no-nit" language.* The school nurse should continue to appraise the other relevant articles from the literature search to address the PICOT question. Once several sources have been appraised, the school nurse would ask the following questions: As a body of evidence, is the practice change recommendation consistent? Does the evidence across the articles align or are there discrepancies? If there are discrepancies, what are they and how do they affect the population of interest (Melnyk & Fineout-Overholt, 2023)?

STEP 4: INTEGRATE THE EVIDENCE WITH ONE'S CLINICAL EXPERTISE AND PATIENT/FAMILY-VALUED PREFERENCES IN MAKING A PRACTICE DECISION OR CHANGE. Once the evidence is evaluated and determined to be appropriate to the PICOT question, the other two components of EBP need to be addressed: population values and clinical expertise (see Fig. 5-1). First, determine whether the intervention is appropriate for the population. For example, if a systematic review or other study being evaluated was focused on elementary schoolchildren and the PICOT population was focused on high school students, the intervention may not be appropriate or may need to be adapted to the high school population (Maughan & Yonkaitis, 2017). At this point in the process, an EBP model is typically chosen to provide a visual framework for the overall process of implementation. One example is the Johns Hopkins EBP model (Fig. 5-4), but like nursing theories in research, the school nurse can choose the model that best fits their needs. Additional examples of EBP models are illustrated in Box 5-4 and included in the Online Materials as OM5-1.

If the intervention is determined to be appropriate for the population, in the next step the school nurse or team must assess whether they have the skills and resources needed to implement the intervention. If the intervention requires an advanced practice nursing degree or a skill the team does not possess, it is not an appropriate intervention. At the same time, if the intervention requires continuous monitoring by a nurse and the school nurse covers multiple schools or does not have the same equipment used in the intervention, consider if it is appropriate to adapt this intervention to your clinical situation. School nurses will find that interventions described in studies of hospital- or clinic-based care will need to be adapted to school situations and replicated with students with similar conditions in schools to grow school nursing knowledge.

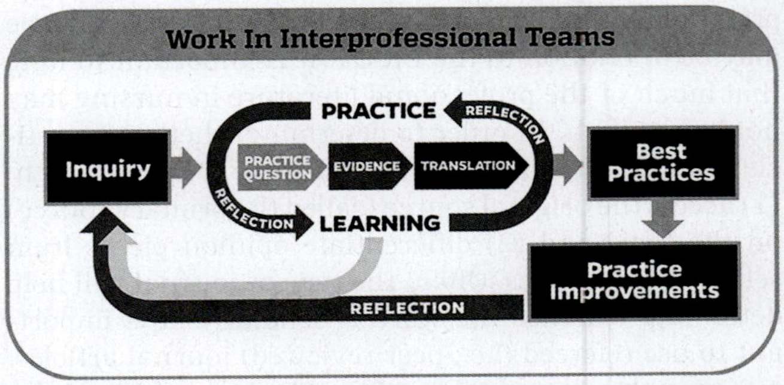

FIGURE 5-4. The Johns Hopkins Evidence-Based Practice Model for Nurses and Healthcare Professionals. *(Dang, D., Dearholt, S., Bissett, K., Ascenzi, J., & Whalen, M. [2022]. Johns Hopkins evidence-based practice for nurses and healthcare professionals: Model and guidelines. 4th ed. Sigma Theta Tau International.)*

BOX 5-4

Additional Evidence-Based Practice Resources

- **ACE Star Model of Knowledge and Transformation** https://uthscsa.edu/nursing/research/resources-scholarly-support/star-model
- **Advancing Research and Clinical Practice Through Close Collaboration Model (ARCC Model)** https://sigmapubs.onlinelibrary.wiley.com/doi/full/10.1111/wvn.12188
- **The Iowa Model Revised: Evidence-Based Practice to Promote Excellence in Health Care** https://uihc.org/iowa-model-revised-evidence-based-practice-promote-excellence-health-care
- **Johns Hopkins Evidence-Based Practice Model** https://www.hopkinsmedicine.org/evidence-based-practice/models-tools.html
- **Promoting Action on Research Implementation in Health Services (PARIHS)** https://implementationscience.biomedcentral.com/articles/10.1186/s13012-016-0398-2

Also see Online Materials OM5-1 to access live links to these resources.

Using the example, we could determine that the exemplar school nurse has the expertise to educate staff, students, families, and school board members regarding the need for practice and policy change. Head lice can be a topic with emotional reactions in the school setting, so education will be crucial in providing the evidence for the best change. The school nurse also has administrator support, which would be an essential resource for this practice and policy change. "No-nit" policies and mass school screenings are often rooted in fear and tradition and not best evidence; gaining buy-in from all key stakeholders will be important for change to happen.

Step 5: Evaluate the Outcome(s) of a Practice Decision or Change Based on Evidence. Once the school nurse has found strong evidence for change, the change fits within the student/population's values and beliefs; the nurse can implement the change, and the practice change is initiated. The implementation should include the identification of specific and measurable outcomes desired because of the change. It is critical to collect baseline data before the change in practice and/or policy begins, and then again following the intervention to see if outcomes were met. Measurable outcomes may be health or academic in nature.

After implementing the change, assess the outcomes of the practice decisions or changes; did the change have the desired impact? *For our example, baseline data would include a retrospective look at the number of screenings for head lice completed in the past 3 months and the number of head lice or nits cases identified from the screenings. The number of cases and number of days absent related to the head lice or nits would also be appropriate data points. Over the first 3 months of implementing the practice and policy change, tracking the number of cases and days absent would be outcome measures. Tracking the number of complaints or specific challenges that arise from implementation would be important for sustainability and assessment of the risks and benefits of the practice change.*

Step 6: Disseminate the Outcome(s) of the EBP Decision or Change. The last step of the EBP process is to share the results with stakeholders. This includes the professional nursing and health-care community, as well as the school community (school administrators, school boards, school staff, students, and families). Many EBP projects would be appropriate to share in a practice journal, such as *NASN School Nurse*, or a scholarly journal, such as *The Journal of School Nursing (JOSN)*. Presenting findings to the school nurses at the district level, at the state's annual school nurse conference, or at the annual NASN conference as a poster presentation or breakout session is imperative in growing the science of school nursing practice. Sharing the experience and journey with a practice change is a valuable opportunity for others to learn and support their inquiry. Sharing results with interprofessional school, district, and state educational stakeholders is also essential to telling your story, especially when you can relate your health outcomes to the academic outcomes. *In our example, sharing the results with school staff and parents would be important in gaining their support for sustainability of the practice and policy change. Linking the head lice screenings to out-of-class time and the no-nit policy to absenteeism is a critical step in addressing the academic outcomes and effects for this example. How did the practice and policy change affect student learning time and absence rates?*

Practice Connection—Quality Improvement

Adverse Event Reporting in Schools

A school nurse used an adverse event from a classroom latex exposure of a student with a latex allergy to implement a quality improvement (QI) plan to reduce future potential of latex exposure in the school environment. This QI plan led to improved communication, knowledge, culture, product labeling in the classroom, and data collection. The QI project also noted that their district and most local education agencies and states do not have requirements or systems to report adverse events. By publishing an article on the adverse event and the need for more system-level reporting mechanisms, the school nurse *disseminated* the results of the QI project and began a conversation on the need to address this issue (Posanka, 2022). See discussion of QI later in this chapter.

CLINICAL PRACTICE GUIDELINES

What Are Clinical Practice Guidelines?

Evidence-based practice is foundational to nursing practice. The amount of new literature and evidence released each year related to health-care delivery is overwhelming and time-consuming to review. Most clinicians, including school nurses, lack the time to review every new article or lack access to the literature. To assist with the translation of evidence into practice, *clinical practice guidelines* (CPGs) are published by several different entities, including professional organizations, as well as federal and state agencies. Clinical practice guidelines (CPGs) provide nurses access to "utilize the principles of EBP in patient decision-making" (Mackey & Bassendowski, 2016, p. 53). Clinical practice guidelines and policy statements are created by experts who synthesize the literature evidence on a specific clinical topic to create standards of care and protocols for providers in clinical practice to access easily and quickly (Melnyk & Fineout-Overholt, 2023). Clinical practice guidelines are reviewed on a regular basis, at least every 5 years, to maintain relevance and keep up with the release of new evidence. As new research and evidence emerge, protocols and guidelines are modified. The updated CPGs synthesize the data so that school nurses need only determine how the guidelines might apply to their specific situation.

Previously, few CPGs specific to school nursing practice were available; however, through collaboration between University of Illinois Chicago (UIC) and NASN, the *Model for Developing Evidence-Based Clinical Practice Guidelines for School Nursing (School Nursing CPG Model)* was developed (Shannon & Maughan, 2020). According to Shannon and Maughan, quality clinical practice guidelines should

- Be authorized by an official professional organization (e.g., medical or nursing specialty association, professional society, government agency, or health-care organization)

- Include a systematic literature search and review of current relevant peer-reviewed evidence
- Contain EBP recommendations, strategies, and information that have been systematically derived to support practitioners in making informed clinical decisions in specific health-care contexts
- Be current or updated within the last 5 years

The *School Nursing Clinical Practice Guideline Model* has been utilized since 2019 by NASN to develop school nursing–specific CPGs to provide school nurses with access to recommendations for best practice. The purpose of developing school nursing–specific clinical practice guidelines is to improve student health and academic outcomes through the implementation of evidence-based school nursing practice (Shannon & Maughan, 2020).

Clinical practice guidelines promote NASN's efforts to support the continuous improvement of school nursing practice in quality and value, which in turn will improve the health and academic outcomes of students and school communities. CPGs outline best practice recommendations and provide the evidence that informs each recommendation. Along with the CPG, an implementation toolkit is also developed as a resource to guide school nurses in implementing the clinical practice guideline. The CPGs represent the *evidence* for the recommendations, and the toolkit represents the *resources* each school nurse can utilize to implement the clinical practice guideline recommendations based on student needs, setting, and nursing judgment. NASN Clinical Practice Guidelines and toolkits can be found in the NASN Learning Center and are free to all members and nonmembers.

What Clinical Practice Guidelines Are Not

Clinical Practice Guidelines are not policies or procedures that must be followed, nor do they outline a specific protocol or checklist. They are evidence-based recommendations for each school nurse to consider when planning, delivering, and evaluating care and clinical decision making (Shannon, 2018). The individual needs of each student, practice setting, and resources available also need to be considered when implementing evidence-based recommendations into practice. Student (patient)–centered care necessitates this relationship between clinical decision making and CPG recommendations on an individual level (Institute of Medicine [IOM], 2011). The *School Nursing Practice Framework* depicts the role of student (patient)–centered care in school nursing (NASN, 2024a). In school nursing, "CPG implementation requires the school nurse to use astute clinical decision-making skills according to the nursing process and individualize care to meet the unique healthcare needs of the given student" (Shannon & Maughan, 2020, p. 415). Therefore, CPGs and implementation toolkits are not prescriptive, but rather provide school nurses with the evidence needed to best apply the recommendations to their students and their setting.

The Role of Clinical Practice Guidelines in Everyday Practice

Utilization of clinical practice guidelines is supported by the *School Nursing: Scope and Standards of Practice* (NASN, 2022b) through Standards 5, 6, 8, and 14, and is a practice component of the Standards of Practice principle within the *Framework*. It is the responsibility of each school nurse to stay abreast of best practice and evaluate their care and student outcomes for gaps and successes (positive outcomes). To fulfill this responsibility, the school nurse should be able to demonstrate the following essential skills related to implementing clinical practice guidelines:

1. Identify NASN's clinical practice guideline resources.
2. Comprehend the state nurse practice act in the state where they practice along with district policies.
3. Use NASN clinical practice guideline implementation toolkits.
4. Evaluate the state nurse practice act and district policies and procedures in relation to CPG recommendations.
5. Assess the students' and school population's needs as they relate to the CPG recommendations.
6. Identify changes in school nursing practice, school procedure, and district policy in relation to clinical practice guideline recommendations.
7. Implement practice, procedure, and policy changes, as needed.
8. Collect data before and after implementing practice, procedure, and policy changes.
9. Evaluate the impact of the practice, procedure, and policy changes.
10. Share experiences, successes, and lessons learned.

Clinical practice guidelines aim to provide a framework for clinical decision making, provide a standard of care, and promote positive patient outcomes. These standards of care are essential in guiding nursing judgment and represent "what a prudent nurse would do." Each level of nursing licensure carries with it an expectation of providing safe, quality, and competent care. Standards of care and state-specific nurse practice acts provide the foundation for these expectations. It is the responsibility of every nurse to stay current with best practices and monitor quality of their nursing care through patient and process outcomes (Young & Smith, 2022).

QUALITY IMPROVEMENT

> *"Of all changes I've observed, about 5 percent were improvements; the rest, at best, were illusions of progress."*
> *(W. Edwards Deming)*

W. Edwards Deming was the pioneer of the quality revolution, first in manufacturing and then in health care. Quality improvement (QI) is a purposeful, systematic approach to change a current process or practice performance to one that more reliably results in a desired outcome (American Academy of Family Physicians, 2023). All industries and businesses strive for the best outcomes possible as defined by their consumers and customers. QI in health care is essential in striving for quality delivery of care and became a focus of health-care institutions, insurance companies, and government bodies following the release of the IOM (2001) report: *Crossing the Quality Chasm.* The Institute for Healthcare Improvement (IHI; 2023b) proposed a QI framework to help optimize health-care systems. This framework, called the Triple Aim, seeks to do three things:

- Improve patient care quality and satisfaction
- Improve the health of populations
- Decrease costs

The U.S. Department of Health and Human Services Agency for Healthcare Research and Quality (AHRQ) published the National Quality Strategy in 2011, which built on the Triple Aim to include the following (AHRQ, 2017):

- **Better Care:** Improve the overall quality by making health care more patient-centered, reliable, accessible, and safe.
- **Healthy People/Healthy Communities:** Improve the health of the U.S. population by supporting proven interventions to address behavioral, social, and environmental determinants of health in addition to delivering higher-quality care.
- **Affordable Care:** Reduce the cost of quality health care for individuals, families, employers, and government.

Since the release of these publications, there have been proposed updates to the *Triple Aim* to include addressing additional aims of clinician burnout and well-being through the *Quadruple Aim* (Feeley, 2017) and health equity through the *Quintuple Aim* (Nundy et al., 2022). Although burnout and clinician mental health are essential priorities in school nursing, this section will focus on the Triple Aim as it focuses on patient outcomes and implementation of best practices by each nurse. Clinician well-being and health equity are critical to quality nursing care, but often require system-level changes outside the direct purview of the school nurse. At this time, the Institute for Healthcare Improvement continues to promote the Triple Aim to focus on better care, healthy people and communities, and affordable care until the aims are achieved. The mental health of school nurses will continue to be a priority area for NASN, and school nurses address health equity daily. Both priorities will continue to be foundational to the advancement of school nursing practice and school nurses' ability to support student health and academic outcomes (Merkle et al., 2022).

The principles of QI also mirror the nursing process, similarly to EBP. See Box 5-2. In the nursing process, school nurses assess and identify the problem and set both nursing and student/family goals for the year. Nurses develop a plan to achieve those goals and develop evaluation measures to determine whether the goals were achieved. Staying current and continually questioning the quality of current practice are key responsibilities of school nurses. QI is based on the principles of using data and the obligation to always improve. It is reflected in the *School Nursing: Scope and Standards of Practice* (NASN, 2022b), specifically:

- Standard 14: Scholarly Inquiry
- Standard 15: Quality of Practice
- Standard 16: Professional Practice Evaluation

NASN's (2024a) *Framework* includes Quality Improvement as one of the key principles, emphasizing the interrelationship between QI and the components of data, documentation, the uniform data set, and performance appraisal and evaluation. As with EBP, research is also a component of QI. Although school nurses are not expected to conduct research, school nurses should use methods of QI to promote the sustainability of best practice (EBP) through measuring outcomes and refining the process.

QI is EBP and the nursing process in action. EBP is the identification of best practices from the literature as it relates to the values of the patient/community, and QI is a means for implementing the best practice through discovery of the best processes. Various models of QI exist, most of which come from business and industry professions. A few of the most common QI models can be found in Box 5-5. The main assumption of QI is that most practice problems are not usually "people problems," but rather issues of *process.* The focus is not on changing people, but on changing the system's process of implementing a best practice more efficiently and

BOX 5-5

Examples of Quality Improvement Models

- **Model for Improvement:** A framework meant to accelerate improvement by addressing three fundamental questions and testing and adapting the changes using the Plan-Do-Study-Act (PDSA) cycle.
- **Lean Model:** Focuses on improving patient care by defining value as what the patient wants and mapping how the identified value gets to the patient. Looks to identify a process that is efficient and cost effective (often combined with Six Sigma).
- **Six Sigma:** A process of improvement that uses statistical thinking to examine existing processes (DMAIC: define, measure, analyze, improve, control) and create new processes (DMADV: define, measure, analyze, design, and verify). (Often combined with Lean Model.)
- **FADE:** Addresses the process and follows steps: Focus (define the process to be addressed); Analyze (collect data to learn of problems); Develop (create a plan of action); Execute and Evaluate (implement and determine whether successful).

Sources: American Society of Quality (2023a, 2023b); HRSA (2011); IHI (2023c).

effectively. In other words, the system is set up to make the right (best) thing to do, the easy thing to do in every situation. School nurses can use QI in all aspects of practice; examples of QI include identifying more efficient ways for sending and receiving vision-screening referrals, or monitoring and communicating immunization compliance.

Like creating a culture of inquiry for EBP, organizations that strive to foster a culture of QI produce the best outcomes (Melnyk & Fineout-Overholt, 2023). A team approach is best with QI projects, as process and system change require cooperation and buy-in from stakeholders. Interprofessional team members share perspectives and ideas that a single person acting alone cannot identify. The National Association of City/County Health Officials (NACCHO) developed a roadmap for institutions seeking to develop a quality culture. See Box 5-6 for additional resources. School nurses will achieve the most success if the school community buys in and participates in the QI process.

BOX 5-6

Additional Quality Improvement Resources

- Agency for Healthcare Research and Quality (AHRQ). https://www.ahrq.gov/
- Community Tool Box. http://ctb.ku.edu/en
- Institute for Healthcare Improvement (IHI). Driver diagram. https://www.ihi.org/resources/Pages/Tools/Driver-Diagram.aspx
- Institute for Healthcare Improvement (IHI). Quality Improvement Essentials Toolkit. https://www.ihi.org/resources/Pages/Tools/Quality-Improvement-Essentials-Toolkit.aspx
- Minnesota Department of Health. Public Health and QI Toolbox. https://www.health.state.mn.us/communities/practice/resources/phqitoolbox/index.html
- NACCHO. (n.d.). QI Roadmap. https://virtualcommunities.naccho.org/communities/community-home/librarydocuments?LibraryKey=2abb346e-3b2b-4fc9-b7d7-0a7fefc1466f
- National Institute for Children's Health Quality (NICHQ). Quality Improvement 101. https://www.nichq.org/resource/quality-improvement-101
- TED talk: How data from a crisis line saves lives. https://www.ted.com/talks/nancy_lublin_the_heartbreaking_text_that_inspired_a_crisis_help_line

Institute for Healthcare Improvement Model of Improvement

The Institute for Healthcare Improvement (IHI, 2023a, 2023c) developed the Model of Improvement Framework that is often used in health-care QI initiatives. See Figure 5-5. The IHI framework includes three questions and the Plan-Do-Study-Act (PDSA) cycle. School nurses can use the model to address QI in their schools starting by asking the following questions.

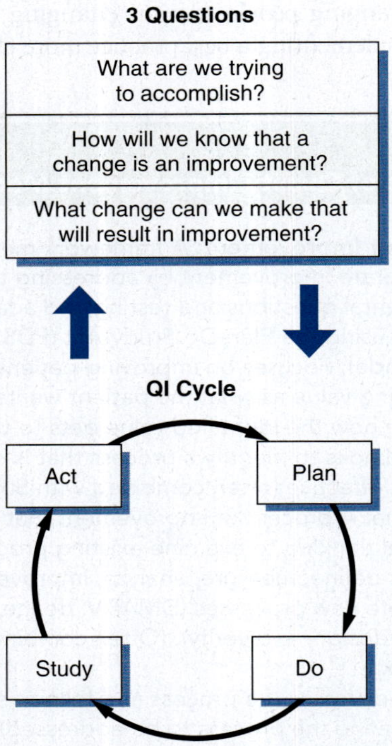

FIGURE 5-5. IHI's 2017 model of improvement. *(From Langley, G. L., Moen, R., Nolan, K. M., Nolan, T. W., Norman, C. L., & Provost, L. P. [2009].* The improvement guide: A practical approach to enhancing organizational performance *[2nd ed.]. San Francisco: Jossey-Bass Publishers; 2009; permission conveyed through Copyright Clearance Center, Inc.)*

Question 1: What Do You Want to Accomplish?

The first step in the QI process is to identify what needs to be changed. The IHI suggests identifying a team and developing an aim statement (IHI, 2023a).

Identifying Your Team. The composition of the team is important when developing the aim. Does the team include the right players? Using the vision compliance example to improve quality for completed vision-screening referrals, consider whether the team members are identified and whether who "owns" each step of the process is clearly communicated. How does the form get to the parent? Who currently receives the forms when they are returned to school? Depending on who is involved, teachers, secretaries, parents, and even students may be important members to include on the team as they have the best knowledge of where the process works and does not work. Team members should include system leaders, those with needed technical expertise, and representation from leaders closest to where the activity is carried out (IHI, 2023a). For vision-screening referrals, the systems leader may be the person who oversees policies on returning forms. If the solution or issue involves electronic submission, the information technology (IT) staff should be included. If there are legal implications or if special wording is needed, include experts from those fields. Leaders in the school whose buy-in is needed should also be included. Often a team has a "champion" or "sponsor," someone who has the authority to support and represent the project to senior leadership (IHI, 2023a).

Developing your Aim. The aim statement clarifies what the group hopes to accomplish and how large a change is required. The statement is grounded in the vision of the group and the organization. The aim statement includes the target population of the project, a time frame for when the change will occur, and how it is measured. Following are examples of aim statements relative to school nursing, including the target population, time frame, and measurability.

- By the end of the school year, the nurse will document 20% more completed vision screening referrals for students in Lillian Wald Elementary School.
- For the next 6 months, all medication administered to students at Brain Middle School will be recorded within 15 minutes.
- By December, the school wellness team will complete five of the seven School Health Index (SHI) modules for Mt. Healthy High School.

Within each aim, the team develops objectives which are smaller steps that break down tasks to address the larger aim or goal. For example, if a family is going on vacation to the beach, to get to the beach, they will pass through a specific town. The beach is the "aim," and passing through the town is one "objective" needed to reach the aim. This is a common process when developing school wellness and school improvement plans. Objectives can be written in many ways, but two common sentence structures are used:

- "[**Who**] will do [**what**] resulting in [**measure**] by [**when**]."
- "By [**when**], [**who**] will do [**what**] resulting in [**measure**]" (Minnesota Department of Health, n.d.).

Returning to the example related to vision-screening referrals, the aim is to increase the number of completed referrals for students by the end of the year. When developing the plan, the aim should be broken down into smaller steps to be completed to reach the destination. Examples of smaller objectives that will help the team reach their larger aim may include the following:

- Nurses will pilot the change in the first grade. If it works well, nurses will expand the service to third graders by November.
- In August, nurses will attend the kindergarten/first grade orientation meetings to explain vision screening to parents, as well as the importance of returning completed referral forms.
- In September, nurses will meet with teachers in grade teams to discuss the goal and obtain buy-in for sending vision referrals directly to the school nurse.
- By October, nurses will create an electronic option for parents of all first graders to return forms. The system will provide reminders to parents to return the form.

Once the aim and smaller objectives are identified it is time to determine how any change will be measured.

Question 2: How Do We Know If the Change Is an Improvement?

One of the important components of an aim statement is that it is measurable. This means that the team must identify which data are critical to determine whether the process change is working (IHI, 2023a; Langley et al., 2009). Measures should be *objective* rather than *subjective* so that the result measures what is *really* happening versus what the team *thinks* is happening. The team identifies measures during the planning process so that all agree on what defines success. If team members are not in agreement, then more discussion and tweaking of the aim statement is needed so all understand the aim and agree with the data points to measure. Once data points are determined, a plan to collect the data is developed.

QI measurement should address outcome, process, and impact. Measures that address each should be identified. Each type is described here:

- **Outcome measures** reflect what the team sets out to achieve. If the aim was to increase completed vision referrals by 20%, the definition of "completed referrals" needs to be clear, the beginning and final totals will need to be collected, and the timeline for collection will need to be described. For example, if the measure is *completed vision-screening referrals*, the definition would be as follows: *A referral form with all questions answered, with the results of the examination, and with the signature of a health-care provider within 3 months of the date of referral.* Data to be collected would be the previous count of completed referrals and the number of current referrals, including the date the referral was sent, the date the completed referral was received, all questions answered, results of examination, and the health-care provider's signature (e.g., met the definition of a completed referral).
- **Process measures** help determine whether the intervention, activities, or process is being implemented as planned. Data on all measures, but particularly process measures, should be reviewed regularly to detect trends and avert problems as they arise. Simple trend charts to plot the data may be useful. Examples of process measures include the following: *Is the electronic return system working? Did parents say it is confusing? Do teachers continue to hold on to referrals before submitting? Do parents prefer the electronic option? Are teachers submitting the completed referral to the nurse on the day they receive it?* Process outcomes and a plan for the means to collect them may need to be developed after completing question 3 (see later discussion).

- **Impact or balancing measures** are the hardest to identify completely. These look at the unintended consequences of the change and address the inputs associated with the process. For example, does implementing the electronic return option of referrals decrease the interaction between nurse and parent, which is how nurses learn the family cannot afford glasses? Just like process outcomes, impact measures should be reviewed and addressed often so that tweaks in the plan can be made in real time to address the situation.

Once measurements are identified, data should be collected to establish the baseline or beginning point. The measures are collected throughout and at the end of the identified time period in order to identify change and improvement. Identifying the outcome, process, impact/balancing measures, and data collection timeline and methods before beginning the QI project ensures the right data are collected at the right times. This allows the most accurate evaluation of the success of the quality improvement project.

One reason that measures must be defined clearly is so that everyone measures the data the same way (reliability). This allows the data from the measures to mean the same thing in each part of the process and mean the same thing over time. Measures should be meaningful, useful, and directly reflect the desired change (aim). Data should not be collected unless there is a plan for using the data. For school nurses, data collection may mean identifying both health and academic measures. Measures can be quantitative (numbers) or qualitative (verbal or text) responses (Health Resources and Services Administration [HRSA], 2011).

Question 3: What Change Can We Make That Would Show an Improvement?

The third question that needs to be asked is "What change can we make to obtain the improvement we would like to make"? This is the actual QI plan that will be put in place. The plan is developed using the steps of EBP as outlined earlier in this chapter, because we want to be sure we use best practices. This is followed by identifying the best process (QI) to implement the best practice in relation to the population, expertise, and setting. The QI practice change is not generalizable, as it is specific to a particular setting and population. This is one of the differences between research and QI; research findings are generalizable. This does not mean the results should not be shared or added to the literature evidence. These results can be replicated in similar situations as evidence to answer future questions.

QI is about a process that needs to be tweaked, so it may be helpful to develop a visual diagram or map of the current process to identify where there may be problems or gaps (IHI, 2023c; Langley et al., 2009). Creating a visual tool such as a flow chart may also be helpful to outline the new process so that everyone is clear on what the new process is and follows it.

Two examples of QI visual maps are flow charts and driver diagrams. **Flow charts** are simple diagrams that describe the process or current flow of events. See Figure 5-6 for an example of a flow chart related to the vision referral process. Flow charts can be useful to see gaps or breakdowns in the process as well as to identify the key players. Another option is to create a diagram of the steps of the process that affect the goal or aim of the improvement. These are called **driver diagrams** and help identify the causes of the problem in the current process (Goldmann, 2023). A driver diagram includes two to five primary drivers or main factors that directly influence the core issue of your aim. For each primary driver, there may be secondary drivers (factors that influence the primary drivers). For example, a primary driver of not receiving completed vision-screening referrals could be that the forms are not returned by parents. A secondary driver would be that the student forgets to give the

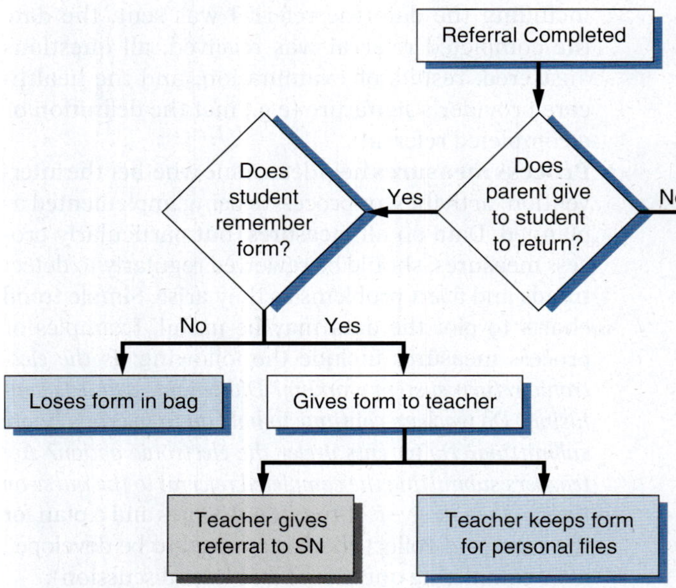

FIGURE 5-6. Example of a flow chart describing the vision-screening referral process.

form to the teacher. Identifying the primary and secondary drivers will help identify gaps in the process where changes need to be made. Figure 5-7 is an example of a driver diagram related to vision-screening compliance.

After identifying the gaps and drivers, the school nurse uses EBP skills to find the best evidence available to address the problem, make sure it is appropriate for the population's culture and beliefs, and ensure that appropriate resources are available to implement the intervention. For QI, it is important that the intervention starts with a pilot of the process—for instance, in one classroom, one grade, or one school, depending on the type of QI project. A pilot allows you to test the process to identify ways it can be improved before it is used system wide as a regular routine or default behavior. It is small in scale and can easily be duplicated; therefore, a pilot is sometimes referred to as a *small test of change.*

Plan-Do-Study-Act

Quality Improvement is not a one-time process, but rather cyclical or continuous in nature (HRSA, 2011). This is best illustrated using the Plan-Do-Study-Act (PDSA) cycle. The PDSA cycle is based on rapid, quick testing of a small change that is part of a larger plan (IHI, 2023c). The time interval could be as short as a week to a month, depending on the intervention. Small increments are critical and become part of a systematic method of improvement (AHRQ, n.d.).

Following is a description of the four steps of the PDSA cycle (AHRQ, n.d.; HRSA, 2011; IHI, 2023a), along with continued examples from the vision-screening referrals completion example. Box 5-7 shares an additional example based on an article published in the *Journal of School Nursing by* Davis et al. (2016) using the PDSA cycle to increase immunization compliance by reducing provisional admittance.

Plan

Each cycle begins by identifying a small change the team wants to address and developing it into a question as discussed earlier. Objectives can help break the plan into measurable tasks as described in question 1 with the development of the aim. A flow chart that outlines the intervention may be helpful to guarantee all apply the intervention consistently. A plan for collecting data should be included as well. Knudsen et al. (2019) found that many who apply the PDSA concept do not use it for small increments and only 27% of QI projects included a description of a specific, quantitative aim. An example of a small increment with the vision-screening referral scenario is *limiting the electronic referral completed returns to first grade to see if it works and how others respond.* Keeping the scope or size of the pilot small is important to make sure that it is implemented as planned, data can be collected, and any problems or gaps can be identified and fixed with limited disruption. This makes it easier to use the process in the larger organization.

Do

Once a plan is developed, the team carries out the plan. The appropriate persons also collect data and take notes of unexpected concerns and process issues or outcomes that arise as they carry out the identified plan. For the vision-screening referral completion scenario, *the first-grade teachers and parents will be informed about their part in the new process and the implementation time period.*

Study (Check)

After gathering the information on the measures identified in the "How Do We Know If the Change Is an Improvement?" section earlier in this chapter, the data are reviewed and analyzed to determine whether the interventions are creating the

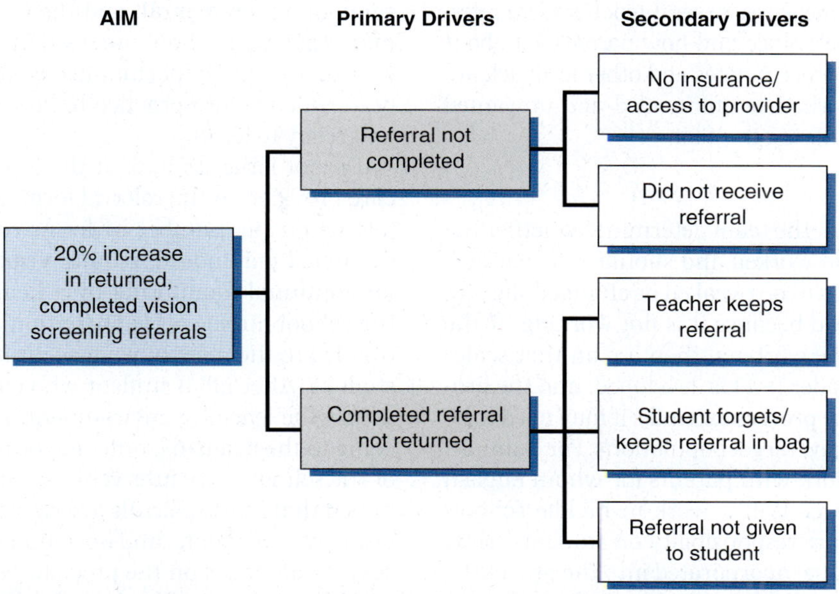

FIGURE 5-7. Example of a driver diagram describing the vision-screening referral process.

BOX 5-7
Example of School Nurses Using Plan-Do-Study-Act (PDSA) Cycle

1. PLAN: **Ask:** ■ Decide your aim ■ Choose your measures ■ Collect baseline data	*Aim:* Improve immunization rates (decrease provisional admittance) by end of the year. *Measurements:* ■ Rates by school, grade, ethnicity ■ School health immunization systems inventory ■ Exemption rates *Identify EBP interventions:* supported by literature, fits community, and have resources
2. DO	■ Maintain comprehensive tracking system ■ Use state registry ■ Increase awareness ■ Document plan for addressing provisional status ■ Engage primary care practices
3. STUDY	■ Monthly reporting ■ Inventory survey of nurses ■ Qualitative responses
4. ACT ■ Expand and repeat; or discard ■ Share results with others	■ Steady decline of provisional admittance ■ Report progress to administrators ■ Standardized processes

Source: Davis et al. (2016).

desired change. As mentioned earlier, data should be reviewed regularly to monitor the new process, not just at the end of the intervention period. Some refer to this step as "check" rather than "study" as it is reflective of the need to regularly assess or check progress. The data should be compared with the initial or baseline data to determine what changes occurred; the results and lessons learned should be summarized. For the vision screen referral scenario, *the team would review the number of referrals received during the pilot period and compare it to the baseline and the initial number of referrals.* During the pilot, data are collected on process measures to see if teachers sent referrals directly to the nurse's office and how parents felt about the change. Finally, the process notes and other feedback are reviewed to determine whether unintended and unwanted consequences occurred during the pilot.

Act

After reviewing the data, the team determines whether the pilot of the intervention worked and should be expanded, if the intervention needs to be tweaked or changed slightly, or if it should be stopped because it is not working. If the intervention seems to be working, then a plan that scales up the process to a broader level is developed, and the process begins again. As the process expands, it may need to be adapted and tested for new target populations. For example, will the new process work with parents for whom English is their second language? Will it work in middle schools where parents place more responsibility on students? How will substitute teachers be incorporated into the process?

Once the intervention is applied to all the areas involved, the evaluation process continues to monitor and measure the outcomes and assess for unintended consequences. Evaluation of the process should continue regularly, and the processes tweaked as needed. New findings in the evidence regarding best practice can also be incorporated using the same measurement process.

Quality Improvement is important to integrate into school nursing culture and practice. School nurses must realize the changes they create can affect other systems. Therefore, changes made in the QI process are meant to be small and incremental, and the QI team needs to include more than just school nurses (HRSA, 2011). Continuous QI processes are important in sustaining the translation of best evidence into practice to keep students healthy, safe, and ready to learn.

Do not forget to look at the feedback from the health-care provider on the referral form; the QI focus should not just be on the number of forms returned. If all children evaluated did, indeed, require visual correction or a plan for continual monitoring by a health-care provider, then the school nurse can validate that his or her assessments that led to the referral were accurate and of benefit to the student. After all, a student who can see better can better access the learning environment. Linking the health outcome to the academic outcome promotes the overall value of the school nurse interventions. If, however, it was determined that most referrals are returned indicating that the vision was adequate, and no action was needed, the QI process should focus on the procedures (and perhaps the skill and knowledge level of those doing the screening) that led to the number of referrals.

PROMOTING EVIDENCE-BASED PRACTICE AND QUALITY IMPROVEMENT IN THE SCHOOL SETTING

Evidence-based practice and quality improvement are both individual and organizational responsibilities (Melnyk & Fineout-Overholt, 2023). EBP (best practice) and QI (best process) complement each other to support and promote the best outcomes for patients, quality improvement (EBQI) in school nursing focuses on improving both student health and academic outcomes. EBQI is particularly relevant to school nursing practice, as it considers the uniqueness of each practice setting and student population as part of the process. This process begins with school nurses gaining access to and staying current with questions that are being asked about nursing and school health, innovations that are being tested, and potential applications of evidence to their practice setting. State school nurse consultants, nurses with research and clinical practice doctorates, and professional organizational initiatives participate in EBQI through the translation of evidence into practice via publications, educational training, project collaboration, and consultation.

School Nursing: Scope and Standards of Practice, Standard 14—Scholarly Inquiry (see Box 5-1) identifies the responsibilities of nurses to stay current and incorporate evidence into practice. When surveyed, school nurses overwhelmingly value EBP and QI; however, less than half feel comfortable evaluating the effectiveness of an EBP or QI interventions (Maughan & Mangena, 2014). A culture change must occur that focuses on producing positive outcomes in the school setting, ensuring that every school nurse has the capacity to work within the EBP model of care (Maughan & Yonkaitis, 2017; Yonkaitis, 2017). This culture change revolves around school nurses gaining confidence and access to the current evidence and reflecting on their current practices to identify gaps and questions. This often begins with data collection to define what the school nurse is currently doing, how it is being done, and whether it is working.

EBP and QI are integral in the implementation and sustainability of clinical practice guidelines (CPGs). The NASN Clinical Practice Guidelines are reviewed every 5 years, and as evidence and practice needs change or emerge. Part of this review process involves the evaluation of implementing CPG recommendations and toolkit resources to support high-quality, student-centered school nursing care. It is an opportunity for school nurses to share experiences related to the implementation of the clinical practice guidelines and identify gaps in practice, process, and knowledge that can inform school nursing research and education. Using the EBQI approach in CPG review engages school nurses not only in the integration of EBP in daily practice but also builds a continuous QI culture.

Quality Improvement is utilized in health care to monitor the quality of care through patient (student) and process outcomes. As school nurses, identifying the processes that guide daily nursing judgment and care provides opportunities to identify data points and student outcomes that represent quality school nursing care (Young & Smith, 2022). The value of a school nurse is often the topic of conversation regarding school nurse staffing models and school district budgets. School nurse value is often measured through data collection and its use to improve processes, student health outcomes, and academic outcomes such as attendance, test scores, graduation rates, and school climate. Sharing EBP and QI experiences using data advances school nursing practice and supports advocacy efforts. For example, school and district level conversations provide school nurses with an opportunity to identify and discuss gaps and successes specific to a shared population and circumstances. Conversations at the regional and state level—including with state school nurse consultants, nursing organizations, and university-based faculty—provide school nurses with an opportunity to identify and discuss gaps and successes in relation to a geographical area and the impact of their state's nurse practice act. On the national level, opportunities may include discussions with peers or experts via national conferences or webinars, NASN's discussion list forum, or school nursing social media. These conversations can result in partnerships for research, development of additional clinical practice guidelines, revision of current CPGs, educational programming, collaboration on EBP and QI projects, or advocacy efforts. EBP and QI efforts benefit from the voice of every school nurse.

STANDARDIZED NURSING LANGUAGE

To successfully measure outcomes, whether as part of a QI, EBP, or other data collection efforts, school nursing care needs to be documented in a consistent, accurate, and retrievable manner. The use of a standardized nursing language ensures that we are all "speaking the same language" and allows the nurse to compare data. The term *standardized nursing language* or *standardized terminology* refers to a universal or commonly understood set of words or terms that describe the nursing process (Rutherford, 2008). School nurses should use standardized nursing language (SNL) to document in health-care records (paper and electronic) and health-care plans.

American Nurses Association (ANA) Approved Standardized Languages

ANA created a means to recognize standardized nursing languages and nursing minimum data sets to quantify nursing contributions to patient care and positive health outcomes (ANA, 2018). To date, ANA recognizes a total of

12 specific terminologies; four of the standardized nursing languages are interdisciplinary terminologies and two are minimum data sets. Table 5-1 has a synopsis of the ANA-recognized standardized nursing terminologies.

Standardized Languages and School Nursing

NASN (2024b) supports the use of standardized nursing language as a part of professional practice. SNLs are a component of the *School Nursing: Scope and Standards of Practice* (NASN, 2022b) as well as the *School Nursing Practice Framework* (NASN, 2024a). However, NASN does not recommend the use of any single SNL for school nursing documentation and data collection. A systematic review suggests that only four SNLs have been studied at the level of implementation: North American Nursing Diagnosis Association International (NANDA-I), Nursing Interventions Classification (NIC), Nursing Outcomes Classification (NOC), and the Omaha System; there is no evidence that any standardized nursing terminology is more effective than another (Tastan et al., 2014). More evidence is needed to determine the influence of SNL on nursing care and health-care outcomes in the school setting.

NANDA International

The most well-known standard nursing language is NANDA International, commonly referred to as NANDA-I. This standardized language for problem identification is evidence-based and was developed inductively based on existing practice. A NANDA-I nursing diagnosis is "a clinical judgment about individual, family, or community responses to actual or potential health problems/life processes. A nursing diagnosis provides the basis for selection of nursing interventions to achieve outcomes for which the nurse is accountable" (Herdman et al., 2021, p. 41). NANDA-I has 281 nursing diagnoses grouped into 13 domains and 47 classes. Nursing diagnoses are written in terms of the client or group experiencing an active problem or a potential problem (at risk) or to promote health (Herdman et al., 2021). School nurses can use nursing diagnoses following their assessment of a student, family, or community. The school nurse can easily determine the number and type of health concerns in a school or district by using NANDA-I to document a student's active or potential problems. These data can also be used to help supply information to school administrators and school boards about school nurse workload and the school's needs.

Nursing Interventions Classification

Following the development of the NANDA-I terminology, a second language addressing nursing interventions was developed at the University of Iowa Center for Nursing Classification and Clinical Effectiveness called *Nursing Interventions Classification,* or NIC. This intervention

TABLE 5-1 ANA-Recognized Standard Nursing Languages

Standardized Nursing Language (SNL)/Terminology	Type of Language (Problem ID, Intervention, or Outcome)	SNL Specifics
NANDA-I	Problem ID	Nursing specific; must be a member of NANDA-I; 234 diagnoses
NIC—Nursing Interventions Classification	Intervention	Interdisciplinary; 554 interventions
NOC—Nursing Outcomes Classification	Outcomes	Interdisciplinary; 490 outcomes
Omaha System	Problem ID, intervention, and outcome	Interdisciplinary, free to use-public domain; LOINC, SNOMED CT, ABC code integrated
Clinical Care Classification System (CCC)	Problem ID, intervention, and outcome	Interdisciplinary
Perioperative Nursing Data Set (PNDS)	Problem ID, intervention, and outcome	Perioperative nursing; cross-mapped with ICNP
International Classification for Nursing Practice (ICNP)	Problem ID, intervention, and outcome	Can cross map with other SNL
SNOMED CT International	Problem ID, intervention, and outcome	Can cross map with other SNL
ABC Coding Solutions	Universal intervention codes	Supplemental codes for nonphysician and alternative medicine health services
Logical Observation Identifiers Names and Codes (LOINC)	Map codes to universal language	Clinical data exchange
Nursing Minimum Data Set (NMDS)	Data set	
Nursing Management Minimum Data Set (NMMDS)	Data set	

ANA (2018).

classification is a "systematic organization of research-based interventions that assigns a label to a group of interventions linked to a NANDA diagnosis and NOC outcomes" (Moorhead & Dochterman, 2012, p. 3). A nursing intervention is "any treatment, based upon clinical judgment and knowledge, which a nurse performs to enhance patient/client outcomes" (Butcher et al., 2018, p. xxi). The NIC seventh edition includes 565 interventions organized in seven domains, and each has its own code. The selection of nursing interventions for an individual client is determined by the nurse's clinical decision making to determine a desired outcome that is reasonable for the setting.

Interventions modify the causative or related factors in the nursing diagnosis. The school nurse determines the nursing intervention based on feasibility, students' preferences, and scheduling of interventions to maximize the student's learning and minimize interruption. These considerations must be consistent with providing evidence-based care. Clear documentation of interventions using standardized language provides comparable and retrievable data, thereby allowing the school nurse and researchers to review the effectiveness of the interventions for individuals or groups.

Nursing Outcomes Classification

Nursing Outcomes Classification (NOC) is another standardized system developed at the Iowa Center for Nursing Classification and Clinical Effectiveness that is used to evaluate the success of interventions (Moorhead et al., 2018). It can also be used to set goals for student care, an important aspect of the nursing process. NOC includes 540 outcomes divided into domains, such as physiological health, psychosocial health, and health knowledge. Each outcome has an associated definition and set of indicators meant to help the nurse assess the client's status as it relates to the outcome. Each of the outcomes is assigned a code number that can be used to track the effectiveness and quality of individual care as well as the effectiveness of interventions in terms of outcomes. These three standard nursing languages (NANDA-I, NIC, and NOC) can work together to provide a clear plan of care and when incorporated into an EHR can be used to collect and compare data on student outcomes and nurse-sensitive interventions.

Omaha System

The Omaha System is a comprehensive research-based interdisciplinary classification system that was originally developed in the 1970s by the Visiting Nurses Association of Omaha (Martin, 2005). The Omaha System has three components: an assessment component called the *Problem Classification Scheme* that includes 42 problems, a care plan/services component called the Intervention Scheme, and an evaluation component called the *Problem Rating Scale for Outcomes.* The interventions are designed to describe multidisciplinary practice to prevent illness; attain, improve, or restore health; decrease deterioration; and/or provide comfort before death. This system provides for four categories of interventions: teaching, treatment and procedures, case management, and surveillance. The outcome schemes use a Likert scale (a scale from 1 to 5) to evaluate knowledge, behavior, and status or condition of a client. The Omaha System is available at no cost to those who wish to use it and has been used across the continuum of health-care services. For example, in 2014 the State of Minnesota recommended that the Omaha System terminologies be used in all EHRs to improve information sharing and accessibility across the state (Martin & Monsen, 2017).

The interdisciplinary nature of many of the standardized nursing languages allows for use by all members of interprofessional teams. Members of student support teams (sometimes called instructional support teams, pupil services teams, student assistance teams, or building resource teams) can easily understand and use the SNLs because they are student-centered and describe the interventions needed and the student's response to more than one health-specific concern. SNL interventions have the potential to describe the team members' roles in providing services needed and can be easily incorporated into many types of student plans. Standardized language can be used in computer databases, providing a means for tracking and analyzing outcome data.

One of the largest barriers to the use of standardized nursing languages by school nurses is that not all electronic health records (EHRs) include standardized nursing terminology in their software. Some EHRs will allow system owners to add or modify health problem lists to meet the individual district's needs. In these cases, nurses within a district should work to ensure that standardized terms are used in EHR documentation. See further discussion on EHRs in the following section.

SCHOOL HEALTH DATA COLLECTION

The value and importance of data collection are echoed in the *School Nursing: Scope and Standards of School Nursing* and the *Framework* (NASN, 2022b, 2024a). Data provide the foundation for research, EBP, and QI and can advance the visibility of school nursing practice. All nurses, regardless of the setting, are required to document the care provided in a legally compliant record. Just as in other health-care settings, the information contained in the school nurse's documentation is valuable information reflecting the health and needs of students. When collected in reports, this information becomes data that are vital in describing the work of school health service personnel, evaluating the care that is delivered, identifying trends, and conducting surveillance of the school community's health. It is essential that once collected, data are sorted, analyzed, and reported to local school and health officials, stakeholders, and policymakers as allowed or required by local and state policies.

Electronic Health Records

Electronic health records are the standard for collecting and managing large student caseloads, for analyzing data, and for producing reports (Johnson et al., 2017b; Lepkowski, 2018). Some school nurses struggle to maintain comprehensive, accurate, and precise documentation of care due to large student caseloads, care provision across multiple school buildings, and, in some cases, lack of investment in EHRs (Bergren, 2016; Bergren et al., 2017). School nurses need to appropriately document, collect (i.e., aggregate), and report on student health data to advocate for their students. School nurses should advocate for appropriate data collection resources, whether electronic or paper, to their supervisor. Box 5-8 provides guidance when selecting an EHR for school health. No matter the circumstance, school nurses must find ways to collect and use pertinent data points in their daily practice.

When available, an EHR can synthesize key data points that a school nurse documents into a report to help identify trends and make decisions. The key to effective usage of an EHR is the school nurse's ability to submit, and retrieve data in meaningful formats, such as reports. In cases where the school nurse is utilizing the health component of a student information system, it may be necessary to work with the district IT team to gain access to the data or customize reports that may be available within the system. It may also be possible to customize the charting screens or dropdown box options to include standardized language and for easier data collection and retrieval. For example, the school nurse could monitor the number of students with asthma; the most common student health office complaints; the number of screenings, referrals, and follow-up documentation; or disease surveillance conducted to identify care trends (Stanislo, 2023b).

Nurses can collect data that support school success. For instance, the *Every Student Succeeds Act* (ESSA; 2015) requires that states collect at least one nonacademic data point. Many states chose chronic absenteeism as their nonacademic data point. The school nurse can contribute to the district data collection of this data point by using the EHR to create a report that documents the

BOX 5-8

Selecting a School Health Electronic Health Record

Electronic health record (EHR) systems allow data to be entered rapidly, analyzed comprehensively from multiple perspectives, and efficiently reported to key stakeholders.

TYPES OF SCHOOL HEALTH RECORD SOFTWARE

- Commercial school EHR systems: Purchased, prepackaged software that records health data and may or may not interface with the district student information system.
- Student information systems: Purchased, prepackaged software that may include components to record transportation, discipline, instruction, schedules, and standardized test scores, as well as student health data.
- District-specific software: Record-keeping database created within the district.

AREAS TO ANALYZE BEFORE PURCHASING/ CREATING AN ELECTRONIC HEALTH RECORD SYSTEM

Security, confidentiality, and privacy

- Is the data secure? Is it password protected?
- Is the software web-based?
- How much control does the software company have over the data that are stored in the cloud?
- Is the system Health Insurance Portability and Accountability Act (HIPAA) and Family Educational Rights and Privacy Act (FERPA) compliant?
- Does the system meet district privacy standards/ guidelines?
- Authentication
- Overwrite protection
- Audit capability
- Partitioning

Ethical use of school health data

- Who owns the data in the EHR? Does it remain with parents/district?
- With whom will the vendor be sharing de-identified aggregated data?
- Refer to the National Center for Education Statistics and the U.S. Department of Education, Privacy Technical Assistance Center for guidelines.

Nursing workflows in the school health office

System capabilities:

- Direct electronic communication with school staff; parents; local, state or federal agencies or health-care providers (interoperability)
- Consistent with the state standards of nursing practice
- Flexible for varying models of practice
- Password protected with individual log-in and passwords, including substitute and unlicensed assistive personnel
- Ability to run queries/reports
- Customizable to include National Uniform Data Set and other data needed for school/district monthly and year-end reports

Adapted from Johnson (2024); NASN (2024b).

absences of students with chronic conditions such as asthma. Once identified, the nurse can support these students and families to decrease asthma-related absences, thereby raising the visibility of their work and demonstrating how nurses can contribute to academic priorities. As an academic priority, attendance is directly linked to school budgets and student learning time. These data, when shared, can be very powerful in supporting the role and value of the school nurse.

If a school nurse does not have an EHR, it is still important to collect data. Collecting data from paper charts, however, can be laborious and time-consuming. School nurses without an EHR are encouraged to start small, collecting and analyzing just a few data points to ease into this change in practice or to illustrate to educators the unique role of school nurses. The use of tally sheets by day or week can be an efficient way to track visit dispositions, number of phone calls, and number of medications administered, among other data points. Using data to tell the story of students' needs and school nurses' efforts to address those needs is powerful and essential for effective school nursing practice; it can also help build the case for an EHR. Regardless of the method by which the data are collected, the key is knowing what data sets are available, how to access them, what to do with them, and how to share them. Tips for getting started are in Box 5-9.

Large Data Sets

Researchers in both health care and education are drawn to large data sets of accurate and comprehensive data for QI, research, and public health policy decision making (Dash et al., 2019; Data Quality Campaign [DQC], 2020; Maughan & Mangena, 2014). "Data is one of the most powerful tools to inform, engage, and create opportunities for individuals along their journeys" (DQC, 2016, para. 1). School health data are not typically included in national education or health data sets, resulting in a dearth of data available to policy makers on school nursing and the amount of health care that takes place in schools each day. Recently, however, there has been interest in incorporating school health data as a necessary component of analyzing larger educational data (DQC, 2020). Most health data are collected nationally through reimbursement systems and billing codes. National data on youth are often obtained

BOX 5-9
Getting Started With Documentation

DOCUMENTATION

Remember that what you document are DATA!

Identify what data will be most important. Review the *Every Student Counts!* data points and definitions.

Are you already collecting it?

If not, how can you start?

- Can you set up an electronic health record (EHR) to run a report?
- Start small
- Make it doable (tracking forms, EHRs)

USING YOUR DATA

Annual presentation to your principal/school board (consider including health and academic outcomes):

- Number of students taking medications
- Number of students diagnosed with type 1 diabetes, type 2 diabetes, severe allergies, seizures disorder
- Number of students with emergency action plans
- Number of students with individualized health-care plans
- Number of special education/504 case conferences attended
- Number of students returned to class, number of times 911 called, number of students sent home
- Number of completed vision/hearing referrals, number of students who required or received glasses/hearing support
- Change in absenteeism or seat time
- Identify and include what is important to your principal/school board
- Use data to illustrate students' health concerns, treatments, blood sugar checks, etc.

Show the complexity of school nursing and the need to

- Change policy (e.g., obesity rates to remove vending machines; increase healthy foods)
- Change procedures (e.g., equipment change/supervision/recess rules to decrease injuries)
- Increase the number of school nurses and/or stop the reduction of school nurses (e.g., identify trends)
- Improve processes (e.g., medication administration)
- Identify students at risk (e.g., social determinants, vulnerable, frequent flyers)

Write a grant or apply for community partnerships/programs

- Include data to demonstrate the need.

WHEN PRESENTING YOUR DATA

- Use charts, graphs, and infographics (more than numbers)
- Use the data to tell a story (not just report facts)
- Have a purpose in sharing your data
- Connect with your audience

Adapted from Stanislo (2023a, 2024).

from parents in a telephone interview (U.S. Census Bureau, 2022)—an expensive and time-consuming process. Even when health data are collected outside of revenue systems, school health services are often omitted. School nurses collect these data regularly in their documentation and it needs to be used meaningfully to provide a more complete picture of health planning for children.

The National Center for Education Statistics (NCES, 2022) collects voluminous data on the education and instruction system in the United States. Billions of data points are collected, tabulated, and published on the number and characteristics of teachers, the number of students in a class, and the structure and composition of schools and school districts. Educational systems in the United States endorse data-driven decision making and policy development (DQC, 2017). With finite resources, school systems require evidence that investments in school health and school nursing services are warranted. However, within these repositories, data on school support services, including school nursing, are limited and incomplete.

The scarcity of school health data collected by NCES undermines the measurement of the impact of school nursing services on child and academic outcomes. Robust data about the health of students, resources to serve those students, and the school health workforce are necessary to make evidence-based decisions about investments in school health. Using standardized data points identified by NASN will promote school nurse–driven identification of NCES data points.

Large data sets are required for the statistical power needed to measure significant differences in outcomes related to school nurse credentials, school nurse caseload, student acuity, and other variables. Systemized data collection in schools is long overdue to measure the impact of school nursing services on student health and academic outcomes.

When armed with many data points and the technology needed to manage the data, scientists use data to not only measure impact but also to predict and identify persons at highest risk. For example, hospitals use predictive analytics to better identify children with asthma who are at risk for repeated hospital admissions so they can intervene earlier, adjust chronic treatment protocols, or make referrals to specialist care (Ardura-Garcia et al., 2018). A crisis text line for youth has used data to better understand students with eating disorders, self-harming tendencies, and depression (Busby et al., 2020). While there are some risks, the potential of using such data for prediction and more proactive intervention is exciting. With school nurses on the front line of student health, their data have the potential to help identify those students and families at risk and provide a new level of prevention and intervention. This creates an opportunity for school nurses to participate in school-level multitiered system of supports (MTSS). As an example, school nurses involved in the NASN School-Based Active Surveillance (SBAS) project identify students who are chronically absent from school and address the health-related needs contributing to the student absences (NASN, 2020). As part of the school team addressing absenteeism, the school nurse is integral in addressing the "whole child," including the needs of individual students and identifying risk factors to address the needs of the school community. For more information, the *School Nurse–Led Active Surveillance Manual* can be accessed through the NASN Web site.

National Standardized Data Set for School Nursing

To address the lack of national systematic school health data collection, NASN and the National Association of State School Nurse Consultants (NASSNC) launched a joint initiative in 2014 to identify a national standardized data set for school nursing. Although several states have aggregated data at the state level, those states' data could not be merged for greater statistical power and comparisons because the terminologies used to collect data were not uniform/identical (Johnson et al., 2012; Selekman et al., 2015). Leaders in school nursing recognized that, before large data sets could be created for school health, it was essential that all school nurses collect data using uniform terminology. The NASN and NASSNC 3-year initiative, *Step Up & Be Counted!*, identified 15 uniform data points that were collected across the United States (Johnson et al., 2017a). The data points can be found in Box 5-10.

The success of *Step Up & Be Counted!* demonstrated that school nurses are motivated to collect the uniform data needed to advance student health. School nurses armed with data collected during the initiative used infographics and slide presentations to advocate for student health, advancing the use of standardized data at the local, state, and national levels (Johnson et al., 2017a). The *Step Up & Be Counted!* initiative laid the foundation for further work on standardized school nursing data collection. In 2018, NASN announced the new data initiative called *Every Student Counts!*, which continues the development of a robust national school health data set. The goals of *Every Student Counts!* are as follows (NASN, 2022a):

- Increase school nurse capacity building for collecting data
- Continue collecting data using uniform data points
- Collaborate with key partners to create a confidential data infrastructure to gather, store, and analyze data

NASN and partners will continue to advance research and evidence for school nurse practice by further developing a national uniform data set (Stanislo, 2023b).

The value of a national uniform data set depends on school nurses' participation at the local and state levels. Essentially, the data collected at the school and district level must be meaningful to the nurses who have collected it. Using data to tell a story to advocate for staffing levels or student needs is just as important as the school nurse utilizing the data on the school or district level to change

BOX 5-10

National Standardized Data Set: *Every Student Counts!* Data Points

STUDENT DEMOGRAPHICS AND WORKFORCE CAPACITY

- Number of students enrolled in district*
- Number of students who are chronically absent during the identified school year
- Percentage of students receiving free/reduced lunch
- Percentage of students whose primary language is not English
- For health services staff serving your student population, please indicate the number who have each level of education (indicate the highest level of education for each member)
- For school nurses serving your student population, please indicate the number who have each of the following credentials

Which of the following statements best describes your model(s) of practice ... School Health Staffing

- Total number of registered nurse (RN) full-time equivalents (FTEs) with an assigned caseload providing services*
- Total number of licensed practical nurse (LPN) FTEs providing direct services*
- Total number of unlicensed assistive personnel (UAP)/ health aide FTEs providing direct services*
- Total number of supplemental/float RN FTEs*
- Total number of supplemental/float licensed practical nurse/licensed vocational nurse (LPN/LVN) FTEs*
- Total number of supplemental/float UAP/health aide FTEs*
- Total number of RNs with special assignment FTEs*
- Total number of LPNs/LVNs with special assignment FTEs*
- Total number of UAP/health aides with special assignment FTEs*
- Total number of RN FTEs providing administrative/ supervisory school health services*
- Total number of LPN/LVN FTEs providing administrative/supervisory school health services*
- Total number of UAP/health aide FTEs providing administrative/supervisory school health services*
- Total number of UAP/health aide FTEs providing administrative support services to RNs or LPNs/LVNs

CHRONIC CONDITIONS

- Number of students enrolled in assigned schools*
- Number of students with a diagnosis of asthma from a healthcare provider*
- Number of students with a diagnosis of type 1 diabetes from a healthcare provider*
- Number of students with a diagnosis of type 2 diabetes from a healthcare provider*
- Number of students with a diagnosis of life-threatening allergy (anaphylactic reaction) diagnosis from a healthcare provider*
- Number of students with a diagnosis of myalgic encephalomyelitis/chronic fatigue syndrome (ME/CFS) from a healthcare provider

SCHOOL-LEVEL DATA: HEALTH OFFICE VISITS—DISPOSITION

- Number of student encounters/health office visits to RNs resulting in the student returning to class during the school year*
- Number of student encounters/health office visits to RNs resulting in 911 being called during the school year*
- Number of student encounters/health office visits to RNs resulting in student being sent home during the school year*
- Number of student encounters/health office visits to LPNs/LVNs resulting in the student returning to class during the school year*
- Number of student encounters/health office visits to LPNs/LVNs resulting in 911 being called during the school year*
- Number of student encounters/health office visits to LPNs/LVNs resulting in student being sent home during the school year*
- Number of student encounters/health office visits to aides/non-RNs, non-LPNs/LVNs resulting in the student returning to class during the school year*
- Number of student encounters health office visits to aides/non-RNs, non-LPNs/LVNs resulting in 911 being called during the school year*
- Number of student encounters/health office visits to aides/non-RNs, non-LPNs/LVNs resulting in student being sent home during the school year*

*Data points developed through joint NASN and NASSNC collaboration for *Step Up & Be Counted!*

Source: NASN (2022a).

practice. These data points provide evidence of patterns, gaps, and improvements. For example, collecting visit disposition data on the school and district level by provider (RN, LPN/LVN, unlicensed assistive personnel [UAP]) can tell a story of how many students are sent home, sent back to class, or required activation of emergency services (911). In a district trying to cut the health services budget and replace the RN with an LPN/LVN or UAP, providing data related to return-to-class rates can be effective in telling the story. If RNs send 90% of students back to class, LPNs/LVNs send 80% of students back to class, and UAP send 70% of students back to class, it is clear the RN supports student learning access and improves attendance rates. Student learning access and attendance are key data points for academic outcomes. Data on chronic conditions of students provide school, district, and state level school nurses with information necessary for advocating for students' needs. The needs may be related to access to services, education, health promotion, or community resources. Data regarding students' needs can be used to advocate for changes in local or state policies or to support grant proposals for program development or research. The overall value of the national data set is supported by local and state level stories that result from its use. The standardized definitions provide the format, but the data collection, submission, and dissemination provide the value when individual stories are combined to tell bigger stories and promote advocacy for systems-level changes. *Every Student Counts!* data points can be reviewed in Box 5-10 and the standardized definitions can be reviewed at https://www.nasn.org/research/everystudentcounts/uniform-data-points.

IMPLICATIONS FOR SCHOOL NURSING PRACTICE

All school nurses have a responsibility to seek and implement best practices. There are specific strategies in which all school nurses can engage regardless of their educational level, exposure to research, or institutional support. These include the following activities:

- *Question school nursing practice.* Much of what school nurses do is based on tradition, intuition, or authority rather than on knowledge garnered through the scientific method. Continuing education or obtaining graduate nursing degrees help school nurses develop expertise in interpreting research evidence. All school nurses need to question if there is evidence for how they practice and the evidence available to support their practices.
- *Stay current in the literature.* In addition to reading *The Journal of School Nursing* and *NASN School Nurse*, school nurses stay abreast of new knowledge by reading original research and evidence-based clinical articles from nursing and related disciplines, such as public health, pediatric nursing, diabetes, or nutrition. Participating in or leading a journal club with school health professionals spurs professional dialogue and partnerships. In some cases, gaining access to this evidence may be difficult for those not currently seeking formal education or collaborating with a university. Attending nursing and interdisciplinary conferences ensures exposure to current school health knowledge and prompts critical questioning of one's current practice.
- *Conduct QI projects.* After questioning current practice and reviewing the literature, school nurses must be change agents to make needed improvements. EBQI provides the guidance needed to make real and lasting changes in school health and daily practice by incorporating the best evidence. Successfully piloting a small project can build the school nurse's confidence to manage larger QI projects and highlight the school nurse's leadership role in school health.
- *Use standardized data and electronic student health records.* It is imperative that school nurses use standardized data points to aggregate the data related to student health needs, the credentials of the health office personnel, and the care that is provided in schools across districts, cities, states, and the nation. It is essential that school nurses document health office data accurately and in a manner that can be used for data collection and research (Hinkle & Maughan, 2019; Taylor, 2020). School nurses must be involved in the decision-making process related to purchasing software and district-wide EHR systems to ensure that the system meets their needs for appropriate documentation and promotes standardization of processes between schools within a district and members of the nursing team (Johnson et al., 2017b; Lepkowski, 2018).
- *Ensure school health policies and protocols are evidence-based and up-to-date.* School health policies and procedures must be reviewed and updated on a regular, planned cycle. The review schedule is determined by how rapidly knowledge is emerging in each area. For example, immunization protocols must be reviewed at least annually, whereas seizure protocols might be reviewed every 2 years and first aid policies reviewed every 3 to 5 years. School nurses can stay abreast of new information by reading recent position statements, policies, protocols, and clinical practice guidelines released by NASN, state and federal agencies, and other professional groups. School health leaders and organizations need to advocate for government resources to compile the latest evidence from a variety of national and international professional health and medical organizations and federal agencies applicable to school health. Maintaining membership with professional school

Focus on the Framework

Quality Improvement

The Framework can be used by school nurses to guide their research and quality improvement projects. Research opportunities flourish in school nursing from evaluation studies to randomized clinical trials. The framework concepts are reflected in current research, but future efforts can be expanded to test school nursing innovations. The goals of school nursing research and the resulting evidence is to enhance students' health, safety, and readiness for learning (Cowell, 2015).

nursing organizations, such as NASN and state school nurse associations, not only provides school nurses access to best practices but also provides support for advocacy efforts by these organizations to improve school nursing practice. Individual school nurses can also advocate for resources and changes in policy to better support student success at the school and district level.

- *Share the "evidence" on topics of interest.* School personnel and parents benefit from research evidence. The school nurse can transform the school culture into one that values and demands evidence by posting articles on faculty and staff bulletin boards, authoring a column in the school newsletter, and contributing to school meetings and staff inservices. School nurses can employ the readability features (literacy level) of word processing programs to ensure that health messages to families and the school community are accessible through reading level and language.
- *Join or support a research team.* School nurses need to proactively facilitate a culture of inquiry and data in school health through research and EBP activities. School nurses can take the initiative to approach schools of nursing to facilitate research studies. Researchers value the school nurse's access to school populations and local knowledge concerning school operations and clinical expertise. School nurses must help shape research to ensure that key research questions address improving student health and school nursing practice through the generation, utilization, and evaluation of evidence.

CONCLUSION

School nurses must base their practice on the best evidence possible and participate in continuous QI projects to implement and sustain best practices into daily school nursing practice. All school nurses are responsible for collecting data and measuring the outcomes of their practice to demonstrate their effectiveness and accountability through student health and academic outcomes. School nurses should partner with experienced researchers to collaborate on research projects and integrate EBP into their practice. No matter where a school nurse works, 21st-century school nursing practice demands that school nurses document, collect, and utilize data and evidence to meet the needs of students and school populations. Each school nurse can utilize their data to tell their story. Contributing data to state and national data sets allows school nurses the opportunity to shape the bigger story of school nursing practice. Every school nurse has a voice and a unique story to share. School nursing is stronger and more effective the more school nurse voices we include.

The editors and authors gratefully acknowledge the work of the previous chapter authors, Janice Selekman, Judith Vessey, Martha Dewey Bergren, and Erin Maughan.

References

Agency for Healthcare Research and Quality. (n.d.). Plan-do-check-act cycle. Tools & Resources. https://digital.ahrq.gov/health-it-tools-and-resources/evaluation-resources/workflow-assessment-health-it-toolkit/all-workflow-tools/plan-do-check-act-cycle

Agency for Healthcare Research and Quality. (2017). About the National Quality Strategy. *Working for Quality.* https://www.ahrq.gov/workingforquality/about/index.html

Agency for Healthcare Research and Quality. (2022). Six domains of healthcare quality. *Select Measure to Report.* https://www.ahrq.gov/talkingquality/measures/six-domains.html

Agency for Healthcare Research and Quality. (2023). Evidence-based center (EPC) reports. *Research Findings & Reports.* https://www.ahrq.gov/research/findings/evidence-based-reports/index.html

American Academy of Family Physicians. (2023). Basics of quality improvement. Managing Your Practice. https://www.aafp.org/family-physician/practice-and-career/managing-your-practice/quality-improvement-basics.html

American Nurses Association. (2018). Inclusion of recognized terminologies supporting nursing practice within electronic health records and other health information technology solutions. [Position statement]. Author.

American Society of Quality. (2023a). What is lean? *Quality Resources.* https://asq.org/quality-resources/lean

American Society of Quality. (2023b). What is Six Sigma? *Quality Resources.* https://asq.org/quality-resources/six-sigma

Ardura-Garcia, C., Stolbrink, M., Zaidi, S., Cooper, P. J., & Blakey, J. D. (2018). Predictors of repeated acute hospital attendance for asthma in children: A systematic review and meta-analysis. *Pediatric Pulmonology, 53*(9), 1179–1192. https://doi.org/10.1002/ppul.24068

Bergren, M. D. (2016). Feasibility of collecting school nurse data. *The Journal of School Nursing, 32*(5), 337–346. https://www.doi.org/10.1177/1059840516649233

Bergren, M. D., Maughan, E. D., Johnson, K. H., Wolfe, L. C., Watts, H. E. S., & Cole, M. (2017). Creating a culture of accurate and precise data. *NASN School Nurse, 32,* 39–41. https://www.doi.org/10.1177/1942602X16682733

Busby, D. R., King, C. A., Brent, D., Grupp-Phelan, J., Gould, M., Page, K., Casper, T. C., Pediatric Emergency Care Applied Research Network. (2020). Adolescents' engagement with crisis hotline risk-management services: A report from the Emergency Department Screen for Teen Suicide Risk (ED-STARS) study. *Suicide & Life-threatening Behaviors, 50*(1), 72–82. https://doi.org/10.1111%2Fsltb.12558

Butcher, H. K., Bulechek, G. M., Dochterman, J. M., & Wagner, C. M. (Eds.). (2018). *Nursing interventions classification (NIC)* (7th ed.). Elsevier.

Cowell, J. M. (2015). Framework for 21st-century school nursing practice: Implications for research. *The Journal of School Nursing, 31*(5), 316–317. https://doi.org/10.1177/1059840515601424

Dash, S., Shakyawar, S. K., Sharma, M., & Kaushik, S. (2019). Big data in healthcare: Management, analysis, and future prospects. *Journal of Big Data, 6*(54). https://doi.org/10.1186/s40537-019-0217-0

Data Quality Campaign. (2016). *Data can help every student excel.* https://dataqualitycampaign.org/resource/data-can-help-every-student-excel/

Data Quality Campaign. (2017). Education data 101: A briefing book for policymakers. *Resources.* https://dataqualitycampaign.org/resource/eddata101/

Data Quality Campaign. (2020). Data linkages enable individual support and shared success. *Resources.* https://dataqualitycampaign.org/resource/data-linkages-enable-individual-support-and-shared-success/

Davis, W. S., Varni, S. E., & Barry, S. E. (2016). Increasing immunization compliance by reducing provisional admittance. *The Journal of School Nursing, 32*(4), 246–257. https://www.doi.org/10.1177/1059840515622528

Engle, R. L., Mohr, D. C., Holmes, S. K,, Nealon, M., Afable, M., Leyson, J., & Meterko, M. (2021). Evidence-based practice and patient-centered care: Doing both well. *Health Care Management Review, 46*(3), 174–184. https://doi.org/10.1097/HMR.0000000000000254

Every Student Succeeds Act (ESSA) of 2015, Public Law No. 114-95. https://www.ed.gov/essa?src=ft

Feeley, D. (2017). The Triple Aim or the Quadruple Aim? Four points to help set your strategy. *Improvement Blog*. https://www.ihi.org/communities/blogs/the-triple-aim-or-the-quadruple-aim-four-points-to-help-set-your-strategy

Gallagher-Ford, L., & Melnyk, B. M. (2022). Evaluating outcomes of evidence-based practice initiatives versus research: Clarifying the confusion with a call to action. *Worldviews on Evidence-Based Nursing, 19*(4), 258–259. https://doi.org/10.1111/wvn.12604

Goldmann, D. (2023). How do you use a driver diagram? *IHI Open School*. https://www.ihi.org/education/ihiopenschool/resources/Pages/Activities/GoldmannDriver.asp

GoWYLD. (2022). GoWYLD—Research & discovery. *Subject Guides*. Wyoming State Library. https://gowyld.libguides.com/?b=g&d=a

Grys, C. A. (2022). Evidence-based practice, quality improvement, and research: A visual model. *Nursing, 52*(11), 47–49. https://doi.org/10.1097/01.NURSE.0000889812.89287.45

Health Resources and Services Administration. (2011). Performance measurement & quality improvement. *Training & TA Hub*. https://www.hrsa.gov/library/performance-measurement-quality-improvement

HEALWA. (n.d.). HEALWA: The on-call library for Washington state practitioners. *University of Washington Health Sciences Library*. https://heal-wa.org/

Herdman, T. H., Kamitsuru, S., & Lopes, C. T. (2021). *NANDA International nursing diagnoses: Definitions and classification, 2021–2023* (12th ed.). Thieme.

Hinkle, D. L., & Maughan, E. D. (2019). Collecting data: Where do I start? *NASN School Nurse, 35*(1), 18–19. https://doi.org/10.1177/1942602X19890049

Hoskote, A. R., Croce, E., & Johnson, K. F. (2022). The evolution of the role of the U.S. school nurses in adolescent mental health at the individual, community, and systems level, an integrative review. *The Journal of School Nursing, 39*(1). https://doi.org/10.1177/10598405211068120

Institute for Healthcare Improvement. (2023a). How to improve. *Resources*. https://www.ihi.org/resources/Pages/HowtoImprove/default.aspx

Institute for Healthcare Improvement. (2023b). Triple Aim: The best care for the whole population at the lowest cost. *Initiatives*. https://www.ihi.org/Engage/Initiatives/TripleAim/Pages/default.aspx

Institute for Healthcare Improvement. (2023c). Science of improvement. *About Us*. https://www.ihi.org/about/Pages/ScienceofImprovement.aspx

Institute of Medicine. (2001). *Crossing the quality chasm: A new health system for the 21st century*. National Academies Press. https://www.doi.org/10.17226/10027

Institute of Medicine. (2011). *Clinical practice guidelines we can trust*. National Academies Press. https://www.ncbi.nlm.nih.gov/books/NBK209527/

The Johns Hopkins Hospital/The Johns Hopkins University. (2022). EBP model. 2022 JHEBP *Tools*. https://www.ijhn-education.org/node/18409

Johnson, K. H. (2024). School health documentation and implications for data collection. In C. A. Resha & V. L Taliaferro (Eds.), *Legal resource for school health services* (2nd ed., pp. 99–122). Schoolnurse.com

Johnson, K. H., Bergren, M. D., & Westbrook, L. O. (2012). The promise of standardized data collection: School health variables identified by states. *The Journal of School Nursing, 28*(2), 95–107. https://www.doi.org/10.1177/1059840511426434

Johnson, K. H., Maughan, E. D., Bergren, M. D., Wolfe, L. C., Cole, M., & Watts, E. S. (2017a). What's up with *Step Up!? Year 2. NASN School Nurse, 32*(2), 100–105. doi:10.1177/1942602X17691808

Johnson, K. H., Maughan, E. D., Bergren, M. D., Wolfe, L. C., & Gerdes, J. (2017b). Step up & be counted! Strategies for data collection. *NASN School Nurse, 32*(6), 355–360. doi:10.1177/1942602X17733241

Knudsen, S. V., Laursen, H. V. B., Johnsen, S. P., Bartels, P. D., Ehlers, L. H., & Mainz, J. (2019). Can quality improvement improve quality of care? A systematic review of reported effects and methodological rigor in plan-do-study-act projects. *BMC Health Services Research, 19*(683). https://doi.org/10.1186/s12913-019-4482-6

Langley, G. L., Moen, R., Nolan, K. M., Nolan T. W., Norman, C. L., & Provost, L. P. (2009). *The Improvement guide: A practical approach to enhancing organizational performance* (2nd ed.). Jossey-Bass.

Lepkowski, A. M. (2018). Unlocking data collection: Practical tips for school nurses. *NASN School Nurse, 33*, 27–28. doi:10.1177/1942602X17744214

Mackey, A., & Bassendowski, S. (2016). Evidence-based practice in nursing education and practice. *Journal of Professional Nursing, 33*(1), 51–55. http://dx.doi.org/10.1016/j.profnurs.2016.05.009

Martin, K. S. (2005). *The Omaha System: A key to practice, documentation, and information management*. St. Louis: Elsevier Saunders.

Martin, K. S., & Monsen, K. A. (2017). *The Omaha System: Solving the clinical data-information puzzle*. http://www.omahasystem.org/index.html

Maughan, E. D., Johnson, K. H., Bergren, M. D., Wolfe, L. C., Cole, M., Pontius, D. J., Mendonca, L. L., Watts, E., & Patrick, K. (2014). Standardized data set for school health services: Part 1—getting big data. *NASN School Nurse, 29*(4), 182–186. https://doi.org/10.1177/1942602X14538414

Maughan, E. D., & Mangena, A. S. (2014). The 2013 NASN school nurse survey. *NASN School Nurse, 29*(2), 76–82. https://www.doi.org/10.1177/1942602X14523135

Maughan, E. D., & Yonkaitis, C. F. (2017). What does evidence-based school nursing practice even mean? Get a CLUE. *NASN School Nurse, 32*(5), 287–289. https://doi.org/10.1177/1942602X17724420

Maughan, E. D., & Yonkaitis, C. F. (2018). What does the evidence say is best for your student? CLUE #3: Appraise. *NASN School Nurse, 33*(2). doi:10.1177/1942602X17753601

Melnyk, B. M., & Fineout-Overholt, E. (2023). *Evidence-based practice in nursing & healthcare* (4th ed.). Wolters Kluwer.

Merkle, S. L., Welton, M., van Zyl, A., Chong, M., Tanner A., Rose, C. E., Hertz, M., Hill, L., Leroy, Z. C., Sifre, K., & Tomas, E. S. (2022). Symptoms of depression, anxiety, and post-traumatic stress disorder, and suicidal ideation among school nurses in prekindergarten through grade 12 schools—United States, March 2022. *The Journal of School Nursing, 39*(2), 114–124. https://doi.org/10.1177/10598405221131048

Minnesota Department of Health. (n.d.). Objectives and goals: Writing meaningful goals and SMART objectives. *Public Health and QI Toolbox*. https://www.health.state.mn.us/communities/practice/resources/phqitoolbox/objectives.html

Moorhead, S., & Dochterman, J. M. (2012). Languages and development of the linkages. In M. Johnson, S. Moorhead, G. Bulechek, H. Butcher, M. Maas, & E. Swanson (Eds.). *NOC and NIC linkages to NANDA-I and clinical conditions: Supporting critical reasoning and quality care*. Elsevier.

Moorhead, S., Swanson, E., Johnson, M., & Maas, M., (Eds.). (2018). *Nursing outcomes classification (NOC): Measurement of health outcomes* (6th ed.). Elsevier.

National Associaton of County and City Health Officials. (n.d.) QI Roadmap https://virtualcommunities.naccho.org/communities/community-home/librarydocuments?LibraryKey=2afb346e-3b2b-4fc9-b7d7-0a7fefc1466f

National Association of School Nurses. (2020). *The school nurse–led active surveillance manual: Guidance and resources to support school nurses' important role in addressing chronic absenteeism*. Author. https://learn.nasn.org/courses/24594

National Association of School Nurses. (2022a). National School Health Data Set: Every Student Counts! *Research.* https://www.nasn.org/nasn/research/everystudentcounts

National Association of School Nurses. (2022b). *School nursing: Scope and standards of practice* (4th ed.). Author.

National Association of School Nurses. (2024a). A contemporary Framework update for today's school nursing landscape: Introducing the School Nursing Practice Framework. *NASN School Nurse, 39*(3), 140–147.

National Association of School Nurses. (2024b). *Electronic health records: An essential school nursing tool for supporting student health.* (Position Statement.) Author.

National Association of School Nurses. (2024c). The National Association of School Nurses research and evidence-based practice priorities. Research Priorities. https://www.nasn.org/research/research-priorities

National Center for Education Statistics. (2022). Digest of education statistics, 2020. *Programs.* https://nces.ed.gov/programs/digest/current_tables.asp

National Institutes of Health. (2021). The impact of COVID-19 on the research community. *Policy & Compliance.* https://grants.nih.gov/policy/natural-disasters/corona-virus/impact-research-community.htm

Nolt, D., Moore, S. Yan, A. C., Melnick, L., Committee in Infectious Disease; Practice and Ambulatory Medicine; Section on Dermatology. (2022). Clinical reports: Head lice. *Pediatrics, 150*(4), e2022059282. https://doi.org/10.1542/peds.2022-059282

Nundy, S., Cooper, L. A., & Mate, K. S. (2022). The Quintuple Aim for health care improvement: A new imperative to advance health equity [editorial]. *JAMA, 327*(6), 521-522. https://doi.org/10.1001/jama.2021.25181

Posanka, B. (2022). Adverse event leads to quality improvement plan: Learning from a classroom latex exposure. *NASN School Nurse, 37*(3), 132–135. https://doi.org/10.1177/1942602X221077234

Rhudy, L. M. (2021). Released before peer review: Why do we care? *Journal of Neuroscience Nursing, 53*(2), 56. https://doi.org/10.1097/JNN.0000000000000583

Rutherford, M. (2008). Standardized nursing language: What does it mean for nursing practice? *OJIN: The Online Journal of Issues in Nursing. 13*(1). https://doi.org/10.3912/OJIN.Vol13No01PPT05

Selekman, J., Wolfe, L. C., & Cole, M. (2015). What data do states collect related to school nurses, school health, and the health care provided? *The Journal of School Nursing, 32*(3), 209–220. doi:10.1177405984051 5606786

Shannon, R. A. (2018). School nursing evidence-based practice guidelines: What they are and are not, and why they matter. *NASN School Nurse, 33*(2), 104–105. https://doi.org/10.1177/1942602X17753602

Shannon, R. A., & Maughan, E. D. (2020). A model for developing evidence-based clinical practice guidelines for school nursing. *The Journal of School Nursing, 36*(6), 415–422. https://doi.org/10.1177/1059840519880938

Stanislo, K. J. (2023a). Data collection: Time to revisit the WHY, WHAT, and HOW. *NASN School Nurse, 38*(6), 310–315. https://doi.org/10.1177/1942602X231199932

Stanislo, K. (2023b). Revisiting the National School Health Data Set: *Every Student Counts! NASN School Nurse, 38*(1), 26–30. https://doi.org/10.1177/1942602X221137519

Stanislo, K. J. (2024). Data sharing: HOW to tell your story. *NASN School Nurse, 39*(1), 21–29. https://doi.org/10.1177/1942602X231214247

Tanner, A. L., & Stanislo, K. (2022). School nursing research and research implementation priorities. *The Journal of School Nursing, 38*(6), 500–501. https://doi.org/10.1177/10598405221123231

Tastan, S., Linch, G. C. F., Keenan, G. M., Stifter, J., McKinney, D., Fahey, L., . . . Wilkie, D. J. (2014). Evidence for the existing American Nurses Association-recognized standardized nursing terminologies: A systematic review. *International Journal of Nursing Studies, 51*, 1160–1170. doi:10.1016/j.ijnurstu.2013.12.004

Taylor, E. (2020). Playgrounds, injuries, and data: Keeping children safe. *NASN School Nurse, 35*(5), 266–268. https://doi.org/10.1177/1942602X20944396

U.S. Census Bureau. (2022). National Survey of Children's Health (NSCH). *Our Surveys & Programs.* https://www.census.gov/programs-surveys/nsch.html

U.S. Preventive Services Task Force. (2023). Recommendation topics. *Home.* https://www.uspreventiveservicestaskforce.org/uspstf/recommendation-topics

Yonkaitis, C. F. (2017). Evidence-based practice and school nurse practice: A review of the literature. *The Journal of School Nursing, 34*(1), 60–67. doi:10.1177/1059840517728108

Yonkaitis, C. F., & Maughan, E. D. (2018). Finding the best evidence to support students with chronic conditions: CLUE #2. *NASN School Nurse, 33*(1), 23–26. doi:10.1177/1942602X17743985

Young, M., & Smith, M. A. (2022). Standards and evaluation of healthcare quality, safety, and person centered care. StatPearls Publishing LLC. https://www.ncbi.nlm.nih.gov/books/NBK430685/

part II

Legal Foundations for School Nursing

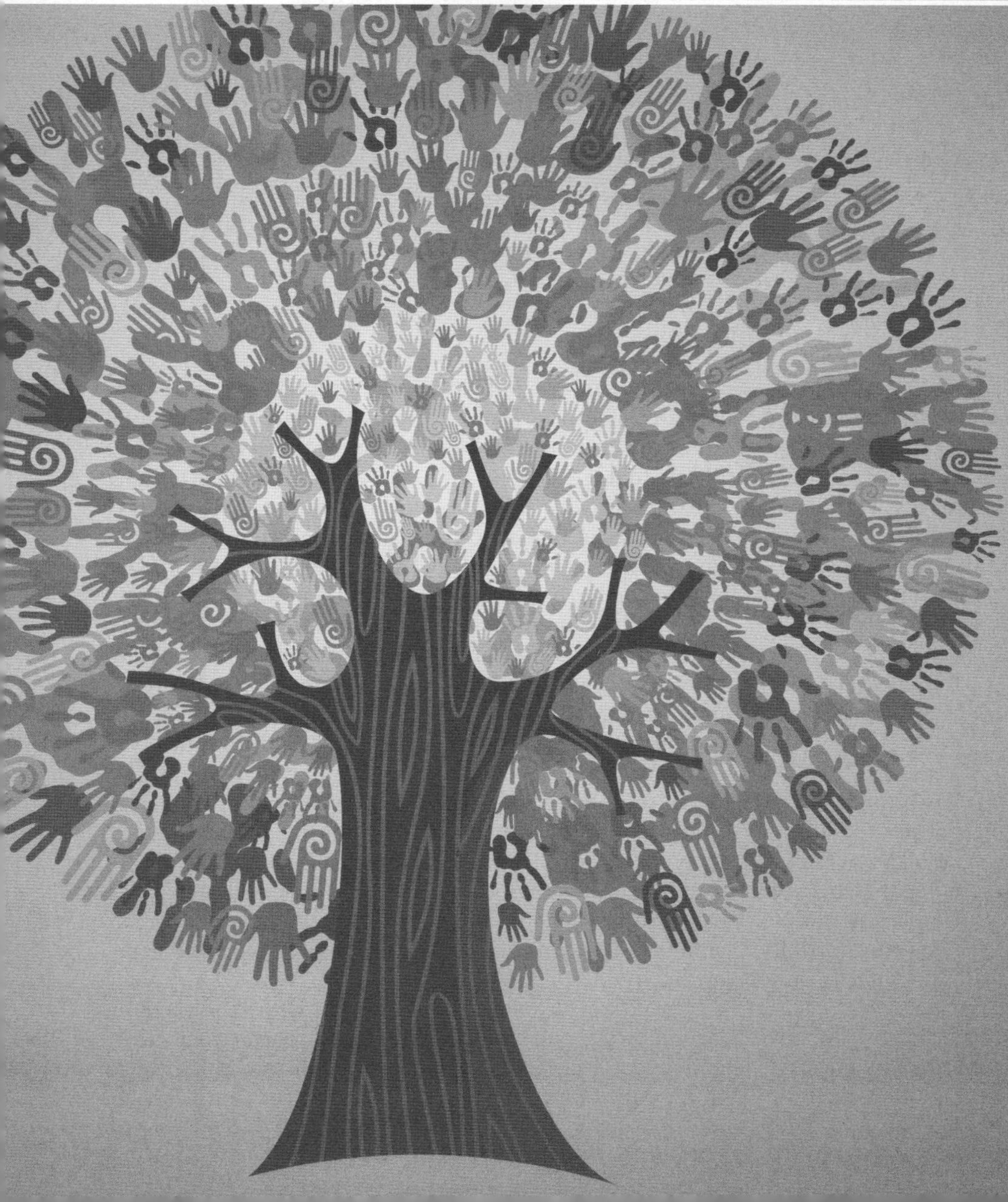

Chapter 6

The Law and School Nursing Practice

Edith Brous

CHAPTER OUTLINE

School nurse practice is subject to laws and regulations. Understanding the sources of law and how the legal system functions can assist the school nurse in practicing lawfully and avoiding legal problems. This chapter is intended to provide an overview of legal and regulatory issues related to school nurse practice. For specific legal advice, school nurses must seek the counsel of an attorney licensed to practice in their state.

OVERVIEW OF THE LEGAL SYSTEM

"This Constitution, and the Laws of the United States which shall be made in Pursuance thereof; ... shall be the supreme Law of the Land" (U.S. Constitution, Article VI). The founding document for the legal structure in the United States is the U.S. Constitution, and it sits at the top of the hierarchy. It is the U.S. Constitution that created a federal government consisting of checks and balances among the three branches: the legislative, executive, and judicial systems. The U.S. Constitution divides power between the federal government and the governments of the individual states. The U.S. Constitution also protects the individual rights and liberties of its citizens. The U.S. Constitution is the supreme law, and all other elements of law-making authority are subordinate to it.

After the U.S. Constitution on the hierarchy are the legislatures at the federal and state levels that enact laws known as statutes. A legislature can only enact laws within the authority granted it by the U.S. Constitution, and any laws it enacts must adhere to the U.S. Constitution. When there is conflict between a federal law and a state law, the federal law prevails unless the state law is more stringent.

Continuing down the hierarchy are the regulatory agencies that promulgate rules, regulations, and procedures to enforce the statutes. Administrative agencies, such as nursing boards, are created by the legislature to enforce laws such as nurse practice acts. In addition to statutes that are enacted by the legislature, laws can also be made by the courts. Known as case law, or common law, court decisions are also a source of legal authority.

The courts also have a hierarchy. At both the state and federal levels, entry level courts (trial courts) hear cases and render decisions. Trial court decisions can be appealed to appeals courts, and appellate court decisions can be appealed to higher courts. The United States Supreme Court (U.S.S.C.) is the court of last resort for all contested state and federal decisions.

Within states, local education agencies (i.e., school boards) develop and pass school board policies that guide the implementation of the rules and regulations of the state concerning education, public health, and safety. School board policies are binding and enforceable. School protocols, practices, and procedures must be compliant with the rule of law at every level: federal, state, and local. Most laws related to education and health are relegated to the states. See Figure 6-1.

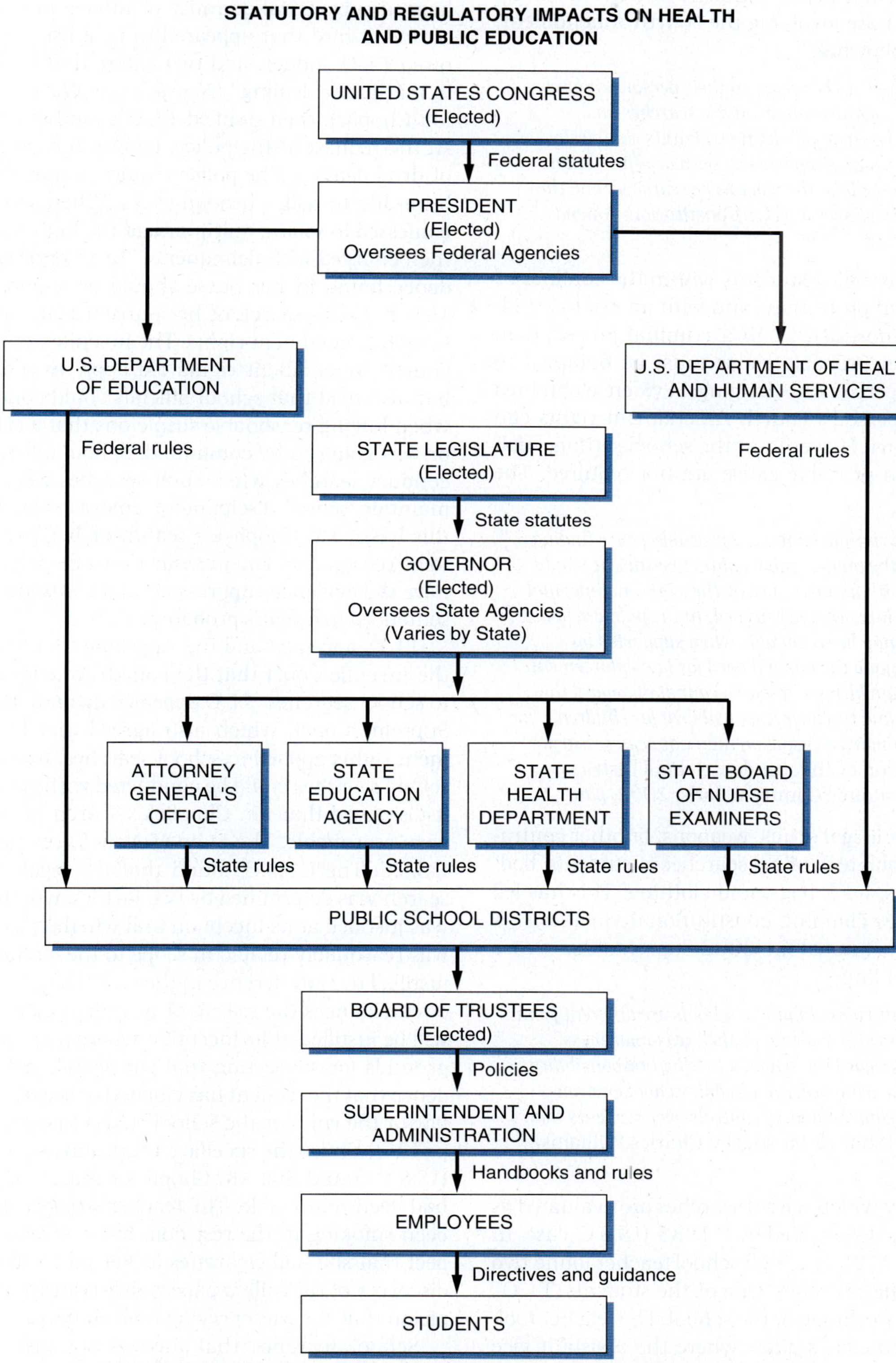

FIGURE 6-1. Statutory and regulatory effects on health and public education.

CONSTITUTIONAL LAWS AFFECTING SCHOOLS

The Fourth Amendment: Search and Seizure

Multiple constitutional issues can arise in the school setting, particularly those involving the Fourth Amendment, which states the following:

> *The right of the people to be secure in their persons, houses, papers, and effects, against unreasonable searches and seizures, shall not be violated, and no warrants shall issue, but upon probable cause, supported by oath or affirmation, and particularly describing the place to be searched, and the persons or things to be seized. (U.S. Constitution, Amendment IV)*

Schools must discipline students within the confines of these constitutional protections and with an eye to avoiding disparities (Amos, 2021). In a criminal prosecution, warrants based on probable cause must be obtained to search a person's person or belongings. Evidence obtained in violation of a person's Fourth Amendment rights can be excluded in court. However, in the school setting, such warrants based on probable cause are not required. The U.S.S.C. noted:

> *In contrast to the criminal context, a probable-cause finding is unnecessary in the public school context because it would unduly interfere with maintenance of the swift and informal disciplinary procedures that are needed. In the public school context, a search may be reasonable when supported by "special needs" beyond the normal need for law enforcement. Because the "reasonableness" inquiry cannot disregard the schools' custodial and tutelary responsibility for children, . . . a finding of individualized suspicion may not be necessary.* (Board of Education of Independent School District No. 92 of Pottawatomie County v. Earls, *2002, para. 2*)

Concerns about illegal drugs, weapons, or other contraband have led schools to conduct searches of students' bodies, lockers, purses, book bags, and clothing. This has led to court challenges claiming constitutional violations. A 2017 Missouri court noted the 2002 Supreme Court case in the following finding:

> *Fourth Amendment rights in public schools are different from those rights possessed elsewhere, as the "reasonableness" inquiry cannot disregard the school's tutelary responsibility for children . . . Securing order in a public-school environment sometimes requires greater controls over students than those over adults.* (State of Missouri v. Charles Williams, *2017, p. 6*)

The standard by which school searches are evaluated as constitutional was determined by a 1985 U.S.S.C. case. In *New Jersey v. T.L.O.* (1985), a high school teacher found two girls smoking in the restroom. One of the students, T.L.O., was a 14-year-old freshman at the school. The teacher took the girls to the principal's office where the assistant vice principal, Theodore Choplick, asked T.L.O. to come into his private office. He demanded to see T.L.O.'s purse. When he found a pack of cigarettes, he accused her of lying when she had claimed she did not smoke. He also found a package of rolling papers in her purse, which he associated with marijuana use.

Further search of T.L.O.'s purse revealed "a small amount of marijuana, a pipe, a number of empty plastic bags, a substantial quantity of money in one-dollar bills, an index card that appeared to be a list of students who owed T.L.O. money, and two letters that implicated T.L.O. in marijuana dealing" (*New Jersey v. T.L.O.*, 1985, p. 328). Mr. Choplick then notified T.L.O.'s mother and the police. At the request of the police, he also turned over evidence of drug dealing. The police requested that T.L.O.'s mother bring her to police headquarters. When she did so, T.L.O. confessed to selling marijuana at the high school. She was then charged with delinquency. T.L.O. argued that the evidence found in her purse should be suppressed because Mr. Choplick's search of her purse was in violation of her Fourth Amendment rights. The Juvenile Court agreed that Fourth Amendment rights did apply to school searches, but also held that school officials could conduct searches when having reasonable suspicions that a crime had been or was going to be committed. School officials could also conduct searches when such searches were necessary to maintain school discipline or enforce school policies. On this basis, Mr. Choplick's search of her purse was found to be reasonable. The Juvenile Court denied her request to have the evidence suppressed. T.L.O. was found guilty and sentenced to a year's probation.

T.L.O. appealed and the Appellate Division agreed with the Juvenile Court that the Fourth Amendment did apply to school searches. T.L.O appealed again to the New Jersey Supreme Court, which also agreed that Fourth Amendment rights applied to school searches. It also agreed that school searches could be conducted without warrants, but it disagreed that Mr. Choplick's search of her purse had been reasonable. The State of New Jersey appealed to the U.S.S.C. The U.S.S.C. found that the legality of a school search was determined by two factors: whether the search was justified at its inception and whether, as conducted, it was reasonably related in scope to the circumstances that justified the interference in the first place. "Under ordinary circumstances the search of a student by a school official will be justified at its inception where there are reasonable grounds for suspecting that the search will turn up evidence that the student has violated or is violating either the law or the rules of the school" (*New Jersey v. T.L.O.*, 1985, p. 325). Under the specific circumstances of this case, the U.S.S.C. found that Mr. Choplick's search of T.L.O.'s purse had been reasonable. The teacher's report that T.L.O. had been smoking in the restroom made it reasonable to suspect that she had cigarettes in her purse. The subsequent discovery of the rolling papers gave rise to a reasonable suspicion that she was carrying marijuana.

School searches that involve not just property, but more intrusive searches of a student's body, require greater scrutiny. In *Safford Unified School District #1 v. Redding* (2009), the U.S.S.C. evaluated the standards set out by *New Jersey v. T.L.O.* within that context. Savana Redding was a 13-year-old student who was called out of class to meet with the assistant principal, Kerry Wilson. Mr. Wilson showed her an unzipped day planner in which there were knives, lighters, and a cigarette. Savana agreed that the planner was hers but denied that any of the items belonged to her, claiming that she had lent the planner to a friend. Mr. Wilson then showed her several nonsteroidal anti-inflammatory drugs (NSAIDs) that she also denied were hers. Mr. Wilson told Savana that he had received reports of her giving these pills to other students. She denied this and allowed him to search her belongings. Administrative Assistant Helen Romero and Mr. Wilson then searched her backpack but found nothing. Upon Mr. Wilson's instructions, Ms. Romero took Savana to the school nurse's office to search her clothes. The nurse, Peggy Schwallier, asked Savana to remove her jacket, socks, and shoes. The nurse then asked her to pull her bra out from under her T-shirt and shake it, then to pull the elastic on her underwear. This exposed Savana's breasts and pelvic area, but the nurse found no pills.

Savana's mother filed a lawsuit against the school, Mr. Wilson, Helen Romero, and Peggy Schwallier, complaining that Savana's Fourth Amendment rights had been violated during the strip search. The defendants attempted to have the case dismissed on the grounds of immunity. The court did dismiss the case on the finding that there had been no Fourth Amendment violation. This was upheld on appeal to the Ninth Circuit Court. The Ninth Circuit appeal had been decided by a panel of judges. When the Ninth Circuit subsequently heard the case *en banc* (before all the judges on the bench), the decision was reversed. The strip search was held to be unjustified under the test set out by *New Jersey v. T.L.O.*, but Helen Romero and Peggy Schwallier were held to be immune because they had not been independent decision makers. The case was then appealed to the U.S.S.C.

The U.S.S.C. found that Mr. Wilson's suspicion was adequate justification for the search of Savana's backpack and outer clothing. With regard to the strip search, however, the Court noted that adolescence intensifies the intrusive nature of such searches, and this requires a higher level of reasonableness to be justified. Noting the *T.L.O.* standard, searches of students' bodies were permissible when "not excessively intrusive in light of the age and sex of the student and the nature of the infraction" (*Safford*, 2009, p. 2642).

To be constitutionally permissible, student searches must be justified at the start by reasonable grounds of suspicion, and the search must be permissible in its scope. In Savana's case, NSAIDs were not dangerous contraband; there was no reason to suspect that she was hiding them in her underwear and there was no indication of danger to other students. The intrusiveness of the strip search was not reasonably related to the circumstances. Although the U.S.S.C. found that qualified immunity applied to all the defendants, it also determined that the search did constitute a constitutional violation. Because Mr. Wilson's suspicions did not justify this level of intrusion, Savana's Fourth Amendment rights had been violated.

School searches and "zero tolerance policies" can be problematic in that they contribute to the criminalization of school policy infractions. Punitive and exclusionary disciplinary practices increase levels of contact with the criminal justice system (Hemez et al., 2020). The school-to-prison pipeline, as it is called, is particularly problematic for students of color and students with disabilities.

Fourth Amendment issues should also be considered in the search of a student's personal device contents. Students generally have an expectation of privacy on their cell phones, laptops, tablets, and other devices. An exception might exist when school staff have a reasonable expectation that content on the device contains information related to safety such as self-harm or harm to others. In *G.C. v. Owensboro Public Schools* (2013), the U.S.S.C. held that

> *[T]he legality of a search of a student should depend simply on the reasonableness, under all the circumstances, of the search. Determining the reasonableness of any search involves a twofold inquiry: first, one must consider whether the action was justified at its inception; second, one must determine whether the search as actually conducted was reasonably related in scope to the circumstances which justified the interference in the first place.*

A teacher confiscated G.C.'s cell phone when he was violating school policy by texting in class. The phone was taken to an assistant principal, who read his text messages. The year previously, G.C. had expressed suicidal ideation and had been treated for mental health issues. At that time his phone has also been checked out of concern for his well-being. This time G.C. brought a suit, claiming that the school violated his constitutional rights by reading his text messages, not because they had a reasonable suspicion of self-harm, but because he violated the school's cell phone policy. The school was successful at obtaining summary judgment at the District Court level, but G.C. appealed to the U.S.S.C., which did not find the search to be reasonable. The U.S.S.C. did not find that general background knowledge of drug abuse or depression was enough to permit the search. Finding that the school did not have reasonable suspicion to justify the search, it reversed the District Court and reinstated the case.

Search of student cars is another area of concern. Searches of students' cars are permitted when acting on reasonable grounds if the car is parked on the school campus. The search must be justified at its inception, meaning there is reason to believe the student is involved in dangerous or illegal activity as per the *T.L.O.* standards.

FEDERAL STATUTES

Civil rights laws are intended to provide equal opportunity to all citizens by removing discriminatory barriers. Federal and state funding is tied to compliance with statutory mandates. Schools engaging in discrimination can lose such funding and subject themselves to lawsuits claiming violations of civil rights. Many federal laws affect school nurse practice. When the U.S. Constitution or federal laws conflict with state constitutions or statutes, the federal law generally prevails. An exception to this is when the state laws are more stringent. A state law can provide stronger protections than the federal law in areas such as constitutional or privacy rights.

Equal Opportunity

The Individuals With Disabilities Education Act

The *Individuals With Disabilities Education Improvement Act* (IDEA) was reauthorized by Congress in 2004 (see Chapter 7). The act allocates funds to assist the states in educating children with specific disabilities. For a state to receive the funds, schools must provide all students with disabilities who qualify under the law with a free and appropriate education (FAPE). FAPE requires that access is provided and is "sufficient to confer some educational benefit upon the handicapped child" (*Board of Education of the Hendrick Hudson Central School District Bd. of Ed., Westchester County, v. Rowley*, 1982, p. 200). Like other federal laws, IDEA sets the minimum standards or the "floor" for compliance. States can exceed those requirements.

States must provide instruction and support systems sufficient to permit the child to benefit educationally. An individualized education program (IEP) must be developed containing goals, benchmarks, annual academic and functional goals, current performance, long-term and short-term objectives, and objective criteria for measuring the student's advance [20 U.S.C. 1400, §614(d)(1)(A)]. IDEA's requirements are met if the state is compliant with the act's procedures and if the IEP is reasonably calculated to enable the child to receive educational benefits. IDEA does provide for a private cause of action, allowing parties to bring civil actions in state or federal court. An example of such a case is *Board of Education of the Hendrick Hudson Central School District Bd. of Ed., Westchester County, v. Rowley* (1982).

Amy Rowley was a deaf student at Furnace Woods School. Her IEP provided for her to be educated in a regular classroom ("mainstreamed"); that she would use a hearing aid; that she would receive 1 hour each day of instruction from a tutor for the deaf; and that she would receive 3 hours a week of instruction from a speech therapist. Her parents insisted that she also be provided with a sign-language interpreter in all her classes. The school determined that she did not need the interpreter and denied this request. The Rowleys then received a hearing before an independent examiner, who agreed with the school. When the examiner's decision was affirmed on appeal, the Rowleys filed a lawsuit in federal court. The court found that denial of a sign-language interpreter constituted a denial of the FAPE required by IDEA. The decision was upheld on appeal. The U.S.S.C. then agreed to hear the case.

The U.S.S.C. reasoned that IDEA did not require states receiving funds to do more than provide "some form of specialized education" (*Board of Education of the Hendrick Hudson Central School District Bd. of Ed., Westchester County, v. Rowley*, 1982, p. 196). The court held that the requirements of FAPE did not mandate the opportunity to achieve full potential commensurate with the opportunity provided to other children. Amy's IEP met the requirement for FAPE without a sign-language interpreter. Other laws that relate to students with chronic conditions that require school accommodations are in Chapter 7.

Every Student Succeeds Act (ESSA)

President Obama signed ESSA into law in December of 2015 as a later version of the No Child Left Behind (NCLB) Act. NCLB created requirements that were difficult for schools to meet. ESSA was an attempt to address those issues while continuing the goal of "upholding critical protections for America's disadvantaged and high-need students" (U.S. Department of Education, 2017). ESSA requires all students to be taught to an academic standard that prepares them for college and careers. ESSA also makes amendments in both IDEA and the McKinney-Vento Act. Like NCLB before it, ESSA still requires standardized tests and school reports on the progress of high-risk students. However, ESSA is less punitive than NCLB, as the emphasis shifted from consequences to accountability. Schools also can design their own plans for addressing failure. The Trump administration repealed many of ESSA's regulations related to accountability and determining compliance such that states are now able to establish their own goals and milestones, but schools are still measured by specific criteria. Congress has provided a detailed explanation of ESSA as amended (Congressional Research Service, 2022).

McKinney-Vento Act

The National Alliance to End Homelessness (NAEH) reports that people in families with children make up 28% of the homeless population. Unaccompanied youth under age 25 account for 6% of the larger group (NAEH, 2022). Homelessness nationwide increased by 6% since 2017. Students who change schools frequently lose academic progress and score lower on tests. Because school stability is difficult for homeless children and youth to achieve, Congress addressed the issue with federal legislation.

The **McKinney-Vento Homeless Assistance Act** was passed in 1987 and reauthorized by ESSA in 2015. The intent

> **Did You Know?**
>
> Undocumented children have a right to attend public schools. Refusal to enroll undocumented children constitutes discrimination and violates the Equal Protection Clause of the Fourteenth Amendment. This right was affirmed by the Supreme Court in *Plyler v. Doe* (1982).

of the act is to ensure that "each child of a homeless individual and each homeless youth has equal access to the same free, appropriate public education, including a public preschool education, as provided to other children and youths" (McKinney-Vento, Sec. 721, Statement of Policy). States must review policies and create procedures related to homeless/unsheltered students through a statewide homeless coordinator, and schools are required to immediately enroll students even if they do not have normally required documents (Institute for Children, Poverty & Homelessness, 2023). The Office of Civil Rights (OCR) enforces the act. School districts receiving federal funds cannot discriminate against homeless children by segregating or stigmatizing them. In addition to educational services, homeless/unsheltered students are entitled to participate in extracurricular activities and to receive medical and dental services. McKinney-Vento funds can also be used for school supplies, glasses, hearing aids, counseling, tutoring, food, clothing, and shoes.

Every local education agency (school district) must appoint a local homeless education liaison to identify and support unsheltered children and youth as outlined in the act.

McKinney-Vento Definition of Homelessness. A homeless child or youth is defined as "someone without a fixed, regular and adequate nighttime residence" (McKinney-Vento Homeless Assistance Act, 1987). This can include the following:

- Sharing housing such as in a motel, hotel, campground, shelter, abandoned in a hospital, or residing in a home they do not rent or own
- Using a public or private place not designed for regular sleeping accommodations
- Living in cars, parks, abandoned buildings, bus or train stations, or similar settings
- Migratory children who live in circumstances as described above

Privacy

Students have privacy rights regarding their educational and medical records. Those rights are protected by federal as well as state statutes. The most relevant federal laws are the Family Educational Rights and Privacy Act of 1974 (FERPA) and the Health Insurance Portability and Accountability Act of 1996 (HIPAA). FERPA applies to all schools that receive federal funding under the U.S. Department of Education. It does not apply to those private schools that do not receive any degree of federal funding. HIPAA does not generally apply to elementary or secondary schools because the schools are not *covered entities* as defined by the statute, or because the records the schools keep are defined as *education records* and thus are covered under FERPA instead of HIPAA.

Family Educational Rights and Privacy Act

FERPA protects the privacy of *educational records* by withholding federal funds from schools that are not compliant with the act's mandates. Educational records are defined as "records, files, documents, and other materials which contain information directly related to a student; and are maintained by an educational agency or institution or by a person acting for such agency or institution" [§1232g(a)(4)(A)]. This does not include *unshared* or *sole possession* medical records that are used only for treatment. Records that are in the sole possession of the person making them and are not accessible or revealed to others are not considered *education records*, subject to FERPA [§1232g(a)(4)(B)]. Treatment records that are only disclosed to other treating providers are also not covered by FERPA. Those treatment records are covered under HIPAA.

FERPA does cover *shared* medical records. School health records maintained by the school nurse and records of students with special needs under IDEA are *education records*. These records are directly related to the student and maintained by the school, subjecting them to FERPA. Immunization records, for example, are *education records* (U.S. Department of Health and Human Services & U.S. Department of Education, 2019). FERPA does *not* cover records maintained by law enforcement units of the school, employment records, peer grading, or evaluations or letters of recommendation written by teachers but not maintained by the school. FERPA also does not cover directory information—information such as name, address, telephone number, attendance dates, field of study, or sports activities. Schools must provide an annual notice of parental rights under FERPA (Box 6-1).

FERPA provides rights to parents that then transfer to the students themselves when they reach the age of 18 or attend a postsecondary school at any age. At this point, the students are referred to as "eligible students." The rights by FERPA include the following:

- The right to inspect and review the student's education records within 45 days after the day the school receives a request for access
- The right to challenge the content of the student's education records to ensure that the records are not inaccurate, misleading, or otherwise in violation of the student's privacy rights
- The right to provide written consent before the school discloses personally identifiable information (PII) from the student's education records unless disclosure is permitted under one of the act's exceptions [§ 1232g(a)]

Subject to specific provisions in the statute, FERPA permits schools to release information about a student's educational records without written permission to the following entities:

- Other school officials with a *legitimate educational interest*
- Officials of other schools where the student is seeking enrollment, or is already enrolled for the purposes of enrollment or transfer

BOX 6-1

Educational Agency or Institution Annual Notification to Parents of Their Rights Under FERPA

Educational agencies or institutions must make annual notifications to parents, legal guardians, and eligible students of their legal rights under FERPA. These notices must inform parents or eligible students that they have the following rights:

1. Inspect and review the student's education records
2. Seek amendment of the student's education records that the parent or eligible student believes to be inaccurate, misleading, or otherwise in violation of the student's privacy rights
3. Consent to disclosure of personally identifiable information contained in the student's education records, except to the extent authorized without consent
4. File with the department a complaint concerning alleged failures by the educational agency or institution to comply with the requirements of FERPA

The notice must include all of the following:

1. The procedure for exercising the right to inspect and review education records
2. The procedure for requesting amendment of records
3. A specification of criteria for determining who constitutes a school official and what constitutes a legitimate educational interest

The notice can be provided by any means that are reasonably likely to inform the parents or eligible students of their rights.

An educational agency or institution shall effectively notify parents or eligible students who are disabled.

An agency or institution of elementary or secondary education shall effectively notify parents who have a primary or home language other than English.

Source: Family Educational Rights and Privacy Act Regulations (20 U.S.C. 1232g; 34 CFR Part 99).

- Authorized representatives of the federal, state, or local government
- Financial aid officials
- Research bodies
- Accrediting bodies
- Parents of eligible students who are dependents for IRS tax purposes
- Child welfare agencies [20 U.S.C. § 1232g(b)]

FERPA also permits disclosure without consent to comply with a lawfully issued subpoena or judicial order or when necessary under a public health and safety exception (U.S. Department of Education, 2023). If disclosure of a student's PII is necessary to protect the health or safety of other students, schools can disclose such information without consent. The health and safety exception is limited to the period of the emergency and restricted to the information required. FERPA compliance is overseen by the U.S. Department of Education's Family Policy Compliance Office (FPCO).

Nonacademic records such as video surveillance footage can also be protected by FERPA, as illustrated in *Bryner v. Canyons School District* (2015). Roger Bryner's middle school child was involved in an altercation with other students. Bryner requested a copy of the school's surveillance camera footage that had recorded the incident. The school district refused, stating that the video was governed by FERPA as an educational record. The school also explained that the video contained personally identifiable information about other students so they could not release it without the written consent of the other parents. Bryner argued with the school that the video was not governed by FERPA because it was not an education record and asked the school to reconsider. When the school continued to refuse to release the video to him, Bryner filed a lawsuit against the school district.

Bryner asked the court to rule that the video was not covered by FERPA as it was not an educational record. He asked the court to find that the video must be disclosed in accordance with his request under Utah's Government Records Access and Management Act (GRAMA). The court reviewed the video in chambers and determined that other students could clearly be identified. Because other students could be identified, Bryner's GRAMA request was subject to FERPA. It found that the school district had been correct in denying his request to release the video. The court ordered the school district to assess the feasibility of redacting student images from the video and the costs of doing so. The school determined that it would cost about $120 to redact the images of the other students. The trial court then ordered Bryner to pay the school that amount within 10 days to receive a redacted copy of the video.

When Bryner did not pay the school within that time, the school asked the court to dismiss his case. The court did so and Bryner appealed. The appeal addressed the issue of whether the video was an educational record subject to FERPA. Bryner argued that the recording was nonacademic, not the kind of record FERPA was intended to protect, and not maintained by the school. It was therefore not an education record subject to FERPA. The school argued that because the video contained information directly related to other students and because it was maintained by the school for disciplinary reasons, it was part of the student's education record. Bryner also argued that the trial court had been wrong to order him to pay the school the cost of redacting the video to receive a copy of it. In considering the interaction between Utah state law and the federal law, the appeals court noted that GRAMA classifies as nonpublic those records "to which access is restricted pursuant to court rule, another state statute, federal statute, or federal regulation, *including records for which access is governed or restricted as a condition of participation in a state or federal program or for receiving state or federal funds* [emphasis added]" (*Bryner v. Canyons School District*, 2015, p. 856).

The court noted that the definition of education records under FERPA was broad and that nothing in the statute limited the application of FERPA to academic records. The court also noted that the district court had relied on guidance from Family Policy Compliance Office and it was FPCO's position that parents were only allowed to view school videotapes if no other students were pictured. Such videotapes were education records for the students involved in the altercation but not for students who had not been involved in the altercation. As such, FERPA did apply to the students involved in the altercation. The court noted that when "an education record contains material or information on more than one student, 'the parents of one of such students shall have the right to inspect and review *only such part of such material or document as relates to such student*'" (*Bryner*, 2015, p. 859). The court held that Bryner had the right to inspect and review the portion of the video that related to his child, but not to the portions of the video in which other students were pictured. Personally identifying information about other students had to be redacted or the school needed the written permission of the other students' parents. The court also held that it was reasonable for the school to charge Bryner for the costs of redaction.

Health Insurance Portability and Accountability Act

HIPAA protects individually identifiable personal *health* information known as protected health information (PHI). The two rules of the act are the Security Rule and the Privacy Rule. Both rules apply to health plans, health-care clearinghouses, and health-care providers, referred to as *covered entities*, who transmit health information in an electronic form. As discussed earlier, generally, HIPAA does not apply to elementary or secondary schools because the schools do not meet the definition of covered entities. HIPAA does apply to school-based health centers located within schools. Their records are kept separate from school records governed by FERPA.

The Security Rule establishes standards for protecting certain health information that is held or transferred in an electronic form. It does not apply to PHI that is transmitted orally or in writing. The Privacy Rule establishes national standards to protect medical records and other PHI. HIPAA specifically excludes *education* records in its definition of PHI. Student health records maintained by educational institutions generally meet the definition of education records under FERPA and are thus exempted from HIPAA coverage. School nurses who engage in HIPAA's covered transactions such as electronic billing for services, however, can be subject to HIPAA. HIPAA permits health-care providers to disclose PHI without consent to other providers for treatment purposes. *Pediatricians, for example, are permitted under HIPAA to disclose PHI to school nurses.*

Like FERPA, HIPAA gives patients the right to review and request corrections in their records. Neither HIPAA nor FERPA provide private rights of action, meaning students cannot sue schools for violation of the acts. The recourse that is available to a student whose HIPAA rights have been violated is to file a complaint with the U.S. Department of Justice. Students whose FERPA rights have been violated can file a complaint with the U.S. Department of Education. Privacy rights might be more stringent at the state level, allowing for lawsuits and monetary damages with violation of the state laws. Determining when FERPA applies and when HIPAA applies can be confusing, and school nurses are advised to seek the advice of the school's legal counsel or compliance officer when specific questions arise regarding disclosure.

Generally, HIPAA does not apply unless the provider is conducting transactions electronically and the records are not otherwise protected by FERPA (U.S. Department of Health and Human Services [USDHHS], 2021a). In all cases, school nurses should be cautious in using social media so that they do not violate student privacy rights and expose themselves to licensure discipline. As the National Council of State Boards of Nursing (NCSBN) notes:

> *"Instances of inappropriate use of social and electronic media may be reported to the Board of Nursing. Laws outlining the basis for disciplinary action by a Board of Nursing vary between jurisdictions. Depending on the laws of a jurisdiction, a Board of Nursing may investigate reports of inappropriate disclosures on social media sites by a nurse on the grounds of:*
>
> - *Unprofessional conduct;*
> - *Unethical conduct;*
> - *Moral turpitude (defined as conduct that is considered contrary to community standards of justice, honesty or good morals);*
> - *Mismanagement of patient records;*
> - *Revealing a privileged communication; and*
> - *Breach of confidentiality."* (NCSBN, 2018a, p. 9)

Child Protection Laws

Beginning in the late 19th century, states and local jurisdictions initiated mechanisms to assist and protect children. Over the past decades, Congress passed significant legislation supporting the states' duty and power to act on behalf of children when parents are unable or unwilling to do so. The *Child Abuse Prevention and Treatment Act* (CAPTA) is the key piece of legislation that protects children. CAPTA was signed into law in 1974 (P.L. 93-247) and was reauthorized several times with amendments expanding and refining the scope of the law. CAPTA was reauthorized in December 2010 (P.L. 111-320) and amended twice: once in May 2015 by the Justice for Victims of Trafficking Act of 2015 (P.L. 114-22) and July 2016 by the Comprehensive Addiction and Recovery Act of 2016 (P.L. 114-198; Child Welfare Information Gateway, 2019).

CAPTA provides federal funding to states in support of prevention, assessment, investigation, prosecution, and treatment activities and also provides grants to public agencies and nonprofit organizations for demonstration programs and projects. In addition, CAPTA identifies the federal role in supporting research, evaluation, technical assistance, and data collection activities. It establishes the Office on Child Abuse and Neglect and mandates the Child Welfare Information Gateway, a Web-based service of the Children's Bureau of the USDHHS Administration for Children and Families that provides access to information and resources to help protect children and strengthen families. CAPTA also sets forth a minimum definition of child abuse and neglect as:

- [A] recent act or failure to act on the part of a parent or caretaker that results in death, serious physical or emotional harm, sexual abuse or exploitation
- An act or failure to act that presents an imminent risk for serious harm (P.L. 111-320)

This definition of child abuse and neglect refers specifically to parents and other caregivers. A "child" under this definition generally means a person who is younger than 18 or who is not an emancipated minor. Although CAPTA defines sexual abuse and the special cases related to withholding or failing to provide medically indicated treatment, it does not provide specific definitions for other types of maltreatment such as physical abuse, neglect, or emotional abuse.

While federal legislation sets minimum standards, each state is responsible for providing its own definition of maltreatment within civil and criminal contexts. Definitions of child abuse and neglect are typically located in two places within each state's statutory code:

- Mandatory child maltreatment reporting statutes (civil laws) provide definitions of child maltreatment to guide individuals who are mandated to identify and report suspected child abuse. The statutes also describe grounds for intervention by state child protection agencies and courts.
- Criminal statutes define those forms of child maltreatment that are criminally punishable (Child Welfare Information Gateway, n.d.).

In addition, areas of state education law, health laws, and corresponding administrative rule may include language to define and direct educators and licensed healthcare providers as mandatory reporters of abuse.

Practice Connection

Official Response to Questions to HIPAA Relevant to School Nursing from U.S. Department of Health & Human Services

1. *Does the HIPAA Privacy Rule allow a healthcare provider to disclose PHI about a student to a school nurse or physician?*

Answer: Yes. The HIPAA Privacy Rule allows covered healthcare providers to disclose PHI about students to school nurses, physicians, or other healthcare providers for treatment purposes, without the authorization of the student or student's parent. For example, a student's primary care physician may discuss the student's medication and other healthcare needs with a school nurse who will administer the student's medication and provide care to the student while the student is at school. In addition, a covered healthcare provider may disclose proof of a student's immunizations directly to a school nurse or other person designated by the school to receive immunization records if the school is required by state or other law to have such proof prior to admitting the student, and a parent, guardian, or other person acting *in loco parentis* has agreed to the disclosure [§164.512(b)(1)(vi)] (USDHHS, 2021b).

2. *Does HIPAA prevent a school administrator, or a school doctor or nurse, from sharing concerns about a student's mental health with the student's parents or law enforcement authorities?*

Answer: In the limited circumstances where the HIPAA Privacy Rule, and not FERPA, may apply to health information in the school setting, the rule allows disclosures to parents of a minor patient or to law enforcement in various situations. For example, parents generally are presumed to be the personal representatives of their unemancipated minor child for HIPAA privacy purposes, such that covered entities may disclose the minor's PHI to a parent [§164.502 (g)(3)]. In addition, disclosures to prevent or lessen serious and imminent threats to the health or safety of the patient or others are permitted for notification to those who are able to lessen the threat, including law enforcement, parents, or others, as relevant [§164.512(j)] (USDHHS, 2022).

3. *When a parent requests that a healthcare provider disclose proof of their child's immunizations to a school so the school can legally admit the child, does the Privacy Rule limit to whom at the school the provider may send the records?*

Answer: No. It is expected that in most cases a school has designated an administrative official or employee, such as a school nurse, to receive and maintain proof of student immunizations to comply with applicable law. Given the designated person may vary from school to school, the Privacy Rule permits the healthcare provider to make the disclosure to whoever at the school is identified in the parent's request or school's instructions to the parent (USDHHS, 2021c).

The CAPTA amendments require states to have specific provisions written into state law. Some of these include the following:

- Immunity from prosecution under state and local laws and regulations for individuals making good faith reports of suspected or known instances of child abuse or neglect [§106 (b)(2)(A)(iv)]
- Procedures or mechanisms to ensure that the state does not require reunification of a surviving child with a parent who has committed certain felonies and that conviction of any one of those felonies constitute grounds under state law for the termination of parental rights of the convicted parent as to the surviving children [§106 (b)(2)(xiii)]
- Authority under state law to permit the child protective services system of the state to pursue any legal remedies, including the authority to initiate legal proceedings in a court of competent jurisdiction, to provide medical care or treatment for a child when such care or treatment is necessary to prevent or remedy serious harm to the child, or to prevent the withholding of medically indicated treatments from disabled infants with life-threatening conditions (§113)

If a state has a law in effect that conflicts with the provisions in any assurance or if the state's statutory definitions of "child abuse and neglect" and "sexual abuse" do not meet the minimum standards in Sections 111 (2) and 111 (4) of CAPTA, it must modify its statute to correspond with the CAPTA requirements.

School Nurses as Mandated Reporters

School nurses are professionals who, in the ordinary course of their work and because they have regular contact with children, are required to report to the appropriate state agency cases of child abuse (physical, sexual, or psychosocial abuse) that are observed or suspected, or when there is evidence of neglect, knowledge of an incident, or an imminent risk for serious harm. *The school nurse MUST report suspected abuse; they CANNOT delegate the reporting to others,* nor can a nurse be ordered by administrators not to report the suspected abuse. Variations exist across states in regard to who else is a mandated reporter, as well as differences in definitions of maltreatment, and standards and procedures for reporting. It is *not* the job of school personnel to investigate cases of suspected abuse.

Each state's statutes can be found on the Child Welfare Information Gateway, a service of the USDHHS Children's Bureau, Administration for Children and Families. The Web site offers an easy way to search the online database for state-specific laws on more than 30 topics regarding child abuse and neglect, child welfare, and adoption. School nurses must familiarize themselves with the laws and rules within their state, as well as the policies and procedures of their school district.

STATE LAWS AND NURSING REGULATION

The constitutional and privacy issues discussed under federal law are mirrored at the state level. State law can exceed the protections offered by federal law but cannot be less stringent. Other regulatory issues are determined solely by the individual states. Nursing law and professional malpractice law, for example, are primarily regulated at the state level.

Nursing Regulation

Nursing boards are created by the state legislatures to *protect the public.* Nurses who violate the standards of practice or the board of nursing (BON) rules and regulations can be disciplined and separated from practice to prevent such harm. School nurses should review their state's nursing regulations frequently. As the NCSBN notes:

> *Every nurse in the U.S. is responsible for knowing the state's NPA [Nurse Practice Act] and regulatory requirements for nursing for every jurisdiction in which they hold a license. Since laws, rules and regulations may change over time, it is also necessary to periodically review the NPA that can be found on each BON's website or at ncsbn.org/npa.htm. (NCSBN, 2018b)*

Nurses frequently have misconceptions about the nursing board's role, thinking it is in place to be an advocate for the nursing profession or to advocate for an individual nurse. It is important to understand that the BON is not in place to benefit nurses. The BON regulates nursing practice to prevent the harm to patients that could be caused by incompetent, unethical, or impaired nurses. The mission statement of the nursing board can generally be found on the BON's Web site.

Nurses also need to know the rules in any state in which they have been issued a license, whether that license is current or lapsed. Many states maintain jurisdiction over licensees, also maintaining the authority to discipline a professional license even when that license is not current. Many states grant licenses for the *lifetime* of the licensee. To continue using that license, it must be reregistered, but allowing a license to lapse does not prevent the holder from being disciplined. Most states also impose discipline on a nursing license when the nurse holds a license in another jurisdiction where the nurse has been disciplined. This is referred to as *reciprocal enforcement.*

It is not only professional misconduct in one state to have been disciplined in another state, it also might be professional misconduct to fail to report such out-of-state discipline within a deadline. It is important to know the self-reporting requirements for any state in which a nurse has been licensed. Nursing boards have the authority to discipline nurses for many things that are not directly related to clinical practice, as discussed later in this chapter. Patients do not have to be harmed for BONs to take disciplinary action. Departures from acceptable practice standards can constitute professional misconduct in the absence of injuries to patients.

The rights one has in criminal prosecutions or in civil lawsuits might not apply to administrative proceedings. Unlike a criminal prosecution, a BON prosecutor does not have to advise the nurse of their rights and is not held to the "beyond a reasonable doubt" standard for conviction. Unlike a civil lawsuit, the nurse in a BON action might not be entitled to "reciprocal discovery" in which the nurse is able to inspect the complaint and all documents related to the investigation.

Disciplinary Process

Nursing boards investigate complaints in different ways, depending on the state. Some states assign investigators to the case who may or may not be nurses. Those investigators can interview the nurse, ask the nurse to complete questionnaires related to the complaint (often referred to as *interrogatories*), make site visits, interview other parties, review documents, and make recommendations. BON prosecutors who also might or might not be nurses can then formally charge the nurse with violations of the NPA. It is important that nurses be represented by counsel at each stage of the investigation and prosecution. BON proceedings are adversarial and license discipline is consequential to one's ability to continue practicing.

Focus on the Framework
Standards of Practice

Nurse Practice Acts

Most states have a statute called the Nurse Practice Act (NPA) that specifies the conduct to which nurses must adhere in the state. Nurses must read and understand the NPA and rules and regulations in any state in which they are practicing to ensure their compliance. Most nursing boards post the statutes, rules, regulations, practice alerts, advisory opinions, or frequently asked questions on their Web sites. Many also participate in social media, posting on platforms such as Facebook or Twitter. The NCSBN provides a link to find your state practice act (NCSBN, 2023). NPAs address the composition and authority of the BON, requirements for licensure, scope of practice, nursing responsibilities, disciplinary procedures, definitions of professional misconduct, professional assistance programs for impaired providers, and educational standards.

Each school nurse's practice is guided by their state's NPA as discussed previously and highlighted in the School Nursing Practice Framework principle of Standards of Practice (National Association of School Nurses, 2024). Along with the NPA, this principle covers several types of regulations and practice and performance standards to ensure school nurses provide the best possible care and outcomes for students.

When the BON determines that a nurse has violated the law, it can then impose discipline. The nurse has a due process right to have notice of the charges, the proposed penalty, and an opportunity to be heard. This can take the form of written submissions, settlement conferences, or formal hearings. Although the investigation is generally confidential, final orders of discipline are usually considered public information and posted on the BON's Web site. BONs can impose a private or public letter of concern, reprimand, censure, or admonition. This might or might not be considered formal discipline, which is public information. BONs can also impose civil penalties, require continuing education or public service, and place nurses on probation. For more serious infractions, BONs can impose practice restrictions or separate a nurse entirely from practice with a period of suspension.

For those infractions that are thought to pose the greatest potential for risk to patients, BONs can revoke a license or request that the nurse voluntarily surrender that license and cease practicing. BONs can also refer nurses to professional assistance programs as an alternative to discipline. Nurses in such programs must be completely compliant with the program requirements to avoid discipline.

Disciplinary Issues

Scope of Practice

Unless a school nurse is a nurse practitioner licensed to diagnose and prescribe, school nurses must stay within their state's scope of practice for registered nurses (RNs). Generally, it is not within the RN scope of practice to administer medications without a physician's order. Some states permit RNs to *recommend* over-the-counter (OTC) medications but not to *administer* them without an order. Maryland (Maryland Board of Nursing, n.d.), for example, allows nurses to recommend OTC medications but holds the nurse accountable to have the knowledge of the product and its interaction with other medications. This includes the duty to educate the student regarding the medication's "use, effects, side effects, contraindications, potential drug interactions of the over-the-counter products, indicators to discontinue using the product and indicators prompting the client to notify [their] primary physician" (para. 3). The nurse recommending OTC medications also maintains the duty to monitor the patient, document care, and communicate with other providers.

Like traditional medications, the nurse's use of complementary, integrative, and alternative therapies such as homeopathic remedies is determined by licensure laws. Some state boards have published statements or position papers that can provide guidance. Minnesota, for example, states the following: "Nurses who employ integrative therapies in their nursing practice to meet nursing care needs and patient goals are held to the same accountability for reasonable skill and safety as they are with the implementation of conventional treatment modalities" (Minnesota Board of Nursing, 2017, p.1). Practice protocols and standing orders can provide protection for the school nurse and should be incorporated into the student's individualized health-care plan (IHP), as well as specific orders prescribed for individual students.

Abandonment

Nurses can subject themselves to nursing board discipline for charges of abandonment under certain conditions. The NPA in each state can define abandonment differently, but generally for a nurse to be charged with abandonment, certain elements must be met:

1. There must be a nurse-patient relationship.
2. The nurse unilaterally severs that relationship while the patient still requires nursing care.
3. The nurse severs the relationship without making provisions for a qualified provider to continue the care.

North Dakota, for example, defines abandonment as

> *accepting the client assignment and disengaging the nurse and client relationship without giving notice to a qualified person. Behavior that demonstrates professional misconduct includes abandoning a client who is in need of or receiving nursing care and may be grounds for disciplinary action. (North Dakota Board of Nursing, 2019, para. 1)*

The New York BON provides specific guidance regarding abandonment charges:

> *Key considerations for determining whether or not a nurse has "abandoned" a patient include: Whether the nurse accepted the patient assignment, which established a nurse-patient relationship; Whether the nurse provided reasonable notice when severing the nurse-patient relationship; Whether reasonable arrangements have been made for the continuation of nursing care by others when proper notification is given. (New York State Education Department, 2023, para. 2)*

Moral Character and Social Media

To maintain one's license in good standing, nurses must be compliant with the moral character requirements as defined by their licensing boards. Criminal convictions, financial improprieties, boundary violations, discipline in other states, falsification of medical or business records, failure to honestly answer application questions, or the misuse of social media can lead to charges of moral character deficiencies. The NCSBN and many individual state boards specifically address the misuse of social media. Texas, for example, notes that "[s]ocial media postings may reflect negatively on individual nurses, the nursing profession, the public's trust of the nursing profession, or the employer and may jeopardize careers" (Texas Board of Nursing, 2022, para. 9).

Similarly, Kentucky reminds nurses that "there are consequences to the inappropriate use of social media. ... The Kentucky Board of Nursing may investigate a nurse after a report of inappropriate use of social media" (Kentucky Board of Nursing, 2017, p. 4).

Misunderstandings about free speech and First Amendment rights can lead school nurses to believe there are no consequences for what they post, but posts that suggest moral character lapses, unlawful conduct, or unethical conduct can lead to BON disciplinary charges.

Professional Boundaries

The nurse-patient relationship is solely for the benefit of the patient. School nurses have intimate and long-lasting relationship with their students, which can lead to a clouding of professional boundaries. Personal relationships with students can be considered inappropriate and unethical. Professional role boundaries must always be maintained. The NCSBN specifically addresses boundaries and the continuum of professional nursing behavior:

- The nurse's responsibility is to delineate and maintain boundaries.
- The nurse should work within the therapeutic relationship.
- The nurse should examine any boundary crossing, be aware of its potential implications, and avoid repeated crossings.
- Variables such as the care setting, community influences, patient needs, and the nature of therapy affect the delineation of boundaries.
- Actions that overstep established boundaries to meet the needs of the nurse are boundary violations.
- Nurses should avoid situations where they have a personal, professional, or business relationship with the patient.
- Post-termination relationships are complex because the patient may need additional services. It may be difficult to determine when the nurse-patient relationship is completely terminated.
- Be careful about personal relationships with patients who might continue to need nursing services (such as those with mental health issues or oncology patients; NCSBN, 2018c).

Licensure Discipline

Discipline on a professional license can cause additional legal issues for nurses. Final orders of discipline are public information and posted on the Internet in many states. Some states also provide the actual legal documents for the public to review. Disciplinary action results in inclusion in the National Practitioner Data Bank (NPDB)—an information clearinghouse containing reports taken against health-care practitioners (NPDB, 2018). As discussed earlier, discipline in one state causes disciplinary action in other states in which the nurse has been licensed through the process of reciprocal enforcement.

Disciplinary action in a state can also result in the loss of a multistate privilege for members of the enhanced nursing licensure compact. Licensure discipline can also cause exclusions from participation in programs such as Medicaid and Medicare, which can make the nurse unemployable. School nurses being investigated by their nursing boards must be represented by attorneys with experience and skill in licensing board issues so potential collateral issues can be explained and prevented when possible.

Licensure Protection

Although most school nurses will never have a legal problem, it is important to take steps to protect one's license as it is the means of making a livelihood. Maintaining clinical competency, exercising caution in the use of social media, belonging to professional organizations, sustaining professional boundaries, adhering to privacy mandates, and accurately documenting nursing care are essential steps. Additionally, *school nurses should maintain their own professional liability insurance policies to provide coverage for licensure defense and out-of-work situations that employer policies do not cover.*

School nurses should also maintain a portfolio. Performance appraisals, thank you letters, continuing education certificates of completion, letters of reference or recommendation, awards or other evidence of professional achievements, volunteer or public interest work, publications and public speaking efforts, and an updated resume or curriculum vitae can all be helpful in a disciplinary defense.

Criminal Charges

A high-profile case of a hospital nurse who was criminally charged for an unintentional fatal medication error made many nurses wonder if this was setting a precedent and if they had to be concerned about being prosecuted for clinical errors. In 2017, registered nurse RaDonda Vaught mistakenly administered vecuronium instead of the ordered Versed to 75-year-old Charlene Murphy. Murphy, who was in the hospital for a subdural hematoma, died shortly after. Although it is unknown if her death was caused by her underlying brain injury or the administration of the vecuronium, Davidson County District Attorney Glenn Funk's office indicted her on charges of reckless homicide and criminal neglect. The case proceeded to trial and a jury found her guilty of neglect of an impaired adult, but not of negligent homicide. After the verdict, the American Nurses Association (ANA) wrote a letter to Judge Jennifer Smith pleading for mercy in the sentencing (ANA, 2022). The letter was entered into evidence and, although Vaught faced 3 to 6 years in prison for neglect, Judge Smith sentenced her to 3 years of probation.

The Vanderbilt Medical Center where this occurred reported the death but attributed it to natural causes and did not report the medication error. The following year, the Centers for Medicaid and Medicare Services (CMS) received an anonymous letter describing the event and multiple system problems that allowed the error to occur (Anonymous Complainant, 2018). CMS conducted an unannounced survey, then issued an immediate jeopardy warning and removing Joint Commission accreditation (Department of Health & Human Services [HHS] & CMS, 2018a). This was accompanied by a 108-page corrective action plan, indicating the organizational responsibility for the error (HHS & CMS, 2018b). In 2019, Vaught was arrested.

The case did not set a precedent, as Vaught was not the first health-care professional to be criminally charged for unintentional clinical error. The Vaught prosecution received the attention it did because social media has made communication easier than was possible in the earlier cases. The important lesson from this case is that adverse events such as fatal medication errors are rarely, if ever, caused by carelessness on the part of a single person. Multiple system and organizational deficiencies contribute to a nurse's ability to make such an error. A full root cause analysis that looks at those contribution factors and takes action to remove them will keep patients much safer than criminally prosecuting a nurse who made a mistake. In fact, fear that mistakes will lead to criminal charges actually harms patients, in that it deters the error reporting that is essential to correcting system deficiencies.

CLINICAL PRACTICE

All nurses must maintain competency and modify their practice to conform to current evidence-based standards of practice. School nurses who work in isolation and report to nonclinical people can find themselves engaging in outdated practices or basing their practice on outdated theories. Belonging to professional organizations, subscribing to professional journals, and attending professional conferences can assist school nurses in staying current, but it is also important to stay connected to general nursing standards and not become sequestered into only focusing continuing education on school nursing issues. It is not a defense in a lawsuit or a nursing board investigation to claim lack of knowledge that practice standards changed since one was taught how to do something. As a professionally licensed nurse, the school nurse will still be held to the current standards of clinical practice for all nurses.

Standards of practice for medication administration, telephone orders, the use of technology, and electronic health records, for example, continue to evolve, and school nurses must participate in continuing education to remain current. In addition to issues specific to school nursing, issues related to cultural competency, recognition of child abuse, scope of practice, proper use of social media, documentation standards, ethical codes, privacy laws, NPA changes, and the nursing licensure compact are examples of critical information school nurses must continue to have.

School nurses can stay current with changing standards by belonging to professional organizations and availing themselves of such association's resources. The National Association of School Nurses (NASN), for example, revised its Scope and Standards of Practice in 2022 and has provided useful position statements, many of which are provided as resources at the end of this chapter. Like the NPA, such documents are dynamic and school nurses must stay current with such standards and policies to maintain competency and compliance with professional standards.

Documentation of Care

From a legal perspective in a health-care setting, if it was not documented, then there is no proof that it was done. The objectives of documentation in school nursing practice are as follows (Johnson, 2024, p. 101):

- Provide a legal record of care
- Provide history of care and the student's needs
- Support communication with other members of the school team
- Support continuity of care
- Allow for evaluation of care

The best documentation of nursing care complies with the *School Nursing: Scope and Standards of Practice* (NASN, 2022) and its position statement on electronic record-keeping (NASN, 2019a) regarding individualized ongoing records of nursing care provided for each student. The confidential records can be kept in paper or electronic formats. The student health records should contain an ongoing record of student demographics, health history, medical diagnoses, medications, allergies, immunizations, health screening results (as mandated in each state), and the nurse's notes reflecting nursing assessments, interventions, and outcomes. Records should also be kept of all nurse visits, with the time and date, the student's reason for the visit, the tests and assessments conducted, the nurse's determination and actions taken, the outcomes/disposition, and the nurse's name (Box 6-2).

In addition, children with IEPs or 504 plans, as well as other students may have IHPs that address medications, interventions, and treatments necessary for the student to attend school. Students whose health-care needs affect or have the potential to affect safe and optimal school attendance and academic performance should have IHPs written and reviewed annually by a school nurse (NASN, 2020). For more information about IHPs, see Chapter 8.

When documenting, terms suggestive of error or speculative conclusions should be avoided, such as "accidentally," "intentionally," or "negligently." Errors in hand-written records should be lined through, initialed, and written correctly. If an entry is made in a wrong file, it should be lined through, and an entry should be made that states "entry recorded in error." Avoid back-dated entries. Note physician telephone consultations and orders, as well as directives to other service providers and school staff, if applicable. Note in the access log any individuals given access to a student's records.

Some school districts determine their own requirements for nurse documentation, often relying on NASN standards when doing so. School nurses must always check with the employing school or district before establishing their own documentation system.

BOX 6-2

Principles of School Nursing Documentation

NASN's basic principles of documentation have been incorporated into state and local board policies. They state that nursing documentation should be accurate, objective, concise, thorough, timely, and well organized.

1. All entries should be legible and written in ink or on a computer. Usually the ink should be black or blue (so that they will copy well, if needed).
2. Computerized records must be secure and password protected.
3. The date and exact time should be included with each entry.
4. Documentation should include any nursing action taken in response to a student's problem.
5. Assessment data should include significant findings, both positive and negative.
6. All records, progress notes, IHPs, and flow charts should be kept current.
7. Documentation should include only essential information; precise measurements, correct spelling, and standard abbreviations should be used.
8. School nursing documentation should be based on nursing classification and include uniform data sets.
9. The frequency of documentation should be consistent over time and based on district policy, nursing protocols, and the acuity of the student's health status.
10. Standardized healthcare plans increase efficiency of documentation and are acceptable to use so long as they are adapted to the individual needs of each student.
11. Student symptoms, concerns, and health maintenance questions (subjective data) should be documented in the student's own words.
12. Only facts (objective data) relevant to the student's care and clinical nursing judgments based on such facts should be recorded; personal judgments and opinions of the nurse should be omitted. For example, "the student is breathing normally" is an opinion, whereas the notation "respirations 20/min; no retractions, rales, or wheezing" provides objective data (Scott & Bubert, 2013, p. 213).

Did You Know?

It is unadvisable for a school nurse to use a personal cell phone to exchange information about a student's health. FERPA only allows the exchange if a FERPA-compliant consent is signed by the parent or guardian. However, even with consent, concerns related to personal information breaches such as unencrypted text messages sent to a wrong number or wireless carriers storing text messages that are then involved in a data breach put the school nurse at risk (Lowrey, 2019).

Electronic Health Records

Electronic health records (EHRs) are intended to replace hand-written records for many reasons. EHRs make it easier to capture charges for reimbursement of services, reduce errors related to misinterpretation of handwritten entries, improve patient safety, facilitate data collection, improve provider-to-provider communication, and are intended to be more efficient for providers. When protected health information becomes available in digital format, however, there are additional concerns for privacy of the records. In addition to FERPA and HIPAA, the federal government requires that the collection or maintenance of such information be compliant with the Children's Online Privacy Protection Act of 1998 (COPPA) and imposes certain requirements on those who collect personal information from a child under age 13 (Federal Trade Commission [FTC], n.d.). Schools contracting with third-party operators to provide services such as online education, after-school Internet programs, and so on must draft their terms of service to be clear that COPPA compliance is the third-party operator's responsibility, not the school's (FTC, 2020).

Additional special considerations for EHRs include the following:

- When possible, school nurses should be involved in the selection and customization of the EHR system to be used.
- EHRs must be set up for compliance with FERPA, HIPAA, and COPPA.
- Complete training on the use of the system must include methods for timing entries, documenting corrections, amendments, late and delayed entries, and multiple users.
- Electronic records time stamp every entry; late or addendum entries must be identified as such.
- Electronic records capture all access to the system and should be reviewed for unauthorized access.
- Hard copy or electronic backup is necessary to avoid loss of data.
- Avoid copy and paste or "cloned entries"—the better practice is to note "no changes from above" or refer to (previous entry).
- Passwords are the least effective privacy and security measures—implement end-to-end encryption and dual authentication measures to prevent unauthorized access.
- Passwords should never be shared.
- Provisions must be made for temporary or substitute personnel to have limited and temporary access to the system.
- School nurses should not use personal devices to receive or transmit protected health information.
- EHRs should have stratified access limiting personnel to access information according to their authorization status.
- Avoid workarounds and overrides.
- Exercise caution with templates and drop-down menus—items inadvertently checked can cause pre-charting or billing fraud.

Delegation

According to the National Council of State Boards of Nursing (NBCSN) and the American Nurses Association (2019), "Delegation is an essential nursing skill" (p. 1). *Delegation* is defined by NASN (2022) as follows:

> *The assignment of the performance of a nursing activity to unlicensed assistive personnel (UAP) or from a registered nurse to a licensed practical/vocational nurse (LPN). The school nurse, after assessment of the UPAs/LPN's capabilities, makes a prudent decision regarding the advisability of delegation. Accountability remains with the registered nurse; state laws and regulations and school regulations must be followed; and standards of school nursing practice must be upheld. The registered nurse may decide against delegation for safety, regulatory, and legal issues; school staffing or student health issues; or UAP/LPN competence or ability. (p. 100)*

Under the right conditions, when permitted by state regulations, and when students have predictable and/or stable health conditions that require routine care, delegation may be an appropriate tool to ensure a student's right to a *free and appropriate public education* (FAPE) as guaranteed under the Rehabilitation Act of 1973 and IDEA (2004). See Chapter 7.

Improper delegation and supervision are issues that can lead to licensure discipline for all nurses. It is critical that school nurses understand the law in their states. Nurse practice acts vary from state to state regarding whether delegation is permitted. When allowed under the RN scope of practice, school nurses must further understand under what conditions delegation is permissible and if there are specific scope of practice stipulations related to delegation in the community setting of schools.

Some states permit the delegation of medications to unlicensed personnel in the school setting. Other states specifically prohibit such delegation; for instance, in Pennsylvania all medications except for emergency medications must be given by a licensed nurse (Pennsylvania Department of Health, n.d.; Pennsylvania Board of Nursing, 2017, §21.14). Many states permit delegation of medications to unlicensed personnel who have the competency to perform the task. Some states provide detailed guidance on delegation. The Texas Board of Nursing (2013) promulgates rules on delegation that provides detailed decision trees to support the school nurse's clinical judgment regarding delegation of medication and special procedures. Other states put specific limits on what can and cannot be delegated. For example, the Illinois nurse practice act limits delegation of medication administration to the following routes only: oral or subcutaneous and topical and transdermal (Illinois General Assembly, 2018).

NCSBN and ANA's *National Guidelines for Nursing Delegation* (2019) emphasize that "The licensed nurse cannot delegate nursing judgment or any activity that will involve nursing judgment or critical decision making" (p. 3). Practically, this means that delegation should be reserved for situations where the student's health condition is routine and stable. Proper delegation requires a comprehensive nursing assessment. The delegatee must accept responsibility to perform the designated health-care task, and the school nurse is responsible for training and monitoring the competence of the delegatee in performing the health-care task.

Some students have a chronic health condition that can episodically present as an emergency that follows a predictable course (e.g., asthma, anaphylaxis, seizures). For these students, the school nurse uses nursing judgment to develop an emergency action plan that outlines in lay terms exactly the steps to a responder should take. See Chapter 8. In the absence of a nurse, the immediate administration of rescue medications by a trained UAP may save a student's life.

NCSBN and ANA (2019) stress that the *nurse maintains responsibility and accountability for the provision of nursing care.* Delegation requires the school nurse to employ nursing judgment, critical thinking, effective communication, and an understanding of the legal parameters in one's own state. See Chapter 31 for further discussion of the principles of delegation.

Field Trips

School-sponsored activities occurring outside of the school setting require guidelines. State law might mandate school districts to provide emergency services at all extracurricular events. Wisconsin, for example, requires school districts to provide emergency nursing services policies and requires that those policies be developed by a nurse. The policy must include "protocols for dealing with pupil accidental injury, illness and administration of medication at all school-sponsored activities including but not limited to curricular, co-curricular and extra-curricular activities and a method to record each incident of service provided" (Wisconsin State Legislature, 2017, Section 8.01[1][g]).

The school nurse's role on field trips can also be regulated by state practice acts. As an example, Connecticut provides specific guidance for field trips that occur both within and outside of the state. Schools in Connecticut are permitted to allow qualified personnel to administer medications during field trips within the state *if deemed safe by the school nurse.* The Connecticut BON also advises school nurses who attend field trips outside of the state to "annually determine the licensure and practice acts in the state or country where the students are visiting" (Connecticut State Department of Education, 2023). Further guidance is also provided by NASN: "If the school nurse determines that medical care cannot be legally or safely delegated, the school nurse will need to determine and coordinate the nursing staff required to accompany the student" (NASN, 2019b).

The NCSBN clarifies that nursing practice does not occur where the *nurse* is, but where the *patient* is: "Practice is where the patient is, and it includes the direct care of patients, telehealth, care via telephone, and distance education of nursing students" (NCSBN, n.d., para. 2). School nurses who are attending out-of-state field trips but are only licensed in their home states must request permission to practice in the other state unless their home state and the state they are going to are both in the enhanced nursing licensure compact and the nurse holds a multistate privilege. If students require nursing procedures or medications and the school nurse is not attending, the school nurse must know what aspects of the care may be delegated and to whom. School nurses must know if the destination state permits nurses from other states to temporarily practice there while on out-of-state field trips and if the destination state permits out-of-state nurses to delegate care when not physically present. It is important to know if the delegation and scope of practice rules in the destination state differ from those of the home state.

The care requirements of students with special health-care needs also need to be considered when preparing for a field trip. The provision of health services while on a field trip should be established through discussion with the parent and written into the student's IHP, IEP, or 504 plan as appropriate. See Chapter 8 for further discussion.

Consent

Generally, parental consent is required to provide care to minors. There are exceptions in which minors have the right to consent to health care without parental approval or notification. These exceptions vary by state. Minors are most likely to have independent authority to make decisions related to reproductive health care, such as treatment for sexually transmitted infections, contraceptive services, and prenatal care, or to mental health services such as drug and alcohol abuse or mental health treatment.

Emancipated Minors

Some minors have the legal authority to make all health-care decisions on their own behalf. Minors can become "emancipated" or freed from parental control, before reaching the age of majority in some circumstances and in some states. A court can declare a minor to be emancipated, and minors can become emancipated in some states by marriage or active military service. Emancipation generally considers issues such as financial independence, employment, and maturity.

Emergencies

A doctrine of *implied consent* or *presumed consent* can obviate the need to obtain parental consent in the event of an emergency. The doctrine is based on the assumption that the person would consent to care if able and that a delay in providing care to obtain full, informed consent can risk loss of life, limb, or organ. Implied consent might also apply to situations where the school nurse suspects child abuse. As with all consent issues, the law varies by state, and school nurses must know the consent laws in their own states.

Malpractice

Although nurses, particularly school nurses, are rarely sued for professional negligence, it is important to understand the elements of a malpractice case:

- *Duty:* For a plaintiff to be successful, they must first establish that the school nurse had a nurse-patient relationship with the student. That relationship creates a *duty* on the part of the school nurse. That duty is the duty of reasonable care, meaning the school nurse acted in a way a reasonably prudent school nurse would have acted in same or similar circumstances.
- *Breach:* The plaintiff must then demonstrate that the school nurse *breached* that duty. This means the school nurse departed from the acceptable standards of practice. The school nurse did something a reasonably prudent school nurse in same or similar circumstances would not have done or did not do something a reasonably prudent school nurse in same or similar circumstances would have done. To establish that the school nurse deviated from acceptable practice, the plaintiff needs to provide the testimony of an expert witness.
- *Causation:* It is not sufficient to prove that a school nurse departed from the standards of care to prevail in a nursing malpractice lawsuit. The plaintiff must also prove that the departure from standards was the *cause* of the student's injury. If it can be proven that a reasonably prudent school nurse would have acted in a manner different from the defendant school nurse, but it cannot be proven that their actions resulted in the student's injuries—that the harm was caused by something else—the case will still not succeed.
- *Harm:* The purpose of a lawsuit is to make a person whole or compensate that person for actual injuries. There must be measurable *harm* for which the person seeks recompense. Damages, costs, injury, and so on must be proven. As stated, even if the school nurse did depart from the acceptable standards of practice, if that departure did not *cause* actual *harm*, the case will not be successful. This differs from nursing board discipline, in which actual patient harm is not necessary to discipline a license for professional misconduct.

Begley v. City of New York (2013) illustrates these elements. The elements of malpractice are italicized in this text to highlight them. Jonathan Begley was an elementary school student with an IEP that addressed severe asthma and extreme allergies. The IEP called for him to attend the Forum School and required an RN to accompany him during transportation to and from the school and to monitor his condition throughout the day. These private nurses were provided by his mother. Additionally, two epi-pens were to be present at all times. When one of Jonathan's teachers expressed concern about the "hovering" of one of the private nurses, the school instituted a new policy that required the nurses to sit outside the classroom.

One of Jonathan's teachers presented a "multisensory" lesson which displayed a basket of blueberries. Although Jonathan was seated at least 5 feet away from the blueberries, and although both the teacher and his nurse did not see him touch the blueberries, Jonathan began experiencing respiratory distress. His private nurse heard wheezing and treated him for an asthma attack. She administered Proventil but his breathing did not improve so she administered another Proventil, then an epi-pen. The school nurse was called to the classroom and asked someone to call 911. She helped stabilize his position and tried to administer oxygen. A second epi-pen, and then a third was administered. The ambulance arrived about 20 minutes after being called. The paramedics intubated Jonathan and transported him to a hospital where he died 2 days later *(harm).*

Jonathan's parents believed his allergic reaction was caused by exposure to the blueberries and brought a lawsuit against the private nurse and the school district. They alleged negligence in allowing Jonathan to be exposed to the allergen and in failing to respond to symptoms of anaphylaxis. The Begleys also alleged that the school nurse should have disinfected the environment; that the first epi-pen given had been expired at the time it was administered; and that the school nurse failed to respond to his anaphylactic reaction appropriately. The Begleys' expert witness provided an opinion that the school nurse *departed from the standard of practice.* It was her opinion that a *reasonably prudent nurse* would have immediately recognized that Jonathan was experiencing an anaphylactic reaction and followed the protocol provided by his pediatrician. She stated that Benadryl should have been administered before the epi-pen and that the first epi-pen administered was probably ineffective because it had expired 7 months earlier. She also stated that the school nurse had an independent *duty* to act in accordance with sound nursing practice regardless of the presence of the private nurse.

The private nurse also provided an affidavit of an expert witness who wrote that the private nurse had not *departed from good and accepted nursing practice.* She stated that the private nurse had no *duty* to prevent allergen exposure and that blueberries were not on the list of known allergies his physician had provided. She also believed that the private nurse's impression that Jonathan was experiencing an asthma attack was consistent with his medical conditions *and within acceptable standards of nursing practice.* She disagreed that Benadryl should have been administered, arguing that it would have been contraindicated to administer a liquid medication during respiratory distress as it would create the risk of aspiration. The school argued that there was no evidence that the blueberries triggered Jonathan's allergic reaction. Additionally, the Begleys could not prove that having the private nurse stationed outside of the classroom was the *proximate cause* of his injury.

The Department of Education (DOE), the Forum School, and the private nurse asked the court to dismiss the case. The court did dismiss the case against the DOE, finding that the private nurse was not an employee of the school, and that the DOE did not exercise day-to-day control over Jonathan at the Forum School. It did not dismiss the case against the private nurse or the Forum School. The private nurse and the Forum School appealed. On appeal, the court found that the school had met its requirements under IDEA by formulating an appropriate IEP. The court reasoned that, "Even assuming that the school's *duty* under the *reasonably prudent* parent standard extended to disinfecting his lunch environment, in the absence of proof as to what triggered Jonathan's reaction, it cannot be concluded that the failure to disinfect the microwave oven used to heat Jonathan's lunch, and to disinfect his lunch table and place mat, *proximately caused* his injuries" (*Begley v. City of New York,* 2013, p. 71). The court also found that the affidavit of the Begley's expert witness was insufficient to demonstrate that the school nurse *departed from good and accepted nursing practice.* The complaints against the Forum School and the private nurse were dismissed.

Immunity

Many nurses have misperceptions or incomplete information about immunity. It is important to understand that immunity does not prevent a school nurse from being named in a lawsuit. Immunity can take many forms but is asserted as a defense in a suit that has already been filed. It does not provide protection from that lawsuit being commenced. Legal arguments about the applicability of immunity statutes can be complex and result in considerable legal expenses even if the lawsuit is ultimately dismissed on immunity grounds.

To dismiss the case on immunity grounds, courts have considered such things as whether an immunity statute applies to the particular circumstances of the case; if the actions by the defendant constituted willfulness, corruption, deliberate indifference, or malice; if the actions taken were ministerial or discretionary; if authority was exercised in bad faith; if the negligence complained of is simple negligence or gross and wanton negligence; if the risks were reasonably foreseeable; if the school is considered a natural person; if the school stands *in loco parentis* under the immunity statute; if the defendants had a fiduciary duty to the plaintiff; if there was an expectation of compensation when volunteering services where the scene of the incident occurred; if the defendants owed a duty to the plaintiff; and if public concerns are involved. Many of the questions are questions of fact that must be determined to establish immunity.

County, City, and Local Law

County, city, and other local laws also affect school nurse practice. Local ordinances, health laws, and school board policies and procedures should be readily available for reference. Failure to abide by employer policies or local laws can lead to licensure discipline and be used as evidence of departure from acceptable standards of practice in a civil lawsuit. Job descriptions and the requirements to hold a position as a school nurse can be evidence of the standard of care and must also be adhered to.

CONCLUSION

School nursing requires specialized skills and presents particular legal challenges. Reporting to nonclinical people can create difficulties in explaining scope of practice limitations or standards of practice mandates. Working in isolation can lead to outdated practice. When represented by collective bargaining units, school nurses are frequently members of teachers' unions that also might not understand the particular employment issues nurses have in an educational setting. The role of school nurses is misunderstood, not only by the general public, but also within the nursing community itself. Education law, health law, and nursing law can be in conflict, requiring the school nurse to be especially vigilant in staying updated with regulatory changes.

Despite the legal challenges, school nurses should take great pride in understanding the contribution they make to health care and the nation. The presence of a school nurse improves the educational level of our population by reducing absenteeism and increasing graduation rates. Better school attendance also improves public health. Students are safer, healthier, and better educated because of school nurses (Allison et al., 2019). School nurses recognize symptoms of serious health problems, manage complex medical conditions, refer troubled students to resources, respond to crisis and emergencies, and serve as the safety net for the country's children. Dealing with school nursing challenges can be stressful. That stress, however, should be balanced by the gratification that comes with knowing that school nurses save lives.

References

Allison, M. A., Attisha, E., & Council on School Health. (2019). The link between school attendance and good health. *Pediatrics, 143*(2). https://doi.org/10.1542/peds.2018-3648

American Nurses Association. (2022, May 5). *Letter to Honorable Judge Jennifer L. Smith.* https://www.nursingworld.org/~49a0c0/globalassets/practiceandpolicy/ethics/vaught-judge-letter-05092022.pdf

Amos, L. (2021, November 18). Eliminating school discipline disparities: What we know and don't know about the effectiveness of alternatives to suspension and expulsion. *Mathematica*. https://www.mathematica.org/blogs/eliminating-school-discipline-disparities-what-we-know-and-dont-know-about-the-effectiveness#:~:text5Discipline%20disparities%20are%20driven%20by,stereotyping%20can%20influence%20these%20referrals

Anonymous Complainant. (2018). *Report to Centers for Medicare and Medicaid Services*. https://www.documentcloud.org/documents/6542003-CMS-Complaint-Intake.html

Child Welfare Information Gateway. (n.d.). *State definitions of child abuse and neglect*. https://www.childwelfare.gov/topics/can/defining/state/

Child Welfare Information Gateway. (2019). *About CAPTA: A legislative history*. https://www.childwelfare.gov/pubs/factsheets/about/

Congressional Research Service. (2022). *The Elementary and Secondary Education Act (ESEA), as amended by the Every Student Succeeds Act (ESSA): A primer*. https://fas.org/sgp/crs/misc/R45977.pdf

Connecticut State Department of Education. (2023). *Field trips: Guidance for school nurses*. https://portal.ct.gov/SDE/Publications/Field-Trips-Guidance-for-School-Nurses

Department of Health & Human Services & Centers for Medicare & Medicaid Services. (2018a, November 16). *Immediate jeopardy letter*. https://www.modernhealthcare.com/assets/pdf/CH1180721128.PDF

Department of Health & Human Services & Centers for Medicare & Medicaid Services. (2018b, November 18). Vanderbilt University Medical Center statement of deficiencies and plan of correction. https://hospitalwatchdog.org/wp-content/uploads/VUMC-PLAN-OF-CORRECTION.pdf

Federal Trade Commission. (n.d.) 16 CFR Part 312, *Children's Online Privacy Protection Act of 1998*, 15 U.S.S. 6501-6505 Children's Privacy. https://www.ftc.gov/legal-library/browse/rules/childrens-online-privacy-protection-rule-coppa

Federal Trade Commission. (2020). *Complying with COPPA: Frequently asked questions*. https://www.ftc.gov/business-guidance/resources/complying-coppa-frequently-asked-questions

Hemez, P., Brent, J. J., & Mowen, T. J. (2020). Exploring the school-to-prison pipeline: How school suspensions influence incarceration during your adulthood. *Youth Violence and Juvenile Justice, 18*(3), 235–255. https://doi.org/10.1177/1541204019880945

Illinois General Assembly. (2018). *Nurse practice act (225 ILCS 65/)*. http://www.ilga.gov/legislation/ilcs/ilcs5.asp?ActID51312&ChapterID524

Institute for Children, Poverty & Homelessness. (2023). *The McKinney-Vento Homeless Assistance Act*. https://www.icphusa.org/mkv/

Johnson, K. H. (2024). School health documentation and implications for data collection. In C. A. Resha & V. L. Taliaferro (Eds.), *Legal resource for school health services* (2nd ed., pp. 99–121). SchoolNurse.com

Kentucky Board of Nursing. (2017). *Advisory opinion statement: Social media for nurses*. https://kbn.ky.gov/KBN%20Documents/aos40-social-media-for-nurses.pdf

Lowrey, K. M. (2019). Data privacy in school nursing: Navigating the complex landscape of data privacy laws (part 1). *The Network for Public Health Law. Robert Wood Johnson Foundation*. https://networkforphl.org/wp-content/uploads/2019/12/Data-Privacy-in-School-Nursing-Navigating-the-Complex-Landscape-of-Data-Privacy-Laws-Part-1-1.pdf

Maryland Board of Nursing. (n.d.). *Over the counter products*. http://mbon.maryland.gov/Pages/practice-over-the-counter.aspx

Minnesota Board of Nursing. (2017). *Statement of accountability for utilization of integrative therapies in nursing practice*. http://www.health.state.mn.us/divs/cfh/program/shn/content/document/pdf/medadmin.pdf

National Alliance to End Homelessness. (2022). *State of homelessness: 2022 edition*. https://endhomelessness.org/homelessness-in-america/homelessness-statistics/state-of-homelessness/

National Association of School Nurses. (2019a). *Electronic health records: An essential tool for school nurses to keep students healthy*. https://www.nasn.org/nasn-resources/professional-practice-documents/position-statements/ps-electronic-health-records

National Association of School Nurses. (2019b). *School-sponsored trips, role of the school nurse* [Position Statement]. Author.

National Association of School Nurses. (2020). *Individualized healthcare plans: The role of the school nurse* [Position statement]. Author.

National Association of School Nurses. (2022). *School Nursing: Scope and Standards of Practice* (4th ed.). Author.

National Association of School Nurses. (2024). A contemporary framework update for today's school nursing landscape: Introducing the School Nursing Practice Framework. *NASN School Nurse, 39*(3), 140–147. https://www.doi.org/10.1177/1942602X241241092

National Council of State Boards of Nursing. (n.d.). *Nurse licensure guidance*. https://www.ncsbn.org/nursing-regulation/licensure/nurse-licensure-guidance.page

National Council of State Boards of Nursing. (2018a). *A nurse's guide to the use of social media*. https://www.ncsbn.org/brochures-and-posters/nurses-guide-to-the-use-of-social-media

National Council of State Boards of Nursing. (2018b). *What every nurse needs to know about state and territorial boards of nursing*. https://www.ncsbn.org/public-files/What_Every_Nurse_Needs_to_Know.pdf

National Council of State Boards of Nursing. (2018c). *A nurse's guide to professional boundaries*. https://www.ncsbn.org/ProfessionalBoundaries_Complete.pdf

National Council of State Boards of Nursing. (2023). *Find your nurse practice act*. https://www.ncsbn.org/policy/npa.page

National Council of State Boards of Nursing & American Nurses Association. (2019). *National guidelines for nursing delegation*. https://www.ncsbn.org/public-files/NGND-PosPaper_06.pdf

National Practitioner Data Bank. (2018). *NPDB guidebook*. https://www.npdb.hrsa.gov/guidebook

New York State Education Department. (2023). *Abandonment of patients who need care*. https://www.op.nysed.gov/professions/licensed-practical-nurses/professional-practice/abandonment-patients-who-need-care-lpn

North Dakota Board of Nursing. (2019). *Practice guidance: Abandonment*. https://www.ndbon.org/Practice/PracticeGuidance/Abandonment.asp

Pennsylvania Board of Nursing. (2017). *Chapter 21. State Board of Nursing, Subchapter A. Registered Nurses: Administration of drugs*. https://www.pacodeandbulletin.gov/secure/pacode/data/049/chapter21/049_0021.pdf

Pennsylvania Department of Health. (n.d.). *School health: Medication administration*. https://www.health.pa.gov/topics/school/Pages/Medications.aspx

Scott, L. R., & Bubert, J. S. (2013). Legal issues related to school nursing practice: The foundation. In J. Selekman, School Nursing: A Comprehensive Text (pp. 196 -224). Philadelphia: F.A. Davis.

Texas Board of Nursing. (2013). *Frequently asked questions: Delegation*. https://www.bon.texas.gov/faq_delegation.asp.html#t13

Texas Board of Nursing. (2022). *Position statement 15.29: Professional boundaries including use of social media by nurses*. https://www.bon.texas.gov/practice_bon_position_statements_content.asp#15.29

U.S. Department of Education. (2017). *Every Student Succeeds Act (ESSA)*. https://www.ed.gov/esea

U.S. Department of Education. (2023, April 12). Know your rights: FERPA protections for student health records. *Student Privacy Policy Office*. https://studentprivacy.ed.gov/sites/default/files/resource_document/file/Know%20Your%20Rights%20-%20FERPA%20Protections%20for%20Student%20Health%20Records.pdf

U.S. Department of Health and Human Services. (2021a). *Health information privacy: Does FERPA or HIPAA apply to elementary or secondary school student health records maintained by a health care provider that is not employed by the school?* https://www.hhs.gov/hipaa/for-professionals/faq/514/does-hipaa-apply-to-school-student-health-records/index.html

U.S. Department of Health and Human Services. (2021b). *HIPAA: Does HIPAA allow a health care provider to disclose PHI about a student to a school nurse*. https://www.hhs.gov/hipaa/for-professionals/faq/517/

does-hipaa-allow-a-health-care-provider-to-disclose-information-to-a-school-nurse/index.html

U.S. Department of Health and Human Services. (2021c). *HIPAA: Does the privacy rule limit to whom at the school a provider may send immunization records?* https://www.hhs.gov/hipaa/for-professionals/faq/1509/does-hipaa-limit-to-whom-at-a-school-a-provider-sends-immunization-records/index.html

U.S. Department of Health and Human Services. (2022). *HIPAA*. https://www.hhs.gov/hipaa/for-professionals/faq/2099/does-hipaa-prevent-school-administrator-or-school-doctor-or-nurse-sharing-concerns-about.html

U.S. Department of Health and Human Services & U.S. Department of Education. (2019). *Joint guidance on the application of the Family Educational Rights and Privacy Act (FERPA) and the Health Insurances Portability and Accountability Act of 1996 (HIPAA) to student health records.* https://studentprivacy.ed.gov/resources/joint-guidance-application-ferpa-and-hipaa-student-health-records

Cases

Begley v. City of New York, 972 N.Y.S.2d 48. (2013). https://scholar.google.com/scholar_case?case5104036854401001994 61&q5Begley1v.1City1of1N.Y&hl5en&as_sdt56,39&as_vis51

Board of Education of Independent School District No. 92 of Pottawatomie County v. Earls, (01-332) 536 U.S. 822. (2002). https://www.law.cornell.edu/supct/html/historics/USSC_DN_0001_0332_ZS.html

Board of Education of the Hendrick Hudson Central School District Bd. of Ed. Westchester County, v. Rowley, 458 U.S. 176. (1982). https://www.law.cornell.edu/supremecourt/text/458/176

Bryner v. Canyons School District, Utah Ct. App. 131, (2015). https://scholar.google.com/scholar_case?case5805613425255912878 9&hl5en&as_sdt56&as_vis51&oi5scholarr

G.C. v. Owensboro Public Schools., 711 F.3d 623, 6th. (2013). https://scholar.google.com/scholar_case?case5164099580722259633 47&q5G.C.1v.1Owensboro1Public.School&hl5en&as_sdt56,39&as_vis51

New Jersey v. T.L.O., 469 U.S. 325. (1985). https://www.law.cornell.edu/supremecourt/text/469/325

Plyler v. Doe., 457 U.S. 202. (1982). https://www.uscourts.gov/educational-resources/educational-activities/access-education-rule-law

Safford Unified School District #1 v. Redding, 129 S. Ct. 2633. (2009). https://www.law.cornell.edu/supct/html/08-479.ZS.html

State of Missouri v. Charles Williams, Mo. Ct. App. East. Dist. Div. 4. (2017). http://caselaw.findlaw.com/mo-court-of-appeals/1866074.html

Laws

Child Abuse Prevention and Treatment Act of 1974 (CAPTA) (Pub. L. No. 93-247; reauthorized in 2010 as Pub. L. No. 111-320). https://www.govtrack.us/congress/bills/93/s1191

Children's Online Privacy Protection Rule. (1998). 15 U.S.C. 6501-6505. https://www.ftc.gov/legal-library/browse/rules/childrens-online-privacy-protection-rule-coppa

Comprehensive Addiction and Recovery Act of 2016 (Pub. L. No. 114-198). https://www.govtrack.us/congress/bills/114/s524

Every Student Succeeds Act (ESSA) of 2015 (Pub. L. No. 114-95, 129 Stat. 1802). https://www.gpo.gov/fdsys/pkg/PLAW-114publ95/html/PLAW-114publ95.htm

Family Educational Rights and Privacy Act of 1974 (FERPA), (20 U.S.C. § 1232g; 34 CFR Part 99). https://www.law.cornell.edu/uscode/text/20/1232g

Health Insurance Portability and Accountability Act of 1996 (HIPAA) (Pub. L. No. 104–191, 110 Stat. 1936). https://www.gpo.gov/fdsys/pkg/PLAW-104publ191/html/PLAW-104publ191.htm

Individuals With Disabilities Education Improvement Act of 2004 (Pub. L. 108-446). https://www.gpo.gov/fdsys/pkg/PLAW-108publ446/content-detail.html

Justice for Victims of Trafficking Act of 2015 (Pub. L. No. 114-22). https://www.govtrack.us/congress/bills/114/s178

McKinney-Vento Homeless Assistance Act of 1987 (Pub. L. No. 100-77, 101 Stat. 482, 42 U.S.C., Title 119, Subchapter 1, § 11301). https://www.govtrack.us/congress/bills/100/hr558

Rehabilitation Act of 1973 (Pub. L. 93-112). https://www.gpo.gov/fdsys/pkg/STATUTE-107/pdf/STATUTE-107-Pg718.pdf

U.S. Constitution, Amendment IV. http://constitution.findlaw.com/amendment4.html

U.S. Constitution, Article VI: Supreme law. https://constitution.congress.gov/browse/article-6/

Wisconsin State Legislature. (2017). Administrative Code, Chapter PI 8, School District Standards, § 8.01(1)(g) Emergency Nursing Services. https://docs.legis.wisconsin.gov/code/admin_code/pi/8/01/2/g

Chapter 7

Federal Laws Protecting Students With Disabilities

Catherine F. Yonkaitis ▪ Elizabeth Crespo

CHAPTER OUTLINE

Together, we must remove the physical barriers we have created and the social barriers that we have accepted. For ours will never be a truly prosperous nation until all within it prosper.

President George H. W. Bush at the signing of ADA Act of 1990

Federal laws provide assurance of educational opportunities, protection, and support for students who have special health needs. School district policies and guidelines for serving students with disabilities must follow the dictates of federal laws. School nurses must understand these laws and the rights of families to best serve and advocate for children with chronic conditions and their families. The school nurse's role and responsibilities in developing health and educational plans to protect the rights and health of students with disabilities is discussed in greater detail in Chapter 8.

HISTORY OF LAWS THAT PROTECT CHILDREN WITH DISABILITIES

The 10th Amendment to the U.S. Constitution states, "powers not delegated to the United States by the Constitution, nor prohibited by it to the States, are reserved to the States respectively, or to the people." Throughout American history, education has been the responsibility of state and local governments, not of the federal government. Mandates for education of children are written into every state constitution; however, in the past, not every child has had access to that education. Therefore, federal laws have been enacted to provide overarching protection to ensure all children have an opportunity to be educated so they can "be prepared to lead productive and independent adult lives, to the maximum extent possible"

(Individuals With Disabilities Education Improvement Act [IDEA], 2004, §01 C.5.A.ii).

The initial impetus to provide special education services in public schools began in the 1950s with the civil rights movement. In 1954, many schools were still racially segregated. The Supreme Court unanimously decided that "separate educational facilities are inherently unequal" and that state laws that established separate schools for black and white students were unconstitutional under the Equal Protection clause of the 14th Amendment of the Constitution (*Brown v. Board of Education*, 1954). Although this ruling may seem far removed from legislation for children with disabilities, it paved the way for using the Equal Protection clause for the civil rights movement and for all forms of integration, including for those with special learning needs.

The 1960s and 1970s were decades that focused on civil rights. The initial focus was on racial equality, then on women's rights and the needs and rights of disabled veterans. The *Civil Rights Act of 1964* (Pub. L. 88-352) made it unlawful to discriminate against persons in the workplace and in public facilities based on race, sex, religion, or ethnicity. The law also strengthened the prohibitions on school segregation and discrimination related to voter registration.

Shortly after the enactment of the Civil Rights Act of 1964, more specific attention to discrimination in schools began when President Johnson signed the *Elementary and Secondary Education Act of 1965* (Pub. L. 89-10). The law supported students in poverty by providing federal monies to underfunded school districts (this was the beginning of "Title" funding). The Elementary and Secondary Education Act is still in place today and has been reauthorized and renamed over the years, first as the *No Child Left Behind Act of 2001* (Pub. L. 107-110) and then as the *Every Student Succeeds Act* of 2015 (Pub. L. 114-95).

During this time, public awareness grew regarding the needs of individuals with disabilities. It is estimated that in the 1960s and 1970s more than half of children with disabilities did not receive an appropriate education. This often occurred because they were misclassified as being "mentally retarded" or "uneducable" or their disability was not detected. Pressure from parents of children with disabilities who were placed in special schools, institutionalized, or denied an education resulted in the enactment of laws to support and protect them (Heward et al., 2022).

Legislation focusing on the education of children with disabilities (then referred to as "handicaps") culminated in the passage of the Education for All Handicapped Children Act of 1975 (Pub. L. 94-142). This landmark legislation mandated that *all* children with disabilities educated in schools that receive federal funds are entitled to a **free and appropriate public education** (FAPE). Congress awarded grants to states to encourage extra educational efforts for rural or underserved areas and for children with "handicapping" conditions. Federal and state oversights to ensure compliance were part of the regulations. As authorized, the Education for All Handicapped Children Act covered only children between the ages of 5 and 18 years.

The purpose of the Education for All Handicapped Children Act of 1975 was to provide children with disabilities an education tailored to their unique needs and abilities in the **least restrictive environment** (LRE). The law as defined in 1998 describes least restrictive environment as

> *(1) to the maximum extent appropriate, children with disabilities, including children in public or private institutions or other care facilities, are educated with children who are not disabled, and (2) that special classes, separate schooling, or other removal of children with disabilities from the regular educational environment occurs only when the nature or severity of the disability is such that education in regular classes with the use of supplementary aids and services cannot be achieved satisfactorily. (34 CFR §300.550)*

The law also ensured that the rights of children with disabilities and their parents or guardians were protected. Up to this point, only some students with "handicapping" conditions were provided access to an education. Those with profound physical disabilities or multiple health-care needs were often centralized at one school in a district or assigned residential placement, rather than being served at their home school (Davis-Alldritt, 2024). These arrangements did not provide all students an education in the LRE as required by the new law.

The Education for All Handicapped Children Act has been amended and reauthorized and in 1997 became known as the *Individuals With Disabilities Education Act* (IDEA). In 2004, significant amendments were made to the act and Congress changed the name slightly to the Individuals with Disabilities Education *Improvement* Act of 2004. Despite the new name, it continues to be referred to as IDEA. In December 2015, IDEA was updated again to maintain technical consistency in terms and language between it and the newly reauthorized *Every Student Succeeds Act* (ESSA; National Center for Learning Disabilities, 2018).

Several significant changes were made to IDEA via the amendments and reauthorizations. One change was the inclusion of children from birth through age 5 years under the law and a mandate that children with potential disabilities be identified and evaluated early and have interventions started before the child entered the school system. Services were also extended to eligible youth until their 22nd birthday. In addition, the focus changed to "person-first" language, meaning that the child was no longer labeled as their condition. The child must come first, so that the "asthmatic" became the "student with asthma." Other language changes included changing the diagnosis of *mental retardation* to *intellectual disability* and changing the word *handicap* to *disability*. Thus, reference to the "handicapped child" became "a student with a disability." School nurses can be role models for using student-first language and the appropriate legal terms.

Today, IDEA has four subsections:

1. *Section A* provides general information about the law, including definitions and the purpose of the law.
2. *Section B* describes the state's responsibility for Child Find and provides information for states on grants (including those for preschools), eligibility, individualized education programs (IEPs), due process, and procedural safeguards for children 3 to 21 years of age.
3. *Section C* addresses the needs of infants and toddlers (children under 3 years of age) who are at risk for developmental delay if services are not provided. This section also requires comprehensive Child Find systems as well as development of individual family service plans, which are similar to IEPs.
4. *Section D* addresses the need to improve special education programs and personnel preparation as well as developing and disseminating research that supports special education (IDEA, 2004).

Many laws have been enacted to protect underrepresented and traditionally marginalized groups. Several have been outlined previously, but four stand out in terms of protection of the rights of children with disabilities: the Rehabilitation Act of 1973: Section 504, The Americans With Disabilities Act (ADA) of 1990, the Every Student Succeeds Act of 2015, and the Individuals With Disabilities Education Improvement Act of 2004.

THE REHABILITATION ACT OF 1973: SECTION 504

The Rehabilitation Act of 1973 banned discrimination against individuals of all ages on the basis of disabilities in programs conducted by or receiving assistance from the federal government. The revision of the Rehabilitation Act in 1973 looked beyond employment (the focus of the prior acts) toward improving the overall lives of persons with disabilities and to addressing the need for research and training with rehabilitation services. The Rehabilitation Act also established affirmative action hiring and the creation of the Rehabilitation Services Administration. Any public school, charter school, or parochial school that receives federal money—such as from the national school lunch program—must adhere to regulations set forth by the Rehabilitation Act.

School nurses are most familiar with Section 504 of the Rehabilitation Act that prohibits discrimination against qualified persons. It reads as follows:

> *No otherwise qualified individual with a disability in the United States, as defined in section 706(8) of this title, shall, solely by reason of her or his handicap, be excluded from participation in, be denied the benefits of, or be subjected to discrimination under any program or activity receiving Federal financial assistance or under any program or activity conducted by any Executive agency or by the United States Postal Service.* (§ 794[a])

The Rehabilitation Act covers all individuals with disabilities, adults and children; therefore, it includes those covered under IDEA and those who are adults. It is a nondiscrimination/civil rights law.

The Rehabilitation Act defines a person with a disability as "someone who (1) has a *physical or mental impairment* that substantially limits one or more *major life activities;* (2) has a record of such impairment; or (3) is regarded as having such impairment." In the Rehabilitation Act, the definition of physical or mental impairment includes the following:

> *Any physiological disorder, or condition, cosmetic disfigurement or anatomical loss affecting one or more of the following body systems: neurological, musculoskeletal, special sense organs; respiratory, including speech organs; cardiovascular; reproductive; digestive; genitourinary; hemic and lymphatic; skin; and endocrine or any mental or psychological disorder such as intellectual disability, organic brain syndrome, emotional or mental illness and specific learning disabilities.* (§ 794, Sec. 504)

The phrase "major life activities" means "functions such as caring for oneself, performing manual tasks, walking, seeing, hearing, eating, sleeping, breathing, *learning,* lifting, bending, speaking, communicating, reading, concentrating, thinking, and working." This law is not age specific and covers any student or staff, including students as they transition into college or the work environment.

There are two primary components of this law. First, it prevents discrimination on the basis of the disability regarding admission, hiring, and participation in the school/job/activity "if otherwise qualified." Second, and most important for the school nurse, it mandates the provision of accommodations so that the student can learn. Often these accommodations are outlined in an individualized accommodation plan to ensure that the student's disabilities will not limit their ability to benefit from the educational program. These are referred to as 504 plans or accommodation plans and are covered in depth in Chapter 8.

Although most schools develop a written 504 plan, it is not required; what is required by the law is that the accommodations be provided. Most school districts have a formal

Did You Know?

Based on the most recent data available from the U.S. Department of Education, Office for Civil Rights (2018), about 2.7% or 1.4 million students have a 504 Accommodation Plan. Disparity in who receives services was identified over a decade ago, but little headway has been made to address the problem. For instance, just over 60% of those with 504 plans were male despite the fact that only about 51% of those enrolled are male. In addition, the majority of students receiving services under Section 504 were white (61%) whereas enrollment of students classified as white was only 47%.

process that reviews each student's needs and determines what accommodations will be made (Tracey et al., 2024). The law stipulates that the accommodations must be *reasonable* and are meant to help the student meet average or passing requirements in a class or grade. The plans are not meant to ensure above average work or participation as some parents might demand.

The Rehabilitation Act covers *all* students and staff with disabilities, including those with chronic conditions. Examples of students who would be covered under Section 504 if their disability impairs a major life activity are students with allergies, inflammatory bowel disease, cystic fibrosis, asthma, obesity, diabetes, and rheumatoid arthritis. School nurses have a responsibility to identify and refer students who may need accommodations due to a physical or mental impairment affecting a major life activity to the 504 team (National Association of School Nurses [NASN], 2023).

Anyone who suspects that a student has a disability that is affecting learning can make a referral for evaluation, including staff, parents, the school nurse, or the student. Schools must establish standards and procedures for evaluation of students and eligibility determination, as well as for planning and evaluation of the efficacy of the accommodations and how to handle appeals. Schools must meet the individual needs of students with disabilities to ensure they have the same access to an education as nondisabled students.

The school nurse should be part of the 504 team and be prepared to determine if and how alterations in major life functions of the student with a disability might interfere with the student's ability to learn. The nurse should be prepared to recommend interventions/accommodations that may assist the student to be successful in the school environment, such as a rest period in the school health office, access to the bathroom at any time without requesting permission, or blood glucose self-testing in the classroom.

Development of a 504 plan must be a collaborative process. The 504 team must include the parents and individuals who are knowledgeable about the student, the disability, and the process to determine both the student's eligibility for accommodations and the accommodations that are necessary. The law was amended in 1992 to ensure that an individual's wishes, strengths, resources, interests, and concerns are also considered (Pub. L. 102-569).

The role of the school nurse in the Section 504 process for a student with a health-related disability may include, but is not limited to, the following:

- Assessment of student health status and communication with the parents and healthcare providers
- Consultation with the classroom teacher and guidance counselor on health issues related to the student
- Development of an individualized healthcare plan (IHP), including student goals and objectives and nursing protocols to meet student-specific health needs while at school
- Development of a list of student-centered health-related 504 plan accommodations
- Monitoring of student progress and initiation of accommodations via the written 504 plan related to health
- Serving as the team liaison to the healthcare community
- Maintaining open communication with the family on the health status of the student

An often-asked question is "Does every child with a disability need a 504 plan?" The answer is no. However, every child with a health-related disability, often a chronic condition, that requires nursing care or special consideration at school needs an IHP. The IHP documents the care the student is expected to receive and informs the 504 plan. See Chapter 8.

The Office for Civil Rights in the U.S. Department of Education enforces Section 504 law in the school setting (Box 7-1). Periodic evaluations are required for Section 504 plans to ensure that the accommodations are being incorporated into the school setting and that they are effective. However, Section 504 does not specify any timelines for the evaluation. There is no federal funding for making accommodations; however, failure to comply with the law can result in withdrawal of future federal funding for other purposes.

BOX 7-1

U.S. Department of Education, Office for Civil Rights (n.d.), Rulings for Students

The U.S. Department of Education's Office for Civil Rights rulings for students so that they may have a free and appropriate education in the least restrictive environment under IDEA and Section 504 include the following:

1. Physical site: All programs must be accessible to a student with disabilities, even if some parts of a school may not be.
2. Program: Education should be in the most integrated setting appropriate, preferably the regular education classroom. Section 504 defines FAPE as regular or special education and related aids and services designed to meet individual educational needs of students with disabilities as adequately as the needs of nondisabled students are met.
3. Eligibility: Under IDEA and 504, the student must be provided with a comprehensive, individualized evaluation, and if eligible, services and periodic reevaluations. For IDEA, a student must have an IEP.
4. Students with disabilities but not in special education must receive assistive technology if needed to reach their full potential.

Practice Connection

Occasionally, the condition of a student with a Section 504 plan changes, and the student is evaluated and found eligible for special education services under IDEA. In these cases, the 504 plan is no longer necessary because the development of the IEP also meets the requirements of FAPE under Section 504 (Yonkaitis & Crespo, 2023).

AMERICANS WITH DISABILITIES ACT

The *Americans With Disabilities Act* (ADA; Pub. L. 110-325), enacted in 1990 and reauthorized in 2008, provided broad civil rights by guaranteeing individuals of all ages who have disabilities equal access to accommodations; they cannot be excluded, segregated, or otherwise treated in a manner different from individuals without disabilities. The ADA picks up where the Rehabilitation Act of 1973 leaves off, as it applies to a wider spectrum of society. The law promotes full participation and integration into society. It stipulates that there will be no discrimination in transportation, education, public services, public accommodations, telecommunications, and employment. The ADA imposed these employment and accessibility laws to private organizations/businesses (of 15 or more employees) and buildings, requiring that reasonable accommodations be made. Schools are included as part of the law.

ADA protects those who have a disability, just as under Section 504, and includes anyone with "a physical or mental impairment that substantially limits one or more major life activities of such individual; a record of such an impairment or being regarded as having such an impairment" (§12102). Major life activities include (but are not limited to) "seeing, hearing, eating, speaking, walking, standing, lifting, bending, speaking, breathing, *learning*, reading, concentrating, thinking, communicating, and working" [§3(2)(A)].

Individuals with a record of a disability, such as a person who has recovered from cancer or mental illness, would be protected from discrimination. ADA also protects individuals who are regarded as having a substantially limiting impairment, even though the impairment may not affect their ability to work or study. For example, an individual who is disfigured after facial burns is protected from being denied employment because an employer might fear negative reactions from customers. ADA does not focus on outcomes; it focuses on the procedures. The intent of the law is to ensure equal *access;* however, it does not guarantee *success.*

In 2008, ADA clarified that an impairment that is episodic or in remission is a disability if it would substantially limit a major life activity when active. The threshold for how limiting a condition must be has been lowered, and courts are encouraged to interpret the ADA broadly. Therefore, with the exception of ordinary eyeglasses and contact lenses, schools can no longer consider the effect of "mitigating measures" such as medication in determining whether someone has a disability. What this means is that even though medication or other measures may help remove barriers for an individual, they still must receive the same benefit of the ADA law.

The ADA does not have the overt impact on students with disabilities in the school as IDEA, although it can be very helpful in facilitating the transition of youth with disabilities into employment positions and higher education. The impact of ADA is more subtle, but ADA is in place to ensure accessibility for all staff, families, and visitors to the school and other rights. Highlights of the ADA are in Box 7-2.

BOX 7-2

Highlights of the Americans With Disabilities Act

Employment: Employers cannot discriminate against a qualified job applicant or employee related to hiring, salary, promotion, benefits, and training opportunities. Existing facilities must be made accessible and usable by individuals with disabilities (i.e., entrances, bathrooms, getting from floor to floor). Reasonable accommodations must be made in all aspects of job attainment and performance to make the disabled on an equal plane with the nondisabled.

Public Services: Qualified individuals with disabilities must have access to all services and programs provided by all forms of government. They must have access to public transportation, including public school transportation (i.e., "school bus vehicles of schoolchildren, personnel, and equipment to and from a public . . . school and school-related activities") (ADA, 2008).

Public Accommodations and Services Operated by Private Entities: Every entity open to the public must be made accessible to those with disabilities. Schools of all forms are included here.

Telecommunication: Telephone companies must furnish telecommunication devices to enable hearing- and speech-impaired individuals to communicate by wire or radio.

Source: Adapted from ADA (2008).

EVERY STUDENT SUCCEEDS ACT

In December 2015, the *Every Student Succeeds Act* (Pub. L. 114-95) was signed into law by President Obama. This law replaced the *No Child Left Behind Act* of 2001 (Pub. L. 107-110) that originated with the Elementary and Secondary Education Act of 1965 (Pub. L. 89-10). The focus of the Elementary and Secondary Education Act as amended by ESSA is to ensure equal opportunity for all students. It provides more flexibility to states and transparency to parents. It also provides grants to under-resourced and underperforming districts by measuring and addressing achievement gaps. The ESSA requires each state to provide a "report card" that is available online and includes data such as test performance in reading, math, and science, as well as information on graduation rates, absenteeism, and teacher qualifications (Office of Elementary & Secondary Education, 2020).

The ESSA shifts the focus in education from standardized testing and uniform teaching styles, as stressed in the No Child Left Behind Act, to meeting the needs of individual learners. This emphasis is made to ensure that students will be prepared to succeed in college and careers. The ESSA requires educators to use evidence-based strategies to improve student achievement [§003, (b) (1) (B)]. The ESSA connects student health and learning by authorizing school nurses or others knowledgeable about student health to provide support for students with health conditions.

The law continues to require each state to develop an accountability plan that includes measures of academic achievement, graduation rates, and other typical academic measures; it also requires a measure that evaluates school quality or school success. Many states are using this last measure to evaluate the whole child, incorporating health and wellness. Twenty-eight states and the District of Columbia have selected chronic absenteeism as their measure of student success (National Center for Education Statistics [NCES], 2018). School nurses are well placed to affect absenteeism, in particular when it comes to students with chronic health conditions. In this way, school nurses, identified as specialized support personnel in the ESSA, can participate in the campaign to improve student outcomes in their schools and affect school, district, and state accountability plans.

INDIVIDUALS WITH DISABILITIES EDUCATION IMPROVEMENT ACT

Defining Disability

The Individuals With Disabilities Education Improvement Act of 2004 (Pub. L. 108-446), more commonly called IDEA, is the primary federal law that governs how all states provide special education and related services to children with disabilities from birth through age 21. IDEA is much more prescribed than other disability laws. The IDEA definition of disability is crucial to determine whether a student qualifies under this law. According to IDEA (Part A, §602), a disability is determined by having one of the following specified categories of conditions:

- Intellectual disability (formerly mental retardation)
- Hearing impairment (including deafness)
- Speech or language impairment
- Visual impairment (including blindness)
- Emotional disturbance
- Orthopedic impairment
- Autism
- Traumatic brain injury
- Other health impairment
- Specific learning disability
- Deaf-blindness
- Multiple disabilities

In addition, IDEA allows states and local education agencies to use one additional disability category termed *developmental delay.* This term may be used for children ages 3 to 9 years who are experiencing delays in "one or more of the following areas: physical development, cognitive development, communication development, social and emotional development, or adaptive development" [§300.8(b)(1)]. All of these conditions have been determined to affect one's *ability* to learn.

While school nurses may work with a child with any one of the IDEA disabilities, it is essential that the nurse be involved with those students who qualify for services under the *other health impairment (OHI)* disability. In 2020–2021, OHI was the third most common disability (15%) behind *specific learning disability* (33%) and *speech or language impairment* (19%) (NCES, 2022). This means more than 1 million students were classified under OHI in 2020 to 2021, whereas in 1990 only 55,000 students were. IDEA describes each of the disabilities in some detail to assist the school team in making disability decisions (§300.8). The process under IDEA includes identification, full and individual evaluation, eligibility determination, IEP development, and placement in the least restrictive environment. Each aspect of the process is discussed in this chapter. Specific responsibilities of the school nurse in special education are further discussed in Chapter 8.

Child Find and Referral

IDEA law is clear that every effort must be given to find and evaluate children with a suspected disability. IDEA mandates that a system be in place to identify children, commonly referred to as **Child Find.** Many know that IDEA requires Child Find for infants and toddlers up to age 3 years in Part C of the law, but the responsibility for seeking children with disabilities also applies under part B, the part of the law that covers school-age children. States and municipalities must seek and evaluate school-age children who may have a disability, including children who attend private schools and public schools, highly mobile children, migrant children, homeless children, and children who are wards of the state. *If school employees know or have reason to suspect that a child has a disability, these school employees have an affirmative duty to act on the child's behalf.* If they fail to do so, they have defaulted in their obligation to identify, locate, and evaluate children with disabilities who need individualized special education programs. If the school district fails to act and the child does not receive the necessary services, then the school district and the state's department of education may be liable for this failure. Anyone (a parent, health-care provider, teacher, school nurse, or other school staff) can refer a student for evaluation under IDEA.

Multitiered System of Supports and Response to Intervention

Multitiered system of supports (MTSS) consists of school-based approaches designed to identify at-risk and struggling students and to provide early intervention to support them. MTSS "is an evidence-based framework for effectively integrating multiple systems and services to simultaneously address students' academic achievement, behavior, and social-emotional well-being" (National Association of School Psychologists, 2017, para. 1). MTSS programs also assist schools to incorporate socially just practices that provide students equitable access to a school's resources (Clark & Dockweiler, 2020). MTSS can be instituted in various ways but it always includes universal identification of high-need students and increasing interventions as needed to support overall student success. MTSS is a similar but broader model than the well-known response to intervention (RTI).

Response to Intervention

What is RTI? It is a multitiered approach to identifying and addressing students who may have learning or behavior needs (National Center for Learning Disabilities, n.d.). As with MTSS, students are usually identified through a universally applied screening process. Once identified, students are provided with supports and interventions with increasing level of intensity to help the student learn or adapt their behavior. The supports may be provided by a variety of personnel, including classroom teachers, special education teachers, school support personnel, and other specialists. Student success must be monitored to determine outcomes and the need for further supports, including referral for evaluation for special education services.

RTI is a school-wide three-level model, with each level providing more individualized support. Schools can use various approaches (e.g., problem-solving, functional assessment) to RTI but, in all cases, the support must be evidence-based.

Tier 1: High Quality Instruction in classroom to ensure that the difficulties are not due to inadequate instruction. Students are evaluated regularly, and if improvements are not seen within 8 weeks the student should be moved to Tier 2.

Tier 2: Targeted Interventions, more intensive instruction usually in small groups as well as in the classroom, is provided. Students continue to be evaluated regularly for as long as a full grading period. As with Tier 1, if progress is minimal then the student should be moved to Tier 3.

Tier 3: Intensive Intervention and Comprehensive Evaluation, individualized interventions are created for the student and students are considered for comprehensive evaluation for special education services under IDEA (2004).

School nurses should keep in mind that even if a student is being supported through an RTI program, IDEA (2004) allows parents to seek a comprehensive evaluation for special education eligibility at any time. *RTI should not be used to delay or deny evaluation under IDEA* (Heward et al., 2022).

RTI and Specific Learning Disability

IDEA allows school teams that evaluate students for specific learning disability (SLD) to use the child's response to scientific, research-based interventions (e.g., RTI) in SLD eligibility determinations (IDEA, 2004, § 300.307). However, each state must determine whether they will use RTI among the options for SLD determination or if they will use alternative data such as severe discrepancy or other alternative research-based procedures.

Full and Individual Evaluation

To qualify for the services guaranteed by IDEA, a student must have a *full and individual evaluation* to determine whether they have a disability as described in the law and whether, because of that disability, the student will need special education, related services, or both. This means that the disability for this child affects their ability to learn. The evaluation is performed by a team of professionals, sometimes referred to as the special education team, child study team, student assistance team, pupil appraisal team, or student resource team. The makeup of this team must

Focus on the Framework
Care Coordination

***Jana K. v. Annville Cleona School District*, 63 IDELR 278 (M.D. Pa. 2014)**

In *Jana K. v. Annville Cleona School District*, the court held the district's knowledge of the student's declining grades, frequent visits to the school nurse, and acts of self-harm were sufficient to trigger the district's Child Find duty. Specifically, the court found the parents never requesting an evaluation or sharing an independent psychological evaluation irrelevant to the district's Child Find failure. Multiple events provided the school with sufficient information that should have resulted in an evaluation.

This case highlights the role of the school nurse to participate in collaborative communication, and direct care, all components of the Care Coordination principle of NASN's School Nursing Practice Framework (NASN, 2024). If the school nurse had been aware of their Child Find duty under IDEA and referred this student for evaluation, the school district may have been able to provide appropriate services to the student and avoided costly legal proceedings.

include individuals within the school who have knowledge regarding the student. These include the parent; at least one regular education teacher (if the child participates in the regular education environment); one special education teacher; someone representing the school, such as an administrator; as well as someone who can interpret the instructional implication of the evaluation results (could be one of members already listed).

In addition, the parent or public agency (school) can include "other individuals who have knowledge or special expertise regarding the child, including related services personnel" [§300.321(a)]. Finally, the student must be included in the meeting whenever transition planning is to occur. Transition planning usually begins around the age of 14 but must start before the student turns 16. Related services personnel can include any of the following: school nurse, psychologist, physical therapist, occupational therapist, speech therapist, social worker, hearing or vision itinerants, and reading specialists. Parents or guardians may request to have a guest or expert present as well.

The evaluation must be sufficiently comprehensive so that all of the student's special education and related services needs are identified. *This evaluation is free to the family.* The team and parent determine what areas require evaluation; this may include academic achievement, functional performance, cognitive functioning, communication status, health, hearing and vision, motor abilities, and social/emotional status. The evaluation of a student's health status should only be done by a health professional, usually the school nurse. The nurse may also be asked to conduct screening of vision and hearing and to collect information from the parent regarding professional hearing and vision evaluations (Yonkaitis & Shannon, 2017).

Any materials used for testing must be nondiscriminatory, meaning that they must be racially and culturally appropriate and must be administered in a nondiscriminatory manner. Families often will provide testing results that have been completed by providers of their choice. Once parental consent has been given for evaluation, the school has 60 days to conduct the evaluation (§300.301). Under IDEA 2004, parents may petition for an independent educational evaluation at the school's expense if they can show that all avenues or evaluations were not used to determine how their child's disability affects learning [§300.502(b)].

Eligibility Determination

Once the comprehensive evaluation of the student has been conducted, the team, including the parent, will meet to discuss the findings and determine whether the student has a disability that is affecting learning under IDEA. For students with health concerns, it is imperative that the nurse be involved. Most often, the school nurse is the only school professional who can interpret medical records for the team, evaluate a student's specialized healthcare needs, and determine what related services may be necessary for the student to benefit from the educational program.

The team's job, under IDEA, is to determine whether the child's condition affects their ability to learn due to academic or functional concerns. This can mean that their condition makes it difficult to learn or that their condition often results in lost class time and in this way impacts their access to learning. Students who qualify for special education services under the other health impairment (OHI) category often experience a mix of these two concerns. In some cases, the evaluation may reveal that the health concern has such a significant impact on the learning and/or behavior that the child may qualify under a disability category other than OHI. For instance, attention deficit-hyperactivity disorder (ADHD) is one of the most frequent health conditions requiring student support with special education services (see Chapter 26). Students with ADHD may qualify as disabled under OHI, specific learning disability, or serious emotional disturbance.

If the evaluation shows that the student does, indeed, have a disability and that because of that disability needs special education, then the child meets the criteria for access to special education and related services. Although the degree of disability needed to meet criteria vary from state to state, this evaluation process enables a school team to discuss the impact of the child's disability on educational performance, identify their strengths and needs, and develop an appropriate individualized education program, for the student. As with the evaluation, the parent must agree to the finding and consent to the development of the IEP for the student. States and local educational agencies have not violated IDEA requirements and are not required to develop an IEP if the parents refuse to consent to special education. However, districts may choose to file due process if they believe that special education is in the child's best interest. A district may also choose not to accept the evaluation of the team or of the independent educational evaluation. In either case, the law spells out a due process protocol that gives families and schools the right to appeal the decisions.

The Individualized Education Program

Disability laws, including IDEA, mandate that all children with disabilities be afforded a free and appropriate education in the least restrictive environment (LRE). FAPE means that

Did You Know?

IDEA (2004) also requires school officials to provide equitable participation in programs carried out under IDEA for children with disabilities who attend private schools. The local education agency with jurisdiction over the district in which the private school is located is obligated to "locate, identify, evaluate, and spend a proportionate share of IDEA funds for equitable services for children with disabilities enrolled by their parents in private, including religious, elementary and secondary schools located in that district" (U.S. Department of Education, 2011, p. 2).

the special education services required for children to learn in school are provided at no cost to the parent. The individualized education program (IEP) is developed by the team and includes the accommodations and curriculum modifications that the student needs to learn. Student strengths and needs are addressed, and achievable goals are written. The IEP also includes what IDEA terms *related services:* those services that make it possible for the child to function in the educational environment of the public school (e.g., nursing care, transportation, etc.). LRE means that the education must be appropriate for the age of the child and should be in the same environment as the child's peers to the fullest extent possible. Every effort should be made to educate a student with disabilities in a regular classroom with supplementary aids and services. When this is not possible, the child should be educated in the next closest environment. See Figure 7-1. The further away from the typical education setting a placement is for a child in special education, the more restrictive the educational environment (Heward et al., 2022). During the process, team members must be aware of the child's and parents' federal civil rights, as well as the special education laws. All children have the following rights:

1. To advance appropriately toward attaining their annual goals
2. To be involved and progress in the general curriculum (e.g., the curriculum used by nondisabled students) and to participate in extracurricular and other nonacademic activities
3. To be educated and participate with other children with disabilities and nondisabled children [§614(d), (1), A. IV]

Developing the IEP

An IEP is required for all students older than 3 years who are eligible for the services of IDEA. It is developed after the IEP team meets and determines that the student has a disability under IDEA and the parent consents. The program is developed by the IEP team, which includes the parents and, depending on their age, the student. IDEA regulations define special education as "specially designed instruction to meet the unique needs of a student with a disability" (§300.39).

The plan should include the following:

1. The student's current level of performance with a statement of how the disability interferes with the child's ability to learn.
2. The strengths of the student and family.
3. Specific goals (short term and long term) to achieve, when they should be achieved, how they will be measured, and who is responsible for them.
4. A statement of the special education to be provided and that it be based on peer-reviewed research to the extent practical.
5. Any related services the student might need.
6. Any supplementary aids and services, program modifications, or other accommodations the student needs.
7. The extent to which the student will not participate with their nondisabled peers in the regular classroom.
8. A statement of any individualized accommodations that are necessary to measure the academic achievement and functional performance of the child on state- and district-wide assessments.
9. Long-range vocational goals and a transition-to-work/continuing education plan (postsecondary goals) by age 16 [§300.320(a)].

Box 7-3 presents an overview of a district's requirements under IDEA.

Each of these steps must be addressed by the IEP team in developing the plan. In addition to the need to provide required services for a student to learn, the district must include a plan to support a student on field trips and extracurricular activities. School nurses are critical to the planning, development, and implementation of appropriate, safe accommodations for students with healthcare needs so that they may participate in the same academic, nonacademic, and extracurricular activities as their peers (NASN, 2023). Once developed, the team and parents sign off on the plan. IDEA requires that the goals be reviewed at least annually, and a case review for eligibility is conducted every 3 years. If a student has difficulty mastering a goal that is set by the IEP team, the team must meet to review, evaluate, and revise the plan to accomplish the goal.

Provision of Related Services

Many interventions provided within the IEP fall under the category of related services. *Related services* refer to the interventions that help children with disabilities benefit from their special education. They are provided by a variety of specialties that assist the student in participating in the

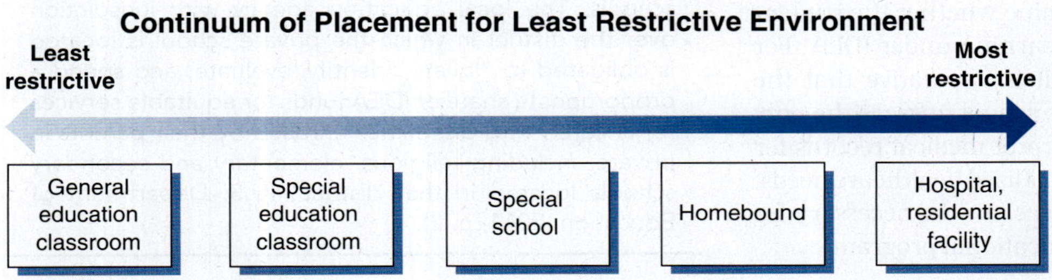

FIGURE 7-1. Continuum of placement for least restrictive environment.

BOX 7-3

District Requirements Under Individuals With Disabilities Education Improvement Act of 2004

Highlights of IDEA (2004) requirements for a school district include the following:

- Defining members of the IEP team—school personnel and parents
- Identifying all children with disabilities, birth through age 21
- Notifying parents of their rights to
  - Participate as a member of the IEP team
  - Approve evaluation and placement
  - Access all records on their child
  - Provide written consent for evaluation, placement, and reevaluation
  - Request an independent evaluation (approval by the district is not automatic)
- Evaluating a student with a multidisciplinary team of professionals knowledgeable in the area of a student's disability; an evaluation must include all areas of a student's unique needs
- Teams may use a process that determines whether a child responds to scientific, researched-based intervention as part of the evaluation of learning disabilities (referred to as Response to Intervention)
- Providing a free, appropriate public education in the LRE
- Preparing IEPs that address the specialized needs of each student, including long-range vocational goals
- Providing for at least an annual review of the IEP
- Developing mediation guidelines between parents and the school district
- Providing a full explanation of all of the procedural safeguards that relate to the presentation and resolution of complaints through due process complaint and state complaint procedures
- Developing disciplinary procedures for students with disabilities and the relationship of a behavior to a disability
- Monitoring by a state agency
- Ensuring that highly qualified teachers are working with the child; teachers must be fully certified in special education, have a bachelor's degree, and demonstrate knowledge of each subject for which they are the primary instructor
- Ensuring that states do not overidentify children with disabilities by race and ethnicity
- Prohibiting states from requiring parents to obtain prescription drugs for conditions, such as stimulant medications for attention deficit-hyperactivity disorder, as a condition of attending school, being evaluated, or receiving special education services

Source: IDEA (2004).

learning environment. According to IDEA, related services can include, but are not limited to, any of the following:

- Speech-language pathology and audiology services
- Interpreting services
- Psychological services
- Physical and occupational therapy
- Recreation, including therapeutic recreation
- Early identification and assessment of disabilities in children
- Counseling services, including rehabilitation counseling
- Orientation and mobility services
- Medical services for diagnostic or evaluation purposes (not for ongoing treatment)
- Transportation
- School nursing services and school health services
- Social work services
- Parent counseling and training (IDEA, 2004, §300.34)

The unique needs of each student determine which, if any, related services are needed and are then delineated in the IEP. School districts are compelled by IDEA to provide related services at no cost to the parent because they are a part of the support provided to the student with an IDEA-defined disability. In the case of students with a health concern, school health or nursing services are often needed. School health services are described in IDEA as "services provided by a qualified school nurse or other qualified person" (§300.34). IDEA describes qualifications for related services as those required by the individual state. Nursing services are usually defined by each state's nurse practice act, which also determines whether any of the services can be delegated to unlicensed individuals.

The school nurse is an integral part of the interprofessional student support team (NASN, 2023). The school nurse's role as the healthcare expert in the school setting is recognized by the American Academy of Pediatrics (2016) and in the language of ESSA (2015). When a student has a known or suspected health condition, the school nurse should be a member of the IEP team. Because it is nearly impossible to determine whether health is affecting learning without an evaluation, it is recommended that when an initial evaluation is conducted on any child suspected of having a disability, that a health evaluation be done (Yonkaitis & Shannon, 2017). Any student who is found to have a disability under OHI or who has a medical diagnosis should have the school nurse on the IEP team. The school nurse will interpret health-related information and assist the team in discerning how the information may impact learning. The nurse may also need to develop an IHP or emergency action plan (EAP). Districts are eligible for state, federal, and third-party reimbursements for the services provided through the IEP (see Chapter 32). Examples of school nursing–related services include gastrostomy tube feedings, suctioning, catheterizations, and medication administration and management.

Assistive technology is another related service. IDEA (2004) requires IEP teams to consider if assistive technology is needed by all children with disabilities based on their unique needs. IDEA defines assistive technology as "any item, piece of equipment, or product system, whether acquired commercially off the shelf, modified, or customized, that is used to increase, maintain, or improve functional capabilities of a child with disabilities" [§1401(1)]. For example, a recording pen for a child who has difficulty taking notes or an augmentative communication device to help a student speak are types of assistive technology. See Chapter 25 for further discussion of assistive technology.

Debate exists as to whether *service animals* are considered assistive devices. They can certainly enhance the child's capacity for functioning by opening doors, retrieving items, and assisting with mobility and are allowable by law to support individuals with disabilities under the ADA (U.S. Department of Justice, 2015). The ADA defines a service animal as "any guide dog, signal dog, or other animal individually trained to provide assistance to an individual with a disability." These animals perform a function that the individual with a disability cannot perform for themselves.

Emotional support, therapy, comfort, or companion animals are not considered service animals under ADA. Some state and local laws allow for emotional support animals, and thus the nurse must be aware of the laws in the school district. However, IDEA and Section 504 laws do allow for animals that do not meet the ADA definition of a service animal in school if the 504 or IEP team deems it is necessary to ensure FAPE for the student (Brennan & Nguyen, 2014).

Practice Connection

Fry v. Napoleon Community Schools

In 2017 the Supreme Court ruled on a procedural case regarding a kindergartener with cerebral palsy, "E. F.," and her service dog Wonder. The school determined that the service dog was excluded from school because the student's needs, as outlined in the IEP, were covered by assistance provided in school. The parents began due process against the school district which they later abandoned when they moved E. F. to a different school district. The parents then filed cases asserting ADA and Section 504 were violated (not IDEA) because the claim was not related to education (FAPE) but to her disability under ADA and Section 504. The case moved through the courts, each denying the parents' claim mainly because the parents had not met IDEA's "exhaustion clause," which requires the parents to move their claim through the IDEA due process system before any other. In *Fry v. Napoleon Community Schools* the Supreme Court ruled in favor of E. F., stating that it was appropriate for the ADA and Section 504 proceedings to proceed without exhausting IDEA due process and referred the case back to the lower court.

The Fry Court focused only on the substance of the complaint rather than giving educators guidance on the plain meaning of the IDEA's exhaustion requirement. A test that would have been more helpful from the Court would have been a test based on the plain language of the IDEA; for example, (1) What relief is the plaintiff seeking? (2) Is that relief available under the IDEA? Fry gave us answers to neither of these questions and did not give lower courts any useful guidance on the exhaustion requirement of the IDEA.

Takeaway: The Fry Court did little to assist lower courts in avoiding procedural challenges and statutory confusion. Despite the uncertainty of the courts on the intersection between federal laws and their requirements, parents and school districts have to continue analyzing under what circumstances students can be accompanied by their service animals in school.

Educational Placement Determination

Once the education services needed have been identified, the team makes a determination of where and how often the student will receive special education services. The number of minutes in and out of the general education setting will be delineated and the LRE will be identified. The team, including parents, must understand the evaluation results and individual needs of the student to thoughtfully determine the LRE. The "least restrictive environment" includes not only the setting but also the services that can be provided in that setting. The team decides which educational setting the student needs to be successful, starting with the general education setting (IRIS Center, 2019). For instance, a student should not be taught outside of the general education classroom if the curriculum can be adjusted to meet the student's learning needs in the classroom. The team should determine the LRE using a standard decision-making process that begins with the general education setting and answers the question, "Can the student be successful with special education and related services in this setting?" Determining whether an educational setting is the LRE to meet the student's needs is sometimes challenging, especially for students who have more profound needs that require intensive related services and equipment.

Did You Know?

If it is determined during the special education evaluation process that a child needs related services but not special education support, the child does not qualify for the services under IDEA. This child would be covered under Section 504 of the Rehabilitation Act and referred for the development of a Section 504 accommodation plan.

Therefore, some districts work together to form special education collaboratives to provide the needed special education services. Likewise, a child should not remain full time in the regular classroom if, despite all efforts, the child is not able to learn in that environment. Safety concerns, especially for students with fragile health or students who might be at risk of harm to self or others, must also be considered. Nevertheless, each student's IEP must allow for the student to be educated with typical peers as much as possible.

Charter schools that are in place specifically to meet the needs of children with special educational needs raise the question of whether these are the LRE, even though they may be a parent's first choice for the educational support provided to a child. In most cases, virtual schools are considered local education agencies (LEAs) and must adopt policies consistent with the state guidance as well as adhere to the standards set out in IDEA Part B, including Child Find, FAPE, proper evaluation, and IEP services (U.S. Department of Education, Office of Special Education Programs, 2016). Schools that exist in cyberspace as "virtual" schools bring to light the question of whether a school must have a physical location to provide the necessary services to a student, a subject that was also explored during school closures for COVID-19 (Marrapese et al., 2021). The success of these placements is mixed in terms of academic achievement reflected in standardized testing scores. One of the concerns about the placement of a student with a disability in a virtual school as a location is whether that school is able to provide appropriate supports for the child and parents and therefore adhere to the requirement of the IEP.

Transition Planning

IDEA mandates transition planning for all students with an IEP. It is important to assess the student's goals, interests, strengths, and desires when planning transition out of high school, whether through graduation or "aging out" at age 22. The law refers to transition services as "a results-oriented process that is focused on improving the academic and functional achievement of the child with a disability to facilitate the child's movement from school to post-school activities" [§300.43(a)]. The purpose of transition planning is to facilitate the transition of students from public school to college or vocational or rehabilitation services, including integrated employment, adult services, and independent living, and to define the financial responsibilities of each agency that provides these supports. IEP teams must begin the process of determining the answers to these questions and to have a plan in place by the time the student is 16 years of age, although some states require that the planning process begin at age 14 years.

It is essential for the student to be part of this process. Transition planning is a good time to assist students to understand the nature of their disability and the accommodations they need to be successful. Curriculum, coursework, and social skills should prepare the student for their next step. The IEP must document progress or the reason for lack of progress. Interagency collaboration is also a part of transition planning. State education agencies are charged with overseeing and coordinating a student's transition plan from school to vocational rehabilitation services; therefore, transition planning in the IEP must include the procedures for coordinating activities between the designated state agency and the school IEP/transition team. Note that a 504 plan can be used throughout life, whereas the IEP terminates at age 22. Therefore, for many youth with IEPs, it may be helpful to develop a 504 plan as they exit the educational system to take with them in their future endeavors.

Procedural Due Process

Due process refers to the rights of all parties to appeal any decision involving the evaluation process, planning, or implementation of measures or provision of FAPE for the child with a disability. Parents or guardians must have these rights explained to them so the process for resolving conflicts and disagreements is understandable. It is also a right that can be exercised by school districts and educators. Due process prevents significant changes to the IEP, such as change of educational placement of a student with a disability without following the process dictated in the law.

There is a 2-year statute of limitations to file due process complaints and a 90-day limit for appeals. The 2-year time limit for filing a complaint is measured from the time the person or the school system "knew or should have known" (§1414) that the child's needs (FAPE) were not being met. The goal is to ensure that students are having their academic needs met in a timely fashion and to ensure that parents are actively involved in their child's education. IDEA does allow exceptions to this requirement if the underlying issue has been resolved or if the local school system has acted in such a manner that parents are prevented from learning of the issue.

Before a due process hearing, the law requires a *resolution session* in an attempt to mediate the conflict between the two parties and come to a solution. A facilitator (neutral party) may be brought in to help both sides (§1415[e]2[f][B][i]). If mediation is unsuccessful, then a hearing is held which is much like a trial where both sides present their cases. A hearing officer is present and functions like a judge. Witnesses may be called to the hearing to give testimony. If indicated, the school nurse could be called and should bring all pertinent documentation. Hearing officers must focus on whether the child has been or is being denied an appropriate education rather than on procedural errors. Lawyers may be liable for filing complaints that courts deem frivolous.

Discipline

Many believe that students with disabilities are not subject to discipline. IDEA does not prohibit the disciplining of students with disabilities; however, it does include safeguards to ensure they are not arbitrarily removed from their educational program and denied FAPE due to their disability. Students with disabilities can be suspended or expelled for the following infractions at school, on school premises, or at a school function, if they

- Violate a school rule or code of conduct that is subject to disciplinary action
- Carry a weapon to (or possess a weapon at) school or a school function
- Knowingly possess or use illegal drugs or sell or solicit the sale of a controlled substance while at school or a school function
- Are substantially likely to injure themselves or others, if left in their current educational placement (§300.530)

To protect students with disabilities, IDEA includes a disciplinary procedure called **manifest determination review.** These reviews are used to determine whether or not the student's behavior that led to the breach of the student code of conduct is linked to his or her disability. It is important to note that IDEA does not require manifest determination meetings if the student is removed for fewer than 10 days and will return to the same education placement. Manifest determination meetings are required any time a change of education placement is desired following a disciplinary infraction.

The manifest determination review meeting is held and includes a school representative, the parent, and relevant members of the child's IEP team. The review meeting will determine either "yes," the conduct was related to the student's disability or the direct result of the school's failure to implement the student's IEP, or "no," the student's disability did not cause the conduct breach or was not the result of the school's failure to implement the IEP. When the finding is "yes," then the child is returned to the educational placement setting and consideration must be made for conducting a functional behavior assessment (FBA) and instituting a behavioral intervention plan (BIP). When the finding is "no," then the school has the ability to apply the same disciplinary procedures as they would to a student without a disability.

Positive Behavioral Support

IDEA (2004) renewed the commitment to provide positive behavioral support for students with disabilities. Any time behavior interferes with learning of the student with a disability or others, IDEA requires that the IEP team "consider the use of positive behavioral intervention and supports and other strategies to address behavior" (§300.324). Schools and IEP teams must be able to demonstrate that the appropriate assessment and intervention took place so as not to impede the student's FAPE. Often **behavioral intervention plans** (BIPs) serve as the legal document that help guide the implementation of behavior intervention strategies; at other times behavior goals within the IEP and associated behavior interventions and supports are sufficient. IDEA requires that schools provide functional behavior assessments and behavior intervention services under the following circumstances: (1) a student's behavior impedes their own or others' ability to learn; (2) behavioral goals in the IEP are not sufficient to address behavior problems; (3) prior or subsequent to a manifestation determination meeting; and (4) a student is placed involuntarily into a more restrictive placement because of behavior [§1414(d)(3)(B)(i)].

Courts have ruled on what constitutes the essential elements of a legally defensible and educationally meaningful behavior intervention plan (*Alex R. v. Forrestville Valley Community Unit School District*, 2004). The six key concepts of BIP planning are behavior functions, situational specificity, behavior change (environment and how to teach or prompt positive behavior), reinforcement tactics, reactive strategies, and team coordination and communication. The nurse on the team may be part of all six components, as well as help monitor the plan. IEP teams must be proactive with their positive behavior interventions and monitoring or decisions by due process officers and the courts will ensue.

As part of the IEP team, the school nurse may be involved in discussions about positive behavior interventions and how they will be evaluated. The school nurse's presence on the team will ensure that the student's healthcare needs are considered when behavior interventions or a behavioral intervention plan is developed and implemented. It will also allow the nurse to understand the student's behavior plan so that it is consistently applied when the student is seen by the school nurse in the health office. The nurse may be a daily participant in the care of students with behavioral problems, especially if they receive daily medication or specialized treatments. The school nurse should adhere to the BIP and can assess whether the behavior the student is exhibiting is consistent with the student's past behaviors, or whether it might be a symptom of disease, distress, or medication, and bring any concerns back to the intervention team. See Chapter 28 for further discussion on student behavior assessment and management.

IDEA Part C: Infants and Toddlers With Disabilities

IDEA Part C requires that infants and young children up to 3 years of age with disabilities be served through early childhood intervention (ECI) programs and permits states to spend up to 15% of federal special education funds on them. State-sponsored Child Find programs identify, evaluate, and provide assistance to families and their infants and toddlers up to age 3 who have disabilities or are at risk for experiencing a substantial developmental delay if services are not provided (§303.5). This is similar to the identification system in place for children and youth ages 3 through 21 under Part B of IDEA discussed earlier.

Once children are identified, parents are to be informed of the evaluation process and that their child may be eligible for special education services. Practitioners evaluate the infant or toddler for deficits or delays in physical, cognitive, communication, social or emotional, or adaptive development (IDEA, 2004). In an ECI program, healthcare practitioners, such as dietitians, nurses, and occupational and physical therapists, as well as speech-language pathologists, social workers, and teachers, conduct an evaluation and provide intervention services to the qualifying child with a disability and their family.

The initial evaluation of the child includes a functional assessment. This includes addressing the family's questions about enhancing their child's development and focusing on each family member's concerns and priorities. Only the information needed for the assessment should be collected, but these data should reflect a complete and accurate picture of the child's strengths, needs, and preferences for activities, materials, and environments. This assessment should be done in a setting familiar to the child, for example, at home, a childcare program, or an outdoor play area (Keilty, 2020).

Individualized Family Service Plan (IFSP)

Infants and toddlers younger than 3 years who are identified as having a disability are eligible for an IFSP under part C of IDEA. Children who are in environmental risk conditions such as homeless, extreme poverty, or abuse or neglect situations can also qualify for early intervention (Heward et al., 2022). The goal is to develop and ensure the implementation of a family-guided plan to enhance the child's development so that he or she is not at a disadvantage when it is time to enter the academic environment. Early intervention services are provided to address five developmental areas:

- Physical development
- Cognitive development
- Communication
- Social or emotional development
- Adaptive development

After the team identifies the outcomes, they assign responsibilities for each of the intervention services needed. Because the family is integral to the child's success, the goals also target the family. The location of services is the home and the natural environment of the community, including public and privately funded childcare centers. The plan needs to facilitate the family's capacity to enhance the child's development (§303.344). Whereas an IEP focuses on learning and school activities, the IFSP focuses on optimizing everyday routines and activities of the family.

The IFSP must be in writing and the family must be involved with the team in developing, implementing, and evaluating the services provided. The plan must be tailored to the specific concerns, priorities, and resources of the family. IFSPs are updated at 6-month intervals or more frequently if needed. As the child nears age 3 years, the plan must include the steps needed to support the child's transition to preschool or other appropriate services [§ 1436(d)(7)].

U.S. Department of Education rules require that non-Part C services needed by a child, such as medical and other services, also be described in the IFSP along with the funding sources for those services. The Early Childhood Intervention program is always the payer of last resort; in other words, if the services are covered under other payers such as public (Medicaid) or private insurance they would be billed first.

Toddlers with disabilities served by an IFSP must have a transition plan developed as they approach their 3rd birthday. If the lead agency believes the child will be eligible for services under IDEA Part B (an IEP), they must notify the local education agency at least 90 days before the child's 3rd birthday so that an evaluation can be conducted. With the parent's consent, an evaluation is performed by the local education agency to determine whether the child has a disability under Part B and is eligible for preschool services. If the lead agency or the local education agency finds that the child is no longer eligible for services and will "age out" of ECI, the team should identify other community services or programs for which the child may be eligible.

Funding Services Under IDEA

In 1975, Congress authorized state funding under IDEA at a rate of up to 40% of the excess cost of educating students in special education. This is based on the premise that a student with disabilities would likely cost about two times as much to educate as a student without a disability. Annual calculations are made, and money is disbursed. However, actual funding percentages are far less than the promised estimated excess cost and vary from state to state (11% to 23%). Special education advocates have introduced "full funding" bills to not only adjust the reimbursement formulas to make the promised 40% achievable but also to

Did You Know?

An IFSP must include the following:

- An assessment of the child's present level of development (physical, cognitive, communication, social, emotional, and adaptive)
- Statement of the family's resources, priorities, and concerns for the child
- A statement of measurable goals/outcomes
- An identification of the support services, programs, and equipment needed by the child and family to achieve those goals (may include preschool)
- The date services will begin
- Identification of the service coordinator
- Transition planning to address child's needs at age 3 (§ 303.344)

address a problem where states with *fewer* resources and *more* children with disabilities receive less money (Kolbe et al., 2022).

The IDEA mandate placed on schools to provide services so that all students can access an education is financially challenging to school districts. Budgets and staffing plans are carefully evaluated when meeting the requirements of IEPs. School nursing services can often generate reimbursement for the service provided it is listed in the student's IEP. Health services provided to students whose health coverage is provided by Medicaid are generally billable. However, each state sets its own rules regarding Medicaid coverage, and the school district must participate in the Medicaid billing program in order to receive funds. Private insurance carried by the student (through the parent) may be another source of reimbursement. District personnel cannot ask parents to use private insurance benefits toward the cost of school care if doing so would decrease the child's lifetime benefits under the insurance plan, if there is a deductible involved, or if the insurance premium would increase (§300.154). See Chapter 32.

SUPREME COURT DECISIONS THAT AFFECT STUDENTS WITH SPECIAL HEALTHCARE NEEDS

State and local education departments have not always agreed with parents on the services needed by their children. Some court cases in which parents have sued an education agency have progressed from local and state courts to the Supreme Court, especially as they and school districts sought further interpretation and clarification of special education and disability laws. When disagreements arise between parents and the school or the school district on eligibility for services and the services required for the child, the law provides a process for hearings at the district level, before state department of education hearing officers, and in the courts. At these due process hearings, both sides present their arguments for or against a program or service according to their interpretation of the law; then a judge or a group of judges makes a ruling.

Judicial rulings may modify, disagree with, or strengthen the law being tested. The subsequent rulings provide *precedent,* which is a previous judicial decision that is taken as a rule for subsequent, similar cases. When a parent requests a due process hearing in a district, the decision affects only that child and that district. An appeal to a state department of education hearing officer or to a state court becomes a precedent for similar cases in school districts in that state. Federal court rulings affect every school district in each state in that court's jurisdiction; a Supreme Court ruling becomes a precedent for every school in the United States. Figure 7-2.

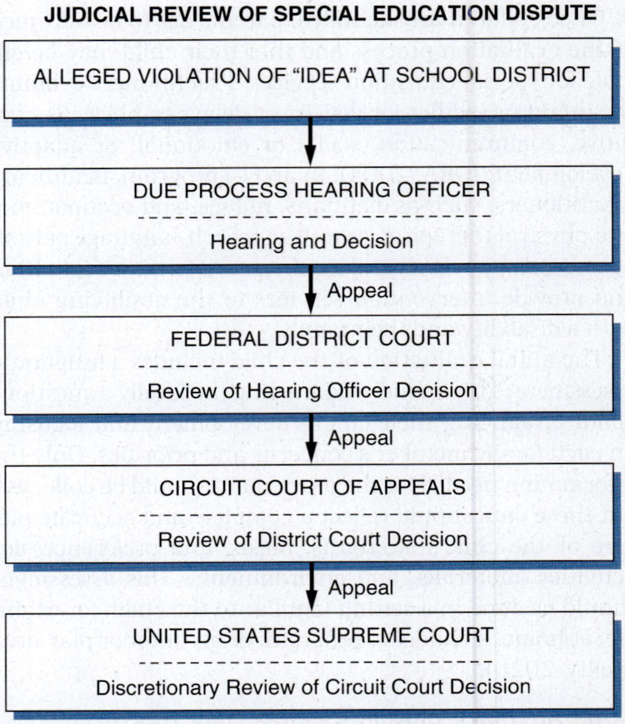

FIGURE 7-2. Judicial review of special education dispute.

As discussed earlier, a child with a disability who requires school health services or school nurse services in order to attend school and receive FAPE must be provided those services by their school at no cost to their parents. These services may be outlined in a child's IEP (governed by IDEA) or 504 plan (governed by Section 504). What follows is an overview of legal decisions that affect special education and related services.

The Rowley Decision

The Rowley decision (*Board of Education of the Hendrick Hudson Central School District v. Amy Rowley,* 1982) resulted in the Supreme Court defining what is meant by the term "related services" in special education. Amy, an 8-year-old student with a hearing impairment, was enrolled in a general education class and doing well. Her parents requested that an interpreter for the deaf be provided for Amy to assist her in school. The school district refused to pay for this service because Amy was achieving at an above average level in the general education setting. A lower court determined that Amy should have an interpreter. The district appealed to the Supreme Court, who agreed that Amy did not need an interpreter. They ruled that Amy's educational program complied with the substantive requirements of FAPE because she performed better than the average child in her class. The Supreme Court concluded that Amy's IEP offered an education equal to that provided to her nonhandicapped classmates. Based on this decision, school districts now determine the need for related services for a student using the "Rowley test." The justices' ruling limited related services to those interventions necessary for the student to learn.

Endrew F. v. Douglas County School District RE-1

The 2017 U.S. Supreme Court case of *Endrew F. ex rel. Joseph F. v. Douglas County School District RE-1* expanded beyond the Rowley decision to consider what a *free and appropriate education* is for students with disabilities educated in a special education setting (Rowley addressed a student educated in the general education setting). The parents of Endrew F., a child with autism, felt his academic and functional performance had stalled in fourth grade. His fifth-grade IEP offered no substantive changes. They withdrew Endrew F. from public school and enrolled him in a private, specialized school where he made significant progress. His parents filed an IDEA complaint with the Colorado Department of Education for the tuition cost of the private school. Their IDEA claim was denied by the Colorado Department of Education, the federal district court, and the Tenth Circuit Court of Appeals. Based on the Rowley precedent, the lower courts agreed that only a low level of academic achievement needed to be demonstrated for students receiving special education services, or in legal terms, that of "merely more than de minimis" (*Endrew F. v. Douglas County School District RE-1*, 2017, p. 992).

The Supreme Court elected to hear the case and they unanimously *rejected* the lower courts' decisions. The court found that "[t]o meet its substantive obligation under the IDEA, a school must offer an IEP reasonably calculated to enable a child to make progress appropriate in light of the child's circumstances." They also stated that "goals may differ, but every child should have the chance to meet challenging objectives" (*Endrew F. v. Douglas County School District RE-1*, 2017, pp. 9–16). The Supreme Court opinion reasoned that the Rowley decision applied "de minimis" to the standard of a general education classroom, not the special education setting. In Rowley, the student was making above average grades, and therefore the courts found she was not entitled to additional special education supports. In other words, the school only needed to provide what was needed to help her achieve passing grades in the general education setting. The Endrew F. ruling clarified that special care must be taken to provide students in special education settings every opportunity for success—whatever that might mean for them. The Supreme Court decision emphasized that the IEP, created by school experts and parents, must address the unique circumstances of the child. School authorities, in the event of a disagreement regarding progress, must be prepared to provide evidence that the IEP is "reasonably calculated to enable the child to make progress appropriate in light of his circumstances" (*Endrew F. v. Douglas County School District RE-1*, 2017, pp. 15–16).

A flood of clarifying litigation followed this decision, but the foundational requirement regarding the quality of the IEP stands as good law (Moran, 2020). However, IEP teams should consult school legal counsel to understand state-level court decisions that may affect the local interpretation of *Endrew F. v. Douglas County School District RE-1*. School nurses should note that for a student's IEP to provide FAPE, the IEP needs to be developed, implemented, and monitored to enable the student to make progress appropriate in light of their circumstances.

Irving Independent School District v. Tatro

The case of *Irving Independent School District v. Tatro* (1984) determined that school health services are a related service under IDEA. Amber Tatro was an 8-year-old student with spina bifida who attended special education classes in Irving Independent School District in Texas. District personnel had prepared an IEP that included speech and physical and occupational therapies, but they refused to provide clean intermittent catheterization every 3 to 4 hours because the district considered it a medical service not covered under IDEA. The parents cited the Education for All Handicapped Children Act (1975), arguing that urinary catheterization is included as a related service under the statutory definition.

In *Irving Independent School District v. Tatro* (1984), the lower courts went back and forth on whether catheterization should be covered, each time the case was appealed. Eventually, the case was heard by the Supreme Court. The Supreme Court cited U.S. Department of Education regulations defining "related services" to include school health services. This ruling made a clarification between those services that can only be provided by a physician and those that can be provided by a nurse. The court determined the definition of a "related service" includes nursing care, but does *not* include medical services, which are services that can *only* be provided by a physician. The Supreme Court established these criteria to determine what are considered required related services, sometimes called the "bright-line test" or the two-step test: a related service must be provided to students if (1) it will assist the student to benefit from special education *and* (2) the service does not have to be performed by a physician (*Irving Independent School District v. Tatro*, 1984).

A subcase in Tatro (*Irving Independent School District v. Tatro*, 1984) was a request by the parents that the district pay legal fees incurred over the 4-year legal contest. Section 504 of the Rehabilitation Act (1973) allows for recovery of attorney fees. The parents claimed discrimination by a program that receives federal funds under the Vocational Rehabilitation Act. The Texas District Court awarded compensatory damages and attorney fees to the parents. The Supreme Court Justices did not agree with the Texas District Court's judgment because the case was decided under the Education for all Handicapped Children Act (1975). Two years later, Congress passed the Handicapped Children's Protection Act (1986) to amend the Education for all Handicapped Children Act to allow parents or guardians to be reimbursed for reasonable legal costs if they prevail.

Cedar Rapids Community School District v. Garret F.

After the Tatro decision, a number of courts ruled that the definition of medical services should also consider complexity, cost, and burden of services to a school. That is, when health services were extremely expensive and complex, they were medical services under IDEA and therefore not the responsibility of the school district. Courts in several states held different opinions on the scope of allowable school health services and medical services (*Detsel v. Board of Education of Auburn Enlarged City School District*, 1987; *Macomb County Intermediate School District v. Joshua S.*, 1989).

The question presented in *Cedar Rapids Community School District v. Garret F.* (1999) was whether a public school district must provide nursing services during school hours for a student who was ventilator dependent. The lower courts agreed that ventilator care should be provided; however, the school district appealed. The Supreme Court found in favor of Garret F., asserting that IDEA covered health services and that included the complex health care a student needs to be able to learn. This decision affirmed the rights of students with complex medical problems to a free and appropriate education in the least restrictive environment.

The justices maintained that the IDEA (1990) definition of related services, the court decision in Tatro (*Irving Independent School District v. Tatro*, 1984), and the overall statutory scheme supported the decision of the lower courts in this case. The decision was based on law, not on the district's broad concerns for the financial burden of providing school health services to one student. The Supreme Court did acknowledge that the school district may have had legitimate concerns about the financial burden of providing the services Garret F. needed and the limit of existing staff; however, cost cannot be considered in determining a required service and this issue was outside the court's authority (*Cedar Rapids Community School District v. Garret F.*, 1999). See Box 7-4.

DISABILITY LAWS AND THEIR IMPACT ON THE PROVISION OF SCHOOL NURSING CARE

School nurses and administrators share a leadership role in fulfilling district obligations to all students, including those with complex health needs covered under IDEA, Section 504, or the ADA. The nurse or health services administrator is also responsible for designing the service delivery system, including staffing patterns, to maintain compliance with the law and with state nurse practice acts regarding delegation of nursing tasks. See Chapter 31.

BOX 7-4

Cedar Rapids Community School District v. Garret F.

Garret Frey, paralyzed in a motorcycle accident when he was 4 years old, was ventilator dependent. Garret required ventilator supervision, tracheotomy suctioning, repositioning every hour, assistance with eating, catheterization, and assessments for respiratory distress and autonomic hyperreflexia (an uncontrolled visceral reaction to anxiety or a full bladder resulting in increased blood pressure and heart rate, and flushing and sweating; *Cedar Rapids Community School District v. Garret F.*, 1999).

Garret successfully participated in a regular education class with assistance. He used a motorized wheelchair operated with a straw and a computer that responded to head movements. During his early school years, Garret's family provided his physical care during the school day through relatives or a licensed practical nurse whose fee was paid by medical insurance.

By middle school, the family requested the district provide a nurse for Garret; the district refused. The family brought their request to a state hearing officer, an administrative law judge (ALJ) at the Iowa State Department of Education. The ALJ determined that the district had to provide all the services the parents requested based on the Tatro bright-line test (*Irving Independent School District v. Tatro*, 1984), state law, and IDEA (1990), including provisions for nursing services for the student. The ALJ concluded that the district cared for other students with needs similar to Garret, except for ventilator dependency. Although Garret needed a greater amount of complicated healthcare services than other students in special education, none were medical procedures that could be provided only by a physician.

The district challenged the decision of the federal court and the court of appeals that agreed with the ALJ. The school district appealed to the Supreme Court on the basis that continuous one-on-one nursing service as a medical service was excluded under IDEA (1990). The Supreme Court reaffirmed its position from the Tatro case (1984) that Garret F. was entitled to "related services" that pertained to the safety and function of his ventilator and other functions, including care of the tracheostomy, suctioning, and assistance with eating and drinking to benefit from special education. Because Garret could not attend school without this one-on-one nursing support, denying him these services would deny him his right to a free and appropriate education in the least restrictive environment.

Source: *Cedar Rapids Community School District v. Garret F.*, 525 U.S. 66 (1999).

The Supreme Court decisions in Tatro (*Irving Independent School District v. Tatro*, 1984) and Garret F. (*Cedar Rapids Community School District v. Garret F.*, 1999) did not address nursing services from the parameters of any state's nursing licensing board. IDEA states that "qualifications of professional personnel serving special education students are consistent with any state-approved or state-recognized certification, licensing, registration, or other comparable requirements that apply to the professional discipline in which those personnel are providing special education or related services" [§300.156(b)]. The law also stipulates that unlicensed assistive personnel need to be appropriately trained and supervised, in accordance with state law, regulations, or written policy. State agency guidelines that address school health services for special healthcare needs may provide additional guidance in areas such as staffing requirements, infection control, medication administration, nursing procedures, classroom modifications, transportation, and policies.

School health and nursing services are varied and determined by the needs of the student and the model of care used in the school or district. School nurses need to not only understand the laws and court ruling but stay abreast of their responsibilities as outlined in *School Nursing: Scope and Standards of Practice* (NASN, 2022) and *The School Nursing Practice Framework* (NASN, 2024). See Chapter 3. Health services may include interpretation of medical records, assessment of the student's symptoms, health interventions, health appraisals, health education, emotional support, use of assistive health devices to compensate for the reduction or loss of a body function, case management, and advocacy. Students with special needs may require medication administration, chronic disease management, intermittent catheterization, tracheostomy care and suctioning, gastrostomy care and feedings, skin assessment, positioning, or equipment monitoring. They may have ventilators, central lines, or mobility technology that may require direct or indirect intervention.

School nurses must be able to clearly understand a student's needs so they may develop a plan and determine the credentials of the persons who may safely provide the care. The responsibilities of the school nurse for the student with a disability include the following:

- Assist in identifying students who may benefit from special education services
- Evaluate students' needs in collaboration with the school team
- Develop IHPs and emergency action plans as needed
- Recommend accommodations and modifications to remove barriers
- Train and supervise assistive personnel as allowed by law
- Provide in-service training on health conditions to teachers and staff
- Participate in transition planning
- Evaluate effectiveness of IHPs, IEPs, and Section 504 accommodation plans

Some students with disabilities may have additional special needs that do not require direct nursing care. In these situations, the school nurse may be requested to coordinate the care and support needed by the student. For example, a student with limited mobility may require a motorized wheelchair to attend school. In addition to monitoring the student for any health-related needs that might occur, the school nurse may be responsible for overseeing issues related to accessibility such as use of an elevator. The school nurse will need to consult with the parents, the healthcare provider, and perhaps a physical therapist to determine a plan of care. For these reasons, it is advisable for the nurse to have consultation minutes on the IEP or continue to be considered a member of the IEP or 504 team whenever a student with a disability has an underlying health condition that does not currently require direct nursing services (see Chapter 8).

CONCLUSION

Special education and educational accommodations have evolved over many decades through the diligent work of students, parents, educators, the court system, and state and federal governments. Terms used in the laws are confusing to the public and to health professionals, and the criteria differ from state to state; thus, the school nurse must understand the terms and concepts to be a cogent member of the team and be a strong advocate for the health needs of students.

The role of the school nurse is to maintain or improve optimum health of all students so that they can participate in their educational programs. Because students with special healthcare needs have unique health considerations, individualized nursing assessment, planning, and intervention are critical to identify appropriate placement and service decisions. Advocacy groups and school nurse leaders have paved the way for the inclusion of school nurses and school health services in the care of students with disabilities. The inclusion of the nurse as a member on 504 and IEP teams is imperative (NASN, 2023). Every school nurse needs to understand past and present legal issues in school health to prepare for the future and ensure that students receive health services needed for them to reach their educational potential. Only by understanding the laws can a school nurse truly be an advocate for the health and education of all children.

The editors gratefully acknowledge the work of the previous chapter author, Lee-Ann Halbert.

References

American Academy of Pediatrics, Council on School Health. (2016). Role of the school nurse in providing school health services. *Pediatrics, 137*(6). doi:10.1542/peds.2016-0852

Brennan, J., & Nguyen, V. (2014). Service animals and emotional support animals. *ADA National Network*. https://adata.org/publication/service-animals-booklet

Bush, G. H. W. (1990). Remarks on signing the Americans with Disabilities Act of 1990. *Public papers of the presidents of the United States, George Bush—Book 2.* Washington, DC: National Archives and Records Administration.

Clark, A. G., & Dockweiler, K. A. (2020). *Multi-tiered systems of support in elementary schools: The definitive guide to effective implementation and quality control.* Routledge.

Davis-Alldritt, L. (2024). Schools' legal responsibility for school health services. In C. A. Resha and V. A. Taliaferro (Eds.). *Legal resources for school health services* (2nd ed., pp. 233–253). SchoolNurse.com

Heward, W. L., Alber-Morgan, S. R., & Konrad, M. (2022). *Exceptional children: An introduction to special education* (12th ed.). Pearson.

IRIS Center. (2019). Information brief: Least restrictive environment (LRE). Peabody College, Vanderbilt University. https://iris.peabody.vanderbilt.edu/wp-content/uploads/pdf_info_briefs/IRIS_Least_Restrictive_Environment_InfoBrief_092519.pdf

Keilty, B. (2020). Assessing the home environment to promote infant-toddler learning within everyday family routines. *Young Exceptional Children, 23*(4), 199–211. https://doi-org.proxy.cc.uic.edu/10.1177/1096250619864076

Kolbe, T., Dhuey, E., & Doutre, S. M. (2022). Unequal & increasingly unfair: How federal policy creates disparities in special education funding. (EdWorkingPaper: 22-578.) https://doi.org/10.26300/ses4-a514

Marrapese, B., Gormley, J. M., & Deschene, K. (2021). Reimagining school nursing: Lessons learned from a virtual school nurse. *NASN School Nurse, 36*(4), 218–225. https://doi.org/10.1177/1942602X21996432

Moran, W. (2020). The IDEA demands more: A review of FAPE litigation after Endrew F. *N.Y.U. Journal of Legislation & Public Policy, 22*, 495.

National Association of School Nurses. (2022). *School nursing: Scope and standards of practice* (4th ed.). Author.

National Association of School Nurses. (2023). IDEIA and Section 504 teams: The school nurse as an essential team member. (Position statement.)

National Association of School Nurses. (2024). A contemporary framework update for today's school nursing landscape: Introducing the School Nursing Practice Framework. *NASN School Nurse, 39*(3), 140–147. https://www.doi.org/10.1177/1942602X241241092

National Association of School Psychologists. (2017). *ESSA and multi-tiered systems of support for school psychologists.* Author. https://www.nasponline.org/research-and-policy/policy-priorities/relevant-law/the-every-student-succeeds-act/essa-implementation-resources/essa-and-mtss-for-school-psychologists#:~:text5analysis%20and%20interpretation.-,Multitiered%20Systems%20of%20Support,needs%20of%20the%20school%20community

National Center for Education Statistics. (2018). *State education practices: Table 5.1. State-level accountability and reporting on Every Student Succeeds Act (ESSA) plans, by state: 2018.* https://nces.ed.gov/programs/statereform/tab5_1-2020.asp

National Center for Education Statistics. (2022). Students with disabilities. *Condition of Education.* U.S. Department of Education, Institute of Education Sciences. https://nces.ed.gov/programs/coe/indicator/cgg

National Center for Learning Disabilities. (n.d.) What is RTI? *RTI Action Network.* http://www.rtinetwork.org/learn/what/whatisrti

National Center for Learning Disabilities. (2018). *IDEA final regulations: Aligning IDEA and ESSA to support students with disabilities.* https://www.ncld.org/archives/action-center/what-we-ve-done/idea-final-regulations-aligning-idea-and-essa-to-support-students-with-disabilities

Office of Elementary & Secondary Education, Department of Education. (2020). *What is the Every Student Succeeds Act?* https://oese.ed.gov/families/essa/

Tracey, C.A., Antonetti, D. P., & Jaquays, J. (2024). Education law for children with disabilities: The Individuals with Disabilities Education Act (IDEA) and Section 504 of the Rehabilitation Act of 1973 (Section 504). In C. A. Resha & V. L. Taliaferro (Eds.). *Legal resources for school health services* (pp. 173–192). SchoolNurse.com

U.S. Department of Education. (2011). *The Individuals With Disabilities Education Act (IDEA): Provisions related to children with disabilities enrolled by their parents in private schools.* Washington DC: Author.

U.S. Department of Education, Office for Civil Rights. (n d.) *Reports and resources.* https://www2.ed.gov/about/offices/list/ocr/reports-resources.html

U.S. Department of Education, Office for Civil Rights. (2018). Civil rights data collection: 2017–2018. *Public use data file.* https://ocrdata.ed.gov/estimations/2017-2018

U.S. Department of Education, Office of Special Education Programs. (2016). *OSEP dear colleague letter regarding education of children with disabilities attending public virtual schools.* https://sites.ed.gov/idea/idea-files/osep-dear-colleague-letter-regarding-education-of-children-with-disabilities-attending-public-virtual-schools/

U.S. Department of Justice, Civil Right Division. (2015). *Frequently asked questions about service animals and the ADA.* https://www.ada.gov/regs2010/service_animal_qa.html

Yonkaitis, C. F., & Crespo, E. (2023). Legal issues 101: Students with disabilities. *NASN School Nurse, 38*(2), 71–74. https://doi.org/10.1177/1942602X221146756

Yonkaitis, C. F., & Shannon, R. A. (2017). The role of the school nurse in the special education process: Part I: Student identification and evaluation. *NASN School Nurse, 32*(3), 178–184. https://doi.orf/10.1177/1942602X17700677

Cases

Alex R. v. Forrestville Valley Community Unit School District #221, 375 F.3d 603 7th Cir (2004).

Board of Education of the Hendrick Hudson Central School District v. Amy Rowley, 458 U.S. 176 (1982).

Brown v. Board of Education of Topeka, 347 U.S. 483 (1954).

Cedar Rapids Community School District v. Garret F., 525 U.S. 66 (1999).

Detsel v. Board of Education Auburn Enlarged City School District, 820 F.2d 587 2d Cir (1987).

Endrew F. v. Douglas County School District RE-1, 580 U.S. (2017).

Fry v. Napoleon Community Schools, 580 U.S. 154 (2017).

Irving Independent School District. v. Tatro, 468 U.S. 883 (1984).

Jana K. v. Annville Cleona School District, 63 IDELR 278 M.D. Pa. (2014).

Macomb County Intermediate School District v. Joshua S., 715 F. Supp. 824 ED Mich. (1989).

Laws

Americans With Disabilities Act of 1990 (Pub. L. 110-325; reauthorized 2008). https://www.gpo.gov/fdsys/pkg/PLAW-110publ325/html/PLAW-110publ325.htm

Civil Rights Act of 1964 (Pub. L. 88-352). https://www.gpo.gov/fdsys/pkg/STATUTE-78/pdf/STATUTE-78-Pg241.pdf

Education for All Handicapped Children Act of 1975 (Pub. L. 94-142). https://www.govtrack.us/congress/bills/94/s6

Elementary and Secondary Education Act of 1965 (Pub. L. 89-10). https://www.gpo.gov/fdsys/pkg/STATUTE-79/pdf/STATUTE-79-Pg27.pdf

Every Student Succeeds Act of 2015 (Pub. L. 114-95). https://www.gpo.gov/fdsys/pkg/PLAW-114publ95/pdf/PLAW-114publ95.pdf

Handicapped Children's Protection Act of 1986 (Pub. L. 99-372). https://www.congress.gov/bill/99th-congress/senate-bill/415/text

Individuals With Disabilities Education Improvement Act of 2004 (Pub. L. 108-446). https://www.gpo.gov/fdsys/pkg/PLAW-108publ446/content-detail.html

No Child Left Behind Act of 2001 (Pub. L. 107-110). https://www.gpo.gov/fdsys/pkg/PLAW-107publ110/html/PLAW-107publ110.htm

Rehabilitation Act Amendments of 1992. (Pub L. 102-569). https://www.congress.gov/bill/102nd-congress/house-bill/5482

Vocational Rehabilitation Act of 1973 (Pub. L. 93-112). https://www.gpo.gov/fdsys/pkg/STATUTE-107/pdf/STATUTE-107-Pg718.pdf

Chapter 8

Health and Education Plans for Students With Special Healthcare Needs

Robin Adair Shannon ▪ Catherine F. Yonkaitis

CHAPTER OUTLINE

The 2019–2020 *National Survey of Children's Health* found that about 19.4% or almost 14.1 million children under 18 years of age have a special healthcare need (Maternal and Child Health Bureau [MCHB], 2022). These data translate into approximately 25% of U.S. households having one or more children with a special healthcare need. Children with special healthcare needs "are children who have or are at increased risk for chronic physical, developmental, behavioral, or emotional conditions." They also "require health and related services of a type or beyond that required by children generally" (MCHB, para. 1). Children and youth with special healthcare needs are a diverse group with at least one of the following needs expected to last for at least 12 months:

- Need or use of prescription medication(s)
- Elevated need or use of medical care, mental health, or education services
- Functional limitation(s) (that limit daily activity)
- Need or use of special therapies (e.g., physical, occupational, or speech therapy)
- Emotional, developmental, or behavioral problem for which treatment or counseling is needed (MCHB, para. 1)

See Figure 8-1 for percentages for types of special healthcare needs experienced by children in the United States.

Additionally, more than one-third of children and youth with special healthcare needs have experienced at least two adverse childhood experiences (ACEs) associated with poor health outcomes (see Chapter 11). Children with special healthcare needs are four times less likely to receive the care they need (e.g., medical, dental, vision, hearing, or mental health care) (MCHB, 2022). The care and support of these students and families

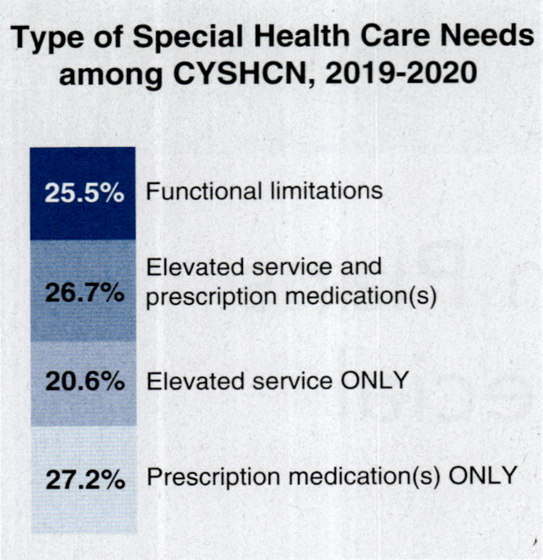

FIGURE 8-1. Type of special healthcare needs among children and youth with special healthcare needs 2019–2020. *(Maternal and Child Health Bureau, 2022, p. 2.)*

is complex and should be planned and provided by the school nurse.

Student health-related plans assist school nurses to provide quality health care in school, account for student safety, protect student rights, and reduce health barriers to learning. It is important to understand the professional, ethical, and legal foundations of student health plans and their impact on federally mandated education plans. The *School Nursing: Scope and Standards of Practice* (National Association of School Nurses [NASN], 2022) and the *School Nursing Practice Framework* (NASN, 2024) guide the school nurse's role in developing, implementing, and evaluating plans that promote student health in the educational setting (see Chapter 3).

As a member of the educational team, school nurses have a responsibility to understand the federal laws that outline the rights of students with disabilities (NASN, 2023b). Importantly, Section 504 of the Rehabilitation Act of 1973 (Pub. L. 93-112) protects against discrimination of students with disabilities by requiring access to the learning environment and mandating that reasonable accommodations be made to assist them in their educational endeavors. The Americans With Disabilities Amendment Act of 2008 (Pub. L. 110-325) further defined and expanded these rights. The Individuals With Disabilities Education Improvement Act (IDEA) of 2004 (Pub. L. 108-446) requires schools that receive federal funds to provide a **free and appropriate public education** (FAPE) to all students in the **least restrictive environment,** including those with disabilities. It also mandates that local education agencies have **Child Find** systems in place to identify children who need special education services. These civil rights laws, along with state laws and court rulings, dictate that children with disabilities must be provided with an education that meets their unique needs and promotes optimal levels of health and learning. See Chapter 7 for more information on laws protecting individuals with disabilities. The purpose of this chapter is to outline the core concepts of the school nurse's vital contributions to student-centered health and education plans.

PLANS FOR STUDENTS WITH SPECIAL HEALTHCARE NEEDS

Student health and education plans foster communication between the student's family, healthcare providers, and teachers and staff to support the student's learning at an optimal level of health. Written plans direct and document the school nurse's pivotal role in providing required care: teaching educational staff to foster safe and optimal learning environments, promoting student self-care, and supporting school health services. There are several types of plans that may benefit students with special healthcare needs: individualized healthcare plans, emergency action plans, Section 504 plans, individualized education programs, transition plans, behavioral intervention plans, and emergency evacuation plans.

Healthcare Plans

The care of students with special healthcare needs requires a comprehensive and systematic approach by the school nurse. The school nurse is the only school professional qualified to develop healthcare plans for students, specifically **individualized healthcare plans** (IHPs) and **emergency action plans** (EAPs; NASN, 2020). Medical management order plans written by licensed prescribers for students with diabetes, asthma, epilepsy, and other conditions need to be interpreted and translated by the school nurse for implementation in the educational setting. IHPs developed by the school nurse serve as the foundation for all school healthcare plans. They are nursing plans of care developed *by* school nurses *for* nurses in accordance with the nursing process, professional school nursing standards, and evidence-based practice (NASN, 2020). EAPs are developed by the school nurse to direct appropriate responses by lay school staff to students in acute situations.

Education Plans

Education plans, such as Section 504 plans and individualized education programs (IEPs), are developed through a multidisciplinary team approach. Education plans for eligible students are mandated by federal civil rights law according to Section 504 of the Rehabilitation Act of 1973 and the Individuals with Disabilities Education Improvement Act of 2004, more commonly called IDEA, the term we will use in this chapter when discussing the law (IDEA, 2004). Section 504 plans and IEPs are legal documents that accompany students across school, district, and state boundaries. Additionally, many states offer guidance related to the responsibilities of local school districts to implement these plans in compliance with federal law.

Section 504 plans protect students with disabilities from discrimination by ensuring *accommodations* that support student learning are implemented in the general curriculum and school environment (Office for Civil Rights [OCR], 2016). An IEP stipulates that special education and related services must be provided for students who need *modifications* for learning or specialized instruction. Remember that the "P" in IEP stands for *program*, not "plan" – a common mistake. Depending on the unique needs of the student, IEPs may include additional components such as behavioral intervention plans or transition plans. Although not responsible for their development, school nurses should also be familiar with **individual family service plans** (IFSPs). These plans outline services provided from birth to the third birthday for children with special needs before entering the public school system (IDEA, 2004). A comparison of the types of plans required for students is outlined in Table 8-1.

Confidentiality and Privacy of Student Health Information

Student health and education plans contain protected health information. The principles of confidentiality and privacy under the **Health and Insurance Portability**

TABLE 8-1 What Health or Education Plan Is Required?

Plan Type	Individualized Healthcare Plan (IHP)	Emergency Action Plan (EAP)	504	Individualized Education Program (IEP)
Student eligibility criteria	School nurse creates an IHP when a student has chronic or significant health needs that require ongoing direct or indirect care from the school nurse.	School nurse creates an EAP to direct specific actions by school staff to intervene for a student in the event of healthcare emergency or situation.	School nurse participates as a team member to develop a 504 Plan when the student has a mental or physical impairment that adversely impacts a major life activity.	School nurse participates as a team member to include health services in the IEP when a student requires specialized instruction.
Plan characteristics	School nurse creates IHP from assessment data and identifies nursing diagnoses, nursing interventions, and expected student outcomes. The IHP is stored as an electronic or hard copy file in the student's health record.	School nurse uses IHP information and medical orders to determine the treatment protocol for school staff to follow. The EAP is distributed to school staff who are responsible for the student.	504 Plan includes health accommodations, aids, and services to provide access to education. The IHP and EAP, when required, should be referenced as "on file in the health office."	The IEP includes specialized instruction, services, accommodations, supplementary aids, and modifications required for a student with a qualifying disability to ensure access and benefit from their IEP. The IEP allocates both direct and indirect health services as "related services." The IHP and EAP, when required, should be referenced as "on file in the health office."
Plan purpose	School nurse uses IHP information to inform the 504 or IEP team regarding student health needs. The IHP documents the nursing process and outlines health services provided at school. The IHP demonstrates compliance with the state nurse practice act and the *Standards of School Nursing Practice*.	The EAP provides other school staff with criteria to identify emergencies and directions to assist the student. The EAP demonstrates compliance with *Standards of School Nursing Practice*.	A 504 Plan provides access to education for students with disabilities. The 504 Plan demonstrates compliance with federal civil rights laws (Section 504) and ADA.	An IEP ensures access and provides a program for educational benefit. An IEP demonstrates compliance with education law (IDEA).

Sampson, C. H., & Will, S. I. (2017). IHP Basics and Using IHPs with Other Educational, Health and Home Care Agency Plans. (Table developed by S. Will & M. Strawhacker.) In S. I. Will, M. W. Arnold, & D. S. Zaiger (Eds.), *Individualized healthcare plans for the school nurse* (pp. 9–10). Forest Lake, MN: Sunrise River Press, with permission.

and Accountability Act (HIPAA) and the **Family Educational Rights and Privacy Act** (FERPA) must be respected (Centers for Disease Control and Prevention [CDC], 2022). When developing a health or education plan, it is often necessary to review student medical records. It is best practice to obtain signed consent from the parent/guardian when requesting medical records from a healthcare provider or covered entity. Under FERPA, it is prudent to obtain parent/guardian agreement before sharing relevant health information with those school personnel who have an educational interest in that information as it pertains to the student's health, safety, and learning.

Not all information collected by the school nurse needs to be shared with school staff, such as reports from healthcare providers and in-depth conversations with parents/guardians. The school nurse should discuss with the parent/guardian what health information they would like to remain private. However, it is helpful to emphasize that sharing educationally relevant health information helps the educational team comprehend the student's unique health and safety needs. For example, parents/guardians should be aware that the Section 504 plan health accommodations and EAPs will be shared with the educational staff responsible for implementing the actions outlined therein. The nurse should be sure the parents/guardians understand that any information shared is confidential and privacy is protected under FERPA to which all school staff must adhere (CDC, 2022).

APPLYING CORE NURSING CONCEPTS TO STUDENT-CENTERED PLANS

The Nursing Process and Standards of School Nursing Practice

The nursing process is defined by NASN (2022) as a

> *circular, continuous, and dynamic critical thinking process comprised of six steps that is client-centered, interpersonal, collaborative, and universally applicable. The six steps are assessment, diagnosis, outcomes identification, planning, implementation, and evaluation. The nursing process encompasses all significant actions taken by registered nurses and forms the foundation of professional nursing decision-making.* (p. 105)

Nurses may think of the nursing process as the background or canvas upon which the art and science of nursing occurs, an underlying and almost automatic approach inherent to nursing intuition. Expert nurses understand that the nursing process is far from linear or intuitive; it is a conscientious exercise that must be carefully considered and actively applied to all aspects of nursing care. As such, the nursing process lays the foundation for all school nurse health and education plans.

The *School Nursing: Scope and Standards of Practice* (NASN, 2022) outlines the nursing process, along with corresponding essential school nurse competencies that guide critical thinking, informed decision making, and evidence-based practice actions (see Chapter 3). The multi-directional dynamic between the constructs of the nursing process and the *Standards of Practice for School Nursing* and the *Standards of Professional Performance for School Nursing* (NASN, 2022) are depicted in Chapter 3, Figure 3-4. Operationalized at the individual student level, the nursing process and the principles of the *School Nursing Standards of Practice* lay the conceptual foundations upon which school nurses build individualized health and education plans for students with special healthcare needs.

Standardized Nursing Language

Standardized nursing language "describes nursing care with uniform, nursing specific terms, and to document and describe nursing interventions" (NASN, 2022, p. 108). The American Nurses Association (2018) supports the use of recognized standardized nursing languages, of which there are several. However, the use of standardized language in school nursing is inconsistent due to several barriers including too many options, high nurse workload, and lack of integration into existing electronic health record software (Office of the National Coordinator for Health Information Technology, 2017). Standardized nursing language has implications for the accurate recording of visits to the health office, communication within healthcare plans, as well as for data collection at the school, state, and national level. When creating a care plan, nurses often use the NANDA-International standardized definitions and taxonomy to compose a nursing diagnosis (Herdman et al., 2021). Such nursing diagnoses help to categorize an area of health concern which improves nursing communication and promotes safe care. See Chapter 5 for a review of standardized language and Box 5-1 for a list of accepted standardized languages, data sets, and universal codes.

INDIVIDUALIZED HEALTHCARE PLANS

Definition and Rationale

An *individualized healthcare plan* (IHP) is defined by NASN (2022) as follows:

> *The individual health plan (nursing plan of care) developed by the professional school nurse that translates student healthcare for the educational setting. The school nurse formulates the IHP in collaboration with the student, parent/guardian, healthcare providers and educational colleagues.* (p. 103)

The IHP is a nursing plan of care developed *by* school nurses *for* nurses and implemented for students with significant health conditions that require direct or indirect nursing services at school (NASN, 2020). An IHP is developed with input from the family, healthcare providers, and educators and combines all the healthcare needs of the student into one document (NASN, 2022). It sets priorities and provides continuity of care as the student progresses through the school system (Sampson & Will, 2017). IHPs are often put in place for students with chronic conditions but are also important for students with significant episodic conditions, such as pregnancy or recovery from physical trauma, or students with potentially life-threatening conditions such as severe allergies to foods, substances (e.g., latex), or insect stings.

IHP development is based on the nursing process and requires nursing judgment. Therefore, creating IHPs is uniquely within the scope of the professional registered school nurse. The school nurse develops each IHP based on the individual needs of the student, including the following:

- Current physical and mental health status
- Medical orders or management plans
- Developmental level
- Educational health accommodations
- Priorities and cultural preferences of the student and family

Although IHPs are nursing plans of care, they should be educationally relevant and aimed at optimizing student instructional time, self-care, and social well-being at school. The IHP informs other health and education plans that are shared with school personnel, such as emergency action plans, Section 504 plans, and IEPs.

The NASN (2020) position statement, *Individualized Healthcare Plans to Support School Health Services*, states that the school nurse

> *initiates and develops an Individualized Healthcare Plan (IHP) for students whose healthcare needs require more complex school nursing services ... It is the responsibility of the school nurse to annually evaluate the IHP, as well as to update the plan if deemed appropriate, to reflect changes in the student's healthcare needs and address nursing interventions and/or student healthcare outcomes. (p. 1)*

Purposes

The IHP details the school nurse-led case management that supports a student with special healthcare needs to attend school and be ready to learn (NASN, 2021). IHPs capture many important school nurse duties that may not otherwise be adequately reflected in health record documentation. The IHP provides legal documentation of evidence-based standards of safe care for students according to nurse practice act stipulations, administrative school code rules and regulations, and school district policies. No less than the minimum standard of care should be documented in the IHP (Galemore & Sheetz, 2015). IHPs have been used in legal proceedings as a standard by which to judge a nurse's conduct. If the appropriate standards of care are not demonstrated in the IHP or not adequately implemented, a school nurse may be at risk for liability (Johnson, 2024).

IHPs are the basis for developing the health portions of the student's Section 504 plan or IEP. The IHP is a dynamic document that may require regular updates as a student's health status changes. In contrast, Section 504 plans or IEPs are intended to cover 1 calendar year. Therefore, school nurses should reference rather than include the IHP in these education plans as evidence of the current care delivered by the school nurse.

When school nurse delegation of health tasks to unlicensed assistive personnel is indicated and allowed by a state's nurse practice act, the IHP outlines the responsibilities of the school nurse and the delegatees (see Chapter 31 for more information on delegation). For students requiring continuous personal nursing services during the school day, the IHP delineates care provided by classroom or contracted nurses in concert with case management services provided by the school nurse.

For school nurses who may be responsible for large caseloads, serve multiple buildings, or travel long distances between schools, IHPs assist in prioritizing interventions and planning for potential emergencies by reflecting the acuity of the students' needs. School nurses can employ IHPs to substantiate to school administration the scope of their professional accountability for the quality of care delivered to students with special healthcare needs (NASN, 2020).

Development

Only a registered nurse should determine whether a student's healthcare needs warrant an IHP. The development of an IHP requires nursing judgment and cannot be delegated to other school support professionals, licensed vocational or practical nurses, or unlicensed school assistive personnel. However, creating IHPs for every student with a health condition is not feasible or necessary. Priority for IHP development must be given to those students with physical or mental health conditions that may result in a health crisis, who receive significant health services at school, and for students with health conditions addressed in a Section 504 plan or IEP.

Focus on the Framework

Within the *School Nursing Practice Framework* (NASN, 2024), the IHP is foundational to the principle of **care coordination** for students with chronic health conditions: "The IHP includes prevention measures; required school-level accommodations; treatment and emergency response; consent for information sharing across sectors; and expectations for recording and communicating incidents to parents/caregivers, community-based healthcare providers, and other partners" (NASN, 2019b, p. 5).

> **Practice Connection**
>
> School nurses must keep in mind that the *I* in IHP stands for *individualized.* IHPs address the unique needs of the specific student, not their medical diagnoses. Although there might be valid examples or templates of IHPs for common health conditions, there is no such thing as a standardized "IHP for diabetes" or an "IHP for seizures." For example: Two students with Down syndrome in the same class may have very different health needs at school resulting in two very different IHPs; whereas a student with Down syndrome might have very similar health needs to a student with traumatic brain injury and thus very similar IHPs.

School nurses may employ different approaches, formats, and templates to write an IHP. Though the format school nurses use is a matter of preference, the nursing process is inherent in every IHP. Some formats outline each step: *assessment, nursing diagnosis, outcomes identification, planning, intervention,* and *evaluation.* Other approaches incorporate the concepts of the nursing process throughout the IHP. Many electronic school health record platforms have IHP templates with drop-down menus to assist in IHP development.

Assessment

Objective and subjective data collection is multifaceted and ongoing—including review of relevant medical and educational records, a health history and appraisal, observation of the student in the classroom and learning environment, as well as input from parents/guardians, teachers, and healthcare providers. Review of the available medical records at school may warrant obtaining parent/guardian consent to request further records or medical orders from healthcare providers. Results of current vision and hearing screening or reports on eye and ear evaluations are always included in objective data collection.

School nurses in the same district often use a standardized interview form to conduct a health history, but the collection of objective and subjective health data should be individualized and developmentally appropriate. Health status questions must be tailored to consider the student's developmental level and solicit answers that are descriptive. Vague answers require further inquiry. For example, if a parent/guardian responds that the stages of development were "normal"—what does that mean? Do their expectations align with typical developmental milestones? An interview about a preschool student should focus on very different questions than an interview for an elementary, middle school, or high school student. If a health history questionnaire is sent home, the school nurse should personally follow up on details. It is also important to inquire about the parent/guardian perceptions of the student's strengths and not just focus on their challenges. The school nurse communicates to the parent/guardian that a nursing physical assessment and review of systems will be conducted in the health office and atypical findings noted.

In addition, collecting information on perinatal, developmental, and physical and mental health history, the school nurse should inquire about environmental factors, past academic history or services, health and dental insurance, access to care, social determinants of health, eating and sleep habits, safety concerns, social connectedness, screen time and social media use, risk-taking behaviors, and exposure to trauma and adverse childhood experiences. The school nurse should review attendance records, keeping in mind that chronic absenteeism is defined as missing more than 10% of school days (days absent divided by the number of attendance days to date; NASN, 2023a). The school nurse should also ask about disciplinary issues. Students with learning or behavior issues should have elevated lead levels ruled out. Questions related to risk for harm or injury at home should be included in the assessment.

It is imperative that the school nurse personally assess the student in the health office and observe the student in the learning environment and social settings, such as the playground or lunchroom. The school nurse should appraise the student's developmental level and understanding of their health condition, as well as the student's capacity or readiness for self-care. When developmentally appropriate, the school nurse may ask the student many of the same questions asked during the parent/guardian interview. When assessing the student, the school nurse should observe carefully for alterations in physical functioning, behavior, academic engagement, and social interaction. A student may act quite differently in the busy milieu of the classroom than during one-on-one interactions with the school nurse in the confines of the health office. See Box 8-1 for a School Nursing Assessment Checklist for students with special healthcare needs. Also see Online Materials OM-S1 for this checklist in downloadable and fillable form.

Nursing Diagnosis

School nurses use critical thinking and nursing judgment to decipher key assessment findings to determine the

> **Did You Know?**
>
> The importance of assessing student safety cannot be overstated. Unintentional injuries are the number one cause of death in children ages 1 to 14 years old. When all children between 1 and 19 years of age are considered, firearm-related injuries become the leading cause of death. The rate of firearm-related deaths has risen nearly 30% from 2019. Drug overdose and poisoning were the third leading cause of death followed by cancer—the leading cause of death from disease in children (America's Health Rankings, 2023).

BOX 8-1

School Nursing Assessment Checklist: Students With Special Healthcare Needs

CONDUCT HEALTH HISTORY

- Parent/student interview and review of records
- Health concern, medical diagnosis, or disability
- Parent/guardian perception of student strengths and opportunities; needs at school
- Social history, parents/guardians, members of the household, support systems, cultural contexts
- Significant family and genetic health history; history of family learning issues
- Pregnancy, birth, and developmental history
- Significant illnesses, injuries, functional impairments, hospitalizations, surgeries, allergies, related treatments, procedures, and/or therapies
- Prior therapeutic or special services received in the home, facility, or at school; alternative therapies
- Behavioral, mental, or social health concerns

CURRENT HEALTH STATUS

- Request and/or review pertinent health records, compliance with physical examination and immunization requirements
- Healthcare access and utilization: insurance, primary and specialty care healthcare providers/contacts; care coordination
- Current medical orders (home and school); medical management plans, medications, special equipment/devices/technology, alternative medicines/therapies
- School nurse health appraisal: physical assessment, review of systems, height/weight/body mass index (BMI), current vision and hearing screening or evaluation, signs/symptoms
- Developmental assessment: cognitive, emotional, social, temperament
- Behavior and mental health concerns
- Health office visits
- Daily functioning and routines: mobility, nutrition, elimination, sleep hygiene, sensory issues
- Vision and hearing status/screening
- Past or current individualized healthcare plan (IHP)

SOCIAL AND CULTURAL CONTEXTS

- School attendance, loss of instructional time, disciplinary actions
- Family strengths/limitations/opportunities: perception of the child's health condition, support systems; health literacy
- Family experiences/perceptions/relationships with past and current health and educational systems
- School engagement and connectedness: friends, extracurricular involvement; exposure to violence/bullying/risk behaviors; social media and screen time
- Cultural and religious health practices and beliefs; alternative therapies
- Student capacity and readiness for self-care: motivation and challenges; decision-making and problem-solving skills
- Risk-taking behaviors; misuse of medications, use of recreational drugs and alcohol

CURRENT ACADEMIC AND SCHOOL FUNCTION

- Observation in the classroom/learning environment
- Consult with teachers, educational team, and other school staff as indicated: interprofessional collaboration
- School staff health literacy and understanding of student health condition
- School staff capacities/readiness to support student health needs
- Past and current student achievement and progress
- Past and current educational plans and services: Section 504, IEP, ECP, etc.
- School/classroom environmental barriers or modifications needed: safety, equipment needs; transportation
- Considerations of privacy, confidentiality, and dignity
- Interagency collaboration

appropriate nursing diagnoses based on the student's individualized needs. According to NANDA International:

> *A nursing diagnosis is a clinical judgment concerning a human response to health conditions/life processes, or a vulnerability for that response, by an individual, family, group or community. A nursing diagnosis provides the basis for selection of nursing interventions to achieve outcomes for which the nurse has accountability.* (2023, para. 1)

The school nurse should prioritize the nursing diagnoses with the highest priority placed on factors that impact student safety, followed by factors that pose health barriers to learning, and then on factors that are considered important to the student, family, and/or educational team. The school nurse should develop nursing diagnoses that can be reasonably addressed at school and will be supported by the student's family (Sampson & Will, 2017).

The nursing diagnosis is a problem statement that focuses on specific health problems, potential health risks, or health promotion strategies (NANDA International, 2023). Note that the nursing diagnosis is different from the student's medical diagnosis that relates to the pathology of the health problem. The nursing diagnosis relates to the student's real experience, potential response, ability to effectively cope with the medical diagnosis, and the educational requirements in the school setting.

The components of a nursing diagnosis include diagnosis label, definition, defining characteristics, risk factors, and related factors (NANDA International, 2023). The following are formats for writing nursing diagnosis statements (Ackley et al., 2021).

Problem-Focused Diagnosis

Problem-focused diagnosis related to (related factors) as evidenced by (defining characteristics).

Example of a student problem-focused diagnosis: Anxiety related to school attendance and academic progress as evidenced by frequent unexcused absences and difficulty completing assignments on time.

Risk Diagnosis

Risk for *(problem)* as evidenced by *(risk factors)*.

Note that no related factors are needed in risk-focused diagnoses as prevention of the potential problem is the goal.

Example of a student risk diagnosis: Risk for injury as evidenced by impulsivity and lack of awareness of environmental safety.

Health Promotion Diagnosis

Readiness for *(improved health outcome)* as evidenced by (defining characteristics).

Note that there is no need for a related factor in health promotion diagnoses.

Example of a student health promotion diagnosis: Readiness for enhanced control of diabetes as evidenced by expressed desire for improving self-care skills at school.

Outcomes Identification

It is important to identify outcomes before IHP interventions can be planned and implemented. Identified outcomes are typically stated in terms of long-range health goals to reach the identified outcome relevant to the school setting. Expected outcomes in an IHP are similar to student-centered health goals in an IEP discussed later in this chapter; outcomes should be evidence-based, relevant, feasible, and measurable. Outcomes are written in terms of what *the student* will do or accomplish within the next year. An example of an identified outcome for a middle school student with diabetes might be stated as follows: ***Increased Self-care:*** *By the end of the school year,* ***the student will*** *participate in 95% of instructional time secondary to adherence to scheduled self-care regimen for diabetes.* The identified outcome will be part of the evaluation criteria documented in the IHP.

Planning and Interventions

Next, the school nurse plans the interventions for the student with special healthcare needs. Nursing interventions should be evidence-based and individualized to the student's unique situation by considering the relevant information from the assessment phase. There may be several appropriate interventions for any given identified outcome.

Nursing interventions guide the school nurse's actions and what healthcare services will be provided for the student. The school nurse determines whether the interventions will be implemented by a registered nurse, a licensed practical or vocational nurse, a classroom or agency nurse, or delegated staff, if state nurse practice delegation rules permit. To continue the example of a middle school student with diabetes, one intervention to improve self-care skills to increase instructional time might read as follows: The school nurse will: *Provide learning opportunities for the student to demonstrate proper techniques for blood glucose monitoring, carbohydrate counting, and insulin administration according to the current diabetes management plan.*

While some interventions will invariably focus on the student directly, other interventions may target what the school nurse will do for the student indirectly. Such interventions include in-servicing school staff on the student's health condition or preparing them to support the student's needs regarding routine, urgent, or emergency care. The school nurse keeps in mind the entirety of the student's school day—including bus transportation, field trips, and after-school activities. The school nurse develops supportive documents as indicated, such as emergency action plans and emergency evacuation plans (discussed later in this chapter), fact sheets, or delegation skills checklists, and staff training materials.

Evaluation

Last, the school nurse evaluates whether the nursing diagnosis and identified student outcomes are appropriate and whether the planned interventions are effective. As with all components of the IHP, the evaluation criteria should be specific, relevant, feasible, and monitored closely. Remember that an IHP is a nursing plan of care written by nurses for nurses. It is not generally shared with lay school personnel, because it is written in nursing language and contains more protected student health information than most school staff have an educational interest in knowing. Therefore, sharing an IHP with lay school personnel is controversial but may be considered if unique circumstances compel. Input from the student's parent/guardian should inform the decision whether to share the IHP and with whom. IHPs should be kept in a password-protected electronic program or in a secure paper file in the health office. Box 8-2 is an example of an IHP for a student with diabetes. Note that the *Outcomes Identification* and *Evaluation* are in the same column in this example because the school nurse wants to monitor progress toward the desired outcomes.

As mentioned earlier, rather than attach an IHP to an education plan as a matter of course, it is best practice to refer to the student's IHP as on file in the health office. There are circumstances where IHP data are used to support administrative decisions by nonnursing supervisors regarding school nurse staffing and performance evaluations. In this case, student personal information could be de-identified. Decisions regarding the sharing of IHPs for students with chronic conditions who are vulnerable to stigma deserve special sensitivity, such as for HIV/AIDS or mental health. When in doubt, school nurses should refer to district policies and protocols and not hesitate to consult

BOX 8-2

Example (Partial) of an IHP for a Middle School Student With Diabetes

ASSESSMENT	NURSING DIAGNOSIS	PLANNING/INTERVENTIONS	OUTCOMES IDENTIFICATION/ EVALUATION
Student is a 7th grader diagnosed with type 1 diabetes 6 months ago. Parent does all diabetic care at home. Student has begun self-care skills for glucose monitoring, carb counting, and insulin administration.	Readiness for enhanced control of diabetes as evidenced by expressed desire for improving self-care skills at school.	The school nurse will provide learning opportunities for the student to demonstrate proper techniques for blood glucose monitoring, carbohydrate counting, and insulin administration according to current diabetes management plan.	By the end of the school year, the student will participate in 95% of instructional time secondary to adherence to scheduled self-care regimen for diabetes.

school nurse administrators, state school nurse consultants, school nursing experts, state school records regulations, or district legal counsel for guidance.

EMERGENCY ACTION PLANS

Many student health conditions have the potential to develop into urgent or emergent episodes requiring immediate response. However, a school nurse may not always be available immediately to provide care. Therefore, when a student's health condition has the potential to develop into a medical crisis, it is the school nurse's responsibility to develop an emergency action plan (EAP). An *emergency action plan* is a "child-specific guide/plan for school staff to facilitate quick and appropriate response for an individual student emergency" (NASN, 2022, p. 101). Note that the term emergency *action* plan is preferred, versus emergency *care* plan, because school personnel are responding to the student with *actions* and not providing nursing *care.* EAPs instruct select faculty and staff how to recognize a health crisis, what actions they must take immediately, and how to get the student under the care of qualified medical professionals quickly (Sampson & Will, 2017). Students with diabetes, asthma, anaphylaxis, seizures, blood disorders, hydrocephalus (ventriculoperitoneal shunts), cardiac disorders, hemophilia, sickle cell disease, adrenal insufficiency, and cardiac conditions are examples of serious health conditions that warrant an EAP.

The school nurse develops the EAP in congruence with medical orders, nursing assessment and judgment, and parent/guardian and student priorities and preferences. Unlike an IHP written in nursing language, an EAP is written in clear and succinct lay terms at a nominal reading and health literacy level. EAPs need to be easily understood by all school staff members who are directly or indirectly responsible for the student's well-being during the school day. Unfamiliar medical terms, acronyms, and nonessential information should be avoided.

Ideally, an EAP is one page and uses a simple format such as "IF YOU SEE THIS *(signs and symptoms),*" then "DO THIS: *(response actions)*." Depending on the health condition and the student's unique needs, the school nurse can organize the symptom recognition (IF YOU SEE THIS) and responses (DO THIS) into categories: NONURGENT, URGENT, and EMERGENCY. This triage strategy is helpful in the absence of a school nurse when lay personnel should take steps to prevent the episode from evolving into an emergency or recognizing a true emergency. Rescue medication, if ordered, must be quickly accessible for use. Emergency contact information should be included for at least two family members or caregivers who will be notified if the EAP is activated.

Careful consideration should be given to the disclosure of sensitive health information on an EAP, while still informing school staff to be alert to the student's risk of a life-threatening event. With parent/guardian consent, it is beneficial to attach a picture of the student at the top of the EAP so that the student can be easily recognized. All EAPs should be clearly labeled "CONFIDENTIAL."

The school nurse distributes the EAP to the appropriate individuals responsible for the student in any capacity, such as administrators, teachers, teaching assistants, office personnel, playground and cafeteria staff, coaches and extracurricular activity leaders, and transportation staff (bus drivers and monitors). Merely distributing the EAP is not sufficient; the school nurse is also responsible for training the recipients on the EAP actions. Group or individual training should be conducted at the initiation of an EAP, at least once a year (preferably at the start of each new school year), and when the EAP is revised. Prudent school nurses have recipients sign a form (either electronically or in hard copy) stating they have received the EAP and understand the actions and responsibilities. Box 8-3 is an EAP example for a student with sickle cell disease. See Online Materials OM 8-2 for a downloadable and fillable EAP template.

School staff must also be prepared to quickly assist students with no known diagnosis who unexpectedly experience a medical emergency at school. Many states mandate

BOX 8-3

Sample Emergency Action Plan (EAP) Student With Sickle Cell Disease

CONFIDENTIAL

Sample Emergency Action Plan (EAP) Student With Sickle Cell Disease

Student: ______________________ ID #: ____________ DOB: ___________

School: __________________ Grade/section: _____________ Date____________

Baseline status: _Student_ has sickle cell disease. Their typical symptom is throbbing pain in the hands, feet, arms, and/or legs. Pain can present anywhere in the body. DO NOT doubt the student. Symptoms can progress rapidly and may be life-threatening.

If (student name) develops symptoms: DO NOT doubt the student. Send the student to the health office, contact the school nurse, notify parent/guardian, and follow these steps.

IF YOU SEE THIS:	DO THIS:
NONURGENT/MILD SYMPTOMS ■ Minor localized pain in extremity ■ Minor injury ■ Feeling of something wrong ■ Tiredness, mild fatigue	■ Provide oral hydration (at least 4 to 8 oz/hr) ■ Allow to rest ■ Contact parent/guardian ■ Trained personnel to administer pain medication as ordered ■ Do NOT apply ice to painful areas ■ Observe and reassess frequently ■ Return to class if feeling better ■ Send home if pain persists or prohibits active learning
URGENT/MODERATE SYMPTOMS ■ Moderate fever ≥100°F (37.8°C) ■ Swelling/tenderness in extremity ■ Mild to moderate pain ■ Increased fatigue	■ Provide oral hydration (at least 4 to 8 oz/hr) ■ Allow to rest ■ Contact parent/guardian to transport student for medical care or home ■ Trained personnel to administer pain medication as ordered ■ Elevate affected extremity ■ Do not put ice on painful area ■ Observe student closely ■ Do not leave unattended
EMERGENCY/SEVERE SYMPTOMS ■ High fever ≥103.1°F (39.5°C) ■ Severe pain in extremities, back, chest, abdomen, or head ■ Seizure ■ Decrease in mental status/alertness ■ Difficulty talking or moving ■ Chest pain, shortness of breath, cough, turning blue ■ Swollen abdomen ■ Paleness, dizziness, fainting, or rapid heart rate ■ Loss of consciousness	**Call 911** ■ Support the student until emergency medical services take over ■ Administer emergency interventions if ordered/indicated (list) ■ Staff member to accompany student to hospital ■ Notify parent/guardian ■ Notify administrator

School Nurse _______________________Signature _______________Date _____

Parent/Guardian _____________________ Signature ______________Date _____

See Contact information attached.

Adapted from Shannon, R. A., & Holman, C. F. (2017). Sickle cell disease. In S. Will, M. J. Arnold, & D. S. Zaiger (Eds.). *Individualized healthcare plans for the school nurse* (pp. 899–914). North Branch, MN: Sunrise River Press, with permission.

general training for all school staff regarding the most prevalent conditions for which an immediate response may be needed, such as asthma, allergies, diabetes, and seizures. These trainings are often offered as online modules by third parties, or they may be provided by the school nurse. While protecting student privacy as much as possible, it is also the responsibility of the school nurse to provide general staff training when a student has a less common serious health condition that might present as a life-threatening emergency. Simple fact sheets without identifying student information about the conditions should be available to all school staff.

Emergency Evacuation Plans

An emergency evacuation plan should be developed for any student who needs extra assistance exiting the school building or campus in the event of a fire drill or other emergency evacuation event. These include students with limitations in physical, mental, or communication capacities, or who are dependent on medical supplies, technology, or electrical and mobility equipment. See Chapter 15 for more information on emergency and disaster preparedness in schools.

> **Practice Connection**
>
> School nurses can conduct classroom drills to practice emergency action and emergency evacuation plans. Walking through what to do in an emergency reinforces the steps to take if the school nurse is not present and prepares teachers and students to react as confidently and calmly as possible.

SECTION 504 PLANS

Civil Rights Protections

Section 504 of the Rehabilitation Act, the Americans With Disabilities Act Amendments of 2008 (ADAA), and the U.S. Department of Education Office for Civil Rights (2010) require all public educational agencies to protect the rights of students with disabilities to a *free and appropriate public education* (FAPE), including extracurricular activities. These laws and regulations protect students with disabilities from being discriminated against at school based on their disability. Schools that receive federal funds must provide aides, services, or accommodations needed for the student to have an *equitable* opportunity to participate in and benefit from the general curriculum and school programs. School districts must inform parents/guardians of these rights. Failure of school districts to comply with the intent of these civil laws may result in significant penalties (see Chapter 7).

The identification and assurance that students with a disability are receiving FAPE is outlined in a Section 504 plan. Any school or family member can refer a student for evaluation if they suspect the student has a disability as defined in the following. The school nurse has an essential role in the development of Section 504 plans for children with special healthcare needs who need support to obtain equitable access to the general curriculum (NASN, 2023b). Interestingly, although a written plan is not mandated by law, implementing accommodations is mandated. Therefore, it is standard practice that schools develop written Section 504 plans. These plans outline individualized student accommodations that ensure participation in learning and facilitate communication among all school staff regarding their responsibilities in implementing the plan.

Section 504 defines a student with a disability as one who

> *(1) has a physical or mental impairment that substantially limits a major life activity; (2) has a record of such an impairment; or (3) is regarded as having such an impairment.* [§705(9)(B), (20)(B); §12102(1)]

Physical or mental impairments are further defined by the U.S. Department of Education as any of the following [§104.3(j)(2)(i)]:

- Physiological disorder or condition
- Cosmetic disfigurement
- Anatomical loss affecting one or more of the following body systems: neurological; musculoskeletal; special sense organs; respiratory, including speech organs; cardiovascular; reproductive; digestive; genitourinary; hemic and lymphatic; skin; and endocrine
- Any mental or psychological disorder, such as mental retardation, organic brain syndrome, emotional or mental illness, and specific learning disabilities

Note that specific diagnoses are not included in the definitions of disability. The emphasis is on the impact on major life activities. The definition of major life activity includes, but is not limited to, the following [§12102(2)(A)]:

- Caring for oneself
- Performing manual tasks
- Seeing
- Hearing
- Eating
- Sleeping
- Walking
- Standing
- Lifting
- Bending
- Speaking
- Breathing
- Learning
- Reading
- Concentrating
- Thinking
- Communicating
- Working

Parent/guardian and educator guidance from the Office for Civil Rights states the following:

> *These lists, however, do not provide every possible major life activity or bodily function; therefore, if an activity or bodily function is not listed in the Amendments Act, it might still be considered a major life activity under Section 504.* (OCR, 2016, p. 5)

The law notes that having an impairment does not apply to impairments that are transitory and minor. These include impairments with an actual or expected duration of 6 months or less [§12102(3)(B)].

Students whose health conditions are in remission or whose treatment regimens are working well may be eligible for accommodations. The ADA states the following:

> *When determining if a person has a disability, a school cannot consider the ameliorative effects of* ***mitigating measures*** *when determining how the impairment impacts the major life activities under consideration. ... The Amendments Act provides a non-comprehensive list of mitigating measures: medications; prosthetic devices (for example, an artificial arm); assistive devices (for example, computer modifications that increase accessibility, wheelchairs, scooters, walkers, canes, and crutches); learned behavior; and adaptive neurological modifications that an individual may use to eliminate or reduce the effects of an impairment.* [OCR, 2016, p. 6; § 12102(4)(E)(i)]

For example, a school cannot consider the use of an asthma rescue inhaler when determining whether a child has a substantial limitation in major life functioning and therefore whether the child has a disability under Section 504.

Accommodations provide eligible students with equal opportunity assistance, such as adapted learning materials, assignments, or tests; transportation to and from school; elimination of physical barriers into or throughout the building; and nursing/health services during school hours and school-sponsored events, including after-school activities. Section 504 plan accommodations do not alter the curriculum the student must follow, but rather support the student's participation and success in learning

Did You Know?

Mitigating Measures

Ordinary eyeglasses and contact lenses are not considered mitigating measures. If a student is able to read typical size font with prescription glasses or contacts, they would not be considered disabled. Conversely, if a student has low vision and requires adaptive vision equipment (e.g., a computer program) to enlarge print because they cannot read typical size font with ordinary eyeglasses or contacts, then the school cannot consider the ameliorating effect of the adaptive vision equipment (mitigating measure). Therefore, the student would be considered to have a disability and is eligible for such accommodations in a Section 504 plan [§12102(4)(E)(i)].

the curriculum they would otherwise access if they did not have a disability that qualifies them for Section 504 plan accommodations.

It is important to note that Section 504 allows for "reasonable" accommodations at school—accommodations that allow students with disabilities to have fair opportunities to participate in learning and school activities (OCR, 2016). Accommodations should not be provided because a parent/guardian feels that the student would "do better" on a test or other academic measure. An accommodation of this sort would give a nondisabled student an unfair advantage; this is not the purpose of a Section 504 plan. Determining reasonable accommodations can be ethically and legally complicated and is a team decision, involving the parents/guardians and the student when developmentally appropriate.

Development

Anyone involved or invested in the education of the student may refer a student to be evaluated for a Section 504 plan. This includes but is not limited to staff, teachers, counselors, school support professionals, the individual student, the family, and—importantly—the school nurse. Parent/guardian consent for evaluation is required by Section 504. If parent/guardians refuse evaluation schools may use the due process to override the refusal (OCR, 2023). A Section 504 coordinator is designated by the school administrator to assemble the appropriate school personnel to form the student's Section 504 team. The school nurse should be a member of the 504 team for students with special healthcare needs.

The following components should be addressed in a Section 504 plan:

1. Description of the nature of the concern
2. Description of the basis for the determination of the disability or impairment
3. Description of how the disability or impairment affects major life activities
4. Description of supplementary aids, services, and accommodations needed
5. Review/reassessment date
6. The names/titles of the evaluation team and the name of the case manager
7. Types of services, aids, and accommodations, as well as the dates when services are initiated and terminated

The evaluation must be complete and accurate to assess the nature of the student's functional capacities at school. The evaluation of the student should not be limited solely to learning but must also consider alterations to any major life activities at school. If the student qualifies as having a disability, a Section 504 plan is developed.

For the school nurse, the evaluation phase of a Section 504 plan parallels that of IHP development described earlier in this chapter. The school nurse develops an IHP to form the basis of the Section 504 plan. Because the IHP is a nursing care plan written in standardized nursing language, the school nurse must translate the information into full sentences and lay terms that educational staff can understand for the Section 504 plan. Such accommodations might address loss of instructional time to visit the health office or the administration of prescribed medications and procedures. The Section 504 plan may indicate changes to the educational environment, such as measures to prevent allergic reactions, plans for evacuation for a student who uses a wheelchair, or provision of special diets. Section 504 plans also should include an EAP for a student with the potential for a health crisis (e.g., peanut allergy or type 1 diabetes). The school nurse is responsible for training school staff on health accommodations identified in a Section 504 plan. The more the educational team is involved in developing the health plan components of the student's Section 504 plan, the more likely they are to follow through.

The 504 team members collaborate to identify accommodations for classroom and school activities, such as alterations in homework assignments, due dates, group participation (classroom/small group), adaptive equipment (writing, computer, augmentative, or sensory access), schedules or routines, alternative transportation, and access to extracurricular activities. The school nurse shares the accommodations related to health that will benefit the student with the 504 team. The 504 plan is implemented once it is agreed on by the team, including by the parent/guardian. A system for continuous evaluation and periodic review is established according to state guidance and district policies. See Box 8-4 for an example of a Section 504 plan for a student with sickle cell disease. See Online Materials OM 8-3 for a sample Section 504 plan for a student with inflammatory bowel disease.

INDIVIDUALIZED EDUCATION PROGRAMS

IDEA (2004) mandates that public schools identify and evaluate children who potentially need special education services and provide those services to those who are eligible. Special education and related services provide *modified* instruction for eligible students who have not made adequate progress or who are not learning optimally in the general curriculum. As defined under IDEA (§300.34, para. 1):

> Related services *means transportation and such developmental, corrective, and other supportive services as are required to assist a child with a disability to benefit from special education, and includes speech-language pathology and audiology services, interpreting services, psychological services, physical and occupational therapy, recreation, including therapeutic recreation, early identification and assessment of disabilities in children, counseling services,*

BOX 8-4

Section 504 Plan for Student With Sickle Cell Disease

The principal will:

- Designate staff member to attend to student's delegated healthcare needs (in accordance with state laws and regulations) in absence of the school nurse.

The school nurse will:

- Train designated school personnel in healthcare tasks (as allowed by state nurse practice act and school administrative code rules and regulations).
- Provide school nurse–led case management services at school according to current medical orders and IHP.
- Develop the health-related components of the student's 504 plan and EAP according to current status, IHP, and medical orders (see current IHP and EAP on file).
- Train need-to-know school personnel to follow the EAP at the beginning of each school year, at least annually, or as changes in status or personnel warrant.

The staff will:

- Allow student shortened homework assignments due to chronic fatigue when requested.
- Not penalize student for late assignments due to pain vaso-occlusive episodes/crisis, complications, or absences due to SCD. A reasonable time for assignment completion will be agreed on among student, teacher, and parent/guardian.
- Permit student to self-modify activity level during physical education according to fatigue and comfort levels.
- Allow student to carry extra water bottle at all times with water, juice, or electrolyte drink to maintain adequate hydration to prevent symptoms.
- Allow student alternative indoor activities during recess on extreme weather days (define temperature parameters).
- Respect student's subjective complaints; requests to visit the health office will be honored.
- Allow student passes to nurse and rest time in the health office when fatigued.

Shannon, R. A., & Holman, C. F. (2017). Sickle cell disease. In S. Will, M. J. Arnold, & D. S. Zaiger (Eds.). *Individualized healthcare plans for the school nurse* (pp. 899–914). North Branch, MN: Sunrise River Press, with permission.

including rehabilitation counseling, orientation and mobility services, and medical services for diagnostic or evaluation purposes. Related services also include ***school health services and school nurse services****, social work services in schools, and parent counseling and training.*

See Chapter 7 for more information about IDEA law.

The school nurse has an important role to play as a member of the interdisciplinary education team, particularly for students with known health concerns (NASN, 2023b). School districts refer to their interdisciplinary professional teams by many different names. For the purposes of this discussion, the following terms will be used to refer to the "team": *student support services team* will be used before a student's qualification for special education; *IEP team* will be used after a student qualifies for special education. The special education process can be viewed as a series of steps. See Figure 8-2.

Child Find and Referral

The identification of students who would potentially benefit from special education services is conducted under the IDEA (2004) mandate called ***Child Find.*** Child Find is a public outreach awareness system to locate and identify children thought to be eligible for special education within the school district's jurisdiction. A public notice through various means (newspapers or other media) provides residents of the school district with information about young children with disabilities who may need special education services. Each state must have policies and procedures to ensure those children are identified and evaluated. The initial evaluation and any reevaluation should be done by those individuals described as qualified professionals (IDEA, 2004). The Child Find mandate to identify children in need of services continues once children are enrolled in school. There are several ways that school districts can identify students:

- Early intervention (EI) programs: identification of children in need of special services between the ages of birth and 5 years. The school nurse is often involved with early childhood assessments as a member of the multidisciplinary assessment team for children 3 to 5 years old.
- Response to intervention (RTI): a multitiered approach to assist students struggling with learning or behavior needs by providing evidence-based interventions to improve student achievement. If the child does not make sufficient progress under RTI, then the child should be evaluated for benefit from special education (IDEA, 2004; see Chapter 7).
- Referral by a parent/guardian, teacher, healthcare provider, school nurse, or any member of the student support services team: referral of any child through their 21st year for evaluation likely to benefit from special education.

Full and Individual Evaluation

After a child is referred to be evaluated for special education services, a *domain meeting,* sometimes called an assessment planning meeting or an initial meeting, is held to determine what categories (domains) need to be evaluated. The evaluation domains include the following:

- Academic achievement
- Functional performance
- Cognitive functioning
- Communication status
- Health
- Hearing and vision
- Motor abilities
- Social-emotional status

The team determines what information is available in each domain, what additional information is needed about the student's ability to perform in school, and which school professional is qualified to collect the needed data (IDEA, 2004).

Once the evaluation domains are identified, the parent/guardian must consent to proceed with the next step: the *full*

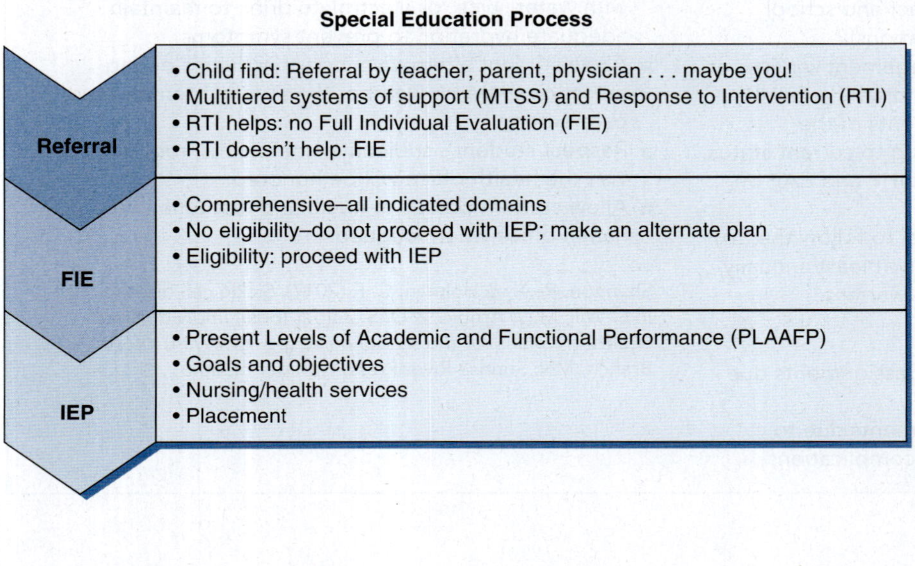

FIGURE 8-2. The special education process.

and individual evaluation (FIE). School districts are required to inform parents/guardians of their and their child's rights in the process as stipulated in the state's special education procedural safeguards. A comprehensive and nondiscriminatory evaluation of the indicated domains must be conducted by a qualified professional. The FIE must use a variety of assessment tools and measures and should be conducted in the child's primary language or mode of communication. Assessment measures must be valid, reproducible, considerate of cultural priorities, and racially unbiased (IDEA, 2004). The multidisciplinary team evaluation results are presented at the IEP eligibility meeting.

In several states, school nurses must hold specific qualifications/certifications to work in a school or to participate in the special education process. In these cases, an RN may conduct the initial assessment and collect data regarding the student's health needs. However, the credentialed school nurse interprets the assessment findings and makes educationally relevant recommendations for the school nursing/school health services.

To avoid delay in collecting pertinent student information for the FIE, it is prudent for the school nurse to obtain consent from the parent/guardian at the domain meeting to request medical records and communicate with treating healthcare providers as appropriate. While a medical diagnosis may indicate the need for a special education evaluation, it does not constitute reason enough for a student to qualify for special education services. The school nurse collects objective and subjective data: review of medical records, a health history interview with the parent/guardian, an observation of the student in the classroom/learning environment, and a nursing assessment of the student, including the student's perception of their health.

Following the collection of assessment data, the school nurse composes a report to be included in the FIE. The FIE school nurse report should be written in full sentences at common reading and health literacy levels for lay people to understand. IDEA (2004) explicitly states that the student's strengths should be emphasized. Medical terms should be explained, and abbreviations and acronyms should be avoided.

The FIE school nurse report should conclude with a concise summary statement of the student's special health care needs that highlights three key points:

1. What the student's health condition is
2. The impact of the health condition on functioning/learning
3. What school nursing/school health services the student receives or requires

A school nurse report summary statement that covers these three key points might read as follows:

> *Student (name) is an active fourth grade student who is struggling with reading and has a diagnoses of asthma. The student has missed significant instructional time due to asthma episodes this school year: absent 15% of school days and 3 to 4 health office visits per week on average for rescue inhaler administration by the school nurse. Asthma triggers include extremes in heat (hot/cold), strenuous exercise during recess or physical education, environmental allergies, and anxiety. The student receives school nurse-led case management services at school according to the current medical orders and individualized healthcare plan on file in the health office.*

Of course, not everything that a school nurse does for a student can be stated in the FIE due to the complexity of care and the frequently changing health status of many students. Remember that an IHP should capture case management activities, such as monitoring of health status; medication administration; serving as a liaison between school, home, and healthcare providers; emergency action plan development and staff training; and teaching asthma self-care (NASN, 2021). Referring to school nurse–led case management in the FIE summary statement is a sound strategy to reflect the comprehensive and holistic care the school nurse provides for the student.

Note that a well-written and concise school nurse summary statement is *not* a summary of the whole FIE school nurse report (which the reader just read). Also note that a well-written and concise school nurse summary statement will directly translate to the *statement of eligibility* for special education services and the *present levels of academic achievement and functional performance* (PLAAFP) in the IEP (discussed later in this chapter). All three statements should include the three key points outlined earlier. See Figure 8-3. See Online Materials OM 8-4 for a template of a school nurse FIE report.

Practice Connection

The School Nurse Is a Vital Member of the Student Support Services and IEP Teams

IDEA (2004) states that for the FIE: "The child is assessed in all areas related to the suspected disability, including, if appropriate, health, vision, hearing, social and emotional status, general intelligence, academic performance, communicative status, and motor abilities" [§300.304(c)(4)]. IDEA mandates that only qualified professionals with appropriate expertise in a given domain conduct the FIE and make educational recommendations for an IEP. School nurses (registered nurses [RNs]) are uniquely qualified to evaluate the health domain and make recommendations for the IEP regarding the health impact on learning and required nursing services. Keep in mind that the decision regarding whether health is an indicated domain requires nursing judgment. Unfortunately, it is common that school nurses are not fully included in the special education process, and other student support team members may be assigned to evaluate the student's health and make decisions regarding the level of nursing/health services. School nurses must advocate for their professional role in the special education process and their rightful position on the interdisciplinary professional teams under IDEA.

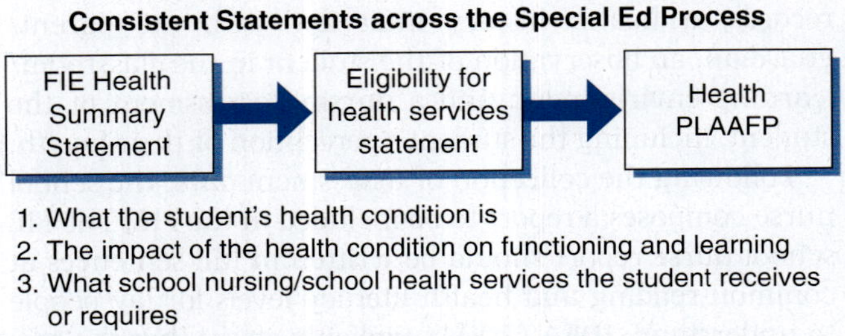

FIGURE 8-3. Consistent school nurse statements across the special education process.

The finalized FIE report with the collective domain evaluation findings from the professionals on the student support team should be shared with the parent/guardian in advance of the eligibility determination meeting, so they are prepared to ask questions and make informed decisions. Each state establishes the timeline and responsibilities for sharing these reports. For families whose primary language is other than English, IDEA is clear that parent/guardian participation must be considered including the "use of interpreters or other action, as appropriate" [§300.322(e)]. Although it does not directly discuss whether the FIE is to be translated, to honor the intent of IDEA, it is best practice to find appropriate means for translation of the report.

Eligibility Determination

Within 60 calendar days of the initial referral, an evaluation and determination of eligibility for special education services must be made (IDEA, 2004). The multidisciplinary student support team meets to review and discuss the FIE findings and determine whether the student is eligible for special education and related services. IDEA clearly defines the required members of the team:

- Parent/guardian of the child
- The child (as appropriate)
- Regular education teacher
- Special education teacher
- Representative of the public agency (school administrator)
- Individual who can interpret instructional implications of evaluation results
- Individuals with special expertise (as appropriate)
  - School nurse
  - Speech-language pathologist
  - Physical and/or occupational therapist
  - Social worker
  - Reading specialist
  - Hearing or vision itinerant teacher
  - School counselor

The team determines whether the student has a disability under one of the 13 disability categories under IDEA (2004, §300.8). See Box 8-5. Note that IDEA also provides the opportunity to use an age-limited eligibility category, *developmental delay* (DD), for children ages 3 to 9. This designation may be applied when a young child demonstrates significant lags in physical, cognitive, or behavioral development qualifies for special education services, thereby giving them a chance to catch up developmentally. However, if special education services are still needed at 9 years of age, then a new appropriate disability category is assigned.

BOX 8-5

IDEA 13 Disability Categories

1. Autism
2. Deafness
3. Deaf-blindness
4. Emotional disturbance
5. Hearing impairment
6. Intellectual disability
7. Multiple disabilities
8. Other health impairment
9. Specific learning disability
10. Speech or language impairment
11. Traumatic brain injury
12. Orthopedic impairment
13. Visual impairment (including blindness)

Developmental delay—special designation for children ages 3 to 9 years.

From *Individuals With Disabilities Education Improvement Act of 2004*, 20 U.S. C. § 1400 (2004). https://sites.ed.gov/idea/regs/b/a/300.8

The school professional responsible for each domain in the FIE recommends whether the student is eligible for special education or related services in that domain. For determination of eligibility in the health domain, the school nurse can directly transpose the FIE school nurse report summary statement (discussed earlier), highlighting three key points: (1) what the student's health condition is, (2) the impact of the health condition on functioning/learning, and (3) what school nursing/school health services the student receives or requires.

Determining eligibility is a serious matter. The decision whether a child needs special education services is one of consensus. Each team member's opinion needs to be heard. It cannot be overemphasized that the parents/guardians are fully participating members of the team whose voice must be respected. Keep in mind that students should be educated in the least restrictive environment and not be assigned services unnecessarily.

The team meets with the parent/guardian, discusses the evaluation findings, and in most cases comes to agreement as to whether the student does or does not have a disability under IDEA—and therefore is or is not eligible for special education services. Students with significant health conditions who do not qualify for special education and related services often have their needs met through

Section 504 plan accommodations or school nurse–led case management.

At times, the student support team is *not* unanimous in opinion about the eligibility determination, and a decision is not reached initially. Any team member can state disagreement with the consensus, the parent/guardian may need more time to decide, or the parent/guardian disagrees with the judgment of the school team. In such cases, a subsequent eligibility meeting needs to be convened. After a subsequent meeting(s), if the parents/guardians and the school are unable to reach agreement, the school district or the parent/guardian have the right to undergo a voluntary mediation process to try to resolve the issue (IDEA, 2004, §300.506). If the parties choose not to go through mediation, or it is not successful, either party has the right to file a ***due process complaint*** as outlined under IDEA (§300.506). Due process is a legal proceeding overseen by a hearing officer (§300.508). If either party is still not satisfied, the case can be moved to the court system to seek a resolution. Several court cases have set important precedents for a student's right to FAPE (see Chapter 7).

Eligibility for special education services must be redetermined every 3 years or sooner if there are significant changes in the student's status, if requested by the parent/guardian, or if required by a state's interpretation of IDEA. A 3-year reevaluation, or triennial evaluation, follows the same process as an initial FIE (IDEA, 2004, §300.303).

IEP Development

Once a student qualifies for special education services, the next step in the special education process (see Fig. 8-2) is the development of the individualized education program (IEP) by the special education team, including the parents/guardians as contributing members. The IEP meeting may take place immediately following the eligibility meeting, or it may be scheduled later—but eligible special education services must be initiated as soon as possible or as stipulated by state guidance.

In preparation for developing the IEP, team members should plan to describe the types of special education and related services that they recommend to benefit the student. Team members will frequently complete IEP forms or enter the proposed plans into an electronic IEP program before the meeting. However, it is a significant procedural error under IDEA [§1415(F)(3)(E)(ii)] if team members *predetermine* special education services without the meaningful participation of the parent/guardian. When tentative plans are entered into the IEP, the team must be open to options and amenable to revisions during the meeting. Effective IEP meetings require leadership, planning, and communication.

IDEA (2004) specifically mandates that the IEP include all of the following:

- The category in the definition under which the student is eligible
- A statement of the student's present level of academic achievement and functional performance (PLAAFP)
- A statement of measurable annual goals
- A statement of how goals will be measured and how progress reports will be made
- A statement of specific education and related services and supplementary aids to be provided
- A description of the extent to which the child will participate in regular education programs and a description of the program to be provided
- A description of the necessary accommodations needed to measure academic achievement and functional performance on state assessments and whether an alternate assessment will be used
- The projected dates for initiation of services and the anticipated duration of services

While the school nurse may play an important role in the development of an IEP for students who qualify for special education under *any* disability category, the school nurse should be involved in the process for students who qualify under the IDEA disability category of ***other health impairment*** (OHI). The definition of OHI is

> *limited strength, vitality, or alertness, including a heightened alertness to environmental stimuli that results in limited alertness with respect to the educational environment; that is due to chronic or acute health problems such as asthma, attention deficit disorder or attention deficit hyperactivity disorder, diabetes, epilepsy, a heart condition, hemophilia, lead poisoning, leukemia, nephritis, rheumatic fever, and sickle cell anemia; and that adversely affects a student's education performance and requires special education. [§300.8(c)(9)]*

Present Level of Academic Achievement and Functional Performance

The ***present level of academic achievement and functional performance*** (PLAAFP) statement is the starting point for the IEP. The PLAAFP statement is written concisely by the qualified related services professionals for each eligible domain. PLAAFP statements describe the student's level of academic achievement, including the student's strengths, challenges, and unique needs. PLAAFP statements also describe the student's functioning, such as the student's ability to participate in activities of daily living and/or self-care skills necessary for independence. This description of present levels provides the baseline data for the next step in the IEP, goal development (IRIS Center, 2019).

The school nurse writes the health PLAAFP. An effective strategy is to use the same or similar statement as in both the FIE school nurse report summary statement and the determination of eligibility statement (discussed earlier). The health PLAAFP should highlight three key points: (1) what the student's health condition is, (2) the impact of the health condition on functioning/learning, and (3) what school nursing/school health services the student receives or requires.

Annual Goals and Objectives

IDEA [§300.320(a)(2) (i-ii)] dictates that an IEP should include the following:

> *(i) A statement of measurable annual goals, including academic and functional goals designed to*
> *(A) Meet the child's needs that result from the child's disability to enable the child to be involved in and make progress in the general education curriculum; and*
> *(B) Meet each of the child's other educational needs that result from the child's disability;*
> *(ii) For children with disabilities who take alternate assessments aligned to alternate academic achievement standards, a description of benchmarks or short-term objectives*

An annual goal is a general statement describing the desired student-centered outcome that addresses the unique needs outlined in the PLAAFP. The IEP must contain documentation of how the goals will be evaluated and a schedule for determining achievement of the IEP goal(s) at least on an annual basis, or sooner if indicated [§300.320(a)(3)]. During this *annual review* process, the IEP team and the parent/guardian(s) assess the student's progress and update the IEP goals and objectives for the coming year.

Although IDEA mandates measurable IEP annual goals, IDEA does not dictate *how* they should be written or evaluated. Therefore, each state's department of education provides guidance for educators and school support personnel, as well as parents, on the IEP process and the development of annual goals. Further, IDEA only specifically requires short-term objectives for students who take alternate assessments [see IDEA (B)(ii) earlier in this chapter]. However, IEP guidance commonly stipulates that progress toward the annual goal should be measured by short-term benchmarks or objectives. It is incumbent upon school nurses to be knowledgeable about their state's IEP guidance. School nurses should develop student-centered goals and objectives for health/nursing services in parity with the other professionals responsible for related services.

The school nurse should bear in mind that the IEP is an *education* program, not a health plan: IEP health goals should be *educationally relevant* and connected to the state's health education learning standards. Goals are typically written as broad statements based on the student's unique needs outlined in the PLAAFP. Health goals are usually functional in nature. Annual goals are educationally relevant when they support a student's right to FAPE. Therefore, the school nurse should focus on the aim of the health/school nursing services provided—such as minimizing loss of instructional time, optimizing participation in the school day, or promoting self-care when developmentally appropriate. Following are two examples of language for student-centered health goals that can be individualized and applied in many cases:

- *By [Date 1 year from present], [Student Name] will experience minimal loss of instructional time secondary to signs and symptoms of [X diagnoses].*
- *By [Date 1 year from present], [Student name] will participate in their [X prescribed treatment] as a beginning step to self-care for [X diagnoses].*

Objectives outline the steps and structure for monitoring of the student's progress toward reaching the annual goal. Objectives should use student-first language and clearly state in quantifiable terms how the student is expected to make progress across the year toward the annual goal. An effective way to write objectives is to use the acronym SMART: *Specific, Measurable, Achievable, Relevant, and Time-bound* (CDC, 2017). SMART objectives are written with positive action words, such as *state, recognize, demonstrate, identify, describe, list.* SMART objectives avoid ambiguous terms that are difficult to measure such as *know, understand, learn,* or *appreciate.* A helpful analogy for goals and objectives is that of a global positioning system (GPS) application that provides directions to a location: the goal is the destination, and the objectives are the steps of the route that keep one from getting lost along the way.

Placement and Service Minutes

The next step is to identify the services guaranteed by the IEP and the amount of time required to deliver those services in terms of *service minutes.* In alignment with the PLAAFP, health/school nursing services include carrying out the student's medical orders and providing school nurse–led case management as outlined in the IHP (NASN, 2021). Careful consideration and documentation of the nursing service minutes are important in seeking Title XIX reimbursement for those students who are Medicaid eligible.

The school nurse should include time in minutes for all aspects of the student's care. It is important not to discount the time needed for consulting with parents/guardians, teachers, and healthcare providers, as well as for IHP and EAP plan development, and health record documentation. For example, although it may only take a few minutes for the nurse to give a student a daily medication, there are many nursing tasks related to medication administration (e.g., transcribing orders; monitoring for effectiveness and side effects; communicating with parent/guardians, teachers, and providers; tracking inventory; and documentation) that take time. A generally accepted time allotment for daily medication administration is 15 minutes. The school nurse should check with the district Medicaid administrator regarding whether billing is appropriate to capture reimbursement for services for Medicaid eligible students. See Chapter 32 for more information on Medicaid funding for schools.

In instances where a student does not require daily nursing services, the school nurse may delineate indirect care or *consult* minutes to allow for aspects of care under case management services, such as care plan development and monitoring of the student's health status. For instance, a student with seizures hopefully does not need the services of the nurse daily, but school nurse–led case management is very involved and should be reflected as consultation minutes.

IDEA (2004) states that *school nurse/school health services* are

> *designed to enable a child with a disability to receive FAPE as described in the child's IEP. School nurse services are services provided by a qualified school nurse. School health services are services that may be provided by either a qualified school nurse or other qualified person. [§1401(26)]*

Therefore, the service minutes should make clear *who* is delivering the services. Sometimes service minutes are divided between a team of nurses. For example, the school nurse serves as the case manager, but a building registered nurse or licensed vocational/practical nurse delivers direct care, or the student requires direct nursing care throughout the school day on an individual basis by a one-on-one or classroom nurse.

School nurses must be familiar with their state's nurse practice act delegation rules that stipulate if unlicensed assistive personnel (UAP) can perform related healthcare tasks for students and under what conditions (see Chapters 6 and 31). If allowed under the state nurse practice act, aspects of health services that might be delegated to UAP would be reflected in the IEP minutes as *health* services minutes, in addition to *nursing* service minutes performed by a nurse. An example of health service minutes might be when a health aide administers a routine medication. The nursing service minutes in this example would cover the school nurse–led case management activities such as time spent training and monitoring the UAP, creating an IHP, communicating with parents, consulting with teachers, and collaborating with providers. The school nurse should ensure that school nursing/health service minutes reflect health care and not time related to nonhealth care tasks or activities of daily living that do not require a nursing license, such as diaper changes or toileting.

The IEP team also determines the *placement* of the special education or related services in the least restrictive environment (LRE). Placement is a misnomer; it is better stated as the best environment for the student to reach their goals. Special education is a set of services; it is not a place. LRE means that students receive their education program with typical peers to the fullest extent possible. The prior steps of IEP development answered the questions regarding "what," "how," and "by whom" services will be provided. The placement step answers the questions of "where" and "when" the student will receive services.

The school nurse has a responsibility to understand the special education process and laws protecting the rights of students. Additionally, the school nurse needs to take a seat at the IEP table as the health expert in the school setting. The importance of the school nurse's role in helping parents/guardians and all the team members understand how the student's health concerns affect learning and their right to school nursing/health services cannot be overemphasized.

See Box 8-6 for a *School Nurse IEP Checklist for Students with Special Healthcare Needs.* Also see Online Materials OM 8-5 for this checklist in a downloadable and fillable form. See Box 8-7 for an example IEP case study for a student with attention deficit hyperactivity disorder (ADHD). See Online Materials for examples of IEP case studies for a student with bipolar disorder (OM 8-6) and a student with seizure disorder (OM8-7).

Early Intervention and Early Childhood Education Services

Each state has a responsibility under Child Find to identify children from birth through 21 years of age who may benefit from special education services. Eligible children from birth to age 3 receive services in the home or at a childcare or therapeutic center. Due to the emphasis on the home and family, an *individualized family service plan* (IFSP) is developed to address the service needs of children in this age group. Individualized family service plans outline the early intervention services that will support the child's development and will assist the family in supporting the child. A service coordinator is assigned to help the family coordinate the services noted in the IFSP.

IDEA (2004) Part C also requires that planning to transition a child from early intervention to early childhood special education services be initiated beginning no less than 3 months before their third birthday. School nurses should be a part of the district early childhood evaluation team. The child is evaluated for early childhood special education services and a meeting is held to determine whether the child is eligible. The team may find that the early intervention services have mitigated the developmental delay, and the child is performing at the appropriate developmental level. Therefore, not all children are found eligible for continued services or to be placed in an early childhood preschool program. However, if the child continues to have a delay or is significantly at risk, the child can qualify for continuing services. At this point, the child transitions from an IFSP to an IEP with services delivered in the school setting. The school nurse should also be aware that some 3- to 5-year-old children may receive single services such as speech and language therapy sessions at a school without attending the full early childhood program.

It is important to note that early intervention services are often more direct and intensive in the home, such as one-on-one occupational, physical, or speech therapy. Whereas for school-age children (3 through 21 years), the focus shifts from therapeutic services to educational services. While a student may still receive some direct therapy service minutes at school, most of the focus is on services in the group classroom setting. School nurses can be instrumental in supporting families and students to understand and navigate this progression. See Chapter 7 for more information on IFSPs.

Behavioral Intervention Plans

IDEA mandates that schools provide positive behavior supports for students with disabilities (§300.324) who display significant behavior problems. The school must conduct a **functional behavioral assessment** and

BOX 8-6

School Nurse IEP Checklist for Students With Special Healthcare Needs

Student's name ____________________

Date of Initial Meeting for Full and Individual Evaluation or 3-Year Reevaluation ________

Date of Eligibility and/or IEP Meeting ____________________

1) School nurse attends the initial Full and Individual Evaluation (FIE) domain meeting as a member of the Student Support Team.

COMPLETED (DATE) | **TASK**

- Briefly review and input student's health data prior to meeting
- The Student Support Team and parent/guardian discuss if an FIE is warranted
- Discuss if *Health* should be a domain of the FIE
- Parent/Guardian signs consent to FIE domains
- Health is an indicated domain
  - **NO:** Consider Section 504 plan accommodations and/or school nurse–led case management
  - **YES:** Obtain parent/guardian consent to obtain medical records. **Proceed to Step 2**

2) School nurse conducts the FIE assessment for the health domain.

COMPLETED (DATE) | **TASK**

Collect subjective and objective student health data:

- Request/review medical records and physicals
- Screen for lead risk and determine if blood lead testing is indicated
- Review attendance and disciplinary records (if any)
- Developmentally appropriate and individualized health history interview with parent/guardian using standardized form
- Observation of the student in the classroom/learning environment
- Health appraisal by the school nurse (height/weight/BMI, review of systems including mental health)
- Recent vision and hearing screening results or evaluation reports within 1 year or conduct needed screenings
- Teacher input
- If the student is transferring in from another district or undergoing a 3-year reevaluation: Review prior IEP records including FIE school nurse reports

Evaluate:

- Student strengths
- Student's health condition
- Impact of the health condition on functioning/learning
- Health/nursing services the student receives or requires (if any)

WRITE A CONCISE "FIE SCHOOL NURSE REPORT" *(SEE ONLINE MATERIALS OM 8-4 FOR DOWNLOADABLE TEMPLATE)*:

- Reason for referral
- Parent/guardian input and student strengths
- School attendance and current special services (if any)
- Family social history and household structure
- Significant family health and educational history
- Gestational and birth history
- Developmental history
- Past health history
- Current health status and school nurse health assessment
- Mental health or behavioral health concerns
- Observation in the classroom/learning environment
- *Compose School Nurse Summary Statement**: Conclude with a brief simple statement of
  1. Student's health condition
  2. Impact of the health condition on functioning/learning
  3. Health/nursing services the student receives or requires (if any)

*The *School Nurse Summary Statement* translates to the *Eligibility Statement* and the health *Present Levels of Academic Achievement and Functional Performance* (PLAAFP).

BOX 8-6

School Nurse IEP Checklist for Students With Special Healthcare Needs—cont'd

NOTE: The School Nurse Report is attached to the FIE (either hard copy or electronic platform). A copy of the team's full FIE is provided to the parent/guardian for review prior to the eligibility meeting.

3) **School nurse attends the *Eligibility* Meeting where Student Support Team determines if the student qualifies for special education and related services.**

COMPLETED (DATE) **TASK**

- Develop the school nurse/health services *Eligibility Statement* and briefly report:
  1. Student strengths
  2. Student's health condition
  3. Impact of the health condition on functioning/learning
  4. Health/nursing services the student requires (if any)
- Parent/guardian and Student Support Team discuss whether the student needs special education and school nursing/school health related services.
- If student is eligible for special education services: The Student Support Team and parent/guardian determine the IDEA disability category(ies):
- Parent/guardians consent to an IEP
  - NO and health is a concern: Consider Section 504 plan accommodations and/or school nurse–led case management.
  - YES: School Nurse participates in the IEP development.

4) **School nurse attends the *IEP Development Meeting* as a member of the IEP Team* and makes educationally relevant student-centered health recommendations.**

COMPLETED (DATE) **TASK**

Develop the health *Present Levels of Academic Achievement and Functional Performance* (PLAAFP)*:

1. Student strengths
2. Student's health condition
3. Impact of the health condition on functioning/learning
4. Health/nursing services the student requires (if any)

Develop student-centered health related goal(s):

- Develop student-centered health related goal(s) to achieve in 1 year.
- Develop *short-term objective(s)* for the health goal.
- State the criteria, procedure, and schedule for determining progress on the objective(s) to meet the goal.

5) **School nurse determines *Educational Services and Placement* with the IEP Team***

COMPLETED (DATE) **TASK**

Identify the school nursing and/or school health services the student requires to meet their health-related goal(s)

Identify the location where the services will be delivered in the *least restrictive environment*

Determine the amount of school nursing and/or school health service delivery *minutes* per week (or appropriate time period; e.g., monthly, per grading period, per semester)

6) **The school nurse develops health plans to support the student's IEP**

COMPLETED (DATE) **TASK**

Develop an *individualized healthcare plan* (IHP) that details the school nurse–led case management for the student's special healthcare needs.

- The IHP remains on file with the student's health record.

For students with potentially life-threatening conditions:

- Develop an *emergency action plan* (EAP) outlining how school staff should respond in the absence of a nurse.

For students who need significant assistance leaving the building:

- Develop an *Emergency Evacuation Plan*.

For students on a timeline to "age out" of special education services:

- The Student Support Team develops a *transition plan*.

Remember: Parent/guardians are integral members of the IEP team.

BOX 8-7

IEP Case Study Example for a 3rd-Grade Student With ADHD

IDEA DISABILITY CATEGORY: OTHER HEALTH IMPAIRED

FIE School Nurse Summary Statement: Student is a social 8 year-old with a diagnosis of ADHD. They have difficulty staying on task and completing assignments. Their teacher reports difficulties with math and reading and frequent displays of disruptive behavior in class. Student has medical orders for medication daily at home and at school to increase concentration and lesson distractibility. They require frequent reminders to visit the health office at lunchtime for medication. They receive school nurse–led case management services for ADHD at school according to current medical orders and individualized healthcare plan on file in the health office.

Determination of Eligibility Statement: Same as FIE summary statement. Disability category: other health impaired

Health PLAAFP: Same as eligibility statement.

Annual Goal* 1: *By (enter Annual review date), Student will experience minimal loss of instructional time secondary to signs and symptoms of ADHD.*

Objective†: *Student will, without adult prompting, come to the health office for daily medication 3/5 days in the first 90 days and 5/5 days by the end of the second 90 days.*

Annual Goal* 2: *By (enter Annual review date), student will demonstrate knowledge of ADHD symptoms and treatment.*

Objective†: Student will name three potential symptoms of ADHD or effects/side effects of ADHD medication at least once a week with 70% accuracy in the 1st quarter, 80% in 2nd quarter, 90% in the 3rd quarter, 100% accuracy in the 4th quarter.

Evaluation and reporting criteria: The student gets to place a sticker on a calendar chart when they meet the objective. Send calendar sticker chart home weekly.

Nursing Service Minutes: School nurse–led case management services for ADHD according to current medical orders and individualized healthcare plan on file in the health office.

Minutes: 15 minutes × 5 days per week = 75 minutes per week

Evaluation: EHR documentation and weekly sticker chart

Reporting: Parent/guardian phone or text contact as needed. Sticker chart sent home weekly.

*Goals and objectives are always based on the unique needs of the individual student: there is no one correct way to write IEP goals and objectives. Goals are target benchmarks for 1 year.

†Objectives should be SMART: (S)pecific, (M)easurable, (A)chievable, (R)elevent, (T)ime-bound. The SMART acronym is intended as a self-check and does not belong in an actual IEP.

institute a **behavioral intervention plan** when the behavior of a student with a Section 504 plan or an IEP significantly affects their ability or the ability of others to learn and participate in the school day (Office of Special Education and Rehabilitative Services, 2022). Behavioral intervention plans (often referred to as BIPs) are also required for students with disabilities who face serious disciplinary actions, such as expulsion or an involuntary change in placement to a different educational setting. Behavioral intervention plans are formal written plans that detail behavioral goals and intervention strategies to reduce barriers to learning and promote student well-being. In essence, behavioral intervention plans should address what the problem behavior is, why it occurs, and strategies to ameliorate the behaviors at school. See Chapters 7 and 28 for more information on behavioral intervention plans.

Transition Planning Within the IEP

The school nurse is an essential multidisciplinary team member that provides care coordination and planning for student with special healthcare needs as they experience a whole host of transitions throughout their school years. Indeed, transition planning is an essential nursing skill (NASN, 2019a). However, the term **transition planning** is specifically outlined in IDEA for students with disabilities. IDEA (2004) requires that all students aged 16 and older who receive special education have transition planning in their IEP before the student graduates or "ages out" on their 22nd birthday, or longer per state policy, to prepare for independence and success in adulthood. States can mandate that transition planning begins as early as 14 years of age. States may require this earlier age to allow adequate time to incorporate transition planning into the IEP and establish achievable transition goals. However, research shows that the majority of families do not have plans to meet their student's future healthcare needs (Anderson et al., 2011).

Transition skills are important steppingstones to allow students to reach their individualized goals related to employment, higher education, and adulthood as independently as possible. According to IDEA (2004), successful transition planning includes the following:

> *(1) Appropriate measurable postsecondary goals based upon age-appropriate transition assessments related to training, education, employment, and, where appropriate, independent living skills; and*
> *(2) The transition services (including courses of study) needed to assist the child in reaching those goals.* [§ 300.320 (b)1]

Transition planning is a collaborative process. The student, family, and outside agencies—such as vocational rehabilitation programs and healthcare providers—should be actively involved with the school team in transition planning (Office of Special Education and Rehabilitative Services, 2020). The process of transition planning should be outcome oriented and guided by the principle of self-determination to facilitate the student's move into adulthood. The key to successful transition is knowing the student's strengths, preferences, and interests. School nurses should be familiar with steps in transition planning. According to the Office of Special Education and Rehabilitative Services (2020, p. 22), when transition planning, schools should do the following:

1. Invite the student.
2. Administer age-appropriate transition services.
3. Determine needs, interest, preferences, and strengths.
4. Develop postsecondary goals.
5. Create annual (IEP) goals consistent with postsecondary goals.
6. Determine transition services, including course of study needed to assist the student in reaching those goals.
7. Consult other agencies, in particular, the vocational rehabilitation agency.
8. Update annually.

In many states, adult programs for individuals with significant disabilities are limited and often underfunded. It is vital that the school social worker collaborates with social services agencies to determine what resources and funding will be available in adulthood, such as insurance coverage, employment or higher education, housing, and other government disability services and assistance programs such as Supplemental Security Income.

Additionally, less than half of all students with special healthcare needs have adequate healthcare transition planning by their providers (Davis et al., 2014). The school nurse, as a member of the school team, should work with students and healthcare providers to create a plan that includes how the student will transition to adult health care and achieve the highest level of self-care possible.

DIFFERENCES BETWEEN A SECTION 504 PLAN AND AN IEP

Section 504 plans and IEPs are needed for different circumstances. However, there is often confusion about whether a Section 504 plan or an IEP is indicated for a student with special healthcare needs. Though the law does not preclude students from having both plans, in practical terms, students qualify for either a Section 504 plan or an IEP—not both (U.S. Department of Health and Human Services & U.S. Department of Education, 2015). To clarify:

- A Section 504 plan is indicated when a student is able to learn within the general curriculum but needs *accommodations* to protect against discrimination based on the disability. Section 504 plans promote an equitable opportunity for academic achievement. Schools do not receive federal or state funding to implement Section 504 plans.
- An IEP is indicated when a student is eligible for special education under one or more of the 13 disability categories specific to IDEA (2004). The student requires *modifications* to the curriculum to meet unique learning needs through special education and related services. Schools receive federal and state funding under IDEA (2004) to support special education services.

For comparison, consider examples of two students with osteogenesis imperfecta (OI). Remember that the school nurse would develop an IHP and an EAP for any student with OI. The first student has a mild form of OI (type I) and is an average student able to learn within the general curriculum. However, the student needs physical education restrictions, environmental safety protections to prevent fractures, and extended time to complete assignments when recovering from fractures. The student's OI causes impairments in major life activities, which qualifies the student for a Section 504 plan. The school does not receive any federal or state reimbursement for these accommodations.

The second student has a more severe form of OI (type III). The student fractures easily, has severe bone deformities and significant hearing loss, and is more than one grade behind in the general curriculum. This student requires specialized instruction, hearing aids, a wheelchair, adaptive equipment, and complex therapeutic regimens (e.g., occupational and physical therapy, mobility, and hearing services). The student's condition needs close monitoring by the school nurse. In this instance, the student's condition fits the IDEA disability category of orthopedic impairment, thus qualifying the student for an IEP. These special education services are supported in part with federal funds.

CONCLUSION

School nurses are responsible for assisting students with special healthcare needs to manage their health conditions at an optimal level of wellness so that they can learn and be successful in school. School nurses are uniquely qualified to provide an interpretation of the impact of a health status on learning and contribute to the development and implementation of quality health and educational plans (NASN, 2023b).

> *It is the position of the National Association of School Nurses (NASN) that the registered professional school nurse (hereinafter referred to as a school nurse) is an essential member of a multidisciplinary education team that identifies, evaluates, and monitors students who may be eligible for services through the Individuals with Disabilities Education Improvement Act (IDEIA) (2004) or Section 504 of the Rehabilitation Act of 1973.* (NASN, 2023b, para. 1)

School nurses strive to promote the development of students with special healthcare needs toward maximal independence by being knowledgeable about all aspects of a student's disability and treatment while empowering students to advocate for themselves. In collaboration with student support and educational teams, healthcare providers, students, families, and school nurses advocate for the civil rights of all students to have equitable opportunities for academic success and physical, social, and emotional well-being at school.

References

Ackley, B. J., Ladwig, G. B., Makic, M. B. F., Martinez-Kratz, M. R., & Zanotti, M. (2021). *Nursing diagnosis handbook: An evidence-based guide to planning care* (12th ed., revised reprint). Elsevier.

American Nurses Association. (2018). *Inclusion of recognized terminologies supporting nursing practice within electronic health records and other health information technology solutions.* [Position Statement.] https://www.nursingworld.org/practice-policy/nursing-excellence/official-position-statements/id/Inclusion-of-Recognized-Terminologies-Supporting-Nursing-Practice-within-Electronic-Health-Records/

America's Health Rankings. (2023). America's Health Rankings analysis of CDC WONDER: Multiple cause of death files. https://www.americashealthrankings.org/explore/health-of-women-and-children/measure/child_mortality_a/state/U.S.

Anderson, L., Larson, S. A., & Wuorio, A. (2011). *2010 FINDS national survey: Technical report part 1: Caregiver survey.* University of Minnesota. http://www.thearc.org/document.doc?id=3673

Centers for Disease Control and Prevention. (2017). *Writing SMART objectives.* https://www.cdc.gov/dhdsp/evaluation_resources/guides/writing-smart-objectives.htm

Centers for Disease Control and Prevention. (2022). Health information & privacy: FERPA and HIPAA. *National Center for State, Tribal, Local, and Territorial Public Health Infrastructure and Workforce,* Public Health Law Program. https://www.cdc.gov/phlp/publications/topic/healthinformationprivacy.html

Davis, A. M., Brown, R. F., Taylor, J. L., Epstein, R. A., & McPheeters, M. L. (2014). Transition care for children with special health care needs. *Pediatrics, 134*(5), 900–908. https://doi.org/10.1542/peds.2014-1909

Galemore, C. A., & Sheetz, A. H. (2015). IEP, IHP, and Section 504 primer for new school nurses. *NASN School Nurse, 3*(2), 85–88. https://doi.org/10.1177/1942602X14565462

Herdman, T. H., Kamitsuru, S., & Lopes, C. (Eds.) (2021). *NANDA International nursing diagnoses: Definitions and classification 2021–2023* (10th ed.). Thieme.

IRIS Center. (2019). *IEPs*: Developing high-quality individualized education programs. https://iris.peabody.vanderbilt.edu/module/iep01/

Johnson, K. (2024). School health documentation and implications for data collection. In C. A. Resha & V. Taliaferro (Eds.), *Legal resource for school health services* (2nd ed., pp. 99–121). SchoolNurse.com.

Maternal and Child Health Bureau. (2022, June). Children and youth with special healthcare needs: NCHS data brief. *Health Resources and Services Administration.* https://mchb.hrsa.gov/sites/default/files/mchb/programs-impact/nsch-data-brief-children-youth-special-health-care-needs.pdf

NANDA International. (2023). *Nursing diagnosis.* https://nanda.org/publications-resources/resources/glossary-of-terms/

National Association of School Nurses. (2019a). *Transition planning for students with healthcare needs* (Position Statement). Author. https://www.nasn.org/nasn-resources/professional-practice-documents/ps-transition

National Association of School Nurses. (2019b). *Translating strategies into actions to improve care coordination for students with chronic health conditions.* https://learn.nasn.org/courses/11191

National Association of School Nurses. (2020). *Individualized healthcare plans to support school health services* (Position Statement). Author. https://www.nasn.org/nasn-resources/professional-practice-documents/position-statements/ps-ihps

National Association of School Nurses. (2021). *A model for school nurse-led case management.* https://learn.nasn.org/courses/33713

National Association of School Nurses (NASN). (2022). *School nursing: Scope and standards of practice* (4th ed.). Author.

National Association of School Nurses. (2023a). *Addressing chronic absenteeism* (Position Statement). Author. https://www.nasn.org/nasn-resources/professional-practice-documents/position-statements/ps-absenteeism

National Association of School Nurses. (2023b). *IDEIA and Section 504 teams—the school nurse as an essential team member* (Position Statement). Author. https://www.nasn.org/nasn-resources/professional-practice-documents/ps-ideia

National Association of School Nurses. (2024). A contemporary framework update for today's school nursing landscape: Introducing the School Nursing Practice Framework. NASN School Nurse, 39(3), 140–147. https://www.doi.org/10.1177/1942602X241241092

Office for Civil Rights. (2010, August). Free appropriate public education for students with disabilities: Requirements under Section 504 of the Rehabilitation Act of 1973. *U.S. Department of Education.* https://www2.ed.gov/about/offices/list/ocr/docs/edlite-FAPE504.html

Office for Civil Rights. (2016). Parent and educator resource guide to Section 504 in public elementary and secondary schools. *U.S. Department of Education.* https://www2.ed.gov/about/offices/list/ocr/docs/504-resource-guide-201612.pdf

Office for Civil Rights. (2023, July 18). Protecting students with disabilities: Frequently asked questions about Section 504 and education of children with disabilities. *U.S. Department of Education.* https://www2.ed.gov/about/offices/list/ocr/504faq.html

Office of Special Education and Rehabilitative Services. (2020). A transition guide to postsecondary education and employment for students and youth with disabilities. U.S. Department of Education. https://sites.ed.gov/idea/files/postsecondary-transition-guide-august-2020.pdf

Office of Special Education and Rehabilitative Services. (2022, July 19). *Questions and answers: Addressing the needs of children with disabilities and IDEA's discipline provisions. U.S. Department of Education.* https://sites.ed.gov/idea/files/qa-addressing-the-needs-of-children-with-disabilities-and-idea-discipline-provisions.pdf

Office of the National Coordinator for Health Information Technology. (2017). *Standard Nursing Terminologies: A landscape analysis.* https://www.healthit.gov/sites/default/files/snt_final_05302017.pdf

Sampson, C. H., & Will, S. (2017). IHP basics and using IHPs with other educational, health, and home care agency plans. In S. Will, M. W. Arnold, & D. S. Zaiger (Eds.). *Individualized healthcare plans for the school nurse: A comprehensive resource for school nursing management of health conditions* (pp. 1–10). Sunrise River Press.

Shannon, R. A., & Holman, C. F. (2017). Sickle cell disease. In S. Will, M. J. Arnold, & D. S. Zaiger (Eds.). *Individualized healthcare plans for the school nurse* (pp. 899–914). Sunrise River Press. With permission.

U.S. Department of Health and Human Services & U.S. Department of Education. (2015). *Policy statement on inclusion of children with disabilities in early childhood programs.* https://sites.ed.gov/idea/idea-files/policy-statement-inclusion-of-children-with-disabilities-in-early-childhood-programs/

Laws

Americans With Disabilities Amendment Act of 2008. (42 U.S.C. § 12101-12102). https://www.ada.gov/regs2016/adaaa.html

Individuals With Disabilities Education Improvement Act of 2004 (Pub. L. 108-446). https://www.gpo.gov/fdsys/pkg/PLAW-108publ446/content-detail.html

Rehabilitation Act of 1973 (Pub. L. 93-112). https://www.gpo.gov/fdsys/pkg/STATUTE-107/pdf/STATUTE-107-Pg718.pdf

part III

Population Health School Nursing Practice

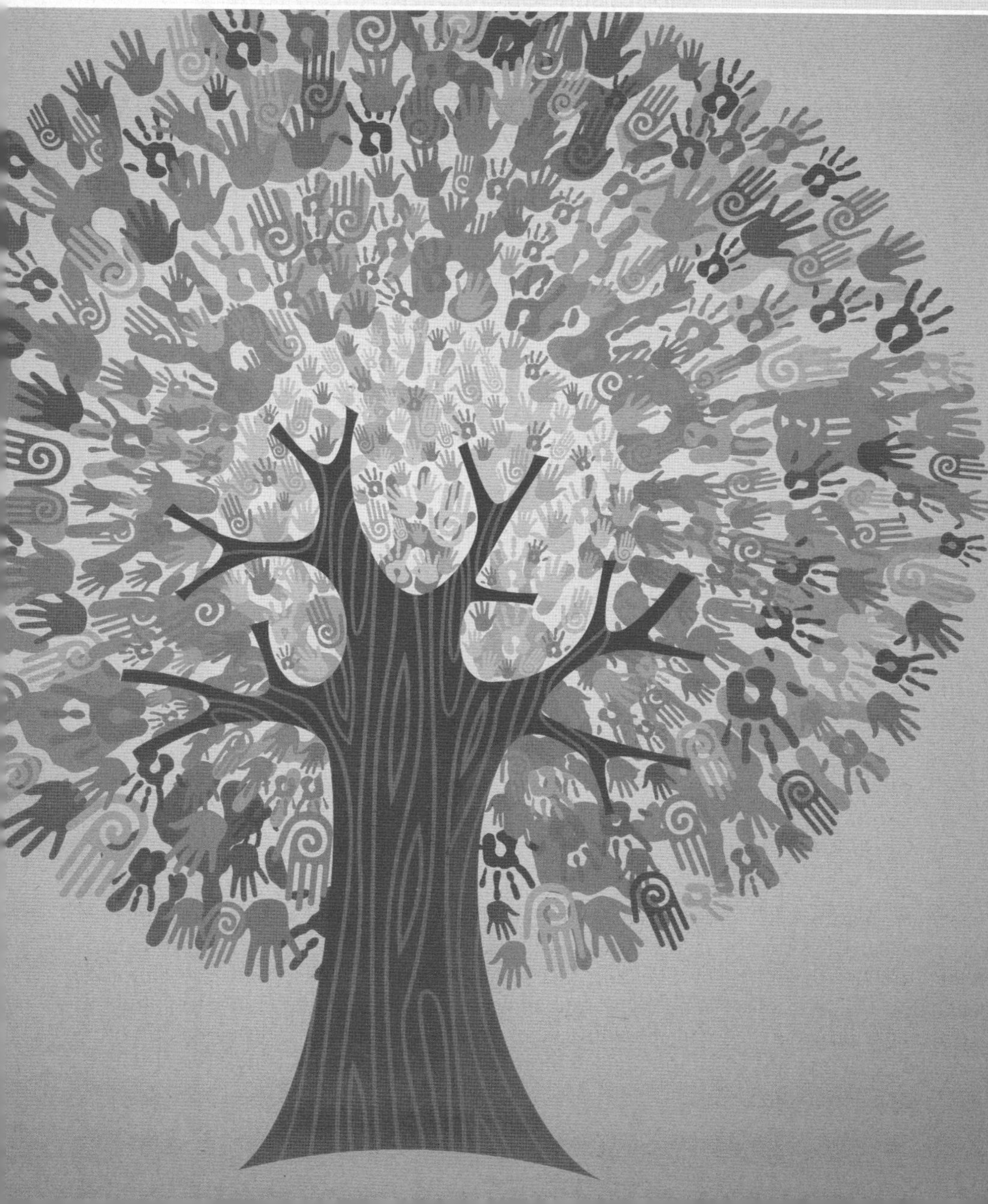

Chapter 9

Growth and Development: Preschool Through Adolescence

Elizabeth Mattey ▪ Jennifer Adams

CHAPTER OUTLINE

Growth and development are the hallmark features of childhood and adolescence. School nurses care for the health and safety of large numbers of students in the school environment and more specifically, the school health office; thus they are the ideal healthcare providers to promote optimal growth and development and identify potential alterations. The growth and developmental milestones expected of children and adolescents are grouped by age into five stages: infancy, toddlerhood, preschool, school-age, and adolescence. This chapter focuses on physical, cognitive, psychosocial, and moral development of school-age children 3 to 18 years of age. However, schools may also include students with special needs until the age of 22. While it is helpful to understand the characteristics expected within each stage, these parameters serve only as a guide because each child is different.

Growth and development encompass many parameters. *Growth* refers to an irreversible increase in the size of an organ or structure. It is a change that can be measured, such as height and weight. *Development* is the maturation of a body or system; it involves the process of acquiring new abilities and skills. The development of language, the ability to process thoughts and reach logical conclusions, and the ability to form social relationships are examples of development. Growth and development are affected by genetics and the environment, including health and nutrition.

School nurses need to understand the specific populations they serve, the families that make up the population, and the developmental expectations within the community. Developmental expectations may vary according to a family's or community's cultural, racial, and social determinants of health. For example, a ninth-grade student may appear to be much smaller than his classmates, but a review of the student's growth and development may indicate that he is within normal limits. Health teaching at an early age must consider that preschoolers may not understand cause-and-effect relationships. By understanding the growth and development of students, school nurses can plan their interactions and interventions to be most effective.

School nurses use their knowledge of pediatric growth and development throughout their careers. Knowledge of the factors affecting growth and development is basic to school nursing and embedded within the principles of the National Association of School Nurses' (NASN's) *School Nursing Practice Framework* (2024). For example, the Framework principle, *Standards of Practice,* calls on the school nurse to ensure their assessment addresses the unique needs of the student and that interventions are evidence-based. Appropriate and effective *Care Coordination* for the growing student requires the school nurse to have a thorough knowledge of developmental milestones and expectations. The principle of *Community and Public Health* is realized when school nurses identify deviations from typical growth and development during health screenings. School nurses who set goals and measure outcomes of health education programs (e.g., nutrition, obesity) are demonstrating the principle of *Quality Improvement.* School nurses practice the fifth principle, *Leadership,* when advocating for policy change to ensure at-risk students receive necessary services in the school environment.

GROWTH

Height and Weight

Children do not grow at a steady rate; they experience periods of rapid growth and times when cognitive development is occurring more than physical growth. The overall picture of a child's increasing height and weight has implications for nutritional needs, developmental expectations, and other physiological changes. The Centers for Disease Control and Prevention (CDC) has developed clinical growth charts for boys and girls to plot percentile curves for the growth of children and adolescents relative to the U.S. population for their age (CDC, 2009). Body measurements for school-age children include stature-for-age, weight-for-age, and body mass index–for–age (BMI). Growth charts are an assessment tool; they are not diagnostic alone of any health conditions. These growth charts for children are available on the CDC Web site (2017). Separate growth charts are available for children with select neurodevelopmental conditions such as Down syndrome.

Children ages 3 to 6 grow an average of 2.75 inches per year, and their weight increases approximately 4 to 5 pounds per year. By age 3½ to 4, the child has doubled his or her birth height. By age 6, children average 45 inches and weigh approximately 45 pounds. Children from age 6 until puberty grow in height approximately 2 to 3 inches per year. Just before menarche, between the ages of 8 and 13, girls reach their peak growth rate then growth slows. Boys show a period of rapid growth during midpuberty, which occurs on average around age 13½. This period of rapid growth levels off within 2 years. Boys may continue to grow but do not show the rapid increase that is seen during puberty (Tanner, 1962).

Girls gain 6 to 8 pounds per year until puberty begins, at which time a gain of 4 pounds per year can be expected as they begin a fast growth spurt and sexual development. Boys average a weight gain of 4 to 6 pounds per year during the elementary years; around age 10, their growth rate increases to add 10 to 12 pounds per year (CDC, 2022a). Children will generally follow their own curve on the growth scale. For example, if a child is identified in the 45th percentile, he or she will likely remain in that percentile during periods of growth.

School nurses should keep in mind that the rate of growth will be affected by a student's stage in the Tanner Scale and may not follow the linear height and age growth charts from the CDC. The rate of growth is accelerated during puberty and the timing of puberty occurs at different ages. The age at which a student reaches puberty is affected by race/ethnicity and can be affected by pubertal disorders (Miller et al., 2020).

Did You Know?

How to Predict Approximate Final Adult Height

$$\text{Girls' height} = \frac{(\text{Father's height} - 5\text{ inches}) + \text{Mother's height}}{2}$$

$$\text{Boys' height} = \frac{(\text{Father's height} + 5\text{ inches}) + \text{Mother's height}}{2}$$

Source: Carswell & Stafford, 2022.

Altered Growth Patterns

An abnormal growth pattern may be the only sign of a growth disorder or a chronic condition. A student should be referred to their healthcare provider to be evaluated for growth failure if the school nurse notes the height or weight measurements cross multiple percentiles.

Overweight and Obesity

Childhood overweight/obesity is a national epidemic. The number of children 6 to 19 years of age who are considered obese has steadily grown since 1998. In 2022, a separate growth chart was added by the CDC for children or youth who measure above the 95th percentile due to the increasing number of obese and severely obese children and youth. These charts provide a more accurate view of progress for clinicians and researchers who are treating these children (CDC, 2022b).

While there has been much attention on the increase in students and youth who are obese, food insecurity, diets high in sugar and fried food, and lack of nutrient-dense foods has contributed to malnutrition and obesity. The COVID-19 pandemic exacerbated this epidemic, with one study showing the rate of children and youth identified as overweight or moderately or severely obese has doubled since the onset of the pandemic (Lange et al., 2021). Of equal concern, additional studies found a larger increase in the BMI of overweight/obese youth during the pandemic among Black and Mexican American youth in all age groups. Experts point to the need to address the disparities that contribute to this imbalance made more glaringly obvious during the pandemic (Stavridou et al., 2021; Wu et al., 2022). Food desserts, lack of physical activity, and decreased opportunities to participate in physical activities must be addressed in communities. Given that youth who are overweight have an increased risk for chronic conditions, such as cardiovascular disease or type 2 diabetes, this is a pressing health issue for our students and youth. Children with obesity are more likely to become obese adults. See Chapter 14.

A drop in weight across percentiles can be the first sign of malnourishment or malabsorption. This is an important finding because once the problem is resolved, a child usually can catch up to their peers, depending on the severity of the problem. Malnourishment occurs when a child's diet does not supply the necessary nutrients needed for normal growth and development. Children living in poverty are at increased risk of inadequate nutrition. Several factors may influence poor dietary choices, including inadequate food intake, inadequate food availability (food insecurity), lack of parental supervision, lack of knowledge about proper nutrition, and the easy availability and use of processed foods, which may be nutritionally inadequate. Malabsorption may occur in children who have celiac disease. Nutritional deficits have been linked to lowered intelligence, poor emotional and mental health outcomes, and a greater rate of childhood illnesses.

An abnormal growth pattern may be related to psychosocial deprivation, a condition where parents/guardians are disconnected from their child, leading to abnormal eating habits. School nurses may notice the student has unusual eating and drinking habits such as scavenging for food. Stunted growth due to psychosocial deprivation can be corrected if the environmental issues are addressed early, which may include removing the child from the environment (Rogol, 2020).

Stature

Students who demonstrate short stature may have delayed growth or a family history of short stature. Students should be referred to their healthcare provider for evaluation for growth failure if the school nurse notes the height or weight measurements cross multiple percentiles. Growth should be evaluated if a student is below the second percentile in height (Collett-Solberg et al., 2019). Short stature may be due to chromosomal disorders. Separate growth charts are available for children with Down syndrome or Turner syndrome. Students with chromosomal abnormalities may also have coexisting conditions such as cardiac anomalies, renal and reproductive disorders, hearing loss, and learning difficulties. Other causes of short stature may be endocrine related and attributed to thyroid hormone deficiency or growth hormone deficiency. Children with Marfan syndrome are typically very tall. Marfan syndrome is a genetic disorder affecting the connective tissues that can cause abnormalities of the heart, blood vessels, bones, joints, and eyes. Abnormalities of the heart and aortic structures can be life-threatening (National Organization of Rare Diseases, 2021).

As students get older, they may be more sensitive about being too tall or too short. For some students with short stature, growth hormone therapy may be considered. Growth hormone therapy may benefit children who have growth hormone deficiency, Turner syndrome, chronic renal insufficiency, Prader-Willi syndrome, and Noonan syndrome. The *2016 Guidelines for Growth Hormone and Insulin-Like Growth Factor-1 Treatment in Children and Adolescents* recommends growth hormone to avoid extreme shortness in children and youth but cautions that the decision to initiate growth hormone should be individualized and the benefits versus risks considered (Grimberg et al., 2016).

School nurses must be alert to the needs of children with altered growth in their schools and provide support when needed. They should plan to educate staff and prepare to manage the additional health and educational issues that may accompany a growth disorder.

Bone Growth

Conversion of cartilage to bone occurs from before birth through adolescence. Linear skeletal growth occurs at the epiphyseal plates at the end of the long bones. The cell layers of the epiphyseal plate are nourished by nutrients in the blood and produce new bone, thus expanding the bone lengthwise. Cartilage cells at the epiphyses are replaced by osteoblasts that deposit calcium. Bones grow in diameter by adding new layers of tissue under the periosteum, the thin tissue that covers the bone. The shorter bones found in the wrist and ankles do not have epiphyseal plates. The ossification occurs from the center of the short bone outwards (Haywood & Getchell, 2020).

Calcium intake during childhood and adolescence is extremely important for providing adequate bone density in adulthood. Phosphate and vitamin D intake are also necessary for the healthy formation of bone. Vitamin D increases the absorption of calcium and phosphate from the intestinal tract.

During adolescence, the growth plate disappears and the epiphysis and diaphysis (the shaft of the bone) fuse. At this point, linear growth is complete. However, old bone is continually replaced by new bone throughout the life span. Children generate new bone faster than the older bone is absorbed; thus skeletal mass increases. As bone formation slows during adulthood, resorption of the bone leads to an eventual overall loss of bone tissue (Haywood & Getchell, 2020).

Skeletal age can be determined by x-ray, referred to as *bone age,* and is used to determine the proportion of total growth completed. The left hand and wrist bones are most commonly used to determine skeletal age because the wrist bones (carpals) ossify in a particular order. The x-ray results are compared with a standard based on the child's chronological age. Bone age can help the healthcare provider determine whether children with short stature will continue to grow and catch up to their expected height percentile (Carswell & Stafford, 2022; Haywood & Getchell, 2020). Bone age also can identify children who grow too fast or too early.

Growing bones are flexible and highly porous. Thus the younger child's bones can absorb a great deal of energy and not sustain a fracture. The bones of children can bend slightly and heal quickly. However, children who suffer damage to the growth plate or epiphyseal plate may have future bone growth affected. This may alter the final length of the growing limb or contribute to a deformity in the joint or the limb (Haywood & Getchell, 2020). It is extremely important injuries to these body parts are adequately assessed and treated so bone deformity does not occur. Scoliosis or similar skeletal changes may occur at this time (see scoliosis screening in Chapter 12). The school nurse needs to be vigilant with these assessments and refer as needed.

Muscle Growth

Muscles grow in length and width to accommodate the growing bones. Muscles grow lengthwise by the addition of sarcomeres, the contractile units of the muscle cell. Multiple sarcomeres make up the muscle cells, also called *myofibrils,* which then make up the individual muscle fibers. A muscle is composed of bundles of muscle fibers. The muscle grows in width based on the activity of the muscles; the more activity, the larger the muscle (Haywood & Getchell, 2020).

Muscle mass in childhood is similar for boys and girls. A marked difference by gender begins at puberty because of the influence of androgens. Girls generally add muscle mass until age 13, whereas boys will continue to add muscle mass until approximately age 17. Muscle mass contributes to approximately 45% of a girl's body weight and 54% in boys (Haywood & Getchell, 2020).

Dentition

Most children entering preschool have all of their primary teeth and will not start losing primary teeth until kindergarten. The permanent teeth develop in the jaw beneath the primary teeth. The roots of the primary teeth gradually are absorbed until the crown of the primary tooth is all that is left. The crowns become loose and fall out, allowing the permanent teeth to erupt. As the child grows, the jaw also grows to allow room for the larger permanent teeth. Eruption of the permanent teeth generally follows a sequential pattern. See Figure 9-1.

During the school-age years, the central and lateral incisors erupt, followed by the second and third cuspids and then the first and second molars. The second molars erupt around age 12 to 13, whereas the wisdom teeth, or third molars, may not erupt until the student has graduated high school (between ages 17 and 21). Because the jaw does not reach its full size until the end of adolescence, early eruption of the wisdom teeth may cause pain and discomfort. This may result in the third molars having to be removed.

Loss of the first tooth generally occurs between ages 5 and 6 and is an important event for a child. Across cultures, it is heralded with fanfare. The American mythical Tooth Fairy promotes a tradition whereby a tooth is left under a pillow and then replaced with money or trinkets. In some cultures a rat or a mouse is said to take the tooth and leave a gift or money. Students need to know losing deciduous teeth is a normal part of development. However, primary teeth may not fall out naturally. If the erupting permanent tooth is visible, a visit to the dentist may be necessary to remove the primary tooth to allow the permanent tooth room to erupt.

Students who lose a tooth in school are often sent to the school nurse, perhaps because of the small amount of bleeding that may occur. Many school nurses have special containers that the student can safely take the tooth home to show family members. Losing the first tooth can lead to a teachable moment and give the nurse the opportunity to discuss brushing and dental hygiene. Unlicensed school personnel can easily assist a student who has lost a tooth.

The American Academy of Pediatric Dentistry (2022) recommends dental services begin around the time of eruption of the first tooth, but at least by 12 months of age. Regular preventive dental care should be continued during

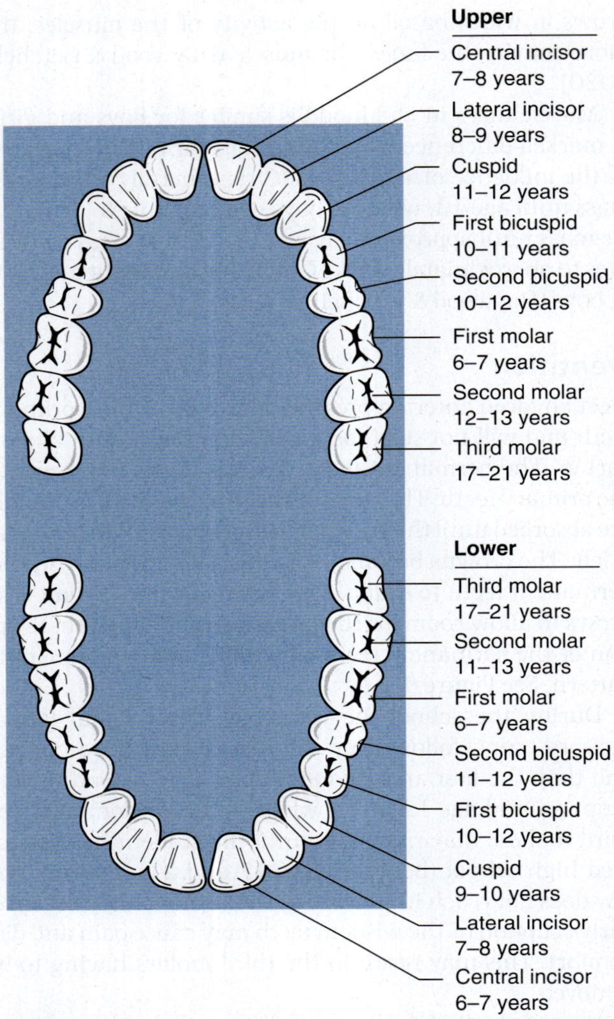

FIGURE 9-1. Eruption of permanent secondary teeth.

the school year with biannual checkups and cleaning or more frequently depending on the need. Health education focused on oral health can help to reinforce the importance of dental hygiene with preschool children. Preschool children can brush their own teeth with some assistance. Some preschool programs make teeth brushing part of the morning ritual.

Oral health is the most common unmet health need among children. *Dental caries are the most common chronic condition in childhood,* affecting almost 46% of children between the ages of 2 and 19 (Krol & Whalen, 2023). Children living 200% below the poverty level have an even higher rate of dental caries. Dental caries are largely preventable, and the pain caused by untreated tooth decay can affect overall health and be a factor in academic performance. The pain from dental caries makes concentrating in class more difficult; eating and sleeping may be affected, which may also affect school performance. Students with poor oral health miss three times as many days as other students, accounting for almost 2 million days of school missed per year (Attendance Works, Healthy Schools Campaign, 2015).

Dental caries are caused by an interaction among bacteria, dietary sugars, saliva, and teeth. The acids produced by the bacteria demineralize the tooth enamel, causing caries. Regular dental visits and proper brushing and flossing can prevent the formation of dental caries. Proper dental hygiene is essential for the development and maintenance of good oral health. Sealants, a clear coating applied by a hygienist or dentist, can prevent up to 80% of decay in the molars and yet up to 7 million children at risk do not have sealants (CDC, 2021a).

The relationship between fluoride and dental caries is well documented. Fluoride gels and varnishes have been shown to be effective in preventing dental caries; fluoride varnish has been shown to be more effective than gels and is easier to apply (Richards, 2015). Fluoride in the water supply is a cost-effective public health approach to maintaining dental health. If fluoride in water is not possible, supplements are available, but care must be taken to consider all possible sources of fluoride in one's diet, including toothpaste (American Academy of Pediatric Dentistry, 2022). However, locations with high fluoride content in the water or swallowing too much fluoride toothpaste can cause mottling of the teeth or white or brownish discolorations.

Unfortunately for many students, professional dental care is not easily accessible or affordable. The social determinants of health (e.g., poverty, lack of transportation, lack of insurance, and food insecurity) can limit a child's access to proper dental care, thus perpetuating continued poor oral health. It has been shown that children living in poverty have more untreated dental caries than those living in homes with a higher income (CDC, 2021b).

School nurses can partner with community and private oral health programs to bring dental services to the school to meet the needs of children at risk. School nurses can coordinate care and identify students at risk who can benefit from school-based oral health treatment, such as students with a history of previous dental caries or who lack access to dental care. Community partnerships are important to leverage dental resources. For example, the school nurse can identify dentists in the community who will accept Medicaid clients, donate toothbrushes for the children, or even volunteer to provide free or reduced fee dental care for children in need. School nurses can keep a dental resource list handy to share with families. Mobile dental services may be available to provide oral screenings and preventative care at school with parent consent and may be covered by Medicaid reimbursement for eligible students. School nurses also can advocate for funding to support school-based health clinics that include dental care so that the barriers preventing students' access to care are removed and equity in the school community is promoted.

Multiple circumstances can affect developing teeth. Malnutrition, illness, and trauma can cause hypocalcification or hypoplasia. Hypocalcification is seen as white opaque patches on the tooth. Hypoplasia results in areas of pitting or loss of enamel. Antibiotic therapy with tetracycline before age 8 can cause brownish yellow discoloration of the teeth (Meissner, 2020). Phenytoin (Dilantin), used to control seizures, and cyclosporine, used to suppress organ rejection, can cause gingival hyperplasia. Meticulous oral hygiene, including brushing, flossing, and frequent dental visits, can help limit the amount of excessive gum growth.

Adolescent high-risk behaviors also may affect the teeth and oral hygiene. Mouth and tongue piercing can cause oral infections, gingivitis, hemorrhaging, and fractures of the teeth. Tobacco use can damage oral tissues, stain teeth, and has been linked to oral cancer. Health education is most effective when offered several years before negative behaviors are likely to occur.

Trauma to the mouth can occur during school hours or during school-sponsored events. Children between the ages of 7 and 11 are more prone to injury, with most sports-related oral injuries occurring in baseball. Bicycle accidents are also a frequent contributor to dental trauma. Rules requiring safety and protective gear in specific school-sponsored sports reduce the incidence of dental trauma in students, but not all sports require a mouth guard or other dental protective gear. School nurses can help by ensuring that students wear the appropriate safety gear and protective mouth guards and by remaining current on the treatment of common oral emergencies. Because of the risk for future complications to teeth, all dental trauma should be referred to a dentist as soon as possible. Avulsion of a permanent tooth is a dental emergency if the tooth is to be saved (see Chapter 17). Trauma to primary teeth can affect the formation of underlying permanent teeth and should be evaluated by a dentist (Day et al., 2020).

Early identification of possible jaw problems or potential problems with teeth eruptions may be easier to correct if identified early. The American Association of Orthodontists (2020b) recommends children have an orthodontic evaluation by age 7. Most children will begin orthodontic treatment between the ages of 9 and 14. The school nurse may need to handle complaints about braces until the student can be seen by their orthodontist. See Table 9-1.

Elementary school children are prime targets for many health promotion habits that can form the foundation for important later values and beliefs. February has been designated National Children's Dental Health Month by the American Dental Association (2024), which offers free flyers and program planning guidance. School nurses can take advantage of numerous opportunities during this time to incorporate dental health lessons into the school day or invite a local dentist or dental hygienist to the school to speak to students. The community/public health component of NASN's School Nursing Practice Framework (2024) can be operationalized through health education, such as teaching students about brushing and flossing; these messages can then be taken home by students and taught to the family members.

TABLE 9-1 Common Problems and Solutions Related to Braces

Problem	Solutions
Food caught between teeth and braces	Dental floss or a toothpick can be used to remove food.
Discomfort	Eat soft foods and rinse mouth with warm salt water.
Ligatures (tiny rubber bands or fine wires) come off	Rubber bands may be replaced using sterile tweezers. Loose wires can be removed with sterile tweezers. (If the wire is sticking out but not loose, use a cotton swab or eraser to bend the wire so that it is not irritating the gums.) Notify parents that the ligature is loose or bent so that they can notify the orthodontist.
Lip/cheek irritation	Keep a supply of nonmedicinal relief wax to create a buffer between the braces and the mouth. A local orthodontist may be willing to supply the school nurse with the wax.
Protruding wire	Bend wire flat against the teeth with a cotton swab or eraser to prevent gum irritation. Use relief wax if the wire cannot be moved to a comfortable position. As a last resort, if the student may not see the orthodontist soon, clip the protruding wire. Wrap the wire in gauze before clipping to prevent the student from swallowing the wire. Notify the parents.
Loose brackets	If brackets are loose, notify the parent so that the orthodontist can determine the best course of action; if the bracket is off center, the adhesive may have failed, and the orthodontist will need to determine the next step.

Adapted from American Association of Orthodontists (2020a).

PHYSIOLOGICAL PARAMETERS

Vital sign parameters change as a child grows. Vital signs are dynamic and fluctuate according to demands on the body. It is important for school nurses to be familiar with the normal ranges of vital signs per age in children and adolescents. The accurate assessment of vital signs assists the nurse to gather objective data about the student's health status and recognize when abnormal variations indicate medical intervention.

Temperature

The normal average body temperature for children and youth is between 97.5°F and 98.6°F when measured orally. The body temperature may fluctuate based on the time of day, type of exercise, excessive clothing, or environmental temperature (Kasbekar et al., 2021). There is no conclusive evidence on the most effective method to measure body temperature in the school environment. Oral electronic thermometers estimate body temperature and are generally accepted as accurate measures for children older than 5 years. The probe should be placed in the posterior sublingual pocket and taken at least 30 minutes after drinking liquids.

There is inconclusive evidence to recommend either a temporal artery scan thermometer or the tympanic membrane thermometer in children ages 3 to 18 years old (Emergency Nurses Association, 2020). Ear-based temperature readings with an infrared sensor reliably measure the temperature in the ear canal, but only if used correctly. During the COVID-19 pandemic, one study of 1,576 patients found the tympanic membrane thermometer to reflect a more accurate reading of fever compared with the infrared forehead thermometer and the temporal scan thermometer (Fong et al., 2020). Accuracy may be affected by the presence of earwax and environmental factors. Some ear-based thermometers commonly used in schools do not measure tympanic temperature and should not be referred to as tympanic thermometers. Whichever method is chosen, care must be taken to follow the instructions for the thermometer consistently. Accessing a rectal temperature is not recommended in the school setting for obvious reasons.

Fever is one of the most common reasons students visit the school health office. Fever is generally considered to be a temperature of greater than 100.4°F (38°C) (Adam, 2020). Most fevers are due to viruses, but they can also be caused by bacterial infections, vaccine reactions, biological agents, tissue injury, malignancy, granulomatous disease, neuroendocrine disorders, metabolic disease, immunological/rheumatological disorders, drugs, and toxins, as well as environmental factors, such as the weather and exercise (Kasbekar et al., 2021). See Chapter 16 for more information on fever.

Heat illness is a potentially serious condition that could result in heat stroke and death if one's core body temperature gets too high. Heat illness also refers to heat exhaustion, heat syncope, heat cramps and heat rash. Exertional heat illness is related to the body's metabolic heat production from increased activity and made worse by a warm climate (Westwood et al., 2021). Many intense school sports are played under conditions that could potentially result in heat illness or heat stroke such as football, cross-country running, soccer, track, tennis, baseball, and softball. Practicing football in full uniform in high heat can increase body temperature significantly. The surface of tennis courts and artificial turf playing fields increases the environmental temperature by 10° to 20°. Factors other than temperature can influence the risk of developing heat illness, including certain medications, hydration, conditioning, obesity, and having a previous history of heat illness (Westwood et al., 2021). Failure to treat symptoms of heat illness can result in reduced performance, stress on the heart and muscles, and the possibility of death.

Students on certain medications, such as anticholinergic drugs, diuretics, certain antibiotics, and antihistamines, are more sensitive to heat and sun exposure, and these children will need special accommodations (Casa et al., 2015). Students taking antipsychotic medications, such as quetiapine (Seroquel), aripiprazole (Abilify), or risperidone, should exercise caution when participating in activities that expose them to excessive heat. Antipsychotic agents may affect the child's ability to regulate body temperature. Other conditions that increase the risk for heat illnesses include obesity, a low fitness level, dehydration, sleep deprivation, sunburn, viral illness, diarrhea, and fever (Westwood et al., 2021).

Extremely cold temperatures also can be dangerous to students. Hypothermia results in the body losing heat faster than it is produced and is a medical emergency. A low body temperature will affect the brain and body's ability to function properly. If frostbite is suspected, the affected area will lose feeling and color due to decreased blood circulation to the area. Until emergency personnel arrive, warm the student with blankets. Frostbitten parts should be immersed in warm (not hot) water. Do not massage the area.

Blood Pressure

Increasingly schools are including blood pressure (BP) screening as part of the annual health screenings. Hypertension is not rare in children and adolescents and can be detected at an early age. According to the National High Blood Pressure Education Program Working Group [NHBPEP Working Group] on High Blood Pressure in Children and Adolescents convened by the National Institutes of Health:

- *Hypertension* is defined as average systolic BP (SBP) and/or diastolic BP (DBP) that is greater than or equal to the 95th percentile for sex, age, and height on three or more occasions.
- *Prehypertension* in children is defined as average SBP or DBP levels that are greater than or equal to the 90th percentile, but less than the 95th percentile (NHBPEP Working Group, 2005, p. 4, para. 1).

Approximately 3.5% of children and youth have hypertension. Boys have a higher incidence than girls, and there is an association between hypertension and increased BMI. It is recommended that healthcare providers screen BP annually for all children older than 3 years (Flynn et al., 2017).

Blood pressure tables now consider age and height when determining normal or high BP. In 2017, the AAP published the *Clinical Practice Guideline for Screening and Management of High Blood Pressure in Children and Adolescents* with new normative BP tables for children of normal weight (Flynn et al., 2017). These tables more accurately screen children and youth for elevated blood pressure but suggest that youth ages 13 or older are at risk if their BP is 120/80 or higher. Table 9-2 provides a quick reference of vital signs for the 50th percentile based on age in the 50th percentile of height; it is to be used only as a guide. In addition to children who are overweight, children with sleep disordered breathing, chronic kidney disease, and a history of low birth weight are also at risk for childhood hypertension (Flynn et al., 2017).

A single high BP reading does not mean the student has hypertension; at least three readings should be taken. Students should be referred for medical evaluation if their BP is consistently above normal range. The school nurse can initiate health education for students with hypertension concerning appropriate nutrition, avoidance of tobacco, preventing excess weight, and regular physical activity. Interventions starting at an early age for individuals identified as high risk can prevent future complications in adulthood.

When measuring BP, care must be taken to *choose the appropriate cuff size.* Using the wrong cuff size will give inaccurate readings. To choose the appropriate cuff size, the width of the bladder in the cuff should be approximately 37% to 50% of the arm circumference measured midway between the olecranon and the acromion. The cuff should cover approximately two-thirds of the upper arm, and the cuff bladder should cover 75% to 100% of the arm circumference (Muntner et al., 2019). Younger students need a pediatric size cuff. Most adolescents need an adult cuff size, and large adolescents may need an extra-large cuff. Several types of BP cuffs are available for measuring BP in children and youth. Aneroid sphygmomanometers have a limited life span and are more easily damaged. Noninvasive

Practice Connection

Blood pressure readings should be taken in the upper right arm with the student/youth sitting and feet and legs uncrossed. The right arm is preferred for consistency and comparison with standard tables unless there is a reason not to use the right arm; the cuff should be at the level of the heart and placed on bare skin. Do not roll up the sleeve because it may be tight around the arm and give a false reading. A cuff that is too small will give false-high readings.

The cuff should be 2 to 3 cm above the brachial artery and antecubital fossa. Support the arm so it is at the level of the right atrium or midpoint of the sternum and legs should be uncrossed. Have the student sit for 3 to 5 minutes without talking or moving for a more accurate reading. If two measurements are taken, wait 1 to 2 minutes before retaking BP. Inflate the cuff 30 mm HG more once the radial pulse disappears. Deflate the cuff at 2 mm Hg per second. Record BP at the onset of the first of at least two consecutive beats and the last audible sound (Muntner et al., 2019).

TABLE 9-2 Median Blood Pressure, Heart Rate, and Respiratory Rate in Youth

>Age	Boys Systolic/Diastolic BP		Girls Systolic/Diastolic BP		Heart Rate	Respiratory Rate
	At 50th Percentile Height and 50th Percentile BP	At Risk of Elevated BP	At 50th Percentile Height and 50th Percentile BP	At Risk of Elevated BP	25th–75th Percentile	Median + or −2 While Awake
3	90/47	101/58	90/50	102/60	102–121	23–27
4	92/50	102/60	92/53	103/62		21–25
5	94/53	103/63	93/55	104/64	96–117	20–24
6	95/56	105/66	94/56	105/67		19–22
7	97/58	106/68	95/57	106/68	90–111	18–22
8	98/59	107/69	97/59	107/69		18–22
9	99/60	107/70	97/60	108/71	84–104	18–22
10	100/62	108/72	99/60	109/72		17–21
11	102/63	110/74	102/61	111/74		16–20
12	104/62	113/75	105/62	114/75	77–97	16–19
13	108/62	>120/80	106/64	>120/80		
14	111/64	>120/80	108/65	>120/80		16–19
15	113/65	>120/80	108/65	>120/80	74–94	
16	115/67	>120/80	109/66	>120/80		16
17	117/68	>120/80	110/66	>120/80		

Adapted from Flynn et al. (2017); O'Leary et al. (2015); Herbert et al. (2020).

automatic BP measurement is acceptable for measuring BP in children and youth due to the sensitivity of the devices (Emergency Nurses Association, 2019).

Initial identification of elevated BP may be made by the primary care provider. The school nurse should collaborate with the provider to monitor BP on a regular basis. Monitoring the student's BP provides the school nurse an opportunity to educate students and families about proper diet and physical activity and to reinforce the education provided by the primary care provider.

Risk factors for hypertension such as family history cannot be changed, but physical activity can be stressed as a method of controlling BP by preventing obesity. A balanced diet high in fruits and vegetables should be encouraged. Diets high in salt, solid fats, and caffeine have been linked to hypertension, as well as use of tobacco and exposure to secondhand smoke. Certain drugs, such as amphetamines and cocaine, can also increase BP.

Heart Rate

Heart rate slows as children age (see Table 9-2). The heart rate should be recorded for a full minute to accurately assess the rate and rhythm. Students may have a normal change in heart rhythm during respiration (i.e., respiratory sinus arrhythmia). The nurse can ask the student to hold his or her breath to evaluate the heart rhythm if there is concern about it being irregular. Peripheral pulses can be used as a measure of heart rate in school-age children and adolescents. The radial pulse is the most frequently used and the most convenient. Rhythm, rate, and amplitude (strength of the beat) should be recorded. Normal amplitude is recorded as 2+.

There are numerous physiological reasons why a student's heart rate may be elevated. The heart rates of most students seen in the school health office will return to within normal limits with rest and hydration. However, the school nurse should refer students for immediate medical evaluation who have prolonged or symptomatic heart rates that are extremely slow, fast, or irregular.

Respiration

Normal respiration should be regular, smooth, and effortless. School-age children have a ratio of inspiratory time to expiratory time of 1:2. The trachea should be midline. Students with chronic respiratory conditions, such as asthma and cystic fibrosis, may have a barrel-shaped chest as a result of air trapping. If this is the case, the fingernails should be checked for clubbing, which is an indication of chronic hypoxia. Breath sounds should be assessed if the student is having difficulty breathing.

When auscultating breath sounds, the school nurse should use the following techniques:

- Place the diaphragm of the stethoscope directly on the student's skin; do not auscultate breath sounds through clothing.
- Instruct the student to take deep breaths in and out; if breath sounds are auscultated during relaxed breathing, then abnormal breath sounds (wheeze, crackles, rhonchi) may be missed.
- Identify whether abnormal, decreased, or absent breath sounds occur during inhalation or exhalation and note the location within the lung fields (Jarvis & Eckhardt, 2024).

Documentation should include symptoms, physical assessment, and the student's status before and after treatments to determine response and next steps (Jakubowski & Perron, 2019). See Chapter 22 for more information on students with respiratory conditions.

PHYSIOLOGICAL DEMANDS

Metabolism

Metabolism refers to all physical and chemical changes in the body. The basal metabolic rate is the minimum energy expenditure of the body at rest. It is affected by many different factors, including age, sex, height, weight, exercise, hormones, and stress. Children and adolescents have higher metabolic rates than adults as needed to produce energy for growth. During periods of exercise or illness the basic metabolic rate increases, whereas during sleep the metabolic rate decreases. With increased metabolic rate, caloric and fluid intake must increase to maintain adequate body function. The presence of fever is an indication that a student should not participate in sports or other physical activity until it is resolved. Increased body temperature puts the student at increased risk for development of a heat-related illness (Casa et al., 2015).

Hydration

Care must be taken to ensure students remain hydrated during the school day. Strenuous physical activity at school during hot weather requires increased fluid intake to maintain adequate hydration and bodily functions. Students should be taught to monitor their fluid intake; they should not be thirsty, and urine should be a light yellow before exercising.

It is especially important for students with some chronic health conditions (e.g., diabetes, sickle cell disease, and migraine headaches) to stay hydrated. These students should have privileges to carry a water bottle during the school day written into their Section 504 accommodations, if not already allowed for all students.

Sleep

Adequate sleep and rest are necessary for restoration and growth, contributing to overall health and well-being. Sleep deprivation can result in decreased cognitive and motor function, inhibiting a child's or youth's ability to concentrate and putting a student at risk for learning difficulties and mood disturbances. Sleep deprivation has been linked to hypertension, obesity, and diabetes (Paruthi et al., 2016; Rigney & Weiss, 2022). Genetics, behavior, health conditions, and environmental influences all contribute to one's overall sleep requirements (Paruthi et al., 2016). Recommendations for sleep during childhood and adolescence depend on multiple factors and change with age (Box 9-1).

There are two main stages of sleep: rapid eye movement (REM) and non–rapid eye movement (NREM). NREM sleep has three cycles: N1, N2, and N3. Children and youth will progress through cycles N1 to N3 sleep within 20 to 30 minutes of falling asleep. Cycle N1 is a light sleep and is just as one is falling asleep. Breathing becomes regular, heart rate slows, and body temperature drops in N2. N3 is the deep stage of sleep, where BP drops, muscles are relaxed, and the restorative properties of sleep occur. It is also when growth hormones are released and blood supply to muscles increases, allowing tissue to repair and grow (National Sleep Foundation [NSF], 2022a). If the child is awakened during this stage, they may experience confusion and disorientation. Nightmares, night terrors, sleepwalking, and bedwetting occur during N3. REM sleep follows the NREM stages. Dreams will occur during the REM stage of sleep and last between 10 and 30 minutes. A sleep cycle lasts approximately 70 to 120 minutes and repeats four to six times a night (NSF, 2022a). By age 4, most children have outgrown the need for a nap during the day. Preschool-age children do not always sleep through the night and may experience periods of nighttime awakening.

Sleep Patterns

It is often important for the school nurse to assess the sleep patterns of students. Children and youth who chronically do not get enough sleep may be irritable and have difficulty concentrating in the classroom, which affects learning. Questions such as, "What was on TV when you went to bed?" may offer an accurate assessment of bedtime. Crowded living conditions and/or turmoil in the home may also affect a child's or youth's ability to sleep and should be investigated. Late-night smartphone and social media use can also lead to inadequate sleep. The school nurse can suggest strategies to ensure a student is getting adequate sleep. These may include finding a quiet place to sleep, bedtime rituals to establish a sleep routine, enforcing quiet time for younger children, an earlier bedtime, no television in bedrooms, and turning off cell phones at night. The ABCs of sleep for children and youth are shown in Box 9-2.

Puberty has been linked with later sleep onset and wake times. School start times that are delayed by a half an hour for adolescents have demonstrated that students sleep more, are more alert, and have shown mood improvements and are supported by the NSF (2022b). The COVID-19 pandemic provided an opportunity for youth to shift to a later sleep time resulting in a better quality of sleep and less daytime sleepiness (Gruber et al., 2020). After-school activities, transportation, and scheduling have all been cited as barriers to delaying school start times for adolescents.

Nutrition

Nutrition is a major component in promoting growth and health and in preventing disease. In order to build healthier communities, nutrition must be considered a high priority for all. Approximately half of all Americans are affected by chronic diseases that can be prevented by a healthy diet, including type 2 diabetes, cardiovascular disease, overweight and obesity, stroke, some types of cancer, and osteoporosis (U.S. Department of Agriculture [USDA] & U.S. Department of Health & Social Services [USDHHS], 2020).

Despite recommendations for healthy nutrition, there is a gap between the knowledge of healthy food choices and behaviors leading to eating a balanced healthy diet.

BOX 9-1

Sleep Recommendations by Age

Age	Recommended Hours of Sleep per 24 Hours
3–5	10–13 hours (includes naps)
6–12	9–12 hours
13–18	8–10 hours

Paruthi et al. (2016).

BOX 9-2

The ABCs of Sleeping Tool

Age-appropriate bedtimes with consistent schedules and routines

- Establish a bedtime routine.
- Maintain consistent wake times.

Location

- The bed should be comfortable and in a quiet location.

Exercise and diet

- Exercise is important but not too close to bedtime.
- Avoid caffeinated drinks or energy drinks close to bedtime.

No electronics in the bedroom or before bed

Positivity, independence, and needs

- The needs of a child should be met during the day, both emotional and physiological.
- Create a positive atmosphere at bedtime that is calming and quiet.
- Encourage independence when falling asleep.
- Do not depend on TV or other devices to fall asleep.

Howlett et al. (2020).

The *Dietary Guidelines for All Americans* (USDA & USDHSS, 2020) provide a broad picture of good nutrition and emphasizes that eating healthy is a lifestyle. A variety of foods and beverages should make up one's overall diet, which should include foods from all food groups: fruits (mostly whole fruits), vegetables (all colors and consistency), grains (at least half from whole grain), protein, low-fat dairy, and oil (USDA & USDHHS, 2020). Foods and beverages should include the vitamins and minerals necessary to support health and prevent disease; these are known as *nutrient-dense foods*. However, many Americans do not obtain adequate recommended amounts of certain vitamins and minerals for good health. See Box 9-3.

Previous USDA guidelines were more prescriptive in the recommendations for a healthy diet, describing the servings and type of food needed at each meal. The current guidelines emphasize healthy eating patterns, meaning a variety of foods and beverages should be consumed over a period of time within the calorie limits recommended for age and activity level. The guidelines now suggest equivalents rather than servings and are dependent on the food type. This new emphasis on eating for nutrition and health offers opportunities for schools to provide nutrition education emphasizing healthy lifestyles to improve overall health. School nurses can educate students on the new recommended nutritional guidelines as part of developing a healthy lifestyle and building a healthy community.

It is important to have healthy choices available to encourage a balanced diet. Students should be encouraged in school to try a variety of foods, because they may prefer certain foods over others. Young children's food preferences may change from week to week. Children who have suspected eating disorders or extremely selective eating patterns should be referred to the healthcare provider to determine whether other evaluations or interventions are warranted (American Academy of Pediatrics [AAP], 2018). See Chapter 28 for more information on eating disorders (e.g., anorexia nervosa, bulimia, avoidant restrictive food intake disorder).

BOX 9-3

Calcium, Potassium, Dietary Fiber, and Vitamin D

The latest Dietary Guidelines for Americans (DGA) identified calcium, potassium, dietary fiber, and vitamin D as nutrients that are underconsumed in the United States and labeled this underconsumption a public health concern.

In addition to bone and tooth health, calcium may reduce the risk of cardiovascular disease, gastrointestinal diseases, and kidney stones. Adequate intake of potassium can lower or control blood pressure. Low potassium has been linked with higher risk of stroke, insulin resistance, and diabetes. Fiber may prevent chronic conditions such as gastrointestinal diseases, obesity, cardiovascular disease, and type 2 diabetes. Vitamin D is recognized as important in maintaining health, beyond its role in bone development and bone health. There is an association between vitamin D, immune deficiency, and the body's inflammatory response and other chronic and severe diseases, such as asthma, cancer, mental health disorders, cardiovascular diseases, and asthma.

USDA & USDHHS (2020).

Healthy Eating at School

Teachers and school nurses can display bulletin boards using *My Plate* (USDA, 2020) to help students visualize portion size and food choices. See Figure 9-2. School nurses across the country lead "garden to table" or "farm to school" activities, helping children grow vegetables in school gardens that are then served in the school cafeteria. Students experience the satisfaction and pride knowing they helped to provide nutritious meals.

Preschool and school-age children enjoy helping prepare meals and are beginning to make snack choices. This is an ideal time to include nutrition education, so children learn about choosing foods with emphasis on assorted colors, especially fruits and vegetables. Nutrition and healthy eating should be incorporated into the curriculum across all grades.

The school health team as part of the *Whole School, Whole Community, Whole Child* (WSCC) model should focus, in part, on nutrition. The child-centered WSCC model encourages collaboration between the school community to keep students healthy, safe, engaged, supported, and challenged. The school nurse is a leader on the WSCC team, which supports appealing and nutritious food choices served in an environment that encourages healthy eating patterns, demonstrating the link between health and education (ASCD & CDC, 2014).

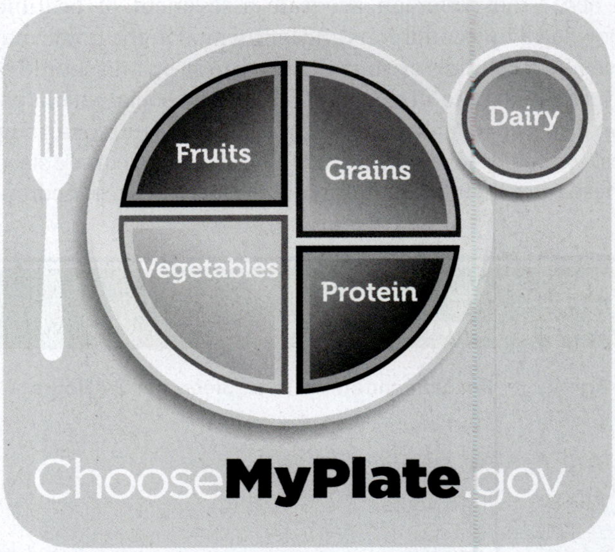

FIGURE 9-2. My Plate. *(U.S. Department of Agriculture, 2020. With permission.)*

The Community Preventive Services Task Force (2018) reviewed interventions in schools to address obesity and nutrition and found that programs that combine physical activity with healthy snacks increased fruit and vegetable consumption and decreased the number of overweight and obese students in schools. This should encourage school nurses to work with partners in physical education and nutrition services to implement similar programs.

The school nurse should collaborate with the cafeteria staff and food vendors to ensure healthy food choices are available at school. Schools that participate in the National School Lunch Program or other federal child nutrition programs are required by federal law to have a school wellness policy giving guidelines on foods served in the school setting, including foods sold at fundraisers and during school-sponsored activities (USDA, 2022c).

Food Insecurity

School nurses are all too familiar with students who have morning hunger pains or headaches due to lack of a nutritious breakfast. Students may come to school hungry because breakfast is overlooked in a rush to get to school, or they may be food insecure. *Food insecurity* describes a lack of access to adequate food at any given time due to a lack of resources (USDA, 2022c). It is important to find out whether the student has adequate food at home and whether the child is eating.

A family may not be officially considered food insecure but may still lack the resources to purchase nutrient-dense food as recommended by the *2020–2025 Food Guidelines.* Fresh fruits and vegetables, such as apples and leafy green vegetables, are nutrient-dense foods, but there may not be a market near the home that sells fresh fruits and vegetables. Foods that are less nutrient dense such as white rice or white bread may be less expensive and stretch further on a tight budget, thus limiting a family's ability to follow the recommended guidelines with nutrient-dense foods.

An astute school nurse seeks to discover the root causes of the problem and addresses the underlying issues causing food insecurity, including a lack of adult supervision, chaotic and/or unsafe living conditions, access to food sources, and poverty. The school nurse should work with the school social worker and refer families to needed community services and resources that assist families to become food secure.

Vegetarian Diets

Vegetarian diets are generally healthy; however, consultation with a dietitian or healthcare provider may be necessary to ensure all nutritional requirements are being met, especially for developing children. Table 9-3 defines different vegetarian diets.

As students enter high school, they may practice food fads and special restrictive diets. Youth who participate in sports and have after-school jobs leading to irregular schedules may also experience alterations in home-prepared family meals, resulting in snacking and eating on the run, often with little thought to nutrition (Kohn, 2022). The recommendations in the 2020–2025 guidelines require more planning by families to achieve healthy eating patterns

TABLE 9-3 Vegetarian Diets

Type of Diet	Food Choices	Supplements That May Be Needed
Semivegetarians	Milk products Limited seafood Limited poultry No red meat	At risk for iron and zinc deficiencies
Lactovegetarians	Milk products No eggs, meat, fish, or poultry	At risk for iron and zinc deficiencies
Ovolactovegetarians	Milk products Eggs No meat, fish, or poultry	At risk for iron and zinc deficiencies
Vegans	Vegetable foods only No foods of animal origin (including fish)	Riboflavin Vitamins D and B_{12} At risk for iron and zinc deficiencies Calcium
Fruitarians	Raw fruit Seeds	Vitamins D and B_{12} At risk for iron and zinc deficiencies Protein

Adapted from Kohn (2022).

that meet the energy needs of active youth. Establishing a link between performance and good nutrition may encourage the student athlete to make healthy dietary choices to maintain a healthy weight. School nurses can advocate for the availability of after-school nutritionally balanced snacks and educate students about nutrient-dense snack foods.

Universal School Meals

Adequate nutrition affects health, behavior, and learning. During the COVID-19 pandemic, U.S. schools offered free meals to all students through a national program, often serving meals in the community. One small study demonstrated during this time that more students participated in the school meal program and there was less stigma associated with eating school meals (Cohen et al., 2021).

Schools that offered free universal breakfast and lunch to all students before the pandemic showed increased participation in the school meal program across all socioeconomic groups, with the largest increase in higher socioeconomic groups. These universal programs improved the nutritional quality for students as well as food security (USDA, 2022b). The link between universal free meals and school attendance showed the biggest improvement in lower socioeconomic groups and in elementary schools with the universal free meals. Overall, academic performance improved in schools where both breakfast and lunch were provided. In the United States, no increase in BMI was noted in the schools where free universal meals were provided to students (Cohen et al., 2021).

During the COVID-19 pandemic, the rate of BMI increase in children and youth (ages 2 to 19) nearly doubled, with individuals with prepandemic overweight or obesity and younger children having the largest increases in BMI (Lange et al., 2021). Government funds helped schools provide free meals to decrease food insecurity during the pandemic. However, the COVID-19 Universal Free Meal Program ended in 2022 and efforts to continue the program at the national level have not been successful. Recognizing the benefits for students, some states (e.g., California, Colorado, and Maine) have adopted a free universal breakfast and lunch program for all students (Butz, 2023). Developing healthy eating with nutrient-dense foods low in sugar, fat, and sodium will provide a healthy foundation for the growing child and youth. Children with chronic conditions may need alterations in the foods they are allowed to ingest and the timing of those meals.

School nurses must continue to educate students, parents/guardians, staff, administrators, and others who are responsible for making decisions about the importance of nutrition and physical activity on the health and well-being of children and adolescents. School nurses also can support the role of the family to be positive role models for their children in developing healthy eating habits.

CHILD DEVELOPMENT

Achievement of developmental tasks at specific ages or stages, or milestones, has always been the standard to measure "typical" development. Development is divided into domains: motor, cognitive, language, psychosocial, and moral.

Motor Development

Gross motor development refers to the development of movement using large muscle groups, and fine motor refers to small muscle groups; both mature and increase strength as the child grows. It is important for the school nurse to be cognizant of the motor skills expected of various age groups. Early identification of possible delays can facilitate access to services to help students reach their potential.

Preschool-Age Children

Balance is important to the overall synthesis of motor coordination and helps with spatial awareness. Balance is well established by the time a child reaches school age. A 3-year-old preschool child can walk up and down steps one foot at a time and climb and runs easily. Throwing, running, and combination movements, such as a hop, skip, and a jump, will continue to be developed through school age (Haywood & Getchell, 2020). A young child can throw a ball using their arm, but an adolescent is able to coordinate the shoulder, leg, and arm to put their body behind the force of the throw.

Children in the preschool years enjoy activities involving gross motor skills, such as marching, hopping, dancing, and traveling around obstacles. They learn to control their body in space and are learning the basics of hand-eye coordination, such as catching and throwing a ball. These activities are simple and require minimal instruction. Very young children do not have the cognitive maturity to understand the rules or strategy involved in many sports. Their coping skills may not be developed to the point where they can deal with stress, disappointment, success, or failure. A child's developmental level is the key to determining the activities in which a child should engage (National Association for the Education of Young Children, 2020). Children's needs for hydration, nutrition, and rest periods should also be considered.

Fine motor skills also continue to develop throughout childhood. By age 3, the child can copy a circle with a pencil, turn book pages, and screw or unscrew lids on a jar. By age 4, children can use scissors, draw a person with two to four body parts, and copy a few capital letters. Children will usually demonstrate a preference for their right or left hand by age 4 (Haywood & Getchell, 2020; Monroe, 2024). Four-year-old children can lace their shoes and by age 6 can tie their shoes, although this skill often occurs later because of the prevalence of Velcro fasteners on shoes.

Young children should have the opportunity to engage in free play. Free play allows children the opportunity to develop the skills necessary to participate in organized sports as they get older. Combining actions such as running, jumping, and kicking are basic skills that will be needed as children move into organized sports (Logan et al., 2019). Children generally express a desire to participate in athletics, anticipating fun and the opportunity to play with their friends. They enjoy being part of a team and the action involved. Parents/guardians frequently encourage their young children to become involved in organized sports, including T-ball, soccer, dance, karate, and gymnastics. This encouragement stems from the belief that enrolling children in a specific program will help develop the physical skills and experience needed to become proficient in that sport, as well as the social sense of commitment and belonging.

Elementary and Early Middle School Children

Most children by age 9 do not often make mistakes in body awareness, such as overreaching for a glass. Children before age 10 are still developing directionality and spatial location; for example, the child may have difficulty when told to throw the ball to the right of the line (Haywood & Getchell, 2020).

The refinement of skills continues throughout the school-age years. Writing and typing skills improve. Children may play a musical instrument, paint, or build models. Between ages 6 and 8, the speed with which messages are relayed to the muscles is significantly increased. This is largely because of an increased production of myelin in the brain. Myelin acts like an insulator around sections of the nerve cells, much like the insulation around an electrical wire. The insulation allows nerve impulses to travel faster, therefore refining fine motor skills. The child's increasing ability to concentrate and focus on a task for prolonged periods also helps fine muscle development.

Young children should have the opportunity to engage in free play. Free play allows children the opportunity to develop the skills necessary to participate in organized sports as they get older. Combining actions such as running, jumping, and kicking are basic skills that will be needed as children move into organized sports (Logan et al., 2019).

Children as young as 6 can participate in organized sports where they focus on enjoyment, participation, and exploration of a variety of sports. The emphasis is on learning basic skills, teamwork, and safety. Children ages 6 to 9 who participate in organized sports show higher motor coordination and higher cognitive performance than those that do not (Logan et al., 2019). Choosing to participate in a particular sport is largely influenced by societal norms and parents/guardians have a strong influence in encouraging participation. Children in elementary school from lower socioeconomic households have been shown to have a lower participation in organized school sports. Transportation may be a factor in younger students' lack of participation because athletic participation in school increases as students age and transportation is provided (Logan et al., 2019). Given the increasing number of children who are overweight or obese, physical activity should be encouraged and supported. Seventy-five percent of adults who participate in sports began their athletic activity by age 8 (Haywood & Getchell, 2020).

Activities should have flexible rules and be entry level so that children can begin to understand the basic idea of the sport. Even young children want to feel competent. Children as young as 5 can compare themselves to others and react to negative feedback from others, which may discourage participation in athletics (Haywood & Getchell, 2020).

Later Middle School and High School

During the period of rapid growth in adolescence, teens may become more awkward because of their rapidly growing extremities. Young adolescents may underestimate the length of their arms or legs and appear awkward or gangly in their movements. They may be clumsy when performing certain activities or misjudge the height of a step based on changing leg lengths. Children who appear clumsy or uncoordinated or are not achieving the milestones expected should be referred to a healthcare provider for evaluation.

School nurses can help parents/guardians and teachers identify types of motor activities that are appropriate for children. They can assess motor development by observing students in both structured classroom settings and unstructured settings, such as recess.

Motor Activity and Safety

Playground Safety

School nurses are often asked to help evaluate playground and gym safety and to make recommendations for equipment that is both safe and promotes development. Hopscotch on the playground during elementary years will help develop motor coordination. A low-to-the-ground balance beam will help a child refine balance and spatial awareness. Climbing can help a child develop body awareness and increase upper body strength; however, children younger than 4 years should not use climbing apparatuses.

Playground equipment is designed for three age groups: children ages 6 months to 23 months, 2 to 5 years, and 5 to 12 years. The National Program for Playground Safety (2015) advocates for separate equipment for children in prekindergarten, kindergarten to grade 2, grades 3 to 4, and grades 5 to 6. Younger children should not play on equipment designed for older children.

A customizable recess planning template is designed to help schools document the details of a recess plan. It identifies strategies schools will use to organize and implement recess at school. It should be written and shared with staff and parents/guardians (CDC, 2016). See Box 9-4 for public playground safety guidelines.

Safety in Farm Communities

In farming communities, children may be performing tasks that may exceed their motor development while working on the family farm. For example, children 7 to 9 years of

BOX 9-4
Playground Safety

PUBLIC PLAYGROUND SAFETY CHECKLIST

1. Make sure surfaces around playground equipment have at least 12 inches of wood chips, mulch, sand, or pea gravel, or are mats made of safety-tested rubber or rubber-like materials.
2. Check that protective surfacing extends at least 6 feet in all directions from play equipment. For swings, be sure surfacing extends in back and front, twice the height of the suspending bar.
3. Make sure play structures more than 30 inches high are spaced at least 9 feet apart.
4. Check for dangerous hardware, like open S-hooks or protruding bolt ends.
5. Make sure spaces that could trap children, such as openings in guardrails or between ladder rungs, measure less than 3.5 inches or more than 9 inches.
6. Check for sharp points or edges in equipment.
7. Look out for tripping hazards, like exposed concrete footings, tree stumps, and rocks.
8. Make sure elevated surfaces, like platforms and ramps, have guardrails to prevent falls.
9. Check playgrounds regularly to see that equipment and surfacing are in good condition.
10. Carefully supervise children on playgrounds to make sure they are safe.

U.S. Consumer Product Safety Commission (n.d., para 2).

BOX 9-5
Car Safety

Age/Weight or Height	Type of Child Safety Restraint
Up to age 4	Rear-facing child safety seat, in the rear seat as long as possible. When child reaches top height or weight limit allowed by car seat's manufacturer, use forward-facing car seat with a harness and tether.
Ages 4–7	Use a forward-facing car seat with a harness and tether in the rear seat until the child reaches the top height or weight limit allowed by the car seat's manufacturer. At that time, use booster seat in the rear seat.
After age 8–12	Use a booster seat in the rear seat where shoulder belt crosses chest and lap belt is across upper thighs. The child can sit on a seat without a booster when the lower belt fits snugly and crosses the body on the upper thighs, not the stomach. The upper belt should fit snugly and cross the shoulder and chest, not the neck or face.

Adapted from National Highway Traffic Safety Administration (n.d.).

age have slower reaction times than older children. This may increase their risk for injury around equipment with moving parts. The *Agricultural Youth Work Guidelines* can help school nurses and parents/guardians determine at what age a child or adolescent is developmentally able to perform various farm tasks (National Children's Center for Rural and Agricultural Health and Safety & National Farm Medicine Center, 2023).

Car Safety

Laws vary from state to state, but all motor vehicle passengers younger than 13 years old should be restrained in the back seat of the vehicle. the National Highway Traffic Safety Administration (n.d.) offers guidelines in an easy-to-remember chart based on age (Box 9-5).

Vehicle safety is important in early childhood settings where children may be transported in school vans or cars. Currently there are no laws requiring seat belts on school buses, but this continues to be discussed nationally.

Gun Safety

In 2020, CDC data identified firearms as the leading cause of death of children and youth between the ages of 1 and 19, surpassing motor vehicle accidents (Goldstick et al., 2022). Forty percent of adults say they live in a household with someone who owns a gun, and 30% say they own a gun (Schaeffer, 2021). One-third of teens who live in a home with guns say they can access a loaded firearm within 5 minutes (Salhi et al., 2021).

Gun violence in America is a public health crisis. Gun control is a very polarizing issue in American discourse. The focus for schools should be on prevention through gun safety education. Guns should be locked in a safe with ammunition stored in a separate safe. Children and youth should not have access to the keys or codes to the locked safe. Students should be taught if they find a gun to leave it alone and get an adult immediately (Byrne et al., 2021). It is important that children and youth understand the danger guns pose and seek adult help. Families may want to work out additional safety measures with their own children. School nurses can work with local public health officials, school administration, and law enforcement to provide gun safety education in a respectful and thoughtful way to keep students and school communities safe.

Cognitive Development

The Brain

Children interpret, adapt, and modify their thinking as they develop. Neural stem cells within the brain develop into the neurons (transmitters) and glia (structure) that make us who we are. As information is received, the brain's neural stem cells divide to become sensory neurons, motor neurons, or interneurons that interpret and transmit the information throughout the brain. The neuron is made up of the cell body, the axon, and dendrites. Information is transmitted from the neuron cell body to the axon and into the dendrites, which transmit information through synapses to receptors. The axon can be long or short depending on where it is transmitting. A myelin sheath covers the axon and acts as a conductor to help messages travel faster and further. Information travels chemically through neurotransmitters or electrically (National Institutes of Health [NIH], 2023). As children experience the environment and social relationships, neural stem cells are divided into more neurons, which continue to interpret and transmit the information to brain cells in a remarkably flexible, growing, and complex system.

As more neurons create pathways, the networks begin to go through a process of "pruning" to remove the pathways no longer necessary or used. In adolescence there is significant pruning in the prefrontal cortex, which sets the stage for a better working memory and the ability to make good decisions based on incoming information. The pruning process may cause certain skills to be learned at a slower rate, but is necessary for optimal cognitive function (Averbeck, 2022).

Theory of Cognitive Development

Jean Piaget's *Theory of Cognitive Development* documented the development of intelligence and cognitive thinking during childhood, as well as the reasons why children form certain beliefs and opinions (Piaget, 1961). He categorized sequential stages of operational thinking, or the way children use mental activity to reach a logical conclusion.

Preschool-Age Children

The preschool child, described by Piaget as ages 2 to 7, is in the *preoperational* stage, having moved on from the sensorimotor stage (Burch, 2024). Preschool children look at what is happening around them as it relates to what they see or hear, and think others see what they see. They have not developed the ability to think logically. They view events from their own perspective and cannot take another's view; thus they are egocentric. Preschool children relate experiences to what they have seen, heard, or felt, and therefore may need preparation before experiences that may bring back fearful memories, such as a visit to the healthcare provider for immunizations. Preschool children cannot always separate the imagined or fantasy from the real world; they engage in magical thinking and believe their thoughts cause events to happen (Monroe, 2024). According to Piaget, young children learn through imagination and play. The use of dolls and puppets can be useful in health promotion teaching.

Elementary and Early Middle School Children

School-age children ages 7 to 12 enter the *concrete operational* stage, where they understand concepts in the concrete form (Burch, 2024). Piaget concluded early school-age children build and hold ideas one at a time; thus ideas will change when presented with different facts. Objects may take on a different view depending on the surroundings. This age group are still egocentric in their thinking but are beginning to think logically. Children in the concrete operations stage understand cause and effect and the concept of time and numbers. They understand the concepts of conservation of matter and reversibility, that is, working backward from a goal to plan steps to reach that goal. They can categorize and classify objects and begin to serialize, that is, arrange objects per category in order. This is the age when they learn to read, write, and work with numbers. During the concrete operational stage, students also begin to understand consequences, and thus make changes based on the expected results.

Later Middle School and High School

The *formal operational* stage usually occurs between the ages of 12 and 15 (Burch, 2024). Teenagers can understand the past, present, and future. They develop abstract thinking and an increased ability to analyze, synthesize, reason, and form logical conclusions. They understand scientific reasoning and benefit from talking about different attitudes and opinions (Piaget, 1961). Early adolescent teens, however, may fluctuate between concrete operations and formal operational thought. As they develop in this stage, adolescents become more confident in their ability to hypothesize, predict, and reflect on the results. Thinking becomes more flexible, and input from various sources can be considered and applied. Adolescents can generate different possibilities from situations and can begin to anticipate potential consequences of actions. Not all adolescents achieve formal operational thought, and many continue to think in a concrete manner. Adolescents want facts and explanations. They learn to identify different alternatives or outcomes based on situational choices. However, their cognitive awareness does not guarantee they will act on new knowledge. Adolescents face many situations as they mature, and even students who have more mature thought processes and are able to analyze the potential results of behavior do not always choose healthy behaviors (Duffy, 2024a). It is well known that adolescents make inappropriate choices, even though they are cognitively aware of the facts.

Myelination in the brain continues throughout adolescence, improving the transmission of neural messages (Duffy, 2024a). Connections between neurons continue to develop in adolescence and into young adulthood. Both the improved efficiency of neural messages and increasing neural connections allow adolescents to expand their cognitive abilities.

Health teaching can be quite effective during the formal operational stage. Youth have an inherent interest in understanding cause and effect and how the body works and stays healthy. Effective health teaching employs visual and experiential learning strategies. Teachable moments can help a student connect their actions with an outcome. When teaching about health and healthy choices, the school nurse should use short-term risks to demonstrate possible consequences of behavior.

Domains of Intelligence

Piaget's theory focuses on the development of linguistic and logical-mathematical intelligence. Howard Gardner (1999) described additional domains of intelligence in which children may have varying levels of competence and comfort. These include the following:

- *Linguistic* intelligence—the gift of language (a strong area for writers and poets)
- *Logical-mathematical* intelligence—strength in problem-solving (a strong area for scientists and mathematicians)
- *Spatial* intelligence: cognitive awareness of spatial relationships (strong for sailors, artists, and engineers)
- *Musical* intelligence: ability to play an instrument, sing, and create music
- *Body-kinesthetic* intelligence: using the body to solve problems or perform (strong among dancers, professional athletes, and craftspeople)
- *Naturalist* intelligence: ability to distinguish between different kinds of animals and different kinds of plants
- *Interpersonal* intelligence: ability to work with people (strong for salespeople, teachers, and politicians)
- *Intrapersonal* intelligence: understanding and using one's own emotions and feelings to guide behavior (Davis et al., 2011)

Students may show strength in one or several areas of intelligence and should be given an opportunity to explore and develop all of their intellectual strengths. Music education, physical education, and art education, as well as traditional cognitive lessons, are important in the overall development of the child (Gardner, 1999). Teaching strategies that incorporate multiple intelligences, such as music, rhymes, games, and humor can help students retain what is taught.

Language Development

Language development reflects cognitive development (Flensborg-Madsen & Mortensen, 2017). Language development is the result of a complex relationship among biological growth, cognitive development, innate ability, and the child's environment (Donnelly & Kidd, 2021).

Preschool-Age Children

Preschool children master language at a rapid rate, forming sentences and developing social conversation. They can speak in sentences and begin to use adjectives in speech. They often ask questions about "who," "what," and "how." An easy rule of thumb to assess language development for children between the ages of 2 and 5 is based on their age. The number range of words in their spoken sentences corresponds to their age plus one; for example, a 3-year-old will construct a sentence using 3 to 4 words (Monroe, 2024).

Adults should be able to understand 90% of a child's speech by age 4 (Hustad et al., 2021). Preschool-age children may have difficulty with pronouns and with pronunciation of certain words. As children develop cognitively, they learn to adjust their language to the situation. For example, a preschool child can adjust their language when talking to a 2-year-old, compared with more formal speech when talking to an adult. Children raised in bilingual homes have the benefit of learning both languages simultaneously. Dual language learners may mix grammar or have a "silent period" where they comprehend more than they express in their nondominant language, but learning a second language does not cause language delays. Students with language delays who are dual language learners would show delays in both languages (American Speech-Language-Hearing Association, 2023b).

Language or speech disorders are frequently identified during preschool education. Parents/guardians may not be aware of speech milestones of their first child, or a child may have older siblings, and a language delay in "the baby" may go unnoticed. Once the child arrives at school, their lack of language development may become obvious in their interactions with others.

Concerns may arise about either *expressive* or *receptive* language. Some children have difficulty expressing what they want to say, even though their actual speaking skills are adequate (i.e., expressive language). Conversely, other children may have difficulty comprehending what is said to them (i.e., receptive language). Language and speech delays may also be due to hearing loss, inadequate stimulation in the home environment, or other developmental delays. Language delays may be the first indication of a developmental delay and should be used as an indicator for early intervention.

Elementary and Early Middle School Children

By age 6, most children have a good vocabulary and are able to communicate clearly (Monroe, 2024). Children ages 6 to 8 can make inferences based on spoken communication and understand more than what was actually said. School-age youth can communicate in code, tell jokes, and communicate nonverbally. They can use the future tense and use nouns, plurals, and possessives. Difficulty pronouncing certain letter sounds (i.e., articulation errors) such as *j, v, r, th, ch,* and *sh* may be noticeable, but this is not necessarily indicative of a larger problem, as these sounds typically are mastered later than other sounds.

Speech therapy is not required for common errors if the difficulty clears by second grade. If there is a concern, a speech and language pathologist can further evaluate the child. By 10 to 12 years of age, students can differentiate formal versus informal speech and can change patterns depending on the audience, for example, parents/guardians

Practice Connection

School nurses should be knowledgeable about typical speech and language development to identify children who need further evaluation for services. These children can be identified during *Child Find* screening and assessment activities as mandated under the *Individuals With Disabilities Education Improvement Act (IDEA) of 2004.* Explore the American Speech-Language-Hearing Association's *How Does Your Child Hear and Talk?* Web site (2023a) for helpful charts on childhood speech articulation, clarity (intelligibility), and vocabulary development.

versus peers. Students also can understand the multiple meanings of words.

Communication in the Health Office

It is often difficult to determine why a young child has arrived at the health office. If students are reserved or have had negative experiences with healthcare providers, they may be reluctant to explain the problem to the school nurse. Other children may feel intimidated by the nurse without the support of a parent/guardian. A visit with the school nurse may be the first independent healthcare interaction a young child experiences.

Deciphering the reason for a health office visit may take creativity and time. It is best to let a child explain what is happening; however, that may not always be possible. A nurse may keep dolls in the office to help children talk about an injury. A picture of different feelings such as "happy," "sad," "angry," and "afraid" may be helpful by allowing the child to point to how they are feeling; the nurse can then ask the child to "point to where it hurts." Pain-rating scales may help determine the severity of pain in a child. Several visual pain-rating scales are available for pediatric use (see Chapter 17).

Psychosocial Development

Erik Erikson (1968) described psychosocial development by identifying certain challenges over the life span that individuals must address to develop healthy personalities and function in society. He called these challenges the *Eight Stages of Man.*

Preschool-Age Children

The preschool and kindergarten years are the stage of *initiative versus guilt;* this follows the earlier stages of trust versus mistrust and autonomy versus shame and doubt. Preschoolers begin to develop a conscience where they are aware of their actions but may feel guilty when their actions or thoughts cause conflict (Erikson, 1968; Monroe, 2024). At this stage children recognize that there is a difference in the sexes and skin color (Erikson, 1968). Preschoolers play *with* other children; they will imitate adult roles in play, such as playing "family" or "doctor." The school nurse can provide the early childhood classroom with health-related equipment to foster imaginative play. Invite the class to visit the health office and describe the role of the school nurse. This early role play can help children see the school nurse as a helper and lessen future anxiety.

Elementary and Early Middle School Children

School-age children enter the stage of *industry versus inferiority,* during which time they gain confidence as they successfully learn new skills. Activities that allow the child to succeed, such as pictures, projects, and recitals, help build self-confidence and thus encourage industry. A supportive environment and positive recognition of accomplishments provides feedback to the child and helps establish a sense of purpose and productivity, in turn, promoting positive self-esteem. Failure at these tasks and criticisms by those around them can lead to feelings of inferiority. This inferiority has a direct impact on the child's self-esteem, and thus the child may feel unable to accomplish tasks. Repeated failures and negative feedback may cause the child to quit trying (Burch, 2024).

The school nurse may need to help a child find success when the school nurse's office becomes an outlet or respite from a stressful academic situation. Musical or artistic talents should be encouraged. A student skilled in interpersonal relationships may be given roles that allow their talent to receive recognition.

Later Middle School and High School Children

Adolescence is identified as the stage of *identity versus role confusion.* Adolescent bodies are growing, maturing, and changing. This stage is highly focused on activities with peers, and adolescents are concerned with how others see them. Peer groups and cliques become important as adolescents try to figure out where they belong and look to others to provide feedback. Acceptance by peers provides a sense of self-worth (Duffy, 2024a; Sherer & Radzik, 2022).

As the adolescent begins to think about where they fit in, they may experiment with different roles and examine different values and norms. This search for identity can lead to some role confusion. Current fads, such as hairstyles, body piercing, ear gauging, and tattoos allow teens to identify with a group and attempt to fit in and belong. This period can be stressful for adolescents and families. Teenagers can be quite cruel to those they perceive as different from themselves. Experimentation with high-risk behaviors, such as tobacco, drugs, and alcohol use, as a way of fitting in can cause conflict with family members and school authority and put the student at risk. Gang involvement may be initiated during this time as a way of fitting in or being accepted by peers (Duffy, 2024a). See Chapter 29 for more information on youth and risk-taking.

School nurses should be aware of this period of confusion and offer guidance and support. Encourage teens to identify strengths and participate in community activities and healthy lifestyles that reflect these strengths. Participating in activities that encourage social responsibility, for example, activities promoting proactive beliefs and behaviors such as cancer awareness or tobacco or substance abuse prevention, can encourage independence.

Late Adolescence

At the end of adolescence, teens enter the stage of *intimacy versus isolation.* A strong connection with peers allows the adolescent to develop relationships that lead to this next stage of development. After developing one's identity, the person is ready to share their identity with others. Thus the search for a significant other begins, as well as exploring different careers for one's future. Adolescent development is discussed again later in this chapter.

Moral Development

Lawrence Kohlberg (1981) examined moral development and identified three levels: Level 1, preconventional morality; Level 2, conventional morality; and Level 3, postconventional morality. According to Kohlberg, most people will remain at the level of conventional morality and not reach the final stage. Kohlberg's theory has been criticized because he studied only male individuals; thus gender differences were not accounted for in the theory (Murphy & Gilligan, 1980).

Preschool-Age Children

The *preconventional level* is where the developing child perceives a rule-based world revolving around rewards and punishments (Kohlberg, 1981). Right and wrong are understood, but the parents/guardians or caregivers, who are in power, judge what is classified as right and wrong. Avoidance of punishment is most important to the child. As the children reach age 4, they begin to examine fairness and sharing, but for the most part they are interested in what they will receive in return and what is the reward. Children at this level can work in groups and be expected to cooperate with each other. They can also be expected to recognize differences in other children, whether cultural, racial, or socioeconomic.

Children at the preconventional level conform to the rules imposed by others and respond to labels such as good or bad. As cultural and familial attitudes are learned by preschool children, many biases and prejudices are also learned as being "good" or "bad." Therefore, care must be taken to expose children to different cultures as a way of learning about differences in others at an early age, without attaching positive or negative labels to the differences.

Elementary and Early Middle School Children

As they enter school, children enjoy helping others because this is "nice behavior;" they enjoy the recognition and praise received for being nice. In school, children are exposed to authority figures other than their parents/guardians and usually believe that the authority figure sets the rules. This stage can be complicated by cultural or familial differences of what is "right" and "nice." Therefore, schools must stipulate the rules of the school. For example, bullying must be defined, and bullying behaviors must be identified.

By age 10, fairness is important, and children consider cooperation and the respect of others when deciding on rules to follow. After age 10, the needs of a group help determine the rules, and children follow the rules to please others and be part of the group.

At the *conventional level,* good behavior is judged by what is generally acceptable by the majority. Rule following and respect for authority are of primary importance. Certain behavior is expected to maintain the social order, such as obeying the rules; most of society functions at this level. Early and middle adolescence also function at the conventional level, where it is important to obey the rules and follow the laws set by society. However, they may question rules that may not seem fair or applied equally. Elementary school students may view the rules differently if presented with a different set of circumstances, exercising moral reasoning (Duffy, 2024a).

Later Middle School and High School Children

The teen has a sense of justice and may have strong feelings about what is right or wrong. The adolescent often look to peers for moral approval rather than to family. Although the teen may believe one way, the teen's behavior and actions may not reflect that belief. School nurses working with teens may find that the story relayed may not always reflect the whole truth. Adolescents may try to save face in front of peers or not be truthful because of potential consequences. Nonjudgmental attitudes can help elicit information, and interactive listening can be an effective tool.

At the *postconventional, autonomous,* or *principled level,* the individual will follow moral principles perceived as transcending society and culture. The values are followed because the individual believes in the rightness of the principles. At this level, one recognizes that laws can be changed if they can be shown to benefit the whole of society. Students can become involved in activities to influence school policies or student government. By late adolescence, postconventional moral values develop, and students are able to look at the laws and rules as they affect society. The older adolescent considers whether the rules fit his or her own inner principles and values.

While Kohlberg focused on justice and moral development, Gilligan (Murphy & Gilligan, 1980) proposed that caring about others is also a consideration when faced with moral decisions. Eventually, one learns to examine these conflicting priorities by understanding the interdependent nature of relationships. In general, females consider a situation based on the care and concern for others more than the justice perspective, whereas males predominantly look at justice overall when faced with moral decisions (Duffy, 2024a).

DEVELOPMENTAL ISSUES: PRESCHOOL CHILDREN, AGES 3 TO 5

Early Childhood Education

Increasing numbers of children are enrolled in early childhood programs in the community or in schools, in either half-day or full-day programs from 2 to 5 days per week (CDC, 2023a). Early childhood education improves cognitive development, academic achievement, behavioral self-regulation, and social-emotional skills.

Federal programs have encouraged the creation of quality preschool programs to meet the needs of children. In 1968, children with disabilities were accepted into Head Start programs. This was followed by the Education for All Handicapped Children Act (later to become the Individuals With Disabilities Education Improvement Act) that mandated public schools offer special education services to eligible 3- to 5-year-old children with disabilities. In 2016, the Child Care and Development Fund Program strengthened the supports that protect the health and safety of children in childcare by requiring agencies to inform parents/guardians about child development and provide access to high-quality childcare, particularly for low-income children (Federal Register, 2016).

Yet disparities remain among children living in poverty where early education can provide the most benefit; over half the children living in poverty did not attend an early childhood program in 2019 (CDC, 2023a). Awareness of programs, transportation issues, and parent/guardian involvement may play a factor in children attending early education programs. Examining and removing the systemic barriers low-income families face due to social determinants of health (e.g., location, transportation, cost, job demands, subsidized extended after-school services) should be considered for the long-term health and productivity of youth.

Children born preterm are at risk for cognitive, motor, speech, language, and sensory delay or impairment. Full-term babies may also exhibit developmental delays. Early intervention and education for these children during the early years when their brains and bodies are rapidly developing can benefit long-term educational and behavioral outcomes.

The U.S. Preventive Services Task Force notes there is a lack of supporting evidence for routine screening of speech and language for asymptomatic children (Siu, 2015). The CDC has a mobile app for parents/guardians to help track development in their child (CDC, 2022a). See Chapter 26 for more information on students with neurodevelopmental disorders.

Prekindergarten

Preschools and prekindergarten (pre-K) programs have been referred to interchangeably; yet pre-K programs are aimed specifically at the 4-year-old population. The goal of pre-K programs is to increase the skill level and develop readiness for entry into kindergarten. Studies have shown that attending a pre-K program can help prepare children for kindergarten when qualified staff are present and use evidence-based curriculum effectively (Pre-Kindergarten Task Force, 2017). Pre-K programs are particularly beneficial for those children living in poverty and non–English-proficient children. Enrollment in publicly funded pre-K programs has increased significantly over the past 30 years. Pre-K continues to be recommended to enhance kindergarten readiness and early grade level success.

Developmental Screening for Pre-K

As mandated by IDEA (2004), school districts must engage in Child Find activities to help identify children of all ages who have developmental issues (see Chapter 7). It is important for school nurses to be familiar with the tools used in the local school community to identify children at risk for developmental delay. Fine motor, gross motor, and language skills expected of the preschool child are listed in Table 9-4.

School nurses need to be sensitive to parents/guardians whose child may have a developmental delay. The diagnostic period can be stressful. Although parents/guardians may suspect that their child is different or slower than other children, having this confirmed by school officials is often upsetting. School nurses should participate in individualized education program (IEP) meetings and other multidisciplinary team meetings where screening results are shared, using knowledge of expected developmental milestones to help translate evaluation results in meaningful ways that families can understand. See Chapter 8 for more information on the school nurse's role in special education.

Toilet Training

Most children entering preschool are toilet trained. Some children with developmental delays may not be toilet-trained on school entry, and the school nurse may be asked to provide guidance. However, toileting students does not require a nursing license, and therefore it is not generally the responsibility of the school nurse. Unlicensed assistive school personnel often are assigned the role of helping students who need assistance with toileting. A bathroom in or near the classroom should be made available to help a child become toilet-trained while at school. A toilet low to the ground or "potty" chair should be available so the child can use it with minimal help from adults.

In a school setting, hygiene and asepsis are essential, especially if staff are asked to change diapers. Effective hand washing is essential for anyone helping a child learn to use the toilet. The use of underpants is considered a badge of success, especially those designed with the child's favorite characters. Parents/guardians should be encouraged to leave an extra set of clothing in the student's cubby in case of accidents. Be sure that wet

TABLE 9-4 Fine Motor, Gross Motor, and Language Skills of the Preschool Child

Age	Fine Motor	Gross Motor	Language and Communication	Self-Help	Play
>3	Copies a circle Strings large beads Puts pegs in pegboard Builds tower of more than six blocks	Runs easily Climbs Walks up and down steps one foot at a time Rides a tricycle	Uses sentences with three or four words Understands biggest/smallest Follows two-step commands Strangers can understand speech Asks questions	Dresses and undresses self Washes hands Brushes teeth with help Puts on shoes Knows gender Helps set table	Role-plays to experiment with adult roles Begins to take turns Usually plays cooperatively with other children but may parallel play Names a friend Plays make believe
>4	Draws 2–4-part person Uses scissors Copies a few capital letters Copies square and traces diamond and cross	Hops and stands on one foot for up to 2 seconds Catches a bounced ball Walks backward Good kicking motion Walks down stairs with alternate feet	Often asks who, what, when, why Uses four- to six-word sentences Communicates effectively Tells stories Knows songs	Dresses self Brushes teeth Laces shoes Buckles belt	Becomes aware of different genders Proud of accomplishments Creative with make-believe play Plays "Mom and Dad" Cooperates with other children
>5	Copies triangle and other shapes Draws six-part person Colors inside the lines Prints some letters or numbers Uses scissors	Hops and may skip Throws and catches a ball Jumps rope Balances on one foot for longer than 10 seconds Walks backward	Communicates feelings Participates in conversation Speaks clearly Uses future tense Says name and address	Covers mouth and nose when coughing or sneezing Uses fork and knife Manners improve More independent and responsible	Plays table games Understands rules Likes to sing, dance, and act Enjoys activities

Adapted from CDC (2022a); Monroe (2024).

or soiled clothes are bagged in a way to avoid contamination with other student materials and to maximize student privacy.

Classroom teachers should ensure toileting is included in the class schedule every 2 hours. They must be alert for signs of the urge to urinate or defecate and usher the child quickly to the toilet. If the child does not show an interest in learning to use the toilet at school, a schedule can be developed. The child can be escorted to the toilet every hour and placed on the toilet for 5 minutes. Attempts and successes should be rewarded with praise and positive reinforcement. It may be helpful to read books about toileting and always work closely with the family to reinforce lessons at home and in school (Duffy, 2024b).

DEVELOPMENTAL ISSUES: ELEMENTARY AND EARLY MIDDLE SCHOOL CHILDREN, AGES 6 TO 12

Skills and Play

The early school-age child is interested in simple board games, cards, music, water, and clay; action games such as tag and hide-and-seek are popular. Young students like to pretend play and will imitate adult behavior. They may play in groups, but the groups are loosely organized. Children are becoming more industrious and may start to take things apart just to put them back together again. They enjoy collecting and sorting items such as cards or stickers; they then trade these with their peers.

Books and pads of paper can occupy the student learning to master skills of reading and writing. As the child develops, games with rules become more important. Group play allows the child to learn cooperation with others, and the rules help form the structure for the games. Social rules are incorporated into play. Winning is important, and although they have an awareness of rules, children may cheat at games to win. Table 9-5 lists the skills the school-age child is expected to accomplish.

School-age children spend much of their day in school, and friends become especially important. A sense of belonging develops as they begin to take part in group activities. Peer group activities help the child to develop interpersonal interactions, self-concept, and gender-role behaviors. Best friends are important at age 8, and children may have a first "best friend" as well as a second "best friend."

During the school-age years, music lessons, swimming lessons, scouts, sports groups, and other organized activities introduce children to multiple aspects of life, as well as build skills and encourage group activities. Schools often promote and may even provide these activities after school

TABLE 9-5 Skills of the School-Age Child

Age	Gross Motor	Fine Motor	Language	Play
6	Easily ties shoelaces Cuts and pastes, draws a person with good detail, and prints	Jumps, skips, and hops Walks a straight line and rides a two-wheeled bicycle Becoming skilled at throwing a ball	Talks in full sentences and use of grammar becomes more correct Tells a simple story	Imaginative play is present Likes table games
7	Writes Reads regular-size type	Jumps with coordination to play hopscotch and skip rope Plays games with balls	Begins to use complex passive sentences and construct conditional sentences	Gender differences in games may surface; for example, boys may be interested in playing ball, whereas girls may be more interested in jump rope Needs more props with play Collects items such as baseball cards, dolls, and coins
8	Increases speed of writing Uses hand tools such as a screwdriver	Adjusts body position to successfully catch a ball Puts right or left foot forward on command	More sociable with improved conversational skills Describes objects in detail	Likes to ride bicycle and participate in organized sports Likes to sort and catalog items
9	Writing looks more mature Continues to refine skills	Catches a ball with one hand Vertical jumping skills improve Balances on one leg with eyes closed	Understands inferences Uses language to persuade and advance an idea	Plays rough and more interested in the game than perfecting skills Takes music lessons and talent becomes evident
10–12			Uses formal and informal speech and can change patterns depending on audience Understands multiple meanings of words Uses sarcasm and puns	Continues to improve at organized sports Enjoys building toys Growth spurts may make body awareness more difficult; thus, some may not participate in sports Time with friends is spent talking Likes to listen and dance to popular music Organized sports important

Adapted from Haywood & Getchell (2020); American Speech-Language Hearing Association (2023c).

hours. The school nurse can recommend these activities to students, especially those who need companionship and increased self-esteem.

Daily activity should be encouraged. Children ages 6 and older can begin to participate in organized sports; however, the emphasis should be on having fun and trying different sports. Children between ages 6 and 10 may have difficulty handling the stress of intense competition or the disappointment of loss or failure, so winning should not be the most important goal. Learning skills and teamwork should be encouraged at this level. Children who cannot physically handle the demands of sport may feel discouraged when they fail and thus not make further attempts.

The development of balance, coordination, and reaction time improves with age; therefore beginning ball sports such as T-ball or noncontact soccer should be encouraged. Children still have short attention spans and are not adept at making quick decisions. Also, their ability to anticipate the projection and direction of a ball may make them appear uncoordinated, but this does improve with age. Improved skills and increasing memory help them remember patterns and plays for sports, which enhance their success and enjoyment. Sports participation can incorporate physical skill-building activities and appropriate socialization, as well as anger management and problem-solving skills. At this age, the importance of developing these skills should be stressed over the need to win. It is important that students have free time for play and not be overscheduled outside of school hours.

The emphasis on daily physical exercise and the link to obesity supports the fact that all children should be encouraged to participate in physical activity. Sport activities should be developmentally appropriate for the child to allow for success in the activity. If the child is successful, it is likely they will continue to enjoy the sport. In addition, the positive feedback achieved from participation will enhance self-esteem.

Head and Neck Changes

The school-age years reflect the continuing development of the immune system. Lymphatic tissue grows until about 9 years of age; excess tonsillar and adenoid tissue may be mistaken for enlargement during an upper respiratory illness and may even interfere with hearing, breathing, and sleep. Once the tissue recedes normally, hearing returns to normal. In addition, the frontal sinuses develop around age 6; thus, students may experience sinus headaches.

Patterns of Elimination

Children ages 6 to 12 normally urinate five to six times within a 24-hour period and defecate more than four times per week; three times a week or less may indicate constipation. Normal patterns of elimination should be encouraged during school, and students should be given easy access to private stall restrooms. Staff education about normal elimination patterns in children, allowing students easier access to restrooms, and ensuring the restrooms are clean and safe decrease the possibility of developing abnormal elimination patterns. The nurse should be alert for abnormal elimination patterns such as incontinence or prolonged holding of urine or feces. Evaluation by a healthcare provider is necessary to rule out a potential physical cause of abnormal elimination, for example, infection or obstruction.

Incontinence/Enuresis

Children may experience urinary incontinence during the day or nighttime bedwetting (nocturnal enuresis). After age 5, bedwetting at night is considered enuresis if it occurs at least once a month over a period of 3 months. Frequent wetting during the daytime means more than 4 times in 1 week (Gontard & Kuwertz-Bröking, 2019). Ten percent of 5-year-old children will have daytime urinary incontinence, which could be caused by an overactive bladder, urinary postponement, or dysfunctional voiding. Daytime urinary incontinence is more common in girls (National Institute of Diabetes and Digestive and Kidney Disease [NIDDKD], 2017). Frequent scheduled voiding may help to alleviate daytime incontinence. It is always helpful to keep a change of clothes in the classroom for young children for the occasional toileting accidents that occur.

Primary nocturnal enuresis occurs in a child who has never been dry at night. Secondary nocturnal enuresis occurs between the ages of 5 and 8 years after the child has been dry at night. Several factors may contribute to nocturnal enuresis. Children of parents/guardians who both have a history of nocturnal enuresis have been shown to have almost a 70% chance of developing nocturnal enuresis (NIDDKD, 2017). Some affected children sleep soundly and do not awaken with the urge to void, whereas others may have a smaller bladder capacity than those who do not wet the bed or have insufficient antidiuretic hormone, interfering with the kidney's ability to concentrate urine.

Children should always be referred to their healthcare provider for a urinalysis and physical examination to rule out an organic cause, such as diabetes or a urinary tract infection. Approximately 20% to 30% of youth who have nighttime bedwetting and 20% to 40% who have daytime wetting have a coexisting mental health concern such as attention deficit-hyperactivity disorder (ADHD), depression, anxiety, or behavioral issues (Gontard & Kuwertz-Bröking, 2019).

Punishment or shaming should never be used to control bedwetting; the child should be encouraged to help change the sheets when wet. To avoid unpleasant odors in the school, the school nurse may be asked to talk with parents/guardians of a child experiencing bedwetting to ensure the child is bathing before coming to school. Parents/guardians can be reassured nocturnal enuresis diminishes as the child gets older. Treatment can begin by keeping a daily calendar of dry and wet nights; 15% of children with enuresis improve by keeping this type of daily calendar (Gontard & Kuwertz-Bröking, 2019).

Functional Fecal Incontinence (Encopresis)

Children beyond the age of toilet training who frequently soil their underwear may have a condition called *functional fecal incontinence (FFI)*, also known as encopresis. FFI is defined as fecal incontinence without underlying conditions in children who completed toilet training. There can be both physiological and psychological aspects to this situation, and it is estimated to affect 1% to 2% of children over the age of 7 (Sood et al., 2023). Shared bathrooms and new routines may serve as triggers.

Most FFI cases (80%) are due to functional constipation with no known medical cause (Sood et al., 2023). Some children hold their bowel movements to avoid the pain they feel when passing hard constipated stool. As the stool builds up in the colon and rectum, water and softer stool leaks around the mass and cannot be withheld by the anus, resulting in soiling. This may be mistaken for diarrhea. The child has no control over this leakage as the sensation of needing to defecate has disappeared due to the stretched anus. Constipation may be due to diet, illness, decreased fluid intake, stress, or limited access to a toilet that is not private. FFI is more common among students with ADHD, autism, anxiety, and depression.

FFI is not usually a behavioral issue or lack of self-control. However, it may result in conflict between the child and parents/guardians or changes to routine, such as starting school; a child may have poor self-esteem and may feel embarrassed. Treatment begins with disimpaction followed by maintenance laxative therapy with a goal of daily soft stools, dietary changes, and behavior modification (Sood et al., 2023). A treatment plan should involve demystifying the condition and having scheduled bathroom breaks, especially after meals, with toilet sitting for 5 to 10 minutes. It may take months for the stretched colon to return to its normal size and the nerves in the colon to become effective again. The family will be encouraged to provide fiber-rich foods, such as fresh fruits, dried fruits such as prunes and raisins, dried beans, vegetables, and high-fiber bread and cereal. An extra set of pants should be kept at school. See Chapter 16 for further discussion of encopresis.

Developing Sexuality and Gender Identity

A child's awareness of their changing body and developing sexuality are important developmental tasks during school-age and adolescent years. From an early age, boys and girls learn what society expects of their birth-assigned gender. Most of society sees gender as binary (male or female), and society responds based on cultural and societal norms. For example, boys may be given baseball gloves and be expected to play with trucks and trains, whereas girls may be dressed in pink, wear dresses, and play with dolls. However, the beliefs that society once held about gender expectations and a healthy sexuality are being expanded beyond the male and female binary definitions.

Sexuality develops over time, and school-age children are curious about their developing bodies, as well as the process of reproduction and the act of sexual intercourse. Young children may imitate the sexual behavior they see at home and in the media; generally this acting out should not be alarming (Monroe, 2024). The school nurse may be asked to talk with the young student who is masturbating or otherwise acting out sexually in class. A frank, nonjudgmental discussion with the student about appropriate behavior in the school setting (including on buses, school trips, dances, and sporting events) may be all that is necessary. The nurse should assess whether a medical problem or problems at home may be causing the behavior. If abuse is suspected, it should be reported to the appropriate agency (see Chapter 11). The school nurse can foster respect and pride in one's body by giving accurate developmentally appropriate information, correct terminology, and reassurance that body changes and interest in sexuality are part of normal growth and development (Ehrensaft, 2016). Children may show preferences for toys, clothes, and games expected of a different sex. Experts recommend allowing the child to explore and play with the toys they enjoy as they grow and learn about their environment.

Sex education in the early school-age years should include factual information at the appropriate developmental level and in consideration of diverse cultural contexts. Sex education should be treated as a normal part of growth and development and can be incorporated into the curriculum in lessons on family life or the study of animals from an early age. Direct, short, factual answers are generally all that is needed during the preschool years (Monroe, 2024). The school nurse may be called on to explain menarche to the 7- or 8-year-old who develops early or sexual maturation to fourth- or fifth-grade classes.

Puberty used to occur primarily during the early teenage years; this was considered the beginning of adolescence. However, many children do begin puberty during elementary school; therefore it is important to introduce body changes and sex education in the early grade-school curriculum. However, because of the earlier maturational development of the female body, a new group has emerged, called *tweens*. These 10- (some say as young as 8-) to 14-year-olds have unique needs because their bodies are developing faster than their cognitive development.

Many programs are available to teach about sexual development and puberty during the latter elementary school years; many of these programs are available in different languages. Families should be informed by the school of the content of the reproductive health or sexuality curriculum. Children and teens with developmental disabilities need appropriate instruction as they begin to experience puberty. See Online Materials OM9-1 and OM9-2 for additional resources on health sexuality and menstruation.

DEVELOPMENTAL ISSUES: LATER MIDDLE SCHOOL AND HIGH SCHOOL STUDENTS, AGES 12 TO 18

Adolescence, also thought of as the teen years, typically starts with the initiation of pubertal changes and includes rapid physiological and psychological changes, as well as the cognitive maturation. Although the biological changes related to hormones occur sequentially, the psychosocial and cognitive changes of puberty may occur at different ages and in nonsequential patterns. School nurses can provide scientific explanations for pubertal changes to help teens understand that the changes they are experiencing are universal.

Puberty

The key hormone responsible for growth is growth hormone (GH). GH released by the pituitary gland stimulates insulin-like growth factors (IGFs) causing bone growth. GH levels increase during puberty resulting in the peak years for physical growth and are linked to the stages of sleep (Carswell & Stafford, 2022). Increases in testosterone and estradiol stimulate linear growth, bone density, and the rate of epiphyseal fusion. See Table 9-6 for hormonal changes during puberty.

Skeletal growth peaks during the adolescent growth spurt, accounting for 20% of the final adult height. Approximately 3 years before menarche girls will start their period of rapid growth and will grow only 1 to 2.5 inches more after reaching menarche (Carswell & Stafford, 2022). The formation of skeletal bone during puberty is extremely important because this is the time when an individual establishes 50% of their skeletal bone mass (Kohn, 2022). The end of bone growth occurs when the epiphyseal plates close.

During adolescence, muscle mass in boys increases rapidly and accounts for 54% of body weight. Boys may experience spurts of increased strength during adolescence, whereas girls have steady increases in strength before leveling off (Haywood & Getchell, 2020). The percentage of body fat decreases in male adolescents and increases in

TABLE 9-6 Hormonal Changes During Puberty

Sex	Changes	Actions
Follicle-Stimulating Hormone (FSH)		
Female	Growth of ovarian follicles Production of estrogen	Estradiols stimulate development of internal and external genitalia and breasts and increase body fat. Estradiols trigger LH production at midcycle, which causes maturation and release of ovum. Estradiols at low levels encourage linear growth and at elevated levels increase the rate of epiphyseal fusion.
Male	Makes cells receptive to testosterone	Testosterone stimulates spermatogenesis. Development of the seminiferous tubules in testes.
Luteinizing Hormone (LH)		
Female	Initiates ovulation Formation of the corpus luteum Production of progesterone	Progesterone, together with estrogen, regulates the menstrual cycle and stimulates breast development.
Male	Promotes maturation and increased size of testicles Development of Leydig's cells in testes, which lead to the production of testosterone Promotes production of small amount of estrogen	Testosterone (1) increases linear growth and rate of epiphyseal fusion and increases muscle mass and bone density; (2) stimulates development of internal and external sexual characteristics and increases libido; (3) increases the size of the larynx, which deepens the voice; and (4) stimulates sebaceous glands to secrete oil. Estradiol increases the rate of epiphyseal fusion and increases bone mineral density.
Adrenal Androgens (Produced by Adrenal Glands)		
Female	Testosterone, estrogen, and progesterone released	Axillary and pubic hair growth and an increase in female libido.
Male	Testosterone released	Axillary and pubic hair growth (influence in puberty is much less than for gonadotropins)

Adapted from Duffy (2024a); Carswell & Stafford (2022).

female adolescents; females may have twice as much body fat as boys.

Facial characteristics become more adult-like as the lips protrude and the nose and jaw become more prominent to accommodate the full set of permanent teeth. The apocrine sweat glands increase their activity, and body odor may become an issue; axillary sweating begins at about the time of axillary hair growth. Sweating can create an environment for tinea infections of the groin or feet.

Middle school and high school are ideal times to promote good overall body hygiene and the use of deodorant. It is common for younger students to be unaware of body odor as they begin pubertal changes, and they may be referred to the school nurse to address unpleasant body odor. Presenting the information in a factual manner by describing normal development and body changes can educate an adolescent in a nonthreatening manner. The school nurse needs to be cognizant of cultural variations regarding hygiene and body odor. The teen may not be aware of the effect their hygiene practices have on others.

An increase in the production of sebum by the sebaceous follicles of the skin in response to increased hormone levels during puberty causes acne. Acne is an inflammation of the sebaceous glands and hair follicles of the skin leading to papules and pustules (see Chapter 18). Stress and genetic factors also influence the development of acne. Washing the face twice daily with mild soap helps wash off excess oil and helps to prevent acne eruptions. Excess cleansing or washing is likely to cause irritation and decrease the effectiveness of medication used to treat acne (Strowd & Krowchuk, 2022). Acne, which may cause scars and alter one's body image, can be treated by the healthcare provider using a variety of topical or systemic medications.

There is a wide variation in individuals within and between sex and racial/ethnic groups. Typically, females begin puberty earlier than males. In general, Black American males experience the onset of puberty earlier than White males, followed by Latino American males (Carswell & Stafford, 2022).

Tanner (1962) described the sexual development of males and females in stages during adolescence in terms of the *sexual maturity rating* (SMR) or Tanner Scale (Carswell & Stafford, 2022). Boys and girls progress through similar stages. See Figures 9-3 and 9-4.

Puberty in Males

In males, the hypothalamus produces gonadotropin-releasing hormone (GnRH) that signals the anterior pituitary gland to release the gonadotropins luteinizing hormone (LH) and follicle-stimulating hormone (FSH) (Carswell & Stafford, 2022). LH causes testicular enlargement and development of Leydig cells in the testes that produce testosterone. FSH stimulates the development of the seminiferous tubules of the testes, leading to spermatogenesis and fertility. Enlargement of the testicles signals the start of puberty in males, but the appearance of pubic hair is often

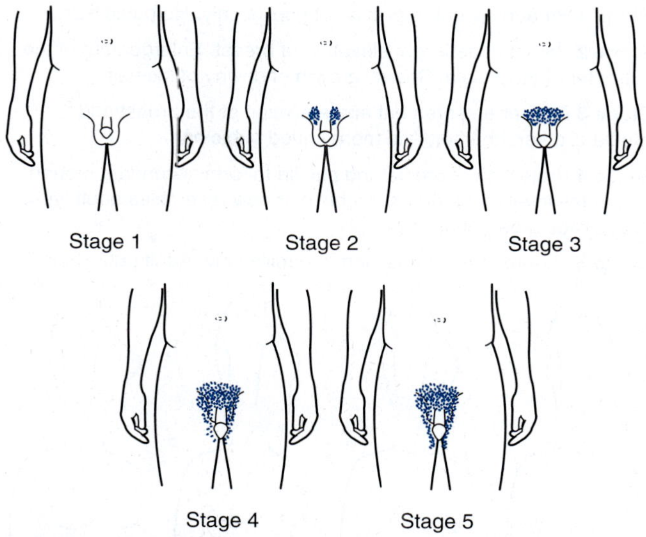

FIGURE 9-3. Male development. *(Art courtesy of Valerie Probst.)*

the first noticeable sign. Voice changes are related to the release of testosterone (Carswell & Stafford, 2022).

The average boy takes about 2 years to go from SMR 2 to 4 and an additional 2 years to progress to SMR 5. Males take about 5 years to complete the pubertal changes.

Spermarche, the onset of sperm emission, generally occurs in midpuberty, which is also the time that height rapidly increases. Facial hair will also appear. Growth of hair on the back and abdomen may continue past puberty (Carswell & Stafford, 2022). Nocturnal emissions, frequently referred to as "wet dreams," are involuntary ejaculations resulting in the release of seminal fluid common during the night. Though sometimes misinterpreted as wetting the bed, nocturnal emissions are normal and cannot be controlled.

Puberty in Females

The appearance of breast buds is the first sign of puberty in girls and is called thelarche (Tanner, 1962). In females, as in males, the hypothalamus produces GnRH that signals the anterior pituitary to release the gonadotropins LH and FSH. The effects of these hormones in girls start the development of secondary sexual characteristics; FSH stimulates ovarian development and estrogen production, whereas estrogen influences the development of most of the other secondary sex characteristics. Pubic and axillary hair are controlled by adrenal androgens.

Menarche, the onset of menses, occurs, on average, between ages 12 and 13, about 2 years after the beginning of breast development (the bud stage). It occurs approximately 3 years after the start of the growth spurt and 1 year after the peak height velocity. Growth after menarche is minimal, and breast development ends shortly after the start of menses (Carswell & Stafford, 2022).

Culture, race, economic status, heredity, and nutrition all influence the age of menarche. Menstrual cycles will become

Stage 1 Preadolescent: elevation of papilla only. No pubic hair.

Stage 2 Breast buds: slight elevation of breast. Enlargement of the diameter of the areola. Sparse growth of downy pubic hair.

Stage 3 Further enlargement and elevation of the breast and areola. Darker, coarser, and more curled pubic hair.

Stage 4 Projection of areola and papilla to form secondary mound above the level of the breast. Pubic hair now resembles adult type, but surface area not as large.

Stage 5 Mature stage: projection of papilla only. Adult pubic hair.

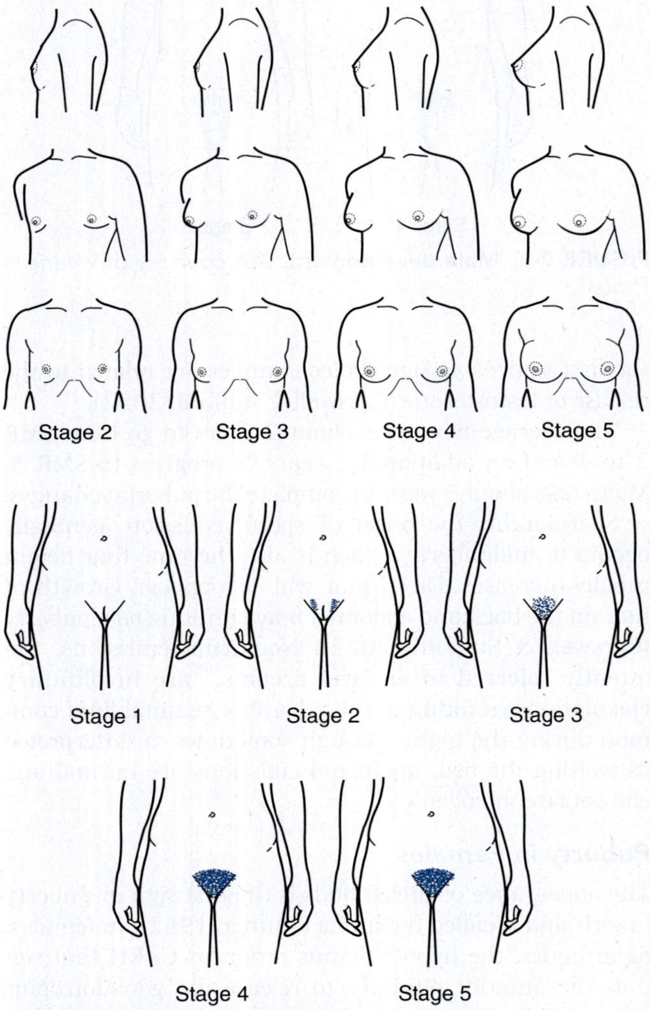

FIGURE 9-4. Female development. *(Art courtesy of Valerie Probst.)*

increasingly more regular 5 to 7 years after menarche (Carswell & Stafford, 2022). Developing a menstrual cycle reflects multiple body processes occurring. It requires a minimum amount of body fat, it results in blood loss, and its absence may indicate multiple endocrine conditions, stress, or medication effects. Studies indicate non-Hispanic black girls have earlier menarche compared with girls of other races (American College of Obstetricians and Gynecologists [ACOG], 2015). Information about a girl's menstrual cycle may be considered a vital sign (ACOG, 2015; USDHSS, 2021).

School nurses should make sure feminine hygiene products are available and accessible for all students in elementary, middle, and high school. A recent study described how adolescents had been taught scientific information about menstruation but when they started menstruating, they did not know how to use a tampon (Secor-Turner et al., 2022). Other concerns identified by students was excusal from class to use the restroom and being allowed adequate time in the restroom to change a pad or tampon. Increasingly, state laws and school policies are mandating that menstrual products be available for free in schools as a matter of health equity. School nurses can advocate for school policies and classroom rules that respect the needs of adolescent females.

Dysmenorrhea, uncomfortable or painful menstrual cycles, can begin 6 to 12 months after menarche. Between 70% and 90% of women have discomfort during their cycle (Sachedin & Todd, 2020). School nurses can recognize and support these students when they come to the nurse's office. A referral to the healthcare provider is needed if students are missing school or activities due to dysmenorrhea. Continued pain requires further investigation to determine whether endometriosis, tissue growth outside of the uterus, may be the cause. Between 6% and 10% of females have endometriosis, which will have a lifelong impact on a woman's health (Mackenzie & Cohn, 2023).

Influences on Puberty

Obesity has an effect on puberty onset. Females who are obese may mature early, but their menstrual cycles are often irregular. Obesity in adolescence can trigger the onset of insulin resistance that affects growth, causing obese youth to be taller than peers due to a spike in growth hormone (Stackpole et al., 2022). Obesity and insulin resistance are risk factors for polycystic ovarian syndrome (PCOS). Excess adipose tissue is a source of estrogen, causing decreased follicle-stimulating hormone (FSH) and an increase in luteinizing hormone (LH). These changes increase the production of androstenedione and testosterone, which are associated with PCOS.

Precocious puberty is when children show signs of early pubertal development. In boys this is younger than age 9, and in girls, before age 8; it may be earlier in black American and Latino American girls (AAP & Pediatric Endocrine Society, 2018). Boys are less likely to have precocious puberty but are more likely than girls to have an underlying pathology as the cause for early puberty (Eimicke & Swartz, 2022). The school nurse should be alert to children who show signs of precocious puberty and recommend them

> **Practice Connections**
>
> Parents/guardians may ask when is the "right" time to have discussions with their daughters about menstruation. Because it takes 2 to 3 years from bud stage to menses, once the bud stage of breast development is noticed, discussions can begin. See Online Materials OM9-2 for resources related to talking about menstruation.

for further medical evaluation. To many youth, however, early signs of puberty are signs of growing up and are seen as desirable.

Later onset of puberty has been noted in larger families, in rural areas, and among those living at higher altitudes (Carswell & Stafford, 2022). Delayed puberty is defined as the development of breast buds after age 13 in girls and in boys, no testicular enlargement by age 14. It is more common in boys and most likely associated with concern over short stature and the lack of muscle development. Most students with delayed puberty have shown a pattern of slow growth throughout life and may have a familial history of delayed puberty. Most youth will eventually catch up to their peers if there is no organic cause. Delayed puberty may also be caused by poor nutrition, perhaps due to an eating disorder; students with a chronic health condition may exhibit symptoms of delayed puberty. A referral to the healthcare provider is advised to rule out any possible organic cause for the delay (Eimicke & Swartz, 2022).

Biopsychosocial Development

Hormonal changes influence both biological and psychosocial growth and development during adolescence. Studies of normal teen brain development indicate the brain continues to change well past the teen years (Carswell & Stafford, 2022). Magnetic resonance imaging has shown the brain develops in stages, from back to front. The prefrontal cortex, which is the area of the brain used in planning, priority setting, organizing thoughts, and recognizing consequences, is the last area to develop. This sequential brain development may partially explain risk-taking and thrill-seeking behaviors during adolescence when the consequences of one's behavior may not be fully considered.

Adolescence has been divided into three stages. Early adolescence occurs between ages 10 and 13, the middle school years; middle adolescence occurs between ages 14 and 17, or the high school years; and late adolescence extends from ages 17 to 20, after high school. Although these categories help to describe the development of adolescent behavior, they are not rigid, and teens may fluctuate among the early, middle, and late behaviors of adolescence. Four main tasks should be achieved during adolescence:

1. Accept a changing body image with a mature and positive self-image
2. Establish independence and separate from parents
3. Plan for future careers
4. Develop a sexual identity

Early adolescents are concrete thinkers; therefore, when thinking about the consequences of their actions, they look at the immediate rather than long-term consequences. They may be rebellious as they test their independence from the family. They may be confused about their changing roles from child to adolescent and may lack confidence and self-esteem. Peers are extremely important; early adolescents look to their friends to determine normal behavior. The focus during this period is on the changes occurring in their bodies.

Adolescents in the middle stage show more abstract thinking and consideration of the long-term consequences of their behavior. Dating and interest in sexual experimentation are common in middle adolescence; thus prevention of sexually transmitted infections and pregnancy become important topics for the school nurse to discuss with students. Teens seek increasing independence from the family and value their privacy. Youth must adapt to their changing bodies; they also experience intense psychological and emotional growth as they become more independent and spend more time with friends than family. This struggle for independence often creates tension with parents. Major conflicts between parents/guardians and teens during adolescence that cannot be resolved are not common but may signal the need for intervention (Sherer & Radzik, 2022).

Late adolescence marks the transition into adulthood, with the young adult taking on increasing responsibility, making independent choices, and attempting to become financially independent. Society expects adolescents at this stage to be thinking about and planning to leave home for college or jobs and establish a relationship with a significant other.

Positive health behaviors are more valued when the adolescent takes part in decision making. If teens see the school nurse as an advocate for their needs and a resource for health services and education, a beneficial partnership can develop. Teens will respect the knowledge and the care and concern with which it is delivered. Nurses need to be prepared to offer accurate and up-to-date healthcare information.

Issues that arise during adolescence require assurance of confidentiality based on local laws. The school nurse should inform teens about what information cannot remain confidential, especially related to suicidal thoughts and abuse. See Online Materials OM9-3 for resources regarding the legal rights of adolescents.

Listening is a valuable tool for the school nurse. A simple request for ice for an injury may uncover a multitude of physical and emotional needs of an adolescent. The key is to take the time to listen in a private, nonthreatening, nonjudgmental environment. Motivational interviewing may help to open dialogue with a student. School nurses can use the principles of motivational interviewing by showing empathy and active listening to help students link behavior and long-term goals (Substance Abuse and Mental Health Services Administration & Health Resources and Services Administration, 2018). Allowing students to explore and discuss possible solutions and scenarios may help to determine a future course of action where positive encouragement and support can lead to a student's self-efficacy.

Sexuality

Developing healthy sexuality is an important task for adolescents. It is during adolescence when relationships and sexual exploration and activity usually begin. Health

Did You Know?

The World Health Organization (2024) defines *sexual health* as

> *a state of physical, emotional, mental and social well-being in relation to sexuality; it is not merely the absence of disease, dysfunction or infirmity. Sexual health requires a positive and respectful approach to sexuality and sexual relationships, as well as the possibility of having pleasurable and safe sexual experiences, free of coercion, discrimination and violence. For sexual health to be attained and maintained, the sexual rights of all persons must be respected, protected and fulfilled.* (para. 4)

professionals must ensure adolescents are getting the information they need to develop a healthy sexuality and identity and healthy relationships.

Early adolescence is the time when youth socialize in mixed-gender groups. Youth may fantasize about a different sex, but little activity is usually initiated. The early adolescent female may daydream of the perfect love interest. Crushes are common and relationships are short-lived. Young adolescents may misperceive "love interests" as extremely significant even though the interaction may be on the phone or in a group setting (Hensel & Beckmeyer, 2022).

Young adolescents need reliable information about sex and comprehensive sexual education, including information about healthy relationships. It is likely early adolescents receive conflicting messages from parents, schools, and the media. Education in early adolescence should include communication, respect for others, and decision making. Gender-specific groups can lead to a more open discussion of sexual activity and concerns of this age group. It may be helpful to have students write questions and concerns on note cards. This allows the educator to address a concern without attributing ownership to one individual.

During middle adolescence, teens get much of their information about sexual activity from peers. Teens start to date, and an increase in sexual activity and experimentation may occur during this period. Intense feelings of infatuation and falling in love may be short-lived but no less real to the adolescent. The breakup of a relationship is quite traumatic, and the teen may benefit from formal or informal counseling at that time. Education can be the key in combating the influence of the media, dispelling myths, offering facts, and reassuring teens.

Data from the 2021 Youth Risk Behavior Survey (YRBS) (CDC, 2023b) indicate 3.0% of all U.S. students had sexual intercourse before the age of 13, and 30% have ever had intercourse. These results indicate a downward trend since 2011. However, one study raised the concern that sexual intercourse among students who attend alternative high schools was almost 3 times higher. Alternative schools educate students at risk of failing in the traditional setting, which may be due to behavioral issues, truancy, and/or substance abuse. Students in both traditional and alternative settings are using condoms less during sexual intercourse than in years past (Johnson et al., 2022).

LBGTQ+ students relate that sex education delivered in school is directed at heterosexual relationships and thus they are not getting the information they need about sexual relationships (Epps et al., 2022). The reluctance of adults to appropriately discuss sexuality with teens often produces misleading and inaccurate information gathered from other sources. The school nurse can help direct youth to appropriate and accurate resources for students, including those who attend school in alternative settings where access to sex education and resources have been shown to be limited for LBGTQ+ students (Epps et al., 2022). School nurses can provide one-on-one education that includes accurate medical information and provide resources and referrals to help all students access the resources they need (Johnson et al., 2022). Placing posters and signage throughout the school is another avenue for teens to access information from legitimate sources (Epps et al., 2022).

Teachable moments may arise when youth come to the school health office with a concern about the risk of a sexually transmitted infection or unintended pregnancy, and the school nurse should have resources readily available to share with students. Discussions should include the importance of mutual respect and trust in all relationships, sexual activity, and sexual decision making. The nurse can educate students about their readiness for sexual activity and the need to say no to unwanted sexual activity. A confidential referral to a healthcare provider for birth control or other issues may be needed.

Unwanted Sexual Activity

Eight percent of female high school students reported they had been forced to participate in sexual activity against their will (CDC, 2023b). Of those youth in a heterosexual relationship, 14% of females compared with 4% of males experienced unwanted sexual activity. The school nurse must be ever alert for signs of sexual harassment, dating violence, sexual abuse of minors, and human trafficking. Students should be referred to professional resources inside and outside of school for help. Proper consent, confidentiality, and mandated reporting protocols must be adhered to regarding unwanted sexual activity. The safety of students and others must be paramount. Signs and/or posters with online resources or local clinic locations can serve as a resource for students who might be reluctant or afraid to discuss any sexual activity. The school nurse should involve law enforcement officials when criminal activity is suspected.

Gender Identity and Sexual Orientation

Gender describes the male or female characteristics, such as behavior, roles, and norms, that are identified and assigned by society. It may be defined differently in different cultures and may change over time. *Gender identity* is part of one's self-concept; it is how one feels and identifies themselves, whether or not it matches the gender a person is assigned at birth (WHO, 2023). Gender identity is an internal sense that can only be described by the individual—it is not a sexual preference or a choice.

While gender identity is how one perceives themself, *gender expression* is how one presents themself to the outside world. One's clothing styles, hairstyles, and behavior all convey expression of gender. The term *cisgender* refers to a person whose gender identity corresponds with their assigned sex at birth (Human Rights Campaign [HRC], n.d.). When one's gender identity and expression differ from their birth gender, the individual is referred to as *transgender.* Youth who identify as transgender may feel "different" at an early age but may not recognize or understand it (Olson-Kennedy, 2022).

Gender nonconforming students may choose to use a preferred name and gender pronouns that are different from their name and gender assigned at birth. He/him/his or she/her/hers are gender pronouns regularly used in the English language, but it is becoming more common for individuals who have a gender nonconforming identity to prefer the personal pronouns they/them/theirs. Individuals may select a pronoun, or neopronoun, that is meaningful to them. Neopronouns include xe/xir/xirs, ze/zir/zirs, and fae/faer/faers (HRC, n.d.). School staff should first ask what name and pronoun a student wants to be called to allow a student to self-identify. This is already done in most classrooms by asking if children have nicknames. When groups are assigned per gender at school, it negates the gender identity of the nonconforming student.

Sexual orientation, one's sexual attraction to or sexual desire for a specific gender, is different from gender identity, or how one feels inside about their gender (HRC, n.d.). Sexual orientation reflects to whom one is sexually attracted: someone of a different sex, someone of the same sex, both, or none. Females sexually attracted to females are generally referred to as lesbian; gay usually refers to males sexually attracted to males. The terms *queer* and *homosexual* may or may not be preferred depending on the individual's personal history and contexts, so it is important that every person have the right to choose their own terms. *Bisexual* refers to individuals who are sexually attracted to more than one gender. Sexual orientation is *not* considered a choice. Physical attraction and emotional attraction are elements that comprise sexual orientation.

The school nurse can provide support and guidance for students to help navigate their emerging sexual orientation. It will help the school nurse to stay abreast of the correct terminology used to describe a student's sexual identity and orientation because the current parlance for sexual identity and orientation is a fluid spectrum. Gender identity, gender expression, and physical and emotional attraction occur across a continuum as depicted by the *Gender Unicorn* in Figure 9-5. Individuals can indicate where they identify along the Gender Unicorn's arrows.

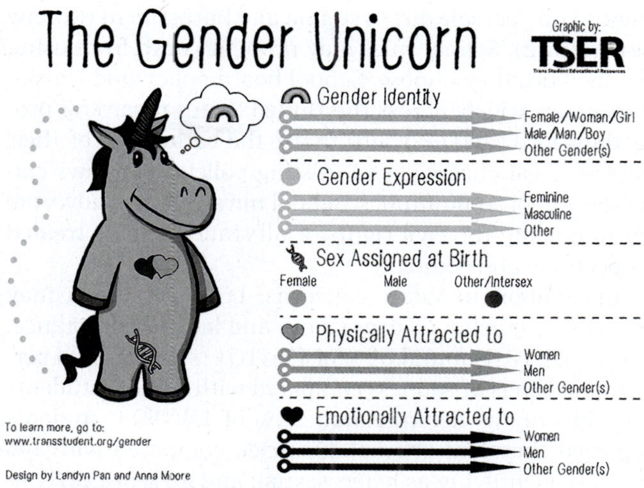

FIGURE 9-5. The Gender Unicorn. *(Trans Student Educational Resources, 2015.)*

Adolescence is often considered a time of experimentation. Sexual orientation encompasses one's sexual identity, sexual attraction, and sexual behavior (Makrides & Fields, 2022). It is not unusual for youth to question where their sexual attractions lie and to experiment to confirm their sexual orientation. Studies of young adults who identify themselves as gay or lesbian report that by age 13, they were aware of their sexual orientation. By age 18, LGBTQ+ youths self-identify and begin to have sexual relationships (Hall et al., 2021). Youth who identify as LGBTQ+ may not have family support and learn that many in society do not approve of or accept their sexual orientation or sexual identity. Teens may hide their feelings and pretend to go along with their peers. School nurses recognize that gender-different youth need care in a nonjudgmental and supportive manner (NASN, 2021).

Safety Concerns of LGBTQ+ Youth

One of the primary concerns for LGBTQ+ youth in the school setting is safety. It has been established that nonbinary students are bullied in school more often, are more likely to experiment with tobacco, have substance use issues, and have a higher incidence of suicide (Makrides & Fields, 2022). A 2021 survey of LGBTQ+ youth found that 68% felt unsafe at school because of their sexual orientation, gender identity, or gender expression; 32.2% missed at least 1 day in the past month because they felt unsafe; 83.1% experienced verbal abuse and harassment because of their sexual orientation; and 76.1% felt harassed because of their expressed sexual orientation, gender identity, or expression. More than 31.2% of LGBTQ+ youth surveyed reported they were physically harassed and 12.5% were physically assaulted in school (Kosciw et al., 2022).

The U.S. Department of Education (2021) prohibits any discriminatory practices in schools based on sex, which includes any discrimination based on sexual orientation or sexual identity. Yet four out of 10 students may avoid bathrooms, locker rooms, or physical education classes because they do not feel safe due to stigma and harassment (Kosciw et al., 2022). School rules may prohibit youth from using the facilities they choose. School board policy and legislation varies widely across the United States regarding protections for LGBTQ+ youth to use the bathrooms of their choice. Legal challenges to existing policies and laws can divide school communities. School nurses should advocate for upholding the civil rights of all students to be treated respectfully and equitably.

In addition to safety concerns, LGBTQ+ youth may experience loneliness, depression, and lack of acceptance. The 2021 YRBS found 69% of LBGTQ+ students had persistent feelings of sadness compared with 35% of students who identify as heterosexual; 22% of LBGTQ+ students reported they had attempted suicide compared with 6% of those identifying as heterosexual; and 45% of LGBTQ+ students seriously considered suicide (CDC, 2023b). Some families do not accept their child's sexual orientation or gender expression and identity. They may ostracize the child from family activities or kick the child out of the home. LGBTQ+ youth may be expelled from the church, prevented from attending sleepovers with their friends, or forced to lie about themselves.

Actions to Promote Safety for LBGTQ+ Youth

These health and safety disparities related to LGBTQ+ youth are alarming and unacceptable. The school community must be accepting of all students; negative comments by teachers and biased policies can send a message of disapproval and lack of acceptance. School nurses can educate school staff so that they may support and affirm the gender identity and sexual orientation of all students. The best predictor of mental health among young LGBTQ+ youth is self-acceptance, which is enhanced by family support. The school nurse can assist the student by contacting social workers or school counselors who can work with the student and family.

School nurses can list their pronouns on e-mail signatures and on online Web conferencing to demonstrate a safe and welcoming environment for students. School nurses should ensure that the school health office is a safe zone; they can do this by placing a rainbow flag decal on the front door and having materials posted that display the diversity of relationships people might have.

All youth need to feel a sense of belonging. One of the most successful resources is a Gay-Straight Alliance or club at school with the support of faculty and administration. It assures these youth they are not alone; it helps them meet others like themselves; it helps them resolve conflicts between who they are and who they are being told they should be; and it allows better communication and understanding by the general school community. Having a Gay-Straight Alliance in school is associated with more positive experiences for LGBTQ+ students, including hearing fewer homophobic remarks, experiencing less victimization because of sexual orientation and gender expression, having less absenteeism because of safety concerns, and enjoying a greater sense of belonging to the school community (Kosciw et al., 2022).

School curriculum should include positive discussions of sexual diversity. Sexual orientation and gender identity can be compared with handedness. Whether one is right- or left-handed does not make one better or worse; it is not a choice. It is the way we respond to others that is the choice. This inclusion gives the message to those youth that it is okay to be who they are. When discussions of safe sexual practices are included in health education curricula, attention must also be paid to safe sex practices for those who are gay, lesbian, bisexual, or transgender.

NASN (2021) promotes school programs that educate both those who discriminate and those who are discriminated against because of their sexual orientation, gender identity, or gender nonconformity. This includes implementing comprehensive antibullying policies, consulting with teachers to develop inclusive curricula, supporting transgender and gender-diverse students, and allowing youth to be themselves. It is important to stress that individuals are *not* their sexuality; it is simply a part of who they are. School can be truly safe only when every student, regardless of sexual orientation, gender identity, and gender expression, is ensured access to an education without fear of harassment, discrimination, or violence.

Technology Use

The youth of today are growing up knowing only a world with social media. Cellphones and Internet use have a significant impact on youth peer relationships. Ninety-five percent of youth 13 to 17 years old have access to a smart phone and 90% have access to a computer (Vogels et al., 2022). Forty-six percent of teens say they spend almost all of their time online, almost double what was reported in 2014–2015.

There are positive and negative consequences of online connectivity. Access to health information and social support for youth are benefits of social media (Moreno & Selkie, 2022). Social networking is important for youth as they develop an identity, an important milestone of adolescence. Teens report they feel more connected on social media and their social network is supportive when they feel they need support. They also say they are able to show their creativity through social media. However, 45% of girls report they are "overwhelmed" by the drama on social media (Anderson et al., 2022). Students who identify as LGBTQ+ (lesbian, gay, bisexual, transgender, queer, plus) have found support from social media. Girls are more likely than boys to use a social networking site such as TikTok, Instagram, and Snapchat, whereas boys play video games more frequently and use YouTube, Twitch, and Reddit. Facebook is no longer a popular choice among teens (Vogels et al., 2022).

Online gaming also can be used to promote physical activity, with various movement activities encouraged in a virtual world. During the COVID-19 pandemic, physical activity was initiated and sustained with daily

> **Practice Connection**
>
> The American Academy of Pediatrics (n.d.) recommends that families develop a *Family Media Plan,* which is a tool designed to help families determine appropriate use and balance of the Internet and social media outlets, available on the AAP Web site.

motivational messaging to students' mobile phones using the app WhatsApp. Once students began to exercise, they continued to be motivated, finding fun ways to exercise and maintain physical activity (Ceylan & Erol, 2022). This is just the beginning of mHealth (mobile health) and an avenue worth pursuing to encourage physical activity in our youth.

School nurses can support teens to use online and social media resources responsibly, while remaining alert and vigilant for youth who are experiencing cyberbullying or problematic Internet use. *Problematic Internet use* can be a concern as youth post inappropriate information or develop social and emotional concerns. Sexting, the act of sharing nude or naked pictures of oneself, could be considered a gateway to sexual activity for teens (Diliberto & Mattey, 2009). However, once these images are shared online, they are forever accessible in cyberspace, often with devastating or long-term consequences—including possible charges of child pornography if the photos are shared.

During the COVID-19 pandemic, Internet connectivity was important for students and youth to remain connected to their friends during lockdown, hence there was a rapid increase in social media and gaming during that time. Parent supervision plays a protective role in preventing negative consequences from social media and online activities. Online gaming addiction occurs when youth give priority to gaming, neglect other activities, are deceptive about gaming, use gaming to escape, and/or continue to game despite negative consequences (Han et al., 2022). Online gaming addiction has been linked with depression, anxiety, and stress, plus social isolation resulting from ignoring other activities.

Internet safety and cyberbullying remain a concern, although teens report they see it more of a problem for others than themselves (Schaeffer, 2021). The messages youth receive from online media often can be misleading and may promote high-risk behaviors. School nurses are in excellent positions to share information and resources to help parents/guardians and children have frank and open discussions about appropriate Internet use. Schools should have policies and procedures to address online bullying, including how to report online bullying (see Chapter 11). School nurses should advocate for school-wide education for both students and parents about cyber safety and lead student support team collaboration to help individual students and families who have been negatively affected by misuse of online media.

CONSIDERATIONS FOR STUDENT ATHLETES

Participation in sports can have positive physical and social benefits for children. However, there are issues that raise concerns related to safety and wellness, including nutrition, hydration, weight management, infection control, and strength training. School nurses and coaches are well placed to identify when a student is engaging in practices that are unsafe and recommend appropriate interventions. This section reviews how to address these concerns and what interventions will best meet the needs of the student athlete and those who exercise intensely.

Middle School

Middle school students are ready for new challenges, both individually and as members of a team. As students mature in their physical ability, they are generally more able to refine their skills and handle the stress of team play and competition. Student athletes may emulate a professional sports figure they admire, which may promote the formation of future sport-related goals. Parents, coaches, and other significant adults can have a major impact on encouraging or dissuading young people in their athletic participation.

Middle school students are still concrete thinkers and live in the moment. They are learning to understand the rules of the game and strategy. Physically, they are beginning puberty, with significant growth in their bones and muscles, as well as changing body proportions. Flexibility may decrease, making them more prone to overuse injury. Injuries increase with the advance of pubertal maturation (Karpinos & Enzinger, 2022).

In middle school, the focus switches from participation to competition, often resulting in students dropping out of athletic activities because they feel that participating is no longer fun (Brenner & Council on Sports Medicine and Fitness, 2016). Fear of performing and feeling they are not good enough can inhibit a student's participation in sports and can be as emotionally destructive as teasing. Dropping out of the sport may influence the child's attitude about physical activity and interfere with the establishment of healthy practices that should carry into adulthood. School nurses can give anticipatory guidance to parents/guardians and children about the psychological effects on those who are not physically gifted or may not have the competitive drive or discipline needed to succeed in a sport.

School nurses can encourage activities beyond team sports that encourage physical activity. Lifetime physical activities, such as running, biking, skating, dancing, walking, martial arts, swimming, and skateboarding, should be encouraged. Schools can organize diverse types of activities to introduce youth to varied physical activities.

High School

In 2021, slightly more than 49% of high school students reported having played on at least one high school or community sports team (CDC, 2023b). School-sponsored athletics offers an opportunity for students to develop their physical and leadership skills, compete with school teams from neighboring communities, and gain peer recognition. School spirit and loyalty provide an opportunity to promote teamwork and to widen the horizons of the student athlete. However, the drive to win may overshadow proper training and reporting of injuries.

The number of students participating in organized sports may decline in high school as the less-talented athletes do not make the teams. Others may drop out because of the time required or intensity of practice sessions, the stress related to competition, or because they are not comfortable with the pressure to win or with the people running the program. Students may experience feelings of frustration and failure when they find themselves on the bench or cut from the team.

Physical activities in which all students can participate should be offered by schools, including intramural sports. Physical education class is a requirement for almost all students at some point during high school. Nationally only 19% of high school students attend physical education class 5 days a week (CDC, 2023b). Students may be encouraged to bike to school or walk around the track during lunchtime or after school. Communal workout rooms and swimming pools are popular in some schools and provide an ideal site for students to see faculty and staff engaging in healthy behaviors.

Nutrition

A key component of health promotion for athletes is an emphasis on good nutrition and appropriate caloric intake needed for the increased activity level of practice and competition (Desbrow, 2021). This is particularly important during adolescence, a time of rapid growth second only to that experienced during infancy. Healthy nutritional practices are particularly challenging at a time when fast-paced family life may make snacks and fast foods more attractive.

Many student athletes come to school early in the day, practice before school, eat during an early lunch period, and practice until dinnertime, which can result in long intervals between meals and snacks. Under these circumstances, the student athlete will require caloric and fluid intake before and during practice, particularly if practice is intense or the weather is hot (Desbrow, 2021). Schools participating in universal breakfast programs may be one way to ensure that all student athletes receive a nutritious breakfast.

Schools that receive federal funding are required that snacks sold in schools meet nutritional standards, that is, *smart snacks* that can be purchased in vending machines, school stores, and snack bars.

Did You Know?

Smart snacks sold in schools outside of breakfast and lunch must follow these standards:

- Be a grain product that contains at least 50% white grains
- The first ingredient be a fruit, vegetable, dairy food, or a protein food
- Be a combination of food that contains at least ¼ cup of fruit and/or vegetable
- Must meet the nutrient standards for calories, sodium, fats, and total sugars (USDA, 2022a)

Schools can make the availability of healthy snacks part of the school wellness plan. Healthy snacks include fresh fruit, cereal bars, sandwiches, milk, fruit juices, or other foods high in protein and carbohydrates needed to provide energy.

There are three basic principles of sports nutrition: hydration, fueling for performance, and recovery. Although student athletes may need more calories because of increased energy expenditure with exercise, they do *not* require a special diet. Caloric requirements will vary with the sport but may exceed the child's baseline intake. Additional carbohydrates for energy and protein for cell repair and endurance are of benefit, but substantial changes in the dietary regimen are not required. A well-balanced diet that includes a variety of foods representing all food groups is critical for maintenance of normal weight and mineral stores and to provide adequate energy during activity (Desbrow, 2021). Fat should make up approximately one-third of an athlete's diet because it provides energy and essential nutrients. Protein consumption will depend on the extent of the activity, but a good rule for a 150-pound student is to eat 102 grams of protein per day.

To promote health and performance, it is important to consider not only the selection of nutrients and fluids but also the timing of a student athlete's intake. During periods of high activity, such as practice or competition, energy and nutrition needs must be met to replenish energy stores, maintain body weight, and repair muscle tissue. The need for nutrients will differ based on whether the activity is a short-term, high-intensity activity, such as diving, which uses anaerobic fuel sources, or longer-term sports, such as basketball, which uses aerobic sources (Desbrow, 2021). Although carbohydrates are needed by all athletes, fats and proteins are primarily needed for those in sports that are aerobic.

Three or more hours before practice or a game, youth athletes should consume a meal or snack to provide carbohydrates necessary for energy, ingest a moderate amount of protein, and drink fluids to maintain hydration. The preparticipation meal needs to be easily digested and low in fat and fiber to reduce gastric distress. Examples are fruit, bread or crackers, peanut butter or low-fat cheese, cereal with low-fat milk, or pasta with tomato sauce. During practice and competition, adequate energy (calories) needs to be consumed to maintain body weight and maximize performance. Inadequate energy reserves during exercise may result in loss of muscle mass, dysfunction, fatigue, injury, or illness. Carbohydrate consumption during exercise (such as low-fat yogurt or raisins) can help maintain blood glucose levels and restore glycogen stores.

After heavy exertion (training, practice, or competition), adequate carbohydrates need to be consumed to replace glycogen stores and to promote rapid recovery, and proteins are needed to repair and build muscles (Desbrow, 2021). Therefore, a meal with a variety of nutrients is recommended after exercise. Student athletes should be offered nutrition education and counseling to assist in maximizing their performance both in the sport and in the classroom. See this textbook's supplemental materials for resources to support nutrition of the student athlete.

Weight Management

Major concern has been expressed about the health of students when weight requirements are a prerequisite for competition, either when weight gain is desired (e.g., football), or when weight is restricted (e.g., rowing, cheerleading, or gymnastics). Wrestling can fall into either category. In sports where weight determines eligibility to compete, athletes may resort to extreme methods to achieve the desired weight goal without regard to the effects such methods may have on their health, as well as their performance. Ideally, weight changes should be accomplished slowly and during the off-season or before the start of competition in consultation with a registered dietitian or healthcare provider.

For athletes who participate in sports that encourage fast weight gain, a well-balanced diet from all food groups is essential. It is important to make sure quality foods are ingested. Diets high in protein help muscle growth, but also may be high in cholesterol. High intake of refined carbohydrates may be detrimental to dental health and provide minimal nutrients.

Coaches may mandate that students attain specific weight limits without regard to the student's percentage of body fat. There has been considerable discussion about the appropriateness of weight restrictions, especially for high school wrestlers, at a time when adolescent growth is expected, and adequate nutrition is essential to support normal physical and sexual development. Practices resulting in rapid weight loss have been common among wrestlers for decades, despite documentation of the potential harmful effects of such practices and the development of guidelines to regulate these practices.

Athletes who participate in sports where maintaining or attaining an unusually low weight for body size is desired need extra care and monitoring to ensure a well-balanced diet. When student athletes restrict energy (caloric) intake, first fat and then lean muscle mass will be used by the body for fuel, resulting in loss of strength and endurance. Students who severely restrict dietary intake may require a multivitamin and mineral supplement to ensure adequate intake of micronutrients. The diets of many adolescents may be deficient in calcium, iron, and zinc.

There is also concern about the effects of repeated weight-loss practices on normal growth and development, academic performance, and immune function. School nurses should play a key role in monitoring the weight and the consequential health status of athletes to ensure safe practices and to educate both athletes and coaches on these practices. School nurses are integral to developing and ensuring that policies or protocols regarding the weight status of players are consistent with state recommendations and national guidelines for athletic participation and followed by coaching staff.

Chronic dietary restriction may result in malnutrition and disordered eating, such as variations of anorexia nervosa and bulimia. This is especially a concern during adolescence when physical and sexual maturation may be affected or when the calcium stores are being laid down in bone. Eating behaviors learned in adolescence can have a lifelong impact on weight management practices in adulthood, as well as on one's perceived body image and self-esteem.

Relative Energy Deficiency in Sport (RED-S)

RED-S refers to low energy availability in both males and females and includes the female athlete triad. RED-S is the underconsumption of calories and nutrients needed to maintain energy output and support overall health. It affects all systems of the body, including metabolic rate, menstrual function in females, bone health, mental health, the immune system, the cardiovascular system, the gastrointestinal system, and more. For many years, low energy availability has been used to describe females and the triad of menstruation dysfunction, altered bone health, and low energy. It is now being recognized that low energy availability affects both male and female athletes (Katzman & Golden, 2022). See Table 9-7 for signs of RED-S.

Low energy availability may occur from inadequate caloric consumption that is not intentional or from disordered eating patterns. Intentional calorie restrictions include restriction of food intake, anorexia nervosa, and bulimia nervosa or from overexercising (Kohn, 2022). Protein deficiency associated with low energy availability can have a negative impact on muscle development and performance. Inadequate caloric consumption also can result in fatigue, dizziness, hair loss, bradycardia, constipation, and cold intolerance. Poor nutrition may result in decreased endurance, strength, speed, and ability to concentrate, and consequently, increase the risk for injury. Not only does physical performance suffer, but there is also psychological morbidity.

Male and female athletes who participate in sports where there is emphasis on appearance, a lean physique, or weight categories for participation, such as dancing, cheerleading, gymnastics, swimming, rowing, cross-country running, middle and long distance running, and wrestling,

TABLE 9-7 Relative Energy Deficiency in Sport (RED-S)

RED-S

Signs, Symptoms, and Contributing Factors

Performance: Fatigue, declining athletic performance

Injuries: Fractures, stress fractures, slow healing

Food behavior: Restricting food, fasting, rigidity around eating, binge eating, intentional vomiting, chewing food but not swallowing, being secretive with food

Excessive exercise: Excessive or compulsive exercising, training while injured

Weight: Weight loss, refusing to weigh or excessive weighing

Behavior: Withdrawal, critical self-image especially with body, restlessness, depression

External factors: Coaches that encourage weight loss, comments from others, peer pressure

Signs That Indicate RED-S	What You Might See
Performance	Fatigue, athletic performance declining
Injuries	Fractures, stress fractures, slow healing
Food behavior	Restricting food, fasting, binge eating, rigidity around eating, intentional vomiting, chewing food but not swallowing, being secretive with food
Excessive exercise	Exercising more than necessary, training while injured, compulsive exercising
Weight	Weight loss, refusing to weigh or excessive weighing, weight loss
Behavior	Withdrawal, critical self-image especially with body, restlessness, depression
External factors	Coaches that encourage weight loss, comments from others

Adapted from Charlton et al. (2022); Katzman & Golden (2022).

are at greater risk for experiencing RED-S. Cross-country runners who were at high risk of having low energy availability were four times as likely to experience a bone fracture (Charlton et al., 2022).

Menstrual dysfunction occurs on a continuum that can include anovulation, oligomenorrhea, or amenorrhea (Weiss Kelly et al., 2016). *Primary amenorrhea* is when menses has not been initiated by the age of 15; *secondary amenorrhea* occurs after at least 3 consecutive months of missed cycles. Females participating in intensive sports generally begin menstruating 1 to 2 years later than their peers, and irregularities are more common in this population. Athletes with menstrual dysfunction generally have low estrogen levels, which contributes to a decrease in bone mass and the third condition of the triad, low bone mineral density.

Both menstrual dysfunction and low energy availability contribute to decreased low bone mineral density. Women reach their peak bone mass between the ages of 20 and 30 with maximal bone mass accumulating in girls between the ages of 10 and 14. Therefore, the female athlete is at risk for future osteoporosis by inadequate nutrition and lack of estrogen. Low bone mineral density may contribute to stress fractures in female athletes.

School nurses need to identify students who are at risk for RED-S to educate them, their families, trainers, coaches, administrators, other healthcare professionals, and the public about the magnitude and seriousness of the health risks involved. All trainers and coaches should receive education about the importance of training that is physically and psychologically sound rather than emphasizing weight or appearance. Female athletes should be monitored regularly by their healthcare provider to evaluate nutritional status, growth and development, and menstrual history for signs of female athlete triad. School nurses should be prepared to recommend community resources for nutritional counseling, as well as medical and psychological evaluations. Treatment should involve a multidisciplinary approach and be individualized to the athlete, with the initial treatment focused on improving energy availability.

Hydration

In addition to good nutrition, adequate hydration is essential to the athlete's health, especially when the temperature and/or humidity is high. Even when practice and competition take place indoors, the temperature in these venues may be higher when students are active. Student athletes need to begin the activity well hydrated and replace fluids regularly during workouts, practice, or competition. Proper hydration not only promotes the health of athletes, but also enhances their performance and endurance. Water breaks should be incorporated into practice sessions and monitored by coaches as young children are often not aware they are thirsty.

Dehydration decreases athletic performance and increases the risk for fatigue, injury, and illness. Hydration requirements vary based on sex, size of the individual, nature of the sport, intensity of the exercise, and environmental conditions. Athletes need to consume sufficient fluids to replace fluid losses. Timing of consumption is critical. During practice or competition, teen athletes should consume approximately 13 mL/kg/hr (Desbrow, 2021). A 150-pound student should then consume approximately 10 ounces of water every 20 minutes during exercise. Adequate hydration after exercise promotes recovery.

Water is the preferred liquid to maintain hydration during short events, but because it has no taste, students often prefer flavored beverages. Athletes who participate in vigorous exercise or compete in extreme weather conditions will benefit from sports/electrolyte drinks. Many sports drinks contain only sugars, sucrose, fructose, and corn syrup that provide energy but do not replace electrolytes lost in sweat. These drinks are not the best choice for extended activity, but the sweetness of energy drinks may be more appealing to students than water and may be helpful in getting the student to consume more fluids.

CONCLUSION

This chapter gives school nurses an overview of the growth and development of the preschool and school-age child and the adolescent. Each student is unique, and individualized approaches based on the specific growth and developmental pattern of the individual student are necessary to effectively support the student. School nurses' expertise and assessment and evaluation skills are critical to identify atypical growth and development patterns to refer appropriately and coordinate care for the child to succeed in school.

School nurses are health leaders in the educational setting. School nurses advocate for removing real and potential barriers to student learning. Educational programs and student interactions must be geared to the developmental level of the students. Partnerships to support the overall well-being of students both at school and in the community enhance optimal student growth and development.

References

Adam, H. (2020). Fever. Quick references. *Pediatric Care Online.* https://doi.org/10.1542/aap.ppcqr.396073

American Academy of Pediatric Dentistry. (2022). Periodicity of examination, preventive dental services, anticipatory guidance/counseling, and oral treatment for infants, children, and adolescents. *The Reference Manual of Pediatric Dentistry,* 253–265.

American Academy of Pediatrics. (n.d.). *Family media plan.* https://www.healthychildren.org/English/media/Pages/default.aspx#home

American Academy of Pediatrics. (2018). *Picky eaters.* https://www.healthychildren.org/English/ages-stages/toddler/nutrition/Pages/Picky-Eaters.aspx

American Academy of Pediatrics and Pediatric Endocrine Society. (2018). *Precocious puberty.* https://pedsendo.org/patient-resource/precocious-puberty/

American Association of Orthodontists. (2020a). *Handling orthodontic issues at home.* www.aaoinfo.org/wp-content/uploads/2020/03/AAO_HandlingOrthoIssuesAtHome_2020.pdf

American Association of Orthodontists. (2020b). When should your child see an orthodontist? https://aaoinfo.org/whats-trending/when-should-your-child-see-an-orthodontist/

American College of Obstetricians and Gynecologists, Committee on Adolescent Health Care. (2015). Menstruation in girls and adolescents: Using the menstrual cycle as a vital sign, committee opinion no. 651. https://www.acog.org/clinical/clinical-guidance/committee-opinion/articles/2015/12/menstruation-in-girls-and-adolescents-using-the-menstrual-cycle-as-a-vital-sign

American Dental Association. (2024). February is National Children's Dental Health Month. https://www.ada.org/en/resources/community-initiatives/national-childrens-dental-health-month

American Speech-Language-Hearing Association. (2023a). How does your child hear and talk? https://www.asha.org/public/speech/development/chart/

American Speech-Language-Hearing Association. (2023b). Learning two languages. https://www.asha.org/public/speech/development/learning-two-languages/

American Speech-Language Hearing Association. (2023c). Social communication benchmarks. https://www.asha.org/practice-portal/clinical-topics/social-communication-disorder/social-communication-benchmarks/

Anderson, M., Vogels, E., Perrin, A., & Rainie, L. (2022). Connection, creativity, and drama: Teen life on social media in 2022. Pew Research Center. https://www.pewresearch.org/internet/2022/11/16/connection-creativity-and-drama-teen-life-on-social-media-in-2022/

ASCD & Centers for Disease Control and Prevention. (2014). Whole school, whole community, whole child model. https://www.cdc.gov/healthyschools/wscc/wsccmodel_update_508tagged.pdf

Attendance Works, Healthy Schools Campaign. (2015). Mapping the early attendance gap: Charting a course for student success. https://www.attendanceworks.org/mapping-the-early-attendance-gap/

Averbeck, B. (2022). Pruning recurrent neural networks replicates adolescent changes in working memory and reinforcement learning. *Proceedings of the National Academy of Science, 119*(22), e2121331119. https://doi.org/10.1073/pnas.2121331119

Brenner, J., & Council on Sports Medicine and Fitness. (2016). Sports specialization and intensive training in young athletes. *Pediatrics, 138*(3), e20162148. https://doi.org/10.1542/peds.2016-2148

Burch, A. M. (2024). Health promotion of the school-age child and family. In M. J. Hockenberry, E. A. Duffy, & K. Gibbs (Eds.). *Wong's nursing care of infants and children* (12th ed., pp. 463–482) [eBook edition]. Elsevier/Mosby.

Butz, L. (2023). States that have passed universal free school meals (so far). Hunter College New York City Food Policy Center. https://www.nycfoodpolicy.org/states-that-have-passed-universal-free-school-meals/

Byrne, A., Hagen, M. G., & Thompson, L. (2021). Gun safety for children. *Journal of the American Medical Association: Pediatrics, 175*(3), 332. https://doi.org/10.1001/jamapediatrics.2020.5989

Carswell, J., & Stafford, D. (2022). In D. K. Katzman, C. M. Gordon, S. T. Callahan, A. Joffe, S. Rosenthal, M. Trent, & R. Chung (Eds.). *Neinstein's adolescent and young adult health care* (7th ed., pp. 35–44) [eBook edition]. Wolters Kluwer Health.

Casa, D., DeMartini, J., Bergeron, M., Csillan, D., Eichner, E., Lopez, R., Ferrara, M. S., Miller, K. C., O'Conner, F., Sawka, M. N., & Yeargin, S. (2015). National Athletic Trainers' Association position statement: Exertional heat illness. *Journal of Athletic Trainers, 50*(9), 986–1000. https://doi.org/10.4085/1062-6050-50.9.07

Centers for Disease Control and Prevention. (2009). CDC growth charts: United States. https://www.cdc.gov/growthcharts/background.htm

Centers for Disease Control and Prevention. (2016). CDC customizable recess planning template. https://www.cdc.gov/healthyschools/physicalactivity/pdf/2016_12_16_customizablerecessplanning template.docx

Centers for Disease Control and Prevention. (2017, June 6). Clinical growth charts. https://www.cdc.gov/growthcharts/clinical_charts.htm

Centers for Disease Control and Prevention. (2021a). Dental sealants. https://www.cdc.gov/oralhealth/fast-facts/dental-sealants/index.html

Centers for Disease Control and Prevention. (2021b). Disparities in oral health. https://www.cdc.gov/oralhealth/oral_health_disparities/index.htm

Centers for Disease Control and Prevention. (2022a). Developmental milestones. https://www.cdc.gov/ncbddd/actearly/milestones/index.html

Centers for Disease Control and Prevention. (2022b). Evaluation of alternative body mass index (BMI) metrics to monitor weight status in children and adolescents with extremely high BMI using CDC BMI-for-age growth charts. www.cdc.gov/nchs/data/series/sr_02/sr02-197.pdf

Centers for Disease Control and Prevention. (2023a). Early childhood education. https://www.cdc.gov/policy/opaph/hi5/earlychildhood education/index.html

Centers for Disease Control and Prevention. (2023b). Youth risk behavior data summary and trends report 2011–2021. https://www.cdc.gov/healthyyouth/data/yrbs/pdf/YRBS_Data-Summary-Trends_Report2023_508.pdf

Ceylan, F., & Erol, S. (2022). The effect of a physical activity program using WhatsApp on adolescents' exercise behavior. *Journal of School Nursing*, 1–13. https://doi.org/10.1177/10598405221132207

Charlton, B., Forsyth, S., & Clarke, D. (2022). Low energy availability and relative energy deficiency in sports: What coaches should know. *International Journal of Sports Science & Coaching, 7*(2), 445–460. https://doi.org/10.1177/17479541211054458

Cohen, J. F., Hecht, A., McLoughlin, G., Turner, L., & Schwartz, M. (2021). Universal school meals and associations with student participation, attendance, academic performance, diet quality, food security, and body mass index: A systematic review. *Nutrients, 13*, 911. https://doi.org/10.3390/ nu13030911

Collett-Solberg, P., Ambler, G., Backeljauw, P., Bidlingmaier, M., Biller, B., Boguszewski, M., Cheung, P., Choong, C., Cohen, L., Cohen, P., Dauber, A., Deal, D., Gong, C., Hasegawa, Y., Hoffman, H., Hofman, P., Horikawa, R., Jorge, A., Juul, A., Kamenický, P., Khadilkar, V., Kopchick, J., Kriström, B., de Lurdes A,. Lopes, M., Luo, X., Miller, B., Misra, M., Netchine, I., Radovick, S., Ranke, M., Rogol, A., Rosenfeld, R., Saenger, P., Wit, J., & Woelfle, J. (2019). Diagnosis, genetics, and therapy of short stature in children: A growth hormone research society international perspective. *Hormone Research in Paediatrics, 92*(1), 1–14. https://doi.org/10.1159/000502231

Community Preventive Services Task Force. (2018). Obesity prevention and control: Meal or fruit and vegetable snack interventions combined with physical activity interventions in schools. https://www.thecommunityguide.org/media/pdf/Obesity-Schools-Meals-PA.pdf

Davis, K., Christodoulou, J., Seider, S., & Gardner, H. (2011). The theory of multiple intelligences. *Multiple Intelligence Oasis.* https://www.multipleintelligencesoasis.org/resources

Day, P. F., Flores, M., O'Connell, A, Abbott, P., Tsilingaridis, G., Fouad, A., Cohenca, N., Lauridsen, E., Bourguignon, C., Hicks, L., Andreasen, J. O., Cehreli, Z., Harlamb, S., Kahler, B., Oginni, A., Semper, M., & Levin, L. (2020). International Association of Dental Traumatology guidelines for the management of traumatic dental injuries: Injuries in the primary dentition. *Dental Traumatololgy, 36*(4), 343–359. https://doi.org/10.1111/edt.12576

Desbrow, B. (2021). Youth athlete development and nutrition. *Sports Medicine, 51*(Suppl 1), S3–S12. https://doi.org/10.1007/s40279-021-01534-6

Diliberto, G., & Mattey, E. (2009). Sexting: Just how much of a danger is it and what can school nurses do about it? *NASN School Nurse, 24*(6), 262–267.

Donnelly, S., & Kidd, E. (2021). The longitudinal relationship between conversational turn taking and vocabulary growth in early language development. *Child Development, 92*(2), 609–625. https://doi.org/10.1111/cdev.13511

Duffy, E. A. (2024a). Health promotion of the adolescent and family. In M. J. Hockenberry, E. A. Duffy, & K. Gibbs (Eds.). *Wong's nursing care of infants and children* (12th ed., pp. 510–536) [eBook edition]. Elsevier.

Duffy, E. A. (2024b). Health promotion of the toddler and family. In M. J. Hockenberry, E. A. Duffy, & K. Gibbs (Eds.). *Wong's nursing care of infants and children* (12th ed., pp. 396–424) [eBook edition]. Elsevier.

Ehrensaft, D. (2016). *The gender creative child.* The Experiment.

Eimicke, T., & Swartz, J. (2022). Abnormal growth and development. In D. K. Katzman, C. M. Gordon, T. Callahan, A. Joffe, S. Rosenthal, M. Trent, & R. Chung (Eds.). *Neinstein's adolescent and young adult healthcare: A practical guide* (7th. ed., pp. 138–150) [eBook edition]. Wolters & Kluwer.

Emergency Nurses Association. (2019). Clinical practice guideline: Non-invasive blood pressure measurement with automated devices. https://media.emscimprovement.center/documents/nibpmcpg.pdf

Emergency Nurses Association. (2020). Clinical practice guideline: Non-invasive temperature measurement. https://enau.ena.org/Users/LearningActivity/LearningActivityDetail.aspx?LearningActivityID=9oIptF2sidDvK%2FI%2Ffr6M%2FA%3D%3D&tab=4

Epps, B., Markowski, M., & Cleaver, K. (2022). A rapid review and narrative synthesis of the consequences of non-inclusive sex education in UK schools on lesbian, gay, bisexual, transgender and questioning young people. *Journal of School Nursing, 39*(1), 87–97. https://doi.org/10.1177/10598405211043394

Erikson, E. (1968). The human life cycle. In S. Schlein (Ed.) (1987). *A way of looking at things: Selected papers from 1930 to 1980* (pp. 595–610). W. W. Norton.

Federal Register. (2016). Childcare and development fund program: A rule by the children and families administration. https://www.federalregister.gov/documents/2016/09/30/2016-22986/child-care-and-development-fund-ccdf-program

Flensborg-Madsen, T., & Mortensen, E. L. (2017). Associations of early developmental milestones with adult intelligence. *Child Development, 89*(2), 638–648. https://doi.org/10.1111/cdev.12760

Flynn, J., Kaelber, D. C., Baker-Smith, C. M., Blowey, D., Carroll, A. E., Daniels, S. R., de Ferranti, S. D., Dionne, J. M., Falkner, B., Flinn, S. K., Gidding, S. S., Goodwin, C., Leu, M. G., Powers, M. E., Rea, C., Samuels, J., Simasek, M., Thaker, V. V., Urbina, E. M, & Subcommittee on Screening and Management of High Blood Pressure in Children. (2017). Clinical guideline for screening and management of high blood pressure in children and adolescents. *Pediatrics, 140*(3), 1–72, e20173318. https://doi.org/10.1542/peds.2017-1904

Fong, W., Yeo, S., Fook-Chong, M., Phang, J., & Sim, E. (2020). Comparison of temperature readings using infrared thermometers at three different sites: Tympanic, forehead and temporal. *Proceedings of Singapore Healthcare, 30*(1), 41–43. https://doi.org/10.1177/2010105820935932

Gardner, H. (1999). *The disciplined mind.* New York: Simon & Schuster.

Goldstick, J., Cunningham, R., & Carter, P. (2022). Current causes of death in children and adolescents in the United States: Letter to the editor. *New England Journal of Medicine, 386*, 1955–1956. https://doi.org/10.1056/NEJMc2201761

Gontard, A., & Kuwertz-Bröking, E. (2019). The diagnosis and treatment of enuresis and functional daytime urinary incontinence. *Deutsches Arzteblatt International, 116*(16), 279–285. https://doi.org/10.3238/arztebl.2019.0279

Grimberg, A., Diall, S., Polychronakos, C., Allen, D., Cohen, L., Quintos, J., Rossi, W., Feudtner, C., & Murad, M. (2016). Guidelines for growth hormone and insulin-like growth factor-I treatment in children and adolescents: Growth hormone deficiency, idiopathic short stature, and primary insulin-like growth factor-I deficiency. *Hormone Research in Paediatrics, 86*, 361–397. https://doi.org/10.1159/000452150

Gruber, R., Saha, S., Somerville, G., Boursier, J., & Wise, W. (2020). The impact of COVID-19 related school shutdown on sleep in adolescents: A natural experiment. *Sleep Medicine, 76*, 33–35. https://doi.org/10.1016/j.sleep.2020.09.015

Hall, W., Dawes, H., & Plocek, N. (2021). Sexual orientation identity development milestones among lesbian, gay, bisexual, and queer people: A systematic review and meta-analysis. *Frontiers in Psychology, 12*, e753954. https://doi.org/10.3389/fpsyg.2021.753954

Han, T., Cho, H., Sung, D., & Park, M. (2022). A systematic review of the COVID-19 pandemic on the game addiction of children and adolescents. *Frontiers in Psychiatry, 13*, 976601. https://doi.org.10.3389/fpsyt.2022.976601

Haywood, K., & Getchell, N. (2020). *Life span motor development* (7th ed.). Human Kinetics.

Hensel, D., & Beckmeyer, J. J. (2022). Adolescent and young adult sexuality. In D. K. Katzman, C. M. Gordon, T. Callahan, A. Joffe, S. Rosenthal, M. Trent, & R. Chung (Eds.). *Neinstein's adolescent and young adult healthcare: A practical guide* (7th. ed., pp. 396–400) [eBook edition]. Wolters Kluwer.

Herbert, A., Pearn, J., & Wilson, S. (2020). Normal percentiles for respiratory rate in children—reference ranges determined from an optical sensor. *Children, 7*(10). https://doi.org/10.3390/children7100160

Howlett, M., Jemcov, A., Adams, A., & Corkum, P. (2020). ABCs of sleeping tool: Improving access to care for pediatric insomnia. *Clinical Practice in Pediatric Psychology, 8*(1), 1–2.

Human Rights Campaign. (n.d.). Glossary of terms. https://www.hrc.org/resources/glossary-of-terms

Hustad, K. C., Mahr, T. J., Natzke, P., & Rathouz, P. J. (2021). Speech development between 30 and 119 months in typical children I: Intelligibility growth curves for single-word and multiword productions. *Journal of Speech, Language, and Hearing Research, 64*(10), 3707–3719. https://doi.org/10.1044/2021_JSLHR-21-00142

Individuals With Disabilities Education Improvement Act of 2004 (Pub. L. 108-446). https://www.gpo.gov/fdsys/pkg/PLAW-108publ446/content-detail.html

Jakubowski, T., & Perron, T. (2019). Asthma assessment in the school health office: Can they stay or should they go? *NASN School Nurse, 34*(1), 37–43. https://doi.org/10.1177/1942602X18803336

Jarvis, C., & Eckhardt, A. (2024). *Physical examination and health assessment* (9th ed.). Elsevier.

Johnson, K., Conn, K., Osborne, C., Wilson, K., & Rew, L. (2022). School-level efforts to address sexual health and risky sexual behavior among students in Texas alternative high schools. *Journal of School Nursing, 38*(3), 299–305. https://doi.org/10.1177/1059840520950438

Karpinos, A., & Enzinger, A. (2022). Guidelines for promoting physical activity and sports participation. In D. K. Katzman, C. M. Gordon, T. Callahan, A. Joffe, S. Rosenthal, M. Trent, & R. Chung (Eds.). *Neinstein's adolescent and young adult healthcare: A practical guide* (7th ed., pp. 229–248) [eBook edition]. Wolters Kluwer.

Kasbekar, R., Naz, A., Marcos, L., Liu, Y., Hendrickson, K., Gorsich, J. C., & Baun, M. (2021). Threshold for defining fever varies with age, especially in children: A multi-site diagnostic accuracy study. *Nursing Open, 8*(5), 2705–2721. https://doi.org/10.1002/nop2.831

Katzman, D., & Golden, N., (2022). Feeding and eating disorders. In D. K. Katzman, C. M. Gordon, T. Callahan, A. Joffe, S. Rosenthal, M. Trent, & R. Chung (Eds.). *Neinstein's adolescent and young adult healthcare: A practical guide* (7th ed., pp. 362–373). [eBook edition]. Wolters Kluwer.

Kohlberg, L. (1981). *The philosophy of moral development.* Harper & Row.

Kohn, M. (2022). Nutrition. In D. K. Katzman, C. M. Gordon, T. Callahan, A. Joffe, S. Rosenthal, M. Trent, & R. Chung (Eds.). *Neinstein's adolescent and young adult healthcare: A practical guide* (7th. ed., pp. 78–84) [eBook edition]. Wolters Kluwer.

Kosciw, J. G., Clark, C. M., & Menard, L. (2022). The 2021 national school climate survey: The experiences of LGBTQ+ youth in our nation's schools. *GLSEN.* https://www.glsen.org/research/2021-national-school-climate-survey

Krol, D., & Whalen, K. (2023). Maintaining and improving the oral health of young children. *Pediatrics, 151*(1), e2022060417. https://doi.org/10.1542/peds.2022-060417

Lange, S., Kompaniyets, L., Freedman, D., Kraus, K, Porter, R., Blanck, H., & Goodman, A. (2021). Longitudinal trends in body mass index before and during the COVID-19 pandemic among persons aged 2–19 years: United States, 2018–2020. *Morbidity and Mortality Weekly Report, 70,* 1278–1283. https://doi.org/10.15585/mmwr.mm7037a3

Logan K., Cuff, S., Council on Sports Medicine and Fitness, LaBella, C. R., Brooks, M. A., Canty, G., Diamond, A. B., Hennrikus, W., Moffatt, K., Nemeth, B. A., Pengel, K. B., Peterson, A. R., & Stricker, P. R. (2019). Organized sports for children, preadolescents, and adolescents. *Pediatrics, 143*(6), e2019099. https://doi.org/10.1542/peds.2019-0997

Mackenzie, M., & Cohn, S. (2023). You can change a girl's life today: The truth about periods and endometriosis. *NASN School Nurse, 38*(2), 85–90. https://doi.org/10.1177/1942602X221127247

Makrides, J., & Fields, E. L. (2022). Sexual minority adolescents and young adults. In D. K. Katzman, C. M. Gordon, T. Callahan, A. Joffe, S. Rosenthal, M. Trent, & R. Chung (Eds.). *Neinstein's adolescent and young adult healthcare: A practical guide* (7th. ed., pp. 401–407) [eBook edition]. Wolters Kluwer.

Meissner, C. (2020). When can doxycycline be used in young children? *AAP News.* https://publications.aap.org/aapnews/news/14899?autologincheck=redirected

Miller, B., Sarafoglou, K., & Addom, O. (2020). Development of Tanner stage-age adjusted CDC height curves for research and clinical applications. *Journal of the Endocrine Society, 4*(9), 1–13. https://doi.org/10.1210/jendso/bvaa098

Monroe, R. (2024). Health promotion of the preschooler and family. In M. J. Hockenberry, E. A. Duffy, & K. Gibbs (Eds.). *Wong's nursing care of infants and children* (12th ed., pp. 425–441) [eBook edition]. Elsevier/Mosby.

Moreno, M., & Selkie, E. M. (2022). Technology and social media. In D. K. Katzman, C. M. Gordon, T. Callahan, A. Joffe, S. Rosenthal, M. Trent, & R. Chung (Eds.). *Neinstein's adolescent and young adult healthcare: A practical guide* (7th. ed., pp. 98–104) [eBook edition]. Wolters & Kluwer.

Muntner, P., Shimbo, D., Carey, R, Charleston, J., Gailiard, T., Misra, S., Myers, M., Ogedegbe, G., Schwartz, J., Townsend, R., Urbina, E., Viera, A., White, W., & Wright, J., (2019). Measurement of blood pressure in humans: A scientific statement from the American Heart Association. *Hypertension, 73*(5), e35–e66. https://doi.org/10.1161/HYP.0000000000000087

Murphy, J. M., & Gilligan, C. (1980). Moral development in late adolescence and adulthood: A critique and reconstruction of Kohlberg's theory. *Human Development, 23*(2), 77–104. http://doi.org/10.1159/000272541

National Association for the Education of Young Children. (2020). Developmentally appropriate practice: A position statement from the national association for the education of young children. https://www.naeyc.org/sites/default/files/globally-shared/downloads/PDFs/resources/position-statements/dap-statement_0.pdf

National Association of School Nurses. (2021). LGBTQ students position statement. https://www.nasn.org/nasn-resources/professional-practice-documents/position-statements/ps-lgbtq

National Association of School Nurses. (2024). A contemporary framework update for today's school nursing landscape: Introducing the School Nursing Practice Framework. *NASN School Nurse, 39*(3), 140–147. https://www.doi.org/10.1177/1942602X241241092

National Children's Center for Rural and Agricultural Health and Safety & National Farm Medicine Center. (2023). Cultivate safety. https://www.cultivatesafety.org/

National High Blood Pressure Education Program Working Group on High Blood Pressure in Children and Adolescents. (2005). The fourth report on the diagnosis, evaluation, and treatment of high blood pressure in children and adolescents. National Institutes of Health. https://www.nhlbi.nih.gov/files/docs/resources/heart/hbp_ped.pdf

National Highway Traffic Safety Administration. (n.d.). Car seat recommendations for children. https://www.nhtsa.gov/sites/nhtsa.dot.gov/files/documents/carseatrecommendationsforchildren.pdf

National Institute of Diabetes and Digestive and Kidney Diseases. (2017). Definition & facts for bladder control problems & bedwetting in children. https://www.niddk.nih.gov/health-information/urologic-diseases/bladder-control-problems-bedwetting-children/definition-facts

National Institutes of Health. (2023). Brain basics: Know your brain. https://www.ninds.nih.gov/health-information/public-education/brain-basics/brain-basics-know-your-brain

National Organization of Rare Diseases. (2021). Marfan syndrome. https://rarediseases.org/rare-diseases/marfan-syndrome/

National Program for Playground Safety (2015). Playground safety handbook. https://cpsc.gov/s3fs-public/325.pdf

National Sleep Foundation. (2022a). What happens when you sleep? https://www.sleepfoundation.org/how-sleep-works/what-happens-when-you-sleep

National Sleep Foundation. (2022b). Would later school start times affect sleep? https://www.sleepfoundation.org/school-and-sleep/later-school-start-times#references-80801

O'Leary, F., Hayen, A., Lockie, F., & Peat, J. (2015). Defining normal ranges and centiles for heart and respiratory rates in infants and children: A cross-sectional study of patients attending an Australian tertiary hospital paediatric emergency department. *Archives of Disease in Children, 100*(8), 733–737. https://doi.org/10.1136/archdischild-2014-307401

Olson-Kennedy, J. (2022). Transgender adolescents and young adults. In D. K. Katzman, C. M. Gordon, T. Callahan, A. Joffe, S. Rosenthal, M. Trent, & R. Chung (Eds.). *Neinstein's adolescent and young adult healthcare: A practical guide* (7th. ed., pp. 408–412) [eBook edition]. Wolters Kluwer.

Paruthi, S., Brooks, L. J., D'Ambrosio, C., Hall, W. A., Kotagal, S., Lloyd, R. M., Malow, B. A., Maski, K., Nichols, C., Quan, S. F., Rosen, C. L., Troester, M. M., & Wise, M. S. (2016). Recommended amount of sleep for pediatric populations: A consensus statement of the American Academy of Sleep Medicine. *Journal of Clinical Sleep Medicine, 12*(6), 785–786.

Piaget, J. (1961). *The growth of logical thinking from childhood to adolescence.* New York: Basic Books.

Pre-Kindergarten Task Force. (2017). *The current state of scientific knowledge on pre-kindergarten effects.* Brookings & Duke Center for Child and Family Policy. https://www.brookings.edu/wp-content/uploads/2017/04/duke_prekstudy_final_4-4-17_hires.pdf

Richards, D. (2015). Fluoride gel effective at reducing caries in children. *Evidence Based Dentristry, 16*, 108–109. https://doi.org/10.1038/sj.ebd.6401131

Rigney, G., & Weiss, S. (2022). Sleep disorders. In D. K. Katzman, C. M. Gordon, T. Callahan, A. Joffe, S. Rosenthal, M. Trent, & R. Chung (Eds.). *Neinstein's adolescent and young adult healthcare: A practical guide* (7th. ed., pp. 293–299) [eBook edition]. Wolters Kluwer.

Rogol, A. (2020). Emotional deprivation in children: Growth faltering and reversible hypopituitarism. *Frontiers in Endocrinology, 11*, 596144. https://doi.org/10.3389/fendo.2020.596144

Sachedin, A., & Todd, N., (2020). Dysmenorrhea, endometriosis, and chronic pelvic pain in adolescents. *Journal of Clinical Research in Pediatric Endocrinology, 12*(Suppl 1), 7–17. https://doi.org/10.4274/jcrpe.galenos.2019.2019.S0217

Salhi, C., Azrael, D., & Miller, M. (2021), Parent and adolescent reports of adolescent access to household firearms in the United States. *Journal of the American Medical Association, 4*(3). https://doi.org/10.1001/jamanetworkopen.2021.0989

Schaeffer, K. (2021). Key facts about Americans and guns. *Pew Research Center.* https://www.pewresearch.org/fact-tank/2021/09/13/key-facts-about-americans-and-guns/

Secor-Turner, M., Huseth-Zosel, A., & Ostlund, R. (2022) Menstruation experiences of middle and high school students in the Midwest: A pilot study. *Journal of School Nursing, 38*(6), 504–510. https://doi.org/10.1177/1059840520974234

Sherer, S., & Radzik, M. (2022). Psychosocial development in normal adolescents and young adults. In D. K. Katzman, C. M. Gordon, T. Callahan, A. Joffe, S. Rosenthal, M. Trent, & R. Chung (Eds.). *Neinstein's adolescent and young adult healthcare: A practical guide* (7th. ed., pp. 45–49) [eBook edition]. Wolters & Kluwer.

Siu, A. (2015). Screening for speech and language delay and disorders in children aged 5 years or younger: U.S. Preventive Services Task Force recommendation statement. *Pediatrics, 136*(2), e474–481. https://doi.org10.1542/peds.2015-1711

Sood, M. R., Li, B. U., & Hoppin, A. G. (2023). Chronic functional constipation and fecal incontinence in infants, children, and adolescents: Treatment. *UptoDate.* https://www.uptodate.com/contents/chronic-functional-constipation-and-fecal-incontinence-in-infants-children-and-adolescents-treatment/print?search=dyfunctional%20elemination&source=search_result&selectedTitle=5~150&usage_type=default&display_rank=5

Stackpole, K. M. W., Crimmins, N., & Xanthakos, S. (2022). Obesity. In D. K. Katzman, C. M. Gordon, T. Callahan, A. Joffe, S. Rosenthal, M. Trent, & R. Chung (Eds.). *Neinstein's adolescent and young adult healthcare: A practical guide* (7th. ed., pp. 354–361) [eBook edition]. Wolters Kluwer.

Stavridou, A., Kapsali, E., Panagouli, E, Thirious, A., Polychronis, K., Bacopoulou, F., Paaliopoulou, T., Tsolia, M., Sergentanis, T., & Tsitsika, A. (2021) Obesity in children and adolescents during the COVID-19 pandemic. *Children, 8*(2), 135. https://doi.org/10.3390/children8020135

Strowd, L. C., & Krowchuk, D. (2022). Acne. In D. K. Katzman, C. M. Gordon, T. Callahan, A. Joffe, S. Rosenthal, M. Trent, & R. Chung (Eds.), *Neinstein's adolescent and young adult healthcare: A practical guide* (7th. ed., pp. 256–262) [eBook edition]. Wolters & Kluwer.

Substance Abuse and Mental Health Services Administration & Health Resources and Services Administration. (2018). Empowering change: Motivational interviewing. https://www.samhsa.gov/homelessness-programs-resources/hpr-resources/empowering-change

Tanner, J. M. (1962). *Growth at adolescence* (2nd ed.). Blackwell.

Trans Student Educational Resources. (2015). The gender unicorn. https://transstudent.org/gender/

U.S. Consumer Product Safety Commission. (n.d.). Public playground safety checklist. https://www.cpsc.gov/safety-education/safety-guides/playgrounds/public-playground-safety-checklist

U.S. Department of Agriculture. (2020). My Plate. https://www.myplate.gov/

U.S. Department of Agriculture. (2022a). A guide to smart snacks in schools. https://fns-prod.azureedge.us/sites/default/files/resource-files/smartsnacks.pdf

U.S. Department of Agriculture. (2022b). Definitions of food security. https://www.ers.usda.gov/topics/food-nutrition-assistance/food-security-in-the-u-s/definitions-of-food-security/

U.S. Department of Agriculture. (2022c). Team nutrition: Local school wellness policy. https://www.fns.usda.gov/tn/local-school-wellness-policy

U.S. Department of Agriculture & U.S. Department of Health and Human Services, (2020). *Dietary guidelines for Americans 2020–2025* (9th ed.). https://www.dietaryguidelines.gov/sites/default/files/2020-12/Dietary_Guidelines_for_Americans_2020-2025.pdf

U.S. Department of Education. (2021). U.S. department of education confirms title IX protects students from discrimination based on sexual orientation and gender identity. https://www.ed.gov/news/press-releases/us-department-education-confirms-title-ix-protects-students-discrimination-based-sexual-orientation-and-gender-identity

U.S. Department of Health and Human Services [USDHSS], Eunice Kennedy Shriver National Institute of Child Health and Development. (2021). Menstrual cycles as a fifth vital sign. https://www.nichd.nih.gov/about/org/od/directors_corner/prev_updates/menstrual-cycles

Vogels, E., Gelles-Watnick, R., & Massarat, R. (2022). Teens, social media & technology overview. *Pew Research Center.* https://www.pewresearch.org/internet/2022/11/16/connection-creativity-and-drama-teen-life-on-social-media-in-2022/

Weiss Kelly, A. K., Hecht, S., Council on Sports Medicine and Fitness, Brenner, J. S., LaBela, C. R., Brooks, M. A., Diamond A., Hennrikus, W., LaBotz, M., Logan, K., Loud, K. J., Moffatt, K., A., Nemeth, B., & Pengel, B. (2016). The female athlete triad. *Pediatrics, 138*(2), e20160922. https://doi.org/10.1542/peds.2016-0922

Westwood, C., Fallowfield, J., Delves, S., Nunns, M., Ogden, H., & Layden, J. (2021). Individual risk factors associated with exertional heat illness: A systematic review. *Experimental Physiology, 106*(1), 191–199. https://doi.org/10.1113/EP088458

World Health Organization. (2023). Health and gender. https://www.who.int/health-topics/gender#tab=tab_2

World Health Organization. (2024). Sexual health: Definitions. https://www.who.int/health-topics/sexual-health#tab=tab_2

Wu, A., Aris, M., Hivert, M., Rocchio, C., Cocoros, N., Klompas, M., & Taveras, E. (2022). Association of changes in obesity prevalence with the COVID-19 pandemic in youth in Massachusetts. *JAMA: Pediatrics, 176*(2), 198–201. https://doi.org/10.1001/jamapediatrics.2021.5095

Chapter **10**

Culturally Effective School Nursing Care

Donna Mazyck ▪ Danielle Guillory

CHAPTER OUTLINE

The 2020 U.S. census reveals more ethnically and racially diverse populations than noted in the 2010 census. The largest increase (276%) was in individuals who identify as two or more races, which grew from 9 million people in 2010 to 33.8 million people in 2020 (U.S. Census Bureau, 2021b). The diversity of people in the United States is noted in schools and communities. Schoolchildren come from diverse cultural, ethnic, and racial backgrounds. People often belong to one or more cultural subgroups that affect the ways they think and behave and what they value. Diversity encompasses all facets between people, including ethnicity and racial identity, physical and cognitive abilities, socioeconomic status and geographical locations, religious and spiritual values, and age (Rose, 2020). Diversity is often referred to in the context of different members belonging to organizations or institutions. Race and ethnicity are often thought to be dominant elements of culture, but the concept of culture is broader.

Respect and equitable practice in school nursing includes self-reflection using a combination of knowledge, skills, and attitudes to work with diverse populations effectively and sensitively with cultural humility and inclusiveness (National Association of School Nurses [NASN], 2022). Culturally effective care requires examining one's own personal beliefs and ensuring such beliefs do not unduly affect the care of others. It also means learning about the cultures with which one works, so that one asks culturally sensitive questions and plans the most appropriate interventions in a manner considered appropriate by the culture. The practice of culturally effective school nursing care starts by realizing the profession of education is a culture, just as is the profession of nursing. Each school building has an organizational culture that needs to be understood.

Recognizing and incorporating cultural beliefs and family values into student-centered multidisciplinary care is essential for safe and effective school nurse interventions.

Becoming culturally effective is an ongoing process. School nurses, who deliver culturally effective care, bridge four cultures: their own, that of the healthcare system, that of the education system, and that of the client (student, family, and school community). School nurses must navigate the process of cultural congruence to connect what students learn about health at school to behavior change outside of the classroom. To be effective practitioners, school nurses must be aware of their biases and learn the nuances of culture that affect health and learning.

School nurses interact with families to provide student-centered care. They use the *School Nursing Practice Framework*™ (NASN, 2024) and the *Whole School, Whole Community, Whole Child Model* (WSCC; Centers for Disease Control and Prevention [CDC], 2018) to focus care on the student, the student's family, and the school community. As the basic social unit of society, families provide students with stability, nurturing, motivation, support, and love. Supporting student health means working with the family. School nurse communication and collaboration with families is integral to keeping students healthy, safe, and ready to learn. School nurses work with students and their families when they conduct assessments, interventions, and evaluations. With the changing demographics of the 21st-century family, it is imperative that school nurses understand the contexts and the interactional processes between families and the school environment. The school nurse must be able to identify family strengths, build rapport, and facilitate therapeutic communication to promote family engagement. School nurses need to understand factors that promote optimal family health and learning, as well as disparities that place students and families at risk for health and education inequities.

The purpose of this chapter is to give school nurses an understanding of culturally effective practice and the critical role of school nurses in cultural responsiveness with students, families, and diverse school communities. This chapter also aims to provide school nurses with a core understanding of the dynamic concepts and contexts of family life that impact student health and well-being at school. Consideration will be given to student and family demographics, family structure, function, family systems theory, and family partnership and engagement.

CULTURAL STANDARDS AND REGULATIONS

Culturally effective school nursing is supported by national standards and regulations. Healthcare providers and organizations, including school nurses and school districts, must adhere to the *National Standards for Culturally and Linguistically Appropriate Services* (CLAS; Office of Minority Health [OMH], 2023). These 15 standards, shown in Box 10-1, delineate specific steps to improve the quality of health care, advance health equity, and decrease health disparities in diverse populations. Understanding these principles guides the interprofessional education team to identify the cultural and language needs of the students and families in the school community.

School personnel must be aware that Title VI of the Civil Rights Act of 1964 prohibits discrimination because of nationality or language. Title VI prohibits the exclusion of a person from participation based on race, color, or national origin in any program or activity that receives federal funds or other federal financial assistance either directly or indirectly, in the types, quantity, quality, or timeliness of program services, aids, or benefits that they provide or the way they provide them. This prohibition applies to intentional discrimination as well as to procedures, criteria, or methods of administration that appear neutral but have a discriminatory effect on individuals because of their race, color, or national origin.

Schools that receive federal funding must uphold Title VI by operating school programs and activities in a nondiscriminatory manner including, but not limited to, admissions, recruitment, financial aid, academic programs, student treatment and services, counseling and guidance, discipline, classroom assignment, grading, vocational education, recreation, physical education, athletics, housing, and employment. Title VI stipulates that schools provide material in languages understood by the school population, including translation and interpretation services. Failure to respect these rights is a reportable offense to the Office for Civil Rights. This office investigates alleged violations and works with school districts to resolve issues of discrimination (U.S. Department of Education, 2023).

DEMOGRAPHIC SNAPSHOTS

School nurses should look carefully at the demographic and socioeconomic backgrounds of their school communities when assessing the needs of the populations they serve. However, school nurses cannot make assumptions about the culture of students and families based on their demographic data; this information should serve as one

Focus on the Framework

NASN's School Nursing Practice Framework (2024) supports the synergistic practice of culturally responsive and effective school nursing practice that focuses on the diverse needs of students through the practice principles of **care coordination, leadership, quality improvement, and public health.** Respectful and equitable school nursing care is woven throughout *School Nursing: Scope and Standards of Practice* with Standard 9, Respect and Equitable Practice, specifically outlining the competencies by which school nurses deliver care to diverse populations (NASN, 2022). Box 10-2 lists the competencies for Standard 9.

BOX 10-1

National Standards for Culturally and Linguistically Appropriate Services (CLAS) in Health and Health Care

The National CLAS Standards are intended to advance health equity, improve quality, and help eliminate healthcare disparities by establishing a blueprint for health and healthcare organizations as follows:

PRINCIPAL STANDARD

1. Provide effective, equitable, understandable, and respectful quality care and services that are responsive to diverse cultural health beliefs and practices, preferred languages, health literacy, and other communication needs.

GOVERNANCE, LEADERSHIP, AND WORKFORCE

2. Advance and sustain organizational governance and leadership that promote CLAS and health equity through policy, practices, and allocated resources.
3. Recruit, promote, and support a culturally and linguistically diverse governance, leadership, and workforce that are responsive to the population in the service area.
4. Educate and train governance, leadership, and workforce in culturally and linguistically appropriate policies and practices on an ongoing basis.

COMMUNICATION AND LANGUAGE ASSISTANCE

5. Offer language assistance to individuals who have limited English proficiency and/or other communication needs, at no cost to them, to facilitate timely access to all health care and services.
6. Inform all individuals of the availability of language assistance services clearly and in their preferred language, verbally and in writing.
7. Ensure the competence of individuals providing language assistance, recognizing that the use of untrained individuals and/or minors as interpreters should be avoided.
8. Provide easy-to-understand print and multimedia materials and signage in the languages commonly used by the populations in the service area.

ENGAGEMENT, CONTINUOUS IMPROVEMENT, AND ACCOUNTABILITY

9. Establish culturally and linguistically appropriate goals, policies, and management accountability, and infuse them throughout the organization's planning and operations.
10. Conduct ongoing assessments of the organization's CLAS-related activities and integrate CLAS-related measures into measurement and continuous quality improvement activities.
11. Collect and maintain accurate and reliable demographic data to monitor and evaluate the impact of CLAS on health equity and outcomes and to inform service delivery.
12. Conduct regular assessments of community health assets and needs and use the results to plan and implement services that respond to the cultural and linguistic diversity of populations in the service area.
13. Partner with the community to design, implement, and evaluate policies, practices, and services to ensure cultural and linguistic appropriateness.
14. Create conflict and grievance resolution processes that are culturally and linguistically appropriate to identify, prevent, and resolve conflicts or complaints.
15. Communicate the organization's progress in implementing and sustaining CLAS to all stakeholders, constituents, and the public.

OMH (2023).

data point in the development of an understanding of the cultures in the school.

When reviewing federally reported data, school nurses should consider how the federal government collects national demographic information as the collection strategies provide context for the data. The U.S. Office of Management and Budget (OMB) developed the *Standards for the Classification of Federal Data on Race and Ethnicity* (Standards) in 1997 and updated them in 2015 to describe groups to which individuals belong. The categories reflect how individuals self-identify; they do not denote scientific definitions of anthropological origins. The designations are used to categorize U.S. citizens, resident aliens, and other eligible noncitizens in the U.S. Census and other government data collection systems (OMH, 2021). The classification standards aim to provide a common language that promotes uniformity in analyzing and comparing aggregate statistical data. Many private organizations employ the same or similar standards in collecting categorical data on individuals and groups.

In March 2024, the Census Bureau updated how the OMB will collect and present race/ethnicity data across agencies (Marks et al., 2024). These updates will be implemented over the next 5 years. Traditionally, respondents have had limited selections for "identity" when entering official demographic data for government agencies. With the update, some of the concerns around how race/ethnicity data are collected were addressed. The first question respondents will be asked has been changed so that it will now be a combined question using both terms, race and ethnicity. When responding, individuals can choose one or multiple race/ethnicity categories. Those who select Hispanic/Latino may indicate this as a complete response. In the past, if Hispanic/Latino was chosen, the respondent had to select a subcategory for country of origin from only three options: Mexico, Puerto Rico, and Cuba. These

BOX 10-2

Standard 9 of the Standards of Professional Performance for School Nursing: Respectful and Equitable Practice

The school nurse practices with cultural humility and inclusiveness.

COMPETENCIES

The school nurse:

9.1 Inventories one's own values, beliefs, cultural heritage, and implicit biases via critical self-reflection to improve culturally congruent practice.
9.2 Identifies the cultural-specific meaning of interactions, terms, and content.
9.3 Engages community partners to identify cultural norms and values.
9.4 Demonstrates respect, equity, justice, cultural humility, and empathy in actions and interactions with all students, families, and the school community.
9.5 Seeks to understand the effects and impact of discrimination and oppression within and among vulnerable cultural groups.
9.6 Respects student and family decisions based on age, tradition, belief and family influence, and stage of acculturation.
9.7 Communicates with appropriate language and behaviors, including the use of professional and competent adult interpreters and translators in accordance with the student's and family's healthcare preferences and state and local regulations.
9.8 Utilizes terminology and salutations, communication characteristics, and written material vetted for the culture, literacy, and language of the population served.
9.9 Engages students, families, key stakeholders, and others in designing and establishing internal and external cross-cultural partnerships.
9.10 Advocates for policies, procedures, programs, services, and practices that promote health, prevent harm, and improve equitable access to care for culturally diverse students and families.
9.11 Advances equitable access to school health services, interventions, health promotion programs, enrollment in research, health and academic education, and other opportunities.
9.12 Promotes equity for students and families by educating nurse colleagues, other professionals, and community stakeholders about cultural similarities and differences of students and families in the school community.
9.13 Models safe, respectful, inclusive, accepting, just, and culturally congruent school nurse practice.
9.14 Collaborates to establish a culture of safety for vulnerable students or groups.
9.15 Documents student's and family's cultural practices, preferences, beliefs, language(s), as well as interventions and outcomes.

Note: Additional competencies for the graduate-level prepared school nurses are also a part of Standard 9 and can be found in its entirety in *School Nursing: Scope and Standards of Practice* (4th ed.).

NASN (2022, pp. 77–78), with permission.

limited choices excluded most of Central America and all of South America for those who selected Hispanic/Latino as their ethnicity.

Next, individuals are asked to indicate one or more race with which they identify. Although the concept of race is increasingly recognized as a social construct without biological or genetic basis, for federal data collection purposes, there are six "races." This is an update from a selection of five races. The 2024 update added Middle Eastern or North African to the category. Individuals may now select from the following six groups: American Indians/Alaskan Natives, black or African American, Middle Eastern or North African, white, Asian, or Native Hawaiian/Other Pacific Islander (Marks et al., 2024). The last two categories have several subcategories that can be selected.

Large categories for "race" in the Standards for the Classification of Federal Data on Race and Ethnicity are problematic (Ulmer et al., 2009). For example, these standards do not recognize that persons from Asia are not all the same race. There are 48 countries with incredibly diverse populations on the continent of Asia, yet only five categories for Asian countries of origin are included (Chinese, Filipino, Japanese, Korean, and Vietnamese). Asia also includes Russia, whose population is predominantly white and typically considered Russian, not Asian. Remarkably, none of the 54 countries of origin in Africa are delineated. Therefore, all persons from arguably the most diverse continent are similarly considered African American. School personnel need to be aware that the unique needs of many "minority" communities are not recognized by state and federal governmental bodies nor represented in official government statistics. Data collected via the Standards for the Classification of Federal Data on Race and Ethnicity are used for the allocation of government funding and resources to meet population-focused needs, including in school and health systems. It does not account for the wide spectrum of diversity and needs that exist in the nation's increasingly transglobal population, thus funding may not be allocated by greatest population need.

Students

School nurses often work with students and families with cultural, ethnic, and racial backgrounds unlike their own. Most recent National Center for Education Statistics (NCES) data reveal a 3% decrease in total enrollment in U.S. prekindergarten through grade 12 public schools following the coronavirus pandemic. Total public school enrollment decreased from 50.8 million students to 49.4 million students between Fall 2019 and 2020 and remained unchanged in Fall 2021 (NCES, 2023b). The drop in enrollment is seen at the elementary level with increases seen at the high school level. An additional 4.7 million students were enrolled in private and parochial elementary and secondary schools (NCES, 2022). The racial/ethnic composition of schools varies significantly. Seventy-seven percent of white students attended schools that had enrollments of no less than 50% white students (NCES, 2023c), whereas 59% of black students attended schools where the enrollment was 75% or more students of color. Hispanic, Asian, American Indian, and Pacific Islander groups experience similar disparity where 61%, 41%, 42%, and 53%, respectively, all attend schools that enroll greater than 75% or more students of color. These data suggest that students who are white are more likely to go to public or private schools where this race is the majority. Students of races other than white are more likely to be in public schools that have increasing diversity. See Figure 10-1.

Many students enrolled are English learners (ELs). The percentage of public school students who are ELs varies greatly across states with the smallest percentage in West Virginia (0.7%) to the highest in Texas (20.1%; NCES, 2023a). For EL students, the language needs of both the student and parents/guardians must be considered. School nurses should consider what resources are needed to assess, plan, implement, and evaluate student care. This includes considering and planning for the use of interpreters. Students should not be asked to interpret for their parents/guardians. See the variability in students who are ELs across states in Figure 10-2.

School nurses should be familiar with the student demographic and educational data available through state, regional, county, and local public education and health authorities. Under the *Every Student Succeeds Act* (2015), state educational agencies (SEAs) and local educational agencies (LEAs) receiving federal funds through Title I (a federal law that provides funding to schools with low-income families) are required to produce publicly available "report cards" with aggregated information on student demographics, performance, and funding. The SEA and LEA "school report cards" typically include de-identified data on academic achievement, graduation rates, mobility, school revenue, and spending per pupil, as well as how well the teaching staff reflects the diversity of the school community. Knowledge of these data points can help inform the school nurse's practice. School nurses can seek additional information to help them understand those they serve from state and local public health departments as well as local health systems. All of these entities collect detailed information about major social, health, and inequity issues.

Families

Students come from families with various configurations. Households with children may experience a variety of stressors related to social determinants of health, such as income, housing, transportation, and food insecurity. In 2023, 71% of children ages 0 to 17 years lived with two parents, 25% lived with one parent, and 4% lived with caregivers other than parents (U.S. Census Bureau, 2023).

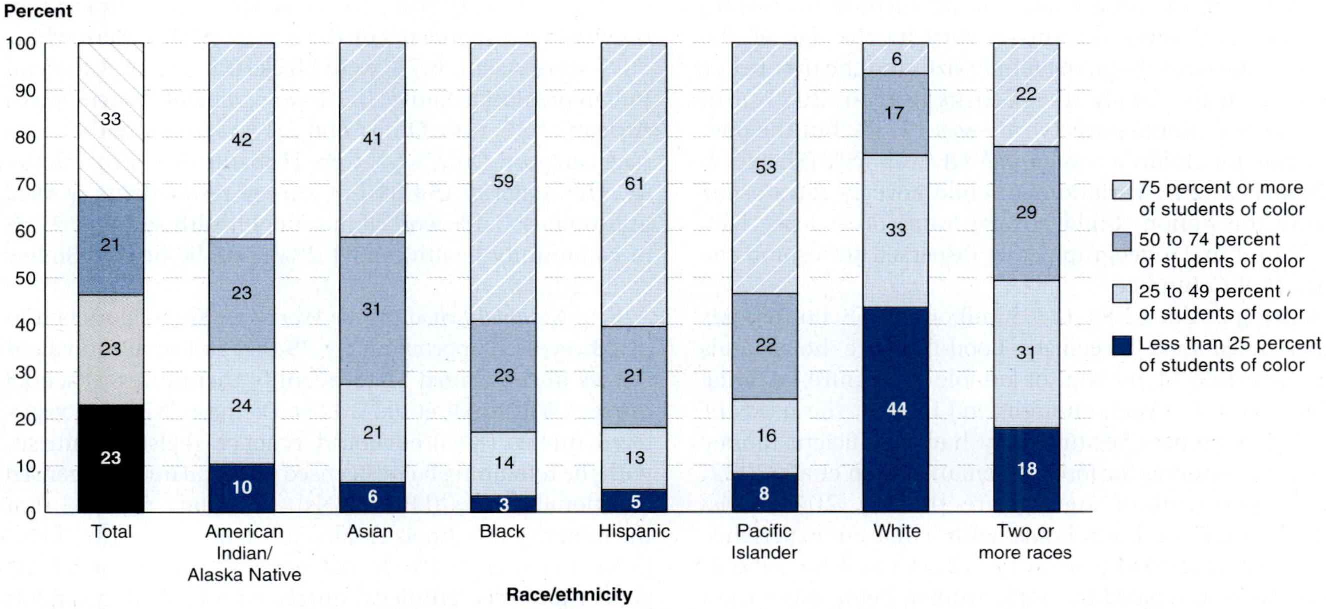

FIGURE 10-1. Percentage distribution of public elementary and secondary school students, by student's race/ethnicity and percentage of students of color enrolled in the school: Fall 2021. *(NCES, 2023c.)*

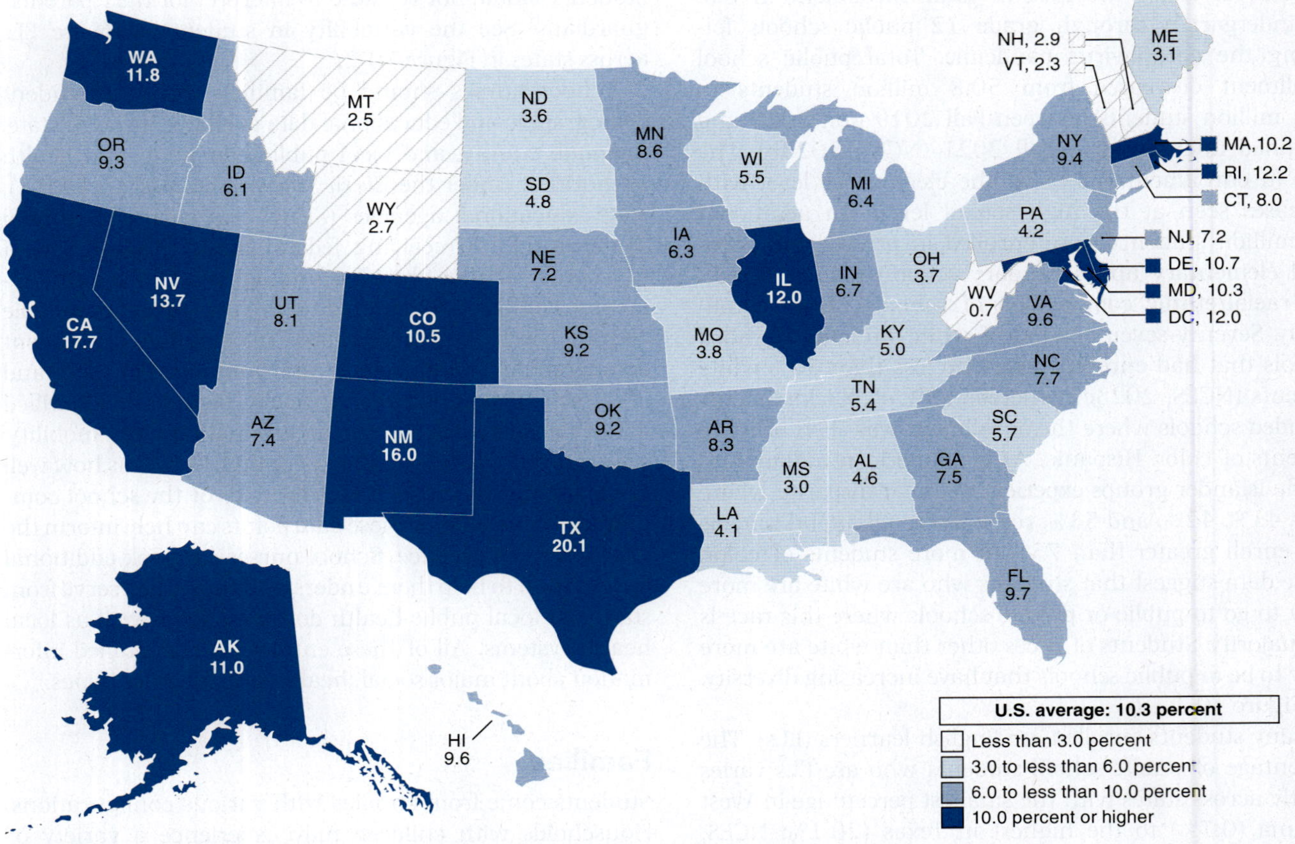

FIGURE 10-2. Percentage of public-school students who were English learners (ELs), by state: Fall 2020. *(NCES, 2023c.)*

Many students and their families live in conditions of poverty. U.S. government surveys measure levels of poverty in families. The determination of poverty standing is calculated by comparing annual income to poverty thresholds. Poverty thresholds vary by the age of the head of the household, the family size, and the number of children in the family (U.S. Census Bureau, 2021c). In 2022, the national poverty rate was 11.5%, but the poverty rate for children (under age 18) was 15% (Shrider & Creamer, 2023). Variations in child poverty rates occur across the nation. Child poverty rates of at least 18% are found in 16 geographically dispersed states and the District of Columbia.

During 2022, 12.8% (13.5 million) of U.S. households experienced food insecurity. Food-insecure households are uncertain of having, or unable to acquire, at some time during the year, enough food to meet the needs of all their members because they had insufficient money or other resources for food (Coleman-Jensen et al., 2022; U.S. Department of Agriculture [USDA], 2023). Disparities exist as households with children experience higher rates of food insecurity (12.5%) and households with children headed by single women being more than twice as likely to experience food insecurity (24.3%). See Figure 10-3.

School Nurses

In 2020, the *National Nursing Workforce Survey* noted the number of registered nurses (RNs) in the United States was 4,198,031 (Smiley et al., 2021). When looking at races represented by respondents of the survey, 80.6% were white, 7.2% were Asian, 6.7% were black, 0.5% were American Indian or Alaska Native, 0.2% were Middle Eastern/North African, 2.3% were Other, and 2.1% were more than one race category. Only 5.6% were Hispanic or Latinx ethnicity. The majority (54.8%) of survey respondents worked in hospitals; 3.1% worked in school health services, 1.7% in community health, and 1.2% in public health (Smiley et al., 2021).

The *National School Nurse Workforce Study* launched in 2023 revealed approximately 79,000 full-time equivalent nurses in the United States identify themselves as school nurses (Willgerodt et al., 2023). Of these, 82% are registered nurses (RNs)/advanced practice registered nurses with the remaining being licensed practical nurses/licensed vocational nurses (LPNs/LVNs). The study revealed that the majority of schools employ full-time nurses (RN/LPN/LVN); however, 6.3% do not employ a nurse at all. By gender and race/ethnicity, nurses who worked in schools are 98.2% female with 91.2% of registered nurses identifying as white, 3.7% black/African American, 1.3%

Prevalence of food insecurity, by selected household characteristics, 2021 and 2022

	Percent of U.S. households 2021	Percent of U.S. households 2022	Percentage point change
All households	10.2	12.8	2.6*
Household composition:			
With children < 18 years	12.5	17.3	4.8*
With children < 6 years	12.9	16.7	3.8*
Married-couple families	7.4	10.7	3.3*
Female head, no spouse	24.3	33.1	8.8*
Male head, no spouse	16.2	21.2	5.0*
With no children < 18 years	9.4	11.0	1.6*
More than one adult	6.9	8.6	1.7*
Women living alone	13.2	15.1	1.9*
Men living alone	12.3	13.8	1.5*
With adults age 65+	7.1	9.1	2.0*
Adults 65+ living alone	9.5	11.4	1.9*
Race/ethnicity of household reference persons:			
White, non-Hispanic	7.0	9.3	2.3*
Black, non-Hispanic	19.8	22.4	2.6*
Hispanic	16.2	20.8	4.6*
Other, non-Hispanic	10.2	11.0	0.8
Household income-to-poverty ratio:			
Under 1.00	32.1	36.7	4.6*
Under 1.30	31.0	35.2	4.2*
Under 1.85	26.5	32.0	5.5*
1.85 and over	5.0	6.8	1.8*
Area of residence:			
Inside metropolitan area	10.1	12.5	2.4*
In principal cities	12.2	15.3	3.1*
Not in principal cities	8.8	10.5	1.7*
Outside metropolitan area	10.8	14.7	3.9*
Census geographic region:			
Northeast	8.8	11.6	2.8*
Midwest	9.9	12.4	2.5*
South	11.4	14.5	3.1*
West	9.7	11.2	1.5*

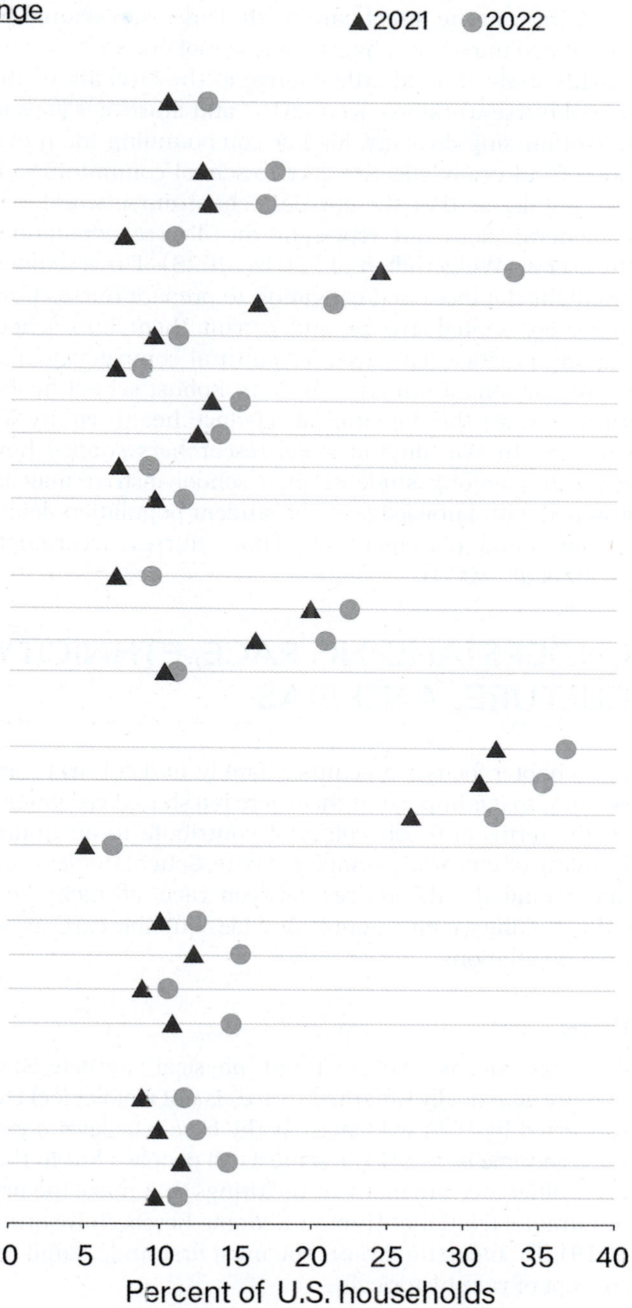

*An asterisk indicates change is statistically different from zero at the 90-percent confidence level (t > 1.645).

Source: USDA, Economic Research Service using data from U.S. Department of Commerce, Bureau of the Census, 2021 and 2022 Current Population Survey Food Security Supplements.

FIGURE 10-3. Trends in food insecurity in the United States. *(USDA, 2023.)*

Asian, 1.6% Hispanic/Latinx, and 2.2% American Indian/Alaskan Native and Hawaiian. It is important to note that NASN (2021) recommends a baccalaureate degree in nursing as the minimal preparation for school nursing practice. Although LPNs/LVNs can play important roles in providing routine direct care to students, they should be considered nurses in schools—not school nurses.

This study showed little change in the diversity of the school nurse workforce from 2017 and illustrates gaps in school nursing diversity, further compounding the provision of culturally effective care to school communities. It also highlights that the current school nurse workforce, in general, does not represent the diverse populations they serve (Willgerodt et al., 2018, 2023). These realities highlight the increased obligation to prepare nurses from underrepresented groups and recruit them into school nursing practice. The need for cultural competency education for school nurses is evident. Robust school health services have the potential to advance health equity for students. In Washington state, researchers studied how disparities among students in a school district may be lessened with knowledge of the student population demographics and placement of school nurses accordingly (Gratz et al., 2023).

UNDERSTANDING RACE, ETHNICITY, CULTURE, AND BIAS

This chapter focuses on culture, family, and cultural competency, so it is important that there is a shared vocabulary on the terms and concepts that contribute to an understanding of culturally competent care. School nurses must understand the differences between race, ethnicity, and culture along a continuum to provide equitable care across their populations.

Race

Although race is associated with physical characteristics that are genetically inherited, "race" is not a biological fact supported by DNA evidence. At the base-pair level a person's genome is 99.9% the same as all people—but in that 0.1% difference are many of the things that make the person unique (National Human Genome Research Institute, 2019). To understand race, one must first understand the concept of race historically.

> *Race is a social construct used to group people. Race was constructed as a hierarchal human-grouping system, generating racial classifications to identify, distinguish, and marginalize some groups across nations, regions, and the world. Race divides human populations into groups, often based on physical appearance, social factors, and cultural backgrounds.* (National Human Genome Research Institute, 2022)

Historically, race has been classified by what a dominant group in power has been conditioned to believe about another group of people who typically represent a minority of the population. Dominant groups have used race to project a sense of inferiority on targeted populations, often leading to widespread subjugation, segregation, injustice, and inequity. Although tremendous strides have been made legally, socially, and economically to correct conditions of inequity, *race* as a concept is not well understood or accepted across American society, and therefore inequality persists.

Using race as a basis for healthcare decisions can create mistrust and marginalization of specific populations within the United States while contributing to negative health outcomes. The healthcare system's historical treatment of populations based on race still impacts families today; the victimization of specific populations is not a history that can easily be forgotten. When working with families, school nurses should take into account that this history is still a burden that some families carry through personal experiences. The school nurse should not minimize the generational trauma experienced by many families. Instead, the school nurse should learn from the family's stories, experiences, and history to provide care that is holistic and relevant so that students/families may feel accepted, included, and safe at school.

Ethnicity

Ethnicity differs from culture by definition. This is important to note because many times these terms are incorrectly used interchangeably. The U.S. Census Bureau considers *ethnicity* to be a person's heritage, nationality, lineage, or country of origin of the person's ancestors (U.S. Census Bureau, 2021a). Ethnicity leads to a more specific identity within a culture. The terms used to describe ethnic groups help identify at-risk groups and track illnesses within the general population and particular groups. This research is vital as it can provide information on diagnoses, outcomes of health conditions, best practices for health conditions, and improvement in health disparities. It is essential to recognize and respect ethnic differences while also not differing care solely based on someone's ethnicity.

Culture

There are many definitions of *culture*, but it is important to understand the general concept on the path to cultural congruency. According to the National Institutes of Health (2021, para. 1):

> *Culture is often described as the combination of a body of knowledge, a body of belief, and a body of behavior. It involves several elements that are often specific to ethnic, racial, religious, geographic, or social groups. This includes personal identification, language, thoughts, communications, actions, customs, beliefs, values, and institutions.*

The Centers for Disease Control and Prevention (CDC) defines culture as "group membership, such as racial, ethnic, linguistic, or geographical groups, or as a collection of beliefs, values, customs, ways of thinking, communicating and behaving specific to a group" (CDC, 2022b, para. 1).

While these two definitions do not fully define all that is encapsulated by one's culture, they give a basis for understanding. It is important to know that culture is more than just identity. Culture can vary even between people of the same race and ethnicity. In addition, culture varies depending on geographical locations, traditions, and life experiences. To practice in a school setting that respects and understands the population's culture, it is essential to remember that culture cannot be established merely on the factors mentioned in the definitions in this chapter. *Culture is not static.* Students are members of multiple cultures based on personal beliefs, religion, ethnicity, and more. Culture can still be diverse within the same ethnicity, race, and geographical location. For example, urban and suburban populations of the same race and ethnicity can be drastically different culturally. At the same time, diverse rural populations may share many culturally similar characteristics due to their isolation, regardless of ethnicity.

Intersectionality

The framework of intersectionality, developed by legal scholar and activist Kimberlé Crenshaw, considers how race and other social identities overlap and influence each other (McRae & Onukwugha, 2021). The concept of intersectionality describes the ways in which systems of inequality based on gender, race, ethnicity, sexual orientation, gender identity, disability, class, and other forms of discrimination "intersect" to create unique dynamics and effects (Center for Intersectional Justice, n.d.). The term *intersectionality* in health care refers to the multiple factors of a person's identity that affect health outcomes.

Using the definitions of race, ethnicity, and culture, one can see how these are similar but also different. Race is a social construct often used to create a structure among certain groups of people that can negatively affect people in general society and healthcare outcomes.

Culture is more personal; race and ethnicity can contribute to culture. Culture is broader because it encompasses not only race and ethnicity but many other factors.

Biases

We live in a time when the United States is becoming increasingly diverse. In less than 30 years, the country will be more diverse than at any other time in history as it is expected that by the year 2050, almost 50% of the United States population will consist of minorities (Nair & Adetayo, 2019). The time to shift thinking away from biases is now. The first step is to recognize how biases can affect health outcomes and student care.

Cultural bias occurs when actions are interpreted through one's own cultural lens. This bias inhibits the ability of the person to fully understand the interaction as they are not considering how the other person's culture may influence that person's actions.

Implicit bias is based on "attitudes and beliefs about race, ethnicity, age, ability, gender, or other characteristics that operate outside our conscious awareness and can be measured only indirectly" (Sabin, 2022, p. 105). Also called subconscious bias, implicit biases are either favorable or unfavorable cognitive assessments of others. Implicit biases are expressed without intent, can affect judgment, and may directly contribute to discrimination (National Education Association [NEA] Center for Social Justice, 2021). According to the National Center for Cultural Competence at Georgetown University (Module 2, n.d.), implicit bias can be triggered by any number of perceived characteristics of others, such as the following:

- Age
- Disability
- Education
- English language proficiency and fluency (including the capacity to speak standard English for native-born English speakers)
- Ethnicity
- Health status
- Disease/diagnosis (HIV/AIDS)
- Insurance
- Obesity
- Race
- Socioeconomic status
- Sexual orientation, gender identity, or expression
- Skin tone
- Substance use (injection drug user)
- Social contact (amount of contact that practitioners have with patient populations)

"***Microaggressions*** are verbal, behavioral, or environmental slights that are the results of an individual's implicit bias. They are often automatic or unintentional and occur on a daily basis. Microaggressions communicate hostile, derogatory, or negative viewpoints" (NEA Center for Social Justice, 2021, para. 4). Calling out, acknowledging, and responding to microaggressions in social, work, and educational environments may create uncomfortable situations that should be handled sensitively and with respect. School staff training on microaggressions is key to providing strategies to create an inclusive and accepting learning environment.

The most widely used tool to measure implicit bias is the Implicit Association Test (IAT; Greenwald et al., 1998). The test asks users to associate an item with an attribute with those selected more quickly being more associated and those that take longer being less associated. This test is taken online with immediate results and provides the user with examples of implicit biases they may hold. While this tool has limitations, it can be used as a starting point to recognize implicit biases within us (Payne et al., 2018). Sample Implicit Association Tests are available in this textbook's online materials. See OM 10-1.

Explicit biases are the attitudes and assumptions that we acknowledge as part of our personal belief systems and can be assessed directly by means of self-report. Explicit and overtly racist, sexist, and homophobic attitudes often underpin discriminatory actions (Sabin, 2022), as does bias rooted in transphobia/transmisia, xenophobia, and religious status (e.g., antisemitism, Islamophobia, etc.). Explicit biases are consciously held and acted out in speech, treatment, and behaviors that can immediately be felt or seen by the target of the explicit bias. Explicit biases that lead to discrimination must be opposed by all parties involved. School nurses must take a firm stand against discrimination, which may not be easy but is essential in the school community.

Cultural blindness can be defined as a lack of recognition of other cultures. This can be intentionally refusing to acknowledge cultural differences or passively ignoring the differences (Center for Substance Abuse Treatment, 2014). Cultural blindness must be recognized by the individual and overcome through active participation in self-reflection and education. This may occur implicitly where the person is not aware of this lack of recognition, or it may be explicit; however, in either scenario, cultural blindness can lead to missing information about a student or family and can result in ineffective or negative health outcomes.

Ethnocentrism can be seen as the strong belief that one's own ethnic group is extremely important. This sense of importance is expressed both subjectively, that is, as being especially important subjectively to the members of an ethnic group, and also objectively, in the grand scheme of things (Bizumic et al., 2020). This view of importance puts one's own culture and experience above another and can be detrimental, leading to negative health and education outcomes.

"A ***stereotype*** is a widely held but oversimplified belief about a particular type of person or group. It happens when someone groups individuals together based on some factor and makes a judgment about them without knowing them" (NEA Center for Social Justice, 2021, para. 5). The resulting stereotype tends to enforce the perception that people of a certain age, gender, or race cannot shift from one social role to a different social role (Eagly & Koenig, 2021). Stereotypes can hinder the care of student populations based on the judgments that are projected onto the specific group.

Prejudice is a favorable or unfavorable preconceived feeling or opinion formed without knowledge, reason, or thought that prevents objective consideration of an idea, individual, group, or thing (Bell, 2013). While this definition does include favorable preconceived feelings or opinions, most prejudices are not viewed from a positive lens. Prejudice historically has had negative effects on the group that is subjected to them. It is hard for anyone to say they do not possess any form of prejudice, but it is key for everyone to identify potentially harmful prejudices they carry.

"***Racism*** is the relegation of people of color to inferior status and treatment based on unfounded beliefs about innate inferiority, as well as unjust treatment and oppression of people of color, whether intended or not" (Braveman et al., 2022, p. 172). Racism has been present in the United States for hundreds of years and often leads to segregation that is still prevalent in many cities and communities. Racism is a driving force of social determinants of health, including housing, education, and employment, and is a barrier to health equity (American Public Health Association, n.d.). Racism is an issue that reaches beyond words such as racial slurs; it is ingrained in systems and institutions.

"***Systemic racism*** emphasizes the involvement of whole systems, and often all systems—for example, political, legal, economic, health care, school, and criminal justice systems—including the structures that uphold the systems" (Braveman et al., 2022, p. 171). Also referred to as structural racism, systemic racism affects the health of populations due to its overwhelming reach into every aspect of life. For example, the implications of systemic racism can be seen in the lack of access to healthy foods due to economic instability among black, Indigenous, and people of color populations. Although systemic racism has been established as a problem for many years, the work to dismantle systemic racism is relatively new. Institutional racism is a term that may be interchanged with structural racism but may also refer to racism within a specific institution (Braveman et al., 2022).

The history of victimization of black, Indigenous, and people of color populations in the United States has engrained systemic racism into the fabric of the country. The identification of systemic racism has been noted as far back as 1900 in writing from W. E. B. Dubois (Braveman et al., 2022). The issues with systemic racism faced today, from police brutality to inequalities within the criminal justice system, show the failure of society to address the issue over time. Systemic racism is rooted in the continued implementation of laws, policies, and prejudices of the past. Systemic racism may be evidenced in school systems by discriminatory policies on dress code or hairstyles. Additionally, ample research has shown that from preschool through high school, black students in comparison to their white peers are disproportionately more likely to be disciplined and/or suspended, more likely to be retained a grade, and more likely to receive special education services. Black students are also less likely to be enrolled in advanced placement courses than their white peers (Shores et al., 2020).

Culturally Effective Care

Culturally effective care stems from the concept of culturally competent care familiar to most healthcare providers. However, culturally effective care is more comprehensive and multidimensional; it incorporates many cultural approaches to providing care that respects diverse and intersectional identities, contexts, experiences, beliefs, practices, and priorities.

Cultural competency is defined as

> *a developmental process in which one achieves increasing levels of awareness, knowledge, and skills along a continuum, improving one's capacity to work and communicate effectively*

in cross-cultural situations. Strategies for practicing cultural competency include:

- *Learning about your own and other's cultural identities,*
- *Combating bias and stereotypes,*
- *Respecting others' beliefs, values, and communication preferences,*
- *Adapting your services to each patient's unique needs, and*
- *Gaining new cultural experiences. (OMH, 2021, para. 3)*

Cultural competence requires school nurses to begin by recognizing what comprises their personal cultural identity. This personal understanding creates the basis for understanding other cultures and being able to work without bias. Cultural competence leads to serving as a student advocate by speaking out against biases and stereotypes. These actions help create an inclusive and welcoming environment for all students.

Cultural competency asks one to work within different cultural contexts and change our practice to meet the needs of other cultural groups (CDC, 2021). This is essential as the work of cultural competency is action based—not just knowledge based. The *NASN School Nursing Practice Framework*™ (2024) puts the student in the center, surrounded by the key principles and components. Focusing on the student requires school nurses to provide care specific to the student's healthcare needs, including cultural needs. Student-focused care requires school nurses to educate themselves about cultures through various methods, including interaction with the student population and populations in the community. Engaging in school and community events will help the school nurse understand cultures within the school while demonstrating a commitment to improving cultural competency. Community involvement allows the school nurse to become a trusted and valuable community member.

Organizational cultural competence requires that organizations do the following:

- Have a defined set of values and principles, and demonstrate behaviors, attitudes, policies, and structures that enable them to work effectively cross-culturally
- Have the capacity to (1) value diversity, (2) conduct self-assessment, (3) manage the dynamics of difference, (4) acquire and institutionalize cultural knowledge, and (5) adapt to diversity and the cultural contexts of the communities they serve
- Incorporate the above in all aspects of policy making, administration, practice, and service delivery, and systematically involve consumers, key stakeholders, and communities (Cross et al., 1989)

Organizational cultural competence is a process that evolves over time. Both the organization and the employees contribute to the work through their awareness, knowledge, and skills. This process is represented on the cultural competence continuum. See Table 10-1. School nurses have a valuable role in developing the cultural competence of any organization. A school nurse can be a member of a committee or group that works to improve cultural competence. These committees and groups are important; however, cultural competence is not the responsibility of only the individuals working within an organization but also of the organization. By neglecting the organizational and systemic drivers of healthcare inequities, individual-level focused interventions toward cultural competency are limited in their ability to impact health inequities (Curtis et al., 2019). An organization needs to support cultural competence in all employees.

Cultural responsiveness is a term commonly used in education but can be used across all disciplines in health care. Cultural responsiveness occurs when differences are viewed as strengths and the environment is safe, just, and equitable for all members (Gatzunis et al., 2022). School nurses serving at the intersection of health and education should view the student's culture in a positive way and consider how that identity can positively influence a

Practice Connections

Cultural Competence: Different but Similar #1

Two school nurses, one in New York City, New York, and one in Jackson, Mississippi, assess their school population and discover that many Spanish-speaking students are struggling with their health maintenance of asthma.

The school nurses in both settings must understand that a commonality between these two student groups could be a language barrier. Another factor to consider is cultural practices, and even though these students live in two very different geographical locations, they may share cultural practices.

Practice Connections

Cultural Competence: Similar but Different #2

The school nurse is assessing her student population and discovers that there are different health practices among African American students. The students all identify as African American and live in the same town but have opposing views on the management of eczema. The families of one group strongly agree with the use of medication. In contrast, the other group strongly distrusts the medications and the healthcare system and chooses to use home remedies to manage their child's eczema.

This population is alike but also different in their views of the healthcare system and medication management of their children's eczema. This can be due to life experiences and family history strongly connected to cultural practices and beliefs.

The school nurse must respect differing strategies of eczema care across families. The nurse should utilize this as a time to build trust with the family that uses home remedies to discuss medication options that can still possibly include their home remedies.

person—leveraging cultural identity for better health and education outcomes.

The concept of ***cultural competence*** is the mainstream concept that has become the standard of culturally competent care. Cultural competence has come under scrutiny as having limitations to its meaning, as the term competence can lead one to believe there is an end, that is, after skills have been learned. The concept of ***cultural humility*** was developed when it became apparent that while cultural competence was needed, there needed to be more to the process to be effective. Cultural humility is a continuing process where there is no end to learning.

> *Cultural humility is a reflective process of understanding one's biases and privileges, managing power imbalances, and maintaining a stance that is open to others in relation to aspects of their cultural identity that are most important to them. Strategies for practicing cultural humility include:*
>
> - *Practicing self-reflection, including awareness of your beliefs, values, and implicit biases*
> - *Recognizing what you don't know and being open to learning as much as you can*
> - *Being open to other people's identities and empathizing with their life experiences; acknowledging that the patient is their own best authority, not you*
> - *Learning and growing from people whose beliefs, values, and worldviews differ from yours (OMH, 2021, para. 4)*

Cultural humility has an emphasis on social justice and has been described as "a lifelong process of learning, self-reflection, and self-critique" (Hussen et al., 2020, p. S536). Cultural competence and cultural humility are practiced in conjunction, not exclusively. Both concepts ask healthcare providers to reflect on their personal biases and seek an understanding of the cultural groups they work with. They also ask the provider to incorporate culture into the care that is provided to diverse populations (Greene-Moton & Minkler, 2019). Cultural competence and cultural humility have their place in culturally effective care. Both concepts should be used to become effective, culturally competent healthcare providers.

> ***Cultural safety*** *is a concept that includes cultural competence but builds upon it as a process. Cultural safety is about acknowledging the barriers to clinical effectiveness arising from the inherent power imbalance between provider and patient. This concept rejects the notion that health providers should focus on learning cultural customs of different ethnic groups. Instead, cultural safety seeks to achieve better care through being aware of difference, decolonizing, considering power relationships, implementing reflective practice, and by allowing the patient to determine whether a clinical encounter is safe. (Curtis et al., 2019, p. 13)*

Cultural safety identifies the differences between cultures and wants to include these differences in the healthcare continuum. Cultural safety offers a leveling of power between students and the school nurse by acknowledging the importance of the student's culture in all health decisions. Ensuring cultural safety is crucial for students to feel comfortable and safe at every interaction with the healthcare system.

Understanding and changing one's biases is work. Creating an environment of cultural safety requires cultural competency and cultural humility, both of which are ongoing processes. Despite the effort involved in these actions, the outcomes for students and families are significant. These actions put the school nurse in a position to be a trusted healthcare provider within the school community.

FAMILY CONCEPTS

Family Structure

Family is a social system of the relationships between two or more individuals (Health Resources & Services Administration, 2023). As society and cultures have changed, so have the definitions of family. Family is a concept, and a family is whoever the family says they are (Shajani & Snell, 2019). Family is defined differently by different contexts of the social sector, including individuals, families, schools, workplaces, communities, and government. The definition of family differs among disciplines in the social sciences (anthropology, counseling, economics, human development, nursing, psychology, public health, religion, and sociology; Kaakinen, 2018). Even within the nursing profession, educators, researchers, and clinicians may not always agree on the definition of family.

The structure of the 21st-century family occurs in many forms of relationships of the members to each other. Households are defined as inclusive of related family members and unrelated people sharing a housing unit; unrelated people could be lodgers, foster children, wards, or employees (U.S. Census Bureau, 2021c). Categorizing families as either traditional or nontraditional is not inclusive; it groups families into categories that defy the definition of family as being whoever they say they are (Shajani & Snell, 2019). Using the term "traditional family" reflects one's own culture and not necessarily the school community. This is a simple example of how the words we use when describing students can create division and discrimination.

Schoolchildren can live in family structures that involve either one or two parents; biological or nonbiological parents; married, unmarried, divorced, or remarried parents; and same- or opposite-sex parents (Payne, 2019). Families may also be headed by guardians when a parent is not primarily involved in raising the children, such as in foster families or when children are cared for by grandparents or other relatives/relations. Many students live in multigenerational family households.

Fifteen states recognize some form of common law marriage as a couple who live together and represents themselves to family, friends, and the community as being married, although they have not had a wedding or obtained a marriage license (Findlaw, 2020). Parents could be living together or apart for many reasons, such as an armed forces deployment, a job out of state, or due to incarceration. A one- or two-parent home does not always guarantee that the parents have the primary responsibility for raising the children, such as when children are mostly cared for by a friend or family member, a childcare provider, or they live at a boarding school. An individual can experience many variations in their family structure throughout their lifetime, and the structure of a family is not an indication of the well-being of the family.

Family Function

Family function is the process that sustains the family. The core functions of families include the exchange of love, affection, and companionship. Family function includes the provision of day-to-day nurturing and care, health care, guidance on commonly held social values, and economic security. Members of the family develop a common sense of identity and belonging. Similar family functions across diverse cultures may include the following:

- Support financially: providing basic needs, such as food, shelter, clothing.
- Support emotionally: providing love, comfort, intimacy, companionship, nurturing, belongingness.
- Socialize children: rearing children, parenting, helping children function to the best of their abilities within their society.
- Reproduce offspring through birth, adoption, fostering, kinship care.
- Provide identity: for example, social class, race, ethnicity, kinship, religion (Lang, 2020).

Multiple variables affect the success of family function. Most important is the provision of unconditional love and respect for the members of the family. Children need to know that someone cares for them and about them. All members of the family must respect each other, each other's belongings, and each other's ideas. The family is a social unit; therefore, communication is essential. Social supports and resilience for parents/guardians yield optimal family functioning and parental sense of child well-being (Gaspar et al., 2022).

It is a fundamental right and responsibility of parents/guardians to protect and raise their children. A minimum standard of that caring established by society is the basis for determining abuse and neglect. See Chapter 11 for information about maltreatment. Factors that affect the quality of family function include the following:

- The health of the child or parent/guardian and access to physical and mental health care
- The socioeconomic resources of the family to provide sufficient nutrition, appropriate clothing, shelter, and quality of life
- The connectedness of the family with others including school and peer groups, cultural groups, and religious groups
- The quality of parenting, including parental monitoring of children, role-modeling appropriate behaviors, setting boundaries, promoting education and life goals, and knowledge of developmental expectations
- The safety of the home, neighborhood, and school

Diversity exists in parenting styles and those styles are influenced by parents'/guardians' cultures. Examples of parenting styles include the following:

- Authoritarian: Parental tendencies: imposes strict rules, has high expectations, leans toward one-way conversations, gives limited nurturing.
- Authoritative: Parental tendencies: gives clear guidelines and supportive discipline; fosters communication and input from child; cultivates close, nurturing relationship; generally can lead to healthiest outcomes for child.
- Permissive: Parental tendencies: provides limited rules, encourages child to figure out things; has open communication; displays warmth and nurture.
- Uninvolved: Parental tendencies: cares for child's basic needs, has limited communication, stays out of the way, is detached, gives limited nurturing (Sanvictores & Mendez, 2022).

When considering parenting styles and the quality of parenting, school nurses must consider that there is minimal training on how to be a parent, and most people's parenting style reflects the parenting they received as a child. Parents/guardians may also affect different parenting styles on different children within the same family. School nurses can provide insight into parenting practice and guidance through a healthcare perspective.

Family Assessment

Family assessment begins during the family's first interactions with the school nurse and is an important component in the development of relevant student health plans. The school nurse develops student-centered health goals based on the needs identified from the family assessment. Student-centered health goals are prioritized with the family's input to ensure the provision of coordinated care of the student within the family, school, and community contexts.

It is important for school nurses to accurately assess family development, structure, and function. The functional assessment of the family examines how family members interact (Shajani & Snell, 2023). Several family assessment models have been developed for use in many different circumstances. While each has strengths and limitations, the *Calgary Family Assessment Model* (CFAM) is perhaps the most applicable for school nurse assessment of a student's family. The CFAM was developed from the integration of systems, cybernetics, communication, and change theories (Shajani & Snell, 2023).

The Calgary Family Assessment Model is consistent with family ecology theory and consists of three major assessment categories: structural, developmental, and functional. Each major category contains subcategories with family assessment questions. Not all categories or questions are applicable to all families at all times, but the CFAM provides guidance for school nursing interviews with parents/guardians or other family members. See

Table OM10-2. The results of the family assessment are used in developing student- and family-centered individualized healthcare plans aimed at reducing health barriers to learning. Careful assessment by the school nurse will reveal the level of a family's engagement in school health services. Barriers and facilitators to family engagement must be explored as family engagement is imperative in developing effective individualized healthcare plans for students, as well as in implementing and evaluating those plans. Family engagement and community partnerships are essential components of supporting the health of children across the home, school, and community contexts as outlined in the Whole School, Whole Community, Whole Child model (CDC, 2018).

In the community context, assessment of the family examines whether resources are culturally and socially essential, equitable, accessible, acceptable, and available to students and families served by the school nurse. The school nurse must be aware of how social determinants of health affect families, including the neighborhood and built environment, social and community contexts, and economic stability, as well as the education and healthcare systems. The school nurse is more equipped to provide holistic health promotion and disease prevention services by assessing students and families across contexts and understanding the interconnectedness between family and community systems.

HEALTH EQUITY

Health care should be a right for all persons. The World Health Organization, through the Declaration of Astana, strongly affirms its commitment to the fundamental right of every human being to the enjoyment of the highest attainable standard of health without distinction of any kind (World Health Organization, 2018, p. 19). Working toward equitable health care is at the foundation of school nursing practice. It is vital that school nurses play an active role in ensuring all populations receive equitable and equal health care. School nurses serve students from multiple populations; it is important that every effort be made to assess student needs in a manner that removes barriers and supports all students and families equitably.

Practice Connections

- The school nurse and school personnel should be mindful that every family may look different. When referencing the adult responsible for the student at home, phrase the inquiries so that it is inclusive of all family types by asking: "With whom do you live?" or when sending things home address letters to "The family of . . ."
- To ensure student safety, school nurses should carefully review the student information card to confirm who can and should be contacted or to whom the child can be released when the child is ill.

Health disparities are preventable differences in the burden of disease, injury, violence, or opportunities to achieve optimal health that are experienced by populations that have been disadvantaged by their social or economic status, geographical location, and environment (CDC, 2022c). Health disparities affect many populations and are not based on race alone. Therefore, recognizing populations affected by health disparities is vital to correcting these disparities and working toward the goal of health equity for all.

Health equity is the state in which everyone has a fair and just opportunity to attain their highest level of health (CDC, 2022c). Not having opportunity to attain the highest level of health results in ***health inequities.*** Health inequities create conditions that often lead to poor health outcomes, that is, health disparities. These conditions are conceptualized as the *social determinants of health* (see Chapter 2). School nurses must advocate for all students' access to equitable education and health care. Working toward the goal of health equity has far-reaching implications for the health outcomes of students and their communities. Achieving health equity requires valuing all people equally with focused and ongoing societal efforts to address avoidable inequalities, historical and contemporary injustices, and the elimination of health and healthcare disparities (CDC, 2022a).

To achieve health equity, multisectoral efforts are needed to address the severe and far-reaching disparities that plague our nation by expanding access and removing the social and economic obstacles that lead to poor health outcomes, including racial discrimination, within organizations—including schools. The Annie E. Casey Foundation (2014) has developed an action guide to help organizations address racial equity and inclusion, which can be downloaded for free from their Web site.

THEORIES GUIDING CULTURALLY EFFECTIVE CARE

Theories have long been used to guide the practice of nursing. Theories are frameworks supported by research, built upon, and updated as practice changes. For school nurses, knowing the theories that affect practice related to culturally competent care and care of the family is a necessity. While numerous theories relate to culturally competent care of students and families, three will be discussed in this chapter.

Did You Know?

Equality = Sameness
Inequality = Unequal
Equity = Fairness
Inequity = Unfair

Purnell Model for Cultural Competence

The *Purnell Model for Cultural Competence* (Purnell model) was created in 1998 and has been used for over 20 years throughout all levels of healthcare practice. School nurses can utilize this model to assess a student's motivation, experiences, and beliefs about health. The Purnell model has a methodology that requires interdepartmental collaboration to achieve cultural competence (Purnell, 2018). This model (Fig. 10-4) consists of four concentric layers; the layers should be interpreted from outer to inner and are then further broken down into 12 pie-shaped pieces representing each of the cultural characteristics and potential topics to cover when assessing these characteristics. The outer circle represents global society, the next layer represents the community, the next layer represents family, and the final layer is the person. The 12 domains include overview/heritage, communication, family roles and organization, workforce issues, biocultural ecology, high-risk behaviors, nutrition, pregnancy, death rituals, spirituality, healthcare practices, and healthcare practitioners. The sawtooth line beneath the circle represents the cultural

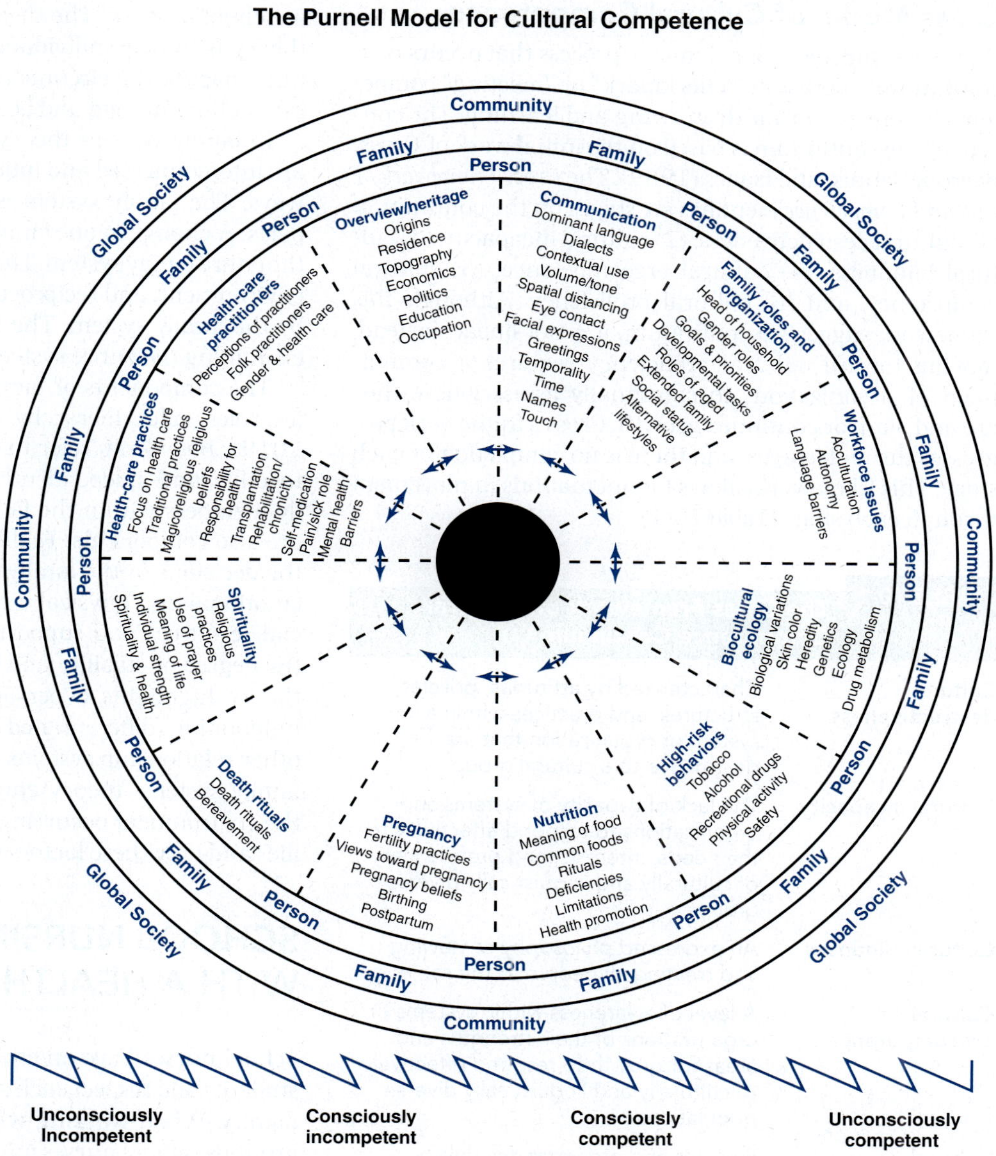

Variant cultural characteristics: age, generation, nationality, race, color, gender, religion, educational status, socioeconomic status, occupation, military status, political beliefs, urban versus rural residence, enclave identity, marital status, parental status, physical characteristics, sexual orientation, gender issues, health literacy, and reason for migration (sojourner, immigrant, asylee, undocumented status)

Unconsciously incompetent: not being aware that one is lacking knowledge about another culture
Consciously incompetent: being aware that one is lacking knowledge about another culture
Consciously competent: learning about the client's culture, verifying generalizations about the client's culture, and providing culturally specific interventions
Unconsciously competent: automatically providing culturally congruent care to clients of diverse cultures

FIGURE 10-4. Purnell Model for Cultural Competence. *(Purnell, 2018.)*

competence and consciousness of the healthcare provider. The blank space in the middle represents all that cannot be or is not known. The original model has been updated to include variant characteristics of culture. The characteristics aim to decrease stereotypes and biases that inhibit positive population health outcomes (Purnell, 2018). School nurses may benefit from using the Purnell Cultural Assessment Tool as they consider their cultural practices. The model can be used to generate culture-specific and culture-general information. See Online Materials OM10-1 for a link to Purnell's cultural awareness tool.

Cross Model of Cultural Competence

Cultural competency is a dynamic process that occurs on a continuum. There is no "checkmark" or "meeting" competency as one is constantly growing and learning. The concept of the continuum is based on the initial work of Cross, Bazron, Dennis, and Isaacs (1989). The *Cross Framework of Cultural Competence* identifies six stages on the continuum: (1) cultural destructiveness, (2) cultural incapacity, (3) cultural blindness, (4) cultural precompetence, (5) cultural competency, and (6) cultural proficiency. Although this framework suggests a continuum, it is not linear; instead, moving toward cultural proficiency requires a commitment of organizations to continually assess where they are and plan for continued growth. Cross's framework progresses through stages, and there is no completion of each stage. This framework allows for fluctuations in movement through each stage (Table 10-1).

TABLE 10-1 The Cross Framework of Cultural Competence Continuum

Cultural destructiveness	Characterized by attitudes, policies, structures, and practices within a system or organization that are destructive to a cultural group
Cultural incapacity	The lack of capacity of systems and organizations to respond effectively to the needs, interests, and preferences of culturally and linguistically diverse groups
Cultural blindness	An expressed philosophy of viewing and treating all people as the same
Cultural precompetence	A level of awareness within systems or organizations of their strengths and areas for growth to respond effectively to culturally and linguistically diverse populations
Cultural competency	Systems and organizations that exemplify cultural competence demonstrates an acceptance and respect for cultural differences
Cultural proficiency	Systems and organizations hold culture in high esteem and use this as a foundation to guide all their endeavors

Goode (2004), with permission.

Family Systems Theory

The family systems theory, developed by Dr. Murray Bowen, provides a framework for school nurses to understand interactions between students and their families. This theory serves as the basis for many other family theories and is used across social science professions. Family systems theory considers the family as a unit or system made up of interacting components that interact among themselves and between the system and the environment (Kaakinen, 2018). It seeks to describe the family response to stimuli from the environment, whether the stimuli are internal stressors or a stressor from an external environment, such as school or work. The therapeutic goal of family systems theory is to help individual members and the family as a unit adapt to the circumstances of life; the focus is on the interactions among and between members of the family.

In family systems theory, all parts of the family system are interconnected and influence each other in predictable ways. The family system is greater than the sum of the parts. A change in one family member in the system affects the entire family system. The family system is affected by the environment, and reciprocally, the environment is affected by the family system. The family can only be assessed by examining the entire system (Kaakinen, 2018).

The components of family system theory are boundaries, roles, rules, hierarchy, climate, and equilibrium (Kerr, 2019). *Boundaries* refer to what a family does and thinks together and independently. The *roles* of the various family members within the family and the rules or the home are also components. *Family hierarchy* denotes who makes the decisions in the family. The *family climate* refers to the emotional and physical environment; this includes financial resources and support systems. *Equilibrium* refers to the degree of stability and balance within the family. This theory highlights a person's emotional and intellectual functioning (differentiated self) in family relationships and other relationship systems (Kerr, 2019). Awareness of the family systems theory enables school nurses to consider the environment occurring within students and their families and how these factors interplay.

SCHOOL NURSING PRACTICE WITH A HEALTH EQUITY LENS

School nurses have an ethical responsibility to care for all students and respect each student's right to be treated with dignity. When working with students from diverse backgrounds, school nurses must always bear in mind that children of marginalized racial and ethnic backgrounds are at greater risk of health inequities and disparities because of discrimination. It is imperative that school nurses are aware of the health and social conditions that affect the diverse aggregates of students in their school communities and work in innovative ways to address disparities. It is known that innovation occurs when professions work at the intersection of multiple disciplines; nurses have functioned as "boundary spanners" in connecting with other professions, organizations, and sectors while coordinating care for individuals (Pittman, 2019).

By professional ethical standards, school nurses are not racist. Obviously, not having racist viewpoints is a good thing—but it is not enough to be "not racist." School nurses should take an active antiracist approach by achieving health equity for students and school communities. An *antiracist* is "a person who opposes and makes efforts to end policies, rules, behaviors, beliefs, etc. that result in a continued unfair advantage to some people and unfair or harmful treatment of others, based on race" (Cambridge Dictionary, 2024). There are immediate steps school nurses can take to reduce or eliminate bias and racism in their schools.

- Review school policies and practices to uncover and eliminate racism, for example:
  - Examine relationships between racial achievement gaps and racial discipline gaps and propose interventions (Pearman et al., 2019).
  - Address racism in bullying and violence policies.
- Advocate for system changes that celebrate diversity, equity, and inclusion:
  - Annually engage school staff in education on cultural diversity, discrimination, and racism.
  - Hire and retain staff with diverse backgrounds.
- Provide evidence-based curriculum that teaches students and families how to recognize implicit bias and address racism.
- Promote empathy by actively listening to lived experience of racism as told by students, families, colleagues, and community members.
- Improve student and teacher interactions to increase students' sense of belonging and connectedness.

As school nurses, it is essential to be aware of how systemic racism is affecting the student population. The work to address and change systemic racism starts with addressing how racism affects individuals. School nurses know that poverty and lack of access to quality health care have negative consequences on the health of student populations. School nurses have first-hand experience with these social inequalities that can be changed through advocacy and challenging those views that continue to reinforce systemic racism (NASN, 2022). School nurses can address systemic racism by identifying and advocating for changes to policies within the school system that uphold racist views.

School nurses advance student health equity as they advocate for policies and practices with school administrators and school-based specialized instructional support personnel, including school counselors, school psychologists, and school social workers. School nurses advance student health equity when connecting students and families to community-based physical and mental healthcare providers and to social agencies for social needs, as well as collaborating with local, regional, and state agencies to address social determinants of health. Access to school nursing services enables advancement of student health equity (National Academies of Sciences, Engineering, and Medicine, 2021).

Health disparities are associated with the social determinants of health factors such as income status, language differences, neighborhood safety, lack of health insurance, accessible transportation, healthy foods, and culturally similar healthcare providers (Schroeder et al., 2018). Students who might benefit most from school health services are students with chronic health conditions and students in communities attending underresourced schools without full-time access to a school nurse. School nurses are equipped to address social determinants of health, which can be complex and incremental and require persistence; this reality needs to be considered as school nurses advocate for workloads that may reduce student absenteeism, increase the time students spend in class, and improve rates of chronic disease education for students (Schroeder et al., 2023). Students benefit from the school nurse's clinical expertise and awareness of social and economic factors that affect student health and well-being (NASN, 2023). Considerations for school nurses in addressing social determinants of student heath include the following:

- Provide care in a culturally effective manner.
- Consider student English language proficiency and literacy.
- Connect students and families to resources.
- Consider family economic resource needs.
- Focus on root causes and policy change (Schroeder et al., 2018).

The COVID-19 pandemic revealed a myriad of health and social inequities. In January 2021, the CDC launched the 2021 *Adolescent Behaviors and Experiences Survey* (ABES), an online survey of U.S. students in grades 9 through 12; over 7,000 students in public and private schools responded to the survey from January to June (Mpofu et al., 2022). Almost 36% of students responded that they had been "treated badly or unfairly in school because of their race or ethnicity during their lifetime (i.e., perceived racism)." Data from the survey showed that among racial/ethnic groups there were higher percentages of perceived racism in students who were Asian (63.9%), black (55.2%), and multiracial (54.5%) compared with those who identified as white. Higher prevalence of perceived racism was reported among students with poor mental health (38.1%); those with difficulty concentrating, remembering, or making decisions (44.1%); and those that did not feel close to persons at their school (40.7%; Mpofu et al., 2022). Promoting healthy and safe school environments requires cultural awareness as well as antiracist and inclusive interventions. The school nurse should be mindful of students who are most at risk for being affected by racism.

Adolescents whose gender identity or expression is different from their sex assigned at birth as well as those who identify as lesbian, bisexual, gay, transgender, queer, plus (LGBTQ+) may experience health disparities related to the chronic stress of stigmatization (Mitchell et al., 2022). School nurses should cultivate healthy and supportive school environments to enable health and well-being for students in these groups. School connectedness has been shown to improve students' perception that peers and school staff care about them, promote healthy behaviors, and increase academic success (McCabe et al., 2022).

Culturally Effective Individualized Healthcare Plans

Individualized healthcare plans (IHPs) are written by the school nurse for the school nurse for students with special healthcare needs (see Chapter 8). However, these plans involve input from the student and family. School nurses should assess any culturally related healthcare practices used by the family and integrate those practices, as appropriate to the school setting, into the IHP. This also includes the type of healthcare provider the family uses and whether traditional healers, such as curanderos or medicine men, are used. Box 10-3 provides guidance for the types of questions that might be asked to elicit information about specific healthcare practices.

After developing an IHP the school nurse should review the document to be sure each of the following questions have been answered:

- What are the dominant cultural beliefs of the child and family? Have these beliefs been accounted for in the care plan?
- Does a copy of the interventions included on the IHP need to be in another language so that the parent/guardian sees what is agreed to?
- Are there culturally responsive healthcare providers in the community who would best fit the needs of the family?
- What is the role of traditional health healers in the care of the child? What traditional remedies are being used and how might this affect treatment?
- How will cultural beliefs affect ability or willingness to follow treatment plans?

When revising care plans, evaluate the impact culture may have on the child's health.

Cultural Competency Professional Development

There are compelling reasons to learn about culturally congruent care. Across cultures and within specific cultures, school nurses will learn how families approach health and education. Cultural competence has been linked with improved satisfaction with care and leads to improved health outcomes (Henderson et al., 2018). Unethical nursing care that results in biased care may inadvertently result from lack of accommodation for unique beliefs, values, and traditions of students and families, resulting in poor communication, nonadherence to instruction, and negative outcomes. This lack of attention to individual needs will lead students and their families to look for services elsewhere, or even worse, ignore available critical services, resulting in increased healthcare costs and worsening health.

School nurses should use caution when using cultural competency training lists that describe cultural traits or cultural health practices of broad ethnic and racial groups. Using a generalized approach or lists of cultural health practices can oversimplify cultural differences and reinforce stereotypes. The complexities of social determinants of health, culture, and family may hinder access to appropriate care with misapplication of stereotypical views. For example, immigrants from Central America may be classified as Hispanic, but they may identify as black or white, may speak Spanish or an indigenous dialect, and may prefer Western allopathic methods rather than traditional homeopathic folk medicine. Assumptions should not be made based on the label a person has related to race, ethnicity, or identity.

A thorough community assessment by the school nurse will reveal what cultural groups make up the school community (see Chapter 2). Additional evidence-based practice resources and culturally relevant information should then be sought from reputable sources to inform contexts of care that can be used as a *starting* point for care. School nurses will want to intentionally interview the families of children with health concerns to assess their specific cultural health beliefs, values, preferences, and practices.

With those concepts in mind, it is helpful to consider how religion, culture, and ethnic customs affect communication and health-seeking behaviors of the students and families in the school community. The *Health Literacy Universal Precautions Toolkit* aims to equip primary care practices to prioritize health literacy by providing guidance on simplifying health communications to increase understanding of health information (Agency for Healthcare Research and Quality, 2020). See Online Materials OM10-1 for a link to the toolkit.

A study of urban and nonurban school nurses in one state revealed differences in professional development on topics relevant to cultural effectiveness over a 3-year period. Results found that nonurban nurses were less likely to have completed continuing education training on topics including reproductive health, diabetes, oral health, sexual identity, suicide prevention (including assessment and screening), and human trafficking. School nurses in nonurban schools were also less likely to have had continuing education training on cultural competency, medical cannabis, and special education laws (Ramos et al., 2022). School nurses should advocate for professional development sessions that are relevant to the populations served at the school with the understanding that professional development on cultural topics allows the school nurse to grow and develop culturally effective school nurse practices.

BOX 10-3

Accounting for Culture When Writing Individualized Healthcare Plans

Several considerations should be assessed before developing a student's care plan. These include the level of acculturation of the child and the child's family to the dominant culture. A school nurse should also assess the cultural beliefs of a child and the child's family. Once this information is gathered, the care plan should be reviewed to see if modifications are needed to ensure the care plan is written in a culturally competent manner.

LANGUAGE AND COMMUNICATION

1. In general, what language(s) does the child (and family) read and speak?
2. What was the language(s) used by parents as a child?
3. What language(s) is usually spoken at home?
4. In which language(s) does the child (and parents) usually think?
5. What language(s) does the child usually speak with friends?
6. In what language(s) are the TV programs they usually watch? Movies?
7. In what language(s) are the radio programs usually listened to?
8. Does the child or family have a cellphone? If so, in what language(s) are text messages?
9. Does the child or family use the Internet? If so, in what language(s)?
10. Do the parents, legal guardian, or emergency contact speak a language other than English? Will they understand English, or will you need a translator? Make note of this information in the care plan. If a translator is needed, a quick reference list of possible translators could be included with the care plan for easy access. Who is the decision maker for the family? This may need to be noted as well, if culturally significant.
11. Does the goal or outcome of the care plan acknowledge any cultural beliefs? For example, obesity among some families is more accepted. Is the weight goal realistic for this population?
12. Each intervention should be reviewed to see if modifications are needed to respect cultural practices or beliefs.
    a. Are certain foods forbidden to eat? [Every preparation done ahead of time to ensure cultural compliance should be done.] *Questions you may ask could include:*
       - *Are there foods you do not eat or are not allowed to eat?*
       - *When your child's blood sugar is low, what foods do you usually give him/her/them?*
       - *At school we like to have an emergency food kit and teach key people what to do. You are welcome to supply food for these kits (depends on district/school). Could we also give these foods, if needed? (In this way you also learn about food familiar to the child, etc.)*

    b. When conducting health education, *be sure to use foods familiar to the students*. For example, when teaching a child with diabetes whose family relies heavily on beans and tortillas about carbohydrate counting, be sure to include foods they eat. Using only examples from the American diet may give the impression that other foods (those more often eaten by the child) do not need to be counted or should be eliminated from the diet.
       - Be sure to review these cultural adaptations with teachers and others.

    c. You may also want to include cultural information regarding eye contact or silence, which may be interpreted incorrectly. For example, some cultures believe it is a sign of respect to remain silent or they may appear to indicate they understand or agree, even if they do not. This could be detrimental in health-related situations.
    d. How does the parent treat fever or respiratory congestion at home?
    e. *What other treatments do you do to help with the condition? (Probe for use of herbs or alternative therapies that may be used.)*
    f. Are there cultural traditions or holidays that may have an impact on a child's health? For example, Ramadan is a month-long fast during daylight hours. The fasting includes refraining from food, liquids, and medications. Children usually do not participate in Ramadan, but adolescent youth may. School nurses should work with families and their care providers to determine how to best comply with such special occasions. *Ask the parent how they wish you to handle situations such as a child who is fasting for religious reasons and comes to the nurse with a headache because the child may not have food until sunset.*

Reflective Practice

A reflective practice approach of professional development can be used to improve the practice of culturally congruent care. This practice is gradually taking the place of the traditional "laundry list" approach of using lectures and handouts about traditional health practices of specific racial or ethnic groups. Reflective practice is the cornerstone of continuous improvement in healthcare practice and is increasingly taught and practiced at prelicensure and graduate levels and in continuing education (Ng et al., 2019).

Reflective practice is an active learning approach based on critical reflection of one's experiences and practices as well as one's personal beliefs and attitudes and how these integrate into professional practice (Hill & Omowale, 2023). Reflective practice asks the nurse to look at a situation with awareness of personal beliefs and values. This awareness allows the school nurse to understand that their personal beliefs and values affect their assessment of a situation. Table 10-2 gives an overview of the stages of reflecting. School nurses have found that the *Think Cultural Health* training provided by the Office of Minority Health provides a strong preparation for facilitation of reflective practice (OMH, n.d.b). Critical reflection includes school nurses' openness to make incremental improvements in their practice settings, which can include challenging the assumptions and harmful interactions in their practices (Ng et al., 2019).

Communication and Health Literacy

Nursing assessment and health promotion are based on two-way communication with the student and parents/guardians. School nurses must familiarize themselves with cultural manners of communication among diverse school groups, including customary differences in nonverbal communication such as eye contact, head nodding (which may be done as a sign of respect and not an indication of understanding of the information), handshakes, personal space, or touching (OMH, n.d.c). Some cultures have a more direct verbal and physical communication style; some feel it is disrespectful to question the suggestions of those in authority.

Communicating with families and students in their primary language is integral to culturally congruent school nursing practice. The availability of a professional interpreter and translation services varies greatly between school districts. School districts need to provide professional interpreter services to eliminate disparities and improve health and academic outcomes for students who are English language learners. It is not appropriate to ask students or family members to interpret for official school communications. Box 10-4 lists tips on how to select and use interpretation services effectively. School staff who can speak a little but are not fluent in a second language may misinterpret and miscommunicate, causing more harm than good, thus should not be used as interpreters. The *National Standards for Culturally and Linguistically Appropriate Services* should serve as a guidepost for communicating with families whose native language is not English (OMH, 2023). Documents should be translated into the primary language at a common reading and health literacy level, which is generally understood to be no higher than 5th grade.

Promoting Family Partnerships and Engagement

School and family partnerships are essential for positive health and education outcomes for students and school communities. The *Whole School, Whole Child, Whole*

TABLE 10-2 Stages of Reflecting

Stage	Action Steps for the School Nurse
What happened?	Think about the situation in detail. Consider the part you played and the result.
How did the situation make you feel?	What feelings were you experiencing during the situation? Were your feelings positive, neutral, or negative?
Why did this situation happen?	What led to this situation happening? Did the situation go well or are there things that should have gone differently?
What could you have done differently?	What did you do well in the situation? Is there anything you could have done differently?
How will this change your practice?	How does the experience you had in this situation affect your future practice? Can this situation be applied to future situations?
Did you change?	As new situations come up, have your practices changed? What worked? What did not work? This stage is a time to refine your practice.

Adapted from Koshy et al. (2017).

BOX 10-4
Tips for Working Effectively With an Interpreter

- Choose an interpreter whose age, gender, and background make it easiest to work with the student and parent. Make sure the interpreter has training in interpretation services.
- Treat the interpreter as a respected healthcare professional.
- Introduce the interpreter to the student and family and get the parent's permission to use an interpreter.
- Position the interpreter behind the student and parent or behind you, not between you and them, so that your attention is focused on the student and parent.
- Speak and look directly at the student and parent, not the interpreter.
- Use first-person language and expect the interpreter to do the same: "Mrs. Smith, I want you to think about when the headaches started."
- Do not speak too long without letting the interpreter interpret.
- Observe the student and parent's nonverbal communication.
- Use simple language that avoids medical jargon.
- Learn basic words from the target languages that you will use often. Asking interpreters about words or comments that have been interpreted prompts attention to detail.
- Come back to an issue if you suspect misunderstanding on the part of yourself or the student and parent.
- If you come across a cultural belief or behavior that is unfamiliar to you, take time later to ask the interpreter about it.

Adapted from Think Cultural Health (n.d.).

Community Framework and *School Nursing Practice Framework*™ recognize that the student and the student's family are the center of a coordinated approach to supporting student success (CDC, 2018; NASN, 2024). It is the school nurse's role to provide school health services and to connect families to healthcare resources, healthcare coverage, and primary care through a medical home. To promote family engagement, the school nurse should focus on student and family strengths using therapeutic communication to establish caring relationships with families.

Parent engagement in schools is defined as parents/guardians and school staff working together to support and improve the learning, development, and health of students (CDC, 2019b). Parent engagement in schools is a shared responsibility in which schools and other community agencies and organizations are committed to reaching out to engage parents/guardians in meaningful ways, and parents/guardians are committed to actively supporting their children's learning and development. This relationship between schools and parents/guardians cuts across and reinforces children's health and learning in multiple settings—at home, in school, in out-of-school programs, and in the community.

It is important to remember that parents/guardians are the primary educators of their children. Students are less likely to engage in poor health habits and more likely to do well in school when they feel supported by their families and parents/guardians (CDC, 2019a). School strategies to engage parents/guardians in school health include having school-wide policies and programs that connect with families in meaningful ways. Schools can collaborate with community organizations to provide parent education classes on healthy child development and parenting strategies. The school nurse can plan school health activities that address the interests or concerns of parents/guardians, such as healthy eating or student health-related risk behaviors. The school health office can serve as a family health resource center with information from local health departments, providers, and healthcare systems.

Some parents/guardians may need special attention as schools seek to engage with them. Special consideration should be given to immigrant and refugee families who have unique educational and social needs. The Institute of Education Sciences of the U.S. Department of Education has developed toolkits to best support educators in welcoming students who are refugees and immigrants (Greenberg Motamedi et al., 2021). One example is *Welcoming, Registering, and Supporting Newcomer Students: A Toolkit for Educators of Immigrant and Refugee Students in Secondary School*, which includes information about collecting health records and conducting physical and mental health assessments upon enrollment.

The school nurse can reach out to families at community events or places of worship with health screenings or workshops. Health programs and activities should be planned with the schedules of busy families and working parents/guardians in mind. Health information must be presented to families in lay terms, at a common health literacy level, and in culturally congruent ways that respect the community being served. When parents/guardians cannot attend school events, alternative ways to communicate important health information should be provided. Examples may include group e-mails and texts as well as recorded phone messages in the parents'/guardians' native language as well as traditional paper messages sent home with the student. Many school nurses have found that a school health–specific Web site is an excellent way to provide families with school health information and expectations (Moss, 2021).

Did You Know?

Engaging parents/guardians in their children's school life is a promising protective factor. Research shows that parent engagement in schools is linked to better student behavior, higher academic achievement, and enhanced social skills. Parent engagement also makes it more likely that children and adolescents will avoid unhealthy behaviors, such as sexual risk behaviors and tobacco, alcohol, and other drug use (CDC, 2019b).

CONCLUSION

Culturally effective school nursing practice means a lifelong commitment to self-evaluation and self-critique to redress power imbalances and to develop and maintain mutually respectful and dynamic relationships with diverse school communities. Culturally meaningful nursing care requires unconventional upstream behaviors and proactive thinking. School nurses who practice culturally congruent care do the following:

- Identify culturally charged institutional barriers at school that prevent student success.
- Consider school and community cultural factors utilizing the social determinants of health model to assess for causes leading to potential or actual student failure.
- Use school district databases to address health disparities by identifying, analyzing, and correcting institutional and systematic ineffectiveness.
- Identify and address cultural, linguistic, and literacy communication gaps among students, families, faculty, and staff.
- Identify available, appropriate, cost-effective, and affordable community resources.
- Provide a warm hand-off when providing referrals and resources.
- Advocate for school and district-wide cultural competency training.
- Advocate for recruitment, hiring, and retention of a diverse school nurse workforce.

- Participate in training modules and webinars in alignment with NASN and the Office of Minority Health principles.
- Collaborate with educational leaders and policy makers to recognize and improve culturally safe institutional and systems improvements.

Ideally, the school environment is organized to promote academic achievement, a safe and caring climate, and positive self-esteem for students. As health experts and leaders on interprofessional educational teams, school nurses are in ideal positions to assess the cultural beliefs and practices of students and staff and to incorporate these into any health encounters. School nurses advocate for population-focused services for underresourced communities and groups. Although it is important to consider culture, it is also important to avoid stereotyping and consider other factors that may affect care. Working in a culturally effective manner is a process, not a static state. The process begins with a self-assessment and continues with limitless possibilities that will benefit the students and families and improve the culture of the school as a community.

The Editors gratefully acknowledge the work of the previous chapter authors Amy Cory, Robin Adair Shannon, Maria Matza, and Jessica Porter.

References

Agency for Healthcare Research and Quality. (2020). *AHRQ health literacy universal precautions toolkit.* https://www.ahrq.gov/health-literacy/improve/precautions/index.html

American Public Health Association. (n.d.). *Racism and health.* https://www.apha.org/topics-and-issues/health-equity/racism-and-health

Annie E. Casey Foundation. (2014). *Race equity and inclusion action guide.* https://cyfar.org/resource/race-equity-and-inclusion-action-guide-7-steps-advance-and-embed-race-equity-and-inclusion

Bell, K. (Ed.) (2013). Prejudice. *Open Education Sociology Dictionary.* https://sociologydictionary.org/prejudice/

Bizumic, B., Monaghan, C., & Priest, D. (2020). The return of ethnocentrism. *Political Psychology, 42*(S1), 29–73. https://doi.org/10.1111/pops.12710

Braveman, P. A., Arkin, E., Proctor, D., Kauh, T., & Holm, N. (2022). Systemic and structural racism: Definitions, examples, health damages, and approaches to dismantling. *Health Affairs, 41*(2), 171–178. https://doi.org/10.1377/hlthaff.2021.01394

Cambridge Dictionary. (2024). *Anti-racist.* https://dictionary.cambridge.org/us/dictionary/english/antiracist

Center for Intersectional Justice. (n.d.). What is intersectionality? *Center for Intersectional Justice.* https://www.intersectionaljustice.org/what-is-intersectionality

Center for Substance Abuse Treatment. (2014). Improving cultural competence: Treatment Improvement Protocol (TIP) series, no. 59. *Substance Abuse and Mental Health Services Administration.* https://www.ncbi.nlm.nih.gov/books/NBK248428/

Centers for Disease Control and Prevention. (2018). *Whole school, whole community, whole child (WSCC) model.* https://www.cdc.gov/healthyyouth/wscc/model.htm

Centers for Disease Control and Prevention. (2019a). *Parent engagement: Strategies for involving parents in school health.* https://www.cdc.gov/healthyyouth/protective/factsheets/parentengagement_overview.htm

Centers for Disease Control and Prevention. (2019b). *Promoting parent engagement: Improving student health and academic achievement.* https://www.cdc.gov/healthyyouth/protective/factsheets/parentengagement_parents.htm

Centers for Disease Control and Prevention. (2021). *Cultural competence in health and human services.* https://npin.cdc.gov/pages/cultural-competence#what

Centers for Disease Control and Prevention. (2022a). CDC core health equity science and intervention strategy. https://www.cdc.gov/healthequity/core/index.html

Centers for Disease Control and Prevention. (2022b). Culture and health literacy. https://www.cdc.gov/healthliteracy/culture.html

Centers for Disease Control and Prevention. (2022c). What is health equity? https://www.cdc.gov/healthequity/whatis/index.html

Civil Rights Act of 1964, 42 U.S.C. § 2000e et seq (1964).

Coleman-Jensen, A., Rabbitt, M. P., Gregory, C. A., & Singh, A. (2022). Household food security in the United States in 2021, ERR-309. *U.S. Department of Agriculture, Economic Research Service.* https://www.ers.usda.gov/webdocs/publications/104656/err-309.pdf?v=5701.7

Cross, T., Bazron, B., Dennis, K., & Isaacs, M. (1989). Towards a culturally competent system of care, volume 1. *CASSP Technical Assistance Center, Center for Child Health and Mental Health Policy, Georgetown University Child Development Center.* https://files.eric.ed.gov/fulltext/ED330171.pdf

Curtis, E., Jones, R., Tipene-Leach, D., Walker, C., Loring, B., Paine, S., & Reid, P. (2019). Why cultural safety rather than cultural competency is required to achieve health equity: A literature review and recommended definition. *International Journal for Equity in Health, 18*(1), 1–17. https://doi.org/10.1186/s12939-019-1082-3

Eagly, A. H., & Koenig, A. M. (2021). The vicious cycle linking stereotypes and social roles. *Current Directions in Psychological Science, 30*(4), 343–350. https://doi.org/10.1177/09637214211013775

Every Student Succeeds Act, 20 U.S.C. § 6301 (2015). https://congress.gov/114/plaws/publ95/PLAW-114publ95.pdf

Findlaw. (2020). *Common law marriage: The basics.* https://www.findlaw.com/family/marriage/common-law-marriage.html

Gaspar, T., Gomez-Baya, D., Trindade, J. S., Botelho Guedes, F., Cerqueira, A., & de Matos, M. G. (2022). Relationship between family functioning, parents' psychosocial factors, and children's well-being. *Journal of Family Issues, 43*(9), 2380–2397. https://doi.org/10.1177/0192513X211030722

Gatzunis, K. S., Edwards, K. Y., Rodriguez Diaz, A., Conners, B. M., & Weiss, M. J. (2022). Cultural responsiveness framework in BCBA(r) supervision. *Behavior Analysis in Practice, 15*(4), 1373–1382. https://doi.org/10.1007/s40617-022-00688-7

Goode, T. D. (2004). Cultural competence continuum. *National Center for Cultural Competence. Georgetown University Center for Child and Human Development.* https://nccc.georgetown.edu/curricula/documents/TheContinuumRevised.doc#:~:text=Systems%20and%20organizations%20that%20exemplify,all%20aspects%20of%20the%20organization

Gratz, T., Goldhaber, D., Willgerodt, M., & Brown, N. (2023). The frontline health care workers in schools: Health equity, the distribution of school nurses, and student access. *The Journal of School Nursing, 39(5)*, 357-367. https://doi.org/10.1177/10598405211024277

Greenberg Motamedi, J., Porter, L., Taylor, S., Leong, M., Martinez-Wenzl, M., & Serrano, D. (2021). Welcoming, registering, and supporting newcomer students: A toolkit for educators of immigrant and refugee students in secondary schools (REL 2021–064). *U.S. Department of Education, Institute of Education Sciences, National Center for Education Evaluation and Regional Assistance, Regional Educational Laboratory Northwest.* https://ies.ed.gov/ncee/edlabs/regions/northwest/pdf/REL_2021064.pdf

Greene-Moton, E., & Minkler, M. (2019). Cultural competence or cultural humility? Moving beyond the debate. *Health Promotion Practice, 21*(1), 1–4. https://doi.org/10.1177/1524839919884912

Greenwald, A. G., McGhee, D. E., & Schwartz, J. L. K. (1998). Measuring individual differences in implicit cognition: The implicit association test. *Journal of Personality and Social Psychology, 74*(6), 1464–1480. https://doi.org/10.1037/0022-3514.74.6.1464

Health Resources & Services Administration. (2023). *Definition of family.* https://www.hrsa.gov/get-health-care/affordable/hill-burton/family#:~:text=Family%3A%20A%20family%20is%20a,as%20members%20of%20one%20family

Henderson, S., Horne, M., Hills, R., & Kendall, E. (2018). Cultural competence in healthcare in the community: A concept analysis. *Health & Social Care in the Community, 26*(4), 590–603. https://doi.org/10.1111/hsc.12556

Hill, M., & Omowale, J. (2023). The value of critical self-reflection in the development of cultural competency. *Teaching and Learning Excellence Through Scholarship, 3*(1). https://doi.org/10.52938/tales.v3i1.2893

Hussen, S. A., Kuppalli, K., Castillo-Mancilla, J., Bedimo, R., Fadul, N., & Ofotokun, I. (2020). Cultural competence and humility in infectious diseases clinical practice and research. *The Journal of Infectious Diseases, 222*(Suppl 6), S535–S542. https://doi.org/10.1093/infdis/jiaa227

Kaakinen, J. (2018). Theoretical foundations for the nursing of families. In J. R. Kaakinen, D. P. Coelho, R. Steele, M. Robinson (Eds.), *Family health care nursing: Theory, practice and research* (pp. 27–51). F.A. Davis.

Kerr, M. E. (2019). *Bowen's theory's secrets: Revealing the hidden life of families.* W.W. Norton & Company.

Koshy, K., Limb, C., Gundogan, B., Whitehurst, K., & Jafree, D. J. (2017). Reflective practice in health care and how to reflect effectively. *International Journal of Surgery Oncology, 2*(6), e20. https://doi.org/10.1097/IJ9.0000000000000020

Lang, D. (2020). *Parenting and family diversity issues.* Iowa State University Digital Press. https://doi.org/10.31274/isudp.8

Marks, R., Jones, N., & Battle, K. (2024, April). What updates to OMB's race/ethnicity standards mean for the Census Bureau. *Within Census Blogs.* https://www.census.gov/newsroom/blogs/random-samplings/2024/04/updates-race-ethnicity-standards.html

McCabe, E. M., Davis, C., Mandy, L., & Wong, C. (2022). The role of school connectedness in supporting the health and well-being of youth: Recommendations for school nurses. *NASN School Nurse, 37*(1), 42–47. https/doi:10.1177/1942602X211048481

McRae, J., & Onukwugha, E. (2021). Why the gap in evaluating the social constructs and the value of medicines? *PharmacoEconomics, 39*(12), 1365–1372. https://doi.org/10.1007/s40273-021-01075-w

Mitchell, K. J., Ybarra, M. L., Banyard, V., Goodman, K. L., & Jones, L. M. (2022). Impact of the COVID-19 pandemic on perceptions of health and well-being among sexual and gender minority adolescents and emerging adults. *LGBT Health, 34,* 42. https://doi.org/10.1089/lgbt.2021.0238

Moss, E. (2021). Enhancing your virtual footprint: The school nurse's professional health office website. *NASN School Nurse, 36*(1), 52–57.

Mpofu, J. J., Cooper, A. C., Ashley, C., Geda, S., Harding, R. L., Johns, M. M., Spinks-Franklin, A., Njai, R., Moyse, D., & Underwood, J. M. (2022). Perceived racism and demographic, mental health, and behavioral characteristics among high school students during the COVID-19 pandemic—Adolescent Behaviors and Experiences Survey, United States, January–June 2021. *MMWR Suppl 2022, 71*(Suppl 3), 22–27. https://dx.doi.org/10.15585/mmwr.su7103a4

Nair, L., & Adetayo, O. A. (2019). Cultural competence and ethnic diversity in healthcare. *Plastic and Reconstructive Surgery—Global Open, 7*(5), e2219. https://doi.org/10.1097/gox.0000000000002219

National Academies of Sciences, Engineering, and Medicine. (2021). *The future of nursing 2020–2030: Charting a path to achieve health equity.* The National Academies Press.

National Association of School Nurses. (2021). *Education, licensure, and certification of school nurses [Position Statement].* Author.

National Association of School Nurses. (2022). *School nursing: Scope and standards of practice* (4th ed.). Author.

National Association of School Nurses. (2023). *Safe, supportive, equitable schools* (Position Statement). Author.

National Association of School Nurses. (2024). A contemporary framework update for today's school nursing landscape: Introducing the School Nursing Practice Framework. *NASN School Nurse, 39*(3), 140–147. https://www.doi.org/10.1177/1942602X241241092

National Center for Cultural Competence at Georgetown University. (n.d.). Conscious & unconscious bias in health care. *Georgetown University Center for Child and Human Development.* https://nccc.georgetown.edu/bias/module-2/2.php

National Center for Education Statistics. (2022). Private school enrollment. Condition of education. *U.S. Department of Education, Institute of Education Sciences.* https://nces.ed.gov/programs/coe/indicator/cgc

National Center for Education Statistics. (2023a). English learners in public schools. Condition of education. *U.S. Department of Education, Institute of Education Sciences.* https://nces.ed.gov/programs/coe/indicator/cgf

National Center for Education Statistics. (2023b). Public school enrollment. Condition of education. *U.S. Department of Education, Institute of Education Sciences.* https://nces.ed.gov/programs/coe/indicator/cga

National Center for Education Statistics. (2023c). Racial/ethnic enrollment in public schools. Condition of education. *U.S. Department of Education, Institute of Education Sciences.* https://nces.ed.gov/programs/coe/indicator/cge

National Education Association Center for Social Justice. (2021). *Toolkit: Implicit bias, microaggressions, and stereotypes resources.* https://www.nea.org/resource-library/implicit-bias-microaggressions-and-stereotypes-resources

National Human Genome Research Institute. (2019, March 13). Human genomic variation. *National Institute of Health, U. S. Department of Health and Human Services.* https://www.genome.gov/dna-day/15-ways/human-genomic-variation

National Human Genome Research Institute. (2022, August 18). Race. *National Institute of Health, U. S. Department of Health and Human Services.* https://www.genome.gov/genetics-glossary/Race

National Institutes of Health. (2021, July 7). *Cultural respect.* https://www.nih.gov/institutes-nih/nih-office-director/office-communications-public-liaison/clear-communication/cultural-respect

Ng, S. L., Wright, S. R., & Kuper, A. (2019). The divergence and convergence of critical reflection and critical reflexivity: Implications for health professions education. *Academic Medicine, 94*(8), 1122–1128. https://doi.org/10.1097/ACM.0000000000002724

Office of Minority Health. (n.d.b). *Think cultural health.* U.S. Department of Health and Human Services. https://thinkculturalhealth.hhs.gov/

Office of Minority Health. (n.d.c). Part 1: Cross-cultural communication skills. Think cultural health: Guide to providing effective communication and language assistance services. *U.S. Department of Health and Human Services.* https://hclsig.thinkculturalhealth.hhs.gov/ProviderContent/Section3/Part1/Section3-1-1.asp?

Office of Minority Health. (2021). CLAS, cultural competency, and cultural humility. Think cultural health. *U.S. Department of Health and Human Services.* https://minorityhealth.hhs.gov/omh/browse.aspx?lvl=2&lvlid=53

Office of Minority Health. (2023). National standards for culturally and linguistically appropriate services in health and health care (CLAS). *U.S. Department of Health and Human Services.* https://thinkculturalhealth.hhs.gov/assets/pdfs/EnhancedNationalCLASStandards.pdf

Payne, K. K. (2019). Children's family structure, 2019. Family Profiles, FP-19-25. National Center for Family & Marriage Research. https://doi.org/10.25035/ncfmr/fp-19-25

Payne, K., Niemi, L., & Doris, J. M. (2018). How to think about "implicit bias." *Scientific American.* https://www.scientificamerican.com/article/how-to-think-about-implicit-bias/

Pearman, F. A., Curran, C.F., Fisher, B., & Gardella, J. (2019). Are achievement gaps related to discipline gaps? Evidence from national data. *AERA Open.* https://doi.org/10.1177/2332858419875440

Pittman, P. (2019). Activating nursing to address unmet needs in the 21st century. *Robert Wood Johnson Foundation.* www.rwjf.org/content/dam/farm/reports/reports/2019/rwjf452706

Purnell, L. (2018). Update: The Purnell theory and model for culturally competent health care. *Journal of Transcultural Nursing, 30*(2), 98–105. https://doi.org/10.1177/1043659618817587

Ramos, M. M., Sebastian, R., Shattuck, D., Acosta, S., & Zamarin, K. (2022). School nursing workforce differences between urban and non-urban areas: Implications for school health services and equity. *The Journal of School Nursing*. Advance online publication. https://doi:10.1177/10598405221119516

Rose, P. R. (2020). *Health disparities, diversity, and inclusion: context, controversies, and solutions* (2nd ed.). Jones & Bartlett Learning.

Sabin, J. A. (2022). Tackling implicit bias in health care. *New England Journal of Medicine, 387*(2), 105–107. https://doi.org/10.1056/nejmp2201180

Sanvictores, T., & Mendez, M. D. (2022). Types of parenting styles and effects on children. In StatPearls. StatPearls Publishing.

Schroeder, K., Malone, S. K., McCabe, E., & Lipman, T. (2018). Addressing the social determinants of health: A call to action for school nurses. *Journal of School Nursing 34*(3), 182–191. https://doi 10.1177/1059840517750733

Schroeder, K., Young, A., Adman, G., Ashmeade, A. M., Bonas, E., Day, S. E., & Konty, K. (2023). The association of school nurse workload with student health and academic outcomes: A cross-sectional study. *The Journal of School Nursing, 39*(4), 305-312. https://doi:10.1177/10598405211012957

Shajani, Z., & Snell, D. (2019). *Wright & Leahey's nurses and families: A guide to family assessment and intervention* (7th ed.). F.A. Davis.

Shajani, Z., & Snell, D. (2023). *Wright & Leahey's nurses and families: A guide to family assessment and intervention* (8th ed.). F.A. Davis.

Shores, K., Kim, H. E., & Still, M. (2020). Categorical inequality in Black and White: Linking disproportionality across multiple educational outcomes. *American Educational Research Journal, 57*(5), 2089–2131. https://doi.org/10.3102/0002831219900128

Shrider, E. A., & Creamer, J. (2023, Sept). Poverty in the United States: 2022. Report no. P60-280. *U.S. Census Bureau*. https://www.census.gov/library/publications/2023/demo/p60-280.html

Smiley, R. A., Ruttinger, C., Oliveira, C. M., Hudson, L. R., Allgeyer, R., Reneau, K. A., Silvestre, J. H., & Alexander, M. (2021). The 2020 national nursing workforce survey. *Journal of Nursing Regulation, 12*(1), S1–S96.

Think Cultural Health. (n.d.). *Working effectively with an interpreter.* https://thinkculturalhealth.hhs.gov/assets/pdfs/resource-library/working-effectively-with-interpreter.pdf

Ulmer, C., McFadden, B., & Nerenz, D. R. (2009). Defining categorization needs for race and ethnicity data. *Race, ethnicity, and language.* Institute of Medicine (US) Subcommittee on Standardized Collection of Race/Ethnicity and Language Data for Healthcare Quality Improvement. National Academies Press.

U.S. Census Bureau. (2021a). *Measuring racial and ethnic diversity in the 2020 census.* https://www.census.gov/newsroom/blogs/random-samplings/2021/08/measuring-racial-ethnic-diversity-2020-census.html

U.S. Census Bureau. (2021b). *Racial and ethnic diversity in the United States: 2010 census and 2020 census.* https://www.census.gov/library/visualizations/interactive/racial-and-ethnic-diversity-in-the-united-states-2010-and-2020-census.html

U.S. Census Bureau. (2021c). *Subject definitions.* https://www.census.gov/programs-surveys/cps/technical-documentation/subject-definitions.html#:~:text=A%20household%20includes%20the%20related,who%20share%20the%20housing%20unit

U.S. Census Bureau. (2023, November 21). Three-quarters of children younger than 6 years old live with two parents. *Census Bureau releases new estimates on America's families and living arrangements.* [Press Release CB23-TPS.116]. https://www.census.gov/newsroom/press-releases/2023/children-families-living-arrangements.html

U.S. Department of Agriculture. (2023, May). Food insecurity in the U.S.: Key statistics and graphics. *Economic Research Service.* https://www.ers.usda.gov/topics/food-nutrition-assistance/food-security-in-the-u-s/key-statistics-graphics/#foodsecure

U.S. Department of Education. (2023). *How to file a discrimination complaint with the office for civil rights.* https://www2.ed.gov/about/offices/list/ocr/docs/howto.html

Willgerodt, M. A., Brock, D. M., & Maughan, E. D. (2018). Public school nursing practice in the United States. *The Journal of School Nursing, 34*(3), 232–244. https://doi.org/10.1177/1059840517752456

Willgerodt, M. A., Brock, D. M., & Tanner, A. (2023). National school nurse workforce study 2.0. https://www.nasn.org/research/school-nurse-workforce

World Health Organization. (2018). *Report of the global conference on primary health care: From alma-ata towards universal health coverage and the sustainable development goals (WHO/UHC/SDS/2019.62).* https://www.who.int/publications/i/item/report-of-the-global-conference-on-primary-health-care-from-alma-ata-towards-universal-health-coverage-and-the-sustainable-development-goals

Chapter 11

Student Exposure to Trauma

Nicole A. DiBattista ▪ Virginia A. Reising

CHAPTER OUTLINE

Trauma is a term used in many different contexts. *Individual trauma* is an event or circumstance that results in physical, emotional, and/or life-threatening harm (Substance Abuse and Mental Health Services Administration [SAMHSA], 2022). These events have lasting effects on a person's mental, physical, and emotional health and/or social or spiritual well-being. The purpose of this chapter is to discuss aspects of trauma and how schools and school nurses can work to prevent and mitigate the effects of trauma on the lives of students.

Trauma can present in the lives of students and affect them in many different ways (SAMHSA, 2022). Students and families can experience trauma in many different forms, including the following:

- Bullying
- Community violence
- Disaster
- Early childhood trauma
- Intimate partner violence
- Medical trauma
- Physical abuse
- Refugee trauma
- Sexual abuse
- Sex trafficking
- Terrorism and violence
- Traumatic grief (National Child Traumatic Stress Network, n.d.b, p. 1)

Traumatic events can be acute in nature or chronic, and reactions are unique to each person experiencing the trauma. There is no single factor that protects or puts children at risk of experiencing trauma. Protective factors against the negative effects of trauma can be both direct and/or buffering factors, including emotional, social, and moral factors, as well as positive peer and familial interactions (Zych et al., 2019).

ADVERSE CHILDHOOD EXPERIENCES

According to the Centers for Disease Control and Prevention (CDC), *adverse childhood experiences* (ACEs) are "potentially traumatic events that occur in childhood (0 to 17 years)" (2023a, para. 1). While the direct impact associated with ACEs takes place during childhood, long-term implications have been associated with a negative impact on physical and psychological health as well as other aspects of social and financial growth into adulthood (CDC, 2023a). ACEs are broken down into the following categories:

- Abuse: emotional, physical, or sexual
- Household challenges: mother treated violently, substance abuse in the household, mental illness in the household, parental separation or divorce, incarcerated household member
- Neglect: emotional or physical (CDC, 2023a)

Prevalence

Adverse childhood events are stressful and common. The first study on ACEs, conducted between 1995 and 1997 in California by the CDC and the Kaiser Permanente Health Appraisal Clinic, brought to light the prevalence of ACEs and the correlation between childhood trauma and adult health and well-being (Felitti et al., 1998). In the *2020 to 2021 National Survey of Children's Health*, 21.6% of children reported experiencing at least one ACE with 17.2% reporting experiencing two or more ACEs (Child and Adolescent Health Measurement Initiative, 2021). However, these data suggest that ACEs are underreported. Approximately 64% of adults surveyed say they experienced at least one ACE before the age of 18; 17% reported experiencing four or more ACEs (Swedo et al., 2023).

ACEs occur across all income, race, and ethnicity groups, although the prevalence of ACEs in Hispanic and black, non-Hispanic children is higher than in white, non-Hispanic children (Child and Adolescent Health Measurement Initiative, 2021). As the number and intensity of ACEs increases, so does the risk to the child for negative health and well-being outcomes across the life span.

ACEs affect neurodevelopment; therefore, the period when the child is initially exposed to ACEs is a significant factor related to the severity of the outcomes. Exposure to repeated trauma or stress may result in dysregulation of the hypothalamic-pituitary-adrenal axis, resulting in hypoarousal or hyperarousal to routine changes or stressful stimuli (Lorig et al., 2022). Dysregulation contributes to the development of behavioral, mental, and physical health problems. The *ACEs Pyramid* (CDC, 2021a) depicts the mechanism by which ACEs influence the trajectory of health and wellness across the life span. See Figure 11-1. Negative outcomes associated with ACEs include the following:

- Depressive disorder
- Chronic obstructive pulmonary disease

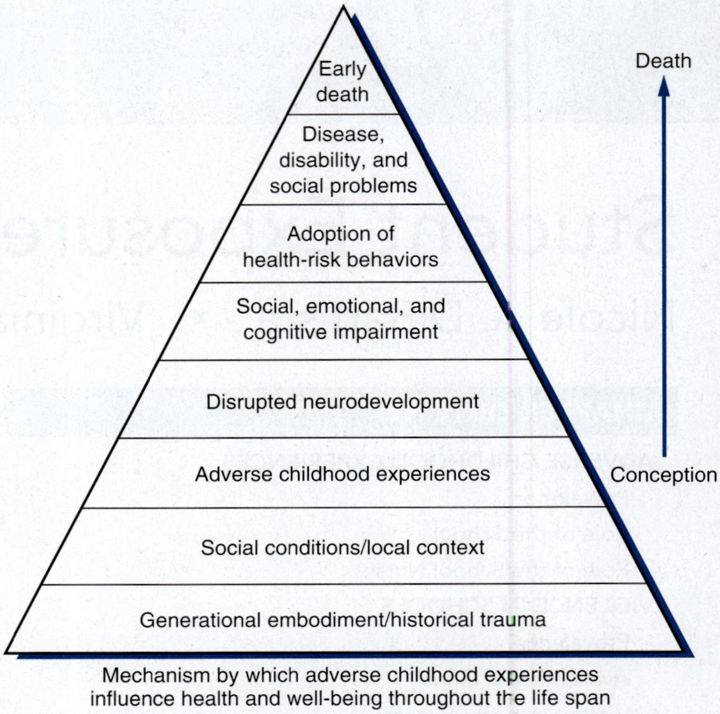

FIGURE 11-1. The ACE Pyramid. *(CDC, 2021a.)*

- Asthma
- Kidney disease
- Stroke
- Coronary heart disease
- Cancer
- Diabetes
- Overweight/obesity
- Smoking
- Heavy drinking
- Unemployment (Merrick et al., 2019)

ACEs are costly. A review by Bellis et al. (2019) found that in North America annual costs associated with ACEs are $748 billion with 75% of these costs associated with people who have experienced at least two ACEs. If exposure to ACEs were reduced by just 10% the United States could see an annual savings of $56 billion (CDC, 2023a).

Role of the School

Despite the prevalence of ACEs, schools can focus on prevention to help reduce the long-term health and social impacts of ACEs (Merrick et al., 2019).

School staff should do the following:

Be aware of the trauma triggers in the environment and minimize these triggers where possible.

- Consider: loud noises, increased activity, unwelcome or unexpected touch

Promote healing by using everyday gestures to support all students.

- Consider: listen, celebrate, collaborate, comfort, and inspire

Adopt trauma-informed assessment and intervention practices.
- Consider: Identify strengths and challenges of each child, engage families, and utilize resources. Further information on trauma-informed care is included later in this chapter.

Make sure to take care of oneself to model resiliency and prevent burnout (Futures Without Violence, 2018).

Role of the School Nurse

The school nurse is often the trusted professional at school to whom students confide their traumatic experiences. School nurses are frontline caregivers and must actively assess students who frequent the school health office for exposure to ACEs. To support students struggling after trauma exposure, school nurses must appropriately recognize and understand the signs and symptoms of traumatic stress in children. Common reactions to traumatic stress include reexperiencing, avoidance, changes in cognition and mood, and hyperarousal (Center for Pediatric Traumatic Stress, 2021). See Box 11-1.

The Center for Pediatric Trauma Stress (2021) recommends that assessment of students consider the "DEFs" in addition to the "ABCs" (airway, breathing, circulation).

- *Distress*—Assess and respond to any pain, fears, worries, grief, and loss.
- *Emotional support*—Consider what and who may support the student and consider any barriers they may face to get to that support.
- *Family*—Consider the distress, stressors, and needs of the rest of the family, including parents/guardians and siblings.

Students who experience ACEs may be affected by symptoms of post-traumatic stress and have difficulty coping with the academic and social demands of school. These students require integrated services through a multitiered system of supports and services (see Chapter 7). They may struggle academically and socially, thus requiring extra services from the interprofessional student support team. The school nurse may notice that these students frequent the school health office with somatic complaints or be chronically absent. The school nurse can be a trusted adult at school who creates a safe and healing space in the health office where students can check in for needed support.

VIOLENCE IN SCHOOLS

Violence crosses sociopolitical, economic, racial, ethnic, and cultural boundaries. Violence is the most common form of victimization in children and a primary category of ACEs. Students may experience violence in forms such as fighting, bullying, electronic aggression, sexual

BOX 11-1

Symptoms of Traumatic Stress in Children

REEXPERIENCING	**Look for:**
■ Experiencing nightmares or reporting "flashbacks" ■ Feelings of distress when thinking or reminded of incident(s) ■ Experiencing intrusive thoughts related to the incident(s)	■ "It pops into my mind." ■ "Every time I smell smoke, I am brought right back to that day." ■ "I feel like it's happening all over again."
AVOIDANCE	**Look for:**
■ Avoiding thoughts or situations that bring about feelings related to the incident(s) ■ Avoid places or activities related to the incident(s)	■ "I block it out and try not to think about it." ■ "I don't drive on that road anymore."
CHANGES IN COGNITION AND MOOD	**Look for:**
■ Overwhelming negative emotions ■ Drastic changes in the way one views themself, others, the world, and future ■ Numbness or detachment from emotions	■ "All people are bad." ■ "Every bad thing that has happened is my fault." ■ "I don't really care what happens, I don't feel anything anymore."
HYPERAROUSAL	**Look for:**
■ Easily startled ■ Irritable ■ Extreme vigilance or always expecting something bad to happen ■ Trouble with concentration and/or sleep	■ "My heart races when I hear loud noises." ■ "Everyone is always bothering me." ■ "I just know that something bad will happen again." ■ "I haven't slept since this happened."

Adapted from Center for Pediatric Traumatic Stress (2021).

victimization, or being threatened with or without weapons. Children may be exposed to violence in the home, school, and community. Violence is constantly depicted and often glamorized across media (e.g., news sources, television, Internet, movies, music, social media, and video games). Violence may also be directed against oneself in the form of self-harm. Regardless of its cause, violence or the threat of violence is highly disruptive to the school environment and interferes significantly with the teaching/learning process, through class disruption or absenteeism.

School violence is a subset of youth violence that affects youth up to age 24. It includes violence on school property, on the way to and from school, during school-sponsored events, or traveling to or from these events. School violence affects learning and has negative outcomes on students and schools (CDC, 2021b). Violence may originate within the school or be brought into the school from outside sources. Young people may be victims, perpetrators, or witnesses of school violence. These distinctions are important when planning interventions. Many national and local agencies are dedicated to the eradication of violence in society. School administrators, law enforcement officers, legislators, and community officials, as well as teachers, families, healthcare providers, and students, need to work together to address exposure to violence and make schools safe spaces for all.

Prevalence

Multiple national reports provide data on the prevalence of violence among high school students and for those ages 10 to 24.

- During the 2020 to 2021 school year the rate of victimization at school was 11 per 1,000 students.
- Approximately 3.5% of high school students carried a gun (5% males; 1.8% females).
- Approximately 3.1% of high school students carried a weapon onto school property at least 1 day (3.9% males; 2.1% females).
- Approximately 6.6% were threatened or injured with a weapon on school property (5.9% males; 7.0% females).
- Approximately 5.8% were in a physical fight on school property at least once in the past year (8.1% males; 3.2% females).
- Approximately 8.7% did not go to school because they felt unsafe at school or on their way to or from school (7% males; 10% females) (CDC, 2021b; Irwin et al., 2022).

In 2023, there were 137 recorded incidents of gunfire on school grounds. These incidents resulted in 42 deaths and 94 injuries (Everytown, 2024).

Five percent of students older than 12 years reported that they avoided place(s) in the school because they were afraid, such as hallways and stairwells, the cafeteria, the restroom, and the entrance to the school building. Fear of being attacked is more prevalent in students of two or more races (11%) and black students (7%) than white (4%) students. Fear in school is highest among 9th graders (Irwin et al., 2022). Although there has been an overall decrease in nonfatal criminal victimization (e.g., theft, rape, sexual assault, robbery, and aggravated or simple assault) in recent years, including during the COVID-19 pandemic, gun violence continues to escalate.

Availability of Guns

In 2021, there were 4,752 deaths related to firearms in children 0 to 19 years old (Roberts et al, 2023). The death rate is significantly higher in males (9.06 per 100,000) compared with females (1.8 per 100,000) and in black children (18.9 per 100,000) compared with white children (3.6 per 100,000). Shockingly, firearms surpassed motor vehicle accidents as the number one cause of death in children in 2019. This is in part due to the wide availability of guns in U.S. society. Forty percent of adults say they live in a house with a firearm. Teens who live in homes with a gun are three times more at risk for suicide than teens who live in homes without a gun (Swanson et al., 2021). In states with more restrictive gun laws, fewer people die by gun violence (Everytown, 2023).

Did You Know?

The presence of gangs has a significant impact on the safety of many schools and communities. A *gang* is "a loosely organized association of three or more persons, whether formal or informal, that has a common name, signs, symbols, or colors, whose members engage, either individually or collectively, in violent or other forms of illegal behavior." (National Center for Education Statistics [NCES], n.d.). The most important criterion in determining whether a group is a youth gang is *group criminality*. Typically, membership includes youth from ages 12 to 24 and is often organized by race, ethnic group, territory, or criminal activity. Groups of young people hanging out together on a street corner or in a park are not necessarily a gang, nor are their behaviors considered gang activity.

Overall, the presence of gangs at schools has decreased, with 9% of students reporting the presence of gangs in their school in 2019. There were higher reports of gang activity in urban areas, among black and Hispanic youth, and in high school students (NCES, 2022c).

Gangs are powerful social networks that young people join for a variety of reasons, including "individual factors, peer pressure, family conditions, lack of school achievement, and community turmoil" (National Crime Prevention Council, n.d., para. 2). Being part of a gang may make the youth feel secure, give them a place to belong, and help them stand up for themselves in the face of aggressive and violent behavior. However, gang activity increases exposure to illegal activities, violence, and the risk of youth becoming involved in the justice system and incarcerated.

Violent Intruder Events

One of the most frightening and potentially lethal events on school campuses is the presence of a violent intruder or active shooter. The U.S. Department of Homeland Security defines an *active shooter* as "an individual engaged in killing or attempting to kill people in a confined and populated area" (n.d.a, para. 1). There is often no specific pattern to victim selection and events occur suddenly without warning.

The National Association of School Psychologists (2021) emphasizes that there is no known profile of a student who will be an active shooter. It is important that school personnel avoid profiling students which can lead to missed identification of students who are at risk of violence. Most students indicate violent intentions before action. Shootings may be motivated by hate or rage, gang activity, or drug activity; retaliation for being expelled; or having a dispute with another student, teacher, or staff member. Potential warning signs of violence are listed in Table 11-1. Many of the warning signs are similar to other risk factors discussed throughout this chapter. School nurses have an opportunity to intervene with students early and/or alert others to potential dangers in time to reduce risks.

It is important to *plan and train* for violent intruder events. The school nurse should work with the school's interdisciplinary safety committee. Many school preparedness resources are available through the U.S. Department of Homeland Security (see Online Materials OM11-1). See Chapter 15 for detailed information about preparing for and responding to an active shooter or violent intruder incident.

TABLE 11-1 Identifying and Addressing Warning Signs of Violence

Be alert to potential warning signs of trouble.	• Escalating behavior that is erratic, unsafe, or aggressive • Expressed feelings of hostility, injustice, or perceived wrongdoing • Change in drug or alcohol use • Withdrawing from friends or colleagues • Changes in school or work performance • Sudden and dramatic changes in home life • Family financial difficulties • Involvement in pending civil or criminal litigation • Known grievances with another student or staff member with threats and plans of retaliation
Appropriate intervention.	• Be observant. Note drastic changes in student attitudes and behaviors toward others. • Be prepared to provide information that may help facilitate intervention and mitigate potential risks to school safety.
Reach out for help.	• Alert others of potential dangers. • Follow your school's policy in reporting concerns about student or staff behavior. Reach out to your principal or nursing supervisor.

Adapted from U.S. Department of Homeland Security (n.d.b).

As with all emergency events, precise planning and preparation are keys to success. The school nurse should take a leadership role in the ongoing protection of students and staff, including preparing for violent intruders (National Association of School Nurses [NASN], 2024). Plans should also be made to assist in coping with the process and the sequelae after the event. Expect and validate emotions, be honest and open, and encourage communication for students and staff to share their fears and concerns (American School Counselor Association, 2024).

Security Measures

Media attention regarding school shootings and other crimes on school property has led the public to question the safety of schools, resulting in increased security measures in schools aimed at protecting students and staff. Before implementing security measures, it is important to conduct a needs assessment of the school community and grounds.

The National Center for Education Statistics (NCES) tracks the use of safety and security measures by school level (primary, middle, and high school). During the 2019 to 2020 school year, 97% of schools limited access to the school during school hours, 91% used security cameras to monitor areas of the school, 77% required faculty and staff to wear badges or picture IDs, 10% required students to wear badges or picture IDs (10%), and 6% used random metal detector checks. All these indicators have increased year by year (NCES, 2022b). In 2019, 99.6% of students reported observing at least one of the security measures at school.

School resource officers (SROs) are sworn law enforcement officers or security guards who work in the school setting (U.S. Department of Justice, Community Oriented Policing Services, n.d.). Training and authority of SROs is not nationally standardized, so the role may vary across districts. SROs may have the authority to arrest students, and most (51.4%) carry firearms. While SROs or police officers may be engaged in discipline at schools, recent

Did You Know?

Although the use of metal detectors in public schools has diminished over time, there continues to be debate on whether they are effective at increasing safety in the school setting. On one hand, metal detectors are a visible reminder of the efforts at safety undertaken by the school, but studies have shown that students feel less safe in schools with visible metal detectors. Evidence has not shown that metal detectors deter violence. There are significant financial costs and staffing needs associated with metal detectors, so it is important for schools to consider their effectiveness before implementation (Schildkraut & Grogan, 2019).

data show that only 41% of principals indicated that their school's policy includes information about the use of firearms by SROs. There appears to be a connection between school size and security practices with sworn law SROs. In large schools with 1,000 or more students, officers carry physical restraints, chemical aerosol sprays, or firearms more often than in smaller schools. In large schools 45% of the officers also report wearing body cameras (Wang et al., 2022). It is important to note that the presence of SROs in schools has been linked to increased exclusions, arrests, and the number of justice-involved youth, especially youth of color (Bleakley & Bleakley, 2018; Cross et al., 2021).

Disciplinary Measures

The most common school response to violence among students is to discipline them, often with suspension or expulsion (LiCalsi et al., 2021). This results in students losing instructional time, which leads to decreased academic performance and creates strain on families. Students who are suspended once are more likely to be suspended again. There are also disparities seen in who is suspended, with one study demonstrating black students making up 55.7% of school suspensions despite representing only 29% of the total population. The relative risk of black students being suspended for more than 4 weeks is 8 times that of white middle school students and 6 times that of white high school students (LiCalsi et al., 2021).

The use of physical restraints and unsupervised seclusion of students has not been found to be therapeutic. These practices pose physical and psychological danger to the students and should not be used. Restraints and seclusion are also more commonly used with students with disabilities, boys, and black students (Prince & Goldberg, 2019). It is the position of the National Association of School Nurses that restraints or seclusion should not be used often and only when a student is at risk of harm to themselves or others (NASN, 2021b). While there is no federal law against these practices in the school setting, the U.S. Department of Education (2012) has a resource document that should be used by schools when developing policies and procedures related to the use of restraints and seclusion.

Violence Prevention and Intervention

For students to thrive in school, they need to feel safe physically, emotionally, and socially. Schools should also be a safe work site for staff, free of crime and violence. It is essential that schools promote a trusting environment where students can feel confident that staff will listen, be vigilant, and act appropriately on their concerns. School nurses must be knowledgeable and work with other members of the school team to develop and implement plans and programs so that students and staff feel safe in the school setting.

In the United States, 96% of public schools have a prevention curriculum, instruction, or training for students that includes conflict resolution, antibullying content, and dating violence prevention. Social-emotional learning principles are integrated into 94.4% of schools. Ninety-two percent of schools offered individual mentoring by adults, and 50.3% offer peer mediation (Wang et al., 2022). The National Center for Injury Prevention and Control recommends universal programming that focuses on helping students develop self-awareness and self-control, problem-solving, and positive community building (David-Ferdon et al., 2016).

More than 90% of schools have written plans describing the procedures to be performed in the scenarios of natural disasters, an active shooter, and bomb threats (Wang et al., 2022). Over 89% have policies about postcrisis reunification of students with their families; 91% have policies regarding a suicide threat or incident; 73% have one regarding chemical, biological, or radiological threats; and 52.7% have one regarding hostages in the school. Of interest, from the 2019 to 2020 data, only 52.7% had written policies on action to take for a pandemic disease (Wang et al., 2022). Policies are only effective when the school community knows what is in the policy and has prepared to implement the policy. Chapter 15 provides more information on policies related to emergencies.

The school team should continually assess for the potential for violence, including the school climate. School nurses can use their assessment skills to better understand the root cause of harmful behavior. It is not only important to know *who* is at risk for violence, but also to find out *why*. Consider the antecedent, behavior, consequence (ABC) model (Meadan et al., 2016; Selekman et al., 2023a, 2023b). The modified ABC model (Fig. 11-2) considers the factors that lead to behavior and the outcomes of the behavior while considering protective and risk factors, as well as emotions and thoughts that lead to behaviors. A clear understanding of the social, psychological, emotional, and physical contexts associated with violent behavior helps guide holistic intervention programs. For example, if a child who is abused at home is lashing out in anger at school, then an important component of the intervention must focus on the child's safety in the home. Another example might be a child who lashes out at others, yet the cause is related to stress and lack of sleep at night due to unstable housing. Working with the school homeless liaison to address the housing issue may ultimately help to resolve the violent outbursts. School nurses can utilize the modified ABC model to help students consider the situation and emotions that lead to unwanted behaviors and problem-solve how to manage those situations and emotions differently.

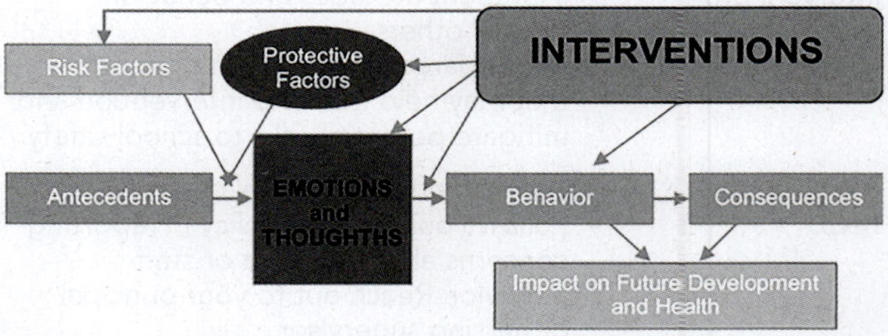

FIGURE 11-2. Modified ABC model. *(Selekman et al., 2023a, 2023b, with permission.)*

There are many risk factors for violence that offer opportunities for prevention. Youth who are disconnected from their families often receive minimal emotional support for what is going on in their lives and have a more challenging time regulating behaviors (CDC, 2021b). School personnel should make special efforts to engage these parents/guardians in school activities, especially activities that promote connections with their children and with the school community. Family-based programs to help families communicate, learn to problem-solve, set limits, and monitor their children can be beneficial. Schools should ensure they are offering these sessions in a manner that meets the scheduling needs of the most families possible (e.g., online or in the evenings). Parents/guardians and students should have input into the development of classroom rules; they should understand them and support them.

Interventions aimed at preventing or decreasing violence can be directed toward a specific student, family, school, or the community at large. Successful strategies should target identified manifestations or risks of violence. Interdisciplinary and coordinated approaches involve proactive school leadership, professional school nurses, the student support team, informed educators and school staff, area stakeholders, and parental engagement and community commitment to a peaceful climate.

School connectedness has been shown to positively affect many risky behaviors, including violence. School connectedness is effective in decreasing risky sexual behaviors, poor mental health, substance use, and violence (CDC, 2022b). School connectedness has also been shown to improve long-term health outcomes into adulthood, including a reduction in emotional distress and adult violence such as victimization or perpetration (Steiner et al., 2019). Effective initiatives for school personnel to increase school connectedness include the following:

- Establishing a climate that promotes and practices respect for others and for the property of others
- Providing caring and support to those who have experienced or witnessed acts of violence
- Creating unambiguous disciplinary policies that are communicated clearly to students, staff, and parents/guardians
- Ensuring that there are no weapons on school property or school buses
- Involving parents in all aspects of school life (CDC, 2022b)

Students who feel adults and peers in their school really "know" them, respect them, and care about their welfare experience better academic achievement then those who lack a sense of belonging. Additional interventions to reduce violence include the following:

- Develop mentoring programs for at-risk youth and families.
- Change the physical and social environment to decrease risk; have faculty and staff on the playground, in the cafeteria, and outside school entrances before and after school.
- Educate students and their parents/guardians on gun safety. (Guns in the home must be locked with trigger guards attached and ammunition stored in a separate location.)
- Teach students how to manage their emotions and develop specific self-calming strategies.

Increasingly, schools are instituting restorative justice practices meant to bring reconciliation between the person who has been harmed with the person or people who harmed them. Restorative justice strives to create resolution as opposed to punishment (Darling-Hammond et al., 2020). In the 2019 to 2020 school year, 60.2% of schools reported having students involved in restorative justice practice (Wang et al., 2022). These practices vary across settings; however, the three main tenets are (1) relationships and their harms, (2) empowerment of all people, and (3) collaboration. Using restorative justice practices in schools requires adults to model the positive behaviors they want to instill in students, including integrity, honesty, respect, and self-control (Darling-Hammond et al., 2020). Alternative nonviolent forms of positive behavioral support should be identified in schools. Evidence suggests that positive behavioral supports in the classroom decrease out-of-school suspensions, specifically in students with disabilities and students who are black (Gage et al., 2019). Box 11-2 offers further interventions to prevent violence in school.

Role of the School Nurse

The school nurse has a key role in both preventing and treating violence in the school setting. The goal is prevention and reduction of violence and ensuring a safe school environment. This is best accomplished by a collaborative

Focus on the Framework

Community/Public Health, Leadership, and Quality Improvement

NASN's *School Nursing Framework* (2024) supports a public health approach to violence prevention in schools. The school nurse can incorporate concepts of the Framework's key principles of **Community/Public Health, Leadership, and Quality Improvement** to understand and address violence within their school community through the following steps:

1. Define and monitor the impact of violence on the community through data collection.
2. Identify risk and protective factors to understand why violence occurs and who it affects.
3. Design and implement interventions to address violence.
4. Evaluate the impact of the intervention to reduce violence within the school community.

The Educational Fund to Stop Gun Violence (2021).

BOX 11-2

Interventions to Prevent Violence in Schools

Develop very clear and specific classroom or school rules.
Remind children of the rules each time they play with each other.
Set clear limits of what is acceptable and what is not. For example:
- Share and take turns.
- Use a quiet indoor voice.
- Keep your hands and feet to yourself.

Discipline in the classroom should be positive and consistent. Develop sensible consequences that fit the situation. (Example: "If you fight over this toy, I will remove the toy for 15 minutes so that no one will use it.")
Teachers should model nonaggressive discipline.
Teach problem-solving techniques and how to resolve problems without violence.
Differentiate assertiveness and aggressiveness; teach skills to be more assertive.
Build self-esteem, especially related to behaviors that enhance learning and build character.
"Catch" children being good, sensitive, and accepting and praise them. All children must feel special and connected to the school environment. Praise children and pay attention to them when they play nicely together.
Decrease access to violent videos and games.
Act immediately and decisively when a child is aggressive or is bullying.
Respect the child's feelings when they express them; just help them redirect how they are expressed.
Have adults in the hallways between classes and at the beginning and end of the school day.

Adapted from National Association of School Psychologists (2015).

environment involving school personnel, including the school nurse, parents/guardians, healthcare providers, and community members. For many students, the school health office can be a reprieve and a place where they seek solace. The school nurse should build authentic relationships with students to detect precursors to violence or signs of victimization (King, 2014).

The school nurse is essential in identifying instances of violence, as well as working in a professional capacity to contribute to policies to prevent and address violence and help resolve the consequences of violence. NASN identifies school violence as one of the issues that makes school nursing more challenging (NASN, 2022). Students may share with the school nurse what they see, hear, or have experienced; this is especially important because some students may have been threatened that they or someone they care about will be hurt if they tell. Therefore, school nurses need to know when confidentiality can and cannot be kept and when they are obligated to share information. In the interest of safety, when a student is at risk of harm to themselves or others the school nurse has a responsibility to communicate this information per district policy and state law.

School nurses need to be aware of school policies regarding how to handle violent behaviors. The local school district's violence plan or the state violence plan can serve as resources for the school nurse and school administrative personnel. If there are no written policies, then the school nurse should work with the school team to develop them. The school nurse can assist in disseminating the rationale for policies and protocols regulating student behavior in school and the relationship between school safety and health. Supporting articles can be shared with parents/guardians and students in health newsletters, on bulletin boards, in classroom presentations, and on the school nurse's Web page. Keeping data about the incidence of intentional injuries as indicated by visits to the health office can help track changes in injury rates and the effectiveness of school safety programs.

BULLYING

Bullying is an adverse childhood experience and a form of violence that can have lasting consequences. Although bullying is not a new phenomenon, the prevalence of school shootings has placed increased focus on studying bullying. The CDC (2023b) endorses the definition of *bullying* as

> *any unwanted aggressive behavior(s) by another youth or group of youths who are not siblings or current dating partners that involves an observed or perceived power imbalance and is repeated multiple times or is highly likely to be repeated. Bullying may inflict harm or distress on the targeted youth including physical, psychological, social, or educational harm (Gladden et al., 2014, p. 7).*

Types of bullying include physical, verbal, relational/social, property damage, and cyberbullying (CDC, 2023b) and can be direct or indirect (Gladden et al., 2014). See Table 11-2. Cyberbullying is a growing concern that affects the well-being of students.

> *Cyberbullying is bullying that takes place over digital devices like cell phones, computers, and tablets. Cyberbullying can occur through SMS, Text, and apps, or online in social media, forums, or gaming where people can view, participate in, or share content. Cyberbullying includes sending, posting, or sharing negative, harmful, false, or mean content about someone else. It can include sharing personal or private information about someone else causing embarrassment or humiliation. Some cyberbullying crosses the line into unlawful or criminal behavior (Stopbullying.gov, 2021b, para. 1).*

A nationally representative survey conducted by the Pew Research Center (2018) found that 95% of teens having access to a smart phone; 45% of teens said they are online "almost constantly"; and 24% of teens said social media

TABLE 11-2 Types of Bullying With Associated Behaviors

Physical	Verbal
• Physical injury (hit, punch, pinch, push, kick, trip, block one's path, hold, throw objects, pull hair) • Damage belongings of others • Threaten with a weapon	• Threaten verbally or with gestures • Make rude gestures or facial expressions • Insult, call names, humiliate
Social	**Cyberbullying**
• Spreading rumors or lies • Teasing • Excluding someone from events or activities	• Hurtful electronic messages • Excluding someone in an online environment • Harass with phone calls, e-mails, texts, etc.

Adapted from Stopbullying.gov (2022b).

has mostly negative effects on them due to online bullying, harming relationships, and unrealistic views of other's lives. It is important to note that 31% reported social media had a mostly positive effective as it helped youth connect with family and friends, creating an avenue to news and information and helping them meet others with common interests (Pew Research Center, 2018). According to the U.S. Surgeon General's Advisory on *Social Media and Youth Mental Health* (2023), the following factors should be considered when assessing whether a person's social media usage is detrimental: the amount of time youth spent on social media platforms, the type of content they consumed or were exposed to, and the degree to which these activities affect activities essential for health (eating, exercising, and sleep).

Prevalence

Bullying is recognized as a serious national public health concern with prevalence varying by population and age. Bullying behaviors can be seen in the preschool years but are not considered bullying until the child reaches a certain level of awareness, intentionality, and empathy and begins to understand the intent to harm another person. However, preschool is a crucial time to work with children on learning prosocial behaviors with peers as this is the first time many children are in social settings without parental oversight (Saracho, 2016). Young children may learn some negative behaviors at this impressionable time from adults who threaten, shame, and punish them rather than set limits and problem-solve.

The incidence of bullying peaks during middle school; 28.1% of 6th graders and 28% of 7th graders reporting being bullied during the school year (NCES, 2022a). There are many reasons why bullying increases during this period, namely the increased importance of friends and increased access to technology. More than 50% of students 12 to 18 years old who reported being bullied at school were bullied three or more days over the school year, indicating the chronic nature of bullying for many students (NCES, 2022a).

High school students report lower overall incidence of bullying. However, they also report increased violence and suicidality related to bullying. In the 2021 Youth Risk Behavior Survey, 15% of high school students reported being bullied on school property and 16% reported being cyberbullied. Female high school students report higher prevalence of bullying on school property (17%) compared with males (13%) and through cyberbullying (20%) compared with males (11%). Lesbian, gay, or bisexual high school students report twice the prevalence of being bullied at school compared with their heterosexual peers (32% compared with 16%) (CDC, 2023b). American Indian or Alaska Natives, white non-Hispanic, and multiracial students were more likely to be bullied on school property and electronically bullied compared with other racial/ethnic groups. However, other studies have demonstrated that black students underreport bullying based on question phrasing. Studies have also shown that non-white youth are more likely to experience negative health and behavioral outcomes related to bias-based bullying (Xu et al., 2020).

Bullying can occur anywhere and is often unseen. Students experienced bullying inside the classroom (47%), in the hallway (39%), in the bathroom or gym locker room (11%), in the cafeteria (26%), outside on school grounds (20%), on the way to or from school (10%), and online or by text (16%) (NCES, 2022a). In addition to prevention activities, schools have a responsibility to intervene any time they are made aware of bullying of or by students or school personnel (NASN, 2023a; Stopbullying.org., 2021c).

Characteristics

Bullying is a violent act. There are characteristics commonly found in students who bully and students who are bullied, as well as bystanders or witnesses of bullying. However, it is important for school nurses to look beyond expected characterizations and instead be alert for any student displaying signs of being affected by violence.

Bullying is an abuse of power. Research has attempted to identify characteristics of and risk factors for becoming a student who bullies others. There are two types of students who are likely to display bullying behavior: (1) those who are popular, socially powerful, like to dominate others, and engage in bullying to increase popularity; and (2) those who are isolated, depressed, or anxious, have low self-esteem, and lack the empathy to identify with the feelings of others (Stopbullying.gov, 2021d). The second group may learn to justify aggressive behavior in response to being bullied themselves. Both groups share negative attitudes about others and have trouble resolving problems with others. Students who bully may manipulate others, lack the ability to perceive or interpret social cues, and/or lack empathy for the needs and desires of others. Students who are more likely to demonstrate bullying behavior are aggressive, have less parental involvement or challenges at home, think badly of others, have difficulty following rules, often have friends who bully, and view violence positively (Stopbullying.gov, 2021d). Students who bully often justify their behavior by blaming their target who they perceive to be annoying or antagonizing.

Students who are bullied may be perceived as weak, depressed, or unpopular, or have difficulty having a good relationship with others (Stopbullying.gov, 2021d). These students should not be referred to as *victims* as this language may imply that the student is helpless, in need of pity, and unable to change the situation (PACER's National Bullying Prevention Center, n.d.). Using the term *students who are bullied* models person-first language.

Students who are bullied may also have characteristics that set them apart from their peers such as height, weight, glasses, clothing, braces, physical disabilities, having a physical or mental health diagnosis, restricted mobility, specific mannerisms, ethnicity, or lack of coordination. Sometimes the difference is not as apparent, such as religious beliefs or sexual orientation. Students who are bullied often experience low self-esteem.

Students who are bullied may not seek adult help because they blame themselves for the situation and/or believe it will make their situation worse by leading to increased harassment. Students who are bullied are more likely to be afraid of an attack or harm, more likely to skip school, and more likely to carry a weapon to school compared with students who are not bullied (NCES, 2022a).

Those who observe bullying are referred to as *bystanders* or *watchers.* Bystanders underestimate the pivotal role they have in promoting or preventing the bullying process; when bystanders intervene, there is 50% reduction in bullying (Padgett & Notar, 2013). Although bystanders may feel uninvolved, they are fueling and facilitating the bully. There are four different roles of bystanders: outsiders, defenders, reinforcers, and assistants. *Outsiders* are exposed to bullying but do nothing to stop it; they stay uninvolved. *Defenders* will intervene to protect the person who is bullied, either privately or publicly. *Reinforcers* encourage the person who bullies through laughing or cheering. *Assistants* will support the person who bullies by getting directly involved with the bullying action (Stopbullying.gov, 2021a). Many people view themselves as defenders but do not intervene due to a variety of reasons. A person is more likely to act as a defender in a bullying situation if they

- Are friends with the person who is being bullied
- Have moral views that bullying is wrong
- Have empathy for the person who is being bullied
- Believe the adults will appropriately address this situation (Barnett et al., 2019; Stopbullying.gov, 2021a)

Consequences

All students are affected by bullying: those who bully, those who are the target of bullying, and those who witness or hear about a bullying episode. Although there may be the risk of physical injury, including death, the more common consequence of bullying is its impact on the emotional and mental health of the bully, the bullied, and the bystanders. Bullying creates a climate of fear and disrespect.

Students who bully or are bullied are more likely to think about or attempt suicide than those who are not involved with bullying (Kim et al., 2020). Students who are bullied are at three times higher risk for depression, anxiety, and nonsuicidal self-injury than those who had not been bullied (Gini & Espelage, 2014). Many of these mental health issues continue into adulthood. Students who experience relational or psychosocial bullying report more emotional distress than do those experiencing physical bullying. The short-term effects are usually psychological in nature, resulting in nightmares and sleep disturbances, lower self-esteem, psychosomatic complaints (abdominal pain, headaches, chest pain), increased incidence of illness (related to chronic stress), impaired concentration, increased stress behaviors (nail biting, comfort measures, and enuresis), loneliness, and depression (Gini & Espelage, 2014; National Academies of Sciences, Engineering, and Medicine, 2016).

The effects of being bullied can interfere with a student's ability to be engaged in the learning process For example, students who are bullied have more difficulty concentrating on their schoolwork and have decreased attendance and performance. These students may fear going to classes, using the school bathroom, riding the school bus, or walking to or from school. The results are lost instructional time, decreased school performance, and decreased participation in certain school activities.

The effects of being bullied do not go away as the student distances themselves or grows up and away from the person who bullied them. Bullying is considered an ACE; there are connections between being bullied and being at higher risk for negative health outcomes during the life course (CDC, 2021c). Studies have shown long-term effects on emotional well-being both for people who were bullied and those who were bystanders to bullying events (Camodeca & Nava, 2022).

Much less is understood about the long-term effects of being a bully. Perpetrators may have a pattern of youth aggression and behavioral problems that may result in increased offending and antisocial behavior in adult life. They may be more likely to experience depression, anxiety, and misuse/abuse of illicit drugs and alcohol (Zych et al., 2019). It is not clear if these characteristics are causal or merely associated with bullying.

Role of the School

Students are less likely to engage in bullying if they feel connected to school, believe the school is fair and trusting, and believe their friends and school personnel are trustworthy and caring (CDC, 2023d; Zych et al., 2019). Schools should have clearly defined policies and protocols related to bullying. Informing students, staff, and families of antibullying policies, what behaviors are expected and are unacceptable, as well as consequences that will occur if bullying occurs provide guidelines for behavior. This sets the tone for expectations in the school community with an aim to create an optimal learning environment. Stakeholders should work together to develop and/or refine antibullying policies and programs within the school. See Box 11-3.

Legal Issues

Although there are no national laws about the prevention of bullying, the U.S. Department of Education has a framework for common components that should be included in local laws and policies (Stopbullying.gov, 2022a). It is important to remember that if bullying involves race or ethnicity, national origin, sex, disability, or religion it can be considered harassment, which schools are required by federal law to address. Bullying can become a law enforcement issue when there is concern about hate crimes, threats of harm, or acts of violence.

There are multiple legal implications to cyberbullying. Courts have ruled that "posting information on the Internet—whatever the subject matter—can constitute speech as surely as stapling flyers to bulletin boards or distributing pamphlets to passersby—activities long protected by the first amendment" (Hudson, 2016, para. 8). According to the Supreme Court, student speech is not protected if it "materially and substantially disrupts the education process of the school environment" (*Tinker v. Des Moines Independent Community School District,* 1969). In other words, if student expression interferes with the work of the school or impinges on the rights of students to learn, then the school has authority and responsibility to act.

Cyberbullying may be considered a crime and reported to law enforcement if it includes threats of violence, child pornography, sending sexually explicit messages or photos, taking a photo of someone in a place where they expect privacy, stalking, or hate crimes. However, criminal prosecution for cyberbullying is rare because the legal landscape is unclear (Hudson, 2016). Litigation against schools by parents/guardians is emerging for failing to keep students safe. School nurses should consult individual state laws to determine the criminality of specific activities.

Prevention and Intervention

Prevention

Prevention of bullying must involve the whole school, as well as families and the community. Schools are placing

BOX 11-3

School Antibullying Policies and Protocols

DEVELOPING SCHOOL ANTIBULLYING POLICIES AND PROTOCOLS

The CDC (2021b) outlines important considerations for school antibullying policies.

Identify Key Players

Key players should include students, school staff, parents/guardians, and community partners.

Define Bullying

The first goal is to have a shared understanding of the definition of bullying that is consistent with state laws. Some states have begun to enumerate or list specific characteristics that could be the basis for bullying such as race, disability, religion, sex or gender, national origin, sexual orientation, ancestry/ethnicity, and gender identity or expressions. Policies should also include language such as "including but not limited to" so all students are protected (CDC, 2021b).

Identify Bullying Behavior

- Identified behaviors must be clear so that students know and understand what and why behaviors are considered unacceptable.
- The policy must be written in respectful language at a level that students can understand.
- Focus must be on *behavior* while also avoiding labeling individual students or groups of students as "targets," "victims," or "bullies."

Develop Consequences for Bullying

- Describe graduated sanctions and consequences for incidents of bullying behaviors, including nonpunitive alternatives.
- Outline a system for identifying, intervening, and reporting incidents of bullying.
- Describe what assistance will be provided to support all students affected by bullying.
- Include a statement of rights and legal recourse.
- Zero-tolerance policies are not considered effective at addressing the needs of a student who was bullied or a student who has bullied.

Integrate the Policy Into the School Culture

Universal training and expectation setting should occur. The policy should be distributed widely to the students, families, educational staff, community partners, and local law enforcement. Policies should be publicly available and shared with local media for publication.

Create a Reporting System

There must be a clear path for students and staff to report bullying behavior, both experienced personally and observed. This system will help schools track patterns of behavior. Data can be used to improve the school climate and environment.

substantial efforts and fiscal resources into bullying prevention programs. Evidenced-based curriculum interventions are the most widely adopted strategies, which rely primarily on social-cognitive behavior changes and improved self-efficacy in students. Preventing bullying requires school administration to be committed to and engaged in identifying and managing bullying and violent behavior. School administrators and personnel are responsible for assessing school safety, which includes the routes to and from school, as well as transportation used by students.

Regardless of selected prevention programs or policies, training of staff on what to look for in bullying, school policy related to bullying, and what to do if bullying is observed is essential. In the classroom, discussions can be held about why people bully, why people watch bullies and do not act, how it feels to be bullied or to bully others, and the effects that bullying has (Box 11-4). Discussions can be held in history classes to explore bullying and prejudice throughout history; civics classes to discuss the law and violence, and what society would be like if bullying was acceptable; and psychology classes to discuss the moral dilemmas faced with bullying and the possible solutions. The questions asked and the responses given during class discussions may provide insight into the types of incidents occurring in the school and the concerns students have about coming forward when bullying takes place. It is essential to listen to what students are saying and to be supportive. Let students know that they have support from school personnel and review the school's antibullying guidelines on how to report bullying.

Intervention

Responding to bullying involves three key steps (Stopbullying.gov, 2021b). The first step is to stop aggressive behaviors immediately whenever and wherever they are reported or observed. It is important to stay calm; separate the students involved, and make sure everyone is safe; and address any medical or mental health needs. Reassure all students involved. Always model respectful behavior for the students.

> **BOX 11-4**
> **Suggested Questions for In-Class Discussions About Bullying**
>
> 1. Why do students say or do "mean" things to other students? Why do they boss other kids around?
> 2. What do people say that make you feel angry, hurt, or not think well of yourself?
> 3. If you saw a student being picked on or made fun of, what would affect whether you stepped in to help or stepped out of the way?
> 4. What happens when students report incidents to teachers/parents?
> 5. Do you feel safe in school (playground, locker area, busses, bathrooms, etc.)?
> 6. What would make you feel safe in school?

The second step is to get the facts and calmly and respectfully determine whether what was reported or observed meets the state's or school's definition of bullying. Keep in mind that not all aggressive behavior is bullying. In bullying there is a power imbalance that results in the negative relationship; other forms of aggression may involve different interventions.

The third step is to support all students involved in the bullying incident. Listen and focus on the student who was the target of bullying. Assure them bullying is not their fault and that the school takes bullying seriously. Ask students what they think would make them feel safe and would not single them out. Maintain open communication; develop a plan that minimizes changes to student routines and include ongoing follow-up.

Make sure students who demonstrated bullying behavior know what specific behaviors are problematic and why this behavior is not acceptable. Try to get the student to take the point of view of the student they bullied, as well as that of their classmates. Explore ways in which students who bully can take responsibility for their actions and make it right with the person who was bullied. It is also important to ensure well-meaning actions do not make the student who was bullied feel uncomfortable, singled out, or unsafe.

Inappropriate responses by adults can make the situation worse for students who are bullied. Advice such as "These experiences build character," "It will help toughen you up for life," "Just ignore them," or "They are just being kids" may make the student feel that they are at fault and that nothing can be done. Advising students to stay away from the student who is bullying them is not a solution. Misinterpreting bullying as just anger and conflict is equally ineffective; conflict is between two or more people of equal standing. Doing nothing is the worst response of all after a student has reported being bullied or feeling scared.

Zero-tolerance policies resulting in suspensions and expulsions are not effective in reducing bullying behaviors and contribute to lower feelings of safety in school from both students and teachers (Huang & Cornell, 2021). It may take more than one attempt to stop an individual from bullying; follow-up and reassurance are required for all students affected. Students who are bullied require a safe environment, emotional support, and freedom from repeated bullying. Students who bully need ongoing support to understand how their actions affect others, develop healthy behaviors to address aggression, and learn how to respectfully interact with classmates. Students who witness bullying behavior require reassurance that school is a safe place to be and that bullying is taken seriously and addressed.

Role of the School Nurse

The school nurse is a member of the school prevention team and is integral in providing leadership in implementing bullying prevention and intervention strategies to promote a positive school climate (NASN, 2023a). School nurses often identify students who bully or are bullied and see the impact of bullying on students' health. Being bullied is stressful; students who are bullied may frequent the school health office with somatic complaints. It is essential for school nurses to differentiate bullying from other forms of aggression or victimization so that students receive the appropriate interventions. Students who witness bullying are also affected and need support. They may not know what they can do to stop bullying and require reassurance that school is a safe place. The school nurse can employ motivational interviewing to foster conversations with students about what they are feeling and what they can do in the future to help stop bullying. The presence of bystanders provides an audience to students who bully, so encouraging these students to walk away and alert a trusted adult are actions that can give them power to stop future bullying.

In a qualitative study to explore the experiences of school nurses in managing bullying incidents, school nurse participants reported that managing bullying incidents was an expected part of their role (Pigozi & Bartoli, 2016). Despite receiving no antibullying training, the school nurses felt prepared to help students in bullying situations but needed information updates and professional development to develop skills in supporting students in bullying situations.

The school health office must be seen as a safe space for students to come when they feel threatened or in danger, a place where they can share their concerns with a trusted individual in private. The school nurse is in a prime position to partner with the interprofessional school team to support students who are experiencing bullying (Kvarme et al., 2020).

> **Practice Connection**
>
> Corporal punishment is when a child is physically punished (including paddling and/or spanking) in a school setting and is considered a form of child abuse. As of 2023, corporal punishment in schools was only banned in 27 states across the United States. While overall reports of corporal punishment are decreasing, there are disparities in students who received corporal punishment, with black students being 2.3 times more likely than white students to receive corporal punishment (U.S. Department of Education, Office for Civil Rights, 2023). The American Academy of Pediatrics' Council on School Health issued the following policy statement in 2023:
>
> *The use of corporal punishment in schools is not an effective or ethical method for management of behavior concerns and causes harm to students. The American Academy of Pediatrics recommends that corporal punishment in all school settings be abolished in all states by law and replaced by alternative forms of student behavior management. (Allison et al., 2023, para. 1)*
>
> School nurses should serve as advocates for the elimination of corporal punishments within their schools and states.

CHILD ABUSE

Child abuse or maltreatment can take many forms. The Child Abuse Prevention and Treatment Act defines *child abuse and neglect* as

> *any recent act or failure to act on the part of a parent or caretaker, which results in death, serious physical or emotional harm, sexual abuse, or exploitation . . . or an act or failure to act which presents an imminent risk of serious harm (U.S. Department of Health and Human Services [USDHHS], 2019, p. 4).*

Neglect occurs when a parent or caregiver fails to meet the basic physical, developmental, or emotional needs of a child. Physical child abuse occurs when a parent/guardian or caregiver intentionally causes bodily injury to a child. Sexual abuse or exploitation occurs when a parent/guardian or caregiver coerces or engages in any sexual conduct with a child. Emotional abuse is when a parent/guardian or caregiver's behavior affects a child's emotional development and self-esteem (Child Welfare Information Gateway, 2022). *Sex trafficking* is defined as the "recruitment, harboring, transportation, provision, or obtaining of a person for the purpose of a commercial sex act" (Child Welfare Information Gateway, 2020). Some states include parental substance use, addiction of the newborn, and abandonment in their definition of child abuse (Child Welfare Information Gateway, 2022). Table 11-3 details types of child abuse.

Prevalence

Child abuse is unacceptably prevalent in the United States and likely underreported. At least one in seven children have experienced child abuse in the past year in the United States (CDC, 2022a). Child protection (or protective) services agencies received an estimated 4.0 million referrals that involved approximately 7.2 million children during 2021 (USDHHS, 2023). Over 3 million children received either an investigation or an alternate response. Of these, there were 600,000 victims and 1,820 fatalities (USDHHS, 2023). The highest rate of victimization occurred in children during their first year of life (25.3 victims per 1,000 children). Rates of victimization vary by race and ethnicity with the rates being lowest in children who are Asian (1.4 per 1,000), white (7.1 per 1,000), and Hispanic (7.8) and highest in children who are black (13.0 per 1,000) and American Indian or Alaska Native (15.1 per 1,000) (USDHHS, 2023). Of all reported cases, 76% of children were victims of neglect, 16% experienced physical abuse, 10.1% were victims of sexual abuse, and 6.4% were victims of emotional abuse (USDHHS, 2023).

TABLE 11-3 Types and Methods of Child Abuse

Type of Abuse	Methods by Which Abuse Is Inflicted
Physical abuse	• Hit/punch/beat with hands or an object/slap/kick • Burn/scald/stab/cut • Poison • Asphyxiate/crush • Shake/throw the child/throw objects at the child • Scratch/pinch/twist/squeeze/grab • Keep in a cage or bound • Refusal to allow a runaway to return home • Expulsion from a home • Engaging in acts that result in physical illness or lie about symptoms that result in invasive medical treatments of the child (Munchausen syndrome by proxy, now called factitious disorder imposed on another)
Emotional/psychological abuse	• Verbally telling a child he or she is not loved, not worth anything, not important, not wanted, ugly • Constantly harshly criticizing, ridiculing • Ignoring the child • Withdrawing affection/lack of warmth and contact • Telling others of child's shortcomings • Ignoring the child's accomplishments • Blaming the child for everything • Threatening harm; terrorizing • Forcing the child to engage in illegal activities (e.g., selling drugs) • Making the child beg (for money or necessities) • Exposure to intimate partner violence • Exploitation
Sexual abuse	• Intercourse (vaginal or anal) • Oral sex • Penetrating with objects or animals • Masturbating in the child's presence or having the child assist • Manually stimulating/fondling of genitals • Sexual comment or conversation • Touching/fondling/kissing in a sexual manner/engaging in indecent exposure • Soliciting a minor over the Internet • Forcing the child to participate in video or photography of sexual acts • Forcing into child prostitution • Coercion of child to assist in any sexually explicit conduct • Exhibitionism • Exposing a child to pornography • Voyeurism (looking at a child's naked body)
Neglect	• Failing to provide adequate or appropriate food, clothing, warmth, shelter, education, or health care (including primary care and dental prophylaxis) • Failing to wash/bathe child or brush teeth • Providing an unsafe environment • Failing to provide adequate supervision • Abandoning the child • Failing to developmentally stimulate a child (failing to interact with the child, provide objects for play, or expose to books) • Failing to ensure that the child attends school and arrives ready to learn

Child Welfare Information Gateway (2022).

Did You Know?

The majority (67%) of all reports to child protection services come from professionals (a person where reporting is part of their job duties). Education personnel are responsible for 15.4% of reports and medical professionals are responsible for 12.2% of reports. It is essential that the school nurse knows how to make a report when abuse is suspected (USDHHS, 2023).

Consequences

There are serious physical, psychological, behavioral, and economic consequences from child maltreatment and child abuse (CDC, 2022a). Death is the most tragic outcome of child abuse/neglect. An estimated 1,820 children died from abuse in the United States during 2021 with most child fatalities (77.7%) involving at least one parent/guardian (USDHHS, 2023). Physical consequences range from bruises, burns, and broken bones to injury or neglect that interferes with brain development.

Child abuse is an ACE with known long-term physical, psychological, behavioral, and societal consequences (Child Welfare Information Gateway, 2019). These consequences may present immediately or manifest in adulthood. Psychological consequences of abuse include depression, anxiety, eating disorders, posttraumatic stress, memory problems, aggression, and suicide-related behaviors.

Role of the School Nurse

By virtue of their longitudinal and predictable presence in the lives of students they work with, school nurses are in a unique position to be a trusted resource for students in times of trouble. Because of this role, school nurses may be more likely to notice signs of abuse and be in a position to help. School nurses are designated as mandatory reporters in all 50 states, the District of Columbia, and the U.S. territories. They are required to report suspected child maltreatment to a child protection services agency (NASN, 2023b). Every state has enacted laws defining child maltreatment and child abuse and the criteria needed for outside intervention. Mandated reporters who fail to report suspected abuse and neglect may be considered an accessory to a crime (see Chapter 6). The mandatory reporting responsibility cannot be delegated to others.

It is the professional and ethical duty of school nurses to comply with mandated reporting requirements according to state laws and regulations, as well as school policies and procedures for reporting suspected child abuse. School nurses should consider the minimum facts needed to make decisions regarding whether to make a report to child protection services or law enforcement and how to keep the student safe. School mandated reporters should *not* take extra measures to investigate or validate the claim or suspicion of child abuse, which is the role of child protection services. In-depth interviewing about explicit details may compound the student's trauma. It is important to record what questions were asked and the responses the student gave, as well as the sources for all information. Document the exact statements used by the student; avoid documenting interpretations of the student's statements. School nurses *must* call the number in their state or county to report suspected abuse. The Childhelp National Child Abuse Hotline (2023) Web site provides a list of phone numbers for local child protective services.

Identification of Child Abuse

It is imperative that school nurses identify possible signs of abuse and neglect. Failing to do so exposes the student to continued risk for abuse that could involve other children in the family. Students experiencing abuse may demonstrate sudden changes in behavior or school performance such as learning problems or difficulty concentrating. They may appear overly compliant, passive, withdrawn, or watchful. Students may also avoid being at home by coming to school or extracurricular activities early and staying late or demonstrating a reluctance to be around a particular person. The school nurse should be attuned to children who seem frightened of their parents or adult caregivers or cry when it is time to go home. These adults may provide conflicting, unconvincing, or inconsistent explanations for their child's injury. They may also be defensive or repeatedly unavailable to discuss injuries or their child's health status with the school nurse. Students who are abused or neglected may lack adult supervision and exhibit physical or medical problems that have not received parental attention.

Students may be hesitant to disclose abuse for fear of being removed from their home, fear that no one will believe them, continued threats from the abuser against the student or their family, or feelings of deep shame. The student's decision to disclose is typically intentional when they have lost hope the abuse will stop without help (Thulin et al., 2020). When a student discloses abuse, it is essential that the school nurse stay calm and listen carefully. Praise the student for sharing and reinforce that what happened was not their fault. The school nurse can assure the student that the school health office is a safe place whenever they need help or want to talk, and that the adults at school care about them. It is essential that the school nurse never promise a student absolute confidentiality. The school nurse should inform the student that it is the school's job is to keep students safe. When the school nurse hears that someone is harming a student, it is their job to take measures to keep the student and/or others safe from harm, which includes telling other adults who can help. If the suspected abuser is a school employee, immediate administrative action should be taken.

The first and most appropriate intervention in a case of suspected child abuse is to treat the presenting problem such as bleeding, burns, or wounds with appropriate first aid, such as ice for areas of swelling, bandages for bleeding, or emotional support as needed. If additional medical attention is needed, steps should be taken to access those services. The primary importance is to protect the safety of the student.

Bruises are the most common sign of physical abuse in children. Therefore, school nurses should assess all bruises carefully. Bruises usually occur when the body encounters a hard object or surface with enough force to cause blood vessel damage and bleeding into subcutaneous tissue. Students who have been physically abused may have more than one bruise; the most common locations include the buttocks or genitalia, cheeks, neck, trunk, head, front of thighs, or upper arms (Johnson et al., 2021). School nurses should consider the student's typical developmental and activity levels when evaluating bruising in relationship to the explanation for the bruising. When assessing bruising in children, it is important to remember that a predisposition to bruising is associated with certain medical conditions. Box 11-5 identifies bruise locations that raise concern.

BOX 11-5

Red Flags When Assessing a Child With Bruising

Always consider age and developmental ability when assessing bruising.

Bruises in babies who are not yet crawling

Bruises located on the
- Ears, neck, feet, buttocks, or torso
- Front of the body and/or overlying bone

Bruises that are
- Unusually large or numerous
- Clustered or patterned (handprints, loop or belt marks, bite marks)

Bruises that do not fit the causal explanation provided by the child or caregiver

Johnson et al. (2021).

Additional signs of potential physical abuse include cuts, burns (especially those caused by cigarettes, hot implements, or scalding), rope burns on the wrists and ankles, missing patches of hair, blackened eyes, loss of or damage to teeth, human bite marks, and guarding of extremities or the abdomen. The quantity, pattern, and appearance of inflicted injuries should be assessed within the scope of the school nurse's practice and without further traumatizing the student. Students seen in the health office should routinely be assessed for malnutrition, body hygiene, and suspicious injuries.

Documentation of assessment and treatment should be included in the child's health record. Body-shaped diagrams assist in the accurate description and location of injuries or complaints. See Online Materials OM11-2 for examples of body-shaped diagrams. Many state reporting forms ask for detailed information and accurate assessment data. One of the hallmarks of abuse is that the stories told by the student or family members often do not match the degree of healing or the placement of injuries.

To conduct proper physical assessments, the school nurse must have appropriate space, equipment, and resources. The school nurse should plan for extra coverage of the school health office to avoid interruptions during the assessment, except for emergencies. The space needs to be private to ensure confidentiality; however, it may be advisable to have a second trusted school professional witness the assessment. The school nurse should use the appropriate assessment tools, including a measuring tape if needed. School nurses should exercise discretion, privacy, and dignity and ask the student permission to assess body parts covered by clothing, such as the back, abdomen, and upper arms and legs. School nurses should not assess beneath undergarments. The right of students to refuse examination should be respected. When injuries of serious concern are reported or suspected, the student should be referred for immediate medical evaluation.

Did You Know?

Factitious disorder imposed on another, previously called "Munchausen syndrome by proxy," is another type of child abuse (American Psychiatric Association, 2022). It involves a parent/guardian or caregiver who falsifies physical and/or psychological signs and symptoms in the child, implying that the child is ill and requires care. The resulting invasive diagnostic tests or treatment modalities by healthcare personnel cause a form of "abuse" to the child. The parent/guardian is often seen as overprotective and caring and thrives on the attention garnered from healthcare professionals. In some cases, harm to the child is fatal or causes permanent damage. There are two diagnoses that result: one for the child and one for the parent/guardian with therapeutic treatment needed for both.

Reporting

Once the assessment and initial treatment is complete, the school nurse should notify only those individuals identified by the school district and the state who need to be informed. The nurse's mandate in all states is to initiate a factual report to child protective services, or equivalent agency as per-state protocol. It then becomes the responsibility of that agency and/or law enforcement agencies to initiate and complete the investigation as to whether abuse exists; it is not the responsibility of the school nurse to conduct the investigation. No one, including school administrators, may absolve the school nurse of the mandate to report abuse.

Usually, a parent/guardian is called when a student appears with an injury or a health need. Should child abuse or neglect be suspected, child protective services may decide to intervene before the parent/guardian is called. If the parent/guardian does call or come for the student, the school nurse needs to note the response of the parent/guardian regarding the injury. Parents/guardians may deny knowledge of the injury or how it occurred; they may trivialize the problem; or they may delay seeking medical assistance. It is never the responsibility of the school nurse to inform parents/guardians that they are suspected of abusing their child. School policy and state law will dictate who needs to be informed. State and district policy will also indicate the form to be used to record the incident; usually documentation about reporting is kept separate from the student's health record whereas assessment and treatment documentation is in the child's health record. Confidentiality of information about both the child and the potential abuser must be maintained.

Student Support

Students who have been abused may believe that the abuse they experienced was deserved; they need to understand that the abuse was not their fault. These students should be praised for sharing and assured that the educational staff and support professionals at school care about them and will make every effort to ensure that school is a safe place for them. Students who have been abused need experiences that build positive self-esteem. School counseling or social work services may be needed to help students learn positive social skills and build a sense of trust with adults. Students can be taught to recognize their own needs and feelings, identify individuals in whom they can confide, and understand that they have the right to food, shelter, safety, love, and affection.

Prevention

In addition to helping students cope and heal after the trauma of abuse, schools should also employ primary prevention strategies to help prevent abuse from happening at all. One approach is to focus on five protective factors: parental resilience, social connections, knowledge of parenting and child development, social and emotional competence of children, and concrete support in times of need (Center for the Study of Social Policy, 2024). School nurses are encouraged to utilize this framework as well as additional education and skills to prevent and address abuse and maltreatment in the lives of the students and families that they work with (NASN, 2023b).

Multiple programs exist for educating children and adolescents about protecting themselves against abuse. It is always best to be proactive rather than reactive. Encouraging children and adolescents to believe that "My body is mine and no one can touch it without my permission" may begin to empower them to say "no." Programs are available for young children to be aware that if a touch doesn't feel right it probably is wrong, how to avoid being tricked by adults, how to fight if an abduction or assault is taking place, that children have a right to personal privacy during toileting or bathing and sleeping, and interventions to build self-confidence and self-esteem. Older children should be informed about how to protect themselves from abuse and about the importance of telling a trusted adult if they have any experiences that concern them.

The school nurse can collaborate with community organizations to raise awareness and reduce the incidence of child abuse and neglect. Parenting seminars might be provided by the school on topics related to developmental expectations of children of specific ages, age-appropriate discipline, and what families can do to prevent or respond to abuse in the household. Parents/guardians can be taught strategies to stay calm when angry or when the child has a temper tantrum, how to provide appropriate supervision and Internet safety, and how to model nonviolent anger management. The school nurse can assist directly by linking students who have been abused and their families to community resources, including securing a medical home. Above all, students and their parents/guardians need to be taught to respect themselves and respect each other.

Legal Issues

There are many issues related to the management of students who are abused or maltreated. Issues regarding where the record of the report is kept and parental access to reports are addressed under Family Educational Rights and Privacy Act (FERPA) laws (see Chapter 6). In 2013, FERPA was amended with the Uninterrupted Scholars Act, which allows education agencies, under specific conditions, to release personal identifiable information to local child welfare agencies or authorized tribal organizations without parental permission for the care and protection of the student (U.S. Public Law 112-278; U.S. Department of Education, Family Policy Compliance Office & Office of Special Education and Rehabilitative Services, 2014).

TEEN DATING VIOLENCE

Teen dating violence is a form of intimate partner violence among adolescents (13 to 18 years old) who are currently or were at one point in a romantic relationship (CDC, 2023c). There are multiple types of intimate partner violence, including physical, sexual, and psychological aggression, and stalking. Teen dating violence is considered an ACE with short-term and long-term effects. The 2019 Youth Risk Behavior Survey data revealed that teen dating violence is prevalent: about 1 in 12 high school students reported physical dating violence and/or sexual dating violence. Female students experience teen dating violence at rates higher than male students. Physical and sexual dating violence is a greater risk for students who identify as lesbian, transgender, queer, nonbinary, or questioning (CDC, 2023c). While there may be less of a power dynamic in teen dating violence compared with adult intimate partner violence, the use of control is common (Rainbow Services, n.d.). See Table 11-4 for a description of manifestations of teen dating violence.

Youth who experience teen dating violence are more likely to experience depressive and anxiety symptoms, engage in risk-taking behaviors, and consider suicide. Additionally, violence in adolescent relationships increases the likelihood that a perpetrator or victim will be involved in violence in relationships later in life (CDC, 2023a). School nurses must be able to identify indicators of dating violence (Table 11-5).

Did You Know?

Some families may have religious beliefs that dictate or restrict what types of health care they seek. This can be construed by some as child maltreatment. Many states have exemptions for parents/guardians who do not seek or follow medical treatment if it conflicts with their religious beliefs. This means that what might be considered neglect in one state is not defined that way in another state. (See Online Materials OM11-3.)

TABLE 11-4 Manifestations of Abuse in Teen Dating Violence

Dimensions of Abuse	Examples
Emotional/psychological	Name-calling via instant messaging; tell partner what they can wear; threaten to spread rumors; threaten to commit suicide if partner tries to leave relationship; damage partner's belongings; treat partner like a servant; insult in public
Social	Monitor cell phone usage; prevent partner from going to school; call or text message multiple times a day to monitor partner's whereabouts; get angry if partner is talking to someone else
Financial	Control what partner can or cannot buy; refuse to pay for things that the abuser insisted the partner purchase
Sexual	Insist on sexual acts; video/record (by cell phone) sexual acts then threaten to put them on the Internet; prevent partner from using birth control; force partner to get pregnant; force partner to use drugs before sexual activity
Physical	Threaten to hit; threaten with a weapon; hurt the partner's pet; hit; slap; kick; choke; restrain

Offenhauer & Buchalter (2011).

TABLE 11-5 Indicators of Teen Dating Violence

Domain/System	Clinical Symptoms and Signs
Social functioning	School failure, disengaged from school activities, lack of friends, lack of hobbies, binge drinking
Constitutional	Frequent headaches, sleep disorders, rapid weight gain or weight loss
Ears, nose, throat	Frequent ear pain (from being slapped); sore throats (forced oral sex); palatal bruising (forced oral sex)
Reproductive health	Multiple requests for pregnancy tests; inconsistent or no contraceptive use; frequent use of emergency contraception; pelvic pain; vaginal discharge; dysuria
Gastrointestinal	Nonspecific abdominal pains; constipation; rectal pain (from forced anal sex); irritable bowel syndrome
Musculoskeletal	Joint or limb pains; neck pain and low back pain; scratches or bruising
Mental health	Poor sleep; sad mood; suicidal ideation; substance use; withdrawn; depressed affect

Miller, E. (2017). With permission from *The Mass General Hospital for Children Adolescent Medicine Handbook* (2017). Goldstein, M. A. (Ed.). Springer International Publishing.

School nurses must be prepared to have sensitive and sometimes difficult conversations with students experiencing intimate partner violence. The school nurse should use the key concepts of trauma-informed care discussed later in this chapter to support students affected by violence and assist them to access the resources they need. Primary prevention practices include a trauma-informed school environment, a curriculum that includes the development of strong social emotional skills, and a school climate that is protective and safe for all students.

YOUTH INVOLVED IN THE JUSTICE SYSTEM

Youth can become involved in the justice system when they are accused or convicted of violating laws before their 18th birthday (U.S. Department of Justice, n.d.). Youth can also get involved with the justice system related to crimes specific to underage youth, including running away, violating curfew, underage drinking, and truancy. Law enforcement agencies, social service agencies, schools, parents/guardians, probation officers, and victims can refer juveniles to the court system through a formal complaint process. Acts committed by youth that violate the law are commonly referred to by law enforcement and the justice system as "juvenile delinquency."

Prevalence

In 2019, there were 696,620 arrests involving youth made in the United States (Puzzanchera et al., 2022). Arrests involving youth accounted for 7% of the total arrests of all individuals made in 2019. Between 2010 and 2019, arrests of youth were reduced by 58%, reflecting updates to the legal system and changes in policing strategies. Despite the overall drop in arrests involving youth, disparities are seen in who was arrested: 63% were white, 34% were black, and 19% were Hispanic. Placement in a correctional setting was more likely for older, male youths; however, the number of arrests involving males is decreasing more quickly than the number of arrests of females. Black youth account for only 17% of the total youth population; yet they were involved in 62% of arrests related to robbery and stolen property and 50% of arrests for motor vehicle theft and murder (Puzzanchera et al., 2022). Such disparities reflect deeper societal inequities in the United States.

In 2019, there were 36,479 youth in residential correctional placements. These settings include detention centers, shelters, group homes, residential treatment centers, and training schools. This represents a 66% decline from the all-time high incidence of 108,802 in 2000. Seventy percent of those who are in residential placement are between the ages of 15 and 17 years old, 33% are white, 41% are black, and 20% are Hispanic (Puzzanchera et al., 2022). Incarceration of a youth costs an average of $588 per youth per day or $214,620 per youth per year

(Justice Policy Institute, 2020), whereas alternative juvenile offender programs typically cost significantly less and include a range of services for both youth and families (American Civil Liberties Union, 2024).

Risk Factors

Before adolescence, parental influence has the highest relation to juvenile delinquency. At adolescence, peer group factors are the strongest known correlate of illegal behavior (Youth.gov, n.d.b.). In addition, adolescents who are involved in the justice system are at higher risk of repeat offenses with 55% being rearrested and 24% being reincarcerated within 1 year (Office of Juvenile Justice and Delinquency Prevention, 2020).

Socioeconomic status is a well-established risk factor for juvenile delinquency. Low socioeconomic status is thought to contribute to involvement with the justice system due to economic deprivation and the resultant impact on neighborhood quality (Rekker et al., 2015). Youths may begin to see criminal activity as an opportunity to increase family resources during times of economic deprivation. Teachers, school nurses, and administrations are often aware when students and their families are experiencing economic hardship; thus assisting families experiencing economic hardship to connect with community resources early may help offset delinquent activity.

Consequences

Being involved in the justice system has long-term effects on educational outcomes; students involved in the justice system are more likely to drop out of school (Rud et al., 2018). There are also high personal and societal costs connected to juvenile delinquency. Adolescents involved in the criminal justice system have a higher likelihood of being unemployed in young adulthood and have a harder time finding a job (Carter, 2019). Imprisoning young people has lifelong negative consequences by removing them from their families, disrupting their education, and exposing them to further trauma and violence. School nurses should be especially aware that adolescents involved in the justice system may be at higher risk of suicide and suicide-related behaviors.

It is essential to remember that youth of color (black and Hispanic) are arrested and incarcerated at disproportionate rates compared with white youth (Sickmund et al., 2021). Thus the long-term consequences of juvenile delinquency will be seen at higher rates in these populations. As a matter of social justice, greater investments in low-income communities of color are needed to reduce inequities in social determinants of health and social determinants of education to provide better opportunities for at-risk youth.

Interventions

There is a strong connection between juvenile delinquency and school dropout. Therefore, it is essential that school-based interventions focus on primary prevention through education and mitigation of risk factors. The Office of Juvenile Justice and Delinquency Prevention recommends multicomponent classroom programs that promote social competence and integrate conflict resolution skills and bullying prevention strategies (Youth.gov, n.d.a.). Model programs are available on the Office of Juvenile Justice and Delinquency Prevention Web site, including school-based prevention programs.

TRAUMA-INFORMED CARE

A trauma-informed approach is recommended to address the needs of all students who have experienced trauma caused by violence inside and/or outside the school setting. *Trauma-informed care* is an interventional approach that addresses childhood trauma and ACEs. It is a framework that provides individuals with a basic understanding of trauma and how trauma can affect families, groups, communities, and individuals. Its emphasis is on physical, psychological, and emotional safety for both the providers and survivors with the hope that the survivors can rebuild a sense of control and empowerment (Substance Abuse and Mental Health Services Administration [SAMHSA], 2014). Trauma-informed care seeks to address the needs of the student population from a primary, secondary, and tertiary level of prevention; thus it can be used comprehensively in schools while also addressing needs of individual students experiencing post-traumatic stress disorder (Lorig et al., 2022). A trauma-informed school is one in which all staff have been trained to recognize and respond to the impact of trauma. School nurses should use the trauma-informed care approach to recognize and address signs of trauma in the students, families, and communities they serve (NASN, 2021a).

There are six key principles of a trauma-informed care approach: (1) safety; (2) trustworthiness and transparency; (3) peer support; (4) collaboration and mutuality; (5) empowerment, voice, and choice; and (6) cultural, historical, and gender issues (SAMHSA, 2014). For the approach to work, students and staff must feel physically and psychologically safe in the physical setting and in interpersonal interactions. This primary prevention approach creates a school climate that is supportive and safe for all students and staff. At the secondary level of prevention, the school nurse may be the first to identify and support students who have been or are being exposed to trauma by building trusting relationships and establishing the school health office as a safe and inclusive place. At the tertiary level of prevention, schools need to provide intensive treatment and wraparound support services for students who have been exposed to trauma. School nurses can be especially supportive in connecting students and families to community resources including behavioral health therapy and support groups. The process of facilitating healing must avoid retraumatization. Trauma-informed care focuses on the strengths and resilience of students, families, and staff to help them move in a more positive direction (SAMHSA, 2014).

Educational professionals, including school nurses, who are close to the experience of trauma happening in students and others may experience *secondary traumatic stress* (National Child Traumatic Stress Network, n.d.a). To prevent secondary trauma, school nurses and other school staff who provide trauma-informed care should promote self-care, maintain adequate support systems, and set clear limits and boundaries both at work and at home.

CONCLUSION

Violence and child abuse are serious problems in society and in the school environment. School staff must be aware of the impact of ACEs on the physical and mental health of students and implement interventions that prevent and reduce harm and promote healing. Adults must be positive role models in managing relationships, resolving conflicts, and managing emotions. They must also teach students the skills needed to promote safety and prevent violence. Emphasizing caring, respect, open communication, and a willingness to help are important factors in creating a culture of safety. Building a climate of tolerance, safety, and respect for others requires a whole school effort. The school nurse plays an integral role in leading these vital efforts.

The Editors gratefully acknowledge the work of previous chapter authors, Shirley Countryman Gordon and Janice Selekman.

References

Allison, M. A., Beers, N., Peterson, J. W., & Council on School Health. (2023, August 21). Corporal punishment in schools. *Pediatrics, 152*(3), e2023063284. https://doi.org/10.1542/peds.2023-063284

American Civil Liberties Union. (2024). *Alternatives to youth incarceration.* https://www.aclu.org/issues/juvenile-justice/youth-incarceration/alternatives-youth-incarceration

American Psychiatric Association. (2022). *Diagnostic and statistical manual of mental disorders: Text revision* (5th ed.). Author. https://doi.org/10.1176/appi.books.9780890425787

American School Counselor Association. (2024.) *Helping students after a school shooting.* https://www.schoolcounselor.org/Publications-Research/Publications/Free-ASCA-Resources/After-a-School-Shooting

Barnett, J., Fisher, K., O'Connell, N., & Franco, K. (2019). Promoting upstander behavior to address bullying in schools. *Middle School Journal, 50*(1), 6–11. https://doi.org/10.1080/00940771.2018.1550377

Bellis, M. A., Hughes, K., Ford, K., Ramos Rodriguez, G., Sethi, D., & Passmore, J. (2019). Life course health consequences and associated annual costs of adverse childhood experiences across Europe and North America: A systematic review and meta-analysis. *The Lancet Public Health, 4*(10), e517–e528. https://doi.org/10.1016/S2468-2667(19)30145-8

Bleakley, P., & Bleakley, C. (2018). School resource officers, "zero tolerance" and the enforcement of compliance in the American education system. *Interchange, 49*(2), 247–261. https://doi.org/10.1007/s10780-018-9326-5

Camodeca, M., & Nava, E. (2022). The long-term effects of bullying, victimization, and bystander behavior on emotion regulation and its physiological correlates. *Journal of Interpersonal Violence, 37*(3–4). https://doi.org/10.1177/0886260520934438

Carter, A. (2019). The consequences of adolescent delinquent behavior for adult employment outcomes. *Journal of Youth and Adolescence, 48*(1), 17–29. https://doi.org/10.1007/s10964-018-0934-2

Center for Pediatric Traumatic Stress. (2021). *Basics of trauma-informed care. Health Care Toolbox, Children's Hospital of Philadelphia.* https://www.healthcaretoolbox.org/

Center for the Study of Social Policy. (2024). *Strengthening families.* https://cssp.org/our-work/project/strengthening-families/

Centers for Disease Control and Prevention. (2021a). *About the CDC-Kaiser ACE study.* https://www.cdc.gov/violenceprevention/aces/about.html

Centers for Disease Control and Prevention. (2021b). *Fast fact: Preventing school violence.* https://www.cdc.gov/violenceprevention/youthviolence/schoolviolence/fastfact.html

Centers for Disease Control and Prevention. (2021c). *Violence prevention. Fast fact: Bullying prevention.* https://www.cdc.gov/violenceprevention/youthviolence/bullyingresearch/fastfact.html

Centers for Disease Control and Prevention. (2022a). *Fast facts: Preventing child abuse and neglect.* https://www.cdc.gov/violenceprevention/childabuseandneglect/index.html

Centers for Disease Control and Prevention. (2022b). *School connectedness helps students thrive.* https://www.cdc.gov/healthyyouth/protective/school_connectedness.htm

Centers for Disease Control and Prevention. (2023a). *Fast facts: Preventing adverse childhood experiences (ACEs).* https://www.cdc.gov/violenceprevention/aces/fastfact.html

Centers for Disease Control and Prevention. (2023b). *Fast facts: Preventing bullying.* https://www.cdc.gov/violenceprevention/youthviolence/bullyingresearch/fastfact.html#:~:text=CDC%20defines%20bullying%20as%20any,highly%20likely%20to%20be%20repeated

Centers for Disease Control and Prevention. (2023c). *Fast facts: Preventing teen dating violence.* https://www.cdc.gov/violenceprevention/intimatepartnerviolence/teendatingviolence/fastfact.html

Centers for Disease Control and Prevention. (2023d). *School connectedness helps students thrive.* https://www.cdc.gov/healthyyouth/protective/school_connectedness.htm

Child and Adolescent Health Measurement Initiative. (2021). *2020–2021 National Survey of Children's Health (NSCH) data query.* Data Resource Center of Child & Adolescent Health. U.S. Department of Health and Human Services, Health Resources and Services Administration, Maternal and Child Health Bureau. www.childhealthdata.org

Childhelp. (2023). *Childhelp national child abuse hotline.* https://www.childhelp.org/hotline/

Child Welfare Information Gateway. (2019). *Long-term consequences of child abuse and neglect.* U.S. Department of Health and Human Services, Administration for Children and Families, Children's Bureau.

Child Welfare Information Gateway. (2020). *Definitions of human trafficking.* U.S. Department of Health and Human Services, Administration for Children and Families, Children's Bureau.

Child Welfare Information Gateway. (2022). *Definitions of child abuse and neglect.* U.S. Department of Health and Human Services, Administration for Children and Families, Children's Bureau. https://www.childwelfare.gov/topics/systemwide/laws-policies/statutes/define/

Cross, S., Gottfredson, D., & Greene, A. (2021). Are effects of school resource officers moderated by student race and ethnicity? *Crime and Delinquency, 68*(3), 381–408. https://doi.org/10.1177/001112872199934

Darling-Hammond, S., Fronius, T. A., Sutherland, H., Guckenburg, S., Petrosino, A., & Hurley, N. (2020). Effectiveness of restorative justice in US K-12 schools: A review of quantitative research. *California School Psychologist, 24*(3), 295–308. https://doi.org/10.1007/s40688-020-00290-0

David-Ferdon, C., Vivolo-Kantor, A. M., Dahlberg, L. L., Marshall, K. J., Rainford, N., & Hall, J. E. (2016). *A comprehensive technical package for the prevention of youth violence and associated risk behaviors.* National Center for Injury Prevention and Control, Centers for Disease Control and Prevention. https://stacks.cdc.gov/view/cdc/43085

Educational Fund to Stop Gun Violence. (2021). *Public health approach to gun violence prevention.* https://efsgv.org/learn/learn-more-about-gun-violence/public-health-approach-to-gun-violence-prevention/

Everytown. (2023). *Gun safety policies save lives.* https://everytownresearch.org/rankings/

Everytown. (2024). *Gunfire on school grounds in the United States.* https://everytownresearch.org/maps/gunfire-on-school-grounds/

Felitti, V. J., Anda, R. F., Nordenberg, D., Williamson, D. F., Spitz, A. M., Edwards, V., Koss, M. P., & Marks, J. S. (1998). Relationship of childhood abuse and household dysfunction to many of the leading causes of death in adults: The Adverse Childhood Experiences (ACE) Study. *American Journal of Preventive Medicine, 14*(4), 245–258. https://doi.org/10.1016/S0749-3797(98)00017-8

Futures Without Violence. (2018). *Childhood trauma: Changing minds.* https://www.futureswithoutviolence.org/wp-content/uploads/Teachers%20English%20.pdf

Gage, N. A., Whitford, D. K., Katsiyannis, A., Adams, S., & Jasper, A. (2019). National analysis of the disciplinary exclusion of black students with and without disabilities. Journal of Child and Family Studies, 28, 1754–1764. https://doi. org/10.1007/s10826-019-01407-7e

Gini, G., & Espelage, D. L. (2014). Peer victimization, cyberbullying, and suicide risk in children and adolescents. *JAMA, 312*(5), 545–546. doi:10.1001/jama.2014.3212

Gladden, R., Vivolo-Kantor, A., Hambuger, M., & Lumpkin, C. (2014). *Bullying surveillance among youths: Uniform definitions for public health and recommended data elements, version 1.0.* https://www.cdc.gov/violenceprevention/pdf/bullying-definitions-final-a.pdf

Huang, F. L., & Cornell, D. G. (2021). Teacher support for zero tolerance is associated with higher suspension rates and lower feelings of safety. *School Psychology Review, 50*(2–3), 388–405. https://doi.org/10.1080/2372966X.2020.1832865

Hudson, D. L. (2016). Is cyberbullying free speech? *ABA Journal.* http://www.abajournal.com/magazine/article/is_cyberbullying_free_speech

Irwin, V., Wang, K., Cui, J., & Thompson, A. (2022). *Report on indicators of school crime and safety: 2021* (NCES 2022-092/NCJ 304625). National Center for Education Statistics, U.S. Department of Education, and Bureau of Justice Statistics, Office of Justice Programs, U.S. Department of Justice. https://nces.ed.gov/pubs2022/2022092.pdf

Johnson, E. L., Lee Jones, A., & Maguire, S. (2021). Bruising: The most common injury in physical child abuse. *Paediatrics and Child Health, 31*(11), 403–409. https://doi.org/10.1016/j.paed.2021.08.001

Justice Policy Institute. (2020). *Sticker shock 2020: The cost of youth incarceration.* Author.

Kim, J., Walsh, E., Pike, K., & Thompson, E. A. (2020). Cyberbullying and victimization and youth suicide risk: The buffering effects of school connectedness. *The Journal of School Nursing, 36*(4), 251–257. https://doi.org/10.1177/1059840518824395

King, K. (2014). Violence in the school setting: A school nurse perspective. *Online Journal of Issues in Nursing, 19*(1). https://doi. 10.3912/OJIN.Vol19No01Man04

Kvarme, L. G., Misvær, N., Valla, L., Myhre, M. C., Holen, S., & Sagatun, Å. (2020). Bullying in school: Importance of and challenges involved in talking to the school nurse. *Journal of School Nursing, 36*(6), 451–457. https://doi.org/10.1177/1059840519846649

LiCalsi, C., Osher, D., & Bailey, P. (2021). An empirical examination of the effects of suspension and suspension severity on behavioral and academic outcomes. *American Institutes for Research.* https://www.air.org/sites/default/files/2021-08/NYC-Suspension-Effects-Behavioral-Academic-Outcomes-August-2021.pdf

Lorig, C. E., Krupina, A., & Varjas, K. (2022). Social justice and trauma-informed care in schools. *International Journal of School Social Work, 6*(2). https://doi.org/10.4148/2161-4148.1080

Meadan, H., Auvazo, S., & Ostrosky, M. (2016). The ABCs of challenging behavior: Understanding basic concepts. *Young Exceptional Children, 19*(1), 3–15.

Merrick, M. T., Ford, D. C., Ports, K. A., Guinn, A. S., Chen, J., Klevens, J., Metzler, M., Jones, C., Simon, T., Daniel, V., Ottley, P., & Mercy, J. A. (2019). Vital signs: Estimated proportion of adult health problems attributable to adverse childhood experiences and implications for prevention—25 States, 2015–2017. *Morbidity and Mortality Weekly Report, 68*, 999–1005. http://dx.doi.org/10.15585/mmwr.mm6844e1

Miller, E. (2017). Adolescent relationship abuse in clinical settings. Opportunities for prevention and intervention. In M. A. Goldstein (Ed.). *The Mass General Hospital for Children adolescent medicine handbook* (2nd ed., pp. 327–334). Springer International Publishing. https://doi.org/10.1007/978-3-319-45778-9

National Academies of Sciences, Engineering, and Medicine. (2016). *Preventing bullying through science, policy, and practice.* The National Academies Press.

National Association of School Nurses. (2021a). *Trauma informed care.* https://www.nasn.org/glossary/trauma-informed-care

National Association of School Nurses. (2021b). *Use of restraint and seclusion in the school setting* (Position Statement). Author. https://www.nasn.org/nasn-resources/professional-practice-documents/position-statements/ps-restraints

National Association of School Nurses. (2022). *School nursing: Scope and standards of practice* (4th ed.). Author.

National Association of School Nurses. (2023a, June). *Bullying and cyberbullying—Prevention in schools* (Position Statement). https://www.nasn.org/nasn-resources/professional-practice-documents/position-statements/ps-bullying

National Association of School Nurses. (2023b). *Prevention and intervention of child maltreatment* (Position Statement). https://www.nasn.org/nasn-resources/professional-practice-documents/position-statements/ps-child-maltreatment

National Association of School Nurses. (2024). A contemporary framework update for today's school nursing landscape: Introducing the School Nursing Practice Framework. *NASN School Nurse, 39*(3), 140–147. https://www.doi.org/10.1177/1942602X241241092

National Association of School Psychologists. (2015). *School violence prevention: Brief facts and tips.* https://www.nasponline.org/resources-and-publications/resources-and-podcasts/school-safety-and-crisis/school-violence-resources/school-violence-prevention#:~:text=Monitor%20school%20parking%20lots%20and,training%20to%20all%20staff%20members

National Association of School Psychologists. (2021). *Behavioral threat assessment and management (BTAM): A school safety and crisis resource.* Author.

National Center for Education Statistics. (n.d.). *Glossary: Gang.* https://nces.ed.gov/programs/coe/glossary#g

National Center for Education Statistics. (2022a). *Condition of education: Bullying at school and electronic bullying.* U.S. Department of Education, Institute of Education Sciences. https://nces.ed.gov/programs/coe/indicator/a10

National Center for Education Statistics. (2022b). *Condition of education: Safety and security practices at public schools.* U.S. Department of Education, Institute of Education Sciences. https://nces.ed.gov/programs/coe/indicator/a19

National Center for Education Statistics. (2022c). *Condition of education: Students' reports of gangs at school.* U.S. Department of Education, Institute of Education Sciences. https://nces.ed.gov/programs/coe/indicator/a08

National Child Traumatic Stress Network. (n.d.a). *Secondary traumatic stress.* https://www.nctsn.org/trauma-informed-care/secondary-traumatic-stress

National Child Traumatic Stress Network. (n.d.b). *Trauma types.* https://www.nctsn.org/what-is-child-trauma/trauma-types

National Crime Prevention Council. (n.d.). *Straight talk about youth gangs: Facts for educators.* http://archive.ncpc.org/programs/teens-crime-and-the-community/publications-1/adult2-pdf.pdf

Offenhauer, P. & Buchalter, A. (2011). *Teen dating violence: A literature review and annotated bibliography.* U.S. Department of Justice. https://www.ncjrs.gov/pdffiles1/nij/grants/235368.pdf

Office of Juvenile Justice and Delinquency Prevention. (2020). *Research central: measuring what works in juvenile reentry.* https://ojjdp.ojp.gov/newsletter/ojjdp-news-glance-novemberdecember-2020/research-central-measuring-what-works-juvenile-reentry

PACER's National Bullying Prevention Center. (n.d.). *Why do we use "target" vs. "victim" and "child who bullies" vs. "bully"?* https://www.pacer.org/bullying/info/questions-answered/target-vs-victim.asp

Padgett, S., & Notar, C. (2013). Bystanders are the key to stopping bullying. *Universal Journal of Educational Research, 1*(2), 33–41. https//: doi.10.13189/ujer.2013.010201

Pew Research Center. (2018). *Teens, social media and technology 2018.* https://www.pewresearch.org/internet/2018/05/31/teens-social-media-technology-2018/

Pigozi, P. L., & Bartoli, J. (2016). School nurse experiences in dealing with bullying situations. *Journal of School Nursing, 32*(3), 177–185. https://doi:10.1177/1059840515613140

Prince, A., & Gothberg, J. (2019). Seclusion and restraint of students with disabilities: A 1-year legal review. *Journal of Disability Policy Studies, 30*(2), 118–124. https://doi.org/10.1177/1044207319854182

Puzzanchera, C., Hockenberry, S., & Sickmund, M. (2022). *Youth and the juvenile justice system: 2022 National Report.* National Center for Juvenile Justice. https://ojjdp.ojp.gov/publications/2022-national-report.pdf

Rainbow Services. (n.d.). *Teen dating violence awareness month.* https://rainbowservicesdv.org/teen-dating-violence-awareness-month-2/

Rekker, R., Pardini, D., Keijsers, L., Branje, S., Loeber, R., & Meeus, W. (2015). Moving in and out of poverty: The within-individual association between socioeconomic status and juvenile delinquency. *PLoS One, 10*(11), e0136461. https://doi:10.1371/journal.pone.0136461

Roberts, B. K., Nofi, C. P., Cornell, E., Kapoor, S., Harrison, L., & Sathya, C. (2023). Trends and disparities in firearm deaths among children. *Pediatrics (Evanston), 152*(3), e2023061296. https://doi.org/10.1542/peds.2023-061296

Rud, I., van Klaveren, C., Groot, W., & van den Brink, H. M. (2018). What drives the relationship between early criminal involvement and school dropout? *Journal of Quantitative Criminology, 34*(1), 139–166. https://doi.org/10.1007/s10940-016-9326-5

Saracho, O. (2016). *Contemporary perspectives on research on bullying and victimization in early childhood education.* Information Age Publishing, Incorporated.

Schildkraut, J., & Grogan, K. (2019). *Are metal detectors effective at making schools safer?* WestEd. https://files.eric.ed.gov/fulltext/ED595716.pdf

Selekman, J., Monforto, K., & Selekman, D. (2023a). Violence toward and by youth. Part I: Looking for the "whys." *NASN School Nurse, 38*(4). https://doi.org/10.1177/1942602X231154549

Selekman, J., Monforto, K., & Selekman, D. (2023b). Violence toward and by youth. Part II: Recommendations for violence interventions in the school setting. *NASN School Nurse, 38*(4). https://doi.org/10.1177/1942602X231154547

Sickmund, M., Sladky, T. J., Puzzanchera, C., & Kang, W. (2021). *Easy access to the census of juveniles in residential placement.* National Center for Juvenile Justice. https://www.ojjdp.gov/ojstatbb/ezacjrp/

Steiner, R. J., Sheremenko, G., Lesesne, C., Dittus, P. J., Sieving, R. E., & Ethier, K. A. (2019). Adolescent connectedness and adult health outcomes. *Pediatrics, 144*(1), e20183766. https://doi.org/10.1542/peds.2018-3766

Stopbullying.gov. (2021a). *Bystanders are essential to bullying prevention and intervention.* U.S. Department of Health and Human Services. https://www.stopbullying.gov/resources/research-resources/bystanders-are-essential

Stopbullying.gov. (2021b). *What is cyberbullying.* U.S. Department of Health and Human Services. https://www.stopbullying.gov/cyberbullying/what-is-it

Stopbullying.gov. (2021c). *Respond to bullying.* U.S. Department of Health and Human Services. https://www.stopbullying.gov/prevention/on-the-spot

Stopbullying.gov. (2021d). *Bullying: Who is at risk.* U.S. Department of Health and Human Services. https://www.stopbullying.gov/bullying/at-risk

Stopbullying.gov. (2022a). *Key components in state anti-bullying laws, policies and regulations.* U.S. Department of Health and Human Services. https://www.stopbullying.gov/resources/laws/key-components

Stopbullying.gov. (2022b). *What is bullying?* U.S. Department of Health and Human Services. https://www.stopbullying.gov

Substance Abuse and Mental Health Services Administration. (2014). *SAMHSA's concept of trauma and guidance for a trauma-informed approach.* HHS Publication No. (SMA), 14-4884.

Substance Abuse and Mental Health Services Administration. (2022). *Trauma and violence.* https://www.samhsa.gov/trauma-violence

Swanson, S. A., Eyllon, M., Sheu, Y.-H., & Miller, M. (2021). Firearm access and adolescent suicide risk: Toward a clearer understanding of effect size. *Injury Prevention, 27*(3), 264–270. https://doi.org/10.1136/injuryprev-2019-043605

Swedo, E. A., Aslam, M. V., Dahlberg, L. L., Holditch Niolon, P., Guinn, A. S., Simon, T. R., & Mercy, J. A. (2023). Prevalence of adverse childhood experiences among U.S. adults—Behavioral Risk Factor Surveillance System, 2011–2020. *Morbidity and Mortality Weekly Report, 72,* 707–715. http://dx.doi.org/10.15585/mmwr.mm7226a2

Thulin, J., Kjellgren, C., & Nilsson, D. (2020). Children's disclosure of physical abuse—the process of disclosing and the responses from social welfare workers. *Northern Ireland Journal of Multi-Disciplinary Child Care Practice, 26*(3), 285–299. https://doi.org/10.1080/13575279.2018.1555139

Tinker v. Des Moines Independent Community School District, 393 U.S. 503. (1969). https://supreme.justia.com/cases/federal/us/393/503/

U.S. Department of Education. (2012). *Restraint and seclusion: Resource document.* Washington, DC: Author.

U.S. Department of Education, Family Policy Compliance Office & Office of Special Education and Rehabilitative Services. (2014). *Guidance document on the Uninterrupted Scholars Act (USA) (Public Law 112-278).* https://studentprivacy.ed.gov/sites/default/files/resource_document/file/uninterrupted-scholars-act-guidance.pdf

U.S. Department of Education, Office for Civil Rights. (2023). *Corporal punishment in public schools.* https://www2.ed.gov/about/offices/list/ocr/docs/corporal-punishment-part-4.pdf

U.S. Department of Health and Human Services, Administration for Children and Families, Administration on Children, Youth and Families, Children's Bureau. (2019). *Child Abuse Prevention and Treatment Act. P.L. 115-271.* https://www.acf.hhs.gov/sites/default/files/documents/cb/capta.pdf

U.S. Department of Health and Human Services, Administration for Children and Families, Administration on Children, Youth and Families, Children's Bureau. (2023). *Child maltreatment 2021.* https://www.acf.hhs.gov/cb/data-research/child-maltreatment

U.S. Department of Homeland Security. (n.d.a). *Active shooter: How to respond.* https://www.dhs.gov/xlibrary/assets/active_shooter_booklet.pdf

U.S. Department of Homeland Security. (n.d.b). *Pathway to violence.* https://www.dhs.gov/sites/default/files/publications/dhs-pathway-to-violence-09-15-16-508.pdf

U.S. Department of Justice. (n.d.). *CRM 1-499, 38. "Juvenile" defined.* Criminal Resource Manual. https://www.justice.gov/usam/criminal-resource-manual-38-juvenile-defined

U.S. Department of Justice, Community Oriented Policing Services (n.d.). *Supporting safe schools.* https://cops.usdoj.gov/supportingsafeschools

U.S. Surgeon General's Advisory. (2023). *Social media and youth mental health.* https://www.hhs.gov/sites/default/files/sg-youth-mental-health-social-media-advisory.pdf

Wang, K., Kemp, J., & Burr, R. (2022). *Crime, violence, discipline, and safety in U.S. public schools in 2019–20: Findings from the School Survey on Crime and Safety* (NCES 2022-029). U.S. Department of Education. Washington, DC: National Center for Education Statistics. https://nces.ed.gov/pubs2022/2022029.pdf

Xu, M., Macrynikola, N., Waseem, M., & Miranda, R. (2020). Racial and ethnic differences in bullying: Review and implications for intervention. *Aggression and Violent Behavior, 50,* 101340. https://doi.org/10.1016/j.avb.2019.101340

Youth.gov. (n.d.a). *Prevention and early intervention.* https://youth.gov/youth-topics/juvenile-justice/prevention-and-early-intervention

Youth.gov. (n.d.b). *Risk and protective factors.* https://youth.gov/youth-topics/juvenile-justice/risk-and-protective-factors

Zych, I., Farrington, D., & Ttofi, M. (2019). Protective factors against bullying and cyberbullying: A systematic review of meta-analyses. *Aggression and Violent Behavior, 4,* 4–19. https://doi.org/10.1016/j.avb.2018.06.008

Chapter 12

Health Promotion and Screening in Schools

Eden J. Donahue ▪ Cynthia Galemore

CHAPTER OUTLINE

Health promotion, screening, surveillance, and outreach activities are practice components within the Community/Public Health principle of the National Association of School Nurses (NASN) *School Nursing Practice Framework* (NASN, 2024); they are essential roles of the school nurse. Health promotion is also a standard of professional school nursing practice. Standard of School Nursing Practice 5B: Health Teaching and Health Promotion states, "The school nurse employs strategies to improve the health and safety of students, family, group, school community, or population" (NASN, 2022a, p. 69). The World Health Organization (WHO) defines health promotion as "the process of enabling people to increase control over, and to improve, their health" (WHO, n.d.a, para. 1), and it involves a purposeful process of assessment and intervention for individuals, groups, and communities focused on improving overall wellness.

Public health initially focused on prevention of disease. However, the past 30 years has seen a shift to an emphasis on health promotion and individual responsibility as evidenced by the *Healthy People* report from the Surgeon General initiated in 1979 (Kleman & Smith, 2022). The WHO further defines health promotion as

> *cover[ing] a wide range of social and environmental interventions that are designed to benefit and protect individual people's health and quality of life by addressing and preventing the root causes of ill health, not just focusing on treatment and cure. (WHO, n.d.a, para. 1)*

The WHO definition aligns with the foundational principles of the *Healthy People 2030* (Office of Disease Prevention and Health Promotion, n.d.a) that include individual and community health and well-being as essential, that the opportunity to reach a state of health must be equitable, and that in order to improve, health prevention must be addressed at all levels and across all sectors. Health promotion includes more than just providing education. Because most children attend school and schools are strategically placed to reach the community, the school is an ideal setting for health promotion activities. Schools are also an ideal place to conduct screenings for prevalent health conditions in the student population.

Health promotion and screening activities entail primary and secondary levels of prevention. For example, primary prevention strives to maintain wellness (e.g., applying dental sealants, promoting dental hygiene), whereas secondary prevention strives for early detection and treatment of health conditions (e.g., identifying dental caries, referring for evalution). In addition to call-to-action reports and goals, such as *Healthy People*, health promotion strategies are directed at the public through the establishment of minimum standards often in the form of laws and regulations such as the Clean Air Act (National Center for Environmental Health [NCEH, 2017). Examples of agencies that establish regulations to protect health in the United States are the Food and Drug Administration and the Environmental Protection Agency. Protection regulations most familiar to school nurses include mandatory immunizations for school attendance. By combining health maintenance and health promotion strategies, school nurses move beyond delivery of health care to a more proactive approach with a focus on population health. While health promotion and health protection involve different strategies, together they provide overlapping support toward improved health (e.g., encouraging annual flu shots and frequent hand washing during disease outbreaks).

School nurses integrate their experience and expertise of working with youth, their extensive knowledge about health, and their understanding of the educational environment to implement evidence-based health promotion strategies within their school and community. School nurses are well positioned to promote health by framing research questions, participating in gathering evidence, and sharing results. The effectiveness of health promotion interventions increases when approached from multiple levels, including the classroom and community. The most effective approach is one that is holistic, varied, and developmentally and culturally appropriate.

CONCEPTS RELATED TO HEALTH PROMOTION

The opportunity to support healthy practices in students is one of many characteristics that draw nurses to the specialty practice of school nursing. Health promotion incorporates the subjective and objective concepts of *health, wellness, illness,* and *disease.* Examining these concepts enhances the nurse's understanding of health promotion and how to effectively promote the health of students, families, and school personnel.

Health

The most commonly used definition of *health* is in the preamble of the WHO Constitution dating back to 1946: "a state of complete physical, mental and social well-being and not merely the absence of disease or infirmity (2020a, p. 1)". Defined in this way, health is a personalized, subjective experience that incorporates the contextual factors of psychological and social health with the objective components of physical health. Kleman and Smith (2022) add to the WHO definition, emphasizing that health is experienced within a developmental context comprised of individual responsibilities and dependent on "collective action to ensure a society and an environment in which people can act responsibly to support health" (p. 6).

The degree of health is usually described as excellent, good, fair, or bad. These modifiers are individualized and subjective based on a variety of factors such as age, sex, race, income, diet, exercise, location of home, accessibility of health care, and health behaviors (Kleman & Smith, 2022; Rector, 2021) and the evaluator's (including oneself or the healthcare provider's) source of comparison. The WHO prerequisites for health are similar, but add the following: "peace, shelter, education, food, income, a stable eco-system, sustainable resources, social justice, and equity" (WHO, n.d.b, para. 5). The degree of health can fluctuate over time and includes adaptation to disease or disability.

Wellness and Well-Being

According to the Global Wellness Institute (n.d.), *wellness* is "the active pursuit of activities, choices and lifestyles that lead to a state of holistic health" (para. 2). This definition highlights two important aspects of wellness: that of it being an *active pursuit* (a capacity to develop) and that of it being *holistic or multidimensional,* going beyond a focus on physical health and including dimensions such as mental, spiritual, emotional, social, and environmental health. Similarly, yet not the same, well-being is agreed on to include the presence of a positive mood, accompanied with feelings of satisfaction, fulfillment, and positive functioning (National Center for Chronic Disease Prevention & Health Promotion [NCCDPHP], 2018a). Wellness can be measured in terms of quality of life—a person's potential to lead a fulfilling and productive life (Rector, 2021) and results in an outcome of optimal well-being (Global Wellness Institute, n.d.). Students model wellness and well-being when they proactively, and with feelings of satisfaction, make healthy choices related to their various roles as student, child, sibling, friend, and classmate.

Illness

Illness is a personalized, subjective experience or response to either a disease or an emotional state and includes a sense of not being in good health. With illness, the individual is in an imbalanced, unsustainable relationship with the environment where there is a mismatch between a person's needs and the resources available to meet those needs (Kleman & Smith, 2022). Obstacles to such resources include limited access to care, insufficient financial resources, inadequate coping skills, language barriers, and limited health literacy, to name a few. Though illness is independently perceived and experienced, it is a signal that the current balance is not working. What constitutes illness for one individual may be a mere inconvenience for another. One student with symptoms of upper respiratory infection will seek out the school nurse for treatment, whereas another student with the same symptoms continues through the day viewing the symptoms as a mere nuisance. Illness is on a continuum from acute to chronic and has social, psychological, and spiritual components.

Disease

Disease and illness are not the same, and disease is not the opposite of health. One can have a disease and be in a state of good health and not be ill. Disease refers to an alteration in normal physiology. Kleman and Smith (2022) define *disease* as "the failure of a person's adaptive mechanisms to counteract stimuli and stresses adequately, resulting in functional or structural disturbances" (p. 6). As such, disease is a medical term and indicates the presence of a recognized deviation in anatomy or physiology—an objective manifestation of pathophysiology that may interfere with typical functioning.

Wellness-Illness Continuum

The *wellness-illness continuum*, also referred to as the health continuum, is a dichotomous depiction between the relationship of health and illness (Kleman & Smith, 2022). Within this continuum, an individual makes either positive, incremental movements from the midpoint going in the direction of wellness, or conversely, negative movements toward illness with a reduction in health beyond the midpoint. Many factors, including the environment, affect movement on the continuum. An individual can have a terminal disease yet reach an emotional state of being prepared for death and, in so doing, display some of the characteristics of high-level wellness (Kleman & Smith, 2022). More simply, how well an individual adapts and has the resources to adapt to internal and external stressors determines one's position on the continuum. Assessments of these internal and external stressors, as well as interventions aimed at reducing or eliminating the stressors, are core components of health promotion.

With the publishing of the Human Genome Project and its resulting scientific application, there are new possibilities to move individuals on the wellness-illness continuum toward greater health. Unlike genetics, which focuses on the function and composition of a single gene, genomics considers the entire set of human deoxyribonucleic acid (DNA) and how these genes interact with each other, the individual's environment, and behaviors (e.g., diet and exercise) to influence health and development (Hold & Amore Jones, 2021; Scott Ricci, 2022). For example, genomics assists in understanding who is more at risk for certain diseases (such as heart disease and cancer), why individuals respond differently to the same treatments, and how to tailor medications through the study of pharmacogenomics. Apart from trauma, such as motor vehicle accidents, "genomic factors play a role in nine of the ten leading causes of death in the United States" (National Human Genome Research Institute, 2018, para. 6). Using genomics, researchers hope to find ways to improve health and target treatments, leading to greater personalization of health care (National Human Genome Research Institute, 2018; Scott Ricci, 2022).

One's overall understanding of health is enhanced by reflecting on the health continuum, as well as the concepts of health, wellness, illness, and disease, with each person seen as a part of a complex, interconnected, biological, and social system (Kleman & Smith, 2022). The understanding of health—as a matter of degree— broadens the scope of nursing practice and, like the vision for *Healthy People 2030*, focuses on each person reaching their full potential to enjoy a sense of well-being throughout their life span (Rector, 2021). Last, health promotion strives to not only decrease disease occurrence, but also to lead to behavior changes that enhance wellness at both the individual and community level.

CONCEPTUAL MODELS AND FRAMEWORKS FOR PROMOTING HEALTH AT SCHOOL

Health promotion program planning at school begins with the identification of an appropriate model or framework. Frameworks and conceptual models provide a layout to build health promotion interventions. Frameworks and conceptual models can help the school nurse throughout the planning cycle. School nurses use models or frameworks in program planning to conduct needs assessments, improve the ability to secure resources, implement programs, and evaluate program outcomes (Todd, 2021). This section describes frameworks and conceptual models that may be utilized for health promotion development and implementation by school nurses.

Health Promotion Model

Pender's *Health Promotion Model* (HPM) provides a model for analyzing health-related behaviors within a nursing and behavioral science context (Murdaugh et al., 2019). See Chapter 2 for additional discussion on social and behavioral theories. The HPM was recently updated to reflect how health behaviors are influenced by others (e.g., family members, healthcare professionals, etc.), as well as technology. The HPM provides a guide to understand, assess, and predict health promotion through an individual's characteristics (prior behavior and personal factors/experiences), behavior-specific understandings and influence, and resulting behavior outcomes (Murdaugh et al., 2019). In other words, it explains why an individual might choose to engage in proposed health promotion activities, including what factors might influence the individual's likelihood of participation (age, sex, knowledge, support, barriers, etc.). Using the HPM, the school nurse can identify predictable factors that can modify the individual's likelihood of engaging in a health-promoting behavior, including health accountability and empowerment, physical activity, nutrition, social support, stress management, and coping skills (Arpaci et al., 2023; Voskuil et al., 2019). School nurses who adopt this model can more easily identify appropriate interventions to address risk factors and health promotion activities for the individual or group.

Socioecological Model

The *Socioecological Model* provides the school nurse with a perspective to understand the individual, family, community, and societal influences that affect health behaviors, choices, and disparities. School nurses can use the socioecological model to develop health promotion plans to support behavior changes across the multiple levels reflected within the school environment (Kleman & Smith, 2022). The Socioecological Model has been used to understand the complexities of the interaction between a student's school performance and their physical, mental, and social well-being (Mann et al., 2021), violence prevention (National Center for Injury Prevention and Control, 2022), and other health disparities. School nurses can successfully use this model to address factors that occur across the individual, relationship, community, and societal levels. The model supports prevention-focused interventions over time rather than a single intervention (National Center for Injury Prevention and Control, 2022).

Public Health Interventions Framework

The *Public Health Interventions Framework* was first conceptualized by public health nurses in Minnesota to provide a language for actions and interventions used to improve population health (Minnesota Department of Health, 2019). This framework identifies public health nursing actions, values, and beliefs, which provide the basis for school nursing practice. The "Intervention Wheel" provides an interrelated composition of five colored wedges that group 17 public health interventions into three levels: individual/family, community, and systems (Minnesota Department of Health, 2019). The individual level includes change of knowledge, attitudes, beliefs, practices, or behaviors of individuals. The community level includes a focus on groups and populations to change community norms, attitudes, awareness, practices, or behaviors. Systems level includes strategizing with departments, organizations, and governments to advocate for collaboration, data collection, or changes to policies or laws. Using a combination of all three levels enhances health quality and equity during routine or emergent school nursing care (Anderson et al., 2018; Flaherty, 2020). See Chapter 2, Figure 2-8, for additional discussion.

School nurses focus on the health of both individuals and populations (Anderson et al., 2018). This might include students, families, school and district staff, and the community surrounding the school. The public health interventions framework articulates the abundant interventions and levels of practice used by public health/school nurses to enhance population health. School nurses can use the public health interventions framework to explain the multifaceted interventions they provide to the school community (Anderson et al., 2018).

Whole School, Whole Community, Whole Child Model

The *Whole School, Whole Community, Whole Child* model (WSCC) combines the coordinated school health model with a focus on the whole child, meaning all students feel supported and are healthy, safe, challenged, and engaged (NCCDPHP, 2023b; see Chapter 3). School nurses who develop health promotion activities using the WSCC model often focus on the health services and employee wellness components of the model; school nurses can also collaborate with other school staff and community members to address the eight remaining components of the WSCC model (NCCDPHP, 2023b). As the WSCC model incorporates aspects of community health and interdisciplinary collaboration, school nurses fulfill an integral role as a user and advocate for the WSCC model in school health promotion activities (Willgerodt et al., 2021).

PRECEDE-PROCEED Model

The *PRECEDE-PROCEED Model* is a comprehensive framework that focuses on the community's perception of needs. The multistep structure of the model resembles the nursing process. The desired outcome and quality of life,

> **Focus on the Framework**
> **Community/Public Health**
>
> During the COVID-19 pandemic, school nurses collaborated with public health departments to provide population-based care to students, families, staff, and community members. School nurses utilized knowledge of the social determinants of health to assist families in accessing both health care and necessities (e.g., food, hygiene supplies). School nurses were also proactive in disease prevention through surveillance, case management, contact tracing, and safety measures/protocols (Flaherty, 2020)

as perceived by the community, is a guiding focus in the development of the plan and evaluation of community-level health programs (Todd, 2021). This model has been applied to several school health promotion programs to address multiple health needs of communities and populations, including nutrition, physical activity, and dental health programs (Bejster et al., 2020; Stewart et al., 2022). PRECEDE is based on the premise that the desired outcome should precede and guide interventions, just as a medical diagnosis precedes a treatment plan. PRECEDE is an acronym for ***p***redisposing, ***r***einforcing, and ***e***nabling ***c***onstructs in ***e***ducational/ecological ***d***iagnosis and ***e***valuation. Predisposing constructs are internal factors that positively or negatively influence a person's ability to change (e.g., knowledge, attitudes, beliefs, values, preferences, skills, self-efficacy). Reinforcing constructs are external factors that provide positive or negative reinforcement of the desired behavior change (e.g., family, friends, community members, leaders, influencers). Enabling constructs are internal and external factors that facilitate motivation to change and sustain behaviors (e.g., psychological, or physical skills, resources, policies; Center for Community Health & Development, n.d.).

PROCEED is an acronym for ***p***olicy, ***r***egulatory, and ***o***rganizational ***c***onstructs in ***e***ducational and ***e***nvironmental ***d***evelopment. This aspect of the model focuses on the variety of systems-level factors necessary to implement and evaluate the interventions (e.g., organizational structure/culture, organizational policies, community/professional regulations) (Todd, 2021). The school nurse can use the PRECEDE-PROCEED model to ensure that interventions are tailored to the needs and cultural values of the community (Stewart et al., 2022).

Social Determinants of Health

The models discussed here acknowledge that health is influenced by many factors. In 2008, the WHO Commission on Social Determinants of Health issued a report to provide evidence about social determinants of health (SDOH) and health equity with an updated report expected sometime in 2025 (WHO, 2024). The WHO Commission emphasized that individual and population health outcomes are a product of SDOH, which are made up of social, political, economic, and physical environments. Individuals and populations have different opportunities and exposures within the SDOH, resulting in health inequity. The SDOH consist of "the structural determinants and conditions of daily life ... and are responsible for a major part of health inequities between and within countries" (Commission on Social Determinants of Health, 2008, p. 1). The Office of Disease Prevention and Health Promotion's (ODPHP's) Healthy People 2030 initiative (n.d.a) and the WHO (n.d.c) incorporate SDOH factors such as housing, education, food security, employment/income, social support, health services, and early childhood development into their goals. The SDOH are "the non-medical factors that influence health outcomes" and "the conditions in which people are born, grow, work, live, and age, and the wider set of forces and systems shaping the conditions of daily life" (WHO, n.d.c).

The *Healthy People 2030* initiative includes a framework for SDOH built around five key areas that encompass health equity:

- Economic stability
- Education access and quality
- Healthcare access and quality
- Neighborhood and built environment
- Social and community context (ODPHP, n.d.c)

Before conducting health promotions programs, the school nurse can assess the social factors (e.g., family support, socioeconomic status, race, culture, education), environmental variables (e.g., neighborhood structure, safety, outdoor and indoor air quality, clean water, exposure to metals), lifestyle practices (e.g., coping skills), early childhood experiences, and healthcare services (i.e., access to and use of). Through this assessment, the school nurse can identify health strengths and risks, develop baseline and outcome measures, and target health promotion programming toward health policy strategies, such as improved quality of life, access to healthcare resources, and education that promotes health and well-being (Schroeder et al., 2018). SDOH are reflected within each community and must be considered when planning health promoting activities (Todd, 2021).

Practice Connections

School nurses can apply the *Whole School, Whole Community, Whole Child* model in their practice. A school nurse took on a leadership role as a facilitator of a Vermont school district's "whole child team," a school-based interdisciplinary team based on the WSCC model. The whole child team included school staff, as well as healthcare providers from the local pediatrician's office. The team utilized quality improvement and evidence-based practice principles to understand issues, identify interventions, and evaluate outcomes. The whole child team members were able to streamline, strategize, and focus their efforts. This approach ensured that the WSCC model was used on projects to address attendance, nutrition, and dental health. Each project was student-focused and involved students, staff, families, and community agencies (Driscoll, 2021).

CONDUCTING HEALTH PROMOTION ACTIVITIES AT SCHOOL

School nurses should be involved in health promotion and disease prevention activities. It is important for the school nurse to remember that each contact with students, parents/guardians, or staff members is an opportunity for health promotion. As discussed in Chapter 13, disease prevention occurs at the primary, secondary, and tertiary levels of prevention. Each of these prevention levels can target individuals, groups, or communities. For the school nurse, individuals could include students, parents/guardians, or school personnel; groups could include groups of students (e.g., classes, clubs, sports teams), groups of school personnel (e.g., staff, faculty), or individuals with similar risk factors or health concerns; and the communities could include families, the school district, and neighborhoods. School wellness teams, mandated for any school receiving federal funds, may also be a driving force behind health promotion activities (U.S. Department of Agriculture, 2022).

Assessment

Promoting health at school begins with identifying what health promotion activities are needed in the school, district, and community. Once the target audience and model or framework has been chosen, the school nurse is better prepared to conduct this initial assessment. A thorough needs assessment at the individual, group, and/or school community level provides the foundation for successful program planning. The assessment may be affected by several variables, including race, ethnicity, culture, primary language, age, developmental status, family structure, socioeconomic status, education level, health status, risk-taking behaviors, lifestyle patterns, communication style, and environment.

Individual and Group Considerations

Needs assessment for individual students or groups will differ from those conducted for a community. For example, a health-risk appraisal tool can be used to help both students and staff identify health promotion opportunities. The school nurse can then use the results to select and design health promotion activities. The school nurse may also consider focusing health promotion efforts on a target group of individuals who share a common health risk or demographic variable, such as students with elevated body mass indexes (BMIs). The student's family can be considered a group when planning health promotion strategies or be incorporated into health promotion activities for their child.

School Community Considerations

Assessment of the broader school community includes many of the variables already listed, but at a systems level. For example, environmental factors at the school and community level might include identifying local health concerns, the role of community-based organizations, transportation options, access to healthy food and exercise opportunities, safety needs, and government priorities. The school nurse may be involved in community needs assessment as part of a team, such as a district wellness committee or other collaborative initiative within the community. See Online Materials OM2-2 for a fillable school community assessment form.

> **Did You Know?**
>
> The Centers for Disease Control and Prevention (CDC) and the UCONN Rudd Center for Food Policy and Health developed the Wellness Policy in Action Tool to help school districts and schools implement wellness policies (CDC & University of Connecticut, 2021).

Compare Your School's Data

As part of the needs assessment process, the school nurse may want to compare the school or district's data to local, state, and national data. Multiple sources of data are available:

- The *National School Health Data Set: Every Student Counts!* is NASN's data initiative that provides resources for school nurses to collect, utilize, and share data; establishes uniform data points with standardized definitions in four data subsets (student demographics and workforce capacity, school health staffing, student chronic health conditions, and health office visit dispositions); and provides a national platform for data submission that also serves as a repository for school, district, state, and national aggregate data (NASN, n.d.b; Stanislo, 2023).
- The *Health Services Assessment Tool for Schools* (HATS) was developed by the American Academy of Pediatrics (AAP) in partnership with multiple agencies, including NASN. This self-scoring online tool assists in identifying areas of strength and weakness, and tracking progress over time to evaluate school health services policies, practices, and infrastructure (AAP, n.d.).
- The *Youth Risk Behavior Surveillance System* (YRBSS) monitors priority health-risk behaviors (e.g., unintentional injuries and violence, behaviors related to unintentional pregnancies and sexually transmitted infections, alcohol and other drug use, tobacco use, unhealthy dietary behaviors, and inadequate physical activity). This includes a national school-based survey of a representative group of 9th to 12th graders called the YRBSS. The survey is conducted by the CDC in schools across the country, with data reported every 2 years (National Center for HIV, Viral Hepatitis, STD, & TB Prevention [NCHHSTP], 2020a).
- *School Health Profiles* is a system of biennial surveys of middle school and high school principals and health teachers that assesses school health policies, health education, and programs in states, large urban school districts, and territories (NCHHSTP, 2022a).
- WHO conducts the *Global School-Based Health Survey,* which measures behavior risk factors and protective factors among 13- to 17-year-olds. The 10 core modules address the leading causes of morbidity and mortality among children and adults worldwide, including alcohol use, dietary behaviors, drug use,

hygiene, mental health, physical activity, protective factors, sexual behaviors, tobacco use, and violence and unintentional injury (WHO, 2022).

Table 12-1 provides examples of additional national data sets available for the school nurse to use.

Planning

In most cases, the needs assessment and analysis will identify far more health promotion opportunities than can be addressed. The school nurse, in consultation with school/district administrators, staff, and related groups (e.g., students, families, community members), must prioritize the needs during the planning phase. Once needs are established, it is important to search for evidence-based programs to promote health. As part of the process, the school nurse and planning team must also consider program logistics, such as when and where the program will be offered. The planning team will also consider the cost to provide the program, including supplies/equipment and salary of the program provider (Rentfro, 2022).

Health Promotion Resources

Many excellent health promotion programs are available for school nurses to use to promote health of students, staff, and community members. Some may be programs

> **Practice Connection**
>
> A research-based assessment tool that the school nurse can use is the CDC's *School Health Index* (SHI), a self-assessment and planning tool to improve school health and safety programs and policies. The school nurse can use the SHI tool to assess the needs of the school, identify the school's strengths in promoting health and safety, and recommend actions the school can take to improve areas of weakness. The SHI was originally designed using the coordinated school health model and was aligned with the WSCC model in 2017. The goal of this resource is to support schools to develop plans to improve student health and engage teachers, students, parents/guardians, and the community in health promotion behaviors through the implementation of health and safety policies and programs.
>
> The CDC SHI is a free electronic resource designed to be completed by a school team and includes 11 assessment modules, along with a comprehensive planning guide. The SHI is available in two versions, one for elementary schools and another for middle and high schools. A school/district team will create a confidential SHI account to enter information, view results, and create plans to improve student health. To learn more, visit the CDC SHI webpage: https://www.cdc.gov/healthyschools/shi/index.htm (NCCDPHP, 2019).

TABLE 12-1 National Health-Related Surveys

Name	Web site	Source	Focus
National Survey of Children's Health (NSCH)	http://www.nschdata.org	Telephone household survey	Physical, emotional, and behavioral child health indicators
Monitoring the Future (University of Michigan)	http://monitoringthefuture.org	Surveys of students in secondary schools (8th, 10th, and 12th grades) annually	Beliefs, attitudes, and behaviors related to substance use, including alcohol, tobacco, vaping, and other drugs
GLSEN National School Climate Survey	https://www.glsen.org/research/2021-national-school-climate-survey	Online survey of a representative sample of LGBTQ+ youth. The 2021 survey consisted of 22,298 participants between the ages of 13 and 21.	Started in 1999, the biannual survey reports on the unique challenges LGBTQ+ students face and identifies interventions that can improve school climate.
National Health and Nutrition Examination Survey (NHANES)	http://www.cdc.gov/nchs/nhanes.htm	Interviews, physical examinations, clinical measurements of children and adults	Health and nutritional status of adults and children in the United States
Search Institute	http://www.search-institute.org	Publishes research findings and provides ongoing surveys for youth programs to promote positive youth development	Developmental assets, student motivation and achievement, developmental relationships, prevention, civic development and service learning, and adult and peer relationships
National Health Interview Survey	http://www.cdc.gov/nchs/nhis.htm	Household interview survey	Health of the nation including health status, healthcare access, mental health, and progress toward achieving national health objectives

provided by the school nurse; others may be provided by community stakeholders. The school nurse's role in health promotion should be proactive and use evidence-based interventions and data when developing a school health promotion program.

The first step in the planning process is to determine program goals and objectives that relate to the information gathered during the assessment process. The school nurse can use *Healthy People 2030* objectives and intervention resources to guide program planning (ODPHP, n.d.a). *The Guide to Community Preventive Services* Web site is another resource that provides evidence-based recommendations for health promotion and disease prevention interventions based on systematic reviews (Community Preventive Services Task Force, 2022). Program topics include adolescent health, oral health, mental health, nutrition, physical activity, SDOH, and other chronic conditions. Another evidence-based resource to support the school nurse's role in health promotion is the U.S. Preventive Services Task Force (USPSTF) recommendations for preventive services and screenings (USPSTF, n.d.). These recommendations provide systematic reviews of clinical research to ensure the accuracy and feasibility of preventive measures, including recommendations for students. School nurse can use the search feature on the Web site to quickly access information related to school screenings.

From a global perspective, the WHO maintains a longstanding commitment to health services and health promotion in the school setting. The WHO published two guidelines related to student health and education: the *WHO Guideline on School Health Services* publication contains information about providing school health services to students (WHO, 2021a), and the *Making Every School a Health-Promoting School: Implementation Guidance* publication contains information about the health-promoting school approach (WHO & United Nations Education, Scientific & Cultural Organization [UNESCO], 2021). *Making Every School a Health-Promoting School: Implementation Guidance* is based on a robust review of evidence related to health promotion in schools (WHO & UNESCO, 2021). The document provides an analysis of the barriers and facilitators to implementing and sustaining a health-promoting school. This information is available in multiple languages and is meant to guide health-promoting school implementation as a global standard.

The ODPHP (2021) is another health promotion resource from the U.S. Department of Health and Human Services (USDHHS). The *National Health Information Center* is a service of ODPHP that maintains a list of information centers and clearinghouses that can be used by professionals. This database includes more than 1,700 national organizations, associations, and governmental agencies; topics include youth violence prevention, dental health, tobacco use, and drug use. Online Materials OM12-1 provides a summary of these, and others recommended by school nurses. In addition to resources identified earlier in this chapter, other programs and resources can be found at local and state health departments, hospitals, or universities. Last, NASN partners with many organizations to provide evidence-based programs ready for implementation in schools (NASN, n.d.a, n.d.c).

During planning, the school nurse must be aware of factors that can affect program success. This primarily involves open communication among all parties affected by the program, including school administrations, teachers, staff, students, families, and other stakeholders who may be involved in the program. For example, competing academic priorities can make teachers reluctant to include health promotion activities in the classroom if instructional time is affected. The school nurse should work to coordinate health promotion content to align with state and national learning standards or health-related measures that are part of the school improvement plan.

Consultation with parents/guardians and other family members will help the school nurse understand if there are any cultural, social, or financial considerations that may affect health promotion efforts (e.g., difficulty with transportation). As health promotion activities/programs focus on enhancing quality of life rather than treating emergent healthcare issues, families may have difficulty prioritizing health promotion activities. With creativity and partnership with community members, there are many opportunities for the school nurse to engage in health promotion at school. See Chapter 2 for ideas for collaborating with the community.

School nurse understaffing can also affect health promotion efforts by limiting the time and resources available to plan and participate in school health promotion activities. Some school nurses may have time to plan and present programs themselves; others may need to function in a collaborative/coordination role as they work with administrators to bring programs into the school from community stakeholders (hospital, community organizations, etc.).

Implementation

The implementation phase of health promotion programming is successful when the assessment and planning phases have been thoroughly conducted. The school nurse implements the evidence-based plan with the identified group. The school nurse may fulfill the role of provider, coordinator, or a combination of both. Program objectives should be reviewed with participants along with a description of the program, time commitment, and any other expectations. Participants should have an opportunity to ask questions. Changes or accommodations to the intervention to meet the unique needs of the individual, group or family should be incorporated before and during the implementation phase. As such, the implementation phase includes characteristics from the assessment, planning, and evaluation phases to reflect the needs of the individual, family, or community (Rentfro, 2022).

Evaluation

The health promotion program should be evaluated on three levels: the process, the structure, and the outcome. Program evaluation often begins with the initial assessment that provided the data that determined the program focus. The data collected (i.e., baseline data) indicated a need within the target group that led to the health promotion activity. The baseline data are used at the evaluation phase to compare program outcomes. Throughout the planning and implementation phases, the school nurse must incorporate and gather additional evaluative data, such as program timelines, resources used (structure evaluation), participation or satisfaction of participants (process evaluation), and the impact or change (outcome evaluation). If the evaluation criteria are carefully identified and are written in measurable terms, the evaluation can provide meaningful insights into lessons learned and areas for program improvement (CDC, 2011).

Evaluation data can be an effective advocacy tool for health promotion activities, particularly when planning for an outcome evaluation to demonstrate behavior changes after school-based health interventions. Outcome data may indicate improved healthy food choices during school meals, decreased high-risk behaviors among students (e.g., decreased smoking), increased use of preventive safety devices (e.g., seat belts or helmets), or increased attendance for students who would have previously been sent home (Simoneau et al., 2020). Additional outcomes might be decreased use of emergency medical services for students at school, increased feeling of connectedness to the school community by students and families, and increased rates of routine healthcare visits for students. Outcome data, whether positive or negative, will help focus future health promotion activities.

To collect meaningful data, the evaluation measures must be planned and incorporated into the health promotion program. The school nurse or health promotion team should review the evaluation results to determine program successes, including needed adjustments and/or whether the program should be expanded or discontinued. Successes and barriers should be shared with stakeholders (e.g., school administrators, staff, families, community stakeholders). Successful program outcomes and lessons should be shared with other nurse colleagues via professional avenues such as poster sessions, presentations, and published articles. See Chapter 4 for additional information on the school nurse's role as an educator.

HEALTH SCREENINGS

Health screenings are key strategies used by the school nurse to promote health and wellness. As mentioned in this chapter's introduction, NASN's School Nursing Practice Framework identifies practice components under the *Community/Public Health* principle as "conducting screenings, surveillance, outreach and immunization compliance activities" (NASN, 2024, p. 156). The AAP Council on School Health also identifies the critical role of the school nurse in providing preventive and screening services (Council on School Health et al., 2016). The term *screening*, as used in community/public health, describes programs that provide disease testing to identify conditions in groups of asymptomatic individuals (Cadena-Malek, 2021). As such, screenings are a sorting tool, though never 100% accurate, "separating people that probably do have a condition from those who probably do not" (WHO, 2020b, p. 3). Screenings target populations who are at higher risk of a health problem or condition so that early treatment and intervention can be offered, with a goal of improving health and decreasing health costs (Kudzma, 2022).

From a public health perspective, it makes sense to perform screenings in schools, as large numbers of children are present in one location. Health screenings performed in the school setting may be directed by state laws and guidelines or by local school policy. The USPSTF (2022a), acting on behalf of Agency for Healthcare Research and Quality (the lead federal agency charged with improving the safety and quality of health care for people in the United States), also provides evidence-based guidance for preventive services and health promotion in primary care settings, some of which are applicable to the school setting. School nurses are the primary individuals coordinating screening programs in schools. They must be knowledgeable about mandated screenings, who conducts the screenings, when during the year various screenings are performed, the required equipment and supplies, which age group or populations are screened, and how referrals and follow-up processes are completed. Screenings, beginning with the prescreening program announcement, provide an opportunity to teach students, parents/guardians, and staff about prevalent health conditions (Cadena-Malek, 2021). Last, it is critical to acknowledge that the screening itself is not diagnostic, but rather a method to determine who requires further medical evaluation or treatment (Cadena-Malek, 2021; National Library of Medicine [NLM], 2019). Thus students displaying symptoms of a condition should be automatically referred for further evaluation.

Principles of Screening

According to the WHO (2020b), the era of modern screening programs dates to 1968, with Wilson and Jungner's publication establishing principles for health screenings. Still to this day, their principles are used to determine whether a screening is likely to improve public health through consideration of the benefits, harm, costs, and ethics of screening programs (WHO, 2020b). First, the screening must address an important health condition, there must be an effective and affordable treatment for the condition, and there must be enough time between detection of the condition and the development of clinical symptoms to allow for early intervention (Cadena-Malek,

2021; WHO 2020b). In addition, consideration is given to the availability of screening tools, the presence of established guidelines for referral and treatment, and the availability and accessibility of referral facilities, healthcare providers, or resources for diagnosis. Last, individuals conducting screenings must examine whether the screening is one that is acceptable to the population being screened, whether the screening will be ongoing, and whether the total cost of the screening program is justifiable compared with the costs of treating the disease or condition if left undetected (Cadena-Malek, 2021; WHO, 2020b).

Screening Tool Criteria

Several criteria exist related to tools used for screening, including availability, safety of the product, ease of use, any discomfort with use, cost-effectiveness, and accuracy (Kudzma, 2022). Variables that measure the accuracy of a screening test, tool, or technique include reliability and validity. ***Reliability*** refers to consistency in yielding the same results when administered on separate occasions by different technicians with the same level of skill performing the test (Cadena-Malek, 2021; Kudzma, 2022). ***Validity*** refers to "the test's ability to accurately identify those with the disease [or condition]" (Cadena-Malek, 2021, p. 235). As perfectly valid screening tools are rare, the measure of validity of a tool is further divided into two components quantifying the margin of error:

- *Sensitivity*—the proportion of individuals *with* a condition who correctly test positive when screened
- *Specificity*—the measure of individuals *without* the condition who correctly test negative when screened (Kudzma, 2022)

When a test has good sensitivity, the number of individuals with the condition who are missed (false negatives) will decrease; similarly, a test with high specificity will rarely refer (false positives) individuals who do not have the condition (Kudzma, 2022). To avoid underidentifying individuals at risk, screening tools should identify a few, but not too many, false positives.

Age appropriateness and equipment maintenance are other important considerations for supporting reliability and validity with screening tools. Vision-screening equipment using LEA SYMBOLS® as optotypes are examples of an age-specific screening tool for preschool-age students. Body weight scales and stadiometers should be age appropriate, and blood pressure (BP) cuffs should be size appropriate for the extremity being measured. Some screening equipment requires calibration on a schedule recommended by the manufacturer (e.g., audiometers for hearing screening); some tools, such as color vision screening plates, require storing considerations (e.g., placed in a dark place such as a file cabinet or drawer when not in use). Thus screening programs should consider both the initial costs required to obtain valid and reliable screening tools and the maintenance and replacement costs encountered over time with the program.

Planning for and Conducting Health Screenings

There are many considerations for conducting health screenings in the school setting, and the planning process should begin several weeks to months before the actual screening date. Start with determining what screenings are mandated and what screenings are optional. For example, vision screening is required for students in 41 states, though there is marked variation in screening methods and criteria, where the screening occurs, and the grade levels that are screened (Wahl et al., 2021). State school nurse organizations, as well state school nurse consultants, can assist new school nurses with this first step. Before conducting screenings, it is important to determine whether training, education, or licensure requirements exist for those providing the screenings. Again, state associations and departments of health and education can assist in clarifying training requirements and locating training offerings.

A collaborative approach involving those affected by the screening is recommended. The school nurse should work with school administration to determine when to schedule screenings with a goal of minimizing time out of the classroom for students. If relying on screeners from outside the school, additional consideration must be given to their schedules. Once the date and time are arranged, the location of the screening must be secured. Providing notice to teachers in advance will allow them to arrange their lesson plans to accommodate the time students will be involved in the screenings.

The school nurse should take steps to educate the staff and parents/guardians about the importance of the screenings and what the screenings will entail. Announcements to parents/guardians should include information about the referral process and how they will be notified of screening results. School newsletters, Web sites, and social media provide avenues for communication, and some schools have systems that can send phone messages, texts, or e-mails out to the whole school or selected groups. Notifications need to include processes for obtaining parental consent, or if consent is not required, parental opt-out options. Parents/guardians electing not to have their student participate in a mandatory screening at school may be responsible for having the screening done elsewhere and providing evidence of completion back to the school. Before the screening, the school nurse should also ensure that students are properly prepared for the screening procedure. Providing students with a brief, developmentally appropriate explanation of the procedure and why it is being done will help to minimize anxiety for the student. The school nurse should also consider any cultural mores that the screening may affect (e.g., personal space, modesty). Students should never be forced to participate in a screening, and all student concerns about participation should be addressed.

As part of the screening process, the school nurse must have a system in place to document the results of the screening in each student's health record. If a student does not pass a particular screening, rescreening might be indicated. If a health condition interferes with the screening, the rescreening should be scheduled as soon as the condition is resolved or as time allows (i.e., a student who needs more time to complete the screening). For example, upper respiratory or ear infections may interfere with a student passing the hearing screening. Students who do not pass the rescreening should be referred to a healthcare provider for further evaluation and follow-up care (NLM, 2019).

Referral forms should follow the principles of health literacy and the health equity guiding principles for inclusive communication to enhance parental understanding and follow-through (e.g., concise content; clarity on actions and the importance of the information; easy to read; uses active voice; follows rules on font size, bullet points, bolding, margins; uses person-first language and preferred terms for select population groups; available in reader's native language) (CDC, 2019). Historically, a common method of distributing referral paperwork to parents/guardians was in paper form, reinforced with phone calls. Technology provides additional options of e-mail, texts, and, in some cases, parent access to their student's electronic health record. No matter the format, notices should consider confidentiality and usability of the information. A sample vision screening referral letter to parents is provided in the Online Materials OM12-2.

An essential role of the school nurse is to not only follow up on referrals, but to also facilitate the referral process, which includes ensuring parents/guardians understand the need for the evaluation and the potential impact to the academic setting. The National Center for Children's Vision and Eye Health at Prevent Blindness (NCCVEH, n.d.a) has resources available in English and Spanish to assist parents/guardians with understanding common vision conditions in children, the importance of an eye examination, and available financial resources. Partnering with school counselors and social workers may be helpful in certain circumstances. Knowledge of resources available in communities, including the location of healthcare providers, sources of transportation, and financial assistance programs, assists in overcoming obstacles to care. Hospital social service departments; primary healthcare providers; and dental, ophthalmology, and optometry professional organizations may be helpful in identifying community resources. Local and state school nurse organizations are additional resources. Table 12-2 lists key considerations for the school nurse when planning and conducting health screenings.

On occasion, the school nurse may identify additional screenings or programs (e.g., dental sealant program) that can be paired with screenings to address health conditions of concern in the student population. The desire to conduct these screenings or programs might be based on data collected in the health office or new evidence-based guidelines. In these cases, the school nurse must obtain administrative and parental permission to conduct screenings and programs outside of state requirements, guidelines, or local policy. Advocating and facilitating local school policy development and revisions to ensure compliance with state mandates, as well as working with state and national governing bodies to ensure screenings are evidence-based, are roles of the school nurse (NASN, 2022a). Some of the most common screenings conducted in schools are described in the remainder of this chapter.

Vision Screening

Many students are unaware they have vision disorders. Routine vision screening, along with comprehensive eye examinations when students do not pass vision screening, is critical to enhancing opportunities for optimal vision outcomes (Prevent Blindness, 2019). Early identification and support of students with vision conditions can improve academic progress, increase focus during lessons, increase participation and classroom interaction, and improve confidence and behavior (Peterseim et al., 2015). When instances of developmental, behavioral, or language concerns present in students, vision screening should be considered as early identification is necessary for treatment or support (Prevent Blindness, 2019). Certain undiagnosed and uncorrected vision disorders can affect a student's educational experience, such as development of early literacy skills and inappropriate classroom behaviors, and lead to permanent vision loss (Bruce et al., 2016; Collins et al., 2017; Johnson et al., 1996; Jonas et al., 2017; National Academies of Sciences, Engineering, and Medicine, 2016; Vision in Preschoolers (VIP)–Hyperopia in Preschoolers (HIP) Study Group et al., 2016). See Chapter 24 for information and discussion of students with vision impairment, including students with low vision and blindness, as well as the related qualifying services in the school setting.

Vision screening at school is important, especially if the student is not under the regular care of an eye care provider. Ages and grades at which vision screening is recommended or mandated vary by state. School nurses should review state law for their state and the Periodicity Schedule from the AAP and Bright Futures for selecting ages appropriate to screen at school (Bright Futures & AAP, 2022). The Periodicity Schedule recommends vision screening during medical well-child visits annually between the ages of 3 and 6 years and again at ages 8, 10, 12, and 15 years. Although these are the Periodicity Schedule recommended ages, the results of one study involving more than 51,000 students found that vision screening in state-mandated grades of prekindergarten, kindergarten, 1st grade, and 8th grade—in addition to nonmandated grades 2nd to 7th—resulted in significantly higher referral rates in nonmandated grades versus mandated grades (Milante et al., 2021). The researchers concluded that screening in only certain grades is inadequate as students in nonmandated grades may go multiple years with visual disorders, especially reduced visual acuity. They also highlighted health equity issues related to vision health

TABLE 12-2 Considerations for Planning and Conducting Health Screenings

Screening	• What qualification is needed to conduct the screening? • Who will conduct the screenings? • Will outside screeners be used? What is the cost? Who will supervise them and ensure that outside screeners use evidence-based tools and procedures? Have they been notified where and when to report? • Are helpers needed to assist with the screening process? • Who will instruct helpers regarding duties and importance of confidentiality?
Announcement and consent	• How will parents/guardians and students be notified regarding the screening date, time, and purpose? • Is parent/guardian consent required? • Has administration approved the consent form? • How will consents be distributed and collected?
Paperwork	• Is all paperwork in an organized format and ready to use? • List of students/classes • Consents • Informational fliers for families • Referral forms • Are written materials culturally appropriate and follow the principles of health literacy and health equity inclusive communication? • Is there a documentation plan in place?
Screening location	• Is the room/area large enough? • Does the room have adequate resources? • Electrical outlets • Tables • Chairs • Trash cans • Screens for privacy • Is the room free of distractions, noise, or glaring light? • Is there a designated break location for the screeners?
Teacher preparation	• Have teachers had input into the schedule to avoid conflicts with other school activities? • Do teachers know how long the screening will take? • Have teachers been given instructions on how to support student attendance at the screening?
Student preparation	• Has the nurse provided classroom instruction, demonstration, or other information about the screening, including its purpose and overview of what will occur? • Will students need name tags? • Are student instructions developmentally and culturally and linguistically appropriate?
Miscellaneous	• Has the time required to get students to and from the screening been considered in the planning? • Who will cover the nurse's office during the screening?
Referrals	• Have resources for referrals been identified? • Is a systematic referral process in place? • Who will follow up on referrals?

as children from low-income communities were more at risk for an incomplete follow-up, potentially due to limited access to eye care providers. A comprehensive vision screening program with trained screeners is necessary to eye health and to support student learning.

Correctly conducted by formally trained and certified individuals, vision screening is a quick and inexpensive method for identifying students who should be referred to an eye care provider for a comprehensive eye examination (Cotter et al., 2015; Donahue et al., 2016; NASN, 2016; NCCVEH, n.d.b). In addition to formal training, initial and ongoing vision screening certification every 3 to 5 years in proper screening techniques and the use of optotype- and instrument-based tools is also recommended (Cotter et al., 2015; NASN, 2016). Information on training/certification and recertification programs may be obtained from state departments of health, state departments of education, Prevent Blindness affiliates, or the national Prevent Blindness program (NASN, 2016; Prevent Blindness, n.d.b).

In some school environments, vision may be assessed only for distance visual acuity; other protocols may also include near visual acuity, color vision deficiency, and eye misalignment screening. Regardless of the assessment conducted, vision screening should begin with an assessment of appearance, behaviors, and complaints (i.e., signs of vision problems).

Initial Assessment

The initial assessment in vision screening includes observing differences in visual appearance of the eyes, behavioral signs, and complaints reported from student, teacher, or parent. Atypical visual appearance signs include unequal pupil size; red-rimmed, encrusted, or swollen eyelids; an obvious strabismus; or a drooping eyelid. Common behavioral signs include squinting or frowning when trying to focus, bringing reading material close to the face, tilting the head to one side most of the time, or avoiding near work or reading. Complaints may include frequent headaches or comments about blurred vision when looking at near objects, or difficulty copying material from a classroom board (NASN, 2016; Prevent Blindness, 2020b).

NASN (2016) and Prevent Blindness (2020b) provide extensive examples of signs of vision problems (appearance, behaviors, and complaints) to monitor. Students expressing complaints or exhibiting appearance and behavioral signs should be referred to their primary healthcare provider or directly for an eye examination, even if the student passes a vision screening (NASN, 2016; Prevent Blindness, 2020b). Similarly, if a teacher or parent has concerns about a particular student's vision, refer that student to the student's primary healthcare provider or directly to an eye care provider for a comprehensive eye examination (Prevent Blindness, 2020b).

Two Approaches to Vision Screening

Vision screening has two approaches: *optotype-based* and *instrument-based* (Cotter et al., 2015; Donahue et al., 2016; NCCVEH, n.d.b; Nottingham Chaplin, et al., 2015). *Optotype-based* screening provides a measurement of visual acuity. "Optotype" is the name of the symbol, letter, or number a student is asked to identify on an eye chart, computer program, or tablet computer application. Visual acuity is the quantifiable measurement of the clearness of vision as determined by the ability to resolve detail at a given distance.

Optotype-based screening is conducted using either threshold or critical line formats. Threshold screening involves beginning at the top of the chart and moving down the chart until reaching the threshold (the line where the majority of optotypes cannot be correctly identified). Critical line charts use only the line of optotypes students should pass according to their age. Critical line screening can be quickly administered, is an effective alternative to threshold screening (Donahue et al., 2016), and can identify students most at risk for a vision disorder who need a comprehensive eye examination.

Instrument-based screening uses automated technology to provide information about the structure of the eyes, such as estimates of refractive error and eye misalignment (Cotter et al., 2015; Donahue et al., 2016; Nottingham Chaplin, et al., 2015). A refractive error occurs when the length of the eyeball or the shape of the cornea prevents light from focusing directly on the retina (Donahue et al., 2016). Refractive errors include hyperopia (farsightedness), myopia (near-sightedness), astigmatism (irregular shape of cornea or lens), and anisometropia (a large difference of refraction between the two eyes). Box 12-1 lists vision disorder definitions, including refractive errors.

BOX 12-1

Vision Disorder Definitions

Amblyopia: A neurodevelopmental disorder, often called "lazy eye," that occurs from abnormal processing of visual images during a critical period of vision development and leads to decreased vision. It typically occurs in one eye but can occur in both eyes, and it can be caused by strabismus, abnormal refractive errors, and cataract.

Astigmatism: Irregular shape of the cornea or lens causing blurred vision at both near and far distances.

Anisometropia: A large difference of refraction between the eyes. For example, one eye may be nearsighted, and the other eye may be farsighted.

Hyperopia: Also called farsightedness, where distant objects are clear and near objects are blurred.

Myopia: Also called nearsightedness, where near objects are clear and distant objects are blurred.

Nystagmus: Involuntary rhythmic movements of the eyes horizontal, vertical, rotary, or mixed.

Refractive error: A refractive error occurs when the shape of the eye prevents light from focusing directly on the retina and is primarily caused by the shape of the cornea or length of the eyeball.

Strabismus: Misaligned eyes where each eye presents different images on the retina, and the brain, depending on the severity, cannot fuse the images from both eyes into one image.

Source: American Association for Pediatric Ophthalmology and Strabismus (AAPOS, 2024).

Vision Screening Methods for Different Age Groups

For school nurses working in early childhood programs serving children from birth to age 3 years, a monitoring questionnaire can be used during a baby's first year of life. An example is the *18 Vision Development Milestones from Birth to Baby's First Birthday* (Prevent Blindness, 2020a). For children ages 1 and 2 years, the joint 2016 guidelines from the AAP, the American Association of Certified Orthoptists (AACO), the American Association for Pediatric Ophthalmology and Strabismus (AAPOS), and the American Academy of Ophthalmology (AAO) recommend instrument-based screening (Donahue et al., 2016). For children ages 3, 4, and 5 years, the joint AAP/AACO/AAPOS/AAO guidance document and the National Expert Panel to the NCCVEH for community-based screening environments recommend *either* optotype- or instrument-based screening approaches (Cotter et al., 2015). For students ages 6 years and older, the joint AAP/AACO/AAPOS/AAO guidance document recommends optotype-based vision screening as the preferred approach; instruments may be used *only* if a student in this older age group cannot participate in optotype-based screening (Donahue et al., 2016). As evidence-based, peer-reviewed research emerges regarding students ages 6 years and older, instrument-based screening may become an alternative recommendation to optotype-based screening for all students.

Evidence-Based Vision Screening Charts and Use of Occluders

Incorrectly designed eye charts can lead to overreferral or underreferral of students with vision disorders (Nottingham Chaplin, 2021). For example, the recommended standardized threshold charts have a 20/32 line instead of a 20/30 line and will not exceed 10 feet as a screening distance. In other instances, wide and linear-spaced threshold charts are not standardized and could result in less accurate visual acuity results. The six characteristics of standardized threshold charts are as follows: (a) optotypes are equally recognizable and legible (i.e., one optotype is not easier to identify than other optotypes), (b) each line has the same number of optotypes, (c) horizontal spacing between optotypes on a line is equal to the width of one optotype on that line, (d) vertical spacing between lines is equal to the height of the optotypes on the next line down, (e) the size of optotypes increases or decreases by 0.1 log units (resulting in 20/32, not 20/30), and (f) optotypes are black on a white background with good lighting (NASN, 2022b; Nottingham Chaplin, 2021). Wide and linear-spaced threshold charts are not standardized and could result in less-accurate visual acuity results. General guidance for optotype-based screening tools is as follows.

- **Optotypes for evidence-based vision screening charts:** For students ages 3, 4, and 5 years, LEA SYMBOLS® or HOTV letters are the recommended optotypes (Cotter et al., 2015; Donahue et al., 2016). Sloan Letters are the preferred optotypes for students ages 6 years and older or when students know letters in random order (Donahue et al., 2016; Nottingham Chaplin, 2021).
- **Optotype format:** For students ages 3, 4, and 5 years, the NCCVEH recommends charts using single optotypes surrounded by four crowding bars at a 5-foot screening distance or booklets with one line of five optotypes per page surrounded by a crowding rectangle at 10 feet (Cotter et al., 2015). Using single optotypes without crowding bars is not recommended because they can lead to underreferrals or to missing students who should be referred because the optotype is easier for the student to identify (Cotter et al., 2015; Donahue et al., 2016). The joint AAP/AACO/AAPOS/AAO guidance document recommends charts with lines of optotypes or single, surrounded optotypes at 10 feet (Donahue et al., 2016). Cotter et al. (2015) state charts with LEA SYMBOLS® or HOTV letters calibrated for 10 feet are acceptable.
- **Nonrecommended eye charts:** Charts *not* recommended for vision screening include the kindergarten "Sailboat" chart, Allen Pictures, the Lighthouse chart (house, apple, and umbrella), Tumbling E, Snellen, or Landolt C (Cotter et al., 2015; Donahue et al., 2016; NCCVEH, n.d.b, 2015). These charts are not standardized and are not well validated in the school screening environment. Some require discrimination of direction and orientation and cognitive skills inconsistently developed in preschool-age students (NCCVEH, 2015; Nottingham Chaplin, 2021).
- **Recommended occluders:** For students ages 3, 4, and 5 years, use adhesive eye patches, 2-inch-wide hypoallergenic surgical paper tape, and specially constructed occluder glasses with opaque or frosted lenses (Cotter et al., 2015; NCCVEH, n.d.b, 2015). Occluder glasses can be used until age 10 years when "lollypop" or "Mardi Gras" occluders can be used. When using lollypop paddle occluders, place the handle toward the temple, not the chin (Prevent Blindness, 2015).
- **Unacceptable occluders:** Do not use students' hands, tissues, paper, or plastic cups because students can easily move the objects and peek at the chart when given responsibility for covering their eyes during the screening (NCCVEH, n.d.b; Prevent Blindness, 2015). It is also unacceptable to have adults hold occluders over younger students' eyes (Cotter et al., 2015).

Optotype-Based Screening Procedures for Distance Vision

The age-dependent line a student should pass for *threshold screening* should be at the student's eye level. Charts in illuminated cabinets with LED lights provide appropriate, even lighting across the chart surface. Normal, even room lighting that does not cause a glare or shadows on the chart surface is also acceptable. Avoid visual distractions, such as gym equipment, near the chart.

Measure the screening distance between the chart and the student's eyes based on the chart's calibration distance—generally 10 feet. Place a line or tape on the floor at the exact end of the screening distance from the optotype-based tool and position students with the arches of their feet on the line or tape to ensure that the end of the screening distance is in alignment with the students' eyes. If using a chair, the back legs of the chair should be on the line and ensure that students sit with their backs against the back of the chair. If students use a matching card for pointing, measure the distance to where their head would be located when bending over the matching card.

- **Prescreening:** To achieve better success when screening preschool-age students or students who do not know letters in random order, tell children that they are playing a game; do not say that they are having a vision screening (Cotter et al., 2015). If using an LEA SYMBOLS® or HOTV chart, use the square "response card" with all four optotypes near the preschool-age or kindergarten student and ask the student to name each optotype to discern how the student will respond during the screening process. Accept the name a student calls an optotype. Students can also point to the optotype on the response card that matches the optotype to be identified on the chart. Some LEA SYMBOLS® or HOTV charts will include four individual cards that can be placed on a tabletop or on the floor in front of the student so the student can point to, or lift, the matching tabletop card, or step on the matching card on the floor. Response cards are also available for Sloan Letters.

- **Screening and recording results:** Occlude the left eye. Starting with the top line on the right side of the chart; as the student faces the chart, ask the student to identify the first optotype on the right side of each line, and move down the chart until the student incorrectly identifies an optotype. When an optotype is misidentified, move up a line and ask the student to identify all optotypes on that line, reading left to right. Continue moving up or down a line until the student correctly identifies three or more optotypes. *The last line on which the student correctly identified the majority of optotypes is the visual acuity value for that eye* (some chart instructions will use three of five as the majority; others will use four of five). Occlude the right eye and follow the same process, using the left side of lines on the left side of the chart, from the student's perspective, and reading left to right. Record the 20/XX number for each eye. Threshold screening requires screening each eye separately to ensure an accurate visual acuity assessment. There is no need to screen distance vision binocularly (both eyes open) as the better-seeing eye usually determines the level of vision acuity, compensating for the other eye with a visual deficit. However, it is acceptable to have both of the student's eyes open for prescreening purposes before screening each eye separately (Nottingham Chaplin et al., 2018b).
- **Critical line screening and recording results:** Use only the visual acuity line a student should pass according to the student's age. Most critical line charts will indicate the age line to use. Critical line charts or booklets are typically held in the screener's hands at the student's eye level. Use the same screening distance measuring method used for threshold screening. Some critical line booklets will include a practice or prescreening line to use with both eyes open when orienting young students to the screening task. To screen, occlude the left eye. Moving from left to right, ask the student to identify each optotype. Occlude the right eye, turn to the next page of the vision screening booklet, and ask the student to identify each optotype on that page, again reading from left to right. To pass, the student must correctly identify the majority of optotypes with each eye individually. Critical line screening results are recorded as pass or refer. Some states may require rescreening the same day; rescreen as soon as possible but not later than 6 months from the initial screen before referring (Cotter et al., 2015; NCCVEH, n.d.b).
- **Pointing at optotypes for threshold and critical line screening:** It is permissible to point to the side of the line of optotypes the student is to identify, but pointing directly at individual optotypes is not permissible (Donahue et al., 2016; WHO, 2003). Isolating an optotype with a finger or pointer, and masking all optotypes but one on a line, can result in missing students who should be referred, because pointing at and masking an optotype makes the optotype easier for the student to identify (Donahue et al., 2016). If a student requires assistance knowing which optotype to identify, briefly point to the optotype and immediately remove the pointer. If using optotypes inside a box of crowding bars or rectangles, stay outside the box when briefly pointing (NCCVEH, 2015).
- **When to refer:** Referral criteria differ across states and eye charts; however, there are two sets of national guidelines that provide referral criteria recommendations. For community settings, including schools, Cotter et al. (2015) recommends referring if the student is *not* able to correctly identify the majority of optotypes on the age-appropriate line: 20/50 for 3-year-old students, 20/40 for students ages 4 and 5 years, and 20/32 for students ages 6 years and older. The 2016 AAP/AAPOS/AAO/AACO joint document for pediatricians recommends referring if the student is unable to correctly identify the majority of optotypes on the age-appropriate line: 20/50 line for 3-year-old students, the 20/40 line for 4-year-old students, and the 20/32 line on standardized charts for students ages 5 years and older (some schools also follow this recommendation; Donahue et al., 2016). When using threshold charts with students ages 4 years and older, the AAP/AACO/AAPOS/AAO joint statement also recommends referring for a 2-line difference of visual acuity between the eyes, even within the passing range (Donahue et al., 2016). An example of a 2-line difference in the passing range is 20/20 in one eye and 20/32 in the other eye.

Optotype-Based Screening for Near Vision

No national guidelines exist recommending near visual acuity screening (Nottingham Chaplin et al., 2018). However, the VIP-HIP Study Group et al. (2016) found that uncorrected hyperopia interfered with acquiring early literacy skills in preschool-age students, and Williams et al. (2005) found comparable results in older students. When school nurses conduct near vision screening (e.g., required or for evaluation purposes), use eye charts with the same optotypes recommended for distance screening, based on student ages.

To maintain the screening distance of 16 inches, eye charts are available with attached cords to place on the orbit bone near the temple (ensure the end of the cord does not touch the eyeball). Keeping the cord taut during screening will prevent the student from moving closer to the chart, which would make the optotypes easier to identify, and result in less-accurate visual acuity results. Near vision screening can be conducted monocularly or binocularly. Follow age-specific distance visual acuity referral criteria when screening monocularly with a threshold near visual acuity chart, or use pass/refer when conducting binocular screening with either a critical line chart or the age-dependent line on a threshold chart.

Plus Lens Testing for Near Visual Acuity Screening

While some state vision screening guidelines recommend plus lens testing as a near visual acuity test (e.g., using +2.50 lenses with the 20/32 line on a distance visual acuity chart), this is *not* a near visual acuity screening test. No national guidelines recommend plus lens testing, and insufficient scientific research is available to support plus lens testing (Prevent Blindness, 2015).

Instrument-Based Screening

Instrument-based screening is quick to administer, requires no response from the student other than looking at the front of the instrument, and is useful in screening students who have difficulty participating in optotype-based screening (Donahue et al., 2016; Marzolf et al., 2017). Instrument-based screening, including photoscreeners and portable autorefractors, provide information about the structure of the eyes and amblyopia risk factors, such as estimates of refractive errors and estimates of eye misalignment.

Devices for instrument-based screening do not measure visual acuity or provide visual acuity values, such as 20/20. Converting a student's estimated refractive error from an instrument into a near or distance visual acuity value is inappropriate (Cotter et al., 2021). If documentation requires a visual acuity value, documentation should be amended to include a pass/refer outcome if instruments are the only vision screening tools used (Cotter et al., 2021).

As new research emerges, instrument-based screening may become appropriate for students of all ages. Currently, instruments approved for students ages 1 to 5 years include the following (Cotter et al., 2015; NCCVEH, n.d.c):

- GoCheck Kids without visual acuity component (ages 3, 4, and 5 years only)
- Plusoptix S12R, S12C, S16 without visual acuity add-on component
- Retinomax (Right Mfg. Co Ltd., Tokyo, Japan)
- Welch Allyn Spot™ Vision Screener

Computer-based vision screening refers to software programs that present optotypes meeting national vision screening guidelines and is acceptable (Prevent Blindness, 2015).

Machines for vision screening using illuminated slides with optotypes to optically simulate distance vision, such as those used at motor vehicle testing facilities, are *not* recommended for students ages 3, 4, and 5 years (Cotter et al., 2015; Furr et al., 2018; Prevent Blindness, 2015). These machines prevent monitoring a student's face and eyes during screening. Additionally, insufficient scientific data exist to support machines for screening the vision of school-age students (NCCVEH, 2015; Prevent Blindness, 2015).

Screening Eye Muscle Coordination

Some vision screening protocols call for testing eye muscle coordination, such as using the cover/uncover or alternate cover test. The National Expert Panel to the NCCVEH discourages cover testing for eye misalignment for students ages 3, 4, and 5 years unless administered by healthcare personnel trained to perform this test and to interpret the results (Cotter et al., 2015).

If mandated to screen for eye muscle coordination, school nurses could conduct stereoacuity screening to determine whether both eyes are working well together to see a three-dimensional object. If the eyes are misaligned and not working well together, the brain is unable to merge separate images from each eye into one image. Stereoacuity screening as a part of mass screening for students ages 3, 4, and 5 years is *not recommended* (Cotter et al., 2015, Prevent Blindness, 2015). If stereoacuity screening is required, Prevent Blindness (2015) and the National Expert Panel to the NCCVEH recommend using the PASS Test 2 (Cotter et al., 2015).

The PASS Test 2 includes a demonstration card with a smiley face, a blank card, a card for students ages 3 and 4 years, a card for students ages 5 years and older, small and medium polarized glasses, and a string to measure the 16-inch screening distance. Screeners hold the blank card and the card with the smiley face in front of a student and the student's task is to point to the card with the smiley face while wearing polarized glasses. The PASS Test 2 includes instructions and pass/refer guidelines. The Random Dot E test, commonly used in the past, is no longer recommended as it showed low testability and sensitivity rates (VIP Study Group, 2006).

Screening for Color Vision Deficiency

No national guidelines are known to recommend color vision deficiency screening at school. If teachers or parents/guardians are concerned that a student may have a color vision deficiency, especially a preschool-age or kindergarten student exposed to a heavily color-coded curriculum, school nurses could conduct color vision deficiency screening on an as-needed basis. When a deficit is identified, the student should be referred for an eye examination (Nottingham Chaplin et al., 2018a). If a classroom concern exists, the student should be referred for a comprehensive eye examination, even if the student passed the color vision deficiency screening.

The eye care provider will confirm whether a color vision deficiency exists, as well as the type and severity of the color vision deficiency. The eye care provider will also talk with parents/guardians about how color vision deficiency could affect learning, life, and career choices (Nottingham Chaplin et al., 2018a). Learning activities may require accommodations to the classroom or learning materials. Career counselors can consult with older students regarding occupation choices that do not rely on color.

Color vision deficiency screening can be conducted with books using pseudoisochromatic test plates with symbols for preschool and kindergarten students and numbers for older school-age students when they know their numbers. An example of a color vision deficiency screening book is the *School Health HRR Color Screening Book* using screening plates from the *HRR Standard Pseudoisochromatic Test, 4th edition.* If younger students require assistance naming symbols on each test plate, the student can use a paint brush or cotton swab to either trace or touch each symbol on each plate. On the plates of some color vision deficiency screening books with symbols, every student will see at least one symbol.

Do not ask the student to trace or point to symbols on pseudoisochromatic plates because the oil from fingertips will desaturate (i.e., fade) colors. Books with pseudoisochromatic test plates should be replaced at least every 5 to 7 years as the colors desaturate over time. Store books in a dark location when not in use. Follow manufacturer instructions and scoring information to administer color vision deficiency screening.

Rescreening

School nurses may be required or want to rescreen students who do not pass vision screening to reduce unnecessary referrals. The National Expert Panel to the NCCVEH (Cotter et al., 2015) recommends rescreening only for untestable students, either the same day or as soon as possible, but not later than 6 months. NASN (2016) recommends rescreening all students who do not pass vision screening within 2 to 4 weeks and no later than 6 months. When rescreening, use the same tools used during the initial screening (NASN, 2016). Refer students who do not pass rescreening for a comprehensive eye examination. When referring students for a comprehensive eye examination, school nurses can work with the student's primary healthcare provider for coordination of the eye examination or refer directly to an eye care provider for a comprehensive eye examination. NASN (2022b) provides information for locating local healthcare providers. The school nurse should consider barriers to care and work with the family to ensure they can access follow-up care.

Other Considerations

Untestable Students. Students may be considered "untestable" for vision screening if they are inattentive, cannot cover one eye, or do not understand the screening instructions. Research suggests that untestable students are at least twice as likely to have a vision disorder as students who pass vision screening (VIP Study Group, 2007). If possible, rescreen untestable students the same day or as soon as possible, but no later than 6 months (Cotter et al., 2015). Difficulty in obtaining a reading when screening a student with an instrument may indicate the need for referral. For example, if 10 or 15 students are screened successfully with an instrument and suddenly the instrument times out before showing screening results and the instrument screen does not show an error message, such as pupils too small, refer the student to their healthcare provider or eye care provider for an eye examination.

Vision Screening Is Part of a Strong System of Vision and Eye Health. Vision screening is only 1 of 12 components of a strong vision and eye health system of care at school (NASN, 2022b; Prevent Blindness, n.d.a). Other components include providing parents/guardians with educational material that respects cultural and literacy needs about the importance of good vision for their child now and in the future; collecting written permission to receive eye examination results for student files to help students follow treatment plans at school and to talk with eye care providers when questions arise about the treatment plan; and evaluating the vision and eye health program annually.

An overall plan for evaluation of the screening program should be conducted annually. The annual evaluation includes comparing screening and eye examination results to determine whether overreferrals are excessive and if screening tools and/or procedures should be reviewed. An evaluation checklist is available as the twelfth component of the Strong Vision Health System of Care on the NASN/NCCVEH *Vision and Eye Health* Web site (NASN, 2022b) and the Prevent Blindness Web site (Prevent Blindness, n.d.a).

Did You Know?

It is recommended that certain students not be screened and, instead, be automatically referred for a comprehensive eye examination or attend a follow-up eye examination if they are currently under the care of an eye care provider. Students with the following conditions or characteristics are more at risk for vision disorders:

- Eye differences, such as misaligned eyes
- Neurodevelopmental disorders, such as autism spectrum disorders or ADHD
- Systemic diseases, such as juvenile idiopathic arthritis
- Family history of first-degree relatives with strabismus, amblyopia, or high refractive error
- History of premature birth and low birth weight (<32 weeks and 1,500 grams birth weight) who are not under the care of an eye care provider
- Parents/guardians who believe their child has a vision problem or have concerns that their children are not reaching age-appropriate developmental or academic milestones (Cotter et al., 2015; NASN, 2022b; Prevent Blindness, 2015; NCCVEH, n.d.c)

School nurses who are mandated to screen students at higher risk should use the same recommended tools used within the vision screening program. If these students pass vision screening, school nurses should inform parents/guardians their children have a higher risk for vision disorders and should still have a comprehensive eye examination.

Hearing Screening

Hearing is one of the senses that prompts the development of communication and language skills. Communication and language are integral to social and learning experiences; therefore it is important to understand the pathways of screening and support so students can use their communication strategies (e.g., signed, spoken, technology-based, written, etc.) to learn and grow. Without timely and appropriate supports, students with hearing loss have a higher risk of difficulties with communication, language, and social skills (Cagulada & Koller, 2020; Guan & Smolen, 2022; National Center on Birth Defects and Developmental Disabilities [NCBDDD], 2022b).

Hearing loss can be present at birth (i.e., congenital) or acquired as when caused by ear infections, loud noises, ototoxic medications, and so on. The prevalence of and risk factors for hearing loss vary across the life span. For example, 2 to 3 of every 1,000 children are born with hearing loss, over 80% of children have had otitis media by age 3, and 13% of people ages 12 years or older have bilateral hearing loss (National Institute on Deafness and Other Communication Disorders, 2021). There are four important components to hearing:

- The ranges and characteristics of sound
- The physical mechanics of how sound enters the ear
- The physical and neural mechanics of the inner ear
- The neural pathways of how the cochlear nerve and brain organize the stimuli

Sound is measured in loudness (decibels [dB]) and pitch (hertz [Hz]). Normal conversational speech is typically 60 dB. For comparison, the sound of a gas lawnmower is 80 dB, and a firecracker 140 dB (NCEH, 2022a). The pitch or tone of sound is measured in hertz, or the frequency of cycles per second. For example, low frequency tones (approximately 250 Hz) include the sound of a bass drum and vowel sounds, such as "oo" and "who"; high frequency tones (approximately 4000 Hz) include the sound of a bird chirping, a whistle, and the consonant sound "s" as in "sun" (American Speech-Language-Hearing Association [ASHA], n.d.e). Typical hearing is between 0 and 20 dB. A person who cannot hear until 20 to 40 dB will have trouble hearing quiet speech, whereas someone who cannot hear until 40 to 60 dB will have difficulty hearing conversational speech. Hearing loss ranges from slight (16 to 25 dB) to profound (91+ dB) (ASHA, n.d.b).

Hearing loss is classified into four categories: conductive, sensorineural, mixed, or auditory neuropathy spectrum disorder. **Conductive hearing loss** occurs when sound cannot travel through the outer canal to the middle ear (e.g., allergic rhinitis, otitis externa, otitis media, perforated eardrum). **Sensorineural hearing loss** occurs due to damage of the inner ear or the cochlear nerve pathway to the brain (e.g., illness, genetics, loud noise). **Mixed hearing loss** occurs when there is a combination of both conductive and sensorineural loss. **Auditory neuropathy spectrum disorder** occurs when the brain is not able to interpret sound due to damage of the inner ear or the cochlear nerve (NCBDDD, 2022a). See Chapter 24 for additional information on the types and degrees of hearing loss.

Although newborn hearing screening programs are established in all 50 U.S. states, either mandated or voluntary, many students will not have another hearing screening until they enter school (ASHA, n.d.c). Students should have access to quality hearing screenings to ensure appropriate referrals and supports are established early. Hearing screenings are usually conducted upon school entry and at specified intervals, such as once every 3 years. To conduct a quality hearing screening program, the school nurse must have the correct training, equipment, setting, screening process, and referral protocols in place (ASHA, n.d.d).

School nurses may need specific certification or training by an audiologist to conduct hearing screenings; information on training programs can be obtained from state departments of health or education. Regardless of the state-specific requirements, school nurses should pursue training on equipment (e.g., audiometers) and protocols before conducting hearing screenings. The school nurse should be familiar with equipment instructions, including the manufacturer suggestions for warm-up periods, equipment checks or calibrations, and temperature-related requirements. Audiometers are the most common way of screening for hearing in the school setting, due to ease of transportation, size, and cost. Audiometers measure both decibels and hertz; as such, this equipment is precise and requires careful handling and annual calibration.

Hearing screenings require a quiet setting for accuracy. If a soundproof room is not available, it is critical to control for ambient noises (e.g., waiting students, ringing phones, flushing toilets, music rooms). A room with acoustical tiles, carpeting, and solid core doors helps to eliminate extraneous noise. The room should be big enough for two chairs and a table to hold the equipment, and it should have an electrical outlet. When preparing for screenings, check each frequency at 20 dB with a person who does not have hearing loss to ensure that the equipment is working and each tone can be heard. If tones of 20 dB cannot be heard, the screening should not be conducted in that environment. It is essential to assess the suitability of a setting before conducting hearing screenings (ASHA, n.d.a).

To conduct the screening, the student's chair should face away from the audiometer at a 45-degree angle so that the student cannot view the examiner pushing the buttons, but so that the examiner can still see the student's face. For the headset to fit correctly, students should remove anything in front of their ears including earrings, headbands, glasses, and hair. Center and adjust the headset so that the speaker is lined up with the student's ear canal; the red earpiece goes on the right ear. Set the decibel level according to state or district guidelines. Twenty decibels is usually the accepted screening level; however, if the environment has a fair amount of extraneous noise, the intensity level can be raised to 25 dB if allowed by state or district guidelines.

The frequencies usually tested are 500, 1,000, 2,000, and 4,000 Hz, but there are recommendations that screening also include 6,000 and 8,000 Hz to ensure complete screening (ASHA, n.d.a; Sekhar et al., 2016).

Tones are pressed for about 2 seconds. Students should be instructed to raise their hand when they hear the tone in the headset; it does not matter which hand they raise. Because students may develop a rhythmic pattern of raising their hand, the examiner should vary the pattern of pressing the tones. For example, wait a longer interval between some tones and have some follow immediately after the last (Subcommittee on Childhood Hearing Screening, 2011). If students do not respond at the recommended frequency (Hz) screening level in either ear, then that constitutes a test failure and further assessment is warranted. Further assessment may include otoscopic inspection to rule out collapse of the eardrum, cerumen impaction, foreign object in the canal, or perforation of the tympanic membrane. In addition, tympanometry (a measurement of middle ear pressure, outer ear volume, and middle ear compliance) may be required by state guidelines for all students or a particular group (ASHA, n.d.a; Subcommittee on Childhood Hearing Screening, 2011). Referral to a healthcare provider should be made immediately if findings include any of the following: drainage of fluid, foreign objects, tympanic membrane perforation, dried blood in the ear canal, foul odor, red tympanic membrane, or report of ear pain (ASHA, n.d.a; Winston-Gerson & Sabo, 2016).

Students that do not pass or complete the initial audiometry screening benefit from rescreening 6 to 8 weeks later (ASHA, n.d.a). The changing health of the conduction and sensory systems of the ear explains why a student may not pass a hearing screening the first time but does pass when rescreened later. A second failed screening triggers a threshold screening—like the initial screening but the screener evaluates the smallest decibel for each hertz where the student hears the tone most of the time. Students who do not pass a threshold screening, but with typical middle ear functioning, are appropriate referrals to an audiologist. As with all screening, the school nurse must document required screening information and referrals. An example of a letter to parents/guardians with the results of hearing screening can be found in the Online Materials OM12-3.

Testing hearing in younger students can include conditioned play audiometry. This involves instructing the student to complete a task, such as dropping a block in a basket when a sound is heard (Bonino & Leibold, 2017; Buz Harlor et al., 2009). Additionally, otoacoustic emission (OAE) testing is a reliable and objective screening method for screening young students, students with disabilities, or students with a different primary language. OAE testing uses auditory stimulation via a microphone device in the outer canal to measure the functionality of the outer hair cells and cochlea. An OAE device resembles an otoscope and provides a printout of the results. OAE screening provides information on the possibility of sensorineural unilateral or bilateral hearing loss (ASHA, n.d.a; Winston-Gerson & Sabo, 2016).

Did You Know?

OAE testing does not actually test hearing. It only provides partial information about the integrity of cochlear and outer hair cell functioning (ASHA, n.d.a; Winston-Gerson & Sabo, 2016).

Students with documented hearing loss who wear hearing devices and/or cochlear implants should not be tested during hearing screenings (Winston-Gerson & Sabo, 2016). School nurses often follow up with the parents/guardians of these students to obtain reports of annual audiograms and, if a school audiologist sees the students, remind the parents/guardians of upcoming appointments.

Dental Screening

The 2000 landmark report from the Surgeon General on *Oral Health in America* brought renewed attention to student dental health (USDHHS, 2000). The report emphasized that dental caries are the single most common chronic childhood disease, with over 50% of children ages 5 to 9 and 78% of 17-year-olds having at least one cavity or filling. The same report called attention to striking disparities in dental disease by income, stating that children from lower income families are more likely to have untreated dental caries, as well as having twice as many dental caries than their peers from higher income families. More recently, Healthy People 2030 reports that between 2013 and 2016, 13.4% of students ages 3 to 19 years had active and currently untreated tooth decay in their primary or permanent teeth, with a target goal of decreasing this to 10.2% (ODPHP, n.d.b).

Fourteen states and the District of Columbia require oral health/dental screenings (Fleming, 2019). Often, the requirement is for an examination at entry into school and then at periodic grade level intervals. Screening most commonly includes a visual observation of the mouth and teeth, observing for both treated and untreated decay and the presence of sealants, as well as identification of students with urgent needs. State regulations may specify who is qualified to perform screenings (e.g., dentists and dental hygienists) and provide specific guidelines for treatment. Moving beyond screenings, schools and school-based health centers are expanding dental services in collaboration with community resources to provide on-site oral health services, including sealants, cleanings, fluoride, and even restorative care. The CDC (NCCDPHP, 2023a) encourages school sealant programs and provides guidance for program implementation. NASN and the American Dental Association provides a list of resources, collaborations, and partnerships surrounding the topic of oral health (Oral Health Connections, n.d.). According to the Association of State and Territorial Dental Directors (n.d.), there are multiple "best" implementation strategies that produce successful oral health outcomes. Examples of success stories and lessons learned are provided on their Web site, along with variables to consider such as available resources, feasibility, and implementation constraints specific to a program's environment.

School nurses often are the ones to identify the need for oral health services for individual students when they present in the health office due to a toothache or other complaint as well as a population/school level need for onsite dental health services. Once an agreement is reached between the district and the oral healthcare provider, the nurse may be responsible for obtaining parental consent and insurance information for the service and for facilitating follow-up dental care for identified students. The school nurse can also be involved in health promotion activities related to oral health, such as teaching lessons on oral hygiene.

Mental Health Screening

School nurses, with an appreciation of the multidimensions of health, are at the forefront of health promotion programs focused on student mental health. At a global level, approximately 14% of youth have mental health conditions (WHO, 2021b). Mental health conditions can be present throughout the life span and include attention deficit-hyperactivity disorder (ADHD), bipolar disorder, anxiety, and depression. In the United States, approximately 9% of students ages 3 to 17 have experienced anxiety, 20% of students ages 12 to 17 years have experienced depression, and 18% of high school students have seriously contemplated suicide (Bitsko et al., 2022). Mental health conditions can affect school attendance, academic performance, social well-being, and risk-taking behaviors (Bitsko et al., 2022; Substance Abuse and Mental Health Services Administration [SAMHSA], 2021; Wickersham et al., 2021). Additional stressors can exacerbate mental health conditions (AlAzzam et al., 2021). Students with mental health conditions, such as anxiety and depression, have an increased chance of future mental health conditions, suicidal thoughts, suicide attempts, and suicide completion, thus early identification and support is essential (USPSTF, 2022b, 2022c).

> **Practice Connection**
>
> *Promoting Oral Health in Schools: A Resource Guide*, 4th ed., can be found on the National Maternal and Child Oral Health Resource Center Web site at https://www.mchoralhealth.org/PDFs/resguideschooloh.pdf. The resource guide is divided into two sections. The first section describes materials, such as brochures, fact sheets, guidelines, curricula, and reports, all published between 2015 and 2019. The second section is a list of resources such as federal agencies, national professional associations, resource centers, and national coalitions (Barzel & Holt, 2019).

Depression screening is recommended during annual well-care visits for students ages 12 to 21 years (Bright Futures & AAP, 2022; USPSTF, 2022c). Anxiety screening is recommended for students ages 8 to 18 years (USPSTF, 2022b). Behavioral/social/emotional screening is recommended yearly for students from birth to 21 years (Bright Futures & AAP, 2022). Despite the recommendation for annual mental health screenings, only 46% of primary healthcare providers ask youth about mental health although 76% of healthcare providers consider mental health screening important (USPSTF, 2022b). This does not account for the lack of mental health screening for youth who do not see or have a primary healthcare provider. This deficit has created conversations about how schools can incorporate mental health screenings into the school health screening programs (Dineen et al., 2022; McCabe et al., 2024).

Mental health screenings, as with other screenings, can be conducted at the individual or school-wide level. Before conducting school-wide mental health screenings, school districts need to have policies specific to mental health screenings, communication with parents/guardians regarding the screening and results, and partnership with community mental health services. Adequate systems of support need to be in place to ensure accurate diagnosis, effective treatment, and appropriate follow-up (McCabe et al., 2024; SAMHSA, 2019; USPSTF, 2022b, 2022c).

School nurses need to be knowledgeable regarding evidence-based screenings, community resources, and appropriate treatment for students at risk for and diagnosed with mental health conditions. The *Screen for Child Anxiety Related Disorders* (SCARED) and the *Social Phobia Inventory* are tools that are appropriate to use for anxiety screening in students (Runyon et al., 2018; USPSTF, 2022b). The *9-Item Patient Health Questionnaire* (PHQ-9) is a depression screening tool appropriate for the school setting (USPSTF, 2022c). Other mental health and neurodevelopmental conditions such as ADHD, bipolar disorder, obsessive-compulsive disorder, and oppositional-defiant disorder require observational data about behavior in various settings, including the school setting. School personnel can assist healthcare providers and counselors by providing data regarding a student's behavior. Often, this is in the form of checklists and rating forms. It is appropriate for the school nurse to coordinate this data collection and communication among the parent, school personnel, and healthcare providers while following school policies, including ensuring that release of information forms are on file. See Chapters 26 and 28 for more information on students with ADHD and other mental health concerns and conditions.

Developmental Screening

Developmental screenings are one of many different approaches to identify children at risk for delays in the following developmental domains: social-emotional, adaptive, cognitive, fine motor, gross motor, language, and communication (Lipkin et al., 2020). Early identification and appropriate supports are important to ensure that students can be successful in their education. Identification happens through surveillance and screenings. School nurses and other school personnel might be involved in developmental surveillance, which is the process of recognizing students at risk for developmental delays (Bright Futures & AAP, 2022). Developmental surveillance includes six components:

- Eliciting and attending to the parent's/guardian's concerns about their child's development
- Obtaining, documenting, and maintaining a developmental history
- Making accurate and informed observations of the child
- Identifying risks and strengths and protective factors
- Maintaining an accurate record of the process and findings
- Sharing and obtaining opinions and findings with other professionals (Lipkin et al., 2020, p. 6)

School nurses, school personnel, and parents/guardians can utilize a variety of documentation tools to track student milestones, such as paper booklets or mobile technology (NCBDDD, 2022c, 2022d).

Developmental screening is the process of using an evidence-based screening tool to identify students with developmental delays. The Individuals With Disabilities Education Act's Child Find process stipulates developmental screenings for children in the United States. States are required to have a screening process to identify and provide services to children with developmental disabilities from birth through age 5, and a general education identification and services process for students from kindergarten through age 21 (IDEA, 2004). These processes are used to locate, evaluate, identify, and coordinate services for students who may be eligible for special education and related resources. When a parent or staff member of a school, preschool, or childcare has developmental concerns, the Child Find process should be initiated by obtaining consent for evaluation from the parent. Once consent is obtained, observations and needed assessments (such as speech, articulation, fine motor, gross motor, behavior, social, emotional, academic, vision/hearing screenings, health information review, and others) are begun. After the initial evaluation, if the student is found to have developmental delays, needs are identified, and a plan is put into place. Depending on the age and needs of the student, an individualized family service plan, an individualized education program, or a Section 504 accommodation plan can be drafted with a collaborative effort by an interdisciplinary team. In the school setting, team members meet to develop a plan. Required team members include the case manager (e.g., classroom teacher or special education teacher), support services provider (e.g., school nurse for health needs or occupational therapist for fine motor needs), school administrator, parents/guardians, and student. Each state has a specific guide with instructions that dictates how this process should be conducted. School nurses should understand their role in providing health assessment information and support to the developmental surveillance and screening process as required by their state and/or the IDEA; see Chapter 7 for more information.

Lead Screening

Lead, a naturally found metal, can be present in air, water, and soil, and it is harmful if inhaled or ingested (Agency for Toxic Substances and Disease Registry [ATSDR], 2020a). Though there has been an overall decline in blood lead levels, exposure remains a significant public health concern for children, as their nervous system is still developing, causing them to be especially susceptible to the harmful effects. Even at lower levels of exposure, the resulting neurotoxicity in infants and children can decrease mental development, affect development and behavior, and lead to hearing loss and speech problems (ATSDR, 2020b). High lead levels have shown a direct impact on the ability to learn, and a connection exists between rising blood lead and worse academic outcomes (Raymond & Brown, 2017). Adding to these concerns, children who swallow large amounts of lead may develop anemia, severe abdominal pain, kidney damage, muscle weakness, and a decrease in physical growth (ATSDR, 2020a).

In 2012, the CDC first established the population-based blood lead reference value (BLRV) to identify children exposed to more lead than most other children in the United States (Ruckart et al., 2021). Children with blood lead levels (BLLs, measured in micrograms of lead per deciliter of blood) at or above the BLRV have BLLs higher than 97.5% of U.S. children (NCEH, 2022b). Although no safe lead level has been determined, the CDC identifies children ages 1 to 5 years with BLLs greater than 3.5 mcg/dL as *at risk,* a change from the former 5 mcg/dL threshold (CDC, 2021; NCEH, 2023).

The most common sources of lead exposure in the United States are lead-based paint and dust (in housing built before 1978), lead-contaminated soil, and lead in water from lead pipes and plumbing fixtures (ATSDR, 2020a). Other sources of lead exposure for children include some toys and jewelry, candy imported from other countries, and lead dust that parents/guardians might bring home on their clothing from the workplace (Ruckart et al., 2021). Students living in housing built before 1978 and neighborhoods serviced by outdated water pipes are at risk for lead exposure (NCEH, 2023; Ruckart et al., 2021). School nurses can assist in informing parents/guardians on actions to take to reduce lead exposure, including becoming more educated about lead hazards; working with a lead-safe certified firm to repair peeling or chipping lead-based paint; replacing lead service lines; frequently washing student's hands, bottles, and toys; and having all family members remove their shoes before entering the home (Ruckart et al., 2021).

The Centers for Medicare and Medicaid Services (2016) requires that all Medicaid-enrolled children be BLL tested at ages 12 and 24 months or at age 24 to 72 months if they have not previously been screened. In addition, some states require BLL screening for students before enrolling in preschool or kindergarten. The BLL is screened by testing venous blood and is usually completed by the primary healthcare provider (NCEH, 2023). The school nurse can support the screening process by checking health records to confirm that a screening was done. School nurses can also collaborate with public health and healthcare providers to develop screening plans responsive to conditions based on local data, with some experts going as far as to recommend universal BLL testing for young children to advance health equity and environmental justice related to preventable lead exposure (Ruckart et al., 2021). Last, school nurses can educate parents/guardians on how to reduce exposure to lead and assist with encouraging parental adherence with care after an elevated blood lead level is detected in a student as early identification can reduce long-term effects from the exposure. Follow-up services include finding and removing lead from the student's environment, encouraging a diet high in iron and calcium, connecting the family to early education services, blood testing, and, for students with very high levels, additional tests and chelation therapy (NCEH, 2022b).

Tuberculosis Testing and Exposure Screening

Tuberculosis (TB) is an infection caused by *Mycobacterium tuberculosis.* Though TB typically involves the lungs, other organs and tissues can become infected (e.g., kidneys, brain, spine). Not everyone infected with TB will have symptoms, and thus there are two classifications for TB-related conditions. In the first, *latent* (or *inactive*) *TB infection* (LTBI), the person infected with TB can fight the infection, though their body still contains the tuberculosis bacteria (NCHHSTP, 2020c). Individuals with LTBI do not have symptoms and *cannot* spread TB to others, but treatment is recommended as the infection can become active if the person's immune system becomes weakened. The second classification is *TB disease* and occurs when the body is not able to fight the infection. A person with TB disease can spread the infection to those with whom they are in regular, close contact (NCHHSTP, 2020c). Like LTBI, TB disease can be treated and cured if medical therapy is followed. Those with TB disease become noninfectious soon after beginning treatment.

The CDC closely monitors TB as part of the global effort to eradicate the disease. The incidence of active TB disease in the United States has steadily decreased since 1992; in 2020 the annual rate of decline was greater than previous years, according to the CDC, likely a result of factors associated with the COVID-19 pandemic (NCHHSTP, 2022b). During 2021, about 7,882 TB cases, a rate of 2.4 cases per 100,000 people, were reported to the CDC compared with 7,171 (rate of 2.2) in 2020 (NCHHSTP, 2022c). As in past years, in 2021 nearly half of all TB cases occurred in California, Texas, New York, and Florida, the most populous states containing about one third of the U.S. population (NCHHSTP, 2022d). TB disease, presented in percent of cases, continues to be higher among marginalized communities in the United States: Asian persons (36.0%), Hispanic or Latino persons (30.6%), black or African American persons (18.0%), and white persons (11.2%; NCHHSTP, 2022b).

Did You Know?

Individuals who are higher risk for TB infection and should be screened include the following:

- People who have spent time with someone who has TB disease
- People from a country where TB disease is common (e.g., Latin America, the Caribbean, Africa, Asia, Eastern Europe, and Russia)
- People who live or work in high-risk settings (e.g., correctional facilities, long-term care facilities, and homeless shelters)
- Healthcare workers who care for patients at increased risk for TB disease
- Infants, children, and adolescents exposed to adults who are at increased risk for latent TB infection or TB disease (NCHHSTP, 2016a)

Screening (testing) for TB is focused on individuals at higher risk for infection. In addition, states may require TB testing for staff upon employment in the school setting. States or local level policies specify testing requirements, if any, for students with a focus on students at elevated risk. Testing in the school setting might also be warranted in the event of disease outbreak following the guidance of local or county public health authorities (Galemore, 2016).

TB testing is accomplished using one of two approved types of tests. The Mantoux tuberculin skin test (TST) involves injecting purified protein derivative intradermally into the forearm producing a wheal (6 to 10 mm in diameter; NCHHSTP, 2020b). The resulting reaction to the skin test is read between 48 and 72 hours after administration. Timing is critical. Inflammation and redness may occur in some individuals before 48 hours and is not a concern. At 48 hours after administration, the specific antibodies to TB, if they are present, will result in an induration (i.e., a hardened, raised palpable area). If not read before 72 hours, the test will need to be repeated. The Mantoux TST is the preferred method for testing children under 5 years of age (NCHHSTP, 2020b). The interferon-gamma release assay (IGRA) screening test, the second option, requires a single venous blood sample. Though more expensive, IGRA screening does not require a follow-up appointment for reading of the test. IGRA is also the preferred test for people with history of receiving the BCG vaccine (NCHHSTP, 2020b) as use of the Mantoux TST will result in a false positive.

School nurses typically do not administer TB testing. They are, however, frequently asked to read a Mantoux TST and report the results to the appropriate healthcare provider. When reading the results, only the area of induration is measured. A large, reddened, but flat area on the forearm is not considered a positive reaction. The diameter of the area of induration is measured in millimeters laterally across the arm. If there is no induration, the result is recorded as a zero (0 mm); do not record it as "negative." Table 12-3 explains how to read a Mantoux TST.

A positive skin test indicates that the person has been infected with TB; it does *not* indicate whether the person has developed TB disease (NCHHSTP, 2016b). Further testing with a chest radiograph and a sputum culture, as part of a physical examination, will help identify whether it is LTBI or TB disease and the course of treatment recommended.

False-positive and false-negative TB results are possible; therefore caution is indicated when providing an interpretation to students and their parents/guardians. Students born outside of the United States may have received a tuberculin vaccine (BCG) before arrival. Although the vaccine's effectiveness is unreliable, a person who has received the vaccine may have a positive Mantoux TST. Finally, it is important to note that live-virus vaccines can interfere with the Mantoux TST; thus the test should be done either the same day as vaccination with the live-virus vaccine or at least 1 month after receiving the live-virus vaccine.

Body Mass Index

The screening of student body mass index (BMI) has been instituted in schools due to concerns about the increasing prevalence of childhood obesity (see Chapter 14; Stierman et al., 2021). The USPSTF (2017) recommends healthcare providers screen for obesity in students 6 years and older annually, and when identified, offer to refer them to comprehensive, intensive behavioral interventions. The evidence around BMI screenings in schools suggests that the laws have not affected the incidence of obesity in students, including those that require student or parental notification regarding student BMI (Churchill, 2024; Poole et al., 2023). Though evidence is still lacking regarding the effectiveness of BMI screening in schools, 25 states require measurement programs (Ruggieri & Bass, 2015). Who to screen, how to screen, and knowledge surrounding the specifics of BMI screenings is essential for school nurses. As with all school screenings, support from administrators facilitates program success.

There are two general types of BMI measurement programs in schools—surveillance and screening. **Surveillance programs** provide de-identified data to determine the percentage of students who are obese, overweight, typical weight, and underweight; identify population trends over time; and monitor the outcomes of interventions. In addition, the aggregate data can be used to create awareness of the problem within the school community; provide information to change policies, practices, and services in schools; and monitor the effects and progress of healthy lifestyle changes. **Screening programs** assess individual students,

TABLE 12-3 How to Read a Tuberculin Skin Test

Degree of Induration	Specific Populations
≥5 mm is considered *positive* in:	People living with HIV
	A recent contact of a person with infectious TB
	People with chest x-ray findings suggestive of previous TB
	People with organ transplants
	Other immunosuppressed people (e.g., patients on prolonged therapy with corticosteroids equivalent to/greater than 15 mg per day of prednisone or those taking tumor necrosis factor alpha antagonists)
≥10 mm is considered *positive* in:	People born in countries where TB disease is common, including Mexico, the Philippines, Vietnam, India, China, Haiti, and Guatemala, or other countries with high rates of TB
	People who abuse drugs
	Mycobacteriology laboratory workers
	People who live or work in high-risk congregate settings (e.g., nursing homes, homeless shelters, or correctional facilities)
	People with certain medical conditions that place them at elevated risk for TB (e.g., silicosis, diabetes mellitus, severe kidney disease, certain types of cancer, and certain intestinal conditions)
	People with a low body weight (<90% of ideal body weight)
	Children <5 years of age
	Infants, children, and adolescents exposed to adults in high-risk categories
≥15 mm is considered *positive* in:	People with no known risk factor for TB

Source: National Center for HIV, Viral Hepatitis, STD, and TB Prevention (2020b).

identify students at risk, and notify parents/guardians of the results so that they can make needed changes and seek additional health services to improve health.

Although the CDC does not recommend for or against the programs, they do provide guidance to schools on what to have in place before implementing either type of program: "a safe and supportive environment for students of all body sizes, a comprehensive set of strategies to prevent and reduce obesity, and a series of safeguards to address the primary concerns raised about such programs" (NCCDPHP, 2022b, para. 3).

Box 12-2 lists evidence-based safeguards provided by the CDC. Eight of the 10 CDC safeguards are applicable to both types of programs, with the last two safeguards also recommended for screening programs. Looking at data from the School Health Policies and Practices Study, researchers measured school implementation of 4 of the 10 CDC safeguards and found that most schools with BMI screening programs had yet to adopt the CDC's safeguards (Sliwa et al., 2019). School nurses, often charged with overseeing and conducting BMI screening programs, are not solely responsible for program implementation, but enhance program effectiveness when collaborating with others to improve adoption and adherence to the safeguards.

Safeguard 1 directs schools to announce the program in advance and to have a process for obtaining parent permission for the screenings. Ruggieri et al. (2020) reinforced the importance of announcing BMI measurement programs to parents/guardians, and that the announcement includes language sharing the school's position as a partner in protecting students' health: "Your child's school wants to keep you aware of all your child's important health information. The BMI measure is a useful screening tool that can tell you if your child's weight is healthy for [their] age, height, and gender" (p. 153). It is also important to inform staff about the screening, including how they can assist in the process.

Students benefit from an advance announcement about the screening, one that establishes a climate for respectful behavior and emphasizes that privacy and confidentiality will be maintained. Safeguard 3 urges that the screening environment ensures measurements are *not* done within the sight or hearing distance of other students (NCCDPHP, 2022b). In addition, limit the viewing of results to the school nurse or other trained and assigned staff performing the screening, and avoid announcing results aloud, even for recording purposes. Maintain anonymity by removing identifying student information from the collection spreadsheet before calculating the BMI, aggregating, and analyzing data for surveillance programs. Final strategies to maintain privacy include having students step up backward on the scale and informing students who request to know the measurements that the information will be shared with parents/guardians. Last, if a student is hesitant to be measured, do not proceed. Instead, inform the parent about the student's hesitancy.

BOX 12-2

Safeguards Needed for School Body Mass Index (BMI) Measurement Programs

Safeguard 1. Introduce the program to parents/guardians, students, and school staff; ensure that there is an appropriate process in place for obtaining parental consent for measuring students' height and weight.

Safeguard 2. *Ensure that staff members who measure height and weight have the appropriate expertise and training to obtain accurate and reliable results and minimize the potential for stigmatization.*

Safeguard 3. *Ensure that the setting for data collection is private.*

Safeguard 4. *Use equipment that can accurately and reliably measure height and weight.*

Safeguard 5. *Ensure that the BMI number is calculated and interpreted correctly.*

Safeguard 6. *Develop efficient data collection procedures.*

Safeguard 7. *Do not use the actual BMI-for-age percentiles of the students as a basis for evaluating student or teacher performance (e.g., in physical education or health education class).*

Safeguard 8. *Evaluate the BMI measurement program by assessing the process, intended outcomes, and unintended consequences of the program.*

Safeguard 9. *Ensure that resources are available for safe and effective follow-up.*

Safeguard 10. *Provide all parents/guardians with a clear and respectful explanation of the BMI results and a list of appropriate follow-up actions.*

Source: National Center for Chronic Disease Prevention and Health Promotion (2022b); Nihiser et al. (2007).

Height

Monitoring growth is an essential part of determining a student's overall health condition and should be assessed at least annually by primary healthcare providers to ensure that students are within expected stature norms (Fenstermacher & Hudson, 2016; Styne et al., 2017). Most states do not mandate height screening in schools. However, school nurses performing BMI measurements will measure both height and weight as part of the process. School nurses should be knowledgeable about typical growth patterns. From ages 3 years to puberty, the typical growth rate is 2 to 2.5 inches/year and weight gain is 5 lb/year (Fenstermacher & Hudson, 2016).

Accurate assessments of height and weight are dependent on precise measurements. Stadiometers are the preferred tool for measuring height and consist of a vertical ruled board with a perpendicularly mounted, movable, horizontal headpiece. They may be wall mounted or attached to a base with a wide, stable platform, and are to be used on a firm, uncarpeted floor. Height attachment arms on beam balance scales should *not* be used as they are frequently inaccurate for measuring height (e.g., the arm is often floppy, not fixed at a right angle, and the student is unable to stand against a flat surface; NCCDPHP, 2022b). If a stadiometer is not available, the school nurse can mount yardsticks to the wall and use a flat headpiece such as a Plexiglas bookend at a 90-degree angle (NCCDPHP, 2021). During measurement, it is critical that students stand tall with their back and feet (shoes removed) to the wall, looking straight ahead without tilting their heads, with arms at their sides and shoulders level (NCCDPHP, 2021). With proper positioning, four points of contact will be visible against the wall: heels, buttocks, shoulders, and head. While in this position, the headpiece is lowered until it firmly touches the crown of the head, applying sufficient pressure to compress the hair (after removal of hair ornaments, buns, braids, or other items interfering with accuracy in measurement). Height should be recorded to the nearest 0.1 centimeter or ⅛-inch increment (NCCDPHP, 2021).

Weight

Recommended scales for measuring weight in students are either quality beam balance or digital scales that can be easily calibrated and allow weight to be measured to the nearest 0.1 kilogram or ¼ pound. The scale should be calibrated on a regular basis according to manufacturer's instructions. Spring-loaded bathroom scales should not be used to weigh students (NCCDPHP, 2022b); the spring counterbalance loses accuracy over time, and they cannot be read accurately to less than half a pound. Reliability is enhanced when all school nurses in the same setting utilize the same measurement technique for growth measurements and growth curves. Students should be measured in lightweight clothes with shoes removed. Screening conducting during warmer seasons or in collaboration with physical education classes will lessen the possibility of heavy and multiple layered clothing compromising accuracy. Record results to the nearest 0.1 kilogram or ¼ pound.

Combined stature-for-age and weight-for-age percentile charts for children can be easily downloaded from the CDC's Web site (National Center for Health Statistics, 2017, 2022). A series of measures over time is valuable in illustrating a student's pattern of growth and is reflective of health. Growth is unique to each student and yet falls within expected norms. Deviations from the student's normal growth pattern may be early warning signs of some illness/disease process or environmental changes. These deviations warrant referral. Notably, a student's height and weight may be measured on an individual basis at any time because of a concern for growth or general wellness.

Body Mass Index Calculation

Once height and weight have been obtained, the BMI can be calculated. BMI is a person's weight in kilograms divided by the square of height in meters and is an inexpensive and commonly accepted measurement for estimating adiposity. A fixed BMI (30.0 or higher) indicates obesity in adults (NCCDPHP, 2022a). BMI calculation in students is a two-step process and is sex-specific, based on age, and reported as a percentile (NCCDPHP, 2022d). Step one is calculating the BMI value, and step two is plotting the BMI value on the sex-specific CDC chart to determine the BMI-for-age percentile, with the percentiles determining whether a student is

- Underweight (<5%)
- Within the normal range (5% to <85%)
- Overweight (85% to <95%)
- Obese (>95%) (NCCDPHP, 2022d)

For example, a 7-year-old male student with a BMI of 19 plots at 95%, meeting the criteria for obesity, whereas a 20-year-old male with a BMI of 19 plots at 5%, almost considered underweight. The CDC provides an online calculator for students ages 2 through 19, as well as a spreadsheet tool to assist with group calculation of BMI such as when performing school screenings (NCCDPHP, 2018b, 2022c). Some school districts have height, weight, and BMI calculations as part of their online documentation system. Although others may be involved in the measurement and recording of the results when implementing school BMI screenings, the school nurse should be the lead person responsible for interpreting the results, as BMI does not consider body composition, such as an athlete with a higher-than-average amount of lean body mass may have a high BMI. In addition, BMI is not as sensitive in measuring body fat in thin students. A more in-depth discussion of obesity is provided in Chapter 14.

Although surveillance allows the school, district, or state to have data on the assessment of the school related to obesity, screening allows individual students to be identified who are overweight, obese, or underweight warranting referral to their primary healthcare provider. Screenings also serve as reinforcers to those who are in the typical range of their status (O'Connor et al., 2017). To prevent perceived bias when conducting a BMI screening program, all parents/guardians should receive the BMI screening results notification, not just those with students falling within certain categories. The notifications should include an easy-to-read explanation of BMI; a simple explanation of how the BMIs were measured (e.g., "The school nurse measured your child's height and weight, while maintaining privacy, and used a formula to calculate the BMI"); recommended follow-up actions; and information about dietary intake, physical activity, and resources in the community to help address these areas and safeguards 9 and 10 (Ruggieri et al., 2020). Hoke et al. (2020) studied the development and use of an electronic notification letter (e-BMI) with the capability to direct parents/guardians to resources and appropriate next steps using embedded links. The electronic notification also reduced costs for translating, printing, and mailing of letters. A sample electronic notification letter is available in the Online Materials OM12-4. Ongoing research is needed to determine parent preferences and acceptance regarding both BMI screening and receiving of results, while also addressing the concerns of parents/guardians least likely to act.

Type 2 Diabetes Risk Factor Screening

Before 1990, type 2 diabetes (T2D) was rarely seen in students. Today, the incidence of T2D continues to increase with students as young as 10 years old being diagnosed, in large part due to increasing obesity rates leading to insulin resistance (CDC, 2022). In addition to being overweight, other factors that put students at increased risk of developing T2D include the following:

- Having a first-degree relative with type 2 diabetes
- Having signs of insulin resistance (acanthosis nigricans)
- Having limited physical activity
- Being born to a mother having gestational diabetes (CDC, 2022)

Some schools incorporate T2D screening as part of their BMI screening program. As many students with T2D are asymptomatic, school nurses can use screening for the presence of acanthosis nigricans to identify students warranting referral to their healthcare provider for assessment.

Acanthosis nigricans is a condition involving a large patch of skin (usually neck, armpit, or groin) that thickens, darkens, and feels velvety to touch. Acanthosis nigricans may also be present on the hands, elbows, and knees (American Diabetes Association [ADA], 2017). While ensuring adequate lighting and privacy for the student, screening is conducted by asking the student to bend the neck forward, lifting long hair if present above the hairline, while the screener observes for color differences in the folds of the skin and feels for textural changes. Students found to have acanthosis nigricans or to be overweight plus one or more additional risk factors should be referred to their primary healthcare provider for additional evaluations. These individuals should also be referred for education on reducing risk factors (ADA, 2017). See Chapter 23 for additional information about T2D.

Blood Pressure Screening

Hypertension occurring in students is separated into two categories:

- Primary—no known cause, but more common in youth with obesity (NCCDPHP, 2023c)
- Secondary—most commonly a result or renal disease, congenital cardiovascular abnormalities, genetic disorders, and endocrine disorders (Flynn et al., 2012; Gartlehner et al., 2020)

In defining elevated BP in this population, the AAP adheres to the definitions revised by their organization in 2017 (Flynn et al., 2017):

- For children ages 1 to 13 years (based on normative distribution in healthy children of normal weight):
  - Elevated BP (previously referred to as prehypertension)—three auscultatory BP measurements between the 90th and 94th percentile based on age, height, and sex, or 120 to 129/<80 mm Hg
  - Hypertension—sustained high BP on three auscultatory BP measurements at three different visits that are either equal to or above the 95th percentile based on age, height, and sex or above 130/80 mm Hg, whichever measurement is lower
- For adolescents 13 years or older, adult guidelines are followed, regardless of sex and height:
  - Stage 1 hypertension—BP measurement of 130/80 to 139/89 mm Hg
  - Stage 2 hypertension—BP measurement above 140/90 mm Hg (Gartlehner et al., 2020; Whelton et al., 2018)

A study by the CDC, using National Health and Nutrition Examination Survey data gathered between 2013 and 2016, found that 1 in 25 youth ages 12 to 19 has hypertension and 1 in 10 has elevated BP (Jackson et al., 2018).

Though the USPSTF has concluded there is insufficient evidence to assess the balance of benefits and harms of screening for high BP in students, the AAP continues to recommend yearly screenings at annual well-child visits beginning at age 3 and at each visit for students with obesity, renal disease, diabetes, or known aortic arch disease (Flynn et al., 2017). As elevated BP is usually asymptomatic, mass assessment of BP is provided in some schools for specific age groups, though not recommended by the USPSTF at this time (Gartlehner et al., 2020). School-based measurement of BP might also be requested to help monitor students with diagnosed hypertension and other related health needs.

Auscultation, using a sphygmomanometer, is the preferred method for measuring BP (Newcombe, 2020). BP should be measured in the right arm with an appropriate size cuff after a resting period from 3 to 5 minutes. For students whose cuff size is difficult to determine, the width of the cuff should be two-thirds the length of the upper arm measuring from the axilla to the antecubital space (Newcombe, 2020). Too large of a cuff can result in a false low reading, and a cuff that is too small can likewise cause a false elevated reading. If the initial BP reading is elevated, the healthcare provider should take three readings at the same visit and average them to determine the BP category. If BP remains elevated after three readings, a referral should be made to the student's primary healthcare provider for formal evaluation (Flynn et al., 2017). BP can be taken for screening purposes, to monitor ongoing health concerns, and to help in the management of medication evaluation. The AAP Clinical Practice Guideline for *Screening and Management of High Blood Pressure in Children and Adolescents* provides detailed instructions for providing BP measurement as well as situations and medications that can affect measurement (Flynn et al., 2017).

School staff members often have hypertension or other health complications that require BP evaluation. Providing school staff BP checks is a convenient way to promote cardiovascular health and wellness. Opportunities to promote a healthy lifestyle along with BP checks can help provide overall optimal health and wellness to the school and district staff.

Posture Screening

The purpose of *posture screenings*, previously called orthopedic or scoliosis screening, is to identify students with possible postural deviations. The most common deviations of the spine are scoliosis, kyphosis, and lordosis.

Scoliosis is a lateral curvature of the spine that exceeds 10 degrees and may be idiopathic (unknown origin), congenital, or associated with other neuromuscular conditions (Hockenberry, 2022). Scoliosis screening is targeted at identifying idiopathic scoliosis, as this form of scoliosis is often recognized in students ages 10 to 18 years (USPSTF, 2018). In the United States, the prevalence of idiopathic scoliosis in youth is 2% to 4% and it affects females more often than males (Szilagyi, 2021). Depending on the severity of the curve, treatment might include observations, bracing, and surgery if severe or worsening, with a goal of halting progression of the curve (Hockenberry, 2022). Severe scoliosis may lead to back pain, psychological effects, cosmetic issues, reduced pulmonary functioning, and reduced quality of life (USPSTF, 2018). Chapter 24 provides an expanded discussion of scoliosis, causes, associated health problems, and treatment.

Kyphosis presents as a rounded back and usually involves the thoracic spine. It is a structural problem of an abnormal fixed posterior convexity of a segment of the thoracic spine mostly seen in older adults. It may be caused by trauma, osteoporosis, congenital conditions, or secondary to surgical treatment of spinal tumors.

Lordosis is an abnormal exaggerated anterior convexity of a segment of the spine, usually the lumbar spine. It is normal in the young toddler who is learning to walk but may occur later because of obesity, pregnancy, or neuromuscular disorders (Hockenberry, 2022).

Since 1996, and most recently in 2018, the USPSTF issued an "I" or insufficient recommendation statement following a systematic review as "the current evidence is insufficient to assess the balance of benefits and harms of screening for adolescent idiopathic scoliosis in students ages 10 to 18 years" (p. 1). The systematic review found no evidence that screening affected health outcomes, but that screening can detect scoliosis. The committee did not find any evidence that screening was harmful, although evidence was limited (USPSTF, 2018). Only a few states require scoliosis screenings in school, although other organizations have expressed varying opinions related to the value of scoliosis screenings (Jakubowski & Alexy, 2014; Timothy Hresko et al., 2015). In a collaborative statement, the Scoliosis Research Society, the American Academy of Orthopedic Surgeons, the Pediatric Orthopedic Society of North America, and AAP state that screening examinations for spine deformity should be part of the preventive healthcare services visit for females at age 10 and 12 years and males once at age 13 or 14 years (Timothy Hresko et al., 2015). The position statement reviewed the available research for screening, diagnosis, and treatment as well as the pros and cons of school screening programs. The statement also called for effective screening systems and stated that inappropriate false-positive screening may lead to unnecessary referrals and radiographs with higher population cost.

If postural screenings are conducted at school, they are most often conducted during middle school, as screening is recommended during early adolescence. Each state determines who can conduct the screening. This may be the school nurse, a physical education teacher, or a nonhealth professional who has been trained to conduct the scoliosis screening (Jakubowski & Alexy, 2014). Because students are often sensitive about exposing their bodies at this age, they need to be prepared by informing them about how the spine develops, why screening is necessary, and how it will be done. It should be stressed that privacy will be provided. Some school nurses recommend that students wear bathing suits under their clothes on the screening day and others recommend screening during physical education classes when students are wearing gym uniforms. Males and females should be screened separately, and precautions taken to preserve privacy. The process takes about 30 seconds per student. Step-by-step instructions for postural screening, including the Adams forward bend test, are provided in Table 12-4. Referral is made or rescreening is scheduled in 3 to 6 months if there is a 5- to 7-degree angle of trunk rotation, which corresponds to a 20-degree curve (Kuznia et al., 2020).

Sports Physical Screening

Preparticipation sport physicals or evaluations are another type of screening routinely recommended for student athletes and required by most state high school athletic associations for participation in school-based sports. According to the CDC (n.d.), as recent as 2019, 57.4% of high school students played on at least one school or community sports team. The primary goal of the sports physical is to ensure an athlete's safe participation through the evaluation of general physical health and the identification of conditions that predispose athletes to injury, illness, or life-threatening conditions, including the risk of sudden cardiac arrest (Macdonald et al., 2021; Polfuss & Davis, 2020). Some additional objectives of sports physicals include (1) provision of an entry point into the healthcare system for those without a primary healthcare provider; (2) promotion of a healthy lifestyle, recommendations for safe ways to improve athletic performance, and education about youth risky behaviors; (3)

TABLE 12-4 Screening Guidelines for Posture

Steps	Observations
1. Ask the student to stand erect with feet slightly apart, weight evenly distributed, hands hanging at sides, and looking forward.	Observe from the front, side, and back: • Is the head midline? • Are the shoulders level? • Are the scapulas level? • Are the spaces between arms and body the same? • Are the hips level? • Are the knees level? • Is there an exaggerated roundness of upper back? • Is there exaggerated arch in lower back?
2. While standing behind the student, have the student bend forward at the waist with arms hanging freely. Ensure that the student's feet are 2 to 3 inches apart and knees are straight. The student's back should be horizontal to the floor. This is called the Adams forward bend test.	• Is one scapula higher than the other? • Is there a prominence or bulge on one side of the back? • Are the hip levels uneven? • Is there a curvature of the spine?* • View from side: Are there spinal humps?
3. Have the student walk away and then turn and walk back.	• Is there symmetry of movement? • Do the knees come together, and the ankles are abducted? (genu valgum—knock-kneed) • Do the knees abduct when the feet are together? (genu varum—bow-legged)

Kuznia et al. (2020).

*Some measure the curvature or degree of rotation using a scoliometer. It can be placed directly across the student's back where the irregularity is most prominent. The "0" should be directly over the top ridge of the spine. Do not press down on the device; any reading greater than 5 to 7 degrees should be rescreened or referred. Referral might also be made if there is asymmetry in two or more areas of visual assessment.

collection of emergency medical data; and (4) provision of anticipatory guidance related to safety and equipment needed for athletic participation (Macdonald et al., 2021; Polfuss & Davis, 2020; Vogt, 2021). A fifth objective might be to assist in the selection of a sport or activity appropriate to the athlete's specific abilities and physical status, as the primary intent of the sports physical is to ensure that students are medically cleared to participate.

The frequency (e.g., annually) and type of sports physical vary from state to state, with some states requiring a general physical examination and others requiring a sport-specific examination. The National Federation of State High School Associations provides a listing of state associations and contact information where information about each state's requirements can be accessed. School nurses should be familiar with state and school district requirements. Completion of the sports physical at least 6 weeks before the first practice allows time to treat any conditions found during the examination, and dependent on state law, are conducted by a physician, nurse practitioner, or physician assistant with clinical training to evaluate and determine medical eligibility of the athlete on a broad range of health issues (AAP, 2022). In 2019, the AAP published the 5th edition of the *Preparticipation Physical Examination (PPE) Monograph* containing consensus recommendations from representatives of multiple stakeholder medical societies (i.e., American Academy of Family Physicians, AAP, American College of Sports Medicine, American Medical Society for Sports Medicine, American Orthopaedic Society for Sports Medicine, and American Osteopathic Academy of Sports Medicine [2019]), and updated template forms based on the guidelines. These templates are available for free online within the PPE 5th edition, on the AAP webpage, and are also endorsed by the National Athletic Trainers' Association and the National Federation of State High School Associations (AAP, 2022).

The Preparticipation Sports Physical Examination consists of multiple components. The first component is the *history section,* which covers both the student's medical history and relevant family history and is often provided in advance to facilitate completion before the physical (AAP, 2022; Conley et al., 2014; Vogt, 2021). Examples of questions related to the student's past and current health conditions include history of asthma, diabetes, or surgeries; current medications, supplements (e.g., use of performance-enhancing substances), or any known allergies; past musculoskeletal and head injuries; missing or damaged organs such as a kidney or an eye; and eating disorders, including attempts to gain or lose weight). With history of past injury, additional questions include inquiry into previous exclusion from sports for any reason, length of time lost from participation, current sequelae of the injury, and any loss of consciousness or amnesia after a head injury (Fenstermacher & Hudson, 2016). Specific to heart health, the American Academy of Family Physicians et al. (2019) preparticipation physical evaluation history form template serves as an example of questions specific to family or student areas of concern:

- Family heart history areas of concern
  - Premature death before age 35 (due to heart disease or because of drowning or unexplained car crash)
  - Any family member with genetic heart problem (hypertrophic cardiomyopathy, Marfan syndrome, arrhythmogenic right ventricular cardiomyopathy, long QT syndrome, short QT syndrome, Brugada syndrome, or catecholaminergic polymorphic ventricular tachycardia)
  - Any family member having a pacemaker or implanted defibrillator before age 35
- Student heart history areas of concern
  - Has had syncope or near syncope during or after exercise
  - Has had discomfort, pain, tightness, or pressure in the chest with exercise
  - Has felt heart race, flutter, or skip beats during exercise
  - Has had doctor tell them that they have a heart problem or has had testing for their heart (e.g., electrocardiography or echocardiography)
  - Has become light-headed or felt shorter of breath than their friends during exercise
  - Has ever had a seizure

More recently, questions to address mental health conditions have been recommended for all athletes. (See American Academy of Family Physicians et al. [2019] History Form inclusion of Patient Health Questionnaire-4 [PHQ-4] addressing anxiety and depression.)

The second part of the preparticipation sports physical examination is the actual *physical examination,* and it is recommended that the evaluation take place in the primary healthcare provider's office rather than in a group setting, as this may be the only encounter the student has with their healthcare provider during the year (AAP, 2022; Vogt, 2021). It is also important to note that many health insurance providers only allow one physical (of any kind) per year. Thus it is a good idea to combine both the annual examination and the sports physical together or to partner with community stakeholders, such as nurse practitioners or medical school programs, to have focused sports physicals offered at no cost onsite. Whether provided in the healthcare provider's office or in a group setting, the sports physical should include a structured physical examination focusing on the cardiovascular, musculoskeletal, and neurological systems; screening for mental health conditions and risk-taking behaviors; and recognition of findings suggestive of nutritional imbalances (MacDonald et al., 2021). Online Material OM12-5 provides a detailed overview of the components of the sports physical examination. Strategies to promote health and prevent injuries (e.g., protective equipment, use of sunscreen), along with the need to balance individual sport and educational goals, should be discussed with both the student athletes and their parents/guardians. The primary healthcare provider can further use the sports physical to discuss health maintenance needs and encourage adherence to recommended immunization schedules (Vogt, 2021).

The AAP's PPE 5th edition provides additional considerations to address the needs and concerns of transgender athletes and athletes with physical and intellectual disabilities (AAP, 2022; MacDonald et al., 2021). The COVID-19 pandemic brought new considerations related to cardiovascular and pulmonary risks after infection with the recommendation to be evaluated by a healthcare provider before returning to play (MacDonald et al., 2021). In 2022, an expert task force from the National Federation of State High School Associations (NFHS) and the American Medical Society for Sports Medicine (AMSSM) reconvened to update guidelines related to cardiac assessment of high school student athletes with prior SARS-CoV-2 infection, and separated the guidance for return to play based on the individual severity of and symptoms associated with the infection (Drezner et al., 2022).

The third and final step of the PPE is the healthcare provider's *medical eligibility statement.* The AAP's medical eligibility form (2022) provides five potential outcomes related to sport participation:

- Cleared to participate in all sports without restrictions
- Cleared to participate in all sports without restrictions with recommendations for further evaluation or treatment (listing the condition[s] of concern)
- Eligible for certain sports as specified
- Not cleared to participate pending further evaluation
- Not medically eligible for any sports

Sports are classified by intensity, with sports such as triathlon events being high intensity and sports such as bowling being of lower intensity, as well as some sports having increased risk of impact (Polfuss & Davis, 2020). Disqualification from participation may be indicated for student athletes with less than optimally controlled chronic health conditions, such as a student with uncontrolled epilepsy not being cleared to participate in weightlifting. Examples where restrictions from sports participation might be considered include student athletes with the following conditions:

- Certain uncontrolled chronic illnesses (e.g., asthma, diabetes mellitus, epilepsy, bleeding disorders, hypertension, or sickle cell disease)
- Unresolved concussion or other head injury
- Cardiac disorders (e.g., cardiomyopathy, arrhythmias, or cardiac infections)
- Enlarged liver or spleen
- Missing limb or organ
- Unresolved previous injury with ongoing symptoms (Polfuss & Davis, 2020)

School personnel, coaches, and parents/guardians should have a shared understanding about the importance of the preparticipation physical examination and its impact on student participation in athletics. In general:

- It is the healthcare provider that "clears" a student to play sports, not the school nurse.
- If a student is not healthy enough to participate in physical education, the student is not healthy enough to participate in a sport.
- The preparticipation physical examination is both a safety measure for students and liability protection for the school district.

The school nurse's role with sports physicals varies. In many school districts, school nurses are responsible for planning and promotion of all logistics involved with sports physicals, including assembling the paperwork, completing the initial screening components (such as height, weight, vital signs, and hearing and vision if applicable), collecting and reviewing completed forms, and ensuring that recommended measures are initiated (e.g., cleared for participating, follow-up appointments). In other districts, coaches or athletic directors take the lead related to sports physical activities and requirements. Regardless, school nurses and athletic directors/coaches should work together to ensure communication about identified student health concerns discovered on a preparticipation sports physical examination to enhance coordination of care and to ensure a safe school environment focused on individualized student health needs.

Cardiac Risks Related to Sports Participation

The student athlete who presents with cardiac concerns during the preparticipation physical examination should be referred to a specialist for clearance to play before participation begins. Cardiac concerns may include personal history of congenital or acquired heart disease. Although rare, sudden cardiac death (SCD) is the leading cause of death among student athletes, occurring in about 0.75 per 100,000 athletes per year and is usually the first sign of an underlying cardiac condition (Fanous & Dorian, 2019; Yow et al., 2022). The most frequent cause of SCD among student athletes is cardiomyopathy, especially hypertrophic cardiomyopathy, and to a lesser extent arrhythmogenic right ventricular cardiomyopathy, both of which are inherited, structural abnormalities of the myocardium that can lead to ventricular arrhythmias and death (Newcombe, 2020). Additional congenital structural, as well as congenital, electrical cardiac abnormalities can lead to SCD, as can causes such as myocarditis, performance-enhancing drugs, and premature coronary artery disease (Newcombe, 2020). Commotio cardis, a blunt, nonpenetrating trauma to the midchest (e.g., baseball, hockey puck), has also been implicated in SCD, and can occur if the blow occurs during the timing of the T wave in the cardiac cycle.

Worldwide, considerable debate continues among the medical community regarding whether electrocardiogram or echocardiography should be part of the preparticipation sports physical examination screening for student athletes (Macdonald et al., 2021). The American Heart Association Cardiovascular Screening Checklist, with its 14 key indicators commonly used in sports physical history-taking templates, and the physical examination (detection of heart murmur, abnormal femoral pulse, physical symptoms of Marfan syndrome, and hypertension), assist in identifying student athletes at risk (MacDonald et al., 2021; Yow et al., 2022). When the history or examination reveals cardiac concerns, electrocardiogram or echocardiogram may be indicated, though routine use of these tests on all athletes has not been widely accepted in the United States (Vogt, 2021). In part, concerns about mass screening involve the sensitivity of the tests (false positives), heightened anxiety to both the athlete and the parents/guardians, and the cost-benefit ratio.

Marfan syndrome is a genetic disorder of the connective tissue that affects approximately 1 in 5,000 people. It often causes structural differences in the heart, blood vessels, bones, joints, and eyes. Aortic enlargement associated with Marfan syndrome can be life-threatening. It should be noted that students with Marfan syndrome can exercise regularly but should have modified physical activity to avoid stress on the aorta, avoid trauma to the chest or eyes, and avoid potential damage to loose ligaments or joints (Marfan Foundation, n.d.). Sudden death in individuals with Marfan syndrome is most often caused by a dissected or ruptured aortic aneurysm and accounts for 1% of the SCD cases (Braverman et al., 2015).

The term *athlete's heart*, or athletic heart syndrome (AHS), describes a condition in endurance athletes that is characterized by both structural and functional remodeling. Structurally there is thickening of the myocardial wall and increase in chamber size. This in turn leads to the functional changes of a lower heart rate, increased cardiac output and oxygen delivery to skeletal muscles, and more rapid heart rate recovery after exercise (Fanous & Dorian, 2019). Though often evident on electrocardiography, these physiological changes that occur in response to systemic engagement in regular exercise are considered normal. In a small percentage of athletes, the degree of structural adaptation may resemble pathological conditions such as hypertrophic cardiomyopathy, spurring further medical evaluation (Fanous & Dorian, 2019).

Athletic eligibility or disqualification is based on the assertion that intense training and competition increase the risk for SCD, and this risk is likely to be reduced by withdrawal from participation. Depending on the cardiac condition, athletes may be recommended to withdraw from participating in competitive sports, with the exception of low-intensity sports. For acquired diseases that may be reversible, athletes may be advised to temporarily withdraw from competition, followed by resumption of the sports activity if resolution is documented.

Although the sports physical provides a useful screening tool for SCD, not all cardiac conditions that pose a risk to athletes will be uncovered. Therefore, school nurses can be involved in the development and implementation of cardiac emergency response plans at their schools. Establishing effective resuscitation protocols and increasing the availability of automated external defibrillators (AEDs) in settings where competitive sport is undertaken are the most effective strategies in helping reduce the incidence of sudden cardiac death among athletes (Bogue et al., 2021; Drezner et al., 2019; Fanous & Dorian, 2019). These should include ensuring that AEDs are easily accessible and properly maintained, ensuring that training occurs for potential responders, and establishing an emergency communication system. The school nurse should also be aware of state laws and high school athletic association rules that delineate the availability of AEDs and trained personnel during physical education and sporting events.

CONCLUSION

The school nurse has multiple roles in the school setting related to health promotion and health screenings. Through participation in many available models, school nurses can lead or assist with the coordination of policies, processes, and practices to achieve improved student health, as well as student educational outcomes. The school environment may be the primary place where many students learn about healthy lifestyles and build health literacy to make positive health decisions. When the school nurse promotes the health and well-being of students, the effect is far-reaching and can be felt by the school staff, families, and the broader school community.

Special thanks for assistance with the vision section of this chapter to P. Kay Nottingham Chaplin, EdD (Education and Outreach Coordinator for the National Center for Children's Vision and Eye Health at Prevent Blindness and contracted education consultant for the Good-Lite Company and School Health Corporation).

The Editors gratefully acknowledge the work of authors on this chapter in the previous edition: Linda Kimel and Graceinda Tedder.

References

Agency for Toxic Substances and Disease Registry. (2020a). *ToxFAQs(tm) for lead.* U.S. Department of Health & Human Services. https://wwwn.cdc.gov/TSP/ToxFAQs/ToxFAQsDetails.aspx?faqid=93&toxid=22

Agency for Toxic Substances and Disease Registry. (2020b). *Toxicological profile for lead.* U.S. Department of Health and Human Services. https://wwwn.cdc.gov/TSP/ToxProfiles/ToxProfiles.aspx?id=96&tid=22

AlAzzam, M., Abuhammad, S., Abdalrahim, A., & Hamdan-Mansour, A. M. (2021). Predictors of depression and anxiety among senior high school students during COVID-19 pandemic: The context of home quarantine and online education. *The Journal of School Nursing, 37*(4), 241–248. https://doi.org/10.1177/1059840520988548

American Academy of Family Physicians, American Academy of Pediatrics, American College of Sports Medicine, American Medical Society for Sports Medicine, American Orthopaedic Society for Sports Medicine, & American Osteopathic Academy of Sports Medicine. (2019). *Preparticipation physical evaluation: History form.* https://downloads.aap.org/AAP/PDF/PPE-History-Form-(English)-rev.pdf?_ga=2.10671799.205390814.1673466475-1334538709.1665364823

American Academy of Pediatrics. (n.d.). *Health services assessment tool for schools.* https://www.schoolhealthteams.org/

American Academy of Pediatrics. (2022). *Preparticipation physical evaluation.* https://www.aap.org/en/patient-care/preparticipation-physical-evaluation/

American Associaton for Pediatric Ophthalmology and Stabismus. (2024). *Glossary: Definitions 2018–2023.* https://aapos.org/browse/glossary

American Diabetes Association. (2017). Children and adolescents. Sec. 12. In standards of medical care in diabetes. *Diabetes Care, 40*(Suppl 1), S104–113. https://doi.org/10.2337/dc17-S015

American Speech-Language-Hearing Association. (n.d.a). *Childhood hearing screening.* https://www.asha.org/practice-portal/professional-issues/childhood-hearing-screening/

American Speech-Language-Hearing Association. (n.d.b). *Degree of hearing loss.* https://www.asha.org/public/hearing/degree-of-hearing-loss/

American Speech-Language-Hearing Association. (n.d.c). *Newborn hearing screening* www.asha.org/Practice-Portal/Professional-Issues/Newborn-Hearing-Screening/

American Speech-Language-Hearing Association. (n.d.d). *School-age hearing screening.* https://www.asha.org/advocacy/state/school-age-hearing-screening/

American Speech-Language-Hearing Association. (n.d.e). *The audiogram.* https://www.asha.org/public/hearing/audiogram/

Anderson, L. J. W., Schaffer, M. A., Hiltz, C., O'Leary, S. A., Luehr, R. E., & Yoney, E. L. (2018). Public health interventions: School nurse practice stories. *The Journal of School Nursing, 34*(3), 192–202. https://doi.org/10.1177/1059840517721951

Arpaci, T., Altay, N., & Copur, G. Y. (2023). Evaluation of the effectiveness of a technology-based psychosocial education and counseling program for adolescent survivors of childhood leukemia: A randomized controlled trial. *Cancer Nursing, 46*(1), 14–28. https://doi.org/10.1097/ncc.0000000000001091

Association of State and Territorial Dental Directors. (n.d.). *Best practice approaches.* https://www.astdd.org/best-practices/#attach

Barzel, R., & Holt, K. (Eds.). (2019). *Promoting oral health in schools: A resource guide* (4th ed.). National Maternal and Child Oral Health Resource Center. https://www.mchoralhealth.org/PDFs/resguideschooloh.pdf

Bejster, M., Cygan, H., Stock, J., & Ashworth, J. (2020). Engaging the school community in a nutrition and physical activity program. *NASN School Nurse, 35*(5), 260–265. https://doi.org/10.1177/1942602X20912747

Bitsko, R. H., Claussen, A. H., Lichstein, J., Black, L. I., Jones, S. E., Danielson, M. L., Hoenig, J. M., Davis Jack, S. P., Brody, D. J., Gyawali, S., Maenner, M. J., Warner, M., Holland, K. M., Perou, R., Crosby, A. E., Blumberg, S. J., Avenevoli, S., Kaminski, J. W., & Ghandour, R. M. (2022). Mental health surveillance among children—United States, 2013–2019. *Morbidity and Mortality Weekly Report, 71*(2), 1–42. http://dx.doi.org/10.15585/mmwr.su7102a1

Bogue, K. A., Idriss, S. F., Sturkey, D., & Derouin, A. (2021). Improving youth sports safety: Implementing an emergency action plan for sudden cardiac arrest. *Journal of Pediatric Nursing, 59,* 81–88. https://doi.org/10.1016/j.pedn.2020.10.001

Bonino, A. Y., & Leibold, L. J. (2017). Behavioral assessment of hearing in 2- to 4- year-old children: A two-interval, observer-based procedure using conditioned play-based responses. *Journal of Visualized Experiments, 119,* e54788. https://doi.org/10.3791%2F54788

Braverman, A. C., Harris, K. M., Kovacs, R. J., & Maron, B. J. (2015). Eligibility and disqualification recommendations for competitive athletes with cardiovascular abnormalities: Task force 7: Aortic diseases, including Marfan syndrome. A scientific statement from the American Heart Association and American College of Cardiology. *Circulation, 132,* e303–e309. https://doi.org/10.1161/CIR.0000000000000243

Bright Futures & American Academy of Pediatrics. (2022). *Recommendations for preventive pediatric health care.* https://downloads.aap.org/AAP/PDF/periodicity_schedule.pdf?_ga=2.257802059.1538049820.1675469022-200829201.1675469021

Bruce, A., Fairley, L., Chambers, B., Wright, J., & Sheldon, T. A. (2016). Impact of visual acuity on developing literacy at age 4-5 years: A cohort-nested cross-sectional study. *BMJ Open, 6*, e010434. http://dx.doi.org/10.1136/bmjopen-2015-010434

Buz Harlor, A. D., Bower, C., Committee on Practice and Ambulatory Medicine, & the Section on Otolaryngology–Head and Neck Surgery. (2009). Hearing assessment in infants and children: Recommendations beyond neonatal screening. *Pediatrics, 124*(4), 1252–1263. https://doi.org/10.1542/peds.2009-1997

Cadena-Malek, Y. (2021). Communicable disease. In C. Rector & M. J. Stanley (Eds.), *Community and public health nursing: Promoting the public's health* (10th ed., pp. 204–241). Wolters Kluwer.

Cagulada, E., & Koller, D. (2020). "It's a hearing world": Parents' perspectives of the well-being of children who are deaf and hard of hearing. *Deafness & Education International, 22*(2), 139–155. https://doi.org/10.1080/14643154.2019.1635297

Center for Community Health and Development. (n.d.). Chapter 2, Section 2: PRECEDE/PROCEED. University of Kansas. https://ctb.ku.edu/en/table-contents/overview/other-models-promoting-community-health-and-development/preceder-proceder/main

Centers for Disease Control and Prevention. (n.d.). *1991–2019 High School Youth Risk Behavior Survey data.* http://yrbs-explorer.services.cdc.gov/

Centers for Disease Control and Prevention. (2011). *Introduction to program evaluation for public health programs: A self-study guide.* U.S. Department of Health and Human Services, Program Performance and Evaluation Office. https://www.cdc.gov/evaluation/guide/CDCEvalManual.pdf

Centers for Disease Control and Prevention. (2019). *CDC Clear Communication Index: A tool for developing and assessing CDC public communication products. User guide.* Office of the Associate Director for Communication. https://www.cdc.gov/ccindex/pdf/clear-communication-user-guide.pdf

Centers for Disease Control and Prevention. (2021, October 28). *CDC updates blood lead reference value for children* [Press release]. https://www.cdc.gov/media/releases/2021/p1028-blood-lead.html

Centers for Disease Control and Prevention. (2022, December 30). *Prevent type 2 diabetes in kids.* https://www.cdc.gov/diabetes/prevent-type-2/type-2-kids.html

Centers for Disease Control and Prevention & University of Connecticut. (2021). *Wellness school assessment tool: 3.0.* https://www.wellsat.org/

Centers for Medicare & Medicaid Services. (2016). *Coverage of blood lead testing for children enrolled in Medicaid and the Children's Health Insurance Program.* U.S. Department of Health and Human Services. https://www.medicaid.gov/sites/default/files/federal-policy-guidance/downloads/cib113016.pdf

Churchill, B. F. (2024). State-mandated school-based BMI assessments and self-reported adolescent health behaviors. *Journal of Policy Analysis and Management, 43*(1), 63–86. https://doi.org/10.1002/pam.22523

Collins, M. E., Mudie, L. I., Inns, A. J., & Repka, M. X. (2017). Pediatric ophthalmology and childhood reading difficulties: Overview of reading development and assessments for the pediatric ophthalmologist. *Journal of American Association for Pediatric Ophthalmology and Strabismus, 21*(6), 433–436, e1. https://doi.org/10.1016/j.jaapos.2017.06.017

Commission on Social Determinants of Health. (2008). *Commission on Social Determinants of Health final report: Closing the gap in a generation: Health equity through action on the social determinants of health.* World Health Organization. https://apps.who.int/iris/rest/bitstreams/65985/retrieve

Community Preventive Services Task Force. (2022, October 13). *The guide to community preventive services.* https://www.thecommunityguide.org/pages/task-force-findings.html

Conley, K. M., Bolin, D. J., Carek, P. J., Konin, J. G., Neal, T. L., & Violette, D. (2014). National Athletic Trainers' Association position statement: Preparticipation physical examinations and disqualifying conditions. *Journal of Athletic Training, 49*(1), 102–120. https://doi.org/10.4085/1062-6050-48.6.05

Cotter, S. A., Cyert, L. A., Miller, J. M., & Quinn, G. E. for the National Expert Panel to the National Center for Children's Vision and Eye Health. (2015). Vision screening for children 36 to <72 months: Recommended practices. *Optometry and Vision Science, 92*(1), 6–16. https://doi.org/10.1097%2FOPX.0000000000000429

Cotter, S. A., Donahue, S. P., & Moore, B. (2021). Position statement on the relationship between visual acuity and refractive error in the context of preschool vision screening using instrument-based technology. *Optometry and Vision Science, 98*(1), 102. https://doi.org/10.1097/01.opx.0000725792.80874.83

Council on School Health, Holmes, B. W., Sheetz, A., Allison, M., Ancona, R., Attisha, E., Beers, N., Pinto, C., Gorski, P., Kjolhede, C., Lerner, M., Weiss-Harrison, A., & Young, T. (2016). Role of the school nurse in providing school health services. *Pediatrics, 137*(6), e20160852. https://doi.org/10.1542/peds.2016-0852

Dineen, J. N., Chafouleas, S. M., Briesch, A. M., McCoach, D. B., Newton, S. D., & Cintron, D. W. (2022). Exploring social, emotional, and behavioral screening approaches in U.S. public school districts. *American Educational Research Journal, 59*(1), 146–179. https://doi.org/10.3102/00028312211000043

Donahue, S. P., Baker, C. N., Committee on Practice and Ambulatory Medicine–Section on Ophthalmology, American Association of Certified Orthoptists, American Association for Pediatric Ophthalmology and Strabismus, American Academy of Ophthalmology, Simon, G. R., Boudreau, A. D. A., Baker, C. N., Barden III, G. A., Hackell, J. M., Hardin, A. P., Meade, K. E., Moore, S. B., Richerson, J., Lehman, S. S., Granet, D. B., Bradford, G. E., Rubin, S. E., ... Granet, D. B. (2016). Procedures for the evaluation of the visual system by pediatricians. *Pediatrics, 137*(1), e20153597. https://doi.org/10.1542/peds.2015-3597

Drezner, J. A., Heinz, W. M., Asif, I. M., Batten, C. G., Fields, K. B., Raukar, N. P., Valentine, V. D., Walter, K. D., & Baggish, A. L. (2022). Cardiopulmonary considerations for high school student-athletes during the COVID-19 pandemic: Update to the NFHS-AMSSM guidance statement. *Sports Health, 14*(3), 369–371. https://doi.org/10.1177/19417381221077138

Drezner, J. A., Peterson, D. F., Siebert, D. M., Thomas, L. C., Lopez-Anderson, M., Suchsland, M. Z., Harmon, K. G., & Kucera, K. L. (2019). Survival after exercise-related sudden cardiac arrest in young athletes: Can we do better? *Sports Health, 11*(1), 91–98. https://doi.org/10.1177%2F1941738118799084

Driscoll, L. (2021). Addressing the whole child: The power of data and teams. *NASN School Nurse, 36*(4), 194–196. https://doi.org/10.1177/1942602X211017533

Fanous, Y., & Dorian, P. (2019). The prevention and management of sudden cardiac arrest in athletes. *Canadian Medical Association Journal, 191*(28), E787–791. https://doi.org/10.1503/cmaj 190166

Fenstermacher, K., & Hudson, B. T. (2016). *Practice guidelines for family nurse practitioners* (4th ed.). Elsevier.

Flaherty, E. A. (2020). School nursing and public health: The case for school nurse investigators and contact tracing monitors of COVID-19 patients in Massachusetts. *NASN School Nurse, 35*(6), 327–331. https://doi.org/10.1177/1942602X20950670

Fleming, E. (2019). *State dental screening laws for children: Examining the trend and impact. An update to the 2008 report.* Children's Dental Health Project. https://cdhp.s3.amazonaws.com/resource/341/attachment_1/original.pdf?1548939615 https://www.cdhp.org/resources/341-state-dental-screening-laws-for-children-examining-the-trend-and-impact

Flynn, J. T., Kaelber, D. C., Baker-Smith, C. M., Blowey, D., Carroll, A. E., Daniels, S. R., de Ferranti, S. D., Dionne, J. M., Falkner, B., Flinn, S. K., Gidding, S. S., Goodwin, C., Leu, M. G., Powers, M. E., Rea, C., Samuels, J., Simasek, M., Thaker, V. V., Urbina, E. M., & Subcommittee on Screening and Management of High Blood Pressure in Children. (2017). Clinical practice guideline for screening and management of high blood pressure in children and adolescents. *Pediatrics, 140*(3), e20171904. https://doi.org/10.1542/peds.2017-1904

Flynn, J. T., Pierce, C. B., Miller III, E. R., Charleston, J. Samuels, J. A., Kupferman, J., Furth, S. L., Warady, B. A., & Chronic Kidney Disease in Children Study Group. (2012). Reliability of resting blood pressure measurement and classification using an oscillometric device in children with chronic kidney disease. *The Journal of Pediatrics, 160*(3), 434–440.e1. https://doi.org/10.1016/j.jpeds.2011.08.071

Furr, B. A., Musch, D. C., Andrews, C. A., & Schumann, R. (2018). Testability study of the Titmus V3 test in pre-school children. *Optometry and Vision Science, 95*(7), 588–593. https://doi.org/10.1097/OPX.0000000000001240

Galemore, C. (2016). Too busy for TB: Managing a case of tuberculosis disease in the school setting. *NASN School Nurse, 31*(2), 83–89. https://doi.org/10.1177/1942602X16628194

Gartlehner, G., Vander Schaaf, E. B., Orr, C., Kennedy, S. M., Clark, R., & Viswanathan, M. (2020). *Screening for hypertension in children and adolescents: Systematic review for the U.S. Preventive Services Task Force.* Evidence Synthesis No. 193. Agency for Healthcare Research and Quality; AHRQ publication 20-05261-EF-1. PMID: 33284560. https://www.ncbi.nlm.nih.gov/books/NBK564973/

Global Wellness Institute. (n.d.). *What is wellness?* https://globalwellnessinstitute.org/what-is-wellness/

Guan, C. Q., & Smolen, E. R. (2022). Visual-motor integration in language learning among deaf and hard of hearing children. *American Annals of the Deaf, 167*(3), 355–371. https://doi.org/10.1353/aad.2022.0032

Hockenberry, M. J. (2022). The child with musculoskeletal or articular dysfunction. In M. J. Hockenberry, D. Wilson, & C. C. Rodgers (Eds.), *Wong's essentials of pediatric nursing* (11th ed., pp. 1005–1046). Elsevier.

Hoke, A. M., Poger, J. M., Lehman, E. B., & Kraschnewski, J. L. (2020). Feasibility of an online, interactive body mass index parental notification letter (e-BMI). *The Journal of School Nursing, 38*(3), 259–269. https://doi.org/10.1177/1059840520930071

Hold, J. L., & Amore Jones, V. (2021). Adult health. In C. Rector & M. J. Stanley (Eds.), *Community and public health nursing: Promoting the public's health* (10th ed., pp. 608–636). Wolters Kluwer.

Individuals With Disabilities Education Act. 34 C.F.R. § 300.111 (2004). https://sites.ed.gov/idea/regs/b/b/300.111

Jackson, S. L., Zhang, Z., Wiltz, J. L., Loustalot, F., Ritchey, M. D., Goodman, A. B., & Yang, Q. (2018). Hypertension among youths—United States, 2001–2016. *Morbidity and Mortality Weekly Report, 67*(27), 758–762. http://dx.doi.org/10.15585/mmwr.mm6727a2

Jakubowski, T. L., & Alexy, E. M. (2014). Does school scoliosis screening make the grade? *NASN School Nurse, 29*(5), 258–265. https://doi.org/10.1177/1942602X14542131

Johnson, R. A., Nottingham, D., Stratton, R., & Zaba, J. N. (1996). The vision screening of academically and behaviorally at-risk pupils. *Journal of Behavioral Optometry, 7*(2), 39–42.

Jonas, D. E., Amick, H. R., Wallace, I. F., Feltner, C., Vander Schaaf, E. B., Brown, C. L., & Baker, C. (2017). *Vision screening in children ages 6 months to 5 years: Evidence report and systematic review for U.S. Preventive Services Task Force.* AHRQ Publication No. 17-05228-EF-1. Agency for Healthcare Research and Quality. https://www.ncbi.nlm.nih.gov/books/NBK487841/

Kleman, C. C., & Smith, Y. M. (2022). Health defined: Health promotion, protection, and prevention. In C. L. Edelman & E. C. Kudzman (Eds.), *Health promotion throughout the lifespan* (10th ed., pp. 1–24). Elsevier.

Kudzma, E. C. (2022). Screening and health promotion. In C. L. Edelman & E. C. Kudzma (Eds.), *Health promotion throughout the lifespan* (10th ed., pp. 226–244). Elsevier.

Kuznia, A. L., Hernandez, A. K., & Lee, L. U. (2020). Adolescent idiopathic scoliosis: Common questions and answers. *American Family Physician, 101*(1), 19–23. https://www.aafp.org/pubs/afp/issues/2020/0101/p19.html

Lipkin, P. H., Macias, M. M., American Academy of Pediatrics Council on Children with Disabilities, Section on Developmental and Behavioral Pediatrics. (2020). Promoting optimal development: Identifying infants and young children with developmental disorders through developmental surveillance and screening. *Pediatrics, 145*(1), e20193449. https://doi.org/10.1542/peds.2019-3449

MacDonald, J., Schaefer, M., & Stumph, J. (2021). The preparticipation physical evaluation. *American Family Physician, 103*(9), 539–546. PMID: 33929170. https://www.aafp.org/pubs/afp/issues/2021/0501/p539.html

Mann, G., Kaiser, K. Trapp, N., Cafer, A., Grant, K., Gupta, K., & Bolden, C. (2021). Barriers, enablers, and possible solutions for student wellness: A qualitative analysis of student, administrators, and staff perspectives. *Journal of School Health, 91*(12), 1002–1013. https://doi.org/10.1111/josh.13092

Marfan Foundation. (n.d.) *Marfan syndrome. What are the key features of Marfan syndrome? Cardiovascular.* https://marfan.org/conditions/marfan-syndrome/#keyFeatures

Marzolf, A. L., Petersheim, M. M., Forcina, B. D., Papa, C., Wilson, M. E., Cheeseman, E. W., & Trivedi, R. H. (2017). Use of the spot vision screener for patients with developmental disability. *Journal of American Association for Pediatric Ophthalmology and Strabismus, 21*(4), 313–315. https://doi.org/10.1016/j.jaapos.2017.04.008

McCabe, E. M., Jameson, B. E., & Strauss, S. M. (2024). Mental health screenings: Practices and patterns of these and other health screenings in U.S. school districts. *The Journal of School Nursing, 40*(2), 144–154. https://doi.org/10.1177/10598405211056647

Milante, R. R., Guo, X., Neitzel, A. J., Kretz, A. M., Mukherjee, M. R., Friedman, D. S., Repka, M. X., & Collins, M. E. (2021). Analysis of vision screening failures in a school-based vision program (2016–19). *Journal of American Association for Pediatric Ophthalmology and Strabismus, 25*(1), 29.e1–29.e7. https://doi.org/10.1016/j.jaapos.2020.09.006

Minnesota Department of Health. (2019). *Public health interventions: Applications for public health nursing practice* (2nd ed.). https://www.health.state.mn.us/communities/practice/research/phncouncil/docs/PHInterventions pdf

Murdaugh, C., Parsons, M. A., & Pender, N. (2019). *Health promotion in nursing practice* (8th ed.). Pearson.

National Academies of Sciences, Engineering, and Medicine. (2016). *Making eye health a population health imperative: Vision for tomorrow.* The National Academies Press. https://doi.org/10.17226/23471

National Association of School Nurses. (n.d.a). *Health and practice topics.* https://www.nasn.org/nasn-resources/resources-by-topic

National Association of School Nurses. (n.d.b). *National School Health data set: Every student counts!* https://www.nasn.org/research/everystudentcounts

National Association of School Nurses. (n.d.c). *Toolkits.* https://www.nasn.org/nasn-resources/toolkits

National Association of School Nurses. (2016). *Principles for practice: Vision screening and follow-up.* Author.

National Association of School Nurses. (2022a). *School nursing: Scope and standards of practice* (4th ed.). Author.

National Association of School Nurses. (2022b). *Vision and eye health.* https://www.nasn.org/nasn-resources/practice-topics/vision-health

National Association of School Nurses. (2024). A contemporary framework update for today's school nursing landscape: Introducing the School Nursing Practice Framework. *NASN School Nurse, 39*(3), 140–147. https://www.doi.org/10.1177/1942602X241241092

National Center for Children's Vision and Eye Health at Prevent Blindness. (n.d.a). *Parent/caregiver resources—Small steps for big vision: An eye health information tool kit for parents and caregivers – Parents need to know.* (2023). https://nationalcenter.preventblindness.org/parents-need-to-know/

National Center for Children's Vision and Eye Health at Prevent Blindness. (n.d.b). *Vision screening guidelines by age.* https://nationalcenter.preventblindness.org/vision-screening-guidelines-by-age/

National Center for Children's Vision and Eye Health at Prevent Blindness. (n.d.c). *Vision screening guidelines by age.* National vision screening guidelines. Instrument-based vision screening. https://nationalcenter.preventblindness.org/instrument-based-vision-screening

National Center for Children's Vision and Eye Health at Prevent Blindness. (2015). *Characteristics of tests of recognition of visual acuity for screening the vision of children ages 3 through 5 years (36 to <72 months).* https://preventblindness.org/wp-content/uploads/2020/04/Characteristics_of_Visual_Acuity_Charts_for_Screening_Children_NO-INSTRUMENTS_0.pdf

National Center for Chronic Disease Prevention and Health Promotion. (2018a, October 31). *Well-being concepts.* Centers for Disease Control and Prevention. https://www.cdc.gov/hrqol/wellbeing.htm

National Center for Chronic Disease Prevention and Health Promotion. (2018b, November 6). *Children's BMI tool for schools.* Centers for Disease Control and Prevention. https://www.cdc.gov/healthyweight/assessing/bmi/childrens_bmi/tool_for_schools.html

National Center for Chronic Disease Prevention and Health Promotion. (2019). *School Health Index.* Centers for Disease Control and Prevention. https://www.cdc.gov/healthyschools/shi/index.htm

National Center for Chronic Disease Prevention and Health Promotion. (2021). *Measuring children's height and weight accurately at home.* Centers for Disease Control and Prevention. https://www.cdc.gov/healthyweight/assessing/bmi/childrens_bmi/measuring_children.html

National Center for Chronic Disease Prevention and Health Promotion. (2022a). *Defining adult overweight & obesity.* Centers for Disease Control and Prevention. https://www.cdc.gov/obesity/basics/adult-defining.html

National Center for Chronic Disease Prevention and Health Promotion. (2022b, August 9). *Body mass index (BMI) measurement in schools.* Centers for Disease Control and Prevention. https://www.cdc.gov/healthyschools/obesity/BMI/BMI_measurement_schools.htm#ui-id-3

National Center for Chronic Disease Prevention and Health Promotion. (2022c, September 1). *BMI percentile calculator for child and teen.* Centers for Disease Control and Prevention. https://www.cdc.gov/healthyweight/bmi/calculator.html

National Center for Chronic Disease Prevention and Health Promotion. (2022d, September 24). *About child & teen BMI.* Centers for Disease Control and Prevention. https://www.cdc.gov/healthyweight/assessing/bmi/childrens_bmi/about_childrens_bmi.html

National Center for Chronic Disease Prevention and Health Promotion. (2023a, February 7). *Oral health.* Centers for Disease Control and Prevention. https://www.cdc.gov/healthyschools/npao/oralhealth.htm

National Center for Chronic Disease Prevention and Health Promotion. (2023b, February 9). *Whole School, Whole Community, Whole Child (WSCC).* Centers for Disease Control and Prevention. https://www.cdc.gov/healthyschools/wscc/index.htm

National Center for Chronic Disease Prevention and Health Promotion. (2023c, February 14). High blood pressure in kids and teens. Centers for Disease Control and Prevention. https://www.cdc.gov/bloodpressure/youth.htm

National Center for Environmental Health. (2017, April 6). *Picture of America: Prevention.* Centers for Disease Control and Prevention. https://www.cdc.gov/pictureofamerica/index.html

National Center for Environmental Health. (2022a, November 8). *What noises cause hearing loss?* Centers for Disease Control and Prevention. https://www.cdc.gov/nceh/hearing_loss/what_noises_cause_hearing_loss.html

National Center for Environmental Health. (2022b, December 2). *Blood lead levels in children.* Centers for Disease Control and Prevention. https://www.cdc.gov/nceh/lead/prevention/blood-lead-levels.htm

National Center for Environmental Health. (2023, January 20). *Testing children for lead poisoning.* Centers for Disease Control and Prevention. https://www.cdc.gov/nceh/lead/prevention/testing-children-for-lead-poisoning.htm

National Center for Health Statistics. (2017, June 16). *Clinical growth charts.* Centers for Disease Control and Prevention. https://www.cdc.gov/growthcharts/clinical_charts.htm

National Center for Health Statistics. (2022, December 15). *CDC extended BMI-for-age growth charts.* Centers for Disease Control and Prevention. https://www.cdc.gov/growthcharts/extended-bmi.htm

National Center for HIV, Viral Hepatitis, STD, and TB Prevention. (2016a, April 14). *Who should be tested for TB infection.* Centers for Disease Control and Prevention. https://www.cdc.gov/tb/topic/testing/whobetested.htm

National Center for HIV, Viral Hepatitis, STD, and TB Prevention. (2016b, April 18). *Diagnosing latent TB infection & TB disease.* Centers for Disease Control and Prevention. https://www.cdc.gov/tb/topic/testing/diagnosingltbi.htm

National Center for HIV, Viral Hepatitis, STD, and TB Prevention. (2020a, August 20). *Youth Risk Behavior Surveillance System (YRBSS) overview.* Centers for Disease Control and Prevention. https://www.cdc.gov/healthyyouth/data/yrbs/overview.htm

National Center for HIV, Viral Hepatitis, STD, and TB Prevention. (2020b, November 2). *Tuberculin skin testing fact sheet.* Centers for Disease Control and Prevention. https://www.cdc.gov/tb/publications/factsheets/testing/skintesting.htm

National Center for HIV, Viral Hepatitis, STD, and TB Prevention. (2020c, December 11). *Latent TB infection and TB disease.* Centers for Disease Control and Prevention. https://www.cdc.gov/tb/topic/basics/tbinfectiondisease.htm

National Center for HIV, Viral Hepatitis, STD, and TB Prevention. (2022a, August 22). *Profiles overview.* Centers for Disease Control and Prevention. https://www.cdc.gov/healthyyouth/data/profiles/overview.htm

National Center for HIV, Viral Hepatitis, STD, and TB Prevention. (2022b, November 9). *Trends in tuberculosis, 2021.* Centers for Disease Control and Prevention. https://www.cdc.gov/tb/publications/factsheets/statistics/tbtrends.htm

National Center for HIV, Viral Hepatitis, STD, and TB Prevention. (2022c, November 9). *Tuberculosis (TB) incidence in the United States, 1953–2021.* Centers for Disease Control and Prevention. https://www.cdc.gov/tb/statistics/tbcases.htm

National Center for HIV, Viral Hepatitis, STD, and TB Prevention. (2022d, November 29). *Reported tuberculosis in the United States, 2021.* Centers for Disease Control and Prevention. https://www.cdc.gov/tb/statistics/reports/2021/state_local_data.htm

National Center for Injury Prevention and Control. (2022, January 18). *The social-ecological model: A framework for prevention.* Centers for Disease Control and Prevention. https://www.cdc.gov/violenceprevention/about/social-ecologicalmodel.html

National Center on Birth Defects and Developmental Disabilities. (2022a, July 18). *Types of hearing loss.* Centers for Disease Control and Prevention. https://www.cdc.gov/ncbddd/hearingloss/types.html

National Center on Birth Defects and Developmental Disabilities. (2022b, July 19). *Hearing loss in children.* Centers for Disease Control and Prevention. https://www.cdc.gov/ncbddd/hearingloss/index.html

National Center on Birth Defects and Developmental Disabilities. (2022c, September 19). *Learn the signs. Act early.* Centers for Disease Control and Prevention. https://www.cdc.gov/ncbddd/actearly/

National Center on Birth Defects and Developmental Disabilities. (2022d, November 25). *Developmental surveillance resources for healthcare providers.* Centers for Disease Control and Prevention. https://www.cdc.gov/ncbddd/actearly/hcp/index.html

National Human Genome Research Institute. (2018, September 7). *Genetics vs. genomics fact sheet.* National Institutes of Health. https://www.genome.gov/about-genomics/fact-sheets/Genetics-vs-Genomics

National Institute on Deafness and Other Communication Disorders. (2021, March 25). *Quick statistics about hearing.* National Institutes of Health. https://www.nidcd.nih.gov/health/statistics/quick-statistics-hearing

National Library of Medicine. (2019). *Benefits and risks of screening tests.* https://www.ncbi.nlm.nih.gov/pubmedhealth/PMH0072602/

Newcombe, J. (2020). Cardiovascular disorders. In D. L. Garzon Maaks, N. B. Starr, M. A. Brady, N. M. Gaylord, M. Driessnack, & K. D. Duderstadt (Eds.), *Burns' pediatric primary care* (7th ed., pp. 700–737). Elsevier.

Nihiser, A. J., Lee, S. M., Wechsler, H., McKenna, M., Odom, E., Reinold, C., Thompson, D., & Grummer-Strawn, L. (2007). Body mass index measurement in schools. *Journal of School Health, 77*(10), 651–671. https://doi.org/10.1111/j.1746-1561.2007.00249 x

Nottingham Chaplin, P. K. (2021). Challenges with commonly used tests of visual acuity (eye charts) for optotype-based screening. [PowerPoint presentation]. https://higherlogicdownload.s3.amazonaws.com/NASN/8575d1b7-94ad-45ab-808e-d45019cc5c08/Uploaded-

Images/PDFs/Practice%20Topic%20Resources/vision_presentation_challenges_with_eye_charts.pdf

Nottingham Chaplin, P. K., Baldonado, K., Bradford, G. E., Cotter, S., & Moore, B. (2018). An eye on vision: 20 questions about vision screening and eye health. *NASN School Nurse, 33*(2), 87–92. https://doi.org/10.1177/1942602X18754320

Nottingham Chaplin, P. K., Baldonado, K., Cotter, S., Moore, B., & Bradford, G. E. (2018a). An eye on vision: Five questions about vision screening and eye health—part 2. *NASN School Nurse, 33*(4), 210–213. https://doi.org/10.1177/1942602X18779801

Nottingham Chaplin, P. K., Baldonado, K., Cotter, S., Moore, B., & Bradford, G. E. (2018b). An eye on vision: Five questions about vision screening and eye health—part 3. *NASN School Nurse, 33*(5), 279-283. https://doi.org/10.1177%2F1942602X18785951

Nottingham Chaplin, P. K., Baldonado, K., Hutchinson, A., & Moore, B. (2015). Vision and eye health: Moving into the digital age with instrument-based vision screening. *NASN School Nurse, 30*(3), 154–160. https://doi.org/10.1177/1942602X15581054

Nottingham Chaplin, P. K., Marsh-Tootle, W., & Bradford, G. E. (2015). *Navigating the path of children's vision screening: Visual acuity, instruments, & occluders.* https://www.schoolhealth.com/media/pdf/NavigatingVisionScreening.pdf

O'Connor, E. A., Evans, C. V., Burda, B. U., Walsh, E. S, Eder, M., & Lozano, P. (2017). Screening for obesity and intervention for weight management in children and adolescents: Evidence report and systematic review for the U.S. Preventive Services Task Force. *Journal of the American Medical Association, 317*(23), 2427–2444. https://doi.org/10.1001/jama.2017.0332

Office of Disease Prevention and Health Promotion. (n.d.a). *Healthy People 2030.* U.S. Department of Health and Human Services. https://health.gov/healthypeople

Office of Disease Prevention and Health Promotion. (n.d.b). Reduce the proportion of children and adolescents with active and untreated tooth decay. *Healthy People 2023.* U.S. Department of Health and Human Services. https://health.gov/healthypeople/priority-areas/social-determinants-health

Office of Disease Prevention and Health Promotion. (n.d.c). Social determinants of health. *Healthy People 2023.* U.S. Department of Health and Human Services. https://health.gov/healthypeople/priority-areas/social-determinants-health

Office of Disease Prevention and Health Promotion. (2021, August 25). *National Health Information Center.* https://health.gov/our-work/national-health-initiatives/health-literacy/resources/national-health-information-center

Oral Health Connections. (n.d.). *Tools and resources.* National Association of School Nurses and American Dental Association. https://www.oralhealthconnections.org/tools-resources

Peterseim, M. M., Papa, C. E., Parades, C., Davidson, J., Sturges, A., Oslin, C., Merritt, I., & Morrison, M. (2015). Combining automated vision screening with on-site examinations in 23 schools: Refocus on children program 2012 to 2013. *Journal of Pediatric Ophthalmology & Strabismus, 52*(1), 20–24. https://doi.org/10.3928/01913913-20141124-01

Polfuss, M. L., & Davis, R. L. (2020). Physical activity and sports for children and adolescents. In D. L. Garzon Maaks, N. B. Starr, M. A. Brady, N. M. Gaylord, M. Driessnack, & K. D. Duderstadt (Eds.), *Burns' pediatric primary care* (7th ed., pp. 700–737). Elsevier.

Poole, M. K., Gortmaker, S. L., Barrett, J. L., McCulloch, S. M., Rimm, E.B., Emmons, K. M., Ward, Z. J., & Kenney, E. L. (2023). The societal costs and health impacts on obesity of BMI report cards in US schools. *Obesity, 31*(8), 2110–2118. https://www.doi.org/10.1002/oby.23788

Prevent Blindness (n.d.a). *Financial assistance information.* https://preventblindness.org/wp-content/uploads/2022/01/IC03_Financial_Assistance13122.pdf

Prevent Blindness. (n.d.b). *Prevent Blindness children's vision screening certification course.* https://nationalcenter.preventblindness.org/prevent-blindness-childrens-vision-screening-certification-course

Prevent Blindness. (2015). *Prevent Blindness position statement on school-aged vision screening and eye health programs.* https://preventblindness.org/wp-content/uploads/2020/05/Prevent-Blindness-Statements-on-School-aged-Vision-Screening-Approved-8-2015-1.pdf

Prevent Blindness. (2019). *Developing a consensus on a systems-based approach to children's vision and eye health.* https://preventblindness.org/wp-content/uploads/2011/08/VSConsensusStatementRev2019.pdf

Prevent Blindness. (2020a). *18 vision development milestones from birth to baby's first birthday.* https://nationalcenter.preventblindness.org/wp-content/uploads/sites/22/2020/05/18-Key-vision-questions-to-ask-in-year-1_version-5.27.2020.pdf

Prevent Blindness. (2020b). *Signs of possible vision problems in children.* https://nationalcenter.preventblindness.org/wp-content/uploads/sites/22/2020/10/5A-Signs-vision-problems-in-children.pdf

Raymond, J., & Brown, M. J. (2017). Childhood blood lead levels in children aged <5 years—United States, 2009–2014. *Morbidity and Mortality Weekly Review Surveillance Summaries, 66*(3), 1–10. http://dx.doi.org/10.15585/mmwr.ss6603a1

Rector, C. (2021). The journey begins: Introduction. In C. Rector & M. J. Stanley (Eds.), *Community and public health nursing: Promoting the public's health* (10th ed., pp.1–23). Wolters Kluwer.

Rentfro, A. R. (2022). Health promotion and the community. In C. L. Edelman, & E. C. Kudzma (Eds.), *Health promotion throughout the lifespan* (10th ed., pp. 202–225). Elsevier.

Ruckart, P. Z., Jones, R. L., Courtney, J. G., LeBlanc, T. T., Jackson, W., Karwowski, M. P., Cheng, P.-Y., Allwood, P., Svendsen, E. R., & Breysse, P. N. (2021). Update of the blood lead reference value—United States, 2021. *Morbidity and Mortality Weekly Report, 70*(43), 1509–1512. http://dx.doi.org/10.15585/mmwr.mm7043a4

Ruggieri, D. G., & Bass, S. B. (2015). A comprehensive review of school-based body mass index screening programs and their implications for school health: Do the controversies accurately reflect the research? *Journal of School Health, 85*(1), 61–72. https://doi.org/10.1111/josh.12222

Ruggieri, D. G., Bass, S. B., Alhajji, M., & Gordon, T. F. (2020). Understanding parents' perceptions of school-based BMI screening and BMI report cards using perceptual mapping: Implications for school nurses. *The Journal of School Nursing, 36*(2), 144–156. https://doi.org/10.1177/1059840518789243

Runyon, K., Chesnut, S. R., & Burley, H. (2018). Screening for childhood anxiety: A meta-analysis of the screen for child anxiety related emotional disorders. *Journal of Affective Disorder, 240,* 220–229. https://doi.org/10.1016/j.jad.2018.07.049

Schroeder, K., Malone, S. K., McCabe, E., & Lipman, T. (2018). Addressing the social determinants of health: A call to action for school nurses. *The Journal of School Nursing, 34*(3), 182–191. https://doi.org/10.1177/1059840517750733

Scott Ricci, S. (2022). The childbearing period. In C. L. Edelman & E. C. Kudzma (Eds.), *Health promotion throughout the lifespan* (10th ed., pp. 387–428). Elsevier.

Sekhar, D. L., Zalewski, T. R., Bieler, J. S., Czarnecki, B., Barr, A. L., King, T. S., & Paul, I. M. (2016). The sensitivity of adolescent school-based hearing screens is significantly improved by adding high frequencies. *The Journal of School Nursing, 32*(6), 416–422. https://doi.org/10.1177/1059840516654004

Simoneau, T., Langton, C. R., Kuo, C. L., Marrero, J., Gherlone, N., Cloutier, M. M., & Hollenbach, J. P. (2020). A school nurse-led asthma program reduces absences: Evaluation of Easy Breathing for Schools. *Academic Pediatrics, 20*(1), 73–80. https://doi.org/10.1016/j.acap.2019.07.007

Sliwa, S. A., Brener, N. D., Lundeen, E. A., & Lee, S. M. (2019). Do schools that screen for body mass index have recommended safeguards in place? *The Journal of School Nursing, 35*(4), 299–308. https://doi.org/10.1177/1059840518758376

Stanislo, K. (2023). Revisiting the National School Health Data Set: Every Student Counts! *NASN School Nurse, 38*(1), 26–30. https://doi.org/10.1177/1942602X221137519

Stewart, R., Pardi, V., Buck, J., Smallwood, O., & Wright, W. (2022). Community-academic partnership to improve the oral health of underserved schoolchildren in rural North Carolina. *Journal of School Health, 92*(3), 325–329. https://doi.org/10.1111/josh.13129

Stierman, B., Afful, J., Carroll, M. D., Chen, T.-C., Davy, O., Fink, S., Fryar, C. D., Gu, Q., Hales, C. M., Hughes, J. P., Ostchega, Y., Storandt, R. J., & Akinbami, L. J. (2021, June 14). *National Health and Nutrition Examination Survey 2017–March 2020 prepandemic data files development of files and prevalence estimates for selected health outcomes.* National Center for Health Statistics (U.S.), NHSR No. 158. National Health Statistics Reports. https://stacks.cdc.gov/view/cdc/106273

Styne, D. M., Arslanian, S. A., Connor, E. L., Farooqi, I. S., Murad, M. H., Silverstein, J. H., & Yanovski, J. A. (2017). Pediatric obesity—assessment, treatment, and prevention: An endocrine society clinical practice guideline. *The Journal of Clinical Endocrinology & Metabolism, 102*(3), 709–757. https://doi.org/10.1210/jc.2016-2573

Subcommittee on Childhood Hearing Screening. (2011, September). *American Academy of Audiology: Childhood hearing screening guidelines.* https://www.audiology.org/wp-content/uploads/2021/05/ChildhoodScreeningGuidelines.pdf_5399751c9ec216.42663963.pdf

Substance Abuse and Mental Health Services Administration. (2019). *Ready, set, go, review: Screening for behavioral health risk in schools.* https://www.samhsa.gov/sites/default/files/ready_set_go_review_mh_screening_in_schools_508.pdf

Substance Abuse and Mental Health Services Administration. (2021). *Key substance use and mental health indicators in the United States: Results from the 2020 National Survey on Drug Use and Health* (HHS Publication No. PEP21-07-01-003, NSDUH Series H-56). Center for Behavioral Health Statistics and Quality, Substance Abuse and Mental Health Services Administration. https://www.samhsa.gov/data/

Szilagyi, P. G. (2021). Children: Infancy through adolescence. In L. S. Bickley (Ed.), *Bates' guide to physical examination and history taking* (13th ed., pp. 935–1082). Wolters Kluwer.

Timothy Hresko, M., Talwalkar, V. R., Schwend, R. M., The Scoliosis Research Society, American Academy of Orthopedic Surgeons, Pediatric Orthopedic Society of North America, & American Academy of Pediatrics. (2015). *Position statement—Screening for the early detection for idiopathic scoliosis in adolescents.* The Scoliosis Research Society, American Academy of Orthopedic Surgeons, Pediatric Orthopedic Society of North America, & American Academy of Pediatrics. https://www.srs.org/about-srs/news-and-announcements/position-statement—screening-for-the-early-detection-for-idiopathic-scoliosis-in-adolescents

Todd, D. (2021). Health promotion through education. In C. Rector & M. J. Stanley (Eds.), *Community and public health nursing: Promoting the public's health* (10th ed., pp. 305–331). Wolters Kluwer.

U.S. Department of Agriculture. (2022, August 15). *Local school wellness policies.* https://www.fns.usda.gov/tn/local-school-wellness-policy

U.S. Department of Health and Human Services. (2000). *Oral health in America: A report of the Surgeon General.* National Institute of Dental and Craniofacial Research, National Institutes of Health. https://www.nidcr.nih.gov/sites/default/files/2017-10/hck1ocv.%40www.surgeon.fullrpt.pdf

U.S. Preventive Services Task Force. (n.d.). *Recommendation topics.* https://www.uspreventiveservicestaskforce.org/uspstf/recommendation-topics

U.S. Preventive Services Task Force. (2017, June 20). *Obesity in children and adolescents: Screening.* https://uspreventiveservicestaskforce.org/uspstf/recommendation/obesity-in-children-and-adolescents-screening

U.S. Preventive Services Task Force. (2018). Screening for adolescent idiopathic scoliosis: US Preventive Services Task Force recommendation statement. *Journal of the American Medical Association, 319*(2), 165–172. https://doi.org/10.1001/jama.2017.19342

U.S. Preventive Services Task Force. (2022a). *Procedure manual.* https://uspreventiveservicestaskforce.org/uspstf/about-uspstf/methods-and-processes/procedure-manual

U.S. Preventive Services Task Force. (2022b). Screening for anxiety in children and adolescents: U.S. Preventive Services Task Force recommendation statement. *Journal of the American Medical Association, 328*(14), 1438–1444. https://doi.org/10.1001/jama.2022.16936

U.S. Preventive Services Task Force. (2022c). Screening for depression and suicide risk in children and adolescents: U.S. Preventive Services Task Force recommendation statement. *Journal of the American Medical Association, 328*(15), 1534–1542. https://doi.org/10.1001/jama.2022.16946

Vision in Preschoolers–Hyperopia in Preschoolers Study Group, Kulp, M. T., Ciner, E., Maguire, M., Moore, B., Pentimonti, J., Pistilli, M., Cyert, L., Candy, T. R., Quinn, G., & Ying, G.-S. (2016). Uncorrected hyperopia and preschool early literacy: Results of the Vision in Preschoolers–Hyperopia in Preschoolers (VIP-HIP) study. *Ophthalmology, 123*(4), 681–689. https://doi.org/10.1016/j.ophtha.2015 11.023

Vision in Preschoolers Study Group. (2006). Random Dot E stereopsis test: Testability and reliability in 3- to 5-year-old children. *Journal of American Association for Pediatric Ophthalmology and Strabismus, 10*(6), 507–514. https://doi.org/10.1016%2Fj.jaapos.2006.08.019

Vision in Preschoolers Study Group. (2007). Children unable to perform screening tests in Vision in Preschoolers Study: Proportion with ocular conditions and impact on measure of test accuracy. *Investigative Ophthalmology & Visual Science, 48*(1), 83–87. https://doi.org/10.1167/iovs.06-0384

Vogt, M. A. (2021). Evidence-based history and physical examinations for sports participation evaluation. In K. Gawlik, B. Melnyk, & A. Teall (Eds.), *Evidence-based physical examination: Best practices for health and well-being assessment* (1st ed., pp. 699–712). Springer Publishing Company.

Voskuil, V. R., Robbins, L. B., & Pierce, S. J. (2019). Predicting physical activity among urban adolescent girls: A test of the health promotion model. *Research in Nursing & Health, 42*(5), 392–409. https://doi.org/10.1002/nur.21968

Wahl, M. D., Fishman, D., Block, S. S., Baldonado, K. N., Friedman, D. S., Repka, M. X., & Collins, M.E. (2021). A comprehensive review of state vision screening mandates for schoolchildren in the United States. *Optometry and Vision Science, 98*(5), 490–499. https://doi.org/10.1097/opx.0000000000001686

Whelton, P. K., Carey, R. M., Aronow, W. S., Casey, D. E., Jr, Collins, K. J., Dennison Himmelfarb, C., DePalma, S. M., Gidding, S., Jamerson, K. A., Jones, D. W., MacLaughlin, E. J., Muntner, P., Ovbiagele, B., Smith, S. C., Jr, Spencer, C. C., Stafford, R. S., Taler, S J., Thomas, R. J., Williams, K. A., Sr., Williamson, J. D., & Wright, J. T., Jr. (2018). 2017 ACC/AHA/AAPA/ABC/ACPM/AGS/APhA/ASH/ASPC/NMA/PCNA guideline for the prevention, detection, evaluation, and management of high blood pressure in adults: Executive summary: A report of the American College of Cardiology/American Heart Association Task Force on clinical practice guidelines. *Hypertension, 71*(6), e113–115. https://doi.org/10.1161/HYP.0000000000000065

Wickersham, A., Sugg, H. V. R., Epstein, S., Stewart, R., Ford, T., & Down, J. (2021). Systematic review and meta-analysis: The association between child and adolescent depression and later educational attainment. *Journal of the American Academy of Child & Adolescent Psychiatry, 60*(1), 105–118. https://doi.org/10.1016/j.jaac.2020.10.008

Willgerodt, M. A., Walsh, E., & Maloy, C. (2021). A scoping review of the Whole School, Whole Community, Whole Child Model. *The Journal of School Nursing, 37*(1), 61–68. https://doi.org/10.1177/1059840520974346

Williams, W. R., Latif, A. H., Hannington, L., & Watkins D. R. (2005). Hyperopia and educational attainment in a primary school cohort. *Archives of Disease in Childhood, 90*(2), 150–153. https://www.ncbi.nlm.nih.gov/pmc/articles/PMC1720267/

Winston-Gerson, R., & Sabo, D. (2016). Hearing loss detection in schools and early child care settings: An overview of school-age hearing screening practices. *NASN School Nurse, 31*(5), 257–262. https://doi.org/10.1177/1942602X16661362

World Health Organization. (n.d.a). *Health promotion.* https://www.who.int/westernpacific/health-topics/health-promotion

World Health Organization. (n.d.b). *Health promotion—the Ottawa charter for health promotion.* https://www.who.int/teams/health-promotion/enhanced-wellbeing/first-global-conference

World Health Organization. (n.d.c). *Social determinants of health.* https://www.who.int/health-topics/social-determinants-of-health#tab=tab_1

World Health Organization. (2003). *Consultation on development of standards for characterization of vision loss and visual functioning.* https://apps.

who.int/iris/bitstream/handle/10665/68601/WHO_PBL_03.91.pdf; jsessionid=D87F2BAC0A45B728501A6BD15F826CDD?sequence=1

World Health Organization. (2020a). *Basic documents* (49th ed.). Constitution. https://apps.who.int/gb/bd/pdf_files/BD_49th-en.pdf#page=6

World Health Organization. (2020b). *Screening programmes: A short guide. Increase effectiveness, maximize benefits and minimize harm.* WHO Regional Office for Europe. https://apps.who.int/iris/bitstream/handle/10665/330829/9789289054782-eng.pdf?sequence=1&isAllowed=y

World Health Organization. (2021a). *WHO guideline on school health services*. https://apps.who.int/iris/rest/bitstreams/1352177/retrieve

World Health Organization. (2021b, November 17). *Adolescent mental health*. https://www.who.int/news-room/fact-sheets/detail/adolescent-mental-health

World Health Organization. (2022). *Global school-based student health survey (GSHS)*. https://www.who.int/teams/noncommunicable-diseases/surveillance/systems-tools/global-school-based-student-health-survey

World Health Organization. (2024). *World report on social determinants of health equity*. https://www.who.int/initiatives/action-on-the-social-determinants-of-health-for-advancing-equity/world-report-on-social-determinants-of-health-equity

World Health Organization & United Nations Educational, Scientific and Cultural Organization. (2021). *Making every school a health-promoting school: Implementation guidance*. https://apps.who.int/iris/rest/bitstreams/1352169/retrieve

Yow, A. G., Rajasurya, V., & Sharma, S. (2022). *Sudden cardiac death*. National Library of Medicine. https://www.ncbi.nlm.nih.gov/books/NBK507854/

Chapter 13

Disease Prevention and Management in Schools

Virginia A. Reising

CHAPTER OUTLINE

Health promotion and disease prevention in both the school and broader community are among the primary functions of school nurses. Health promotion activities support behaviors conducive to achieving and maintaining health (World Health Organization [WHO], 2021). Disease prevention focuses on keeping people healthy, but more specifically, it addresses reducing the risk of developing health-related problems. Disease prevention is categorized as primary, secondary, and tertiary levels (see Chapter 2).

The school nurse's role in disease prevention is achieved through collaboration with students, families, teachers, school staff, school administrators, healthcare providers, and community partners. School nurses can develop and enforce school health policies and prepare or adapt health educational programs and materials. These activities align with the Community/Public Health principle of the *School Nursing Practice Framework* (National Association of School Nurses [NASN], 2024) and are clearly delineated in the 4th edition of *School Nursing: Scope and Standards of Practice* (NASN, 2022b). Although the school nurse's role has expanded over the years, the overarching goal remains the same: promoting student health to facilitate learning (NASN, 2018). While the school nurse can prevent disease through a wide range of strategies, this chapter focuses on the school

> **Focus on the Framework**
> **Community/Public Health**
>
> "Teaching health promotion, health literacy, and disease prevention" is a key concept in the *School Nursing Practice Framework's* principle of **Community/Public Health.** School nurse effort to prevent disease supports healthy and safe school communities, which are essential for optimal health and academic success (NASN, 2024).

nurse's role in infection control, promoting a healthy environment, and communicable disease prevention.

INFECTION CONTROL MEASURES IN SCHOOLS

Infection control is an important component of the school nurse's role. The roots of school nursing were formed when nurse Lina Rogers went into schools and homes to manage and eradicate infections so that students could return to school (see Chapter 1). That role continues today. Infection control as applied to school nursing includes implementing guidelines for the following:

- Proper hand hygiene and cough/sneeze etiquette
- Bloodborne pathogens in the school setting
- Assessment of children in the school setting
- Attendance/exclusion of sick children
- Immunization surveillance

Frequent and proper hand hygiene is one of the best ways to prevent the spread of disease (Centers for Disease Control and Prevention [CDC], 2024c), as is proper cough and sneeze etiquette.

Hand Hygiene

Hand Washing

Hand washing is an easy opportunity to prevent the spread of gastrointestinal and respiratory illnesses. Hand washing has been demonstrated to reduce the number of people who get sick with gastrointestinal and respiratory illnesses (CDC, 2024e). The nurse can serve as an exemplar of hand hygiene when washing their own hands and by offering education.

Nurses should wash their hands before and after providing care to students, before and after giving medications, and after contact with infectious materials. The use of gloves is not a substitute for washing one's hands. School nurses should encourage students to wash their hands when they are seen in the school health office for medication administration or other health concerns. This practice reinforces the importance of hand washing and allows the nurse to assess whether proper technique is being used. In the school community, students and staff should be encouraged to wash their hands before and after meals, after toileting (or changing diapers), after disposal of used tissues, after coughing, sneezing, or blowing one's nose, and after playing outside (CDC, 2024b). Students and staff alike should be reminded that hand hygiene is also recommended before preparing foods, after handling uncooked food such as meat and poultry, after contact with animals or cleaning their cages, after handling trash/garbage, and after playing in sandboxes or on playgrounds (CDC, 2024b).

While those who work in health care are instructed to use alcohol-based hand sanitizers due to the nature of the germs they encounter, the CDC guidelines for hand washing at home, at play, and in the community encourage washing hands with soap and water whenever available (CDC, 2024e). Students and staff should be taught to effectively wash their hands by following these simple directions: *wet, lather, scrub, rinse, and dry*. This process should take 40 to 60 seconds. The CDC Web site has many resources available to help schools develop hand washing campaigns, including videos and posters, many of which are in multiple languages.

Hand Sanitizer

Although recommended for hospitals and other healthcare settings, alcohol-based sanitizers are not the primary recommendation for community settings, including schools. It is easy to make hand sanitizer available throughout the school, but hand sanitizers are less effective than soap and water against bacteria such as *Clostridium difficile* and viruses such as the norovirus; both are known causes of severe diarrhea in children and adults. Studies show that using hand sanitizer on visibly soiled hands is ineffective and does not remove harmful contaminants such as pesticides or heavy metals.

When washing with soap and water is not possible, CDC guidelines (2024d) support the use of alcohol-based hand sanitizer. Alcohol disrupts the coating of the virus and bacteria particles, thereby deactivating them. These products come in multiple forms and the ingredients in hand sanitizers vary greatly. The school nurse should work with other school personnel to determine which products are ordered and ensure they contain at least 60% alcohol and are U.S. Food and Drug Administration (USFDA) approved (USFDA, 2023). The use of hand sanitizer by children should always be supervised to prevent misuse, fire, or alcohol poisoning. School nurses and wellness teams need to advocate for the use of soap and water whenever possible. However, when hand sanitizers are used, the following simple procedure should be followed (CDC, 2024d):

- Put enough sanitizer on your hand to cover all surfaces.
- Rub the gel over all surfaces of your hand and fingers until your hands are dry—this should take around 20 seconds. Do not rinse or wipe off the sanitizer before it is dry.

Figures 13-1 and 13-2 show the proper procedures for hand hygiene using soap or hand sanitizer.

Environmental Infection Control Measures

The school nurse's environmental infection control responsibilities vary by federal, state, and school district mandates; however, all school nurses should be familiar with basic environmental control measures. School nurses must be familiar with the mission and mandates of the Occupational Safety and Health Administration (OSHA) to prevent work-related injuries, illnesses, and deaths, which include protection from occupational exposure to infection from bloodborne pathogens (BBPs), specifically HIV and hepatitis B or other potentially infections materials. Occupational exposure is defined as any "reasonably anticipated

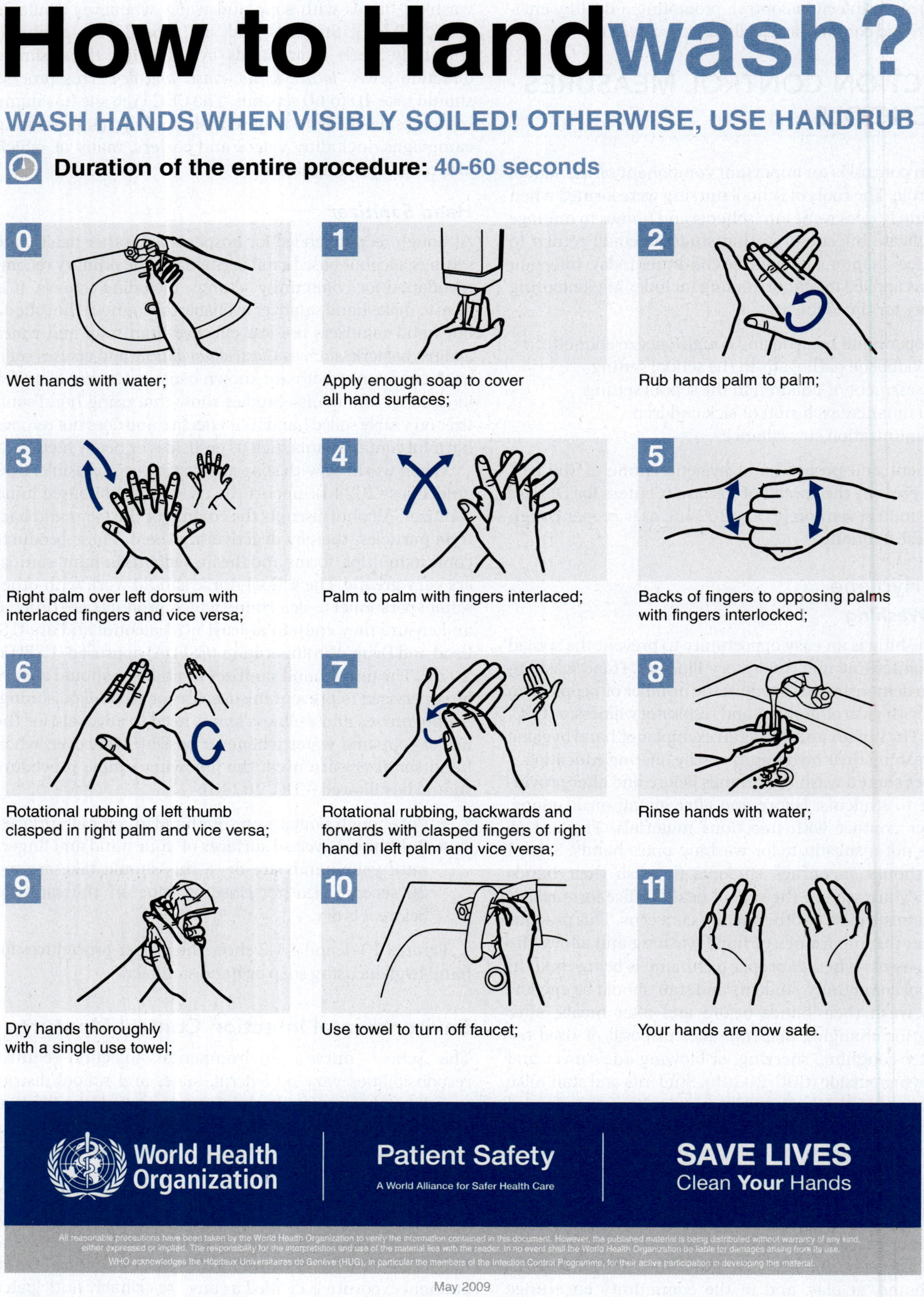

FIGURE 13-1. Hand hygiene technique: hand washing. *(Reproduced with permission of the World Health Organization. [2009b]. https://www.who.int/docs/default-source/patient-safety/how-to-handwash-poster.pdf?sfvrsn=7004a09d_2)*

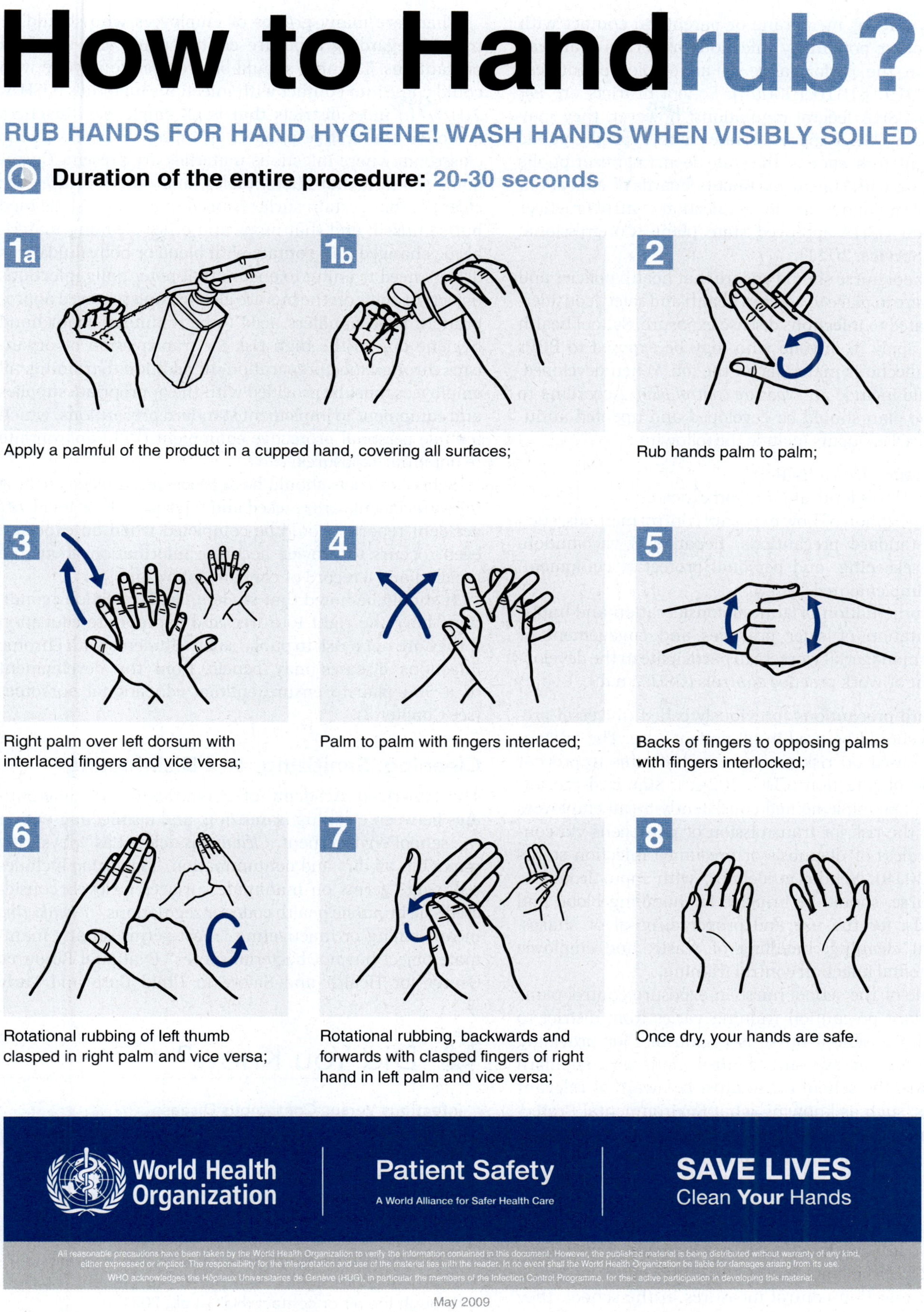

FIGURE 13-2. Hand hygiene technique: hand rub. *(Reproduced with permission of the World Health Organization. [2009a]. https://cdn.who.int/media/docs/default-source/integrated-health-services-(ihs)/infection-prevention-and-control/how-to-handrub-poster.pdf)*

skin, eye, mucous membrane or parenteral contact with blood or other potentially infectious materials that may result from the performance of an employee's duties" [OSHA, 2019, §1910.1030(b)]. School districts are *not* subject to OSHA federal regulations; however, they may be covered by OSHA-approved state plans. Typically, public health regulators, such as the state departments of public health along with state departments/boards of education, will provide guidance on school infection control practices based upon OSHA-approved state plans (Congressional Research Service, 2021).

The school nurse should ensure that health policies and protocols are in place to address health and safety considerations related to infectious disease exposure. School health protocols apply to anyone who may be exposed to BBPs or other infectious materials on the job. When developed, they should include an *exposure control plan.* According to OSHA, the plan should be developed and updated annually; required elements include the following:

1. Exposure determination
2. Procedures for evaluating an exposure
3. A description of how exposure control methods, such as standard precautions, hepatitis B vaccination, housekeeping, and personal protective equipment, are implemented
4. Documentation of annual consideration and implementation of safer practices and engagement of nonmanagerial workers to participate in the development of work practice controls (OSHA, n.d.)

Standard precautions (previously called universal precautions) should be used in all patient care. The precautions are based on risk assessment that aims to prevent the spread of infection (CDC, 2024u). Standard precautions are to be implemented consistently by all employees to reduce the risk for transmission of pathogens via contact regardless of diagnosis or presumed infection status (OSHA, 2019). School guidelines, with input from the school nurse, should be in place for handling blood and body fluids, for the use and proper disposal of sharps, equipment cleaning, handling of waste, and employee environmental infection control training.

The role of the school nurse in exposure control plans and standard precaution training varies from district to district. If the school nurse is responsible for providing staff training on exposure control plans and standard precautions, the school nurse must be aware of relevant guidelines, such as knowing what Environmental Protection Agency (EPA) registered disinfectants are approved for cleaning BBPs and how to handle expired medications. School nurses have a role in providing evaluation and guidance following an exposure to a student, staff, or visitor. Although the ultimate responsibility for training lies with the school district, the *School Nursing Standards of Practice* (NASN, 2022b) dictate that if the school nurse notices a breach in infection control measures in the school, they should try to mitigate the effects of that breach.

There are many groups of employees who should be trained regarding exposure control plans and standard precautions. Training should be provided to anyone who could come into contact with infectious materials (OSHA, 2019). In most districts that is all employees. Teachers are often the first responders to injury or illness in the classroom where infectious materials are present. Custodians see to it that floors, tables, and other surfaces are cleaned; that certain surfaces need to be not just cleaned but sanitized; and that mops and other cleaning materials be changed if in contact with blood or body fluids. Bus drivers need training to ensure that potentially infectious objects or spills on the bus are cleaned and removed appropriately. Food handlers need to be reminded about hand hygiene due to the high risk for transmission of organisms through food preparation. In addition to training, all employees must be provided with the appropriate supplies and equipment to implement standard precautions, which include personal protective equipment (PPE) appropriate to potential exposures.

School districts should have processes in place for how injury/accidents are tracked and reported. These incident/accident reports should be completed when an exposure event occurs to provide accurate information about the incident and a record of care and follow-up.

It should be noted that students with infectious conditions have the right to a free and appropriate education if they are not a risk to public safety. Students with chronic infectious diseases may benefit from the development of a 504 plan to ensure optimal educational outcomes (see Chapter 8).

Cleaning, Sanitizing, and Disinfecting

The American Academy of Pediatrics (AAP) differentiates between cleaning, sanitizing, and disinfecting within the school environment. *Cleaning* is defined as "physically removing all dirt and contamination." *Sanitizing* includes reducing "germs on inanimate surfaces to levels considered safe by public health codes or regulations." *Disinfecting* means killing or inactivating "most germs on any inanimate object but not bacterial spores" (National Resource Center for Health and Safety in Child Care and Early

Did You Know?

Infectious Versus Contagious Disease

Infectious diseases are transmitted by viruses or bacteria but do not necessarily spread from person to person. For example, tetanus spreads through toxin-contaminated material entering a wound or from ingesting food contaminated with tetanus.

Communicable and contagious diseases are essentially synonymous terms that refer to the transmission of an infectious agent from person to person, usually through the air or contact (Hall et al., 2021).

Education, 2022). Only U.S. Environmental Protection Agency (USEPA)–labeled cleaning products should be used; these products are labeled as to their type (e.g., sanitizing, disinfecting) and whether they are *green* or environmentally safe (USEPA, 2015). Districts should select only a few products to lessen the chance of confusing the types of cleaners. The USEPA has a Safer Choice webpage and search engine to help identify products that meet the Safer Choice standard (USEPA, 2024b). During outbreaks, school nurses are encouraged to contact their local health department for guidance as to which specific EPA-approved cleaning product to use.

The Occupational Safety and Health Administration's (OSHA's) Hazard Communication Standard (OSHA, 2012a) requires that employers maintain **safety data sheets** for all hazardous chemicals. This rule applies to cleaning products and other chemicals used in schools. The safety data sheets must always be readily accessible to employees (OSHA, 2012b). Safety Data Sheets are divided into 16 sections that include information such as the composition of the product, handling and storage, exposure controls, personal protective equipment to be used, and first-aid measures should an exposure occur. The school nurse should know where the safety data sheets are stored in case an exposure occurs and emergency treatment is needed. School nurses should ensure that proper cleaning procedures are used on surfaces and equipment in the health office. In addition, the school nurse should use surveillance data related to student or staff absences to make suggestions about sanitizing and disinfecting classrooms and common areas within the school.

If EPA-approved products are not available, a solution using bleach can be used. Bleach solutions (Box 13-1) made by the school nurse or other school staff must be appropriately labeled and kept out of the reach of students (Aronson & Shope, 2020). This solution should be made daily because chlorine evaporates and is weakened by sunlight and heat. To sanitize, the bleach solution should be left on the surface as indicated by the bleach product before wiping it off, or it can be air-dried (CDC, 2024w).

BOX 13-1

Bleach Solution Recipe

- Add ⅓ cup household bleach to 1 gallon of room temperature water OR 4 teaspoons of bleach to 1 quart of water.
- Apply solution to the surface with a cloth.
- Let stand 3 to 5 minutes.
- Rinse the surface with clean water.
- The solution should be remade every 24 hours as the bleach will lose its potency over time when mixed with water.

Source: CDC (2024w).

PROMOTING SAFE AND HEALTHY SCHOOL ENVIRONMENTS

The school environment is vitally important to student health and safety, yet it is often overlooked. School environmental health and safety are *not* regulated by the federal Department of Education or the Department of Health and Human Services, and the few school environment–related federal laws and regulations that do exist fall under the U.S. Environmental Protection Agency. The USEPA (2023b) estimates that children spend 90% of their time indoors, mostly in schools. Children from low-income and under-resourced communities experience higher exposures to multiple environmental concerns and are at increased risk for associated health risk (USEPA, 2023a). Researchers have found that schools that implement healthy school environment policies can positively affect school attendance and academic performance and decrease costs related to unhealthy environments (USEPA, 2023a).

The USEPA stresses that every school and district should implement a comprehensive and sustainable school environment health program that embraces preventive measures and appropriately maintains school buildings and grounds. They have developed the State School Environmental Health Guidelines to assist schools in developing their environmental health programs (US EPA, 2023a).

Since the responsibility for most school environment health and safety regulations rests with the states, each state sets its own laws and regulations on topics such as mold, radon, CO_2, building ventilation, vehicle idling, indoor air quality management plans, green cleaning, and integrated pest management. The laws and regulation vary considerably from state to state but best practices are highlighted on the EPA Web site.

A school environmental health program should include five key components:

1. Practice effective cleaning and maintenance.
2. Prevent mold and moisture.
3. Reduce chemical and environmental contaminant health.
4. Ensure good ventilation.
5. Prevent pests and reduce pesticide use (USEPA, 2022a).

These components are complex and require team-based approaches and include community and governmental stakeholders. School nurses can identify and address issues related to a healthy school environment through the use of the CDC's *School Health Index* (2022c), which is designed to help school teams improve their health and safety policies and programs. The USEPA has developed the *Sensible Steps to Healthy School Environments*, which is an assessment tool that can help schools understand their current environmental health (USEPA, 2017). This tool also provides helpful insights about common hazardous exposures seen in the school environment.

The School Building

Federal and state capital investment in school infrastructure is underfunded, and low-resourced schools are often the ones that suffer the greatest consequences (Filardo, 2021). It is up to school administrators and school boards to make proactive decisions to improve school environments; however, school nurses are important advocates for their school community. Surveillance and data collection activities around student illness and school grounds injury, including the playground, collected by the school nurse can help identify issues within the school building.

Noise

Noise pollution is a concern in school buildings as noise interferes with the intelligibility of speech and affects language development, memory and reading, and auditory word discrimination (CDC, 2024k). Schools located near airports, busy highways, train tracks, and loud factories may have increased noise levels in the school.

Research indicates that prolonged or repeated sounds above 85 A-weighted decibels (dBA) can cause hearing loss. A jet flying over a building is about 100 dB, a lawn mower is 85 to 94 dB, a diesel locomotive at 50 feet is 87 to 103 dB, and freeway noise is about 87 dB (National Institute on Deafness and Other Communication Disorders [NIDCD], 2022). Practical actions that school nurses can advocate for within the school building to improve classroom acoustics include the following:

- Using carpets on the floors
- Hanging curtains or blinds from the windows
- Hanging soft items on the walls, including corkboards (American Speech-Language-Hearing Association, n.d.)

Indoor Air Quality

The EPA has found cases of exposure to indoor air pollution that are two to five times greater than the exposure to outdoor pollutants. Typical sources of indoor air pollutants are described in Figure 13-3. Poor indoor air quality (IAQ) has been demonstrated to exacerbate asthma and other respiratory illness for students and school staff. IAQ is improved by control of airborne pollutants, adequate outdoor air, and temperature and humidity control (USEPA, 2023b). The USEPA webpage has an *Indoor Air Quality Tools for Schools Action Kit* that includes best practices, industry guidelines, sample policies, and IAQ management plans ready to put in place; the tools are available in paper form and a mobile device application (USEPA, 2022).

> **Practice Connection**
>
> The National Institutes of Health has a program called "It's a Noisy Planet: Protect Your Hearing" that provides educational materials for educators, health professionals, parents, school-age children, and adolescents to assist in addressing noise pollution in schools and communities (NIDCD, 2016).

The key components to effective school IAQ programs are communication, continuous assessment of the environment, addressing structural and behavior issues, and evaluating the results for continuous improvement (USEPA, 2018). These components should be directed toward solutions that can lead to effective IAQ management for the following:

- Quality Heating/ventilation/air conditioning (HVAC)
- Strong integrated pest management
- Effective cleaning and maintenance
- Control of moisture and/or mold
- Smart materials selection
- Aggressive source control
- Integrated energy management solution (USEPA, 2018)

The Environmental Law Institute (2022) maintains a database of state indoor air quality laws that directly relate to schools. They recommend that the state education code be checked to determine whether and how often it requires that schools be inspected to ensure minimal health and safety criteria. Nurses should be familiar with these regulations to advocate for implementation in their school while also collecting illness surveillance data to identify environmental causes for student illness.

Bus and Car Idling

The EPA encourages schools to develop an idle reduction policy as bus and car idling affects health both outside and inside the school as the diesel exhaust can enter the school through air intakes, doors, and open windows. Diesel exhausts contain particulate matter that enters the heart and lungs and can lead to death, asthma and allergy exacerbation, and decreased lung function (USEPA, 2024c). The EPA provides a sample policy that can be used by schools to address bus idling; however, training and enforcement will be needed. (See Online Materials OM13-1 for a sample bus idling policy.)

Indoor Environmental Contaminants

Toxic hazards can be related to pest control, cleaning methods and materials, and chemical exposures. These hazards should be addressed as part of a comprehensive IAQ and environmental management plan. Discussion of the impact of airborne chemicals and metals is important since they may go undetected and may affect cognitive function and behavior. Figure 13-3 provides examples of common indoor air pollutants that affect the IAQ of a school.

Lead

One of the most well-known chemical exposures is lead. Although lead in paint was banned in 1978, lead paint and lead pipes can still be found in school buildings built before 1978. Lead is also found in plastic, which is used to create some toys and jewelry, as the use of lead in plastic has not been banned. Cases of lead poisoning have been linked to

TYPICAL SOURCES OF INDOOR AIR POLLUTANTS

OUTDOOR SOURCES	BUILDING EQUIPMENT	COMPONENTS/ FURNISHINGS	OTHER POTENTIAL INDOOR SOURCES
Polluted Outdoor Air • Pollen, dust, mold spores • Industrial emissions • Vehicle and nonroad engine emissions (cars, buses, trucks, lawn and garden equipment) **Nearby Sources** • Loading docks • Odors from dumpsters • Unsanitary debris or building exhausts near outdoor air intakes **Underground Sources** • Radon • Pesticides • Leakage from underground storage tanks	**HVAC Equipment** • Mold growth in drip pans, ductwork, coils, and humidifiers • Improper venting of combustion products • Dust or debris in ductwork **Other Equipment** • Emissions from office equipment (volatile organic compounds (VOCs), ozone) • Emissions from shop, lab, and cleaning equipment	**Components** • Mold growth on or in soiled or water-damaged materials • Dry drain traps that allow the passage of sewer gas • Materials containing VOCs, inorganic compounds, or damaged asbestos • Materials that produce particles (dust) **Furnishings** • Emissions from new furnishings and floorings • Mold growth on or in soiled or water-damaged furnishings	• Science laboratory supplies • Vocational art supplies • Copy/print areas • Food prep areas • Smoking lounges • Cleaning materials • Emissions from trash • Pesticides • Odors and VOCs from paint, caulk, adhesives • Occupants with communicable diseases • Dry-erase markers and similar pens • Insects and other pests • Personal care products • Stored gasoline and lawn and garden equipment

FIGURE 13-3. Typical sources of indoor air pollutants. *(Reproduced with permission of the U.S. Environmental Protection Agency. [2009]. https://www.epa.gov/sites/default/files/2014-08/documents/reference_guide.pdf)*

traditional ceramicware used for preparing or serving food and drink (USFDA, 2017). The high lead blood levels are known to decrease the body's ability to make hemoglobin, increase blood pressure, interfere with nerve conduction, and damage the kidneys. Higher blood lead levels build up in the brain and can lead to lowered intelligence, decreased attention, and poor school performance (CDC, 2024a). Healthy People 2030 includes two objectives related to lead: reduce exposure to lead and reduce blood lead levels in children 1 to 5 years old (Office of Disease Prevention and Health Promotion, n.d.). Exposure to lead is very connected to the community in which one lives, and non-Hispanic black children, those in low-income households, and immigrants/refugees have higher exposures to lead (Ruckart et al., 2021).

There is no safe blood lead level in children; however, any lead level of 3.5 mcg/dL or higher is considered a level of concern and warrants referral to identify and mitigate the cause (CDC, 2024a). Because lead is absorbed into the blood, bones, teeth, and soft tissues and the half-life of lead is at least 1 month it can take more than a year to reduce blood lead levels. Early screening is important as no treatment effectively reverses the developmental effects of high lead levels (CDC, 2024a).

The issue of lead exposure and poisoning is still prevalent. The Flint water crisis, exposed in 2015, brought the issue of lead poisoning into the news. This example illustrates our built environments' impact on health outcomes in communities. In 2014, Flint, Michigan, switched its municipal water source from Lake Huron to the Flint River; this change caused the water pipes to corrode and leach lead into the water. The lead in the water resulted in a public health emergency whereby residents were told not to drink tap water unless filtered and a spike was seen in childhood blood lead levels. As the situation was shared via news and other outlets, an outcry regarding public safety resulted in much scrutiny of municipal water systems throughout the country (CDC, 2024h). The nurse is responsible for being aware of the effects of lead poisoning and assessing students who may be at increased risk for lead exposure.

Mercury

Mercury is a natural metal that comes in three forms that can be toxic when a person comes in contact with it.

Mercury poisoning can affect the nervous system, lungs, and kidney. Although mercury has been removed from most schools, it may still be found in science labs, glass thermometers, barometers, and thermostats. Schools should have a mercury policy in place in case of spills, as it should be scooped up and discarded in a hazardous waste container and not poured into drains or toilets. Both an audit checklist and sample policy can be found on the Agency for Toxic Substances and Disease Registry webpage (2018; see Online Materials OM13-2 for the link). The nurse should be aware of items containing mercury and be involved in the development of the school policy related to mercury so they can respond in case of a spill.

Radon

Radon is a radioactive gas that can seep from the soil through cracks in the foundations. Radon is known as the leading cause of lung cancer among nonsmokers. The USEPA conducted a national survey of schools and found that nearly one in five has at least one classroom with a short-term radon level of concern (USEPA, 2024a). It is recommended that all schools test for radon and develop mitigation plans.

Animals in the School Setting

The CDC, National Science Teachers Association, and others recommend animals in school settings as valuable science teaching aids (CDC, 2024j). Classroom animals present an opportunity to discuss care and responsibility of animals and other aspects of social-emotional learning (Herbert & Lynch, 2017). However, animals in the classroom can also be a source of potential allergy, infection (especially *Salmonella* and *Escherichia coli*), and injury. The CDC has issued guidelines for animals in the schools, including the importance of hand washing and safe enclosures for the animals. In addition, they have animal-specific guidelines as well as a list of animals that are not recommended in school settings, especially reptiles, amphibians, chickens, rodents, and ferrets for children under age 5 years; any animal likely to spread rabies; stray animals; and those that are venomous or toxin producing (CDC, 2024j).

Service animals in schools are increasing in prevalence; these animals are working animals and not pets. They are helpful to students or staff who have physical, sensory, psychiatric, intellectual, or other mental disabilities and are covered by the Americans With Disabilities Act (Americans With Disabilities Act National Network, 2024). Another student's fear of or allergy to animals is not a reason to exclude the animal from the school setting. The animal must be housebroken and vaccinated according to state laws. The care and supervision of the animal are the responsibility of the "handler," and the animal may not disrupt (i.e., barking) or threaten (i.e., growling) the other students in the class (Brennan & Nguyen, 2014). For detailed information on policy development regarding service animals in the school setting, refer to the Online Materials OM13-2. The school nurse should be involved in all conversations about animals in the school setting as they are best able to support the health needs and concerns of the students.

IMMUNIZATIONS

Immunizations have reduced vaccine preventable disease by more than 90%; thereby reducing disease morbidity and mortality in students, their families, and school staff (CDC, 2021b). Achieving high vaccination rates among students protects the entire school community through herd immunity when a critical proportion of the community is protected so that those who cannot be vaccinated will have less risk of communicable disease exposure (Hall et al., 2021). Herd immunity becomes ever more important when infectious outbreaks occur. The ease of international travel and the migration of persons from countries with endemic infections is an additional rationale for keeping immunization levels high. The quarantine and isolation rules during the COVID-19 pandemic led to many missed routine vaccine appointments both in the United States and abroad. The lower vaccination rates threaten herd immunity, leading to increased concern about the spread of communicable diseases in the future.

School Immunizations Compliance

All states require some vaccination as a requirement for school entry (Barraza et al., 2017). The school nurse must be knowledgeable about how vaccines work, the diseases they prevent, state regulations regarding the vaccine schedules, and district exemption and exclusion policies. As much of this information changes over time, the school nurse should be familiar with the Advisory Committee for Immunization Practices Web site, where the most current information can be found. School nurses are expected to conduct communicable disease surveillance, collect immunization compliance data, and evaluate programmatic success. The school nurse's role in immunization compliance includes developing evidence-based vaccination strategies to improve the number of students and families who receive mandated vaccinations. School nurses can use their position as health advocates to educate students, staff, and families about vaccines and dispel immunization myths (NASN, 2020).

Did You Know?

Immunization Versus Vaccination

Vaccination refers to the administration of a vaccine, usually as an injection, whereas *immunization* refers to how the body responds by developing protection. Protection can also be acquired after recovering from certain infectious diseases. Therefore vaccination is a strategy for achieving immunization (CDC, 2021b).

All states have access to immunization information systems. These computerized databases record immunization data from participating providers (CDC, 2019). These systems have greatly improved the tracking of vaccinations but are only as good as the data that are entered into them and the access to which the data is available. School nurses should maintain an easily accessible reference list of unvaccinated students in the event of a communicable disease outbreak. This list can be used to quickly notify parents, administrators, and local health departments if certain children need to be more closely monitored or, in some cases, excluded from school. School nurses must work in conjunction with the local health department any time there is a suspected outbreak.

Students Without Vaccination Records

The student's healthcare provider should be consulted if the parent/guardian cannot present an immunization record to the school. If records are not retrievable, vaccinations need to be administered by a healthcare provider using the CDC's *Catch-Up Immunization Schedule* (CDC, 2024m). There are many reasons why immunization records might not be readily available, including students who have moved frequently, have lost a home due to fire or natural disaster, are homeless, or are in foster care. The school nurse should take into consideration these determinants when communicating with parents or guardians and take a collegial, active, and communicative approach with families and healthcare providers that supports the family to meet immunization requirements. Parents who do not submit immunization forms may need informal or formal reminders, such as telephone calls or form letters (Maurer et al., 2016). Each district needs to evaluate the best way to share information and alert students and families about immunization compliance.

> **Practice Connection**
>
> The transfer of student health information to schools can become a point of contention when healthcare providers are unfamiliar with the stipulations of the Health Information Portability and Accountability Act (HIPAA). HIPAA allows immunization records to be shared between healthcare providers (e.g., primary care providers and school nurses or school physicians) for the purpose of protecting public health (U.S. Department of Health and Human Services, 2019). However, a relationship between the school nurse and local provider, as well as the parents, needs to be transparent and collaborative. Although state regulations vary, school nurses are encouraged to share the information linked in online materials OM 13-2 with providers. The school nurse should also be open to pursuing a release of information from the parent if it becomes clear that the immunization records will not otherwise be released by the provider.

Types of Vaccines

There are several classifications of vaccines: live attenuated (weakened), inactivated (killed) vaccines, and polysaccharide and recombinant vaccines that actively stimulate the immune system to make protective antibodies (Hall et al., 2021). It is important for the vaccine provider to evaluate the health history of the individual before any type of vaccination and follow any recommended contraindications and precautions.

Live attenuated vaccines are viral or bacterial agents modified in a laboratory to decrease the risk of causing disease. They provide active protection identical to the immune response of someone who had a natural case of the disease. Students who are immunocompromised are at increased risk of contracting the communicable disease if vaccinated with live attenuated vaccines. This may also be true for the siblings and other family members of those who are immunocompromised. Examples of live attenuated vaccines include measles, mumps, rubella, varicella, and rotavirus.

Inactivated vaccines are created from bacteria or viruses grown in a laboratory and then inactivated with heat or chemicals. Inactivated viruses cannot replicate and therefore do not cause the disease, even in immunosuppressed individuals (Hall et al., 2021). Because inactivated vaccines stimulate a weaker immune response, multiple booster doses are recommended throughout life to maintain protection. Inactivated vaccines include diphtheria, tetanus, polio, and hepatitis A.

Polysaccharide and recombinant vaccines are produced with components or subunits of the pathogen; they are also incapable of causing the actual disease. Examples of these vaccines include hepatitis B, influenza (injectable), pneumococcal, meningococcal, human papillomavirus (HPV), and COVID-19.

Vaccine Additives

Vaccine production involves the use of chemicals, often referred to as additives and adjuvants. Adjuvants are ingredients that improve the vaccine's effectiveness and include preservatives and stabilizers such as albumin and antibiotics such as neomycin to prevent bacterial growth (CDC, 2022f). These additives, while only in small amounts, inactivate the organism and stabilize the vaccine to ensure potency over time. Thimerosal, a product used to prevent unwanted growth of bacteria and fungi in multidose vials, has not been used in pediatric vaccines since 2001 and there is no link between thimerosal and autism (CDC, 2020). Nevertheless, some parents may have concerns about vaccines and school nurses should have evidence-based information to dispel this and other myths that pose barriers to immunization.

Vaccine Schedules

The Advisory Committee on Immunization Practices (ACIP) annually reviews the latest research and presents recommendations to the CDC regarding recommended vaccines and administration schedules. Upon review and approval by the CDC and the Department of Health and Human Services, updated immunization schedules are published annually. Schedules for all age groups are available in various formats from the CDC Web site, *Immunization Schedules.* This includes a catch-up schedule for persons 4 months through 18 years who start late, miss doses, or who are more than 1 month behind with vaccinations (CDC, 2024m). While student immunization compliance is the primary focus, it is important for school nurses to also be informed about adult immunizations to ensure that adults in the school setting are appropriately educated and protected.

The CDC immunization schedules are just recommendations; at the state level these recommendations are reviewed, legislated, and/or regulated. Every state requires children to receive certain vaccines before attending public school. Specific requirements may also apply to children attending day care or private schools (National Center for Immunization and Respiratory Disease, 2023b).

General Immunization Principles

For school nurses to provide information and support to school administrators, staff, and parents, they must remain up to date regarding timing and spacing of vaccines. Many people are not well informed about immunizations, and there are many myths about vaccines that have been disproven through extensive scientific research but still create hesitancy. Following are some general rules about vaccines (Hall et al., 2021).

General Rules

- Generally, all vaccines for which the child is eligible can be administered at the same visit (except for children with functional or anatomic asplenia).
- If two live parenteral vaccines are given less than 4 weeks apart, the vaccine given second should be repeated.
- Vaccines may not be mixed together unless they come combined by the manufacturer (e.g., measles, mumps, rubella [MMR] or diphtheria and tetanus toxoids and acellular pertussis [DTaP]).
- Multiple vaccines given at the same time should be given in different sites.
- *Increasing* the interval between doses of a multidose vaccine does *not* diminish the effectiveness of the vaccine; however, decreasing the interval will result in decreased antibody response.
- Vaccine doses administered up to 4 days before the minimum interval or age can be counted as valid.
- All documented immunizations count, no matter how long ago they were given. There is *no need to start over,* even if a long interval occurred between doses (Hall et al., 2021).

Adolescent Vaccines

Much focus has been put on vaccination between birth and 6 years old; however, the ACIP recommends several vaccinations be given to older children and adults (CDC, 2024m). Annual influenza vaccination is recommended. Starting at age 9, the HPV vaccine can be given. This vaccine, the first to prevent cancer, prevents cervical, penile, oropharyngeal, and anal cancers due to HPV and related infections. The vaccine is recommended for both males and females. At age 11, a Tdap booster (a full dose of tetanus, a reduced dose of diphtheria, and a reduced dose of acellular pertussis) is recommended due to pertussis outbreaks in adolescents. A four-strain meningococcal conjugate vaccine, including strains A, C, W, and Y, is recommended due to severe morbidity and mortality from meningococcal meningitis prevalent in the mid-to-later adolescent years.

Travel Vaccines

Global travel, both personal and school-sponsored, might put students at risk for exposure to communicable diseases. The CDC recommends vaccination depending on endemic infections in the host country, duration of stay, and specific areas of travel in that country (CDC, 2023d). In addition, the host country might require proof of certain vaccines. It is recommended that the CDC Web site be checked at least 4 to 6 weeks before travel to ensure timely receipt of recommended or required vaccines. School nurses should make administrators, staff, and families aware of these requirements when discussing school-sponsored trips.

Postexposure Prophylaxis or Prevention

When a nonprotected person is exposed to a serious preventable disease, treatment with vaccines, immune globulin, antibiotics, or antiviral medication can reduce illness severity and infection transmission (Bader & McKinsey, 2013). Examples of postexposure treatment include tetanus immune globulin, varicella-zoster immune globulin, hepatitis B immune globulin, and rabies vaccine (Hall et al., 2021). The immunoglobulins provide passive immunity; they give the individual the already-made antibodies for immediate protection. However, they do not stimulate the immune system, do not provide extended protection, and protection is cut in half in 28 days. In addition to vaccinations, individuals exposed to bacterial infections such as meningitis can be treated with antibiotics and persons exposed to viruses such as HIV can be treated with antiretroviral treatment.

Vaccine Adverse Reactions

Vaccine adverse reactions, sometimes known as side effects, are unwanted effects caused by the vaccine. Federal law requires that parents be provided with a **Vaccine Information Statement** before administration that includes a description of the disease, who should get the vaccine and when, a list of the possible risks and reactions, what to do in case of a reaction, and how to learn more about the vaccine (CDC, 2023e). School nurses can find Vaccine Information Statements in English and other languages on the CDC's Web site (CDC, 2023e).

Vaccine adverse reactions are classified as local, systemic, or allergic. **Local reactions** are minor, such as

Did You Know?

Endemic—refers to the amount of disease present in the community or a baseline. This is not necessarily a desired level but may be regarded as an expected level. To learn more about endemic, epidemic, and pandemic visit https://www.lung.org/blog/epidemic-pandemic-endemic-covid (American Lung Association, 2022).

redness, pain, and swelling at the site of the injection that may emerge within hours of vaccination and go away within a few days (Hall et al., 2021). **Systemic reactions** are also typically mild and include fever, headache, muscle aches, anorexia, and malaise. For live attenuated vaccines (e.g., MMR and varicella), systemic events may occur 3 to 21 days later and generally present as fever and a mild rash that mimics the disease against which they were given. These symptoms also resolve within days, and the child is not contagious.

More significant adverse reactions include the following:

- Allergic reactions: Allergic reactions to the vaccine antigen or to vaccine ingredients are extremely rare. Severe reactions include hives, swelling of the mouth and throat, difficulty breathing, wheezing, hypotension, or shock. According to a CDC study, the incidence of anaphylaxis is 1.3 per million doses (American Academy of Allergy, Asthma, and Immunology, 2019).
- Syncope (fainting): Syncope is also rare and most commonly occurs among adolescents, generally occurring moments after the vaccine injection. To prevent syncope, the CDC recommends that adolescents be seated while vaccinated and observed for 15 minutes after vaccination (2022e). If symptoms develop, have the student sit or lie down and remain under observation until the symptoms resolve. It is important to make clear to the parents that research has shown that the vaccination is not generally what harms the patient but rather the injury that results from fainting.

Vaccine Adverse Event Reporting System

The Vaccine Adverse Event Reporting System (VAERS) was developed in 1990 and is a voluntary reporting system to monitor vaccine safety by accepting reports from healthcare professionals, vaccine manufacturers, and the general public (VAERS, n.d.). Reports signal the CDC and the Food and Drug Administration (that oversees vaccine manufacturers) to monitor and report vaccine reactions ranging from mild to severe. Online and written reporting forms for healthcare providers are located on the VAERS Web site.

Contraindications for Vaccine Administration

There are valid circumstances when vaccines should not be given. Many are temporary and the vaccine(s) should be given when the contraindication no longer remains. A **precaution** is a condition that might increase the chance or severity of a serious adverse reaction, but the risk of injury is less than with a contraindication. Moderate to severe illness with fever is considered a precaution to vaccination as it would be difficult to discern whether the fever was due to a vaccine reaction or the original illness. Typically, vaccines should be administered when a precaution is present unless the benefit of the vaccine outweighs the risk of the vaccine (CDC, 2023f). A **contraindication** is a condition that increases the likelihood of a serious adverse reaction; when these conditions are present a vaccine should not be administered.

Did You Know?

The National Vaccine Injury Compensation Program

The National Vaccine Injury Compensation Program, administered by the Health Resources and Services Administration (HRSA), compensates individuals who experience certain health events following immunization on a "no fault" basis; the person filing a claim is not required to prove negligence on the part of either the healthcare provider or manufacturer to receive compensation. Healthcare providers should provide information regarding the National Vaccine Injury Compensation program to patients who may have had an adverse effect from their vaccine (HRSA, 2024). Claims may be made based on the Vaccine Injury Table, which is amended regularly to reflect current scientific evidence.

Examples of contraindications include the following:

- Severe allergic reaction (anaphylaxis) to a vaccine component or to a previous dose of vaccine
- Pregnancy (no live vaccines)
- Immunosuppression (no live vaccines)
- Encephalopathy not due to another identifiable cause occurring within 7 days of a pertussis vaccination (no inactivated vaccine)
- If a child had a temperature of 105°F or higher within 48 hours of a dose of pediatric DTaP, collapsed in a shock-like state within 48 hours of a dose, had persistent inconsolable crying lasting 3 or more hours within 48 hours of a dose, or had a seizure within 3 days of a dose. In these cases, further doses of pediatric DTaP are withheld during childhood (Hall et al., 2021)

Invalid contraindications to vaccination include the following:

- Mild illness
- Antimicrobial therapy
- Disease exposure or convalescence
- Pregnant or immunosuppressed person in household
- Allergy to products not present in vaccine
- Allergy that is not anaphylactic
- Family history of adverse events
- Tuberculin skin test

Although there are limited true contraindications and precautions, it is important that the vaccine provider screen patients for each vaccine being given at the time of administration (Immunization Action Coalition, 2023b). Box 13-2 includes screening questions to rule out contraindications.

Immunization Exemptions

Exemptions, formerly known as waivers, refer to an allowance as per state law for temporarily or permanently opting out of one or more vaccines. Medical exemptions, which can be temporary or permanent, are based upon contraindications or precautions. medical exemptions are allowed across all states and the District of Columbia (CDC, 2022d). Currently many states allow nonmedical exemptions (religious or philosophical); however, leading medical organizations, including the American Nurses Association and National Association of Pediatric Nurse Practitioners, are seeking to eliminate these nonmedical exemptions as decreased rates of vaccination put those who are unable to be vaccinated at greater risk (Immunization Action Coalition, 2023a). State vaccination laws include an application process for exemptions. During an outbreak, students who are not fully immunized for that disease are excluded from school.

BOX 13-2

Screening Checklist for Contraindications to Vaccines for Children and Teens

- Is the child sick today?
- Does the child have allergies to medications, food, latex, or any vaccine?
- Has the child had a serious reaction to a vaccine in the past?
- Has the child had a health problem with asthma, lung disease, heart disease, kidney disease, metabolic disease such as diabetes, or a blood disorder? Are they on aspirin therapy?
- If the child is between 2 and 4 years old, has a health provider told you that the child has wheezing or asthma in the past 12 months?
- If the child is a baby, have you been told they have intussusception?
- Has the child, a sibling, or a parent had a seizure; has the child had a brain or other nervous system problem?
- Does the child have cancer, leukemia, HIV/AIDS, or any other immune system problem?
- Does the child have a parent, brother, or sister with an immune system problem?
- In the past 3 months, has the child taken medication that could affect the immune system?
- In the past year, has the child received a blood or blood product transfusion or been given immune globulin or an antiviral drug?
- Is the adolescent pregnant or is there a chance they could become pregnant in the next month?
- Has the child received vaccinations in the past 4 weeks?
- Does the child have cancer, leukemia, AIDS, or any other immune system problem?
- Has the child taken cortisone, prednisone, other steroids, or anticancer drugs, or had x-ray treatments in the past 3 months?
- Has the child received a transfusion of blood or blood products or been given a medicine called immune (gamma) globulin in the past year?
- Is the person pregnant or is there a chance she could become pregnant during the next month?
- Has the child received vaccinations in the past 4 weeks?

Source: Immunization Action Coalition (2023b).

Philosophical reasons for refusal to vaccinate include the perceived danger of the vaccine and/or the belief that the parent, not a state law, should determine healthcare services for their child. It is important for the school nurse to be aware of the reasons for refusal to vaccinate and to collaborate on immunization strategies that will help close the immunization gap so that all children are adequately protected. Vaccine refusal or vaccine hesitancy may stem from safety concerns or just a need for more information from the healthcare provider. A recent study found that 1 in 15 parents are hesitant about routine childhood vaccines and more than 1 in 4 are hesitant about annual influenza vaccines (Kempe et al., 2020). It is important to be sure the refusal is not related to something the school nurse may be able to address, such as an inability to pay for the vaccine or challenges in locating vaccination facilities.

When parents present worries or reluctance to vaccinate, it is important for the nurse to listen to the overt message and underlying fears. Presenting an attentive manner and asking questions about their concerns may help. Examples include the following: Tell me more about your concerns. Did your child ever have a bad experience with vaccination? Have you expressed your concerns to the pediatrician? What have you heard or read that concerns you? Does your health insurance cover vaccination? Questions like these will not only help discern what the parents already know and discover underlying fears, but also convey to the parent that you care about their child and their concerns (CDC, 2021c). If the parent has not spoken to the primary care provider, encourage that conversation. Box 13-3 lists resources, in English and other languages, for nurses and parents regarding vaccination concerns.

Parents or guardians may also be concerned about their children receiving too many vaccines too often. There is little danger to simultaneous vaccinations per ACIP recommendations (Hall et al., 2021). Some families are concerned about the pain or trauma of administering many concurrent injections during one visit, informally known as the "pincushion effect," but studies document that children can receive as many vaccines during a visit as are age appropriate with no correlation between sequelae and the number of injections given nor does it interfere with the antibody production to each of the antigens (Hall et al., 2021).

BOX 13-3

Resources for Nurses and Parents Regarding Vaccination Concerns

There are many educational materials in English and other languages that can help to explain the value of vaccinations and address the more common concerns.

For School Nurses:

Provider Resources for Vaccine Conversations With Parents. https://www.cdc.gov/vaccines/hcp/conversations/conv-materials.html

Q and As: Diseases and Vaccines. https://www.immunize.org/handouts/vaccine-questions.asp

For Parents:

Vaccines for Your Children. https://www.cdc.gov/vaccines/parents/index.html

Childhood vaccines, in 12 languages. https://medlineplus.gov/languages/childhoodvaccines.html

Although multiple vaccinations during a visit may seem daunting, healthcare providers should take advantage of every opportunity to vaccinate. Vaccinating according to schedule increases immunization coverage and protects against serious vaccine-preventable disease. Children entering the school system should receive all age-appropriate recommended vaccines before the first day of class. Exclusion for lack of immunizations and physicals is dictated at the state level and varies considerably.

School-Located Vaccination

Because most students are vaccinated through primary care providers or school-based health centers, school nurses are not generally expected to administer routine vaccinations. However, school nurses may be recruited or required to administer vaccinations at school during outbreaks or when a new vaccination law is implemented. The Immunization Action Coalition (2024) has developed easy-to-follow administration guidelines that are available on its Web site.

The nurse also serves as a leader in the development of school-located vaccine clinics and identifies students who could be best served by these services. School-located vaccine clinics eliminate some of the barriers to care that some families face as they seek to access health care, including transportation and work schedules that do not allow time off for medical appointments (NASN, 2022a).

When considering school-located vaccine clinics, it is important to consider what equipment and supplies are needed and to ensure there is adequate vaccine storage. Some vaccines require refrigeration whereas others, such as MMR and varicella, require freezer units. The CDC has developed a toolkit (CDC, 2024i) for vaccine storage and handling that school nurses should consult if they must store vaccines on site. The *NASN School Nurse* journal published a supplemental issue on the topic of school-located vaccine clinics in January 2022 that includes an overview of policies, practices, and lessons learned during the COVID-19 pandemic.

Special Populations

It is important that the school nurse assess the needs of all students in the building to make sure they are best able to meet state requirements related to vaccines. Additionally, there are populations that the school nurse should be especially aware of when considering protection from communicable diseases.

Children Who Are Immunocompromised

Children who are immunocompromised are at higher risk of communicable disease and may have contraindications for vaccination due to their immunocompromised status. However, being immunocompromised is not a blanket reason for a child not to be vaccinated. Considerations by the healthcare provider will need to be made on when and what vaccines are administered. The Advisory Committee on Immunization Practices (ACIP) provides vaccination recommendations for people experiencing altered immunocompetence (ACIP, 2023).

Children Experiencing Homelessness

It is estimated that 2.42% of all students enrolled in public schools are homeless (National Center for Homeless Education, 2022). The McKinney-Vento Homeless Assistance Act of 1987 is federal legislation that removes barriers to school enrollment for children who are homeless. This Act defines homeless as those who "lack a fixed, regular and adequate night-time residence." This includes children who are sleeping in shelters, living unsheltered in cars or parks, living in hotels or motels, and those who are living with another family. The Act seeks to protect these children and ensure that they receive the same education as their housed peers. It is important for the school nurse to note that these children cannot be kept from registering for or excluded from the school setting due to lack of medical records. School nurses should work with these children and families to assist them in accessing the care that is needed; parents who are experiencing homelessness may have logistical challenges that prevent them from accessing their children's medical care (Gennaro et al., 2021). Assistance may involve connecting the families to primary care providers to initiate care or contacting previous medical providers to obtain health records.

Children Who Have Recently Arrived From Outside the United States

The school nurse may be one of the first healthcare providers the newly arrived student and family interacts with in the United States. Newly arrived children are at increased risk of tuberculosis, HIV, hepatitis C, malaria, and vaccine-preventable diseases in general related to undervaccination

(Shetty, 2019). These families have often undergone traumatic situations to arrive in the United States and the nurse should engage with them in an open manner to best assist them with accessing health care. Vaccine requirements vary by country so it is possible that the child may have been up to date on requirements in their previous home but are now in need of vaccination. It is important that the school nurse explain the requirements to the parents and support them in seeking care in a system that may be unfamiliar. The catch-up immunization schedule should be referred to when administering vaccines (CDC, 2024m). The American Academy of Pediatrics (n.d.) has an Immigrant Child Health toolkit that is a helpful resource for school nurses.

COMMUNICABLE DISEASES AND VACCINES

Due to the success of immunization efforts, most healthcare providers, including school nurses, have never seen the signs and symptoms associated with vaccine-preventable diseases. An overview of communicable disease and, when relevant, the vaccines recommended by the ACIP that prevent the disease is included here to assist the school nurse in the care of schoolchildren and families. It is important to note that many communicable diseases occurred less often during the COVID-19 pandemic. Many of the precautions set in place to protect populations from COVID-19 also protected people from communicable diseases. However, the COVID-19 pandemic also created disruptions in children receiving routine childhood immunization. Disruptions were seen across all populations but were most pronounced in non-Hispanic Black children (DeSilva et al. 2022). The school nurse should work with their school population to ensure children who fell behind with immunizations are caught up.

Refer to the Advisory Committee on Immunization Practice Vaccine Recommendations and Guidelines for the most updated vaccine-specific recommendations (CDC, 2022e).

Notification of Communicable Disease Outbreak

The CDC and the state and local health departments have policies and processes for reporting communicable diseases. At the national level, the CDC maintains the National Notifiable Diseases Surveillance System (NNDSS) and the National Outbreak Reporting System (NORS). The NNDSS is a national collaborative to share information about state and nationally reportable infectious and noninfectious diseases and outbreaks by case or person (CDC, 2024r). NORS is a web-based reporting platform where health departments can report cases of water- and food-borne disease and enteric disease outbreaks (CDC, 2023b). Both sites can inform the school nurse regarding infectious disease and outbreaks at the population level. Each state and local health department can assist the school nurse with identifying and reporting infectious diseases. Regular review of the local health department policies regarding communicable illness will help the school nurse prepare for outbreaks. Keeping the lines of communication between the school district administration, the nurse, and the health department is essential.

When one or more cases of serious contagious disease are identified (e.g., one student with pertussis or tuberculosis), typically the local public health department, in coordination with the healthcare provider of the ill student, leads investigations and follow-up, and can assist in preparing appropriate communication to the school community and/or public. Students who report to the health office with a known or suspected serious contagious disease need to be isolated to prevent transmission. The school nurse should notify the parents to take the student home or to a medical provider as soon as possible. School administration should be kept informed.

Per health department guidance, it may be necessary to inform the student's classroom contacts, or a wider group, such as the grade level or entire school, of the outbreak. The health department can provide guidance in preparing appropriate communication to the school community and/or public. It is wise to obtain a confirmed diagnosis before communicating to staff, parents, and students. The accuracy of diagnosis prevents misinformation or, at worst, unwarranted panic in the school and larger community.

Many school nurses prepare a district template letter for use in these situations that can be adapted to reflect the specifics of the disease. For privacy and protection, *the student's name is not included*. The letter might include information about the disease, steps to reduce or prevent transmission, and steps to follow if symptoms appear. The school nurse will have to consult school-wide medical records and make specific exclusion notifications for those students who are not immunized against the disease.

Students or staff who are ill with contagious conditions should remain at home to prevent further disease transmission and fully recover. The number of days that a student should remain at home will vary widely depending on their level of immunity and general health. The district or local health department will have guidelines regarding the recommended number of days that a student should remain at home due to illness, including communicable diseases. Collaboration by the school nurse with the child's healthcare provider and family can assist in supporting the student in recovery and return to school.

To prepare for medical situations such as outbreaks or pandemics, every district and school should have a school emergency operations plan that includes pandemics. This should include a Continuity of Operations Plan (see Chapter 15). The plan can be adapted for school-wide medical crises. The National Education Association (NEA) has developed a guide for developing a school crisis plan (NEA, 2018). Depending on the size of the school district and existing infrastructure, the school nurse might be expected to coordinate activities among the school or district administration and local public health officials.

Diphtheria, Pertussis, Tetanus

Diphtheria

Diphtheria is caused by bacteria that proliferate in the respiratory tract and multiply on dead tissue in the throat, producing toxin across the respiratory tract at the back of the throat; this results in a mechanical airway obstruction and respiratory distress. Diphtheria is spread through droplets, typically person to person, and has an incubation period of 2 to 5 days. The disease is more serious in infants and may cause renal, cardiac, and peripheral nervous system damage; however, it can affect individuals of any age (CDC, 2024g).

Before vaccinations, diphtheria was one of the most common causes of death in school-age children, peaking in 1921 with 207,000 cases in the United States. Immunization has been highly effective; in the United States between 1996 and 2018 there were 14 reported cases of diphtheria reported with only one fatality (Hall et al., 2021).

The full dose of diphtheria vaccine, noted by the capital *D*, is part of the DTaP (diphtheria and tetanus toxoids and acellular pertussis vaccine) or DT (diphtheria and tetanus toxoids) doses given to children younger than 7 years. After the age of 7, as the risk of the sequelae of diphtheria decreases, all subsequent boosters have a smaller dose of diphtheria, noted by the lowercase *d* in Td (tetanus and diphtheria toxoids) or Tdap (tetanus and diphtheria toxoids and acellular pertussis vaccine; Hall et al., 2021).

Pertussis

Pertussis, commonly called *whooping cough*, is caused by the toxin from bacteria that proliferate in the respiratory tract. The toxin causes inflammation, which inhibits clearance of pulmonary secretions. Pertussis is highly contagious, transmitted person to person by aerosolized respiratory droplets or direct contact with secretions, and has an incubation period of 4 to 21 days (CDC, 2024s). The clinical course of pertussis is divided into three stages: the *catarrhal stage* is characterized by symptoms of a common cold such as runny nose, sneezing, and a mild cough; the *paroxysmal stage* has spasms or paroxysms of numerous rapid coughs followed by a high-pitched whoop; and the *convalescent stage*, which can last weeks to months. Pertussis may be contagious during the incubation period before the cough begins but is most infectious during the catarrhal stage.

Coughing associated with pertussis can be severe, with restricted breathing during the spell of coughing, followed by vomiting, cyanosis, and even loss of consciousness. Bacterial pneumonia is the most common complication and cause of death.

Following the implementation of pertussis vaccination, the incidence of pertussis decreased to about 1 per 100,000 population; however, certain populations remain at higher risk and incidence is gradually increasing. Infants are at greatest risk with the rate of incidence at 73.2 per 100,000 in infants younger than 6 months old compared with 1.4 per 100,000 in people 20 years or older. There is an increasing incidence among fully vaccinated children between the ages of 11 and 18 with a rate of 13.1 per 100,000 population (Hall et al., 2021). Increased attention and public awareness have helped to lower these rates; however, much work needs to be done. The CDC recommends that pregnant women be immunized between their 27th and 36th week in order to protect themselves and their infants. In 2022, there were 2,388 cases of pertussis in the United States; about half (1,298) were under the age of 20 years (National Center for Immunization and Respiratory Disease, 2023a).

Tetanus

Tetanus is a neurological disorder caused by anaerobic, spore-forming bacteria that produce an exotoxin; it lives in soil and animal feces. The bacteria enter the skin through puncture wounds, lacerations, and abrasions and travel to the axons of the nerves, causing involuntary muscle contraction, muscular rigidity, and painful paroxysmal seizures. The incubation period is 8 days. While there are three different forms of tetanus, generalized tetanus is the most common. It starts with trismus (lockjaw) and difficulty in swallowing, and can cause laryngospasm, respiratory distress, intramuscular hemorrhage, and death. Spasms continue for 3 to 4 weeks (Hall et al., 2021).

Before the development of vaccines for tetanus, 500 to 600 cases were reported in the United States annually; however, since 2000, there have been less than 50 cases reported annually. In 2022, 28 cases were reported with no deaths. Because protective titers are maintained for only about 10 years, boosters are recommended every 10 years throughout life. The school nurse's responsibility includes caring for any wound by providing good wound care and assessing for risk of tetanus by checking the student's immunization record and referring to a healthcare provider for prompt follow-up if vaccination is lacking (CDC, 2024v).

Students should be informed that body piercing and tattooing may expose them to tetanus if supplies and equipment are not sterilized. The school nurse should take the opportunity to review the immunization records of students with new piercings or tattoos to check for receipt of a tetanus booster and offer anticipatory guidance.

Diphtheria and Tetanus Toxoids and Acellular Pertussis (DTaP) Vaccine

DTaP is almost always given as a combination vaccine. It is recommended at 2, 4, and 6 months, with boosters between 15 and 18 months and again between 4 and 6 years. That means children should have five doses before entering first grade. The fifth dose is not necessary if the fourth dose was given after the fourth birthday (Hall et al., 2021). Tdap, which contains the same ingredients as DTaP but with a lesser dose of diphtheria and pertussis, was developed in 2005 as a booster dose for people who have completed the DTaP when they are 10 years or older. Side effects of the DTaP vaccine include pain and redness at the injection site. Fever was reported in less than 5% of children (Hall et al., 2021). Contraindications to the DTaP vaccine include severe allergic reaction to a vaccine component or following a prior dose or encephalopathy, not related to another cause, within 7 days after a prior dose.

Measles, Mumps, and Rubella

Measles

Measles (rubeola), a respiratory tract virus, is one of the most contagious of the vaccine-preventable diseases, with an incubation period of 11 to 12 days. It starts with a high fever, a rasping cough, conjunctivitis, coryza, and Koplik spots on the buccal mucosa, described as blue-white spots on a bright red background. The rash presents as a red maculopapular rash that begins at the hairline and then involves the face as it moves cephalocaudally. The rash lasts for 5 to 6 days. There is a high risk for consequences of this infection, including bacterial super-infections, causing diarrhea; pneumonia; otitis media; encephalitis, often with permanent brain damage and intellectual disability; seizures; and death. The virus can be transmitted to others 4 days before to 4 days after the rash occurs (Hall et al., 2021). The incidence of measles has declined precipitously since developing a vaccine and initiating a second MMR dose. However, outbreaks continue to be reported, most notably in underimmunized communities. In 2023, there were only 53 cases of measles, but as of May 2024, there have been 10 outbreaks resulting in 142 cases (National Center for Immunization and Respiratory Disease, 2024a).

Mumps

Mumps (parotitis) is caused by a virus that infects the respiratory tract and usually causes swelling of the parotid glands, unilaterally or bilaterally. The incubation period is 16 to 18 days. Mumps is often asymptomatic or initial complaints are nonspecific and may include pain, fatigue, headache, and low-grade fever. Typically, there will be swelling of the parotid glad (parotitis) that lasts for 5 days. The possible consequences of this infection include aseptic meningitis, orchitis in older men, and deafness (Hall et al., 2021).

Since the development of the vaccine and the introduction of a second dose in 1989, the number of cases was less than a thousand a year until 2006. In 2006, there were over 6,500 cases of mumps. In subsequent years, the number of mumps cases ranged from 229 to 6,366 cases per year (National Center for Immunization and Respiratory Disease, 2024b). With the onset of the pandemic, the cases of mumps have dropped to below 450 per year. Most of these cases occurred in vaccinated populations who were in close contact settings (Hall et al., 2021).

Rubella

Rubella is a virus spread by respiratory droplets. It is often called *German measles* to differentiate it from the rubeola virus. The incubation period is 14 days. In young children, it usually starts with a pink maculopapular rash, spreading in a cephalocaudal pattern. Older children and adolescents may start with low-grade fever, lymphadenopathy, and upper respiratory symptoms. However, up to 50% of infected cases are subclinical and asymptomatic (Hall et al., 2021). Individuals who contract this disease are not very ill or uncomfortable, but they are moderately contagious from 7 days before to 5 to 7 days after the rash appears. Serious but rare adverse effects include transient arthralgia and arthritis in adults, thrombocytopenic purpura, and encephalitis.

The greatest danger of contracting rubella is congenital rubella syndrome, which affects the fetus of a pregnant person (Hall et al., 2021). Congenital rubella syndrome, usually contracted during the first trimester, affects virtually all organ systems, and may lead to miscarriage, stillbirth, or birth defects.

Rubella was eliminated from the United States in 2004; however, it is present in other parts of the world. Since 2012, all rubella cases in the United States have occurred in people infected outside the United States (Hall et al., 2021).

Measles, Mumps, Rubella (MMR) Vaccine

Two doses of MMR are recommended at 12 to 15 months and then again between 4 and 6 years of age. However, the second dose can be given at any age, as long as it is at least 28 days after the first dose. Only doses administered after the first birthday count as part of the series (Hall et al., 2021). Contraindications to the MMR vaccine include severe allergic reaction to a vaccine component or following a prior dose, severe immunocompromise, systemic high-dose corticosteroid therapy for more than 14 days, a family history of congenital or heredity immunodeficiency, and pregnancy (Hall et al., 2021).

Parents have been known to voice concerns related to the MMR vaccine. One concern relates to children with an egg allergy since the measles and mumps vaccines are grown in an egg embryo medium. However, research shows that the MMR vaccine is safe for those with severe egg allergies (Gastanaduy et al., 2021). The live virus can also be given to those with mild immunosuppression. Another concern is that the vaccine exacerbates tuberculosis. This is untrue; however, as a live virus vaccine, MMR may temporarily suppress tuberculin reactivity and cause a tuberculin skin screening test to read negative when, in reality, it may be positive. Therefore, tuberculosis skin testing should be done during the same visit as the measles vaccine is given; otherwise, TB skin testing should be delayed at least 4 weeks (Hall et al., 2021).

Poliomyelitis

Polio is caused by an enterovirus that spreads via the fecal-oral route from person to person or is transmitted by indirect contact with contaminated saliva, feces, sewage, or water. The polio virus replicates in the gastrointestinal tract and then enters the blood and spreads to the central nervous system. While 95% of individuals infected with polio are asymptomatic, those who do become symptomatic get a stiff neck and muscle pains followed by nerve damage and asymmetrical flaccid paralysis. The incubation period is 3 to 6 days for nonparalytic polio and 7 to 21 days for paralytic polio.

Polio affected more than 21,000 people each year in the United States until the advent of immunization in the 1950s. A polio eradication program conducted by the Pan American Health Organization (PAHO) helped to eliminate wild polio from the Western Hemisphere by 1994 (Hall et al., 2021). In 2022, there was a case of paralytic polio in New York that was found to be vaccine-derived poliovirus type 2. Because of this case, PAHO reassessed the regional risk to be high and encouraged anyone unvaccinated to get vaccinated for polio as there is no cure for the sequelae associated with the virus (CDC, 2022a).

Polio Vaccine

The current polio vaccine is a trivalent enhanced potency inactivated Salk polio vaccine. It requires three doses during the first 18 months of life and then a booster between 4 and 6 years of age. The vaccine is effective at producing immunity with 99% immune after three doses (Hall et al., 2021). Contraindications to the polio vaccine include severe allergic reaction to a vaccine component or following a prior dose.

Varicella

Varicella (chickenpox) is caused by the varicella-zoster virus (VZV) and is transmitted by respiratory droplets. The incubation period is 14 to 16 days after exposure. VZV is a member of the herpes virus group and is highly contagious. Varicella is diagnosed by a vesicular, pruritic rash, with each clear-filled vesicle surrounded by a reddened area that begins on the trunk and progresses cephalocaudally and proximodistally. Ultimately, the lesions develop a scab. The lesions are 1 to 4 mm in diameter and can be found in all stages simultaneously (macular rash, vesicle, scab), with most on the trunk; children usually have 200 to 500 lesions (Hall et al., 2021). Lesions can also occur on the mucous membranes of the throat, eyes, and vagina. Complications associated with varicella include bacterial infection of the skin lesions, pneumonia, and Reye syndrome.

Since the introduction of the varicella vaccine, incidence as declined significantly; however, a student suspected of having varicella with papular or vesicular lesions should be excluded from school immediately. Breakthrough varicella is possible even in those vaccinated, although it is typically milder (CDC, 2022b). Refer to Online Material OM13-3 for a varicella break through factsheet with graphics detailing varicella. When all the lesions become crusted, the student is no longer contagious and may return to class, as the scabs are *not* infectious. Individuals infected are contagious from 1 to 2 days before the initial appearance of a rash to 4 to 5 days after (Hall et al., 2021); infected students whose rash appears during school hours have been contagious for at least 24 to 48 hours.

Varicella Vaccine

Varicella vaccine is a live attenuated vaccine. Like the MMR, varicella vaccine is not given until after the first birthday. Two doses at least 4 weeks apart are recommended for children. The second dose increases vaccine effectiveness from 82% to 92%. Varicella vaccine is 98% effective in preventing moderate to severe disease, defined as having fewer than 50 lesions, and 82% effective in preventing all forms of varicella (Hall et al., 2021). Contraindications to the varicella vaccine include severe allergic reaction to a vaccine component or following a prior dose, severe immunosuppression, and pregnancy.

Hepatitis

Hepatitis is an inflammation of the liver most often caused by a virus. Individuals can experience brief bouts of hepatitis or can have the condition in chronic forms. The chronic forms can lead to scarring of the liver, cirrhosis, or liver cancer. Hepatitis A, hepatitis B, and hepatitis C are the most common forms of hepatitis (CDC, 2023g).

An infected person may be asymptomatic. However, common symptoms of hepatitis in adults include jaundice, fatigue, nausea and vomiting, bleeding disorders, and dark urine. Many children with infectious hepatitis do not present overt symptoms, making diagnosis difficult.

Hepatitis A

Hepatitis A is spread through the fecal-oral route and can live in the environment for months. Following ingestion, the virus multiplies in the liver and is excreted in the bile and then through the stool (Hall et al., 2021). The incubation period is from 15 to 50 days. The period of infectivity peaks during the 2 weeks before symptoms appear and for about a week after jaundice develops. While most infected persons no longer excrete virus in the feces by the third week of illness, children may excrete longer. In most cases, children infected with hepatitis A are asymptomatic. Lack or inadequate hand hygiene before food preparation, after toileting, or after changing diapers can result in transmission. School nurses and school personnel who are in contact with very young children requiring toileting assistance or diapering should always reinforce proper hand hygiene to prevent fecal-borne illnesses, including hepatitis A (CDC, 2024l). In 2021, there were 5,728 cases of hepatitis A. The cases are related to food-borne outbreaks as well as exposure among people who use drugs and those experiencing homelessness (National Center for HIV, Viral Hepatitis, STD and TB Prevention, 2023a).

Hepatitis A Vaccine

Children between 12 and 23 months of age should receive two doses of the inactivated whole-virus hepatitis A vaccine 6 months apart. The vaccine is also recommended for older children living where they are at increased risk of infection (Hall et al., 2021). Contraindications to the hepatitis A vaccine include severe allergic reaction to a vaccine component or following a prior dose (Hall et al., 2021).

Hepatitis B

Hepatitis B virus (HBV) is much more serious than hepatitis A and can be found in all body secretions, including blood, saliva, semen, and vaginal secretions. The greatest risk of contracting HBV is through blood or serous fluids. Individuals may contract HBV through human bites, shared toothbrushes, tattooing and body piercing, sexual intercourse, intravenous drug use, acupuncture, and even exposure to cuts and scrapes during contact sports. HBV can remain infectious for a week on room temperature surfaces (Hall et al., 2021). The incubation period is 60 to 90 days with most infected children and up to 50% of infected adults being asymptomatic. Hepatitis B symptoms start with nausea, vomiting, anorexia, and other prodromal symptoms, as well as right upper quadrant abdominal pain. The urine becomes dark (due to the excess bilirubin being excreted through the kidneys) 1 to 2 days before the onset of jaundice. Jaundice lasts 1 to 3 weeks. Additional symptoms are light clay-colored stools, hepatomegaly and tenderness, and fatigue that can last for weeks (Hall et al., 2021). Infants and children who are infected are at high risk for developing chronic hepatitis B infection. People with the chronic infection are carriers of the virus and can infect others and experience complications including cirrhosis, hepatocellular carcinoma, fulminant hepatitis, and death (Hall et al., 2021). In 2021, the incidence of chronic hepatitis B was 5.9 per 100,000 cases with non-Hispanic Asian/Pacific Islander persons being infected at 14 times the rate among non-Hispanic white persons (National Center for HIV, Viral Hepatitis, STD and TB Prevention, 2023b).

Hepatitis B Vaccine

There are several formulations and combinations of recombinant vaccines for HBV, meaning that an antibody response is generated, but there is no risk of the vaccine causing infection. The ACIP recommends three doses given intramuscularly over a 6-month period (dose two 1 month after dose one, and dose three 5 months after dose two). A nonimmunized individual who is exposed to hepatitis B is eligible to receive hepatitis B immune globulin and the first of the three-shot series of hepatitis B immunization within 24 hours of exposure. Contraindications to the HBV vaccine include severe allergic reaction to a vaccine component or following a prior dose and a history of hypersensitivity to yeast (Hall et al., 2021).

Hepatitis C

Like hepatitis B, hepatitis C virus (HCV) is transmitted through exposure to infected blood or contaminated equipment during medical procedures. In rare cases, HCV can be transmitted through sexual contact or perinatally (CDC, 2023a). Individuals infected with HCV are generally asymptomatic. However, left untreated, HCV often leads to cirrhosis and cancer. HCV infection is the leading cause of liver-related death and the primary reason for liver transplant in the United States. About 30% of HCV infections resolve on their own; 95% of the remaining cases can be cured with antiviral medications. HCV is extremely rare in children, but the incidence of cases begins to increase between ages 15 and 19 (CDC, 2023a). School nurses who work in high schools or with any age group that might be using intravenous drugs should counsel students on the risks of contracting HCV. Currently there is no vaccine for hepatitis C.

Pneumococcal Disease

Pneumococcal disease is a major cause of pneumonia, bacteremia, and meningitis in children and adults (Hall et al., 2021). *Streptococcus pneumoniae,* also known as pneumococcus, is an encapsulated, gram-positive polysaccharide with 90 different serotypes. In the United States, seven of the serotypes account for 80% of invasive disease in children younger than 5 years and 50% in older children and adults. *S. pneumoniae* is carried in the nose and throat of healthy people and spread from person to person by respiratory droplet; 20% to 60% of school-age children are carriers of the bacteria. The incubation period is 1 to 3 days, and symptoms appear abruptly. The very young, the elderly, and those with chronic conditions are most at risk for infection and its sequelae (Hall et al., 2021). Before the routine use of pneumococcal conjugate vaccine (PCV) for children, there were an estimated 17,000 cases of invasive disease each year. The vaccine has been very effective at preventing invasive disease caused by the 13 serotypes covered by the vaccine (CDC, 2024t).

Pneumococcal Vaccine

The ACIP recommends four doses of PCV13 for all children 24 to 59 months of age (CDC, 2024m). This vaccine protects against 13 serotypes of the bacteria. For children older than 5 years who are considered high risk, the 23-valent polysaccharide vaccine can be administered. Although it is an effective vaccine, multiple strains of *S. pneumoniae* are not covered by the vaccine; therefore, the vaccine does not eradicate pneumococcal disease. Contraindications to the pneumococcal vaccine include severe allergic reaction to a vaccine component or following a prior dose.

Meningococcal Disease

Meningococcal disease is an acute illness caused by 5 serotypes (A, B, C, W, and Y) of the bacteria *Neisseria meningitidis. N. meningitidis* is spread through respiratory droplets; however, transmission is rarely through casual contact but can occur in households or among persons living in close proximity, such as dormitories. The incubation period is 2 to 10 days, and the infected person remains contagious for at least 24 hours after starting antibiotics. Symptoms of meningococcal meningitis include a severe headache, stiff neck, fever, nausea, and vomiting. Sensitivity to light and sleepiness may also be present. In rare cases, symptoms progress to confusion, seizures, altered consciousness, coma, and, in 10% to 15% of cases, death. Even among survivors, as many as 20% experience negative outcomes, such as hearing loss, neurological damage, scarring, or limb loss (Hall et al., 2021). For persons in direct contact with an infected student or staff member, antibiotics can be administered to prevent transmission. Case fatality rates of invasive meningococcal disease are 9% to 12%, even with appropriate antibiotic therapy (Hall et al., 2021).

Rates of meningococcal disease have been dropping in the United States; in 2023 there were 422 cases reported with cases mainly caused by serogroup Y, which is prevented by the vaccine (CDC, 2024p). Although the greatest incidence is in infants, the disease declines in early childhood and increases again during adolescence and early adulthood. College students living in a dormitory are at higher risk due to the communal living setting; thus vaccination during high school is very important and should be reinforced by the school nurse.

Meningococcal Vaccine

ACIP recommends the four-strain meningococcal conjugate vaccine (Men ACWY) to all children 11 to 12 years of age, with a booster at age 16; if not previously vaccinated, one dose is given between ages 13 and 15, and a booster dose is given between ages 16 and 18 (CDC, 2024m). An additional vaccine was developed to cover serogroup B and is recommended for 16- to 18-year-olds who take certain immunosuppressive drugs or who have spleens that are damaged or that have been removed (Hall et al., 2021). Contraindications to the meningococcal vaccine include severe allergic reaction to a vaccine component or following a prior dose.

Human Papillomavirus

Human papillomavirus (HPV) is the most common sexually transmitted infection in the United States. HPV accounts for 37,300 cases of cancer each year (CDC, 2021a). HPV is associated with cervical cancer in women and anogenital cancers in both sexes, including cancers of the vulva, vagina, penis, and anus. HPV infection typically occurs soon after onset of sexual activity; 40% are infected 24 months after their first sexual intercourse (Hall et al., 2021). Therefore it is important to vaccinate young men and women before their first sexual encounter.

There are 200 different serotypes of HPV. Forty are associated with cervical cancer, with type 16 causing 50% of the cases and type 18 causing another 16% (Hall et al., 2021). Types 6 and 11 cause less serious health problems, such as warts. Not everyone infected with the virus develops cancer; most who are infected are asymptomatic. If the infection is not resolved, the risk for cancer increases within a few years. The most common symptom is anogenital warts. Because there is no specific treatment for an HPV infection, prevention with vaccination, before sexual onset, is imperative.

Human Papillomavirus Vaccine

The ACIP recommends HPV vaccination for all adolescents at 11 or 12 years of age, though vaccination can start as young as age 9. Depending on the age at which the vaccine is given, the child or adolescent will need a series of two or three vaccinations administered at least 6 months apart. Catch-up vaccination is also recommended for youth ages 13 through 26 years (CDC, 2024m). *Gardasil-9* is the HPV vaccine distributed in the United States and it contains 6, 11, 16, 18, and five additional serotypes. It is important to note that this vaccine is effective only at preventing cancer caused by these serotypes; it does not protect against all of the serotypes that cause infection. Therefore, education regarding barrier methods is important before the child becomes sexually active. HPV vaccine has been associated with syncope among adolescents. To avoid injury, it is recommended that adolescents be seated during all vaccine doses and observed for 15 to 20 minutes after vaccination (CDC, 2022e). Contraindications to the HPV vaccine include severe allergic reaction to a vaccine component or following a prior dose.

Influenza

Influenza is generally considered a moderate to severe illness of inconvenience due to the lost school or work time while ill and convalescing; some outbreaks result in higher levels of morbidity and mortality from influenza. Human influenza is generally either type A or type B. Type A is usually more severe and can infect humans in any age group as well as other animals. Type B is usually a milder disease and is most often the cause of influenza in children (Hall et al., 2021).

Influenza A has 18 subtypes defined by their surface antigens: H for hemagglutinin and N for neuraminidase (Hall et al., 2021). Hemagglutinin helps the virus attach to and enter the cell; neuraminidase helps the new virus exit the cell to affect other cells. Therefore, all type A influenza viruses have markers for one type of H and one type of N. However, even within these categories, there are multiple variations. In general, the antigenic markers on influenza exhibit a gradual change referred to as antigenic *drift.* Although the general population develops some immunity because of exposure or past influenza vaccines, a new vaccine is required each year to address the mutations caused by antigenic drift. Every 10 to 40 years a second type of influenza change occurs called *antigenic shift.* When an antigenic *shift* occurs the influenza viruses mutate quickly and are so different from previous years that the general population, especially those younger than 20, are infected. An example is the 2009 H1N1 pandemic that caused 12,500 deaths in the United States, with 90% of deaths in persons younger than 65 years; those over 65 had developed immunity because of prior exposure to variants of H1N1. This finding was in contrast with typical influenza season when 90% of deaths occur among those over 65 (Hall et al., 2021).

Influenza is spread by respiratory droplets with a short incubation period of 1 to 4 days. Children can be infectious for up to 10 days (Hall et al., 2021). Symptoms may include fever, achiness, headache, nonproductive cough, sore throat, rhinitis, otitis media, nausea, and vomiting; fever typically lasts 3 to 4 days but can last up to a week. Aspirin should *not* be administered to children with flu symptoms because it is correlated with Reye syndrome (Hall et al., 2021). Complications of influenza include pneumonia and secondary bacterial infection.

Because coughing, sneezing, and touching infected objects are the primary ways the virus is spread, empirical data support that frequent hand hygiene and cough/sneeze etiquette decrease transmission (CDC, 2024n). The CDC Web site contains educational resources and tools for flu prevention, specifically in schools. Cleaning and disinfecting of the school facility should also be undertaken to slow the spread of flu (CDC, 2024x). In the event of a major outbreak, the local public health department will provide guidance with such issues as communicating with parents, school staff, and the wider community and offering school-based immunization clinics.

Directions to parents of children with influenza-like illness typically include the following (CDC, 2024n):

- Stay home from school until 24 hours after the fever returns to normal without the use of antipyretics.
- Encourage plenty of fluids.
- Give acetaminophen or ibuprofen if needed; do not give aspirin.
- Wash your hands; cover your nose and mouth with a tissue or use the forearm when you sneeze or cough; do not share food or drink; and rest.
- Call the primary care provider if symptoms get worse, appear to disappear and then reappear, or if there is any trouble breathing.

Influenza Vaccine

Each year, the CDC projects which types of influenza A and B viruses are likely to circulate throughout the United States during the next flu season. Pharmaceutical companies then manufacture a vaccine that contains two strains of type A and one of type B influenza.

The current recommendation to prevent seasonal influenza is annual vaccination for all persons 6 months of age and older (CDC, 2024m). Children younger than 8 years who receive injected flu vaccine for the first time will need a second dose 28 days after the first (CDC, 2024m). After that, only one dose per year is needed.

Flu vaccines can be trivalent (protects against three different flu viruses) and quadrivalent (protects against four different flu viruses). In addition, there is a high-dose (adjuvanted) flu vaccine that contains four times the amount of antigen than a regular flu vaccine to create a stronger immune response; this vaccine is for use by those 65 years and older. There are two egg-free flu vaccines available, a cell-based vaccine and a recombinant vaccine. The trivalent inactivated and quadrivalent influenza vaccines are administered intramuscularly. Live attenuated influenza vaccine is a nasal spray approved for those ages 2 to 49 years who are in good health. Overall, the vaccine is 40% to 60% effective, depending on how accurate the projections were regarding which type of influenza might be prevalent. Contraindications to the inactivated influenza vaccine include severe allergic reaction to a vaccine component or following a prior dose. Contraindications for the live attenuated vaccine include severe allergic reaction to a vaccine component or following a prior dose, severe immunocompromise, concurrent aspirin or salicylate-containing therapy, and children ages 2 to 4 years with a diagnosis of asthma or asthma-like symptoms in the previous year.

Coronavirus

The SARS-COV-2 (COVID-19) pandemic that started in 2020 disrupted life as most knew it. Many schools ceased in-person learning for a period as they assessed and prepared for safely educating their students during a pandemic. School nurses were essential champions for health and safety during this time. COVID-19, a highly contagious coronavirus, spreads through respiratory droplets; thus precautions for coronavirus are similar to those used to prevent influenza. Schools should ensure proper cleaning procedure and good ventilation in the school building, encourage coronavirus vaccination, encourage students and staff to stay home when sick, and promote hand hygiene and respiratory etiquette. Masking with a well-filling mask, although not recommended universally, should be done by anyone with COVID-19–like symptoms or exposure to someone who is positive for COVID-19. As guidance for coronavirus continues to evolve it is important for school nurses to stay up to date with current guidance from the Centers for Disease Control and Prevention (CDC, 2023c).

As of May 2024, there had been almost 112 million cases of COVID-19 reported in the United States with almost 1.2 million deaths (CDC, 2024f). Disparities are seen in those most seriously affected by COVID-19 with higher rates of death seen among people who are black or Hispanic compared with those who are white.

Coronavirus Vaccine

The ACIP recommends vaccination for all people over the age of 6 months (CDC, 2024o). There are four vaccines approved for use by the Food and Drug Administration; two are mRNA vaccines (Pfizer BioNTech and Moderna), one is a protein subunit vaccine (Novavax), and one is an adenovirus vector vaccine (Janssen). The Janssen vaccine is not recommended for people under 18 years old. These vaccines were developed and implemented during a global pandemic and thus are not on the ACIP 2022 Child and Adolescent Immunization Schedule; however, they are recommended by ACIP with the information included in the Interim COVID-19 Immunization Schedule for Persons 6 Months of Age and Older (CDC, 2024o). Dosing includes two vaccines with boosters recommended at least 8 weeks following the second dose. Contraindications to the COVID-19

Practice Connection

NASN has developed COVID-19 reference materials that are designed to support school nurses as they navigate the ongoing COVID-19 pandemic. These resources, found on the NASN webpage, include information across a variety of topics and relate to broader communicable disease prevention activities (NASN, n.d.).

vaccine include severe allergic reaction to a vaccine component or following a prior dose.

SUN EXPOSURE

Ultraviolet (UV) radiation from sun exposure has been linked to skin cancer. Although a small amount of sun exposure is necessary for vitamin D production in the body, students should exercise caution to avoid unnecessary sun exposure. Sun safety measures can be implemented to limit outdoor activities when the sun's UV waves are most harmful. The American Academy of Dermatology (AAD; 2023) and the American Medical Association (AMA; 2016) support allowing students to bring and carry sunscreen in school without a healthcare provider order. The AAD notes sunscreen is safe, and there are no harmful effects of its use. Para-aminobenzoic acid (PABA) has been banned from sunscreen in the United States since 2019 due to the potential for allergic reactions and damage to marine life (Guan et al., 2021). Parents/guardians should be encouraged to apply sunscreen before sending their student to school. An analysis of sun safety practices in schools showed 47% of schools allowed time for students to apply sunscreen, but only 13% of schools supplied sunscreen (Jones & Guy, 2017). Despite the link between sun exposure and skin cancer, sunscreen use among youth in grades 6 to 12 remains low, averaging from never to sometimes (Rajagopal et al., 2021). School policies can also encourage students to wear protective clothing (long-sleeve shirts, lightweight pants, hats, visors, and sunglasses) when in the sun. Posters, social media posts, and educational programs on sun safety for students and youth should be promoted. See Chapter 18 for more information on sun exposure.

CONCLUSION

The COVID-19 pandemic revealed how unprepared many schools were to manage a health crisis. Conversations about cleaning procedures and indoor air quality became front of mind for school administrators as they sought to safely provide in-person education during a pandemic. The school nurse played a key role in managing student health during this pandemic and highlighted the school nurse's expertise in case surveillance, vaccination advocacy, and education.

School wellness policies are some of the best weapons against the transmission of infectious diseases and help to prepare for unexpected communicable disease outbreaks. School nurses can support hygienic school environments through participation in policy development; implementation of standard precautions; education of students, staff, and families; and advocacy for facilities that are appropriately built, cleaned, and disinfected. School nurses ensure compliance with state immunization requirements by listening closely and providing accurate information in a sensitive manner to reluctant parents and assisting families who need support to obtain immunizations for their children. School nurses collaborate quickly and appropriately with parents, healthcare providers, school administrators, and departments of health to reduce disease transmission and risk. As public health champions, school nurses serve as leaders and champions in the campaign for disease prevention to promote the highest level of wellness for students and the school community.

The Editors gratefully acknowledge the work of the previous chapter authors, Lynda Boyer-Chu and Catherine F. Yonkaitis.

References

Advisory Committee on Immunization Practices. (2023). *Altered immunocompetence.* https://www.cdc.gov/vaccines/hcp/acip-recs/general-recs/immunocompetence.html

Agency for Toxic Substances and Disease Registry. (2018). *Mercury in your school.* https://www.atsdr.cdc.gov/dontmesswithmercury/mercury_school.html

American Academy of Allergy, Asthma, and Immunology. (2019). *Reported anaphylaxis in the United States after vaccination, 1990–2016.* https://www.aaaai.org/Tools-for-the-Public/Latest-Research-Summaries/The-Journal-of-Allergy-and-Clinical-Immunology/2019/vaccination

American Academy of Dermatology. (2023). *Position statement on access to sunscreen and sun protective clothing in schools and summer camps.* https://www.aad.org/forms/policies/uploads/ps/ps-access%20to%20sunscreen_sun%20protective%20clothing.pdf

American Academy of Pediatrics. (n.d.). *Immigrant Health Toolkit.* https://downloads.aap.org/AAP/PDF/cocp_toolkit_full.pdf?_ga=2.202278993.1946412567.1673539932-46040723.1672660405

American Lung Association. (2022). *Epidemic, pandemic and endemic what's the difference?* https://www.lung.org/blog/epidemic-pandemic-endemic-covid

American Medical Association. (2016). *Permitting sunscreen in schools [H-440.841].* https://policysearch.ama-assn.org/policyfinder/detail/sunscreen?uri=%2FAMADoc%2FHOD.xml-0-3857.xml

American Speech-Language-Hearing Association. (n.d.). *Classroom acoustics.* https://www.asha.org/public/hearing/classroom-acoustics/

Americans With Disabilities Act National Network. (2024). *Taking a service animal to school.* https://adata.org/service-animal-resource-hub/school.

Aronson, S. S., & Shope, T. R. (Eds.). (2020). *Managing infectious diseases in child care and schools: A quick reference guide.* American Academy of Pediatrics.

Bader, M., & McKinsey, D. (2013). Post-exposure prophylaxis for common infectious diseases. *American Family Physician, 88*(1), 25–32.

Barraza, L., Schmit, C., & Hoss, A. (2017). The latest in vaccine policies: Selected issues in school vaccinations, healthcare worker vaccinations, and pharmacist vaccination authority laws. *Journal of Law, Medicine, and Ethics, 45*(S1), 16–19. https://doi:10.1177/1073110517703307

Brennan, J., & Nguyen, V. (2014). *Service animals and emotional support animals.* https://adata.org/publication/service-animals-booklet

Centers for Disease Control and Prevention. (2019). *About immunization information systems.* https://www.cdc.gov/vaccines/programs/iis/about.html

Centers for Disease Control and Prevention. (2020). *Vaccine safety: Thimerosal and vaccines.* https://www.cdc.gov/vaccinesafety/concerns/thimerosal/index.html

Centers for Disease Control and Prevention. (2021a). *Human papillomavirus (HPV).* https://www.cdc.gov/hpv/

Centers for Disease Control and Prevention. (2021b). *Immunizations: The basics.* https://www.cdc.gov/vaccines/vac-gen/imz-basics.htm

Centers for Disease Control and Prevention. (2021c). Provider resources for vaccine conversations with parents. https://www.cdc.gov/vaccines/hcp/conversations/conv-materials.html

Centers for Disease Control and Prevention. (2022a). *CDC news room: United States confirmed as country with circulating vaccine-derived poliovirus.* https://www.cdc.gov/media/releases/2022/s0913-polio.html

Centers for Disease Control and Prevention. (2022b). *Chickenpox (varicella): For healthcare professionals.* https://www.cdc.gov/chickenpox/hcp/

Centers for Disease Control and Prevention. (2022c). *Healthy schools: School health index.* https://www.cdc.gov/healthyschools/shi/index.htm

Centers for Disease Control and Prevention. (2022d). *State school immunization requirements and vaccine exemption laws.* https://www.cdc.gov/phlp/docs/school-vaccinations.pdf

Centers for Disease Control and Prevention. (2022e). *Vaccine recommendations and guidelines of the ACIP preventing and managing adverse reactions.* https://www.cdc.gov/vaccines/hcp/acip-recs/general-recs/adverse-reactions.html

Centers for Disease Control and Prevention. (2022f). *Vaccine safety: Adjuvants and vaccines.* https://www.cdc.gov/vaccinesafety/concerns/adjuvants.html

Centers for Disease Control and Prevention. (2023a). *Hepatitis C.* https://www.cdc.gov/hepatitis-c/about/index.html

Centers for Disease Control and Prevention. (2023b). *National outbreak reporting system (NORS).* https://www.cdc.gov/nors/about.html

Centers for Disease Control and Prevention. (2023c). *Operational guidance for K-12 schools and early care and education programs to support safe in-person learning.* https://www.cdc.gov/coronavirus/2019-ncov/community/schools-childcare/k-12-childcare-guidance.html

Centers for Disease Control and Prevention. (2023d). *Traveler's health: Travel vaccines.* https://wwwnc.cdc.gov/travel/page/travel-vaccines

Centers for Disease Control and Prevention. (2023e). *Vaccine Information Statements (VISs): Instructions for using VISs.* https://www.cdc.gov/vaccines/hcp/vis/about/required-use-instructions.html

Centers for Disease Control and Prevention. (2023f). *Vaccine recommendations and guidelines of the ACIP: Contraindications and precautions.* https://www.cdc.gov/vaccines/hcp/acip-recs/general-recs/contraindications.html

Centers for Disease Control and Prevention. (2023g). *What is viral Hepatitis?* https://www.cdc.gov/hepatitis/abc/index.htm

Centers for Disease Control and Prevention. (2024a). *Childhood lead poisoning prevention.* https://www.cdc.gov/lead-prevention/about/?CDC_AAref_Val=https://www.cdc.gov/nceh/lead/default.htm

Centers for Disease Control and Prevention. (2024b). *Clean hands: About handwashing as a healthy habit in the kitchen.* https://www.cdc.gov/clean-hands/prevention/about-handwashing-a-healthy-habit-in-the-kitchen.html?CDC_AAref_Val=https://www.cdc.gov/handwashing/handwashing-kitchen.html

Centers for Disease Control and Prevention. (2024c). *Clean hands: Hand hygiene in school and early care and education.* https://www.cdc.gov/clean-hands/prevention/about-hand-hygiene-in-schools-and-early-care-and-education-settings.html?CDC_AAref_Val=https://www.cdc.gov/handwashing/handwashing-school.html

Centers for Disease Control and Prevention. (2024d). *Clean hands: Hand sanitizer guidelines and recommendations.* https://www.cdc.gov/clean-hands/about/hand-sanitizer.html?CDC_AAref_Val=https://www.cdc.gov/handwashing/hand-sanitizer-use.html

Centers for Disease Control and Prevention. (2024e). *Clean hands: Handwashing facts.* https://www.cdc.gov/clean-hands/data-research/facts-stats/index.html

Centers for Disease Control and Prevention. (2024f, May 20). *COVID data tracker.* https://covid.cdc.gov/covid-data-tracker/#datatracker-home

Centers for Disease Control and Prevention. (2024g). *Diphtheria.* https://www.cdc.gov/diphtheria/about/index.html

Centers for Disease Control and Prevention. (2024h). *Flint water crisis.* https://www.cdc.gov/nceh/casper/pdf-html/flint_water_crisis_pdf.html

Centers for Disease Control and Prevention. (2024i). *Healthcare providers/professionals: Vaccine storage and handling toolkit.* https://www.cdc.gov/vaccines/hcp/admin/storage/toolkit/index.html

Centers for Disease Control and Prevention. (2024j). *Healthy pets, healthy people: Resources for schools and daycare.* https://www.cdc.gov/healthy-pets/schools-daycares/?CDC_AAref_Val=https://www.cdc.gov/healthypets/specific-groups/schools.html

Centers for Disease Control and Prevention. (2024k). *Hearing loss in children: About.* https://www.cdc.gov/hearing-loss-children/about/?CDC_AAref_Val=https://www.cdc.gov/ncbddd/hearingloss/facts.html

Centers for Disease Control and Prevention. (2024l). *Hepatitis A basics.* https://www.cdc.gov/hepatitis-a/about/index.html

Centers for Disease Control and Prevention. (2024m). *Immunization schedules: For healthcare providers.* https://www.cdc.gov/vaccines/schedules/hcp/index.html

Centers for Disease Control and Prevention. (2024n). *Influenza (flu): Key facts about influenza (flu).* https://www.cdc.gov/flu/about/keyfacts.htm

Centers for Disease Control and Prevention. (2024o). *Interim COVID-19 immunization schedule for persons 6 months of age and older.* https://www.cdc.gov/vaccines/covid-19/downloads/COVID-19-immunization-schedule-ages-6months-older.pdf

Centers for Disease Control and Prevention. (2024p). Meningococcal disease: Cases are increasing in the United States. *National Center for Immunization and Respiratory Distress.* https://www.cdc.gov/ncird/whats-new/meningococcal-disease-cases-increasing-us.html

Centers for Disease Control and Prevention. (2024r). *National Notifiable Diseases Surveillance System (NNDSS).* https://www.cdc.gov/nndss/

Centers for Disease Control and Prevention. (2024s). *Pertussis.* https://www.cdc.gov/pertussis/about/index.html

Centers for Disease Control and Prevention. (2024t). *Pneumococcal disease: surveillance and reporting.* https://www.cdc.gov/pneumococcal/php/surveillance/?CDC_AAref_Val=https://www.cdc.gov/pneumococcal/surveillance.html

Centers for Disease Control and Prevention. (2024u). *Standard precautions for all patient care.* https://www.cdc.gov/infection-control/hcp/basics/standard-precautions.html?CDC_AAref_Val=https://www.cdc.gov/infectioncontrol/basics/standard-precautions.html

Centers for Disease Control and Prevention. (2024v). *Tetanus: Tetanus surveillance and trends.* https://www.cdc.gov/tetanus/php/surveillance/index.html

Centers for Disease Control and Prevention. (2024w). *Water, sanitation, and environmentally related hygiene (WASH): Cleaning and disinfecting with bleach.* https://www.cdc.gov/hygiene/about/cleaning-and-disinfecting-with-bleach.html?CDC_AAref_Val=https://www.cdc.gov/hygiene/cleaning/disinfecting-bleach.html

Centers for Disease Control and Prevention. (2024x). *When and how to clean and disinfect a facility.* Water, sanitation, and environmentally related hygiene (WASH). https://www.cdc.gov/hygiene/about/when-and-how-to-clean-and-disinfect-a-facility.html?CDC_AAref_Val=https://www.cdc.gov/hygiene/cleaning/facility.html

Congressional Research Service. (2021). *OSHA jurisdiction over public schools and other state and local government entities: COVID-19 issues.* https://crsreports.congress.gov/product/pdf/IF/IF11619

DeSilva, M. B., Haapala, J., Vazquez-Benitez, G., Daley, M. F., Nordin, J. D., Klein, N. P., Henninger, M. L., Williams, J. T. B., Hambidge, S. J., Jackson, M. L., Donahue, J. G., Qian, L., Lindley, M. C., Gee, J., Weintraub, E. S., & Kharbanda, E. O. (2022). Association of the COVID-19 pandemic with routine childhood vaccination rates and proportion up to date with vaccinations across 8 US health systems in the vaccine safety datalink. *Archives of Pediatrics and Adolescent Medicine*, 176(1), 68–77. https://doi.org/10.1001/jamapediatrics.2021.4251

Environmental Law Institute. (2022, March). *Database of state indoor air quality laws*. https://www.eli.org/sites/default/files/files-pdf/Final%20 2022%20Schools_2.pdf

Filardo, M. (2021). *State of our schools: America's PK–12 public school facilities 2021*. 21st Century School Fund. https://resources.wellcertified.com/tools/2021-state-of-our-schools-report/

Gastanaduy, P., Haver, P., Rota, P.A. & Pate, M. (2021). Epidemiology and prevention of vaccine-preventable diseases. Measles. In E. Hall, A.P. Wodi, J. Hamborsky, V.Morelli, & S. Schillie (Eds.), *Epidemiology and prevention of vaccine-preventable diseases* (14th ed.). Public Health Foundation.

Gennaro, E., Caleb, S., Torres, R., Alexander-Parrish, R., Thoburn, E., McLaughlin, J., & Fu, L. (2021). Parental beliefs, logistical challenges, and improvement opportunities for vaccination among children ages 19-35 months experiencing homelessness. *Journal of Pediatrics, 236*, 246–252. www.doi.org/ 10.1016/j.jpeds.2021.04.029

Guan, L., Lim, H., & Mohammad, T. (2021). Sunscreens and photoaging: A review of current literature. *American Journal of Clinical Dermatology, 22*, 819–828. https://doi.org/10.1007/s40257-021-00632-5

Hall, E., Wodi, A., Hamborsky, J., Morelli, V., & Schillie, S. (Eds.). (2021). *Epidemiology and prevention of vaccine-preventable diseases* (14th ed.). Public Health Foundation.

Health Resources and Services Administration. (2024). *National vaccine injury compensation program*. https://www.hrsa.gov/vaccine-compensation

Herbert, S., & Lynch, J. (2017). Classroom animals provide more than just science education. *Science and Education, 26*(1–2), 107–123. www.doi.org/10.1007/s11191-017-9874-6

Immunization Action Coalition. (2023a). *Leading medical organizations endorse strong school and childcare vaccination requirements and elimination of non-medical exemptions*. https://www.immunize.org/catg.d/p2071.pdf

Immunization Action Coalition. (2023b). *Screening checklist for contraindications to vaccines for children and teens*. https://www.immunize.org/catg.d/p4060.pdf

Immunization Action Coalition. (2024). *Clinic tools: Administering vaccines*. https://www.immunize.org/clinic/administering-vaccines.asp

Jones, S., & Guy, G. (2017). Sun safety practices among schools in the United States. *Journal of Medical Association Dermatology, 153*(5), 391–397. https://doi.org/10.1001/jamadermatol.2016.6274

Kempe, A., Saville, A. W., Albertin, C., Zimet, G., Breck, A., Helmkamp, L., Vangala, S., Dickinson, L. M., Rand, C., Humiston, S., & Szilagyi, P. G. (2020). Parental hesitancy about routine childhood and influenza vaccinations: A national survey. *Pediatrics, 146*(1), 1–12. https://doi.org/10.1542/peds.2019-3852

Maurer, M., Warren, K. E., & Pohl, C. (2016). The postcard initiative: Personal communication from students can increase timely compliance with health requirements. *NASN School Nurse, 31*(3), 147–149. https://doi.org/10.1177/1942602X15619757

McKinney-Vento Homeless Assistance Act of 1987. (Pub. L. No. 100-77, 101 Stat. 482, 42 U.S.C., Title 119, Subchapter 1, §11301). https://www.govtrack.us/congress/bills/100/hr558

National Association of School Nurses. (n.d.). *COVID-19 reference*. https://schoolnursenet.nasn.org/covid19ref/home

National Association of School Nurses. (2018). *Healthy communities—The role of the school nurse* (Position Statement). Author.

National Association of School Nurses. (2020). *Immunizations* (Position Statement). Author.

National Association of School Nurses. (2022a). *School-located vaccination* (Position Statement). Author.

National Association of School Nurses. (2022b). *School nursing: Scope and standards of practice* (4th ed.). Author.

National Association of School Nurses. (2024). A contemporary framework update for today's school nursing landscape: Introducing the School Nursing Practice Framework. *NASN School Nurse, 39*(3), 140–147. https://www.doi.org/10.1177/1942602X241241092

National Center for HIV, Viral Hepatitis, STD, and TB Prevention. (2023a). *Hepatitis A outbreaks in the United States*. Division of Viral Hepatitis. https://www.cdc.gov/hepatitis-a/outbreaks/ongoing/?CDC_AAref_Val=https://www.cdc.gov/hepatitis/outbreaks/hepatitisaoutbreaks.htm

National Center for HIV, Viral Hepatitis, STD, and TB Prevention. (2023b). *Hepatitis B surveillance in 2021*. Division of Viral Hepatitis. https://www.cdc.gov/hepatitis/statistics/2021surveillance/hepatitis-b.htm#:~:text=During%202021%2C%2047%20states%20reported, again%20by%2C14%25%20in%202021

National Center for Homeless Education. (2022). *National overview*. https://profiles.nche.seiservices.com/ConsolidatedStateProfile.aspx

National Center for Immunization and Respiratory Disease. (2023a). *2022 Provisional Pertussis Surveillance Report*. Division of Bacterial Diseases: Centers for Disease Control and Prevention. https://www.cdc.gov/pertussis/downloads/pertuss-surv-report-2022_provisional.pdf

National Center for Immunization and Respiratory Disease. (2023b). *Vaccine-specific requirements: State laws and requirements by vaccine*. Immunize.org. https://www.immunize.org/official-guidance/state-policies/requirements/

National Center for Immunization and Respiratory Disease. (2024a). *Measles cases and outbreaks*. Centers for Disease Control and Prevention. https://www.cdc.gov/measles/data-research/index.html

National Center for Immunization and Respiratory Disease. (2024b). *Mumps cases and outbreaks*. Centers for Disease Control and Prevention. https://www.cdc.gov/mumps/outbreaks.html.

National Education Association. (2018). *NEA's school crisis guide*. https://www.nea.org/sites/default/files/2020-National Resource Center for Health and Safety

National Institute on Deafness and Other Communication Disorders. (2016). It's a noisy planet: Protect their hearing. *U.S. Department of Health and Human Services*. https://www.noisyplanet.nidcd.nih.gov/

National Institute on Deafness and Other Communication Disorders. (2022). Noise-induced hearing loss. *U.S. Department of Health and Human Services*. https://www.nidcd.nih.gov/health/noise-induced-hearing-loss

National Resource Center for Health and Safety in Child Care and Early Education. (2022). *Caring for our children: Routine cleaning, sanitizing and disinfecting* (3.3.0.1). https://nrckids.org/CFOC/Database/3.3.0.1

Occupational Safety and Health Administration. (n.d.). Quick reference guide to the bloodborne pathogens standard. *U.S. Department of Labor*. https://www.osha.gov/bloodborne-pathogens/quick-reference

Occupational Safety and Health Administration. (2012a). Occupational Safety and Health Standard, No. 1910.1200: Hazard communication, *U.S. Department of Labor*. https://www.osha.gov/laws-regs/regulations/standardnumber/1910/1910.1200

Occupational Safety and Health Administration. (2012b). *OSHA brief: Hazard communication standard: Safety data sheets*. https://www.osha.gov/publications/osha3514.html

Occupational Safety and Health Administration. (2019). Occupational Safety and Health Standard, No. 1910.1030: Bloodborne pathogens. U.S. Department of Labor. https://www.osha.gov/laws-regs/regulations/standardnumber/1910/1910.1030#:~:text=Occupational%20Exposure%20means%20reasonably%20anticipated,performance%20of%20an%20employee's%20duties

Office of Disease Prevention and Health Promotion. (n.d.). Healthy People 2030. Environmental health. Reduce exposure to lead—EH-08. *U.S. Department of Health and Human Services*. https://health.gov/healthypeople/objectives-and-data/browse-objectives/environmental-health/reduce-exposure-lead-eh-08

Rajagopal, G., Talluri, R., Chuy, V., Chengm A., & Dali, L. (2021). Trends in sunscreen use among U.S. middle and high school students, 2007–2019. *Cureus, 13*(7), e16468. https://doi.org/10.7759/cureus.16468

Ruckart, P. Z., Jones, R. L., Courtney, J. G., LeBlanc, T., Jackson, W., Karwowski, M., Cheng, P., Allwood, P., Svendsen, E., & Breysse, P. (2021). Update of the blood lead reference value—United States, 2021. *Morbidity and Mortality Weekly Report, 70*(43), 1509–1512. http://dx.doi.org/10.15585/mmwr.mm7043a4external icon

Shetty, A. K. (2019). Infectious diseases among refugee children. *Children (Basel, Switzerland), 6*(12), 129. https://doi.org/10.3390/children6120129

U.S. Department of Health and Human Services. (2019). *Does the HIPAA privacy rule allow a health care provider to disclose protected health information (PHI) about a student to a school nurse or physician?* https://www.hhs.gov/hipaa/for-professionals/faq/517/does-hipaa-allow-a-health-care-provider-to-disclose-information-to-a-school-nurse/index.html

U.S. Environmental Protection Agency. (2009). *Indoor air quality for schools: Reference guide.* https://www.epa.gov/sites/default/files/2014-08/documents/reference_guide.pdf

U.S. Environmental Protection Agency. (2015). *Safer Choice standard.* https://nepis.epa.gov/Exe/ZyPURL.cgi?Dockey=P1013LWM.txt

U.S. Environmental Protection Agency. (2017). *Sensible steps to healthier school environments.* https://www.epa.gov/sites/default/files/2017-06/documents/sensible_steps_final_may2017_web.pdf

U.S. Environmental Protection Agency. (2018). *The indoor air quality tools for schools approach: Providing a framework for success.* https://www.epa.gov/sites/default/files/2018-08/documents/iaq_2018_management_framework_success_3page_508_final_2.6.18.pdf

U.S. Environmental Protection Agency. (2022). *Indoor air quality tools for schools action kit.* https://www.epa.gov/iaq-schools/indoor-air-quality-tools-schools-action-kit

U.S. Environmental Protection Agency. (2023a). *Healthy school environments: Executive summary of State School Environmental Health guidelines.* https://www.epa.gov/schools/executive-summary-state-school-environmental-health-guidelines

U.S. Environmental Protection Agency. (2023b). *Indoor air quality in schools: Why indoor air quality is important to schools.* https://www.epa.gov/iaq-schools/why-indoor-air-quality-important-schools

U.S. Environmental Protection Agency. (2024a). *Radon in schools.* https://www.epa.gov/radon/radon-schools

U.S. Environmental Protection Agency. (2024b). *Safer Choice: Safer products that meet the Safer Choice standard.* https://www.epa.gov/saferchoice/products

U.S. Environmental Protection Agency. (2024c). *School bus idle reduction.* https://www.epa.gov/dera/school-bus-idle-reduction

U.S. Food and Drug Administration. (2017). *Environmental contaminants in food: Questions and answers on lead-glazed traditional pottery.* https://www.fda.gov/food/environmental-contaminants-food/questions-and-answers-lead-glazed-traditional-pottery#:~:text=Lead%20may%20be%20present%20in,or%20served%20in%20the%20dishes

U.S. Food and Drug Administration. (2023). *Safely using hand sanitizer.* https://www.fda.gov/consumers/consumer-updates/safely-using-hand-sanitizer

Vaccine Adverse Event Reporting System. (n.d.). About VAERS. *Centers for Disease Control and Prevention, U.S. Food and Drug Administration, and U.S. Department of Health and Human Services.* https://vaers.hhs.gov/index.html

World Health Organization. (2009a). *How to handrub?* https://cdn.who.int/media/docs/default-source/integrated-health-services-(ihs)/infection-prevention-and-control/how-to-handrub-poster.pdf

World Health Organization. (2009b). *How to handwash?* https://www.who.int/docs/default-source/patient-safety/how-to-handwash-poster.pdf?sfvrsn=7004a09d_2

World Health Organization. (2021). *Health promotion glossary of terms 2021.* https://www.who.int/publications/i/item/9789240038349

Chapter 14

Prevention and Management of Childhood Obesity in Schools

Judy E. Harkins

CHAPTER OUTLINE

Overweight and obesity have been established as among the most challenging health concerns facing children today. Obesity is a complicated disease that places strains on students and their families and puts children at risk for long-term complications such as heart disease, diabetes, depression, anxiety, and certain cancers (Centers for Disease Control and Prevention [CDC], 2022a). An objective of *Healthy People 2030* is to reduce obesity in children to 15.5% (Office of Disease Prevention and Health Promotion, n.d.). Despite efforts from many governmental and private sectors, there has been a steady increase in childhood obesity rates; between 2016 and 2020, rates of obesity rose from 17.8% to 19.7% (U.S. Department of Health and Human Services [USDHHS], 2022). These historically high rates are especially concerning in school-age children within marginalized communities where populations tend to be more affected by the obesity epidemic and its consequences (Loren et al., 2022). Childhood obesity is not only a health concern—it is also expensive. Compared with children of healthy weight, medical costs for children with obesity are estimated to cost $166 more annually and almost twice that for children with severe obesity (CDC, 2024a).

School closures during the COVID-19 pandemic negatively impacted obesity among school-age children. School closures limited many families' access to healthy food options, and the shutdown of school-based physical activity and sports programs led to decreased activity levels in students. Yet food insecurity persists after the height of the pandemic; in February 2023, over 14% of families with children reported food insufficiency (Food Research and Action Center, 2023b; Hoffman & Miller, 2020).

School nurses are on the front lines of implementing primary, secondary, and tertiary level prevention strategies aimed at both individual students and communities. School nurses' frequent contact with and assessment of students at risk are key to the management of the obesity crisis. This chapter discusses the school nurse's role in the assessment, prevention, and management of students who are overweight and obese from the perspectives of students, families, and school communities.

> **Focus on the Framework**
>
> The National Association of School Nurses' (NASN's) *School Nursing Practice Framework* (NASN, 2024) includes the principle of **Community/Public Health.** School nurses can provide population-focused leadership on their school's Wellness Committee to address the epidemic of obesity. School nurses understand that implementing prevention programs must "address cultural sensitivity, social determinants of health, and education for health promotion and disease prevention" (p. 145).

DEFINITIONS

Definitions of overweight and obesity vary slightly, and criteria may differ depending on ethnicity and geographical region. The World Health Organization (WHO) states that "*overweight* is a condition of excessive fat deposits" (2024, para. 2) and "obesity is a chronic complex disease defined by excessive fat deposits that can impair health" (WHO, 2024, para. 3). The CDC states "weight that is higher than what is considered healthy for a given height is described as overweight or obesity" (CDC, 2022b, para. 3). The American Academy of Pediatrics (AAP) supports a change in language from *obese children* to *children with obesity* and *children with overweight* to align with person-first language (Hampl et al., 2023).

The current standard of defining overweight or obesity requires measurement of body mass index (BMI). BMI is calculated by dividing a person's weight in kilograms by square of height in meters (CDC, 2023a). Height and weight must be measured accurately. A child's BMI is expressed as a percentile because of the variations that occur in children's bodies by age and sex. Measurements are then plotted on an appropriate growth chart for age and sex (often referred to as BMI-for-age). The child's age is located on the horizontal axis of the chart, and BMI on the vertical access; the point of intersection provides the student's BMI-for-age. BMI can be calculated manually or through user-friendly calculators that are readily available online, such as the CDC's *Child and Teen BMI Calculator Widget* (CDC, 2023a). Among children of the same age and sex, a normal BMI ranges from above the 5th percentile to below the 85th percentile. At or above the 85th percentile is considered overweight, and at or above the 95th is considered obese (CDC, 2022c). BMI for children is differentiated into four categories: *underweight, normal weight, overweight,* and *obese* (Box 14-1).

The rates of children with obesity in the United States have risen significantly over the last several decades, from 5% in 1978 to 19.7% in 2020. Rates of obesity are rising the fastest among 2- to 5-year-olds. This highlights the need for prevention programs and early intervention with preschool and early school-age children (Anderson et al., 2019). Kindergarten students who are overweight are 4 times more likely to have obesity by 8th grade than students who are not overweight in kindergarten (CDC, 2022a). As children age, the rate of obesity increases with the highest rates seen in students between 13 and 19 years old (Table 14-1).

TABLE 14-1 Obesity Among Children and Adolescents by Age Group

Population	2013–2016	2017–2020
2–5 years	11.6%	12.6%
6–11 years	17.9%	20.9%
12–19 years	20.6%	22.1%

Adapted from National Center for Health Statistics (2023).

There are disparities in the prevalence of obesity across populations. Children of color are disproportionately affected by obesity, with the highest rates of obesity seen in Hispanic children (25.6%) and non-Hispanic black children (24.2%), followed by white children (16.1%) and Asian children (8.7%; CDC Healthy Schools, 2022a).

CAUSES

The causes of the overweight and obesity epidemic in children are recognized as being complex parts of a dynamic process, rooted in one's genetics and influenced by psychosocial, economic, and environmental factors. Some factors are considered modifiable, such as environment, portion size, and activity levels; other factors, including side effects of medications, genetics, and hormonal influences, are more difficult to overcome (Lin & Li, 2021).

Social Determinants of Health

Two major themes have been consistent with the examination of risk factors associated with pediatric obesity: lack of physical activity and poor-quality dietary intake. However, there are other influences that are strongly related to calories consumed and energy expelled, such as economics, community safety, school, and the child's built environment, all of which influence the ability to exercise and eat healthy foods. The impact of *social determinants of health,* where people live, learn, work, and play, have clear connections to rates of overweight and obesity and contribute to the disparities seen across populations (CDC, 2022a). See Chapter 2 for more information on social determinants of health.

BOX 14-1

CDC Body Mass Index Percentile Calculator for Child and Teen

Example of BMI calculation for a 5-year, 6-month-old boy

Height: 4 feet 2 inches
Weight = 55 pounds
BMI = 15.5

Based on the information entered, the body mass index (BMI) is 15.5. This child's BMI-for-age is at the 53rd percentile, which means that this child's BMI is greater than the BMIs of 53% of 5-year, 6-month-old boys in the reference population used to create CDC's growth charts. This child's BMI falls into the Healthy Weight category, defined as a BMI that is at or above the 5th to less than the 85th percentile for sex and age.

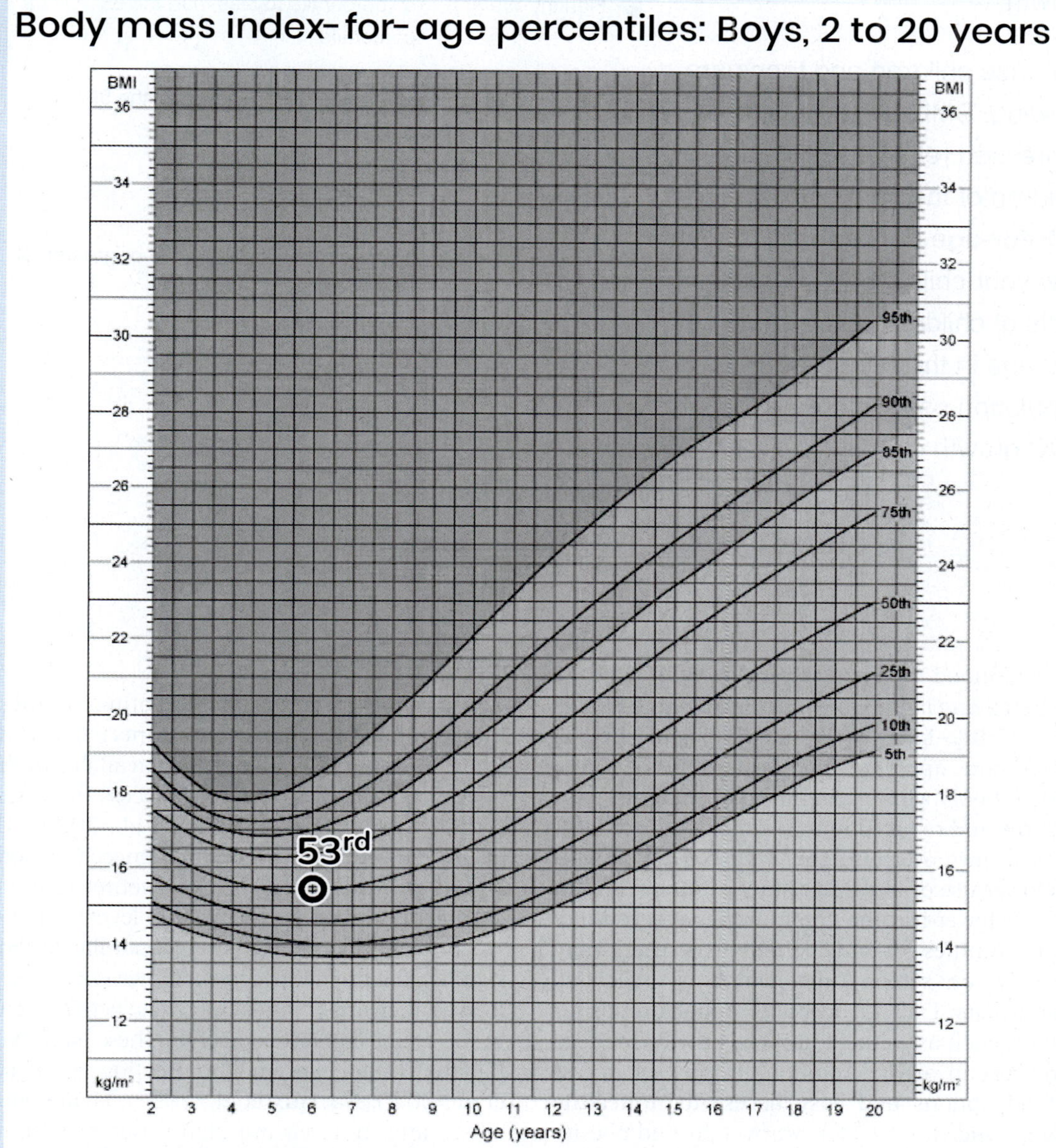

Body mass index for age percentile: boys 2 to 20 years.

Continued

BOX 14-1

CDC Body Mass Index Percentile Calculator for Child and Teen—cont'd

What does this mean?

BMI is a calculated measure of weight relative to height. BMI is used to assess a child's physical growth.

Because children and teens are growing, BMI values must be expressed relative to other children of the same sex and age. **BMI-for-age percentiles** indicate how your child's BMI compares to BMIs of children of the same sex and age in the reference population used to create the CDC growth charts.

BMI Category	BMI Range
Underweight	Less than the 5th percentile
▶ Healthy Weight	5th percentile to less than the 85th percentile
Overweight	85th percentile to less than the 95th percentile
Obesity	95th percentile or greater
Severe Obesity	120% of the 95th percentile or greater OR a BMI of 35 kg/m or greater

BMI: What does this mean?

CDC (2023a).

Rates of childhood obesity are inversely related to income; children living in low-income households have the highest rates (25.8%) followed by middle-income households (21.2%) and upper-income households (11.5%; CDC, 2024a). Schools where a higher percentage of students receive free and reduced lunch, an indicator of family income level, have overall higher BMI compared with schools with lower use of free and reduced lunch (Amram et al., 2019). In lower-income communities where there are fewer opportunities for outside activities, there may be more reliance on screen time, which is associated with exercise deficits. Lack of access to opportunities for physical activity, such as walkable streets, may be reduced in low-income urban areas. Additionally, lack of access to healthy food options and easy access to unhealthy fast foods compound the risks for overweight and obesity (Venturelli et al., 2019).

Conversely, conscientious neighborhood planning can reduce noise, increase safety, improve air quality, and enhance overall quality of life, leading to increased opportunities for activity. One example, *Play Streets*, involves systematic closing of streets in targeted neighborhoods, which leads to an increased sense of community and increased physical activity levels (Umstattd Meyer et al., 2019).

Family Patterns

The home environment and the eating routines and dietary intake of family members are connected to a child's health. The amount and quality of food available in the home will affect the foods a student has access to outside of school (Jansen et al., 2020; Naviaux et al., 2020). The presence or lack of family mealtimes influences the food consumed. Family physical activity levels, whether sedentary or physically active, influence the activity levels of the child.

Emotional factors and parent/guardian feeding styles hold significant influence over a child's weight. Consistently using food as a reward or punishment can activate reward systems in the brain; similar to addiction, these patterns can become habitual leading to emotional eating as an adult (Jansen et al., 2020; Naviaux et al., 2020). Living within a family where anxiety levels are high raises the risk of childhood obesity (Davodi & Ahadi, 2021). Food insecurity can further exacerbate stress levels while reducing the variety of food choices a family has (Lappan et al., 2019). Alternatively, living within a higher-income, higher-educated family lessens the risk of obesity significantly (Davodi & Ahadi, 2021).

Chronic adversity within the child's environment can have a negative effect on obesity rates and general nutrition. Students who experienced adverse childhood events (ACEs), live in low-income families, live in single parent/guardian households, and/or have dual working parents are at higher risk of becoming obese. Busy schedules frequently contribute to quick meal preparation, using calorie-dense foods, and unhealthy food choices overall (Lappan et al., 2019).

Parents/guardians also can positively influence their children through role modeling, such as limiting their own screen time, or by maintaining adequate sleep. Role modeling has also been correlated with increased physical activity levels for children. Parents/guardians can promote physical activity through family activities and behaviors, engagement within the community using outdoor spaces, and available play areas and through the promotion of organized sports. This is especially effective for students who live in two-parent households (Rhodes et al., 2020). Parents/guardians and children are more likely to develop healthy eating habits through shared conversations and decision making related to food choices. Additionally, hands-on learning activities for children, such as participating in the preparation of foods, can have a positive influence on future food choices. However, it is important to note that parental influence begins to wane at age 12, making changes later in adolescence more challenging (Perdew et al., 2021).

Dietary Patterns

The CDC provides guidance and statistics on dietary patterns in the United States; there has been a steady increase in calories consumed since 1970 with the largest increases occurring since 1990. Additional facts related to the dietary intake of children and youth include the following:

- Approximately 40% of total caloric intake for American children comes from high-energy, high-density calories from fats and added sugars (CDC Healthy Schools, 2022a).
- From 2009 to 2019, the percentage of adolescents who consume sugary beverages trended down. However, in 2019, 15.1% of teens consumed soda at least once per day; 10.6% consumed at least one sports drink per day (Merlo et al., 2020).
- On a given day, 36% of children and adolescents consumed fast food. The percentage of calories consumed from fast food increases during adolescence and differs by race and ethnicity of the groups surveyed (Fryer et al., 2020). Note that many races and ethnicities are not specifically identified in these data. See Figure 14-1.
- In the 2021 Youth Risk Behavior Survey (YRBS), 9.3% of high schoolers reported not eating a vegetable (excluding potatoes) over the previous 7 days, and 7.7% reported not eating a fruit or drinking 100% fruit juice over the previous 7 days (CDC, 2023b).

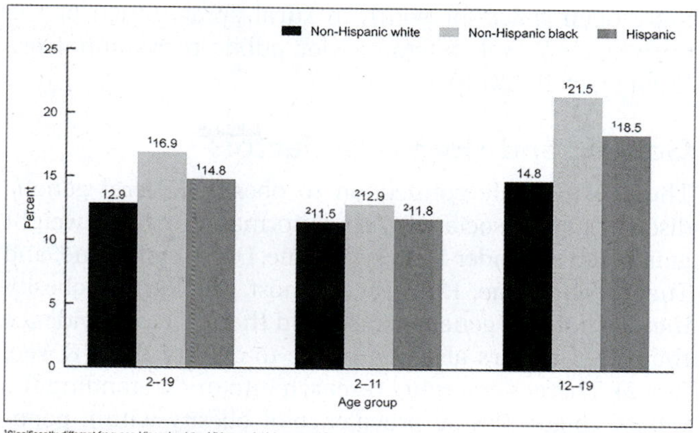

[1]Significantly different from non-Hispanic white children and adolescents of the same age group.
[2]Significantly different from those aged 12–19 years.
NOTE: Access data table for Figure 3 at: https://www.cdc.gov/nchs/data/databriefs/db375-tables-508.pdf#3.

FIGURE 14-1. **Mean percentage of calories from fast food on a given day among children and adolescents ages 2 to 19 by race and Hispanic origin and age: United States, 2015–2018.** *(Fryer et al, 2020.)*

Physical Activity Patterns

While calorie consumption has increased, calorie expenditure has declined. Physical activity levels have decreased in recent decades, primarily due to increased use of electronic devices and screen time (CDC, 2022a). There is nearly unanimous agreement globally that children between 5 and 17 years old should participate in 60 minutes of physical activity per day (Parrish et al., 2020). Yet less than 25% of children in the United States participate in the recommended 60 minutes of physical activity daily. Marked decreases in physical activity typically occur between the ages of 9 and 15. According to the 2021 YRBS, only 23.9% of adolescents were participating in recommended levels of activity (CDC, 2023b). School-age children are becoming more sedentary over time, with 40% reporting 3 or more hours of television per day.

The Role of the School

Physical education (PE) provides students with life-long skills on how to be active through adulthood and have a positive effect on their mental well-being. Although 74% of states require some type of PE programs, many are observed as inadequate. Typical programs require less than 90 minutes per week associated with structured PE. Only six states require a minimum of 150 minutes per week in elementary schools, and two that hold the same standard for high school students (Piekarz-Porter et al., 2020). In the 2021 YRBS, only 19% of high school students reported attending PE class on all 5 days of the school week (CDC, 2023b).

The Role of the School Community

Physical environment and community play a role in physical activity levels. Children who have open spaces, such as parks, are more likely to engage in physical activity. Those without access demonstrate screen time averages over 4 hours per day and are more likely to become obese (Reuben et al., 2020). In the United States, 24% of children live in low-income, urban areas that lack park spaces. In communities where parks are available, it is important they are considered safe so people will use them. Despite more open space for youth in rural areas, much of the open space is not designated for public recreational use (Reuben et al., 2020).

Genetic and Hormonal Factors

There is a family connection to obesity. Several genetic disorders are associated with abnormal, increased weight gain, such as Prader-Willi syndrome, Down syndrome, and Turner syndrome. However, in most people with obesity there is not one genetic cause, and there is clear evidence that other drivers also contribute to obesity (Loos & Yeo, 2022). There is emerging research into understanding the role of epigenetics on prevalence of obesity within populations. *Epigenetics* is the study of how behavior and environment affect how genes work (CDC, 2024c). Examples of environmental exposures that may influence how genes work include environmental toxins, nutrition, maternal stress , smoking, and alcohol use (King & Skinner, 2020). It is important to remember that epigenetic changes are not necessarily permanent.

Hormonal fluctuations and interactions may also account for increased body fat leading to overweight and obesity. For example, subclinical hypothyroidism (elevated thyroid-stimulating hormone with normal levels of thyroxine, also known as T_4) is present in up to 14% of children who are obese (Kumari et al., 2021).

Leptin and ghrelin are the two most important hormones involved with human appetite regulation and energy balance (Klok et al., 2007). Their receptors in the hypothalamus create a negative feedback system. Both hormonal pathways are disrupted in the case of obesity. *Leptin* is secreted by adipose tissue and signals the brain on how much energy is available and when to suppress appetite. Blood levels of leptin are increased in obesity. Ghrelin is produced in multiple peripheral tissues and the gastrointestinal tract. *Ghrelin* signals hunger and reverses the inhibitory effects of leptin; therefore ghrelin increases before meals and lowers after. It also assists in the regulation of other hormones (Klok et al., 2007). Elevated levels of insulin, caused by overeating, and chronically elevated levels of leptin produced by an abundance of adipose tissue are believed to cause physiological resistance to both hormones. Research has shown that restoration of normal hormonal rhythms may occur with weight loss (Hernández Morante et al., 2020).

CONSEQUENCES

As obesity rates rise, the consequences and complications also increase. Children who become obese by age 6 are more likely to be obese with the onset of adolescence, and adolescents are more likely to be obese into adulthood. Obesity in early adulthood increases the risk of mortality through the connection to chronic disease, such as hypertension and diabetes, and nearly every organ is affected by the consequences of obesity (Deal et al., 2020). Many of the diseases now being seen in children who are overweight or obese were traditionally seen only in adults over the age of 30. Treatment of childhood illnesses and diseases is made more complicated by obesity because medications used in pediatric populations are typically dosed according to weight. The metabolic and pharmacokinetic changes that occur due to decreased lean muscle mass, increased adipose tissue, and changes in blood volume make accurate dosing more difficult (Matson et al., 2017).

Metabolic Syndrome

The physiological changes that occur because of overweight and obesity during childhood have potentially devastating effects that last well into adulthood. Of highest concern is the risk for *metabolic syndrome*, a constellation of symptoms that increase the risk of cardiovascular events such as stroke and myocardial infarction. Chronic oxidative stress and its associated inflammation causes a *pro-inflammatory state*, which is a major contributor to atherosclerosis (Čolak & Pap, 2021). The American Academy of Pediatrics has identified five major risk factors in the development of metabolic syndrome in children:

- Central obesity (large waist circumference)
- High blood pressure
- High blood sugar
- High overall cholesterol levels
- High triglyceride levels (Magge, 2021)

Hypertension

The CDC estimates that 1 in 25 children between 12 and 19 years old have hypertension (HTN); 1 in 10 children have higher than normal blood pressure, formally known as "prehypertension" (CDC, 2024b). Though specific reasons for hypertension in youth are unknown, there is a clear link to overweight and obesity during childhood as the rise of both have paralleled each other. This is challenging for families to understand because hypertension is not thought of as a pediatric disease. Early-onset hypertension is a significant concern due to its long-lasting effects and risk factor for end-organ damage, including kidney failure (Wühl, 2018).

The American Academy of Pediatrics recommends that blood pressure (BP) screening be part of routine pediatric care:

- BP should be measured annually in children and adolescents greater than or equal to 3 years of age.
- Trained healthcare professionals in the office setting should make a diagnosis of HTN if a child or adolescent has auscultatory-confirmed BP readings greater than or equal to 95th percentile at three different visits (Flynn et al., 2017).

Students with obesity can be screened periodically in the school nurse's office. Any child presenting with consistent high BP readings in the school nurse's office should be referred by the school nurse to their primary care provider. See Chapter 12.

Did You Know?

Due to their increased amount of adipose tissue, children with obesity may need a larger size sphygmomanometer cuff (based on midarm circumference) to measure blood pressure. Using a cuff that is too small may result in a false reading of high blood pressure (Brady, 2017). The school nurse ensures that there are appropriately sized BP cuffs to accommodate all students in the school building.

Dyslipidemia

Dyslipidemia, or abnormal lipid levels, interferes with epithelium, creating the origins of cardiovascular events such as stroke and myocardial infarction. The major function of the epithelium layer of a blood vessel wall is to provide a protective layer against damage that occurs during inflammatory processes. Of highest concern is the buildup of low-density lipoproteins (LDLs) within the epithelium of the blood vessel wall. The body's defense is the circulation of high-density lipoproteins (HDLs), which tend to "clean up" the walls of the blood vessel by transporting excess LDLs away from the walls (Beverly & Budoff, 2020).

The total cholesterol level should be less than 170 mg/dL. Findings of 170 to 199 mg/dL are considered borderline, and anything more than 200 mg/dL is considered high. LDLs should be less than 110 mg/dL, with borderline being 110 to 129 and high being anything greater than 130 mg/dL (de Ferranti & Newburger, 2023).

Lipid disorders are more likely to be observed in individuals who are overweight or obese with rates increasing as the BMI reaches the 99th percentile. Thirty-nine percent of children with obesity have overall cholesterol increases, with 13% having high LDL levels. This *combined hyperlipidemia* results in thickening of arterial walls and other structural changes. Triglyceride levels also rise, further increasing the risk for metabolic syndrome (de Ferranti & Newburger, 2023).

The American Academy of Pediatrics recommends regular monitoring of fasting lipid levels in children starting between 9 and 11 years of age (Sleeth et al., 2020). Screening is especially important in children with strong family histories of hyperlipidemia. Early detection is important because children with high cholesterol levels tend to maintain higher levels as adults, increasing the risk for cardiovascular events later in life. Dietary measures remain the mainstay of early treatment in children.

Diabetes Mellitus Type 2 and Insulin Resistance

Formerly a disease only found in adults, diabetes mellitus type 2 (T2D) has risen steadily in American youth over the last 2 decades. Obesity is the number one risk factor for T2D in children (Castorani et al., 2020). Of notable concern is that the rates of T2D in white children doubled between 2001 and 2017, and the rates among black and Hispanic children rose at an even higher rate (Bendor et al., 2020).

Initial screening for T2D differs between adults and children; hemoglobin A1c is more commonly used in adults whereas fasting glucose levels are used in children (Lawrence et al., 2021). For children, fasting glucose levels of 126 mg/dL with follow-up hemoglobin A1c at greater than or equal to 6.5% is diagnostic for the disease (Bendor et al., 2020).

T2D begins with insulin resistance and beta-cell dysfunction, both of which occur more rapidly in children than in adults. Insulin resistance occurs when there is reduced glucose uptake despite high insulin levels (Castorani et al., 2020). In addition to elevated blood glucose levels, early physical symptoms of insulin resistance may include hyperinsulinemia and acanthosis nigricans characterized by thick, velvety, darkened plaques of skin commonly found in the neck and axillary areas (Leung et al., 2023). See Figure 14-2. As insulin resistance progresses to T2D, microvascular damage leads to increased arterial wall thickness. People diagnosed with T2D at younger ages are at a highest risk for more aggressive progression of symptoms, sequelae, and higher mortality rates (Bendor et al., 2020).

Asthma

In the United States, asthma occurs in 7% of the general pediatric population. However, in what has been described as a "dual epidemic," children who are obese have rates of asthma up to 20% (Wong et al., 2022). In students who are obese and have asthma, daily control and prevention of exacerbations can be more complicated than their normal-weight peers. When exacerbations occur, children who are obese have a higher risk of severity and hospitalization and poorer outcomes (Wong et al., 2022). Underlying chronic inflammation caused by obesity could be a contributor—enhancing airway inflammation, systemic response, and changes in immune responses (Reyes-Angel et al., 2022). Further, the child's larger body demands more metabolically during asthma exacerbations, and a larger chest mass

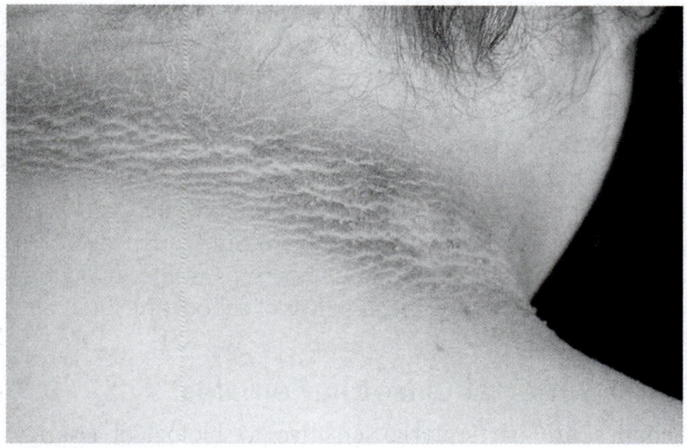

FIGURE 14-2. **Acanthosis nigricans.** *(Dermatology Online Journal, with permission.)*

creates lower lung volumes with each breath and increased work of breathing (Bhammar & Babb, 2021). See Chapter 22 for more information on students with asthma.

Sleep Disorders

Insufficient sleep not only creates daytime sleepiness and decreased academic performance but can also increase the risk of obesity in students (Chehal et al., 2021). Inadequate sleep alters the balance of leptin and ghrelin, resulting in increased hunger. Children who are overweight often sleep fewer hours per night and experience more sleep disruptions. Children who are overweight or obese are at higher risk for sleep disorders, including obstructive sleep apnea (Bhatt et al., 2021). Obstructive sleep apnea occurs in as many as 40% of children with obesity and carries its own risks of increased chronic inflammation, insulin resistance, and, later, cardiac events.

Musculoskeletal Disorders

Children who are overweight and obese experience injury and recovery at slower rates than their normal-weight peers (McGregor et al., 2022). They tend to be less stable on their feet and less flexible leading to increased musculoskeletal injury, including fractures. Additionally, Blount's disease and slipped capital femoral epiphysis are two orthopedic conditions associated with obesity, fractures, and poor recovery.

Blount's disease can have an early onset, before age 6, or a later onset, during adolescence (Janoyer, 2019). *Blount's disease* is characterized by bowing of the lower extremities and joint instability and youth will complain about knee pain or instability. In the United States, Blount's disease is most associated with obesity and is found most commonly in black non-Hispanic children. Obesity further exacerbates the condition both by applying heavier loads on already unstable joints and by increasing the risk of thrombosis.

Slipped capital femoral epiphysis is an orthopedic emergency with the first symptoms being the onset of pain originating in the groin that presents as thigh and/or knee pain on the affected side (Aprato et al., 2019). The injury occurs when the femoral head moves, or *slips,* out of its normal position in the hip joint. Typical age of onset is between 8 and 15 years, with higher incidence in Polynesian, black, and Hispanic children. Though the cause of slipped capital femoral epiphysis is unclear, the mechanical forces and metabolic changes seen in children who are obese are connected to its development. Though not common, the condition can become chronic, requiring multiple surgeries, and cause chronic pain issues and joint stability issues into adulthood. Subsequent decreased activity can further exacerbate obesity, as well as affecting a child's academic status through loss of school time.

Early Pubertal Onset in Females

Females are particularly sensitive to biological changes related to obesity, which is connected to early pubertal onset (Tenedero et al., 2021). The timing of puberty occurs through a mechanism known as the hypothalamic-pituitary-adrenal and hypothalamic-pituitary-gonadal axes. Fat cells can manufacture estrogen, leading to early and increased production in girls who are obese. Obesity also complicates the staging of puberty; adipose tissue on the breasts may lead a clinician to stage for puberty based on breast development.

The biological changes of puberty occur an average of 0.3 years earlier in girls who are obese (Itriyeva, 2022; Tenedero et al., 2021). Early onset of puberty has additional consequences, including shorter stature, risk for polycystic ovarian syndrome, hyperinsulinism, abnormal uterine bleeding, and significant psychosocial concerns. Additionally, early onset of puberty due to obesity raises all-cause mortality rates in adulthood.

Psychosocial and Mental Health Issues

Psychosocial needs are greater for students who are overweight or obese, related to the higher incidence of depression, anxiety, disordered eating, and feelings of social isolation and low self-esteem. Students who are obese report being bullied at higher levels and have lower quality-of-life scores than nonobese peers (Raynor et al., 2022). Weight stigma and weight-based discrimination can arise due to implicit bias among students and staff. Stressors related to weight bias and bullying from peers can lead to binge eating and self-isolation, creating psychological distress and increasing the risk of depression (Hampl et al., 2023).

These experiences also affect communication between students with obesity and school nurses. Sensitivity to the mental health and physical challenges for the student with obesity can improve the relationship between nurse and student. Students who are obese are likely to experience feelings of shame and embarrassment, while facing simultaneous physical challenges with school seating, bathroom stalls, and physical education classes. Concerns such as these may extend to the home; parents/guardians may be hesitant to take children out into public spaces to protect them from harmful psychosocial experiences (Haqq et al., 2021).

ASSESSING STUDENTS FOR OVERWEIGHT AND OBESITY

The U.S. Preventive Services Task Force (2017) recommends that all children 6 years and older be screened for obesity. Though screening processes vary from state to state, school nurses can play a pivotal role in addressing childhood obesity, starting with proper assessment during screenings. Monitoring growth patterns should occur as a partnership between schools, parents/guardians, and primary care providers, and is the first step in obesity prevention. The most common method of screening for overweight and obesity in the school setting is using height and weight to calculate BMI.

Though BMI measurement is a useful tool, it is not an exact measurement of body fat, but rather an estimate of such. For instance, lean muscle mass is not differentiated in a BMI measurement, and research has demonstrated that ethnicity may play a role in the accuracy of BMI measurements (Chen et al., 2018; Jackson et al., 2018). Additionally, students with early onset of puberty show higher BMIs; but when adjusted for early maturity, up to 31% will fall into a lower weight category (Gillison et al., 2021).

There are more accurate ways of measuring body fat content, such as skin fold thickness measurements and densitometry (underwater weighing). Alternative measurements, such as waist to height ratio and waist circumference, have shown some predictability for metabolic syndrome and future cardiovascular risk (Ma et al., 2022). However, studies using these measurements on children are limited and are not feasible in the school setting. Thus BMI calculation is the most common and practical measurement for a pediatric population.

Student comfort with school-based weight and growth measurements varies, and children who are unhappy with their weight may find the assessment experience distressing. However, despite feelings of apprehension, research shows us that students have a higher comfort level when measurements are conducted by a school nurse, rather than another staff member (Altman et al., 2022). A judicious level of privacy is essential to the student's comfort level, yet on average, only 30% of students find that privacy during height and weight screening is treated as a priority. To date, there is no conclusive evidence that school-based BMI surveillance programs reduce obesity rates significantly. The CDC (2022c) does not make a recommendation for or against school-based BMI screening programs. Nevertheless, if not conducted with a high level of sensitivity, the BMI assessment process could be construed as increased pressure to control weight and contribute to an environment of stigma. Careful planning and effective communication can mitigate concerns. The CDC provides guidance on surveillance with 10 safeguard provisions for schools to prevent unintended negative consequences of school-based screenings (CDC, 2022c). Guidance regarding how to screen for height, weight, and BMI is detailed in Chapter 12.

When conducting school-based BMI screenings, school nurses should implement evidence-based practices related to height and weight measurement, as well as procedures for thorough documentation. Accuracy is essential; weights should be calculated to the nearest quarter of a pound and height should be to the nearest one-eighth inch. The difference of an inch in height or a pound of weight may cause an inaccurate BMI. Accuracy with interpretation of BMI scores is also important. Once height and weight have been obtained, the BMI can be calculated using an online BMI calculator or other method (CDC, 2022c). See Online Materials OM14-1 for a link to the CDC's BMI calculator. State and local districts may mandate BMI screening, including when to screen, who to screen, and the mechanism for notifying parents/guardians of students who are overweight and obese. However, it is incumbent on the nurse to ensure the BMI screenings and policies are evidence-based and up to date. School nurses should advocate for changes when needed in order to support students and families.

Practice Connection

An 11th-grade football player eats nutritionally balanced meals, exercises regularly, and lifts weights to prepare for his role on the school team. He is 16.5 years of age, with a height of 69 inches, and weighs 210 pounds. He has virtually no body fat, yet his BMI would be 30.1. Although his BMI percentile is greater than the 95th percentile, care must be taken to ensure that he is not mislabeled as obese. The school nurse should consider what, if any, communication should be sent home from a school-based BMI screening program to this family.

Reporting BMI Results to the Family

A mechanism for reporting positive screening results and a follow-up component should be maintained as part of the school record. Reports to parents/guardians may be included with other health screenings completed at school, such as vision and hearing, creating an opportunity to include suggestions for healthy and safe lifestyle changes. Although routine assessments allow for valuable information to be communicated such as reinforcement of normal weight values and risks for the underweight individual, the emotional element needs consideration when notifying families that a child is found to be overweight or obese.

Communication about an elevated BMI should be provided with respect and empathy with emphasis placed on the child's overall health, not just the BMI. Parents/guardians who are engaged in a meaningful way and allowed to reflect on information provided are more responsive to information. Parents/guardians can be reluctant to discuss obesity, and some prefer the word *overweight* in conversation due to the stigma and blame that can be associated with having a child who is obese. Parents/guardians also prefer emphasizing *health*, rather than weight. Lack of information or an inability to answer questions can be discouraging for parents/guardians. Conversely, telling a parent/guardian something they already know can be perceived as not paying attention to prioritized needs. Culture can also play a role in what is healthy and what is not, or what is spoken of and what is not (Eli et al., 2022). If communication must occur by sending a letter home, parents may have more difficulty understanding and following up appropriately. If BMI screening results are sent home in paper form with the students, all students should receive a letter, not just those who have an elevated BMI.

In general, parents/guardians want to be informed of screening processes before the screening and expect accurate, timely information on findings (Ames et al., 2020). Finally, they expect that all information will be kept private throughout the process, as well as being communicated in a nonjudgmental way. See Chapter 12 for more information on screening and surveillance of overweight and in schools. See Online Materials OM12-4 for an electronic, interactive BMI parental notification letter template.

PREVENTION APPROACHES IN THE SCHOOL SETTING

Prevention of overweight and obesity requires holistic prevention strategies involving primary care providers, families, schools, and communities. This approach recognizes that people's needs must be met throughout the life span and in multiple aspects of their lives with a focus on developing self-determination. The broad spectrum of social determinants of health that contribute to overweight and obesity must be addressed through public policy. Schools, where most school-age children spend significant time, are a priority setting for obesity prevention efforts with regular opportunities for physical activity and nutritious foods. School nurses are poised to provide significant contributions in the prevention of childhood obesity.

As schools consider prevention approaches, the CDC's School Health Index (SHI) is a useful tool to assess the school's strengths and weaknesses as it relates to providing an environment that promotes health and reduces risk of overweight and obesity (CDC, 2019b). The School Health Index is a self-assessment tool that allows schools to plan and focus resources on areas most in need; there are sections that specifically address physical activity and education and nutrition. Ideally, the School Health Index should be completed by a team of stakeholders with the school nurse as a team member (See Chapter 2).

Environment, diet, and activity are the most important components of any obesity prevention plan. The creation of a healthy school community provides opportunities for engagement among families, schools, healthcare providers, and municipalities. Concepts such as increasing water intake, eating more fruits and vegetables, and increasing physical activity should be introduced within the school environment as part of a comprehensive prevention approach.

Dietary Approaches

Dietary recommendations for school-age children are based on the culmination of data from multiple sources. The *Dietary Guidelines for Americans* (Dietary Guidelines) are updated every 5 years and contain recommendations across the life span. In addition to recommendations on dietary intake, the Dietary Guidelines provide information on how communities can organize their efforts to promote healthy eating patterns and resources on how to elicit help from local government, schools, and parents/guardians (U.S. Department of Agriculture [USDA] & U.S. Department of Health and Human Services [USDHHS], 2020). The *Dietary Guidelines for Americans 2020–2025* emphasize that food choices should be customized to reflect individual cultures and budgetary restraints. Diets should prioritize nutrient-dense foods, rather than low-nutrient, high-calorie, processed foods. The current Dietary Guidelines contain the following significant elements for children and adults:

- Meals and snacks should include a wide variety of fruits and vegetables, including from their subgroups, such as dark leafy greens, starchy vegetables, and legumes. Fruits and vegetables that are bright in color are emphasized and recommended due to their variety of nutrients.
- Whole fruits are recommended, excluding those that are processed, canned, or jarred or those with added sugar.
- A variety of grains, at least 50% of which are considered whole grain.
- Dairy products should be fat-free or low-fat, including yogurt, milk, and fortified soy products.
- Lean proteins, such as seafood, lean meats, poultry, eggs, nuts, and legumes, are preferred to high-fat proteins.
- Limits are set on fats, especially saturated fats (less than 10% of total calories), added sugars (10% or less of total calories), and sodium (2300 mg per day). Attempts should be made to eliminate trans fats (USDA & USDHHS, 2020).

The Dietary Guidelines are important to discuss with families as they consider nutrition outside of school. While students are in school, they are most affected by the guidelines set forth by the Healthy, Hunger Free Act of 2010 (Act). Through this Act public and private schools administer a federally subsidized meal program, known as the National School Lunch Program, and the School Breakfast Program. The Act requires the USDA to update nutrition standards on a regular basis while creating a safety net for children, including limits on sodium, unhealthy fats, and sugary foods (USDA, 2013). In 2023, public comment was being requested on revisions to the school nutrition standards to better align them with the Dietary Guidelines. The key areas of update are related to added sugars, milk, whole grains, and sodium (USDA, 2023a).

Research suggests that students who eat breakfast, eat at least one fruit or vegetable per day, drink milk, avoid sugary beverages, and demonstrate better academic outcomes compared with those who do not (Scaglioni et al., 2018). Students consume 30% to 50% of their daily calories through foods provided by school-based programs, thus these programs are valuable tools in the prevention of overweight and obesity in children. Studies have shown that students reach a higher *Healthy Eating Index* when they are in school, participating in the school food programs (Frisvold & Price, 2019; Valizadeh & Ng, 2020).

School nurses support students' nutrition habits through health education and individual counseling with students. Helping students understand the Dietary Guidelines and how to make healthy food choices when presented options is essential in prevention efforts. Some students skip meals, most commonly breakfast; however, food restriction approaches have been connected to obesity because they may decrease a child's level of self-control and ability to select healthy foods (Koletzko et al., 2020; Wicherski et al., 2021).

Sugary Beverages

Research has shown that adolescents consume at least 17% of their calories from added sugars as a conservative estimate, and at least half of those come from sugary beverages (Muth et al., 2019). Nationally there have been several cities and municipalities that have attempted to restrict sugary beverage intake through reduction in the number of ounces that can be served, or by inducing "sugar taxes" on soft drinks, such as local sales taxes and excise taxes on manufacturers. In 2019, the AAP addressed the issue, citing that the Dietary Guidelines for sugar intake (i.e., limiting beverages to 10% of overall calories) is an inadequate approach to preventing obesity (Muth et al., 2019). The AAP recommends that schools serve water, unflavored milk, or 100% fruit juice as it has been shown that when schools limit access to sugary beverages, adolescents are less likely to consume calories through beverages.

Physical Activity

Recognizing that exercise plays a key role in long-term health outcomes, the AAP has updated its physical activity guidelines, which are in line with the *2018 Physical Activity Guidelines for Americans* (Lobelo et al., 2020; USDHHS, 2018). One of the key recommendations is the importance of physical activity during preschool, starting with encouraging physical activity through play with parents/guardians at age 3, then continuing throughout childhood with age-appropriate activities. The key points of the *2018 Physical Activity Guidelines for Americans* include the following:

- School-age children should get 60 minutes or more of aerobic physical activity daily, with vigorous activity 3 times per week.
- Activity can include a mix of light or moderate activity with more intense activities.
- Activities can be structured or unstructured.
  - Structured: muscle strengthening activities (e.g., lifting weights or resistance bands) or bone strengthening activities (e.g., basketball, tennis, jumping rope)
  - Unstructured: climbing trees or playground equipment, running, jumping, hopscotch (USDHHS, 2018)

Data suggest that nearly 75% of children are not meeting these recommendations (Merlo et al., 2020). The CDC's *Increasing Physical Education and Physical Activity: A Framework for Schools* (2019a) addresses the physical education and physical activity components of the *Whole School, Whole Community, Whole Child* (WSCC;CDC, 2021a). The model includes the following key components:

- Physical education
- Physical activity during school, and physical activity before and after school
- Staff involvement
- Family and community engagement

Each component has a strategy guide that can be used by schools to improve their programming. See Online Materials OM14-2 for links to specific strategies.

Schools should consider creative ways to integrate physical activity into the school day. Classroom teachers have found that integrating classroom-based physical activity allows for "brain breaks." Classroom-based activity has been shown to positively contribute to students meeting the goal of 60 active minutes per day and increases time on task behavior (Masini et al., 2020).

Schools should guarantee students opportunities for safe and robust physical activity. In 2020, researchers examined the potential effects of the COVID-19 pandemic on childhood obesity rates. Applying the data on over 15,000 children to a microsimulation model, researchers were able to project that the loss of physical activity associated with school closures during the pandemic would result in an approximately 10% weight gain for children of school age with most effects seen in children living in areas with limited outdoor spaces and in low-income urban environments. Further, the research suggested that the longer the lock-down period, the higher the prevalence of weight gain (An, 2020).

School Staff Health Promotion

In 2018, the National Association of Chronic Disease Directors (NACDD) developed the *Healthy School, Healthy Staff, Healthy Students* guide. The aim of the initiative was to bring awareness to the mental, physical, and emotional well-being of school employees, while providing step-by-step instructions for schools interested in developing a staff wellness program. Wellness programs allow school employees to serve as health role models for students and families and can be led by school wellness teams.

School staff can promote resilience, physical health, and mental health among the school community. School nurses are poised to lead school wellness teams and can enhance such programs by organizing exercise activities or mindfulness sessions to reduce stress and anxiety, and providing health education, while helping to recognize healthy milestones (CDC, 2021b). See Chapter 33 for detailed information about supporting school staff wellness.

National Initiatives

The U.S. government has committed resources to preventing and addressing childhood obesity through a variety of programs.

Choose MyPlate

The USDA (n.d.) developed *MyPlate* in 2011 to replace the food guide pyramid. MyPlate uses simple visual aids for children and families to use as a guideline for what a typical meal plate should look. See Figure 14-3. Fruits and vegetables cover half of the plate, with the remainder being filled with whole grains and proteins. Research has revealed some barriers to including MyPlate instruction in the classroom such as time constraints and lack of awareness; yet overall, teachers recognize the need for basic nutrition knowledge because students often ask questions about what it means to eat healthy (Hastert et al., 2022). Education materials and family-based tools are easily accessible through the MyPlate.gov Web site.

5-2-1-0 Healthy Habits

The *5-2-1-0* approach from Canada is an easy to remember mnemonic that emphasizes key strategies that every family can do to promote healthy lifestyles for their children (Childhood Obesity Foundation, n.d.). With 5-2-1-0, families follow four simple rules:

- **5** servings of fruits and vegetables per day
- No more than **2** hours of screen time per day
- Engage in at least **1** hour of physical activity per day
- Drink **0** sugary beverages per day

Further emphasis is placed on avoiding processed foods, including highly refined grains, watching portion sizes, exercising, and ensuring adequate sleep.

Racial and Equity Approaches to Community Health

The *Racial and Ethnic Approaches to Community Health* (REACH) program is a CDC-funded program that aims to assist communities in the prevention of chronic illness by first addressing health inequities schools (Trust for America's Health, 2022). REACH provides funding for locally developed programs that address modifiable risk factors. Projects have led to improvements such as local farmers accepting electronic benefits transfer (EBT) cards as payment for fresh fruits and vegetables and assisting local communities with providing healthier beverages.

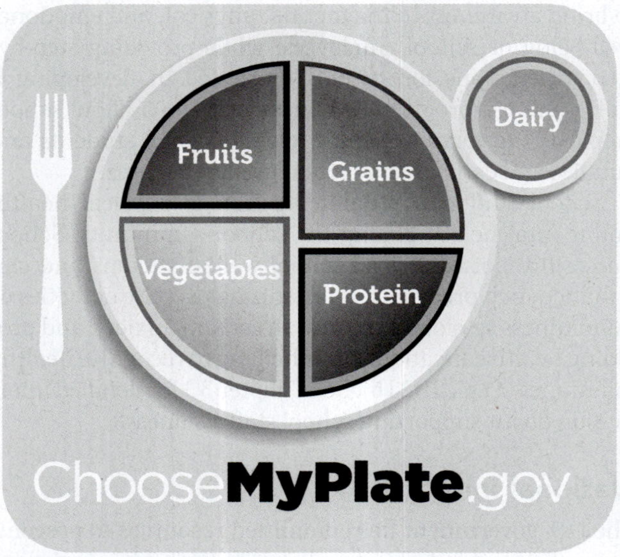

FIGURE 14-3. My Plate. *(U.S. Department of Agriculture, 2020, with permission.)*

MANAGEMENT OF OBESITY IN THE SCHOOL SETTING

Since 2013, the American Medical Association has recognized that obesity is a disease process. Classifying obesity as a disease with a diagnostic code has helped track prevalence of obesity and led to the development of evidence-based interventions to prevent onset and complications (Garvey & Mechanick, 2020). Recognizing that obesity is a disease, the American Academy of Pediatrics also encourages the use of a chronic care model where evidence-based care is provided in partnership with children and families. Care considers cultural and social factors of influence, and children should be treated within a medical home (Hampl et al., 2023). Yet only about half of school nurses surveyed feel confident in the treatment of students with obesity (Thompson et al., 2021).

The use of diet and physical activity to treat obesity is well documented and remains the mainstay of obesity treatment (Tak & Lee, 2021). Addressing obesity in the school setting is important as children spend much of their awake time in the school setting. Obesity has an impact on educational outcomes; students who struggle with obesity may also struggle with low levels of self-esteem and may be subject to negative peer interactions and bullying at school (Ho et al., 2021). School-based treatment interventions have demonstrated improvement in levels of self-esteem compared with interventions only implemented in a clinical setting.

While primary care providers are responsible for diagnosing obesity in children, school nurses have a key role in addressing this disease; school-based interventions are a valuable addition to any treatment plan. School nurses should be involved beyond anthropometric screening. They are key participants in the development of school policies and programs that address nutrition and physical activity for the students. Successful school-based interventions occur when there is consistency between the home and school setting and when interventions are holistic, including information about nutrition, physical activity, and short behavioral intervention sessions (Ho et al., 2021). School-based interventions require both personnel and financial commitment, which can be difficult to achieve in underresourced schools.

The school nurse understands the concept of developmental readiness and the logistics of treatment options within the school setting. School nurses can provide education for students and their families, reinforce healthy behaviors, supervise treatment plans, and follow up when referral for medical evaluation is required (McCabe, 2020). Managing obesity requires daily intervention but also a degree of self-management. The school nurse should bear in mind that school-age children are capable of self-management. Self-management does not put the onus on a child who is not developmentally ready, but is a collaborative approach, involving families and healthcare providers.

School nurses may work with students who participate in weight loss programs, which can include behavioral therapy, pharmacological therapy, and surgical interventions. These types of programs are often intensely monitored and multidisciplinary.

Behavioral Approaches

The U.S. Preventive Services Task Force recommends intensive behavioral interventions in the treatment of obesity. While these interventions cannot be conducted solely in the school setting, the school nurse plays a valuable role in the behavioral therapy process (Grossman et al., 2017). School nurses can serve as role models, mentors, and support during school hours (Coupe et al., 2022). Behavioral interventions can be placed into several categories, including behavior modification, peer-to-peer, and family-based sessions. Family-based interventions can be expanded to include group sessions to create additional support. They are particularly successful in children 6 years old and older when tailored to the level of motivation of the child and family (Di Figlia-Peck et al., 2020). Studies show that when families work together and receive the support of peers, weight reduction is greater than when interventions involve children alone. The AAP guidelines for the treatment of children with obesity describe optimal plans as including at least 26 hours of counseling over the course of 2 to 12 months (Hampl et al., 2023).

When developing a behavioral treatment plan, it is best to determine modifiable behaviors and prioritize accordingly. When treating adolescents, the *Healthy Habits Questionnaire (Ages 10–18)* can be a helpful tool to start with. The tool gathers information related to the 5-2-1-0 Healthy Habit Goals while also integrating motivational interviewing questions to understand what the student is motivated to change (Camp et al., 2020). See Online Materials OM14-3 for a link to this questionnaire. School nurses can utilize motivational interviewing strategies to help students set short- and long-term personal goals. A stepwise approach increases the chance of success because it allows adolescents and their families to get used to changes in dietary plans gradually and allows for optimal learning (Di Figlia-Peck et al., 2020).

Any behavior modification plan should include a total lifestyle approach from the perspective of the family, including physical activity, the importance of choosing healthy foods while avoiding processed foods, working on issues surrounding low self-esteem and depression, and addressing concerns with peers. A well-rounded behavioral approach should also include goals to reduce screen time. In addition to behavioral therapy, medical nutrition therapy (MNT) administered through a registered dietitian may enhance obesity treatment programs (Calcaterra et al., 2021; Siopis et al., 2020). Studies have shown behavioral interventions have an impact on obesity-related illnesses such as diabetes and polycystic ovarian syndrome.

Practice Connection

The *Healthy Options and Physical Activity Program* (HOP) is a school nurse–led obesity intervention and was implemented with 1,054 New York City students during the 2012–2013 school year (Schroeder et al., 2017; Schroeder & Smaldone, 2017). This program was modeled after 5-2-1-0 Healthy Habits. Although HOP did not result in significant reduction in obesity of the participants, it shed light on important components of school nurse–led interventions.

1. Parental/guardian engagement is key to success. The school nurse must consider barriers and facilitators to parental participation.
2. School nurses should receive specific professional development about obesity treatment and motivational interviewing.
3. School nurses need to carve out time to deliver interventions for specific students. They need support from other staff and school administration to make this possible within the daily demands of the health office.
4. Low-intensity programs do not address the complex needs of a child with obesity. Successful programs are multifaceted and involve an interdisciplinary team.
5. The school and community environment have a large influence on the quality of food available to children.
6. Stigma, real or perceived, has an influence on how students will engage in a program related to obesity. The school nurse should consider how to mitigate stigma.

Pharmacological Approaches

The pharmacological approach to treatment in children remains limited, and any pharmacology used to treat obesity should be combined with lifestyle measures. Weight loss drugs are more commonly used in the treatment of adults. Many providers decline the option of pharmacological treatments for children due to lack of knowledge, limited studies, lack of insurance coverage, concerns for safety, or simply not being in favor (Borzutzky et al., 2020). There are two FDA-approved medications for children with obesity over the age of 12, *orlistat* and *liragutide;* both are used sparingly and have side effects (Raman & Foster, 2021). Metformin remains the most common form of drug treatment in obese children, closely followed by topiramate.

Neither drug has an official FDA approval for weight loss management, though studies have shown modest success when used off label in combination with physical activity, dietary management, and behavioral therapy.

Many providers believe that the epidemic of pediatric obesity requires more aggressive measures and pharmacological treatments should be considered. Johnson et al. (2021) describe a "call to action," with recommendations for considering pharmacotherapy in patients with a BMI of greater than 30, or greater than 95th percentile, and at least one comorbidity related to obesity. Advances in pharmacological research and weight loss medications are continually being introduced into the healthcare market.

Surgery

Recently, the discussion regarding using bariatric surgery as a tool for treating pediatric obesity has broadened, especially when obesity-related comorbidities exist. Bariatric surgery has been shown to reduce insulin levels, blood pressure, lipid levels, and ventricular wall thickness. However, it is typically reserved for adolescent patients (Mustafa & Chernoguz, 2021). As surgical intervention becomes more common, referrals will occur earlier, possibly curtailing life-threatening obesity-related health conditions. However, bariatric surgery programs have strict protocols that some families may have difficulty following, due to lack of knowledge, transportation concerns, or limited financial means. Children and their families are expected to commit to a long-term program, typically 6 months or longer, which includes psychiatric care and multidisciplinary support. Children with severe psychiatric disorders or diagnosed eating disorders, those with alcohol or drug addiction, and those who are pregnant are not typically acceptable for surgical treatment (Till et al., 2021).

The American Society for Metabolic and Bariatric Surgery supports consideration of weight loss surgery for children and youth younger than 18 years old with a BMI of 35 kg/m^2 (120% of the 95th percentile) *and* a comorbidity, or a BMI of 40 kg/m^2 (140% of the 95th percentile; Eisenberg et al., 2022). Bariatric surgery for adolescents has become more common, partially due to the lack of success in standard lifestyle management, as well as increasing numbers of providers who can manage complex pediatric patients. Both laparoscopic sleeve gastrectomy and Roux-en-Y gastric bypass cases have increased, and recent studies are showing their success in reducing comorbidities (Till et al., 2021). However, surgery is not without risk. Malabsorption disorders, especially vitamin deficiencies and electrolyte imbalances, will often need long-term, if not life-long, management. Vitamin D, thiamine, and vitamin B_{12} are the most common.

Reducing Weight Bias

Most nurses agree that it is important to treat all students with respect and empathy. Yet when asked, many school nurses refer to students with obesity as noncompliant and difficult. Stereotyping is common, as well as the inclination to believe students with obesity lack motivation (Thompson et al., 2021). In addition to weight bias, many nurses feel unqualified to treat students with obesity. Nurses who have obesity may also express weight bias and be less apt to believe interventions will work. However, more positive attitudes toward treatment emerged when school nurses work more frequently with students who are overweight or obese.

Students who are obese are more likely to be impacted affected by bullying both physically and emotionally. They often develop low self-esteem and feelings of embarrassment that affects them in the classroom and can lead to depression and anxiety (Ciloglu & Yilmaz, 2022). Students were more likely to pick a non-obese child as a friend, providing evidence for the isolation that many children with obesity may experience. Chapter 11 provides information for the school nurse on assessing and managing bullying in the school setting.

Individualized Healthcare Plans

Individualized healthcare plans (IHPs) are developed for many chronic conditions commonly seen in the school setting, including for students who are identified as overweight or obese. When students are overweight/obese and their condition compromises their well-being, safety, or ability to learn in school, an IHP is warranted. The success of any intervention for the student is dependent on the student's motivation and commitment to follow a plan as well as family engagement and support.

It is especially important for the school nurse to develop an IHP for students returning to school after bariatric surgery to ensure close monitoring for fluid and electrolyte imbalances in the early recovery period. Long-term follow-up with a multidisciplinary team approach to address the health and psychosocial needs of the student is recommended. Each plan must be individualized to the student's developmental level, particular needs, and unique situation. An appropriate management plan for an overweight 6-year-old may not be effective or appropriate for an overweight 16-year-old. See Chapter 8 for more information on developing IHPs.

Practice Connection

Opportunities exist to reduce weight bias through antibullying policies and continuing education. School nurses must recognize that bias can be prevented when diversity, equity, and inclusion education is integrated throughout professional development, including nursing school curriculums. Chapter 10 provides more information about explicit and implicit bias and the impact these biases have on health outcomes.

POLICIES AIMED AT REDUCING OVERWEIGHT AND OBESITY IN SCHOOLS

Trust for America's Health, a nonprofit health policy organization, produced a report called the *State of Obesity 2022: Better Policies for a Healthier America,* which outlined policy priorities surrounding the obesity epidemic. The report cited 19 states with obesity levels greater than 35% of the population, an increase of three states compared with the previous year. The report focused on the underlying causes of obesity with an understanding that there are longstanding inequities that contribute to the disparities in rates of obesity across populations. The report recommends several policy initiatives, including the following:

- Focus on and commit federal resources to efforts that reduce obesity-related disparities.
- Decrease food insecurity while improving nutritional quality of available foods.
- Change the marketing and pricing strategies that are connected to obesity and lead to health disparities.
- Make physical activity and the built environment safer and more accessible for all.
- Close disparities between healthcare and community settings.

The CDC's *Whole School, Whole Community, Whole Child* framework (2021a) provides opportunities for school nurses to advocate, organize, and lead at the policy level. These strategies stand as strong examples of how the alliance between school, parents/guardians, healthcare providers, and school nurses can lead to active and healthy children, giving them the best chance at academic achievement. The components of the program represent the 10 most pressing issues facing school policy, encompassing the underlying need for students to reach optimal health, while feeling safe, engaged, supported, and challenged (CDC, 2021a). Obesity prevention is addressed in several of the components, including the following:

- Emphasis on health education, which provides students with instruction on mental health, safety, and the importance of physical activity and healthy eating.
- Promotion of meaningful family and community engagement, which supports children by providing healthy eating and activity reinforcement outside of the school environment. This may include safe walking spaces and opportunities for physical activity equipment use.
- Support for social, emotional, and mental health within the school environment, recognition of the social barriers to health, and policy support for protection against bullying and bias.
- Attention to nutrition environment and services, which allows for students to engage in healthy eating education, allows for opportunities to advertise healthy eating throughout the school environment, ensures that school nutrition staff receive professional development, and training annually that supports healthy eating.
- Maintaining high-quality physical education programs characterized by planned curriculums based on national standards that engage students in healthy, active living, while improving cognitive skills, self-efficacy, and emotional intelligence.

Data to support school-based policies to prevent obesity are difficult to relate directly to reducing students' BMIs. Over physical activity policies, school-based nutrition policies may have the greatest impact on reducing BMIs over time (Ickovics et al., 2019). In 2003, the state of Arkansas attempted to reduce adolescent obesity through legislation that required elementary schools to restrict access to vending machines, increase PE and nutrition education, and screen for BMI annually. Results were disappointing as there was no overall impact on BMI (Gee, 2018). This highlights that school-based policies in isolation are not enough to improve rates of overweight and obesity. School-based strategies should be combined with home- and community-based prevention strategies to yield optimal outcomes.

Cost-effectiveness is another underlying concern when implementing obesity prevention programs. School district budgets must include monies to support the infrastructure necessary for school-based obesity prevention programs to be successful (Barkerman et al., 2022). With the implications of the human capital required to create and maintain an effective weight reduction program, budgets should be carefully considered. When researchers examined the financial factors associated with school-based obesity programs through systematic review, results demonstrated that comprehensive school-based obesity interventions are both cost effective and result in overall cost saving (Xu et al., 2020).

Every 5 years, the Child Nutrition and WIC Reauthorization Act is reviewed for renewal (Food Research and Action Center, 2023a). This Act includes funding for school breakfast and lunch programs, summer food programs, school-based wellness programs, and maintenance of nutrition standards in schools. The school nurse can take a lead role

Did You Know?

September is *National Childhood Obesity Prevention Month.* Schools can boost obesity prevention policies through engaging in awareness and prevention activities during this time (Health.gov, 2018). The U.S. Department of Agriculture (2023b) offers web-based resources on how parents/guardians and schools can provide games and simple activities that reduce screen time, encourage healthy eating with recipes, and assist with learning to use MyPlate.

in how such programs are implemented by collaborating with administration, nutrition services, students, families, and decision makers.

Policy-making processes should include gathering local data and evidence from agencies such as the CDC and Trust for America's Health, among others. See Online Materials OM14-4 for a list of resources from a variety of organizations to help inform programs and policies. Input from parents/guardians and community members informs the process and improves accountability. Policy also provides clear avenues for communication on specific actions within the school community. School policy takes into consideration the health and well-being of both students and staff, and school nurses should play an active role in health policy development and implementation.

CONCLUSION

School nurses contribute to developing a school climate that engages children and families in forming healthy communities. School nurses play vital roles in the prevention and treatment of child and adolescent overweight and obesity. By encouraging a culture of health within the school and community, including a balance of quality nutrition and physical activity, school nurses promote habits that last a lifetime.

As students in the United States struggle with overweight and obesity, governments at the federal, state, and local level and community agencies search for answers to this pressing public health crises. Schools will continue to play a significant role by assessing children for overweight and obesity, being a main source of food and nutrition for many students, and providing a foundation of support for families. School nurses have the expertise and longitudinal relationships with students who are overweight or obese necessary to build the trust that underpins effective treatment and management. School nurses must work as partners with families, schools, and communities at large to prevent obesity and its related comorbidities.

The editors gratefully acknowledge the work of the previous chapter authors, Janice Selekman, Denise Buffin, and Nancy Mosca.

References

Altman, E., Linchey, J., Santamaria, G., Thompson, H. R., & Madsen, K. A. (2022). Weight measurements in school: Setting and student comfort. *Journal of Nutrition Education and Behavior, 54*(3), 249–254. https://doi.org/10.1016/j.jneb.2021.11.007

Ames, H., Mosdøl, A., Blaasvær, N., Nøkleby, H., Berg, R. C., & Langøien, L. J. (2020). Communication of children's weight status: What is effective and what are the children's and parents' experiences and preferences? A mixed methods systematic review. *BMC Public Health, 20*(1). https://doi.org/10.1186/s12889-020-08682-w

Amram, O., Amiri, S., Lutz, R. B., Crowley, A., & Monsivais, P. (2019). The association between obesity, socio-economic status, and neighborhood environment: A multi-level analysis of Spokane public schools. *Journal of Community Health, 45*(1), 41–47. https://doi.org/10.1007/s10900-019-00714-w

An, R. (2020). Projecting the impact of the coronavirus disease–2019 pandemic on childhood obesity in the United States: A microsimulation model. *Journal of Sport and Health Science, 9*(4), 302–312. https://doi.org/10.1016/j.jshs.2020.05.006

Anderson, P. M., Butcher, K. F., & Schanzenbach, D. W. (2019). Understanding recent trends in childhood obesity in the United States. *Economics and Human Biology, 34*(August), 16–25. https://doi.org/10.1016/j.ehb.2019.02.002

Aprato, A., Conti, A., Bertolo, F., & Massè, A. (2019). Slipped capital femoral epiphysis: Current management strategies. *Orthopedic Research and Reviews, 11*, 47–54. https://doi.org/10.2147/orr.s166735

Barkerman, S. S., Weaver, M., & Scarton, L. (2022, January 5). School health infrastructure and students' elevated body mass index. *Journal of School Nursing, 40*(2). https://doi.org/10.1177/10598405211068

Bendor, C. D., Bardugo, A., Pinhas-Hamiel, O., Afek, A. & Twig, G. (2020). Cardiovascular morbidity, diabetes and cancer risk among children and adolescents with severe obesity. *Cardiovascular Diabetology, 19*(1). https://doi.org/10.1186/s12933-020-01052-1

Beverly, J. K., & Budoff, M. J. (2020). Atherosclerosis: Pathophysiology of insulin resistance, hyperglycemia, hyperlipidemia, and inflammation. *Journal of Diabetes, 12*(2), 102–104. https://doi.org/10.1111/1753-0407.12970

Bhammar, D. M., & Babb, T. G. (2021). Effects of obesity on the oxygen cost of breathing in children. *Respiratory Physiology & Neurobiology, 285*, 103591. https://doi.org/10.1016/j.resp.2020.103591

Bhatt, S., Guleria, R., & Kabra, S. K. (2021). Metabolic alterations and systemic inflammation in overweight/obese children with obstructive sleep apnea. *PLOS ONE, 16*(6), e0252353. https://doi.org/10.1371/journal.pone.0252353

Borzutzky, C., King, E., Fox, C. K., Stratbucker, W., Tucker, J., Yee, J. K., Kumar, S., Cuda, S., Sweeney, B., Kirk, S., & on behalf of the POWER Work Group. (2020). Trends in prescribing anti-obesity pharmacotherapy for pediatric weight management: Data from the power work group. *Pediatric Obesity, 16*(1). https://doi.org/10.1111/ijpo.12701

Brady, T. (2017). Obesity-related hypertension in children. *Frontiers in Pediatrics*, 5, 1–7. doi:10.3389/ped.2017.00197

Calcaterra, V., Verduci, E., Cena, H., Magenes, V., Todisco, C., Tenuta, E., Gregorio, C., De Giuseppe, R., Bosetti, A., Di Profio, E., & Zuccotti, G. (2021). Polycystic ovary syndrome in insulin-resistant adolescents with obesity: The role of nutrition therapy and food supplements as a strategy to protect fertility. *Nutrients, 13*(6), 1848. https://doi.org/10.3390/nu13061848

Camp, N. L., Robert, R. C., & Kelly, K. P. (2020). Healthy habits questionnaire feasibility and utility for high-risk children. *Clinical Pediatrics, 59*(11), 978–987. https://doi.org/10.1177/0009922820927030

Castorani, V., Polidori, N., Giannini, C., Blasetti, A., & Chiarelli, F. (2020). Insulin resistance and type 2 diabetes in children. *Annals of Pediatric Endocrinology & Metabolism, 25*(4), 217–226. https://doi.org/10.6065/apem.2040090.045

Centers for Disease Control and Prevention. (2019a). *Increasing physical education and physical activity: A framework for schools*. https://www.cdc.gov/healthyschools/physicalactivity/pdf/2019_04_25_PE-PA-Framework_508tagged.pdf

Centers for Disease Control and Prevention. (2019b). *School health index*. https://www.cdc.gov/healthyschools/shi/index.htm

Centers for Disease Control and Prevention. (2021a, March 23). *Components of the whole school, whole community, whole child (WSCC)*. https://www.cdc.gov/healthyschools/wscc/components.htm

Centers for Disease Control and Prevention. (2021b, April 28). *Tips for promoting school employee wellness*. https://www.cdc.gov/healthyschools/tips_employee_wellness.htm

Centers for Disease Control and Prevention. (2022a, May 13). *Overweight and obesity: Helping young children thrive*. https://www.cdc.gov/obesity/strategies/early-care-education/helping-young-children-thrive/index.html

Centers for Disease Control and Prevention. (2022b, June 3). *Healthy weight, nutrition, and physical activity: Assessing your weight*. https://www.cdc.gov/healthyweight/assessing/index.html

Centers for Disease Control and Prevention. (2022c, August 9). *Body mass index (BMI) measurement in schools.* https://www.cdc.gov/healthyschools/obesity/bmi/bmi_measurement_schools.htm

Centers for Disease Control and Prevention. (2023a, September 14). *BMI percentile calculator for child and teen.* https://www.cdc.gov/healthyweight/bmi/calculator.html

Centers for Disease Control and Prevention. (2023b). *1991–2021 high school youth risk behavior survey data.* http://yrbs-explorer.services.cdc.gov/

Centers for Disease Control and Prevention. (2024a, April 2). *Childhood obesity facts.* https://www.cdc.gov/obesity/php/data-research/childhood-obesity-facts.html

Centers for Disease Control and Prevention. (2024b, May 15). *About high blood pressure in kids and teens.* https://www.cdc.gov/high-blood-pressure/about/about-high-blood-pressure-in-kids-and-teens.html?CDC_AAref_Val=https://www.cdc.gov/bloodpressure/youth.htm

Centers for Disease Control and Prevention. (2024c, May 15). *Epigenetics, health, and disease.* https://www.cdc.gov/genomics-and-health/about/epigenetic-impacts-on-health.html?CDC_AAref_Val=https://www.cdc.gov/genomics/disease/epigenetics.htm

Centers for Disease Control and Prevention Healthy Schools. (2022a, August 5). *Childhood nutrition facts.* https://www.cdc.gov/healthyschools/nutrition/facts.htm#:~:text=The%20Dietary%20Guidelines%20for%20Americans,and%20low%2Dfat%20dairy%20products

Chehal, P., Shafer, L., & Cunningham, S. (2021). Examination of sleep and obesity in children and adolescents in the United States. *American Journal of Health Promotion, 36*(1), 46–54. https://doi.org/10.1177/08901171211029189

Chen, Y., Zhang, Y., & Wang, L. (2018). Low diagnostic accuracy of body mass index-based and waist circumference-based references of childhood: overweight and obesity in identifying overfat among Chinese children and adolescents. *Biomed Research International, 2018.* https://doi.org/10.1155/2018/4570706

Childhood Obesity Foundation. (n.d.). *What every family can do: The 5-2-1-0 rule.* https://childhoodobesityfoundation.ca/families/simple-steps-families-can-take/

Ciloglu, H., & Yilmaz, M. (2022). Attitudes and self-perception of 10- to 14-year-old students toward obese children. *The Journal of School Nursing, 38*(3), 279–286. https://doi.org/10.1177/1059840520933341

Čolak, E., & Pap, D. (2021). The role of oxidative stress in the development of obesity and obesity-related metabolic disorders. *Journal of Medical Biochemistry, 40*(1), 1–9. https://doi.org/10.5937/jomb0-24652

Coupe, N., Peters, S., Ayres, M., Clabon, K., Reilly, A., & Chisholm, A. (2022). Educators' experiences and perspectives of child weight discussions with parents in primary school settings. *BMC Public Health, 22*(1). https://doi.org/10.1186/s12889-022-13210-z

Davodi, A., & Ahadi, A. (2021). The moderating effect of parental feeding style in relation to familial psychosocial risk factors and childhood obesity. *Journal of Nutrition and Food Security.* https://doi.org/10.18502/jnfs.v6i3.6826

Deal, B. J., Huffman, M. D., Binns, H., & Stone, N. J. (2020). Perspective: Childhood obesity requires new strategies for prevention. *Advances in Nutrition, 11*(5), 1071–1078. https://doi.org/10.1093/advances/nmaa040

de Ferranti, S. D. & Newburger, J. W. (2023). *Dyslipidemia in children and adolescents: Definition, screening and diagnosis.* UpToDate. https://www.uptodate.com/contents/dyslipidemia-in-children-and-adolescents-definition-screening-and-diagnosis#H66231589

Di Figlia-Peck, S., Feinstein, R., & Fisher, M. (2020). Treatment of children and adolescents who are overweight or obese. *Current Problems in Pediatric and Adolescent Health Care, 50*(9), 100871. https://doi.org/10.1016/j.cppeds.2020.100871

Eisenberg, D., Shikora, S. A., Aarts, E., Aminian, A., Angrisani, L., Cohen, R. V., de Luca, M., Faria, S. L., Goodpaster, K. P. S., Haddad, A., Himpens, J. M., Kow, L., Kurian, M., Loi, K., Mahawar, K., Nimeri, A., O'Kane, M., Papasavas, P. K., Ponce, J., Pratt, J. S. A., … Kothari, S. N. (2022). 2022 American Society of Metabolic and Bariatric Surgery and International Federation for the Surgery of Obesity and Metabolic Disorders Indications for Metabolic and Bariatric Surgery. *Obesity surgery, 33*(1), 3–14. https://doi.org/10.1007/s11695-022-06332-1

Eli, K., Neovius, C., Nordin, K., Brissman, M., & Ek, A. (2022). Parents' experiences following conversations about their young child's weight in the primary health care setting: A study within the stop project. *BMC Public Health, 22*(1). https://doi.org/10.1186/s12889-022-13803-8

Flynn, J. T., Kaelber, D. C., Baker-Smith, C. M., Blowey, D., Carroll, A. E., Daniels, S. R., de Ferranti, S. D., Dionne, J. M., Falkner, B., Flinn, S. K., Gidding, S. S., Goodwin, C., Leu, M. G., Powers, M. E., Rea, C., Samuels, J., Simasek, M., Thaker, V. V., Urbina, E. M., & Subcommittee on Screening and Management of High Blood Pressure in Children. (2017). Clinical practice guideline for screening and management of high blood pressure in children and adolescents. *Pediatrics, 140*(3), e20171904. https://doi.org/10.1542/peds.2017-1904

Food Research and Action Center. (2023a). *Child nutrition reauthorization.* https://frac.org/action/child-nutrition-reauthorization-cnr

Food Research and Action Center. (2023b). *Food insufficiency during COVID-19.* https://frac.org/foodinsufficiencycovid19

Frisvold, D., & Price, J. (2019). The contribution of the school environment to the overall food environment experienced by children. *Southern Economic Journal, 86*(1), 106–123. https://doi.org/10.1002/soej.12371

Fryer, C.D., Carroll, M.D., Ahluwalia, N., & Ogden, C.L. (2020, August). *NCHS data brief, No. 375.* U.S. Department of Health and Human Services, Center for Disease Control, National Center for Health Statistics. https://www.cdc.gov/nchs/data/databriefs/db375-h.pdf

Garvey, W., & Mechanick, J. I. (2020). Proposal for a scientifically correct and medically actionable disease classification system (ICD) for obesity. *Obesity, 28*(3), 484–492. https://doi.org/10.1002/oby.22727

Gee, K. A. (2018). Leveraging the public school system to combat adolescent obesity: The limits of Arkansas's statewide policy initiative. *The Journal of Adolescent Health, 63*(5), 561–567. https://doi.org/10.1016/j.jadohealth.2018.06.006

Gillison, F. B., Grey, E. B., Cumming, S. P., & Sherar, L. B. (2021). Does adjusting for biological maturity when calculating child weight status improve the accuracy of predicting future health risk? *BMC Public Health, 21*(1). https://doi.org/10.1186/s12889

Grossman, D. C., Bibbins-Domingo, K., Curry, S. J., Barry, M. J., Davidson, K. W., Doubeni, C. A., Epling, J. W., Kemper, A. R., Krist, A. H., Kurth, A. E., Landefeld, C., Mangione, C. M., Phipps, M. G., Silverstein, M., Simon, M. A., & Tseng, C.-W. (2017). Screening for obesity in children and adolescents. *JAMA, 317*(23), 2417. https://doi.org/10.1001/jama.2017.6803

Hampl, S. E., Hassink, S. G., Skinner, A. C., Armstrong, S. C., Barlow, S. E., Bolling, C. F. Avila Edwards, K. C., Eneli, I., Hamre, R., Joseph, M. M., Lunsford, D., Mendonca, E., Michalsky, M. P., Mirza, N., Ochoa, E. R., Sharifi, M., Staiano, A. E., Weedn, A. E., Flinn, S. K., Lindros, J., & Okechukwu, K. (2023). Clinical practice guideline for the evaluation and treatment of children and adolescents with obesity. *Pediatrics, 151*(2). https://doi.org/10.1542/peds.2022-060640

Haqq, A. M., Kebbe, M., Tan, Q., Manco, M., & Salas, X. (2021). Complexity and stigma of pediatric obesity. *Childhood Obesity, 17*(4), 229–240. https://doi.org/10.1089/chi.2021.0003

Hastert, M., Chrisman, M., Endsley, P., Skarbek, A., & Marchello, N. (2022). Familiarity and use of MyPlate: An online focus group exploration among midwestern K–12 teachers. *Journal of Nutrition Education and Behavior, 54*(12), 1125–1131. https://doi.org/10.1016/j.jneb.2022.08.017

Health.gov. (2018). *TOOLKIT: National childhood obesity awareness month.* U.S. Department of Heath and Human Services, Office of Disease Prevention and Health Promotion. https://health.gov/news/news-and-announcements/2018/09/toolkit-national-childhood-obesity-awareness-month

Healthy, Hunger-Free Kids Act. S. 3307, 111th Cong. (2010). https://www.congress.gov/bill/111th-congress/senate-bill/3307

Hernández Morante, J., Díaz Soler, I., Muñoz, J., Sánchez, H., Barberá Ortega, M., Martínez, C., & Morillas Ruiz, J. (2020). Moderate weight loss modifies leptin and ghrelin synthesis rhythms but not the subjective sensations of appetite in obesity patients. *Nutrients, 12*(4), 916. https://doi.org/10.3390/nu12040916

Ho, T., Cheng, L., & Lau, Y. (2021). School-based interventions for the treatment of childhood obesity: A systematic review, meta-analysis and meta-regression of cluster randomized controlled trials. *Public Health Nutrition, 24*(10), 3087–3099. https://doi.org/10.1017/s1368980021001117

Hoffman, J. A., & Miller, E. A. (2020). Addressing the consequences of school closure due to Covid-19 on children's physical and mental well-being. *World Medical and Health Policy, 12*(3), 300–310. https://doi.org/10.1002/wmh3.365

Ickovics, J. R., O'Conner Duffany, K., Shebl, F. M., Peters, S. M., Read, M. A., Gilstad-Hayden, K. R., & Schwartz, M. B. (2019). Implementing school-based policies to prevent obesity: Cluster randomized trial. *American Journal of Preventive Medicine, 56*(1). e1–e11. doi:10.1016/j.amepre.2018.08.026

Itriyeva, K. (2022). The effects of obesity on the menstrual cycle. *Current Problems in Pediatric and Adolescent Health Care, 52*(8), 101241. https://doi.org/10.1016/j.cppeds.2022.101241

Jackson, M., Fatahi, F., Alabduljader, K., Jelleyman, C., Moore, J. P., & Kubis, H.-P. (2018). Exercise training and weight loss, not always a happy marriage: Single blind exercise trials in females with diverse BMI. *Applied Physiology, Nutrition, and Metabolism, 43*(4), 363–370. https://doi.org/10.1139/apnm-2017-0577

Janoyer, M. (2019). Blount disease. *Orthopaedics & Traumatology: Surgery & Research, 105*(1), S111–S121. https://doi.org/10.1016/j.otsr.2018.01.009

Jansen, P. W., Derks, I. M., Mou, Y., Rijen, E. M., Gaillard, R., Micali, N., Voortman, T., & Hillegers, M. J. (2020). Associations of parents' use of food as reward with children's eating behavior and BMI in a population-based cohort. *Pediatric Obesity, 15*(11). https://doi.org/10.1111/ijpo.12662

Johnson, V. R., Bowen-Jallow, K. A., & Stanford, F. (2021). A call to action: Multi-disciplinary care and treatment of obesity in pediatrics. *Pediatric Investigation, 5*(1), 1–2. https://doi.org/10.1002/ped4.12245

King, S. E., & Skinner, M. K. (2020). Epigenetic transgenerational inheritance of obesity susceptibility. *Trends in Endocrinology & Metabolism, 31*(7), 478–494. https://doi.org/10.1016/j.tem.2020.02.009

Klok, M. D., Jakobsdottir, S., & Drent, M. L. (2007). The role of leptin and ghrelin in the regulation of food intake and body weight in humans: A review. *Obesity Reviews, 8*(1), 21–34. https://doi.org/10.1111/j.1467-789x.2006.00270.x

Koletzko, B., Fishbein, M., Lee, W. S., Moreno, L., Mouane, N., Mouzaki, M., & Verduci, E. (2020). Prevention of childhood obesity: A position paper of the global federation of international societies of pediatric gastroenterology, hepatology and nutrition (FISPGHAN). *Journal of Pediatric Gastroenterology & Nutrition, 70*(5), 702–710. https://doi.org/10.1097/mpg.0000000000002708

Kumari, R., Chachar, S., Ashfaq, M., Nisa, B., Bai, S., & Hussain, W. (2021). Functional status of thyroid among children with obesity. *Rawal Medical Journal, 46*(2), 378–380.

Lappan, S. N., Parra-Cardona, J., Carolan, M., & Weatherspoon, L. (2019). Risk and protective factors associated with childhood obesity in a sample of low-income, single female, parent/guardian households: Implications for family therapists. *Family Process, 59*(2), 597–617. https://doi.org/10.1111/famp.12440

Lawrence, J. M., Divers, J., Isom, S., Saydah, S., Imperatore, G., Pihoker, C., Marcovina, S. M., Mayer-Davis, E. J., Hamman, R. F., Dolan, L., Dabelea, D., Pettitt, D. J., & Liese, A. D. (2021). Trends in prevalence of type 1 and type 2 diabetes in children and adolescents in the US, 2001-2017. *JAMA, 326*(8), 717. https://doi.org/10.1001/jama.2021.11165

Leung, A. K., Lam, J. M., Barankin, B., Leong, K., & Hon, K. (2023). Acanthosis nigricans: An updated review. *Current Pediatric Reviews, 19*(1), 68–82. https://doi.org/10.2174/1573396318666220429085231

Lin, X., & Li, H. (2021). Obesity: Epidemiology, pathophysiology, and therapeutics. *Frontiers in Endocrinology, 12*. https://doi.org/10.3389/fendo.2021.706978

Lobelo, F., Muth, N. D., Hanson, S., & Nemeth, B. A. (2020). Physical activity assessment and counseling in pediatric clinical settings. *Pediatrics, 145*(3). https://doi.org/10.1542/peds.2019-3992

Loos, R. F., & Yeo, G. H. (2022). The genetics of obesity: From discovery to biology. *Nature Reviews Genetics, 23*(2), 120–133. https://doi.org/10.1038/s41576-021-00414-z

Loren, D. M., Rea, E. M., Harber, K. A., & Bohnert, A. M. (2022). An ecological model of weight gain among school-age children. *Health Psychology, 41*(3), 193–203. https://doi.org/10.1037/hea0001163

Ma, Y.-L., Jin, C.-H., Zhao, C.-C., Ke, J.-F., Wang, J.-W., Wang, Y.-J., Lu, J.-X., Huang, G.-Z., & Li, L.-X. (2022). Waist-to-height ratio is a simple and practical alternative to waist circumference to diagnose metabolic syndrome in type 2 diabetes. *Frontiers in Nutrition (Lausanne), 9*, 986090. https://doi.org/10.3389/fnut.2022.986090

Magge, S. N. (2021). *5 Ways to protect your kids against metabolic syndrome: AAP report explained.* Healthy Children.org, America Academy of Pediatrics. https://www.healthychildren.org/English/health-issues/conditions/obesity/Pages/Ways-to-Protect-Your-Kids-Against-Metabolic-Syndrome.aspx?_ga=2.205060116.589045128.1673369726-456064477.1669750353&_gl=1*1afxsyz*_ga*NDU2MDY0NDc3LjE2Njk3NTAzNTM.*_ga_FD9D3XZVQQ*MTY3MzQ1MjMwNC41LjAuMTY3MzQ1MjMwNC4wLjAuMA

Masini, A., Marini, S., Gori, D., Leoni, E., Rochira, A., & Dallolio, L. (2020). Evaluation of school-based interventions of active breaks in primary schools: A systematic review and meta-analysis. *Journal of Science and Medicine in Sport, 23*(4), 377–384. https://doi.org/10.1016/j.jsams.2019.10.008

Matson, K. L., Horton, E. R., & Capino, A. C. (2017). Medication dosage in overweight and obese children. *The Journal of Pediatric Pharmacology and Therapeutics, 22*(1), 81–83. https://doi.org/10.5863/1551-6776-22.1.81

McCabe, E. M. (2020). School nurses' role in self-management, anticipatory guidance, and advocacy for students with chronic illness. *NASN School Nurse, 35*(6), 338–343. https://doi.org/10.1177/1942602x20906534

McGregor, P. C., Lyons, M. M., Wozniak, A., Linko, K., Fishman, F., & Cappello, T. (2022). The effect of obesity on pediatric tibia fractures. *The Iowa Orthopaedic Journal, 42*(1), 41–46.

Merlo, C. L., Jones, S., Michael, S. L., Chen, T. J., Sliwa, S. A., Lee, S., Brener, N. D., Lee, S. M., & Park, S. (2020). Dietary and physical activity behaviors among high school student—Youth Risk Behavior Survey, United States, 2019. *MMWR Supplements, 69*(1), 64–76. https://doi.org/10.15585/mmwr.su6901a8

Mustafa, L., & Chernoguz, A. (2021). Running the obstacle course: Improving the utilization of bariatric surgery in adolescent obesity. *Clinical Therapeutics, 43*(7), 1154–1161. https://doi.org/10.1016/j.clinthera.2021.06.006

Muth, N. D., Dietz, W. H., Magge, S. N., Johnson, R. K., Bolling, C. F., Armstrong, S. C., Haemer, M., Rausch, J., Rogers, V., Abrams, S. A., Kim, J., Schwarzenberg, S., Fuchs, G., Lindsey, C., & Rome, E. S. (2019). Public policies to reduce sugary drink consumption in children and adolescents. *Pediatrics, 143*(4). https://doi.org/10.1542/peds.2019-0282

National Association of School Nurses. (2024). A contemporary framework update for today's school nursing landscape: Introducing the School Nursing Practice Framework. *NASN School Nurse, 39*(3), 140–147. https://www.doi.org/10.1177/1942602X241241092

National Center for Health Statistics. (2023). *Health, United States, 2020–2021: Annual perspective.* https://dx.doi.org/10.15620/cdc:122044

Naviaux, A.-F., Janne, P., & Gourdin, M. (2020). Pediatric obesity, addiction and family dynamics: concept of co-obesity. *International Journal of Recent Advances in Multidisciplinary Research, 7*(9), 6172–6178.

Office of Disease Prevention and Health Promotion. (n.d.). Overweight and obesity. Healthy People 2030. *U.S. Department of Health and Human Services*. https://health.gov/healthypeople/objectives-and-data/

browse-objectives/overweight-and-obesity/reduce-proportion-children-and-adolescents-obesity-nws-04/data

Parrish, A.-M., Tremblay, M. S., Carson, S., Veldman, S. C., Cliff, D., Vella, S., Chong, K., Nacher, M., del Pozo Cruz, B., Ellis, Y., Aubert, S., Spaven, B., Sameeha, M., Zhang, Z., & Okely, A. D. (2020). Comparing and assessing physical activity guidelines for children and adolescents: A systematic literature review and analysis. *International Journal of Behavioral Nutrition and Physical Activity, 17*(1). https://doi.org/10.1186/s12966-020-0914-2

Perdew, M., Liu, S., & Naylor, P.-J. (2021). Family-based nutrition interventions for obesity prevention among school-aged children: A systematic review. *Translational Behavioral Medicine, 11*(3), 709–723. https://doi.org/10.1093/tbm/ibaa082

Piekarz-Porter, E., Lin, W., Leider, J., Turner, L., Perna, F., & Chriqui, J. F. (2020). State laws matter when it comes to school provisions for structured PE and daily PE participation. *Translational Behavioral Medicine, 11*(2), 597–603. https://doi.org/10.1093/tbm/ibaa013

Raman, V., & Foster, C. M. (2021). Metformin treatment of pediatric obesity. *Pediatrics, 147*(3). https://doi.org/10.1542/peds.2020-044982

Raynor, H. A., Robson, S. M., & Griffiths, L. A. (2022). Translating the recommended multicomponent intervention for childhood overweight and obesity into practice: Implementation challenges. *Journal of Contemporary Psychotherapy*. https://doi.org/10.1007/s10879-022-09554-7

Reuben, A., Rutherford, G. W., James, J., & Razani, N. (2020). Association of neighborhood parks with child health in the United States. *Preventive Medicine, 141*, 106265. https://doi.org/10.1016/j.ypmed.2020.106265

Reyes-Angel, J., Kaviany, P., Rastogi, D., & Forno, E. (2022). Obesity-related asthma in children and adolescents. *The Lancet Child & Adolescent Health, 6*(10), 713–724. https://doi.org/10.1016/s2352-4642(22)00185-7

Rhodes, R. E., Guerrero, M. D., Vanderloo, L. M., Barbeau, K., Birken, C. S., Chaput, J.-P., Faulkner, G., Janssen, I., Madigan, S., Mâsse, L. C., McHugh, T.-L., Perdew, M., Stone, K., Shelley, J., Spinks, N., Tamminen, K. A., Tomasone, J. R., Ward, H., Welsh, F., & Tremblay, M. S. (2020). Development of a consensus statement on the role of the family in the physical activity, sedentary, and sleep behaviours of children and youth. *International Journal of Behavioral Nutrition and Physical Activity, 17*(1). https://doi.org/10.1186/s12966-020-00973-0

Scaglioni, S., De Cosmi, V., Ciappolino, V., Parazzini, F., Brambilla, P., & Agostoni, C. (2018). Factors influencing children's eating behaviours. *Nutrients, 10*(6), 706. https://doi.org/10.3390/nu10060706

Schroeder, K., Jia, H., Wang, Y. C., & Smaldone, A. (2017). Implementation of a school nurse-led intervention for children with severe obesity in New York City schools. *Journal of Pediatric Nursing, 35*, 16–22. https://doi.org/10.1016/j.pedn.2017.02.030

Schroeder, K., & Smaldone, A. (2017). What barriers and facilitators do school nurses experience when implementing an obesity intervention? *The Journal of School Nursing, 33*(6), 456–466. https://doi.org/10.1177/1059840517694967

Siopis, G., Wang, L., Colagiuri, S., & Allman-Farinelli, M. (2020). Cost effectiveness of dietitian-led nutrition therapy for people with type 2 diabetes mellitus: A scoping review. *Journal of Human Nutrition and Dietetics, 34*(1), 81–93. https://doi.org/10.1111/jhn.12821

Sleeth, C. M., Peterson, A. L., & Hokanson, J. (2020). Pediatric dyslipidemia screening by pediatricians and family medicine physicians: Current practices and future directions. *Pediatrics*, 636–637. https://doi.org/10.1542/peds.146.1MA7.636

Tak, Y., & Lee, S. (2021). Long-term efficacy and safety of anti-obesity treatment: Where do we stand? *Current Obesity Reports, 10*(1), 14–30. https://doi.org/10.1007/s13679-020-00422-w

Tenedero, C. B., Oei, K., & Palmert, M. R. (2021). An approach to the evaluation and management of the obese child with early puberty. *Journal of the Endocrine Society, 6*(1). https://doi.org/10.1210/jendso/bvab173

Thompson, N., Adams, E. L., Tkacz Browne, N., & Bean, M. K. (2021). Pediatric surgery and school nurse attitudes regarding children with obesity. *Journal of Pediatric Nursing, 59*, 75–80. https://doi.org/10.1016/j.pedn.2021.01.007

Till, H., Mann, O., Singer, G., & Weihrauch-Blüher, S. (2021). Update on metabolic bariatric surgery for morbidly obese adolescents. *Children, 8*(5), 372. https://doi.org/10.3390/children8050372

Trust for America's Health. (2022). *The state of obesity: Better policies for a healthier America.* https://www.tfah.org/wp-content/uploads/2022/09/2022ObesityReport_FINAL3923.pdf

Umstattd Meyer, M., Bridges, C. N., Schmid, T. L., Hecht, A. A., & Pollack Porter, K. M. (2019). Systematic review of how play streets impact opportunities for active play, physical activity, neighborhoods, and communities. *BMC Public Health, 19*(1). https://doi.org/10.1186/s12889-019-6609-4

U.S. Department of Agriculture. (n.d.). MyPlate. https://www.myplate.gov/

U.S. Department of Agriculture. (2013, November 20). *Healthy, hunger-free kids act*. USDA Food and Nutrition Service. https://www.fns.usda.gov/cn/healthy-hunger-free-kids-act

U.S. Department of Agriculture. (2023a). Proposed updates to the school nutrition standards. https://www.fns.usda.gov/cn/proposed-updates-school-nutrition-standards

U.S. Department of Agriculture. (2023b). *Nutrition education and food safety*. Food and Nutrition Service. https://www.fns.usda.gov/nutrition-education

U.S. Department of Agriculture & U.S. Department of Health and Human Services. (2020). *Dietary guidelines for Americans, 2020–2025* (9th ed.). www.dietaryguidelines.gov

U.S. Department of Health and Human Services. (2018). *Physical activity guidelines for Americans* (2nd ed.). https://health.gov/sites/default/files/2019-09/Physical_Activity_Guidelines_2nd_edition.pdf

U.S. Department of Health and Human Services. (2022). *Reduce the proportion of children and adolescents with obesity—data.* Office of Disease Prevention and Health Promotion. https://health.gov/healthypeople/objectives-and-data/browse-objectives/overweight-and-obesity/reduce-proportion-children-and-adolescents-obesity-nws-04/data?group=Age+group%E2%80%A0+%C2%A7&state=United+States&from=2013&to=2020&tab=data-table&populations=#edit-submit

U.S. Preventative Services Task Force; Grossman, D. C., Bibbins-Domingo, K., Curry, S. J., Barry, M. J., Davidson, K. W., Doubeni, C. A., Epling, J. W., Kemper, A. R., Krist, A. H., Kurth, A. E., Landefeld, C., Mangione, C. M., Phipps, M. G., Silverstein, M., Simon, M. A., & Tseng, C.-W. (2017). Screening for obesity in children and adolescents. *JAMA, 317*(23), 2417. https://doi.org/10.1001/jama.2017.6803

Valizadeh, P., & Ng, S. W. (2020). The new school food standards and nutrition of school children: Direct and indirect effect analysis. *Economics and Human Biology, 39*, 100918. https://doi.org/10.1016/j.ehb.2020.100918

Venturelli, F., Ferrari, F., Broccoli, S., Bonvicini, L., Mancuso, P., Bargellini, A., & Giorgi Rossi, P. (2019). The effect of public health/pediatric obesity interventions on socioeconomic inequalities in childhood obesity: A scoping review. *Obesity Reviews, 20*(12), 1720–1739. https://doi.org/10.1111/obr.12931

Wicherski, J., Schlesinger, S., & Fischer, F. (2021). Association between breakfast skipping and body weight—a systematic review and meta-analysis of observational longitudinal studies. *Nutrients, 13*(1), 272. https://doi.org/10.3390/nu13010272

Wong, M., Han, Y.-Y., Rosser, F., Acosta-Pérez, E., Canino, G., Forno, E., & Celedón, J. C. (2022). Persistent overweight or obesity, lung function, and asthma exacerbations in Puerto Rican youth. *Annals of Allergy, Asthma & Immunology, 128*(4), 408–413.e2. https://doi.org/10.1016/j.anai.2022.01.004

World Health Organization. (2024). *Obesity and overweight.* https://www.who.int/news-room/fact-sheets/detail/obesity-and-overweight

Wühl, E. (2018). Hypertension in childhood obesity. *Acta Paediatrica, 108*(1), 37–43. https://doi.org/10.1111/apa.14551

Xu, H., Li, Y., Du, S., Zhang, Q., Liu, A., Sun, J., & Ma, G. (2020). Cost–utility and cost–benefit analyses of school-based obesity prevention program. *BMC Public Health, 20*(1). https://doi.org/10.1186/s12889-020-09718-x

Chapter **15**

Emergency and Disaster Preparedness and Response for Schools

Robin Adair Shannon ▪ Kathy L. Reiner

CHAPTER OUTLINE

Emergencies and disasters can occur at any time, causing large scale damage and disruption to communities. Some emergencies and disasters may be preceded by advance notice, such as hurricanes or pandemics, but many strike without warning, such as earthquakes or hazardous materials release. The scope and effect of an emergency or disaster can be limited to a small locality, like a school, or be more widespread, such as bioterrorism attacks or pandemics. The Federal Emergency Management Agency (FEMA) holds that the *whole community* should be involved in coordinated emergency and disaster preparedness efforts:

> *Preparedness is a shared responsibility; it calls for the involvement of everyone—not just the government—in preparedness efforts. By working together, everyone can help keep the nation safe from harm and help keep it resilient when struck by hazards, such as natural disasters, acts of terrorism, and pandemics. (FEMA, 2020b, paras. 1–2)*

The whole community includes residents, community stakeholders and organizations, and institutions, as well as private and government agencies, including schools (FEMA, 2020b).

Nurses, and importantly school nurses, play critical roles in emergency and disaster preparedness and response, especially in underresourced communities. The *Future of Nursing 2020–2030 Report* states the following:

> *The increasing frequency of natural and environmental disasters and public health emergencies, such as the COVID-19 pandemic, reveals in stark detail the critical importance of having a national nursing workforce prepared with the knowledge, skills, and abilities to respond to these events. COVID-19 has revealed deep chasms within an already fragmented U.S. health care system, resulting in significant excess mortality and morbidity, glaring health inequities, and the inability to contain a rapidly escalating pandemic. Most severely—and unfairly—affected are individuals and communities of color, who suffer from the compound disadvantages of racism, poverty, workplace hazards, limited health care access, and pre-existing health conditions resulting from the foregoing factors. As other disasters and public health emergencies threaten population health in the decades ahead, articulation of the roles and responsibilities of nurses in disaster response and public health emergency management will be critical to the nation's capacity to plan for and respond to these types of events. (National Academies of Sciences, 2021, p. 11)*

School nurses are uniquely qualified for leadership roles before, during, and after an emergency or disaster by virtue of their professional education, expertise, perspectives, and attitudes. Furthermore, the National Association of School Nurses (NASN) Position Statement, *Emergency Preparedness* (2019), highlights that school nurses are leaders in planning for emergency events and multiple casualty incidents and educating staff. School nurses are first responders who provide emergency triage and treatment, as well as long-term physical and emotional first aid to students, staff, and the school community during recovery.

Yet dealing with emergencies and disasters can be one of the most anxiety-provoking roles of the school nurse. Preventing and preparing for, responding to, and recovering from a variety of emergencies and disasters presents many challenges for school communities. The purpose of this chapter is to assist school nurses in their leadership role before, during, and after emergencies and disasters. See Chapter 17 for content on school nursing care for individual students in emergent situations.

EMERGENCIES AND DISASTERS

The terms *emergency* and *disaster* are often interchanged. Although they have many common characteristics, emergencies and disasters are not the same. There is no official U.S. government definition for an emergency, but it is widely understood that an ***emergency*** is a dangerous event potentially affecting many people that can be managed at the local response level. A ***disaster*** is defined by the U.S. Department of Homeland Security (USDHS) as

> *an adverse condition or occurrence that requires coordinated action across multiple entities and/or levels of government to resolve and may be natural, technological, or human-caused; may cause multiple deaths/multiple injuries, property damage/loss, and/or destruction resulting in a serious disruption of the functioning entity; exceeds the ability of the affected entity to cope without outside assistance. (2017b, p. 178)*

Emergencies and disasters present crisis situations; the terms *crisis, critical incident,* and *critical event* are often used in reference to an emergency or disaster situation.

There are a wide range of emergencies and disasters that may present threats and hazards to schools. Threats and hazards represent risks or dangers that are potential precursors to an emergency or disaster. ***Threats*** include human-caused emergencies, such as crime, or violence. ***Hazards*** include natural disasters, disease outbreaks, and accidents (U.S. Department of Education [USDOE] et al., 2019). These have the potential to widely affect schools and surrounding communities. Some incidents, such as explosions or earthquakes, generally cause more localized effects. Local hazards, at first considered an emergency, can evolve into national or even global disasters that require a high level of planning, coordination, and response (FEMA, 2021). The COVID-19 pandemic in 2020 is an example of this. See Table 15-1 for types and examples of threats and hazards.

TABLE 15-1 Threat and Hazard Types and Examples

Type	Examples
Natural Hazards	• Earthquakes • Tornadoes • Lightning • Severe wind • Hurricanes • Floods • Wildfires • Extreme temperatures • Landslides or mudslides • Tsunamis • Volcanic eruptions • Winter precipitation
Technological Hazards	• Explosions or accidental release of toxins from industrial plants • Accidental release of hazardous materials from within the school, such as gas leaks or laboratory spills • Hazardous material releases from major highways or railroads • Radiological releases from nuclear power stations • Dam failure • Power failure • Water failure
Biological Hazards	• Infectious diseases (pandemic influenza, tuberculosis, *Staphylococcus aureus*, meningitis, etc.) • Contaminated food outbreaks (*Salmonella*, botulism, *E. coli*, etc.) • Toxic materials present in school laboratories
Adversarial, Incidental, and Human-Caused Threats	• Fire • Active shooters • Criminal threats or actions • Gang violence • Bomb threats • Domestic violence or abuse • Cyberattacks • Dangerous animals • Suicide • Kidnapping, missing student • Bus accident • Riot/student demonstration

USDOE (2022d), para. 3.

Focus on the Framework

Community/Public Health

The National Association of School Nurse's *21st Century Framework for School Nursing Practice* (2016) identifies the school nurse's connection to **community/public health** as one of the founding principles of school nursing practice. As public health nurses, school nurses are integral to emergency and disaster planning and management.

Regardless of the extent of the critical incident, the degree of community vulnerability and response readiness directly affects the outcomes. The ability of a community to adequately prepare is greatly affected by the available resources, local infrastructure, social determinants of health, and the exposure to existing hazards and threats. In low-income and/or historically marginalized communities, inequities in these capacities often lead to increased vulnerability, disproportionate disruptions, and disparities in recovery (Raju et al., 2022).

In addition, climate change is causing some hazards, such as hurricanes, wildfires, and heat waves, to become more frequent, severe, and longer lasting, resulting in disasters (FEMA, 2021). Disasters often disrupt basic services that are essential to human health and safety, such as water service or electric power. Utility disruptions can be brief and easy to mitigate; but more severe incidents can interrupt services for many weeks or months. This reality necessitates a tiered response with some incidents managed at the local level, while others require state and even federal support to repair services. Underresourced communities are also particularly vulnerable to the risk, multiplying the effects of climate change (Raju et al., 2022).

EMERGENCY AND DISASTER FRAMEWORKS AND PLANNING

In response to the terrorist attacks on September 11, 2001, President George W. Bush signed the first presidential directive to establish the *National Preparedness Goal:* "A secure and resilient Nation with the capabilities required across the whole community to prevent, protect against, mitigate, respond to, and recover from the threats and hazards that pose the greatest risk" (USDHS, 2015, p. 1). The National Preparedness Goal seeks to actively help communities, regions, states, tribes, insular areas, and the nation prepare for emergencies and disasters in five mission areas and across 32 core capabilities. The mission areas are as follows:

Prevention: Prevent, avoid, or stop a threatened or actual act of terrorism.

Protection: Protect our citizens, residents, visitors, and assets against the greatest threats and hazards in a manner that allows our interests, aspirations, and way of life to thrive.

Mitigation: Reduce the loss of life and property by lessening the impact of future disasters.

Response: Respond quickly to save lives, protect property and the environment, and meet basic human needs in the aftermath of a catastrophic incident.

Recovery: Recover through a focus on the timely restoration, strengthening, and revitalization of infrastructure, housing, and a sustainable economy, as well as the health, social, cultural, historic, and environmental fabric of communities affected by a catastrophic incident (FEMA, 2020a, p. 1).

To reach the National Preparedness Goal, *Presidential Policy Directive 8,* signed by President Barack Obama, established the ***National Preparedness System*** in 2011. The National Preparedness System includes the *National Response Framework* (FEMA, 2019) and the *National Incident Management System* (FEMA, 2017). These two guides are meant to work together to provide a model of emergency preparedness that is locally executed, state managed, and federally supported (FEMA, 2019). Federal, state, and local governmental agencies—including local education agencies and private sector and nongovernmental agencies—need to coordinate to prepare for a wide range of events that exceed the capabilities of any single entity (FEMA, 2021). Effective preparation requires the use of recognized concepts, standardized terms, and a unified coordinated national approach.

National Response Framework

The *National Response Framework* describes best practices for efficiently and effectively managing all types of emergencies or disasters. It provides the basis for decision makers and responders to mount a unified and integrated response by outlining standardized command management structures, processes, and protocols (FEMA, 2019). The National Response Framework discusses how entities, such as schools, can work together with communities, states, the federal government, and private partners when responding to emergencies or disasters. The guiding principles are as follows:

- Engaged partnership
- Tiered response
- Scalable, flexible, and adaptable operational capabilities
- Unity of effort
- Readiness to act

National Incident Management System

The *National Incident Management System* (NIMS) reinforces the National Response Framework and details a comprehensive national approach to incident management (FEMA, 2017). It establishes a flexible framework for coordinating, planning, and response activities among all jurisdictions and organizations, regardless of incident cause, size, or complexity. The components of the NIMS are resource management, command and coordination, and communication and information management.

The *Incident Command System* is an element of the command and coordination component of NIMS. Integrating the concepts of NIMS and the Incident Command System into a school emergency operations plan (often referred to as an EOP) ensures common terminology and processes, integration of resources, coordination of planning efforts, and continuous quality improvement among schools and their community partners (USDOE, 2022b).

Developing School Emergency Operations Plans

In 2013 in response to several devastating disasters involving schools, the Obama White House issued a call to the United States Departments of Education, Justice, Health and Human Services, and Homeland Security to develop emergency planning guidance for schools. This directive acknowledged that although most schools had emergency plans in place, many plans were ineffective and did not coordinate with local community partners.

The *Guide to Developing High Quality School Operations Plans (School Guide)* (USDOE et al., 2013) and the companion, *The Role of Districts in Developing High-Quality School Emergency Operations Plans: A Companion to the School Guide* (USDOE et al., 2019), translate Presidential Policy Directive 8 to the school setting, supporting a coordinated response to emergencies in the National Preparedness System's five mission areas of prevention, protection, mitigation, response, and recovery. These guides separate the five mission areas by time frames associated with the incident, before, during, and after. See Figure 15-1.

In addition, the Office of Safe and Supportive Schools administers the *Readiness and Emergency Management for Schools (REMS) Technical Assistance Center* where schools can access support and resources to enhance their emergency operations responsibilities (USDOE, 2022f). Schools are advised to incorporate the planning principles represented in Figure 15-2 to develop a comprehensive school emergency operations plan.

Practice Connection

Healthy People 2030 includes an Emergency Preparedness objective to "Increase the proportion of parents and/or guardians aware of the emergency or evacuation plan in their child(ren)'s school, including the evacuation location and how to get information about the child in the event of a disaster" (PREP-DO1). Explore the Healthy People 2030 to learn more about data-driven objectives to improve the health of the nation (Office of Disease Prevention and Health Promotion, n.d.).

Steps in the Planning Process

According to this guidance from the U.S. Department of Education (2022f, para. 2), there are six steps in the planning process. See Figure 15-3.

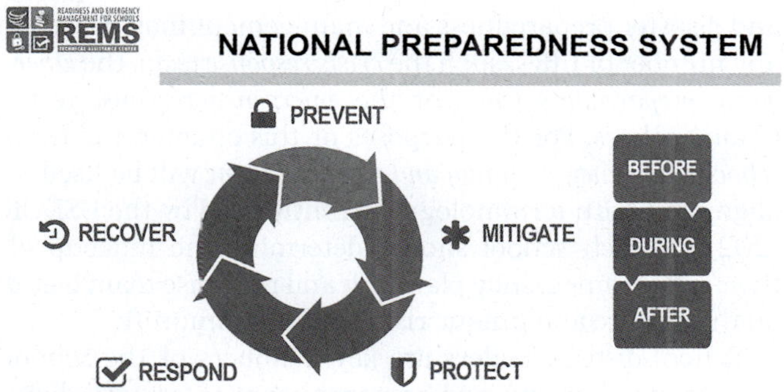

FIGURE 15-1. The National Preparedness System before, during, and after phases. *(From Sullivan et al., 2021 Slide 10.)*

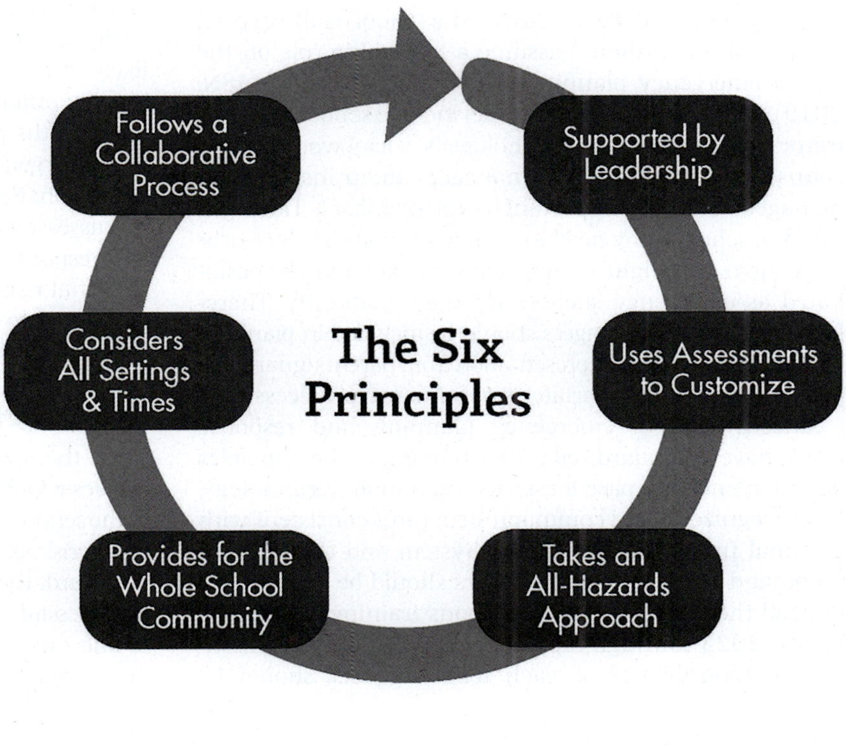

FIGURE 15-2. School emergency operations planning principles. *(USDOE, 2022a, p. 6.)*

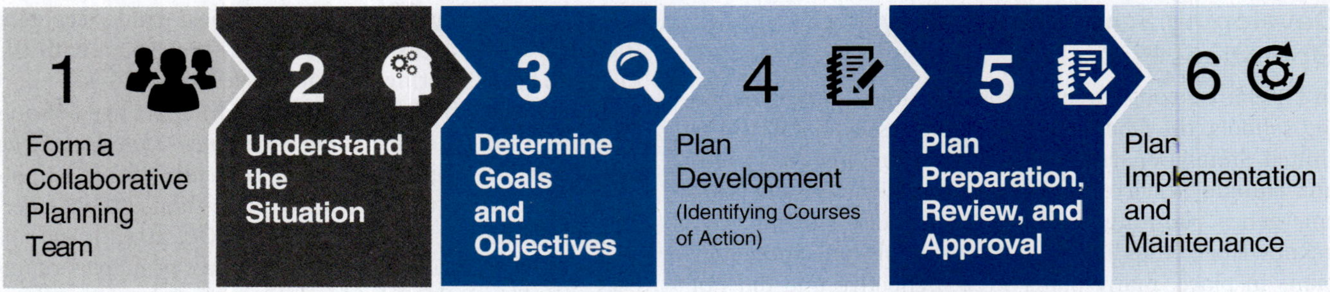

FIGURE 15-3. **K-12: Six steps in school emergency operations planning.** *(USDOE, 2022a, p. 12.)*

Step 1: Form Collaborative Planning Team

Emergency and disaster preparedness means that schools must prepare themselves before, during, and after a critical incident that may involve large numbers of injuries and possibly deaths. The team responsible for school emergency and disaster preparedness and management may be called any number of titles, such the *crisis response team*, the *emergency preparedness team*, or the *emergency response team*, among others. For the purposes of this chapter, the term *school emergency planning and response team* will be used in alignment with terminology currently used by the USDOE (2022a). Each school should determine the makeup of their school emergency planning and response team based on the culture and unique risks of the community.

School district leaders are key members of the school emergency planning and response team to ensure alignment with district priorities and demonstrate commitment to the plan. Involving first responders (e.g., emergency medical services (EMS), fire and police departments, and public and mental health experts) as members of the planning team is essential to provide expertise in emergency management, including knowledge of the Incident Command System (USDOE 2022a). As the school health expert, the school nurse should assume a leadership role on the school emergency planning and response team (NASN, 2019). Other key school personnel include school administrators, teachers, school psychologists, social workers, and counselors. School facilities managers and transportation managers are also important team members. During a disaster, schools may need to shelter students in place over the course of a night or even days, or they may be designated as emergency shelters for the community. Therefore food services managers should be included in planning (USDOE et al., 2019). Representation from parents/guardians and students, as appropriate, is paramount to success.

Effective school emergency planning and response teams have a standardized understanding of the principles of emergency preparedness, use common terminology, and recognize shared command structures consistent with National Incident Management System and the Incident Command System. Team members should be encouraged to avail themselves of the numerous trainings offered by FEMA (2023) through the Emergency Management Institute. Responsibilities of each team member should be clearly defined and communicated. All team members need to take time to learn what their teammates are accountable for and attend regularly scheduled planning meetings (USDOE et al., 2019).

Step 2: Understand the Situation

An effective school emergency operations plan accounts for all possible threats and hazards and is dependent on understanding the unique situation of the school (USDOE et al., 2019). Identifying all potential threats and hazards requires that the school emergency planning and response team share their own knowledge of past, current, or potential threats and hazards, and seek threat and hazard data from local, state, and federal agencies. Strengths and vulnerabilities should be evaluated, including buildings and structures, electrical systems, water and food supplies, and information technology and communication systems. The evaluation should explore four important domains: (1) site assessment, (2) culture and climate assessment, (3) school threat assessment, and (4) capacity assessment.

Once potential threats and hazards and the strengths and vulnerabilities unique to the school community are identified, the team completes a risk assessment to determine the probability that the specific threat or hazard will occur; the likely effects and severity; the time between warning and impact; and the duration of possible events. A risk assessment of the potential hazards and threats helps to prioritize emergency operations planning efforts and resource allocation. See Table 15-2 for a sample school community risk assessment worksheet. The school emergency planning and response team can use this basic format to identify the potential risks in their community and determine numerical ranges to indicate the risk priority of potential threats. Higher scores indicate greater risks (USDOE et al., 2019).

Step 3: Determine Goals and Objectives

Next, the school emergency planning and response team decides which of the potential threats and hazards to address in the school emergency operations plan based on the findings of the risk assessment (USDOE et al., 2019). For each threat or hazard, the team develops goals and objectives to achieve a successful outcome. Goals are broad, general statements of the outcomes that need to be achieved. Objectives are measurable actions or steps to take to achieve the goals.

TABLE 15-2 Sample Risk Assessment Worksheet

Hazard	Probability	Magnitude	Warning	Duration	Risk Priority
Fire	4. Highly likely	4. Catastrophic	4. Minimal	4. 12+ hr	High
	3. Likely	3. Critical	3. 6–12 hr	3. 6–12 hr	Medium
	2. Possible	2. Limited	2. 12–24 hr	2. 3–6 hr	Low
	1. Unlikely	1. Negligible	1. 24+ hr	1. <3 hr	
Hazardous material spill outside the school	4. Highly likely	4. Catastrophic	4. Minimal	4. 12+ hr	High
	3. Likely	3. Critical	3. 6–12 hr	3. 6–12 hr	Medium
	2. Possible	2. Limited	2. 12–24 hr	2. 3–6 hr	Low
	1. Unlikely	1. Negligible	1. 24+ hr	1. <3 hr	

USDOE et al. (2019), Table 4.

See Chapter 8 for more information about writing goals and objectives. Typically, there will be at least one goal and set of objectives per identified threat or hazard in three time frames, before, during, and after the incident. An example of goals and objectives for the high-priority risk of fire is in Figure 15-4.

Additionally, the team considers specific activities, or *cross-cutting functions,* that pertain to multiple threats or hazards, such as communication, evacuation, and continuity of operations (USDOE et al, 2019). This approach allows teams to clearly identify functions that are common across hazards and threats. Understanding these functions assists the school emergency planning and response team to develop an efficient and effective emergency operations plan.

Step 4: Plan Development

The next step is to develop a plan that identifies the courses of action to accomplish the goals and objectives identified in Step 3 (USDOE, 2022a). *Courses of action* are protocols and procedures that address who, what, where, when, and how for each threat, hazard, and function. The school emergency planning and response team typically uses *scenario-based planning* to determine the course of action, which includes the following four steps:

1. *Depict the scenario.* Create a potential scenario based on the threats and hazards identified and prioritized in Step 2.

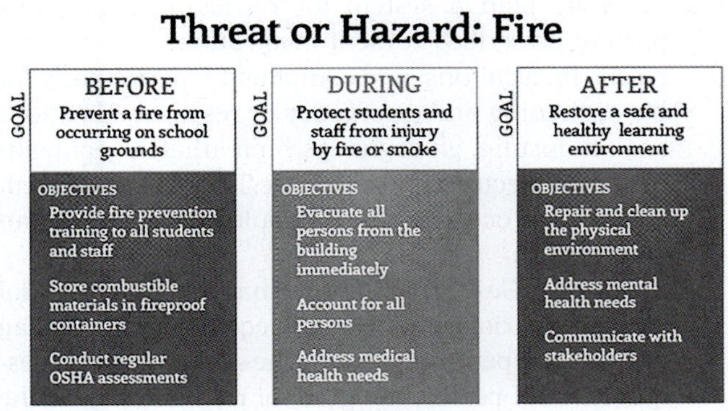

FIGURE 15-4. Threat or hazard: fire. *(USDOE, 2022a, p. 4)*

2. *Determine the amount of time available to respond.* This will vary based on the type of threat or hazard and the scenario. For example, in the case of a hurricane, the school might have days or hours to respond before the storm makes landfall, whereas the school may have to respond in minutes during an armed assailant situation.
3. *Identify decision points.* Decision points indicate the place in timeline, as threats or hazards unfold, when leaders anticipate making decisions about a course of action. Walking through each scenario in detail will help identify the relevant decision points for each threat or hazard, such as whether to evacuate, shelter-in-place, or lockdown.
4. *Develop courses of action.* Planners develop courses of action to achieve their goals and objectives by answering the following questions (USDOE et al., 2019, pp. 34–35):
    - What is the action?
    - Who is responsible for the action?
    - When does the action take place?
    - How long does the action take, and how much time is actually available to perform the action before the school is confronting the hazard?
    - What must happen before a potential emergency?
    - What happens after a potential emergency?
    - What resources are needed to perform the action?
    - How will this action affect specific populations, such as individuals from religiously, racially, and ethnically diverse backgrounds; individuals with limited English proficiency; individuals with cognitive and/or physical disabilities; individuals with mental health needs; and individuals with other access or functional needs? What resources are needed to best support these individuals? The district should work with school core planning teams to develop customized, site-specific courses of action for addressing the goals and objectives that the schools have selected from the district's master list of threats, hazards, and functions. (USDE et al., 2019, pp. 34–35)

Step 5: Plan Preparation, Review, and Approval

In this step, the team writes the school emergency operations plan, obtains official approval and shares the plan with the school staff and community partners, such as first responders, local EMS officials, and other stakeholders (USDE et al., 2019). The plan should be written in clear, understandable language using a logical and consistent format. The plan should summarize all essential information, including checklists and visual aids, such as maps and flowcharts, and equipment and supplies.

A school emergency operations plan traditionally has three sections:

1. The *basic plan*
2. *Functional annexes* that address cross-cutting functions, such as evacuation and reunification
3. *Threat- and hazard-specific annexes* that identify how the school will handle specific threats or hazards, such as an active shooter or a tornado (USDOE et al., 2013)

Table 15-3 lists suggested criteria for evaluating a school emergency operations plan. See Box 15-1 for an outline of a traditional school emergency operations plan.

Health and medical plans, including the school nurse's roles and responsibilities, are included in the *Functional Annex* section of the emergency operations plan. The school nurse should anticipate what is needed in an emergency and prepare needed resources and supplies, including medical supplies and student medications, and ensure they are stocked, stored properly, and accessible. Conducting scenario-based planning, as discussed in Step 4, can identify resources and supplies needed to respond to specific threats and hazards. The school nurse can utilize the findings of the capacity assessment completed in Step 2 to identify available resources both within the school and from community partners. The school nurse should also consider the following actions related to necessary emergency equipment and supplies.

- Maintain and inspect all equipment and supplies at appropriate intervals.
- Avoid items with expiration dates as much as possible. When it cannot be avoided, monitor and replace items when expired. If budget constraints limit replacing expired items, consider whether keeping expired supplies is better than no supplies, depending on the type of supply. Seek professional advice if unsure about a specific supply shelf-life.

Did You Know?

School emergency operations plans should align with state and local requirements, rules, and regulations. Explore the U.S. Department of Education's *Readiness and Emergency Management Technical Assistance Center* Web site for links to each state's laws and regulations related to school safety and emergency preparedness (USDOE, 2022c).

TABLE 15-3 Criteria for Evaluation of a School Emergency Operations Plan

The plan is adequate if it:	• Identifies and addresses critical courses of action • Accomplishes the assigned function • Includes valid assumptions
The plan is feasible if:	• The school can accomplish the assigned function and critical tasks
The plan is acceptable if it:	• Meets the requirements driven by a threat or hazard • Meets costs and time limitations • Is consistent with the law
The plan is complete if it:	• Incorporates all needed courses of action • Integrates the needs of the whole school community • Provides a complete picture of what should happen, when, at whose direction • Estimates times for achieving objectives • Identifies success criteria • Conforms to the planning principles in this guide
The plan is compliant if it:	• Adheres to applicable state and local laws

USDOE et al. (2019), Table 8.

- Place all general emergency equipment in an unlocked office or cabinet to expedite emergency care.
- Medications, nursing equipment, and other healthcare equipment must be easily accessible. Depending on state and local laws and school policy, emergency/rescue medications may be kept in an unlocked but secure location, and nonemergency medications are kept in a locked location. If locked, keys must be readily accessible by authorized staff.
- Clearly mark the location of emergency equipment and supplies on the school site floor plans.
- Keep bleeding control kits with tourniquets in the automated external defibrillator (AED) cabinets.
- If the supply budget does not cover all items, purchase at least a portion of each category of material.
- Carefully plan a system for retrieving and transporting prescribed student medications, emergency/rescue medications, and equipment—particularly for life-sustaining and emergency or rescue medications such as insulin, glucagon, asthma inhalers, epinephrine autoinjectors, and naloxone. Hard copies of medication or procedure orders should be available in an emergency.
- Maintain a *Go Bag*, or Go Box, that includes essential emergency triage and response equipment. A Go Bag is a portable pack or case that the school nurse or designated staff person can grab (or roll) and take to the scene as soon as an emergency is declared.

BOX 15-1

Traditional Format for School Emergency Operations Plans (EOPs)

BASIC PLAN

1. Introductory Material
   1.1 Promulgation Document and Signatures
   1.2 Approval and Implementation
   1.3 Record and Changes
   1.4 Record and Distribution
   1.5 Table of Contents
2. Purpose, Scope, Situation Overview, and Assumptions
   2.1 Purpose
   2.2 Scope
   2.3 Situation Overview
   2.4 Planning Assumptions
3. Concept of Operations
4. Organization and Assignment of Responsibilities
5. Direction, Control, and Coordination
6. Information Collection, Analysis, and Dissemination
7. Training and Exercises
8. Administration, Finance, and Logistics
9. Plan Development and Maintenance
10. Authorities and References

FUNCTIONAL ANNEXES

Note: This is not a complete list, but it is recommended that all EOPs include at least the following annexes:

1. Communications
2. Evacuations
3. Shelter in Place
4. Lockdown
5. Accounting for All Persons
6. Reunification
7. Continuity of Operations
8. Security
9. Recovery
10. Health and Medical

THREAT- OR HAZARD-SPECIFIC ANNEXES

Note: This is not a complete list, but it is recommended that all EOPs include at least the following annexes:

1. Hurricane or Severe Storm
2. Earthquake
3. Tornado
4. Hazardous Materials Incident
5. Mass Casualty Incident
6. Active Shooter
7. Pandemic or Disease Outbreak

USDOE et al. (2019), p. 19.

- Determine a system for documentation during the critical event. The Go Bag should include a notebook or a clipboard with paper and pen to keep an extemporaneous temporal log of assessments, interventions, and dispositions of individuals until more formal documentation can be completed.

See Online Materials OM15-S1 for *NASN Emergency Resources, Equipment, and Supplies.*

Effective communications plans must also be considered and prepared. This includes ensuring that communication devices used during an emergency or disaster are compatible internally and externally with community partners and local responders (USDOE, 2022b). Note that when using a wireless phone, text messaging is more likely than a voice call to go through and less likely to overload the cellular system (Federal Communications Commission, n.d.). Text messages can also be conveyed silently when hiding from an armed assailant. Two-way radios—commonly known as "walkie talkies"—must be able to cover the distance needed but should not be used in the event of explosion hazards because they can detonate some devices. Additional suggestions for means of communication include intercoms, bullhorns, ham radios, or runners.

Step 6: Plan Implementation and Maintenance

With the plan ready to be implemented, several activities need to take place to ensure the effectiveness of the plan. The school nurse has an important role to play in coordinating the implementation of the plan (NASN, 2022). Everyone involved in the plan—including school staff, students, volunteers, and community stakeholders—must be trained on their roles and responsibilities before, during, and after an actual emergency or disaster occurs (USDOE, 2022a). The key components of training are as follows:

- *Hold a meeting.* At least once a year, educate all parties on the plan. Go through the plan to familiarize these stakeholders with it.
- *Visit evacuation sites and other key locations.* Show involved parties not only where evacuation sites are located but also where specific areas, such as reunification areas, media areas, and triage areas, will be located.
- *Provide relevant literature.* Give involved parties appropriate and relevant literature on the plan, policies, and procedures. It may also be helpful to provide all parties with quick reference guides that remind them of key courses of action.
- *Post key information throughout the building.* It is important that students and staff are familiar with and have easy access to information such as evacuation routes and shelter-in-place procedures and locations. Ensure that information concerning evacuation routes and shelter-in place procedures and locations is effectively communicated to the whole school community (students, staff members, families and guardians, visitors with disabilities and other access and functional needs, and individuals with limited English proficiency) by producing accessible information in multiple languages, in Braille, and in electronic formats in compliance with disability laws.
- *Familiarize students and staff with the plan and community partners.* Bringing community partners who have

emergency response roles (e.g., law enforcement officers, fire officials, and EMS personnel) into the school to talk about the plan will make students and staff feel more comfortable working with these partners.

- *Train staff on the skills necessary to fulfill their roles.* School personnel with any role in emergency preparedness, incident management, or response should complete National Incident Management System training (USDOE, 2022b) in addition to any training related to their roles in the plan that require specific skills such as first aid, cardiopulmonary resuscitation/AED training, threat assessment, and provision of personal assistance services for students with disabilities and others with access and functional needs. Training exercises and drills based on the specific needs and context of each school and its surrounding community will help staff work through possible emergency or disaster scenarios. Training can be done in collaboration with community partners to share the details of the plan, increase positive working relationships, and allow for more realistic practice. A regular schedule of drills will provide staff with consistent practice and identify gaps and weaknesses. Consider others who should be trained on the plan and their role such as substitute staff (USDOE, 2022a).

Emergency and disaster preparedness activities include tabletop exercises where the plan is discussed in small groups, drills where key personnel practice responding to potential emergencies or disasters on the school campus, and systems exercises where more full-scale responses involving participating agencies are practiced (USDOE, 2022b). A continuous cycle of review, revision, and practice of the school emergency operations plan is essential to success. A schedule for reviewing and revising portions of the plan regularly will keep the plan updated and avoid the overwhelming task of reviewing and revising the whole plan all at once (USDOE et al., 2019). Preparing the school community can save lives, prevent injury, and minimize property damage in the moments of a crisis.

Planning for Students With Special Healthcare Needs

Students with special healthcare needs may experience especially unique challenges in an emergency that require extra care and coordination, depending on the student's health condition and developmental level. Challenges might include difficulty communicating, understanding the situation, moving, or transitioning quickly. Quick access to medications and treatment, dependence on medical equipment and power, or heightened mental and behavioral health issues may pose additional challenges in an emergency situation (CDC, 2021).

The school nurse should take a leadership role in ensuring that emergency operations planning equitably addresses the unique needs and vulnerabilities of children with special healthcare needs before, during, and after an emergency. As mentioned earlier, health and medical plans, including the school nurse's roles and responsibilities, are included in the Functional Annex section of the emergency operations plan. The school nurse utilizes the nursing process and collaborates with students, families, and the interprofessional team to develop individualized plans, including individualized healthcare plans (IHPs) and emergency action plans for students with special healthcare needs (see Chapters 8 and 20). These plans should include provisions for emergency and disaster preparedness such as the following:

- Information and supplies needed for at least a 72-hour period, including healthcare provider orders, and provisions for medications, special procedures, prescribed diets, supplies, and equipment
- Emergency evacuation plans for students with physical, mental, or communication limitations (e.g., visually and/or hearing impaired, students with autism, and "English as a second language" students)
- Emergency plans for students with special healthcare needs should be readily accessible and updated at least once per year or as changes in status warrant.

In addition, the school nurse can ensure the plan includes the following:

- A system for retrieving and transporting medications and supplies to areas of lockdown or evacuation
- Education of all staff members/substitutes responsible for the child with special healthcare needs on student-specific emergency plans, outlining specific roles and responsibilities to be taken during a disaster
- An alarm system for students with auditory and/or visual needs
- Battery power sources and backup batteries are always fully charged for students who are dependent on electrically powered medical equipment, such as ventilators.

Role of Volunteers

Many parents/guardians and others, including those affiliated and unaffiliated with a voluntary organization, will come to the school and want to help during a critical incident. This presents many challenges and opportunities. The school emergency planning and response team needs to consider how to manage and organize volunteers before, during, and after the event and include this information in the emergency operations plan. In addition to the need for background checks and confidentiality agreements, volunteers must be trained and their roles carefully coordinated with paid staff before they are allowed to assist (USDOE et al., n.d.a). See Online Materials OM15-2 for a fact sheet with detailed information to guide schools in managing volunteers.

THE SCHOOL NURSE'S ROLE IN RESPONSE

When a critical incident occurs, it is time to put the school emergency operations plan into action. The primary role of the school nurse during an emergency or disaster is to follow the communication directives and to provide triage and immediate first-aid care to injured students, staff, family, and community members. The school nurse must be ready to respond as soon as it is safe to do so. Some high-level assessment and treatment tasks should be accomplished only by nurses or EMS. However, school nurses may delegate many basic first aid and simple healthcare tasks to trained personnel as allowed by state nurse practice acts and as outlined in the school emergency operations plan. See Chapters 30 and 31 for more information on school nurse delegation.

Response Protocols

As soon as an emergency or disaster is identified, the response begins by activating the Incident Management System via predetermined signals, codes, or modalities. There is no universally accepted format or language that school districts should use. School districts should be aware that some response protocols must be purchased as products or services and that some proprietary services pertain only to specific scenarios, such as active shooters. Collaboration and agreement with local agencies are recommended before instituting the standard response protocol into the school emergency operations plan.

One commonly adopted format is the *Standard Response Protocol*, which was first developed for kindergarten through 12th-grade schools in 2009 and has undergone several updates (I Love U Guys Foundation, 2022). The Standard Response Protocol is a uniform guideline for school and classroom responses to any critical incident scenario (e.g., severe weather, fires, floods, environmental accidents, violent intruders, and other threats). This protocol represents a synthesis of common crisis procedures used by emergency service providers, law enforcement agencies, and schools.

The Standard Response Protocol uses five clear actions typically communicated over the school public address system. Each action in a given scenario includes a simple directive to be performed by the event participants such as school staff, students, and first responders. Once the scene is safe or at least stable, schools must clearly communicate when the situation is "all clear" and provide specific next step directions. See Box 15-2 for the five Standard Response Protocol actions.

Triage

The goal of emergency first aid is to provide the greatest good for the greatest number of victims through the principle of *triage*, a French word meaning to sort by priority of life-threatening injury. Triage is a basic competency of registered nurses. Triage of multiple or mass casualties at the scene during a critical incident takes special training, which school nurses should have (NASN, 2019). The goal of emergency triage is to sort victims according to acuity and

BOX 15-2

Standard Response Protocol

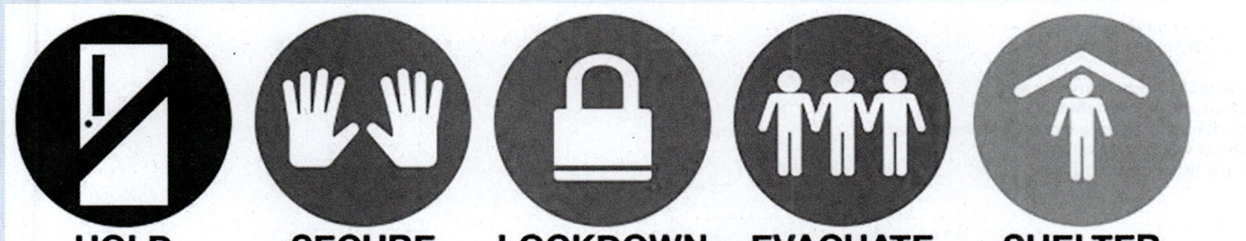

Standard response protocol.

- **Hold** is followed by "In Your Room or Area. Clear the Halls" and is the protocol used when the hallways need to be kept clear of people.
- **Secure** is followed by "Get Inside, Lock Outside Doors" and is the protocol used to safeguard students and staff within the building.
- **Lockdown** is followed by "Locks, Lights, Out of Sight" and is the protocol used to secure individual rooms and keep students quiet and in place.
- **Evacuate** may be followed by a location, and is the protocol used to move students and staff from one location to a different location in or out of the building.
- **Shelter** is always followed by the hazard and a safety strategy and is the protocol for group and self-protection.

From I Love U Guys Foundation (2023), para. 6.

prioritize those in most need of medical help, as well as identify victims who cannot be helped under the circumstances.

During a critical incident involving multiple victims, safety of the responders is the highest priority. Therefore the first assessment that school nurses and first responders must make is scene safety to prevent placing more people in harm's way. Triage begins only when the response protocol indicates that the situation is all clear and the risk of further harm is acceptable. Triage is an ongoing dynamic process because victims who are initially triaged to be stable or have nonurgent injuries can quickly deteriorate to an urgent or emergent status due to evolving acute injuries or serious medical conditions.

The U.S. government recommends a triage system called the *SALT Mass Casualty Triage Algorithm* (Chemical Hazards and Emergency Medical Management [CHEMM], 2022b). SALT stands for *Sort, Assess, Lifesaving interventions, Treatment/Transport.* This triage system is applicable regardless of the age of the victim. See Figure 15-5.

The first triage step is global sorting of victims according to their capacity to move or respond. The second step is to assess individual victims prioritized by acuity. Victims who are not moving or who have obvious life-threatening injuries are assessed first and assigned the triage code RED. Examples of life-threatening injuries include severe head injuries, massive hemorrhage, evisceration, symptomatic shock, and collapsed lung. Significant respiratory distress, loss of consciousness, and exposure to hazardous material are also considered emergent. Lifesaving interventions are implemented immediately as indicated, such as controlling severe bleeding, securing an open airway, giving rescue breaths, starting chest compressions, or administering rescue medications. The victims who are most likely to survive given the treatment and resources at the scene are prioritized for rapid EMS transport to the closest hospital equipped to handle the extent of the injuries (CHEMM, 2022b).

Victims who can wave or are moving purposefully are assessed next. Victims with injuries that are not immediately life-threatening but are serious enough to require urgent medical care are assigned a YELLOW triage code. Delayed transportation to a hospital is not expected to place

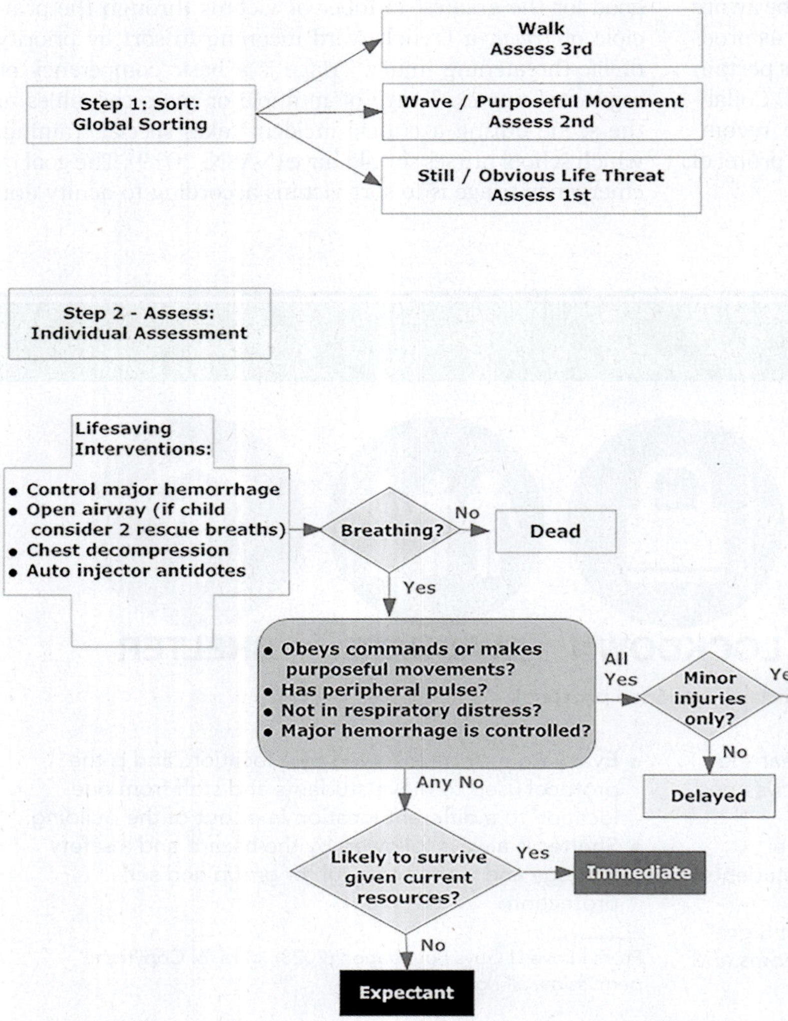

FIGURE 15-5. SALT mass casualty triage algorithm. *(CHEMM, 2022b, p. 1.)*

the victim in jeopardy (CHEMM, 2022b). Examples include extremity fractures, abdominal or facial trauma without shock, moderate blood loss, and moderate burns.

Victims who can walk are assessed last. Those found to have minor injuries needing minimal care and do not require EMS transport other than for convenience (i.e., the *walking wounded*) are assigned a GREEN triage label (CHEMM, 2022b). Examples of nonurgent injuries include minor burns, lacerations, possible joint injuries, and abrasions.

Victims who are legally dead or are not expected to survive due to catastrophic injury are assigned a BLACK triage label. Examples of injuries incompatible with life include exposed brain material, cardiac arrest, respiratory arrest unresponsive to opening the airway, severed trunk, and decapitation (CHEMM, 2022b).

Two other triage system algorithms called *START* and *JumpSTART* are also commonly used in mass casualty scenarios (CHEMM, 2022a, 2022c.). Like SALT Mass Casualty Triage, both START and JumpSTART are effective triage systems for school mass casualty scenarios because complex skills are not required, the assessment is rapid, no specific diagnosis is made, quick stabilization is provided (i.e., airway and major bleeding), and it is easy to teach, learn, and remember. START stands for *Simple Triage And Rapid Treatment* and is applied to triaging adult victims. START can be used if the victim "looks like an adult" (CHEMM, 2022c).

The *JumpSTART Pediatric Multiple Casualty Incident Triage* (CHEMM, 2022a) complements START but is based on the known differences in causes of respiratory arrest between children and adults. Traumatic respiratory failure in adults usually follows circulatory failure or catastrophic head injury, whereas in children, circulatory failure typically follows respiratory failure. JumpSTART also recognizes that some older children can be the size of adults and some children with disabilities can be smaller than usual. JumpSTART can be used if the victim "looks like a child." See Online Materials to reference the START (OM15-3) and JumpSTART (OM15-4) algorithms.

Provide Continuity of Care

Providing effective emergency care in mass casualty incidents is dependent on the ability of the school nurse to prioritize interventions with ill or injured students, staff, and community members. The school nurse should monitor how emergency first aid is being administered to the injured and maintain good communication with EMS. The school nurse should provide as much detailed student-specific information as possible when transferring care to EMS (e.g., diagnoses, medications, allergies).

Did You Know?

NASN (2023) offers an online professional development program called *School Emergency Triage Training* (SETT). "The purpose of SETT is to provide school nurses with the knowledge, skills, and training resources to lead school-based Disaster Response Teams and perform triage in response to mass casualty incident (MCI) events" (para. 5). School Nurses can ask their district to cover the cost of attending this invaluable educational offering.

Document

Documentation may be difficult during a chaotic event but is vitally important. Following an emergency or disaster, the school nurse can use their extemporaneous notes taken during the event to more accurately and formally document the triage and care provided at the scene. Documentation of the incident must be comprehensive, consistent, and completed in a timely manner. Documentation according to the nursing process and standards of practice provides continuity of care and a legal record of events either on paper or electronically. Incident reports must be thorough and accurate, describing the incident, care provided, and actions planned or taken. Notations of agency coordination and resources utilized are important.

Reunify

During and after a large-scale emergency or disaster, students can become separated from the school or their families, such as when they run off school grounds to escape or due to separation during a natural disaster (e.g., tornado, fire, flood, etc.) or human-caused threat (e.g., terrorist attack, school shooting or bombing). Panicked parents/guardians, family members, and caregivers of students and staff will flock to the site of the critical incident to find their child or loved one. According to the Readiness and Emergency Management for Schools (REMS) Technical Assistance Center:

> *As guardians of children, K-12 schools and districts may have a significant role to play in reuniting children with their families. This is especially true when a disaster occurs during normal school hours, before-school programs, after-school programs, or summer programs. In some cases, families may be able to reunite with their children immediately following the disaster. In other cases following a disaster, however, it may take a few days or longer to reunite a child with their family because of a variety of factors that may include: communication challenges with legal guardians, custodial disputes (e.g., those that require evidence of legal guardianship, which may have been destroyed in the disaster), the inability to track or locate children (e.g., lack of registration process or other human tracking tools), deceased legal guardians, wandering or abduction, and long-distance displacement that results in the transfer of people to out-of-state shelters. The task of reuniting children with their families is important, as the risk of trauma or danger experienced by children increases with the time that they remain separated from their family. (USDOE, n.d.b, para. 2)*

The school emergency operations plan must include *courses of action* to account for all persons before, during, and after a critical incident and designate an assembly area (USDOE et al., 2019). The school emergency response team should carefully consider the following:

- How to inform families and guardians about the reunification process in advance, and how to clearly describe their roles and responsibilities in reunification
- How to verify that an adult is authorized to take custody of a student
- How to facilitate communication between the parent check-in and the student assembly and reunion areas
- How to ensure students do not leave on their own
- How to protect the privacy of students and parents from the media
- How to reduce confusion during the reunification process
- How frequently families will be updated
- How to account for technology barriers faced by students, staff, parents, and guardians
- How to effectively address language access barriers faced by students, staff, parents, and guardians (USDOE et al., 2019, p. 69)

In some cases, school emergency response reunification of staff and students with their loved ones may not be immediately possible. The team and community law enforcement and health officials must predetermine how, when, and by whom families will be notified in case individuals are missing, injured, transported off-site, or confirmed dead. Parents/guardians and loved ones must be assured of receiving information related to an active shooter incident in a timely and compassionate manner. See Online Materials OM15-S5 for guidance on post-disaster reunification in the school setting.

Communicate

Communications infrastructure may be disrupted during an emergency or disaster. As outlined in the school emergency operations plan, the school team must communicate clearly and frequently with and to the school community. Schools must have multiple modes of information technology (e.g., phone, computer, two-way radios) to keep the lines of communication open. Interoperability of communication channels between the school and local responding agencies is of paramount importance. The school nurse is typically the communications liaison with healthcare systems and providers. Parents/guardians of injured students or students with special healthcare needs need clear and regularly updated information from the school nurse during a crisis. It is wise to set up clear expectations and lines of communication to avoid misunderstanding and confusion. Schools are wise to consider using social media channels and the school Web site to update the school community as the situation evolves during and after the event to minimize misinformation and disinformation from spreading.

Debrief

Debriefing after the event is an essential component for all involved. The debriefing should be conducted as soon as possible to ensure that the events are fresh in the emergency response team's mind. It is a way to evaluate the school's response, including the delivery of first aid and emergency care. It also allows the team to evaluate the emergency operations plan. Debriefing allows the team to discuss the physical and mental status of students, staff, and responders. This can be a difficult time for the team as they too have just experienced the critical incident being discussed. The mental health of members of the school emergency response team and educational staff is a primary concern. The debriefing should be guided by a skilled facilitator (not the school nurse or other team members involved in the event). During the debriefing, group norms are agreed to; everyone is given a chance to speak, but individuals may elect to pass. The debriefing should be considered a "safe space" and confidentiality ensured, unless the facilitator feels a group member is in danger of hurting themself or others (see Recovery section later in this chapter).

POTENTIAL EMERGENCIES OR DISASTERS AFFECTING SCHOOLS

It is not feasible to cover all potential threats and hazards that may affect school communities. Select scenarios will be discussed as exemplars for emergency preparedness in schools.

Pandemics

The U.S. government defines a *pandemic* as "a disease outbreak that spans several countries and affects a large number of people. Pandemics are most often caused by viruses, like Coronavirus Disease 2019 (COVID-19), which can easily spread from person to person" (Ready.gov, 2022, para. 1). Pandemics are caused by exposure to a novel (new) or quickly mutating virus. Therefore few people will have immunity against a pandemic virus, and a vaccine might not be developed or widely available allowing rapid community spread. The number of people who become sick and how sick they become will depend on the characteristics of the virus, whether people have any immunity to that virus, and the health and age of the persons being infected.

In the history of modern health care, the threat and impact of a pandemic has never been more acutely experienced in the United States and globally than during the COVID-19 pandemic. First declared as a public health emergency in the United States on January 31, 2020, the United States recorded over 1 million deaths attributable to COVID-19 by May 12, 2022 (CDC, 2022a). As discussed throughout this textbook, the implications for public health, education, students, families, and communities related to the pandemic are profound and continue to unfold, particularly for students living in low-income households and under-resourced, historically marginalized communities.

Major lessons learned during the COVID-19 pandemic are applicable to any emergency and disaster that entails a long recovery time or the restoration of infrastructure (power, phone and Internet, roads, and school buildings). For example, schools need to have a *Continuity of Operations* (COOP) annex in their emergency operations plan (USDOE, 2022e). Continuity of operations plans anticipate short- and long-term periods of widespread student and staff absences, school dismissals and/or closures, including the urgency of dissemination of health guidelines and the transfer of student learning to online platforms with technology support. See Chapter 13 for more information about COVID-19.

School nurses should be ever vigilant in anticipating outbreaks of novel viruses in school populations and work closely with public health authorities to prevent and mitigate spread through communities. In 2009, it was a New York parochial school nurse, Maria Pappas, who recognized the first school outbreak of the novel influenza A (H1N1) virus when scores of her high school students fell ill on the same day. She immediately brought it to the attention of the health department (Pappas, 2011). During the winter of 2023, the United States experienced a *tripledemic* in which three respiratory viruses, COVID-19, influenza, and respiratory syncytial virus, were in high circulation at the same time. Children were especially affected, and the pediatric hospital bed capacities in many states were overflowing (Stein, 2022).

School communities need to be prepared not only for large numbers of ill people but also for a depleted workforce and the possibility of disruption of the community's infrastructure. Recommendations from the CDC may change frequently based on new data. It is critical that school nurses keep up to date on the current information and be able to change practices on the spot as new directives are given by the CDC, as well as state and local health departments.

The school emergency operations plan should contain a *Continuity of Operations Plan Annex* that addresses which staff are cross-trained to fill in for team members who may become ill and need to quarantine or who have been exposed and need to isolate. The school nurse should lead pandemic planning efforts that include members of the health department, key community stakeholders, and medical professionals. The continuity of operations plan should also include how the school can carry out mass immunization at school-located vaccination clinics, with support of the school nurse and public health officials (Park et al., 2021). School-located vaccination clinics may be especially important in rural states without large organized public health infrastructures. See Chapter 13 for more information on school-located vaccination clinics.

The school nurse's role includes collaborating with local health departments on novel virus surveillance. This includes alerting the health department of unusually high numbers of student and staff absences or health office visits due to respiratory virus symptoms, which can indicate an outbreak. Once an outbreak is suspected or confirmed, students with symptoms should be isolated in a separate area away from asymptomatic persons. Appropriate personal protective equipment should be worn by nurses or school staff that supervise students who are symptomatic. Parents/guardians should be notified that they will be expected to make arrangements to pick up their children if they become ill. Healthcare systems and practitioners need to be notified if large numbers of patients with influenza-like illness will be sent to them.

Extreme Weather Events

Extreme weather events, such as heat waves and severe storms, are occurring more often and causing more devastation. Rising global average temperatures associated with human-caused (i.e., anthropogenic) climate change is associated with increasing intensity and frequency of extreme weather (U.S. Environmental Protection Agency, 2022). In 2022, the United States experienced 18 separate weather and climate disasters that cost an estimated $165 billion and caused 474 deaths, including a winter storm and cold wave, wildfires, drought and heat waves, flooding, tornado outbreaks, hurricanes, and severe weather/hail events (National Oceanic and Atmospheric Administration, 2023).

The risks of climate or weather-related emergencies and disasters are often amplified and cascade in the context of human vulnerability (Raju et al., 2022). Increasingly, tornadoes surprise communities in the Midwest and South during winter. Intense hurricanes evolve in rapid succession, devastating coastal communities. Severe and lasting seasons of drought lead to massive wildfires, destroying forests and homes. Heavy rains or snowmelt in the wake of fires can cause flooding and mudslides. Power outages damage and disrupt communications, vital services (police, fire, health care), and infrastructure. The wake of such extreme weather events furthers the cycle of vulnerability, especially for children who are English language learners, live with a disability or in low-income households, or belong to historically marginalized groups (U.S. Government Accountability Office, 2022).

As discussed earlier, schools should conduct threat and hazard assessments that consider both the risks and the vulnerabilities so school communities can prepare and respond to mitigate the most harm (USDOE, 2022d). The impact may be short term (hours or days) or long term (weeks, months, years). Schools need to coordinate with emergency and disaster authorities to prepare *continuity of operations plans* for potential scenarios (USDOE, 2022e). How will the district respond if the school or surrounding infrastructure is physically damaged or if the community loses essential utilities for an extended period (e.g., power, communications, Internet, sewer, water)? How and where could families be relocated, or how can the school itself become a safe place for families to reunite, shelter, and receive needed food, donations, and recovery services? Teams must consider how learning could continue at alternate sites or how to switch to virtual learning. Continuity of operations plans should be included as an annex to the main school emergency operations plan (USDOE, 2022e).

School Shootings

In 1999, when two students killed 19 people at Columbine High School in Colorado, the nation was shocked (Aster, 2017). Since then, school shootings have become alarmingly frequent across the United States. In 2020, firearm-related injuries replace motor vehicle crashes as the leading cause of death in children and adolescents (Goldstick et al., 2022). The shootings at Sandy Hook Elementary School in Newtown, Connecticut, left 20 students and six adults dead and two adults wounded on December 14, 2012 (USDOJ, FBI, 2018). In 2018, a lone shooter at Marjory Stoneman Douglas High School in Parkland, Florida, killed 17 students and staff and injured another 17. On May 24, 2022, in Uvalde, Texas, a shooter entered Robb Elementary School in Uvalde, Texas, and killed 19 students (ages 7 to 10 years) and two teachers; an additional 18 students and staff were wounded. In 2022 alone, there were 51 school shooting incidents resulting in 140 casualties, 39 of whom were killed, including 32 children (Blad et al., 2022). See Figure 15-6 for statistics on school shootings.

Such grim societal realities necessitate that an effective all-hazards approach must include response to an armed assailant or active shooter on school property. The U.S. Department of Homeland Security defines an *active shooter* as an "individual who is engaged in killing or attempting to kill people in a confined and populated area; active shooters use firearms(s) and there is no pattern or method to their selection of victims" (FEMA, 2018, para. 2). School shooting incidents are unpredictable and unfold quickly. The common reaction in a crisis is panic or fear. Armed assailant preparedness training can save lives and should be conducted in coordination with local law enforcement agencies (USDHS, 2017).

It is essential to instill a culture of vigilance and readiness throughout the school. However, realistic drills involving props (e.g., guns), noises, or physical interactions can be traumatizing for any age participant and should not be conducted (National Association of School Psychologists [NASP] et al., 2020). Schools should practice armed assailant drills that are developmentally appropriate, options-based, and nonsensorial, meaning that the drill is conducted "by calmly walking and talking through the procedures, with no simulation of a real-life event" (NASP et al., 2020, p. 2).

The school's armed assailant response plan must indicate what means will be used to communicate that there is an active shooter in the school. The accepted standardized response protocol discussed earlier in this chapter and specific directives should be used to inform the students and staff of what is happening in the immediate situation (I Love U Guys Foundation, 2022). Code words should not be used as they do not give enough direction to the school community (Selekman & Melvin, 2017).

Federal and local law enforcement agencies recommend three possible tactics individuals can take to increase the chance of survival during an active shooting: *Run, Hide, or Fight* (FBI, 2020). Table 15-4 describes these tactics. Running means escaping through the nearest exit or escape route and continuing to run with hands up until reaching safety. Hiding includes blocking the door with every piece of office/classroom furniture available and remaining quiet, including silencing cell phones. When it is not possible to run or hide, one should fight "for their life," ideally using a coordinated attack with any improvised weapon available (e.g., fire extinguishers, blunt objects; FBI, 2020).

At the same time the school emergency operations plan is activated to alert others of an armed assailant, the area Incident Command System is put into effect. Armed teams of police officers will arrive wearing protective equipment. Their priority is to locate and stop the assault, not to assist

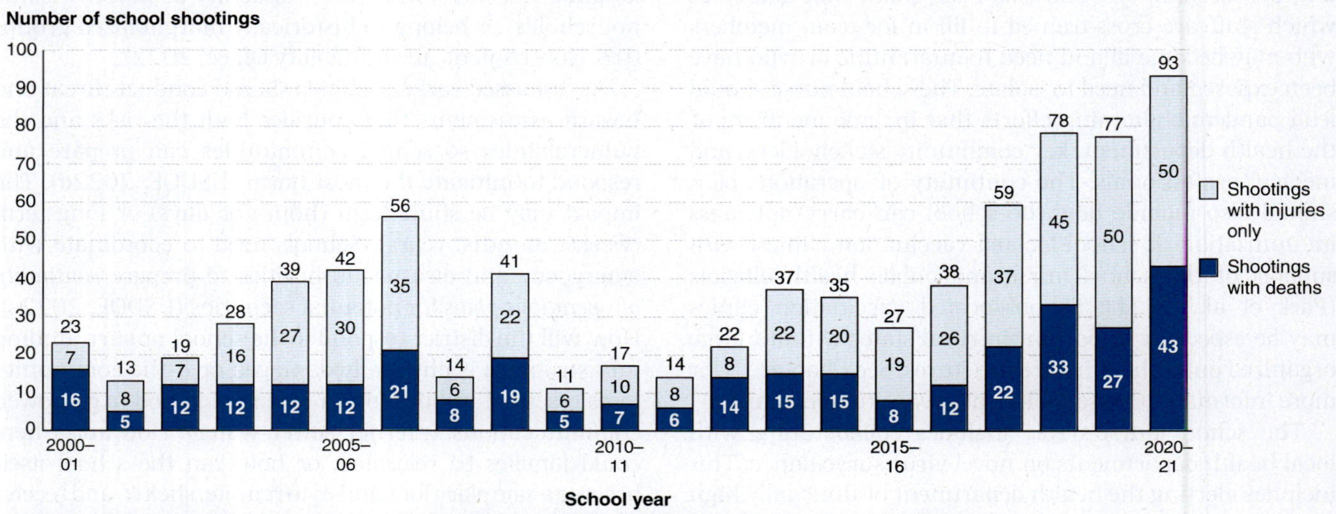

FIGURE 15-6. School shootings with casualties: 2000–2021. *(National Center for Education Statistics, 2022, para. 6.)*

TABLE 15-4 Run, Hide, Fight

Response	Important Note: More Than One Response May Be Required
Run/escape if possible	Have an escape route and plan in mind.
	Leave your belongings behind.
	Evacuate regardless of whether others agree to follow.
	Help others escape, if possible.
	Do not attempt to move the wounded.
	Prevent others from entering an area where the active shooter may be.
	Keep your hands visible.
	Call 911 when you are safe.
Hide if escape is not possible.	Hide in an area out of the shooter's view.
	Lock door or block entry to your hiding place.
	Silence your cell phone (including vibrate mode) and remain quiet.
Fight only as a last resort.	Fight as a last resort and only when your life is in imminent danger.
	Attempt to incapacitate the shooter.
	Act with as much physical aggression as possible.
	Improvise weapons or throw items at the active shooter.
	Commit to your actions ... your life depends on it.
When law enforcement arrives	Remain calm and follow instructions.
	Drop items in your hands (e.g., bags, jackets).
	Raise hands and spread fingers. Keep hands visible at all times.
	Avoid quick movements toward officers, such as holding on to them for safety. Avoid pointing, screaming, or yelling.
	Do not ask questions when evacuating.

FBI (2020).

injured victims, who will be tended to by first responders once the scene is safe. Students and staff should expect to hear loud noises, including shouting and gunshots. It is important that students and staff remain calm and follow the instruction of police officers and school authorities (FBI, 2020).

Once the scene is safe after an active shooter event, the school nurse takes a lead role—possibly being the first on the scene to assess and assist victims according to the triage algorithms described earlier. The school nurse is a role model in calming others and enforcing the emergency operations plan.

RECOVERY

Emergencies and disasters are traumatic events for children and adults alike. Victims of trauma or loss will react based on a variety of influences: life history, personality, social support systems, previous losses, proximity to the critical incident, coping strategies, age, and developmental stage (National Education Association [NEA], 2018). Trauma may change the way individuals view the world and make them feel less secure.

As a central source of community support after an emergency or disaster, schools are often among the first agencies to reopen, sometimes at an alternate site if the school has been damaged or is inaccessible. As quickly as possible after an emergency or disaster, it is essential to return to school routines to establish a sense of resiliency and healing. There are four recognized areas of recovery from a natural disaster or emergency: emotional, academic, financial, and physical. See Figure 15-7.

After a traumatic event, it is common for both children and adults to experience a sense of grief and loss, as well as guilt or self-blame that they should have done more to prevent harm (NEA, 2018). People often feel a loss of control, hopelessness, anxiety, and/or depression. Some individuals may inappropriately turn to drugs, alcohol, or food for comfort. Others may experience sleep disturbances, numbness, withdrawal, or somatic complaints. It may be difficult to concentrate and continue with daily responsibilities and routines of school due to an increased sense of responsibility and worry about safety (NEA, 2018).

Some children may process their emotions related to a crisis within a few days to weeks, while others take much longer to recover. Limiting exposure to media coverage and social media about the critical event is recommended to reduce exposure to triggering events and mitigate retraumatization. It is imperative that the school nurse and all members of the crisis team understand reactions to trauma. According to the National Association of School Psychologists, the following reactions are typical:

- *Preschoolers*—thumb sucking, bedwetting, clinging to parents, sleep disturbances, loss of appetite, fear of the dark, regression in behavior, and withdrawal from friends and routines
- *Elementary school children*—irritability, aggressiveness, clinginess, nightmares, school avoidance, poor concentration, and withdrawal from activities and friends
- *Adolescents*—sleeping and eating disturbances, agitation, increase in conflicts, physical complaints, delinquent behavior, and poor concentration (NASP, 2017, para. 11)

Teachers and school staff, including the school nurse, may feel especially responsible for student well-being, while simultaneously being concerned for their own safety and that of their families. Adults at school may have difficulty concentrating, calming emotions, and carrying out daily

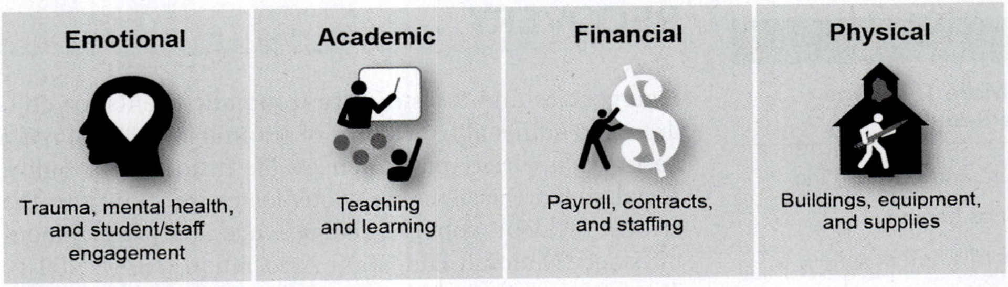

FIGURE 15-7. Key aspects of school recovery from a natural disaster or emergency. *(U.S. Government Accountability Office, 2022, p. 1.)*

routines. Children will pick up the anxiety of adults, so it is important that adults receive the psychological support they need. School personnel may benefit from external mental health resources or accessing employee assistance services available through district employee assistance programs (NEA, 2018).

It is imperative that school nurses take a leadership role in an interdisciplinary team approach to address the immediate and long-term mental health needs of the students and staff. The school nurse may see increased health office visits for students with somatic complaints or an increase in chronic absenteeism related to stress, anxiety, or depression. It is important for school staff to understand how to support students appropriately after trauma. However, teachers and school support personnel, including the school nurse, should not be expected to provide counseling, mental health treatment, or grief support for individuals who have difficulty coping, display maladaptive behaviors, or are overwhelmed by loss. Teams of experts should be brought in from outside to provide the needed professional services (NEA, 2018). Schools must offer sufficient mental health resources to help the students and school community recover and to minimize the risk for vulnerable individuals to experience secondary trauma and/or post-traumatic stress disorder (PTSD) for lack of proper intervention.

The school nurse and school mental health team should connect students to mental health services for evaluation and treatment who exhibit significant, inappropriate, or prolonged reactions. Individualized support and services should be given to children who

- Have loved ones that have been killed or injured, or are missing
- Must continue to live in or relocate from devastated communities
- Have survived other natural disasters
- Are grieving a recent death of a parent/guardian or family member
- Have preexisting trauma or mental/behavioral health concerns (NEA, 2018).

There is much the school staff can do to support the emotional well-being of the student body and staff during and after an emergency or disaster. Teachers can provide developmentally appropriate classroom activities to help students process the event and feel positive about the future. A widely accepted approach is *Psychological First Aid for Schools (PFA-S), which is*

> *an evidence-based intervention model to assist students, families, school personnel, and school partners in the immediate aftermath of an emergency. PFA-S is designed to reduce the initial distress caused by emergencies and to foster short- and long-term adaptive functioning and coping. (Brymer et al., 2012, p. 3)*

Psychological First Aid for Schools is not to be confused with treatment from mental health professionals; it can be implemented by any school staff person with Psychological First Aid for Schools provider training as soon as it is safe to do so, sometimes while the incident is still evolving. The goal of PFA-S is to promote a sense of resilience and normalcy and identify those most in need of further help. PFA-S should be culturally sensitive and consider the needs of students with special healthcare needs and disabilities. There are eight core actions of PFA-S.

1. *Contact and engagement.* Goal: To initiate contacts or to respond to contacts by students and staff in a nonintrusive, compassionate, and helpful manner
2. *Safety and comfort.* Goal: To enhance immediate and ongoing safety and provide physical and emotional comfort
3. *Stabilization (if needed).* Goal: To calm and orient emotionally overwhelmed or disoriented students and staff
4. *Information gathering: current needs and concerns.* Goal: To identify immediate needs and concerns, gather additional information, and tailor PFA-S interventions to meet these needs
5. *Practical assistance.* Goal: Offer practical help to students and staff in addressing immediate needs and concerns
6. *Connection with social supports.* Goal: To help establish brief or ongoing contacts with primary support persons or other sources of support, including family, friends, teachers, and other school and/or community resources
7. *Information on coping.* Goal: To provide information about stress reactions and coping to reduce distress and promote adaptive functioning
8. *Linkage with collaborative services.* Goal: To link students and staff with available services needed at the time or in the future (Brymer et al., 2012, p. 17)

Did You Know?

Explore the *National Child Traumatic Stress Network* Web site (n.d.) for a wealth of information about child trauma, trauma types, populations at risk, trauma treatments, and screening and assessment, as well as other resources.

CONCLUSION

Natural and human-caused emergencies and disasters test the school's ability to effectively respond and protect the well-being of students, staff, and the school community. Well-planned and well-practiced school emergency operations are essential across all areas of emergency and disaster preparedness: *prevention, protection, mitigation, response,* and *recovery.* Schools provide safe haven for the students, staff, their families, and the community by disseminating information, identifying environments and individuals at risk, providing prehospital care, restoring teaching and learning, linking individuals to services, and supporting long-term recovery.

Preparing schools for crises can save lives, prevent injury, and minimize property damage in the moments of a crisis. As trusted and respected health professionals, it is incumbent on school nurses to take leadership roles before, during, and after emergencies and disasters affecting schools.

The Editors gratefully acknowledge the work of authors on this chapter in previous editions: Janice Doyle, Betty Fitzpatrick, and Patricia Guilday.

References

Aster, M. (2017). Columbine shocked the nation. Now mass shootings are less surprising. *The New York Times.* https://www.nytimes.com/2017/11/10/us/columbine-texas-mass-shooting.html

Blad, E., Baker, L., Kim, H., & Peele, H. (2022, December 31). *Education week.* https://www.edweek.org/leadership/school-shootings-this-year-how-many-and-where/2022/01

Brymer, M., Taylor, M., Escudero, P., Jacobs, A., Kronenberg, M., Macy, R., Mock, L., Payne, L., Pynoos, R., & Vogel, J. (2012). *Psychological first aid for schools: Field operations guide* (2nd ed.). National Child Traumatic Stress Network. https://www.nctsn.org/sites/default/files/resources//pfa_schools.pdf

Centers for Disease Control and Prevention. (2021, January 6). *Children and youth with special healthcare needs in emergencies.* https://www.cdc.gov/childrenindisasters/children-with-special-healthcare-needs.html

Centers for Disease Control and Prevention. (2022a, August 16). *CDC Museum: COVID-19 timeline.* https://www.cdc.gov/museum/timeline/covid19.html#:~:text=January%2031%2C%202020&text=The%20Secretary%20of%20the%20Department,outbreak%20a%20public%20health%20emergency

Chemical Hazards and Emergency Medical Management. (2022a, November 16). *JumpSTART Pediatric Triage Algorithm.* U.S. Department of Health and Human Services, Administration for Strategic Preparedness and Response. https://chemm.nlm.nih.gov/startpediatric.htm#more

Chemical Hazards and Emergency Medical Management. (2022b). *SALT mass casualty triage algorithm (Sort, Assess, Lifesaving interventions, Treatment/Transport).* U.S. Department of Health and Human Services, Administration for Strategic Preparedness and Response. https://chemm.hhs.gov/salttriage.htm

Chemical Hazards and Emergency Medical Management. (2022c.). *START adult triage algorithm.* U.S. Department of Health and Human Services, Administration for Strategic Preparedness and Response. https://chemm.hhs.gov/startadult.htm

Federal Bureau of Investigation. (2020, September 21). *Run. Hide. Fight: FBI training video.* https://www.fbi.gov/video-repository/run-hide-fight-092120.mp4/view

Federal Communications Commission. (n.d.). *Tips for communicating in an emergency.* https://www.fcc.gov/reports-research/guides/tips-communicating-emergency

Federal Emergency Management Agency. (2017, October). *National incident management system.* U.S. Department of Homeland Security. https://www.fema.gov/sites/default/files/2020-07/fema_nims_doctrine-2017.pdf

Federal Emergency Management Agency. (2018). *Be prepared for an active shooter.* U.S. Department of Homeland Security. https://www.fema.gov/media-library-data/1523561958719-f1eff6bc841d56b7873e018f73a4e024/ActiveShooter_508.pdf

Federal Emergency Management Agency. (2019). *National Response Framework.* U.S. Department of Homeland Security. https://www.fema.gov/sites/default/files/2020-04/NRF_FINALApproved_2011028.pdf

Federal Emergency Management Agency. (2020a, July 20). *Mission areas and core capabilities.* U.S. Department of Homeland Security. https://www.fema.gov/emergency-managers/national-preparedness/mission-core-capabilities

Federal Emergency Management Agency. (2020b, October 6). *Whole community.* U.S. Department of Homeland Security. https://www.fema.gov/glossary/whole-community

Federal Emergency Management Agency. (2021). *National preparedness report December 2021.* U.S. Department of Homeland Security. https://www.fema.gov/sites/default/files/documents/fema_2021-national-preparedness-report.pdf

Federal Emergency Management Agency, Emergency Management Institute. (2023, March 1). *Welcome to national preparedness: Online course catalog.* U.S. Department of Homeland Security. https://training.fema.gov/

Goldstick, J. E., Cunningham, R. M., & Carter, P. M. (2022). Current causes of death in children and adolescents in the United States. *The New England Journal of Medicine, 386*(20), 1955–1956. https://doi.10.1056/NEJMc2201761

I Love U Guys Foundation. (2023). The standard response protocol K12 schools and districts: Operational guidance for implementing the standard response protocol in a K12 environment. https://iloveuguys.org/The-Standard-Response-Protocol.html

National Academies of Sciences, Engineering, and Medicine; National Academy of Medicine; Committee on the Future of Nursing 2020–2030. (2021). *The future of nursing 2020-2030: Charting a path to achieve health equity.* National Academies Press. https://www.ncbi.nlm.nih.gov/books/NBK573904/

National Association of School Nurses. (2016). Framework for 21st century school nursing practice. *NASN School Nurse, 31*(1), 45–53. https://www.doi.org/10.1177/1942602X15618644

National Association of School Nurses. (2019). Emergency preparedness (Position Statement). Author. https://www.nasn.org/nasn-resources/professional-practice-documents/position-statements/ps-emergency-preparedness

National Association of School Nurses. (2022). *School nursing: Scope and standards of practice* (4th ed.). Silver Spring, MD: Authors

National Association of School Nurses. (2023). School emergency triage training (SETT). https://learn.nasn.org/courses/9102

National Association of School Psychologists. (2017). Large-scale natural disasters: Helping children cope [handout]. https://www.nasponline.org/resources-and-publications/resources-and-podcasts/school-safety-and-crisis/natural-disaster-resources/large-scale-natural-disasters-helping-children-cope

National Association of School Psychologists, Safe and Sound Schools, & National Association of School Resource Officers. (2020, April). *Best practice considerations in armed assailant drills in schools.* https://www.nasponline.org/resources-and-publications/resources-and-podcasts/school-safety-and-crisis/systems-level-prevention/best-practice-considerations-for-armed-assailant-drills-in-schools

National Center for Education Statistics. (2022). Violent deaths at school and away from school and school shootings. *Condition of education.* U.S. Department of Education, Institute of Education Sciences. https://nces.ed.gov/programs/coe/indicator/a01/violent-deaths-and-shootings?tid=4

National Child Traumatic Stress Network. (n.d.). *What is child trauma?* https://www.nctsn.org/what-is-child-trauma/trauma-types/disasters

National Education Association. (2018). *School crisis guide: Help and healing in a time of crisis.* https://www.nea.org/resource-library/neas-school-crisis-guide

National Oceanic and Atmospheric Administration. (2023, January 10). *Record drought gripped much of the U.S. in 2022: Nation struck with 19 billion-dollar disasters.* https://www.noaa.gov/news/record-drought-gripped-much-of-us-in-2022

Obama, B. (2011, March 30). *Presidential policy directive. PPD-8L: National preparedness.* The White House, Office of the President. https://www.dhs.gov/xlibrary/assets/presidential-policy-directive-8-national-preparedness.pdf

Obama White House. (2013, January 16). The time is now: The President's plan to protect our children and our communities by reducing gun violence. The White House, Office of the President. https://obamawhitehouse.archives.gov/sites/default/files/docs/wh_now_is_the_time_full.pdf

Office of Disease Prevention and Health Promotion (OASH). (n.d.). *Emergency Preparedness – Healthy People 2030.* health.gov. https://odphp.health.gov/healthypeople/objectives-and-data/browse-objectives/emergency-preparedness

Pappas, M. (2011). From local school nurse to national advocate. *NASN School Nurse, 26*(3), 180–182. https://www.doi.org/10.1177/1942602X11404559

Park, K., Cartmill, R., Johnson-Gordon, B., Landes, M., Malik, K., Sinnott, J., Wallace, K., & Wallin, R. (2021). Preparing for a school-located COVID-19 vaccination clinic. *NASN School Nurse, 36*(3), 156–163. https://www.doi.org/10.1177/1942602X21991643

Raju, E., Boyd, E., & Otto, F. (2022). Stop blaming the climate for disasters. *Communications Earth & Environment, 3*(1). https://doi.org/10.1038/s43247-021-00332-2

Ready.gov. (2022, November 17). Pandemics. Ready.gov. https://www.ready.gov/pandemic

Selekman, J., & Melvin, J. (2017). Planning for a violent intruder event. *School Nurse, 32*(3), 1–5. https://doi.org/10.1177/1942602X16686140

Stein, R. (2022, December 5). *CDC updates the status of the "tripledemic."* [Podcast]. NPR. https://www.npr.org/2022/12/05/1140806412/cdc-updates-the-status-of-the-tripledemic

Sullivan, M., Clark E., Hughes, J. W., & Curtis A. (2021, August 10). Understanding the role of school nurses in supporting school safety before, during and after an emergency. [Webinar.] REMS Technical Assistance Center. https://rems.ed.gov/webinardetail?id=70

U.S. Department of Education. (n.d.a). *Managing donations and volunteers as a part of education agency emergency management.* Readiness and Emergency Management for Schools (REMS) Technical Assistance Center. https://rems.ed.gov/docs/Donations_Volunteers_FactSheethttps://rems.ed.gov/docs/Donations_Volunteers_FactSheet_508C.pdf

U.S. Department of Education. (n.d.b). *Post-disaster reunification and K-12 schools.* Readiness and Emergency Management for Schools (REMS) Technical Assistance Center. https://rems.ed.gov/docs/Post-Disaster_Reunification_Fact_Sheet_for_compliance_508C.pdf

U.S. Department of Education. (2022a, April). *Building blocks to school safety: A toolkit for K-12 schools and school districts for developing high-quality school emergency operations plans.* Office of Safe and Supportive Schools. https://rems.ed.gov/docs/BuildingBlocksToSchoolSafety_508C.pdf

U.S. Department of Education. (2022b, September 21). *National Incident Management System.* Readiness and Emergency Management for Schools (REMS) Technical Assistance Center. https://rems.ed.gov/AboutUs.aspx

U.S. Department of Education. (2022c, September 30). *State emergency management resources.* Readiness and Emergency Management for Schools (REMS) Technical Assistance Center. https://rems.ed.gov/stateresources.aspx

U.S. Department of Education. (2022d, October 5). *Threat- or hazard-specific annexes.* https://rems.ed.gov/K12ThreatAndHSAnnex.aspx

U.S. Department of Education. (2022e, October 6). *Ensuring continuity of operations and learning during and after emergency incidents.* Readiness and Emergency Management for Schools (REMS) Technical Assistance Center. https://rems.ed.gov/Resources/Specific?Topic=COOP

U.S. Department of Education. (2022f, October 13). *About us. Readiness and Emergency Management for Schools (REMS) Technical Assistance Center.* https://rems.ed.gov/AboutUs.aspx

U.S. Department of Education, U.S. Department of Health and Human Services, U.S. Department of Homeland Security, U.S. Department of Justice Federal Bureau of Investigation, & Federal Emergency Management Agency. (2013). *Guide for developing high-quality school emergency operations plans.* https://rems.ed.gov/docs/REMS_K-12_Guide_508.pdf

U.S. Department of Education, U.S. Department of Health and Human Services, U.S. Department of Homeland Security, U.S. Department of Justice Federal Bureau of Investigation, & Federal Emergency Management Agency. (2019). *The role of districts in developing high-quality school emergency operations plans: A companion to the school guide.* https://rems.ed.gov/docs/District_Guide_508C.pdf

U.S. Department of Homeland Security. (2015, September 5). *National preparedness goal.* https://www.fema.gov/sites/default/files/2020-06/national_preparedness_goal_2nd_edition.pdf

U.S. Department of Homeland Security. (2017). *Instructional manual 262-12-001-01: DHS lexicon terms and definitions.* https://www.dhs.gov/sites/default/files/publications/18_0116_MGMT_DHS-Lexicon.pdf

U.S. Department of Justice, Federal Bureau of Investigation. (2018). *Active shooter incidents in the United States from 2000–2018.* https://www.fbi.gov/file-repository/active-shooter-incidents-2000-2018.pdf/view

U.S. Environmental Protection Agency. (2022, August 1). *Climate change indicators.* https://www.epa.gov/climate-indicators/weather-climate

U.S. Government Accountability Office. (2022, January). *Disaster recovery: School districts in socially vulnerable communities faced heightened challenges after recent natural disasters.* https://www.gao.gov/assets/720/718505.pdf

part IV

Caring for Students with Episodic Conditions

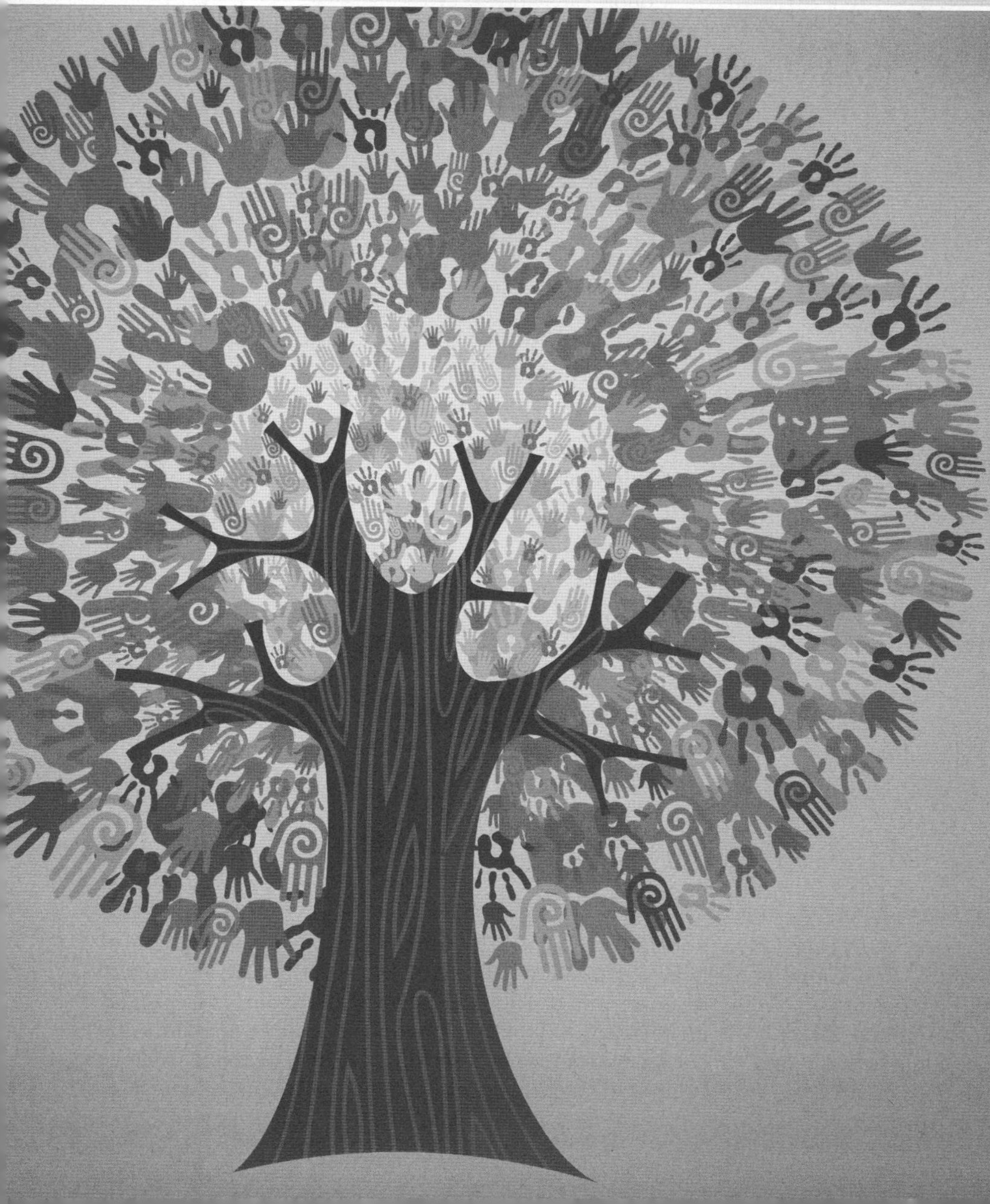

Chapter 16

Students With Common Health Complaints

Tami L. Jakubowski ▪ Sarah Curtis

CHAPTER OUTLINE

A major responsibility of the school nurse is to care for students visiting the school health office with common pediatric health complaints. Although school nurses are part of a multidisciplinary team, they are often the only healthcare professional in the educational setting and the most accessible touchpoint with health care. It is imperative that school nurses create an atmosphere of health and safety where students feel they are valued and taken seriously. The purpose of this chapter is to provide an overview of common childhood health complaints and a systematic approach for school nursing care of students visiting the health office.

GENERAL PRINCIPLES OF SCHOOL NURSING CARE OF STUDENTS WITH COMMON HEALTH COMPLAINTS

The school nurse needs to be knowledgeable about how to collect key health history data and how to assess, triage, and treat students with common health complaints. With each student visiting the health office, the school nurse uses the *nursing process* to conduct a nursing *assessment*, make accurate nursing *diagnoses*, identify appropriate outcomes for the student, *plan* and *implement* focused *interventions*, and *evaluate* their effectiveness. A rapid generalized assessment surrounding the presenting complaint, symptom, or incident is done to determine the areas that need more focused assessment and interventions as discussed in the following sections according to body area or system. In addition to common physical complaints, the school nurse must keep in mind that social, mental, and behavioral health issues are also prevalent reasons that students visit the health office for help. School nurses systematically and thoroughly document each school health office encounter.

> **IMPORTANT NOTE:** The sections that follow regarding *focused history, focused assessment*, and *focused interventions* of specific common student health complaints are intended to provide *guidance* to school nurses caring for students presenting to the school health office. The information contained in these sections is not all inclusive and is *not* intended to replace nursing judgment in the care of individual students.

History

When a student presents in the health office, the school nurse collects a history, assesses the problem, and implements care using the most current scientific evidence available in the treatment and/or referral of students. Each encounter begins with questioning the student. The school nurse should use a systematic process for history taking when a student presents with a health concern. Of the multiple formats for history taking, the acronym *PQRST* can guide the school nurse to gather relevant data for the presenting problem:

P: factors that *p*revent, *p*romote, *p*recipitate, or *p*alliate the symptom
Q: the *q*uality and *q*uantity (duration) of the symptoms
R: the *r*egion of the complaint (what part of the body) or whether it *r*adiates
S: the *s*everity (diminishing or increasing), *s*etting in which symptoms occur, or *s*imultaneous symptoms
T: any *t*emporal factors relating to when the student became aware of the problem, such as onset, duration, interval, frequency, recurrence, or changes over time (Aggarwal, 2021)

Some student health information may be known to the school nurse or may be accessible in the health record. Questions should be individualized to the specific student and current situation. For significant issues, the school nurse contacts the parent/guardian for further information. Using the *PQRST* format, the school nurse should find out relevant information, including (but not limited to) the following:

- Subjective presenting complaint: the nature of the symptom, illness, injury, or incident; location of pain or discomfort, or onset of signs and symptoms relating to specific body systems
- Current diagnoses and comorbidities
- Patterns of school health office utilization: frequency, time of day, association to class schedule
- Medications: routine scheduled and/or as-needed medications at home and at school; medication effectiveness and side effects
- Family structure: responsible and/or available adult contact, members of household, siblings at school
- Health literacy: language level and preferences
- Cultural health beliefs and practices, including complementary or alternative therapies
- Pain: onset, precipitating factors, frequency, radiation, alleviating factors
- Daily habits or routines: eating and elimination habits, sleep hygiene, hydration, screen time (e.g., TV, computer, gaming, phone, social media)
- Changes in functionality: alterations in mood or affect, activities of daily living, or signs of mental status impairment
- Healthcare utilization: primary care, specialists, emergency department visits, hospitalizations, surgeries, diagnostic evaluations
- Mental, behavior, or social health concerns: peer interactions
- Activity before onset of symptoms
- Developmental considerations
- School function: loss of instructional time (attendance, tardiness, truancy), academic concerns, recent changes in grades, discipline issues
- Adverse childhood experiences (ACEs): trauma; abuse; victimization; family strife; exposure to violence, poverty, discrimination (see Chapter 11)
- Access to health care, healthy foods, and transportation; affordable housing, neighborhood safety, and recreation (social determinants of health)

Students will provide an accurate history to varying degrees depending on age, developmental level, verbal skills, experiences with illness, relationships with others, family experiences, and religious and cultural norms.

Assessment

In addition to a brief general health history, a rapid physical assessment contributes to the triage data and illuminates the need for further focused assessment. Initial assessment data commonly include vital signs, particularly temperature and heart and respiratory rates, depending on the presenting complaint. A head-to-toe scan will reveal signs of injury, changes in breathing, skin color or integrity, and other alterations in normal status. It is important to remember that students may not be able to localize complaints well; therefore the school nurse should evaluate above and below the area of complaint. For example, if a student reports abdominal pain, it is possible the pain is caused by a problem in the lungs, hips, or genitalia.

Interventions

Often, students will arrive at school with a health concern. The school nurse, in collaboration with the school district administration, should help parents/guardians and educational staff to understand the criteria by which students should be kept home and those that will result in the child being sent home from school. These guidelines should be easily accessible in school handbooks and on school webpages (Box 16-1).

Nursing judgment based on triage data and school protocols determines whether and how parents/guardians should be contacted regarding student health office visits for minor issues when students are safely able to return to class. For example, schools may have guidelines that bumps to the head, even when minor, require that a parent/guardian be contacted. When students are unwell and sent home, the school nurse needs to communicate specific instructions regarding what to watch for and when to contact the provider, seek further medical care in an emergency department, or activate emergency medical services (i.e., call 911). For health issues that are considered *urgent*, students must be picked up from school to seek health care within 2 hours. *Emergent* health issues require that the student be transported immediately to the nearest hospital emergency department (Illinois Emergency Medical Services for Children & OSF HealthCare Children's Hospital of Illinois, 2022).

The school nurse may discuss the student's health concern with teachers and other staff if the situation relates to class activity, student responsibility, learning, or the school environment, as allowed by the Family Education Rights and Privacy Act (FERPA) (see Chapter 7). A multidisciplinary team approach is needed for students with significant physical or mental/behavioral health concerns that affect learning over time. Such students should be evaluated for a Section 504 plan or an individualized education program (IEP) with school nursing as a related service (see Chapter 8).

BOX 16-1

General Reasons Students Should Be Kept Home or Sent Home From School*

Students should generally be kept home from school if they exhibit any of the following within the last 24 hours:

1. Temperature 100.4°F or higher or as stated in school health policy
2. Uncontrolled cough or difficulty breathing
3. Vomiting and/or repeated diarrhea
4. Severe headache, especially with fever
5. Red eyes with discharge; discolored nasal discharge
6. Severe ear pain
7. Rash accompanied by fever, drainage, or blistering
8. Sore throat accompanied by fever, rash, or difficulty swallowing
9. Psychological or physical issues affecting academic performance

*Parents/guardians should be encouraged to consult their primary care provider to determine whether their child's condition warrants further evaluation and treatment.

Documentation

It is important to document the time of the arrival to and departure from the health office to quantify the amount of lost class time, particularly if the student is frequently seen in the health office. Accurate and timely documentation of even minor health office visits contributes to the database that informs school decision makers (administrators and school boards) of the need for school nursing services and, if indicated, the need for additional staffing and resources. The use of electronic medical records systems can help to ease documentation burdens and facilitate the reporting of collective data reports regarding health office utilization (see Chapter 5). Focused assessments and interventions for specific common health office visit presentations are discussed in the following sections.

FREQUENT HEALTH OFFICE VISITORS

Students who visit the school health office with various subacute and frequent complaints must be taken seriously. First and foremost, school nurses must carefully assess and refer frequent visitors for medical evaluation to rule out underlying organic causes as indicated. In the absence of physical reasons for the symptoms, school nurses need to understand the basis for somatic complaints (i.e., recurrent physical complaints that cannot be attributed to any specific medical condition). Somatization in children is common and can take the form of acute, chronic, or recurrent experiences of physical pain or discomfort (Boerner et al., 2020). A subset of children with vague or unexplained medical symptoms, also referred to psychosomatic complaints, tend to use school health services disproportionately and therefore are often labeled as *frequent flyers*. This term is stigmatizing and trivializes the student's lived experience. School nurses should avoid this stigmatizing term and model objective language for teachers and school staff, such as the term *frequent visitors*.

The most common somatic complaint of students is stomachache followed by headache (Boerner et al., 2020). Other common complaints include neck pain, shoulder pain, low back pain, feeling tense, feeling nervous, complaining of fatigue, difficulty sleeping, dizziness, irritability, and increased frequency of other illness or stress-related symptoms (Armitage, 2021). Underrecognized psychosocial variables may be contributing factors. Increased stress is linked to somatic complaints; somatic complaints are associated with mediating the relationship between emotions, including anxiety and depression, and pain (Boerner et al., 2020).

A thorough history and examination can provide the school nurse with valuable information. Frequent school health office visitors should be screened for bullying and victimization, exposure to violence, heightened and/or chronic stress, mental and behavior health concerns, and other adverse experiences of childhood (ACEs). The *Pediatric Symptom Checklist* is one valid, easy to use, and free instrument that school nurses can use to identify and refer students for appropriate evaluation and intervention (American Academy of Pediatrics [AAP], 2022) (see Chapter 28). The school nurse can employ motivational interviewing to provide students with an opportunity to share causes of stress in their lives (Reinauer et al., 2021). It is important that school nurses establish therapeutic relationships with students with somatic complaints and work with the family and school support team to support their well-being at school and minimize loss of instructional time.

FEVER

Fever is one of the most common presenting problems in school nursing practice. Normal temperature varies in children and adolescents depending on age, sex, time of the day, ambient air temperature, and anatomical site measurement (Kasbekar et al., 2021). Most fevers are due to viruses, but they can also be caused by bacterial infections, vaccine reactions, biological agents, tissue injury, malignancy, granulomatous disease, neuroendocrine disorders, metabolic disease, immunological/rheumatological disorders, drugs, and toxins, as well as environmental factors, such as the weather and exercise (Kasbekar et al., 2021). Most sources indicate fever as being greater than 100.4°F (38°C) (Adam, 2020).

> **Focus on the Framework**
> **Care Coordination**
>
> Students who visit the school health office are often seeking direct care. According to the National Association of School Nursing's (NASN's) *School Nursing Practice Framework* (2024), direct care includes student-centered interventions to address acute, urgent, or chronic health needs. Under the Care Coordination principle of the Framework, school nurses serve as liaisons between the student, family, healthcare providers, and school to optimize health and learning.

Having a fever in the presence of a pathogen is a positive physiological response; the inflammatory response causes an elevation of the hypothalamic set point in the central nervous system. Increased body temperature helps the inflammatory cells work more efficiently. To help the body generate heat, the muscles contract, causing shivering, and the vessels constrict, causing heat conservation. Clinically, a child's heart rate increases 10 to 15 beats/min for each elevation of degree centigrade (°C); the respiratory rate increases 3 to 5 breaths/min for each elevation of degree centigrade (Rhoads & Petersen, 2021) (1°C equals 1.8°F). Tachycardia occurs when the pulse rate is elevated out of proportion to the child's temperature.

While fever is usually a sign of illness, it may not necessarily indicate that a significant health problem exists; the fever pattern does not reliably distinguish the cause. The child's clinical appearance is more important than the degree of fever, and every sign and symptom expressed by the child must be further evaluated (Barbi et al., 2017). Some children, such as those with a deficient immune system, may not be able to mount a normal fever response, yet they still may be quite ill.

In addition to illness, other causes of fever include the following:

- Heat production exceeding heat loss (overheating)
- Defective heat loss caused by a genetic defect (ectodermal dysplasia) or poisoning via anticholinergic drugs

Fever should be differentiated from a heat illness (e.g., hyperthermia, heat stroke). See Chapter 17. Fever is a very specific response to an endogenous pyrogen, but heat illness occurs when the body temperature is elevated despite a normal setting in the hypothalamus. Heat illness occurs when the body produces more heat than it loses because of extrinsic factors, such as an extreme air temperature around the body, or intrinsic factors, such as spinal cord or brain injury or hyperthyroidism.

Measuring Body Temperature

The school nurse should use a consistent method to measure temperatures to avoid variation in readings related to method. Proper technique is also important to avoid inaccurate readings. If multiple types of thermometers are available in the health office, the type of thermometer used should be documented as the temperature reading can vary between physiological sites (Kasbekar et al., 2021). The options in the school setting include sublingual, axillary, tympanic, temporal artery, and infrared forehead scanning. The ranges of normal body temperature via these routes vary; temperature can be affected by diurnal factors (peaks later in day), menses, exercise, and age (Jarvis, 2020). There are advantages and disadvantages to each method (Table 16-1).

TABLE 16-1 Normal Temperature by Route

Route	Normal Range	Average
Axillary	94.46°F to 99.14°F (34.7°C to 37.3°C)	97.52°F (36.4°C)
Sublingual (oral)	96.4°F to 99.1°F (35.8°C to 37.3°C)	98.6°F (37.0°C)
Tympanic	96.26°F to 99.86°F	97.88°F (36.5°C)
Temporal	95.4°F to 98.1°F (35.2°C to 36.72°C)	97.6°F (36.4°C)

Jarvis (2020).

The axillary method has the poorest correlation with core temperature (Rhoads & Petersen, 2021). This method is affected by sweating, may be low due to peripheral vasoconstriction, requires a longer period of time to register, and the thermometer is often not placed in the correct location in the middle of the axilla. The sublingual route using battery-operated thermometers is appropriate only for children with a developmental age older than 5 years. The readings are affected by tachypnea, mouth breathing, hot and cold drinks, exercise, and the position of the thermometer under the tongue. Oral thermometers should be positioned in the posterior sublingual pocket on the side of the frenulum; the teeth should not be on the probe. The oral route is slower than the tympanic and temporal route but can be used if there are no contraindications.

Temperature measurement using the tympanic membrane is reflective of core body temperature because both the tympanic membrane and hypothalamus in the brain share their blood supply from the internal carotid artery (Jarvis, 2020). The tympanic thermometer is inserted toward the tympanic membrane just as an otoscope is inserted once the ear canal is straightened by pulling the pinna up and back on anyone older than age 3 years (down and back for a child under age 3). The probe handle should be rotated toward the jaw to form a firm seal around the probe and prevent ambient temperature from altering the reading. When the thermometer tip does not fit securely or is improperly angled, the probe may measure the temperature of the ear canal, skin, or cerumen (Jarvis, 2020). If the student has been out in the cold or has been swimming, it may be necessary for the nurse to wait for approximately 20 minutes before taking the student's temperature via the tympanic route. If the device is used correctly, the tympanic route can be rapid, convenient, and relatively risk free.

The newest noninvasive method to measure temperature in the school setting is the temporal artery route. Studies show this method to be accurate (Jarvis, 2020). The infrared sensor tip that detects temporal artery blood flow is placed on the middle of the student's forehead and swept across the forehead and behind the ear (Jarvis, 2020).

Focused History

- Onset of fever: Did they have the fever at home? How was the temperature taken? How high did it go?
- Analgesics taken and their effect on temperature
- Other symptoms: headache, cough, diarrhea, nausea, vomiting, myalgia, pain with urination, ear or throat pain, stiff neck
- Last oral fluid intake; last voiding
- Chronic health conditions
- Recent immunizations
- Recent exercise or being in a hot environment
- Travel in the past 6 months

Focused Assessment

- Vital signs
- Skin: sweating, moisture, temperature, turgor, rashes, or petechiae
- Signs or symptoms of infectious disease: lymphadenopathy, rash, pharyngitis, otitis, cough, abdominal pain, stiff neck
- Rash: macular, papular, vesicular, scarlatina form, petechial, purpura

Focused Interventions

- Emergency medical transport is required for fever accompanied by extreme lethargy, cyanosis, unusual drowsiness, an altered level of consciousness, stiff neck, or purpura.
- Notify parents/guardians that the student has a fever and needs to go home or for further evaluation.
- Provide comfort and nursing care until the student is picked up by parents/guardians.
- Minimize the amount of clothing to improve heat loss via the skin without causing shivering.
- Keep diaphoretic student dry; change clothes as needed.
- Apply cool compresses to the forehead if the fever is 104°F or higher.
- Encourage cool fluids to replace insensible loss and to cool the body, as appropriate.
- Anticipate the possibility of febrile seizures if fevers are repeatedly untreated (Barbi et al., 2017).
- Administer antipyretics (e.g., acetaminophen or ibuprofen) if there is a healthcare provider order and parental/guardian permission, as per school policy and the state's nurse practice act. Acetaminophen and ibuprofen inhibit prostaglandin synthesis thus lowering the body temperature about 1°F to 2°F within 2 hours of administration. If medications are given, and if the student is still in school, it is important to check the temperature 30 to 60 minutes later when the medication peaks to note whether it was effective (Vallerand & Sanoski, 2020).

Did You Know?

Brain damage from a fever generally will not occur until the fever is greater than 107.6°F (42°C) (MedlinePlus, 2022).

> **Practice Connection**
>
> The normal dose of acetaminophen for children is 10 to 15 mg/kg/dose every 4 to 6 hours (650 mg/dose for adults), not to exceed five doses in 24 hours; the normal dose of ibuprofen for children is 5 to 10 mg/kg/dose every 6 to 8 hours (400 mg/dose for adults) (Vallerand & Sanoski, 2020). Do not give aspirin to children experiencing flu-like illness because of the risk for Reye syndrome. All medications, even over-the-counter medications, given in the school setting require licensed prescriber orders and parental/guardian authorization.

EYE PROBLEMS

Problems related to the eye can be due to altered vision, illness (e.g., conjunctivitis, chalazion), or injury to the eye or surrounding area.

Vision

Students often present to the school nurse for an eye screening after the teacher, the parent/guardian, or the student has identified visual concerns. It is possible for a student's vision to change during the school year or to have a pathological cause. The school nurse can provide an initial screening when a student presents with a vision concern (see Chapter 12) and the student can be referred for a comprehensive evaluation by an eye health professional if needed.

To determine whether a vision screening or referral is needed, the nurse can start by observing the student in the office while the student is waiting to be seen. Having age-appropriate reading and picture books available can help the nurse observe the student's visual skills. The average 3-year-old has a visual acuity of 20/40; for a 4-year-old, 20/30 is typical. By 6 or 7 years of age, children normally have 20/20 visual acuity (Jarvis, 2020). Peripheral vision, ocular muscle control, and color discrimination are fully developed by age 7 (Jarvis, 2020).

Focused History

- When did vision problem start? Is it bilateral or unilateral? Sudden onset or gradual?
- Is vision blurred, double? Is photophobia present? Is vision present and equal in all visual fields?
- Precipitating factors: trauma, eye fatigue after close work or looking at chalkboard, insect/dirt/sand in eye
- History of vision/eye concerns, corrective lens, diabetes; does the student wear contact lenses, and how long do they keep them in? Do they wear their prescribed glasses?
- Recently entered puberty? Visual complaints can begin because the length of the eye also changes during this period.

Focused Assessment

- Vital signs: blood sugar for student with diabetes
- Eye assessment: symmetry, redness, trauma, pupil size and reaction, tearing, direction of gaze (Table 16-2)
- Conduct an age-appropriate vision screening.

Focused Interventions

- Share vision-screening results with a parent/guardian.
- Suggest further evaluation by primary care provider, ophthalmologist, or optometrist, as indicated.
- Request a written follow-up and directions/guidance from healthcare or vision provider.
- Arrange classroom accommodations such as preferential seating, improved lighting, larger-print materials.

Conjunctivitis

The most common cause of red eyes among students is *conjunctivitis,* which is inflammation and redness of the conjunctiva. Conjunctivitis can be classified as infectious or noninfectious and as acute, chronic, or recurrent (Johnson et al., 2022). Infectious conjunctivitis includes viral or bacterial conjunctivitis (i.e., pink eye). The types of noninfectious conjunctivitis are allergic, mechanical/toxic, immune mediated, and neoplastic (Woo, 2020). The school nurse conducts a focused history and physical assessment, which are needed to triage the complaint effectively.

The most common cause of a red eye is inflammation due to viral or bacterial causes. Bacterial conjunctivitis is spread by direct contact with discharge from an infected eye or by touching contaminated surfaces (Varu et al., 2019). A history of crusty eyelids and physical findings of purulent discharge are highly predictive of bacterial infection requiring ophthalmic antibiotic therapy. The American Academy

TABLE 16-2 Evaluating Pupils

Evaluating Pupillary Light Reflex	Technique
	Note pupil size, shape, and if equal (normal is round, regular, and equal size, 3–5 mm in adult).
Direct pupil response	Darken room, have child gaze into distance.
	Move penlight in from side, observing response of pupil.
Consensual light reflex	Observe for simultaneous constriction of opposite side pupil.
Variation in Pupils	
Anisocoria	Normal variant in 20% of people, pupils of unequal sizes. If pupillary difference is >1 mm, consider central nervous system injury if new finding.

Adapted from Hoersting & Mullen (2017).

of Pediatrics (2021) recommends that *once the appropriate therapy is started, the student can return to school.* There is no longer the need to wait 24 hours unless the child has other symptoms that qualify for exclusion. Viral conjunctivitis is self-limiting and does not require topical medication.

Allergic conjunctivitis is a localized allergic condition frequently associated with rhinitis, asthma, and atopic dermatitis (Bielory et al., 2020). Allergic conjunctivitis may be seasonal or year-round and can be itchy or stinging with bilateral watery discharge (Bielory et al., 2020). While avoidance of the allergen is the most effective preventive intervention, students often require treatment with topical antihistamine ophthalmic drops or a mast cell stabilizer; oral antihistamines minimally decrease symptoms. Students should not be excluded from school for allergic conjunctivitis because it is not contagious. Although it is often appropriate to request the student be evaluated by a healthcare provider to determine the cause of the conjunctivitis, once it is determined that a student has the allergic type, repeated trips for evaluation are not necessary unless symptoms indicate otherwise.

Sometimes a red eye can be a brief event that occurs from simply rubbing the eye. If the student looks well, has no complaints, no discharge, and normal vital signs, allow the student to lie down with eyes closed for a few minutes to see if the redness disappears so they may return to class. Cool compresses may also help to alleviate mild irritation due to benign causes.

Focused History

- When did redness, pain, itch, or discharge start? Bilateral or unilateral? Is there pain/tenderness around the eye (bones of eye socket or sinuses)?
- Vision: blurred, double, photophobia
- Discharge: continuous or on awakening, color of discharge
- History of vision/eye concerns, use of corrective lens, diabetes, allergies
- History of trauma: splash of chemicals, soap, makeup
- Signs of systemic illness, especially respiratory infection

Focused Assessment

- Vital signs
- Eye assessment: symmetry, redness, trauma, pupils, tearing, gaze, signs of allergy (allergic shiners, boggy pale nasal mucosa)
- Discharge: bilateral, color of discharge, present only in the morning or throughout the day

Focused Interventions

- The focus is on alleviating symptoms and preventing the spread of infection.
- Encourage the student not to rub or touch the eye.
- Apply warm compresses to loosen the crust that accumulates on the eyelids overnight (Johnson et al., 2022).
- Clean discharge by wiping from the nose to the outer part of the eye.
- Apply cool compress to relieve the itch associated with allergic conjunctivitis.
- Switch from contacts to glasses until the condition is resolved.
- Request cleaning staff disinfect doorknobs, faucets, and surfaces that students touch.
- Stress the importance of hand washing (Centers for Disease Control and Prevention [CDC], 2022a).
- Keep classroom environments free of potential allergens.
- Teach the student and parent/guardian to disinfect areas frequently touched by children and not to share towels.
- Refer to the primary care provider immediately if there is a change in vision or change in pupil size. For suspected conjunctivitis, students should be evaluated for the need for antibiotics.
- When administering eye drops for bacterial conjunctivitis, remove all dried debris and mucous before administration, and wash hands before and after administration.

Periorbital Edema

Swelling around the eye, or *periorbital edema*, can result from local or systemic problems. Students may not experience pain initially from the cause or injury. The cause of swelling may be related to a local reaction, such as an insect bite, trauma, or infection. The area around the eye has a looseness of tissue and excess skin, so the edema may be larger than expected, especially first thing in the morning. Systemic diseases that cause edema in various parts of the body may also cause periorbital edema, such as nephrotic syndrome (Elliott, 2020).

Focused History

- Onset and location of swelling: Is it bilateral or unilateral?
- Length of time: Is there more swelling in the morning than later in the day?
- Respiratory symptoms, fever, impaired vision
- History of allergies, contact lenses, face creams or ointments, bug bites, trauma
- History of systemic disease (cardiac or renal)
- Current medications
- Pain, itching

> **Practice Connection**
>
> **Eye Irritation/Injury**
>
> Prevent rubbing of the eye. If dirt or an eyelash is visualized, either irrigate with clean water or a sterile saline eye irrigant. Blink several times. If the problem is not resolved, refer to an ophthalmologist. A corneal abrasion can be caused by fingernails, contact lenses, and foreign bodies. There is pain, redness, tearing, possible photophobia, and a foreign body sensation. Corneal abrasions require evaluation and treatment. Never remove an intraocular foreign body or projectile (Varu et al., 2019).

Focused Assessment

- Vital signs, including blood pressure
- Eye assessment: redness, swelling under the eye, trauma, pupils, tearing, gaze deviation
- Insect bite
- Discharge: bilateral or unilateral, color and amount
- Systemic symptoms, including urine output; other areas of edema, especially ankles; respiratory symptoms, signs of allergy

Focused Interventions

- Encourage the student not to rub or touch the eye.
- Apply cool compress to the eye.
- Keep head elevated.
- Refer to primary care provider.

EAR PROBLEMS

Earache

Earache (i.e., otalgia) is a common complaint in pediatrics. The usual cause is an inflammation of the external ear (i.e., otitis externa) or middle ear (i.e., otitis media). Other causes outside the ear include problems with the teeth, temporomandibular joint, or pharynx (Earwood et al., 2018). The causes of otalgia within the ear can be related to infection, trauma, allergy or inflammation, lymphadenopathy, eustachian tube dysfunction, impacted ear wax, or, rarely, tumor.

It is imperative to assess not only the ear but also the head and neck region to help determine the cause of ear pain. Most children have at least one episode of acute otitis media in childhood (Paul & Moreno, 2020). Although the diagnosis of otitis media can be challenging, common symptoms include tugging at ears, irritability, restless sleep, and headache (Danishyar & Ashurst, 2022). A majority of these patients also present with a fever, which is typically low-grade (Danishyar & Ashurst, 2022). In the AAP clinical guidelines on otitis media, the definition of acute otitis media requires the presence of three equally important elements: acute onset (less than 48 hours) of signs and symptoms, a middle-ear effusion, and signs and symptoms of middle-ear inflammation (Lieberthal et al., 2013).

Otitis media is generally painful, and treatment with nonopioid analgesics is indicated and provides pain relief within 24 hours with or without antibiotic treatment (Danishyar & Anhurst, 2022). Following evaluation by a healthcare provider, a careful decision will be made as to whether antibiotics should be prescribed; antibiotics are not always indicated because some cases of otitis media are self-limited or nonbacterial. Students should receive treatment for pain because otalgia interferes with learning.

Did You Know?

A *stye* (i.e., hordeolum) is usually a bacterial infection of a blocked oil gland or hair follicle on the eyelid resulting in a lump. A *chalazion* is a cyst-like nodule inside the eyelid, also caused by a blocked oil gland; it is a healed noninfectious stye. A stye is more painful than a chalazion. Both are treated with warm compresses (American Academy of Ophthalmology, 2023).

Focused History

- Onset and location of ear pain: unilateral or bilateral?
- Length of time, pain (rate), pain while chewing and swallowing
- Hearing: muffled, ringing, popping, buzzing
- History of otitis, hearing loss, cerumen; dental, throat, or craniofacial concerns; trauma; swimming history
- Current medications, myringotomy tubes
- Did the student put anything in the ear, including cotton swabs?

Focused Assessment

- Vital signs
- Ears: pain on gently pulling the pinna, mastoid, ear canal redness (swimmer's ear/otitis externa), ear canal blocked with cerumen or foreign body, drainage, trauma
- Eyes: otoscopic assessment (see Practice Connection)
- Respiratory: breath sounds, nose, lips, mouth, throat, and lymph nodes, especially behind the ear. Ear pain can be referred from the throat.
- Teeth and mouth: caries, gums (gingivitis), halitosis
- Balance, dizziness
- Signs of systemic illness: fever, cough, rhinitis, stiff neck, headache

Focused Interventions

- Administer analgesics for pain, if medical orders are in place or if permitted by policy and protocol.
- Provide dry warmth to help relieve ear pain.
- Have child lay with affected ear down.
- Avoid use of ear plugs, including headphones.
- Educate parents/guardians that exposure to passive smoking increases the risk for otitis media (Tarhun, 2020).
- Review the importance of completing prescribed course of antibiotics even though symptoms are improved.
- Keep the ear dry until pain free, about 7 days when treating otitis externa.

Hearing Disturbances

Hearing loss may be congenital or acquired. The different types of hearing loss and the issues related to hearing loss are discussed in Chapter 24. The school nurse, however, may see students who present with sudden hearing loss or decreasing ability to hear. Many nurses are qualified to

Practice Connection

Examining the ear with an otoscope:

Caution: If the external canal is red and painful, do not insert an otoscope.

Be cautious putting the otoscope into the ear as it can push any foreign body into the ear canal; look first before inserting.

Inspect for impacted cerumen or foreign objects as you gently place the otoscope into the ear canal. Ear wax is normally sticky/waxy or flaky and ranges from light yellow to dark brown.

Inspect the tympanic membrane (eardrum), noting color.

Inspect for scarring of the tympanic membrane; may be due to chronic otitis media or prior history of myringotomy tubes.

Inspect light reflex and bony landmarks. Distortion of the bony landmarks and an abnormal light reflex with a bulging, red, and poorly mobile tympanic membrane are indicative of acute otitis media. Clear fluid behind the drum without any redness indicates serous otitis media.

Observe for retraction of the eardrum (appears pulled in on itself).

provide an initial screening when a student presents with a hearing concern (see Chapter 12).

Regardless of the cause of hearing loss, early identification and intervention can make a huge difference in the student's ability to communicate and achieve academically (Shojaei et al., 2016). Over 98% of infants in the United States are screened for hearing at birth; however, many babies identified with hearing loss are lost to follow-up (CDC, 2023). Mild-to-moderate hearing loss in young students is easy to miss because they may not realize their hearing is impaired. The school nurse is an advocate who can identify early, refer for evaluation, and remediate impairments in the educational setting. Even mild hearing losses are educationally and medically significant.

Hearing loss can result from damage to structures and/or nerve fibers in the middle or inner ear from head trauma, brain infections, chemotherapy, or ototoxic drugs given for a variety of reasons. The National Institute for Occupational Safety and Health (NIOSH) reports that approximately one in eight youth between the ages of 6 and 19 has some level of hearing loss (Sliwinska-Kowalska & Davis, 2012). One of the most common causes of hearing loss in children is noise-induced hearing loss caused by exposure to excessively loud sounds. Loud music from concerts, clubs, personal audio systems, and headphones is a potentially dangerous source of recreational noise; other sources of loud noises include loud traffic, farm equipment for rural youth, and continuous close exposure to other musicians for student musicians (Sliwinska-Kowalska & Davis, 2012). Noise-induced hearing loss cannot be surgically corrected.

Cerumen or foreign bodies can also cause hearing impairment. Sudden hearing loss can follow trauma or problems with circulation. Hypersensitivity to sound, or hyperacusis, may also be a complaint that brings the student to the health office. These students may complain that the classroom is too loud and may complain of a headache. These students need to be evaluated by their primary care provider.

Focused History

- Onset of hearing loss, unilateral or bilateral
- Duration and intensity of pain
- Hearing: hearing devices used; muffled, ringing, popping sounds
- History of otitis, hearing loss, cerumen, upper respiratory infection
- Current medications, myringotomy tubes
- History of noise exposure at school or play; use of ear phones for listening to music or playing video games

Focused Assessment

- Vital signs
- Hearing screening
- Ear assessment: trauma, pinna, mastoid, external ear canal, drainage, foreign body, cerumen
- Otoscopic assessment (see Practice Connection)
- Respiratory assessment: breath sounds, nose, lips, mouth, throat, and lymph nodes
- Balance, dizziness
- Consultation with teacher and observation of the student in a classroom setting; tilting of head toward the speaker; frequent requests to repeat questions

Focused Interventions

- Share hearing screening results with a parent/guardian.
- Suggest further evaluation by healthcare provider or audiologist, if indicated.
- Request a written follow-up and directions/guidance from provider.
- Arrange classroom accommodations such as preferential seating, decrease ambient noise, note taker.
- Educate students about how noise and personal listening devices can affect their ability to hear; volume should be audible but not loud.
- Discuss sources of loud noise at home, school, and work, and how to avoid or protect against loud noise.
- Initiate measures to address noise in the school, such as in the gymnasium, machinery (lawn equipment outside of school windows), or band.

Ear Trauma

Students who present with ear trauma can have damage to the outer, middle, and inner ear and may present to the school health office after a traumatic event. Auricle trauma is more common in certain sports such as wrestling or boxing. Bleeding into the cartilage of the auricle with hematoma formation requires medical assessment and may require drainage to prevent perichondritis, which could result in cartilage loss.

Focused History

- Cause and location of trauma
- Pain: duration, intensity, radiating, drainage from the ear or nose
- Hearing: muffled, ringing, popping
- New-onset hearing loss
- Complaint of headache

Focused Assessment

- Vital signs, pain
- Ear assessment: trauma to ear canal or tympanic membrane, foreign body, crepitus, drainage. (NOTE: If the drainage is clear, it may be cerebrospinal fluid [CSF].) If sugar dipsticks are available, use one to test clear drainage for CSF (positive sugar indicates CSF).
- Facial/head trauma: palpate skull bones for pain
- Balance, dizziness (especially if inner ear is involved)
- Facial nerve palsy
- Inspect for mastoid ecchymosis (Battle's sign)
- Inspect for "raccoon eyes" or hematomas around the eye

Focused Interventions

- Keep the student comfortable.
- Apply cool compress.
- Cover ear with gauze if drainage is present and position with the affected ear down.
- Refer student to primary care provider for further evaluation.

NASAL PROBLEMS

Rhinitis

Students commonly present with complaints of nasal congestion and rhinitis caused by allergic rhinitis or upper respiratory infections. *Rhinitis* is inflammation of the nasal mucosa. Allergic rhinitis is among the most common chronic conditions in school-age children (see Chapter 21). Students may complain of itching of the nose and eyes, nasal congestion, or sneezing. Rhinitis can be seasonal, intermittent, or persistent. Upper respiratory infections (URIs) or colds are caused by viruses, the most common of which is rhinovirus (Thomas & Bomar, 2022). It is normal for children to have four to seven URIs a year. The largest concentrations of URI viruses are found in the nose; therefore it is important that students wash their hands after wiping their noses (Jefferson et al., 2023). The highest concentration of the virus is not found in secretions from coughing or saliva; some viruses can survive on a fomite (a nonliving surface) for several days and on hands for 2 hours (DeGeorge et al., 2019). The incubation period for the common cold is 2 to 14 days; an infected individual is usually contagious a few days before symptoms appear and while the rhinorrhea persists (DeGeorge et al., 2019). Symptoms are often present for 7 to 10 days and start to subside after the first week.

Foreign bodies in the nose may also present with mucopurulent discharge and be mistaken for infection or allergy, but these symptoms are almost always unilateral (Zavdy et al., 2021). Nasal irritation and even trauma to the septum can be caused from nose picking and inhalation/huffing of recreational drugs. Nose piercing and tattooing can also lead to infections and scarring (Das, 2018).

Focused History

- Onset of nasal discomfort, length of time
- URI, epistaxis, nose picking, drug use, piercings
- History of allergies, asthma or eczema, allergy testing
- Triggers: exposure to cold air, tobacco smoke, environmental allergens
- Family history of environmental/seasonal allergies
- Current medications
- History of nasal trauma
- Close contacts with URIs

Focused Assessment

- Vital signs
- Nasal assessment: exterior and interior swelling, foreign body, discharge; septum should be midline
- Respiratory assessment: breath sounds, nose, lips, mouth, throat, and lymph nodes
- Associated symptoms: fever, cough, headache, muscle aches, sore throat, and gastrointestinal complaints
- Palpate frontal sinuses (press up under eyebrows) and maxillary sinuses (below cheekbones)

Focused Interventions

- Remind the student not to forcibly blow the nose.
- Increase fluids, rest, and humidification of the air.
- Encourage medicine compliance for allergies or infection, including at school.
- Evaluate the classroom and school environment to identify irritating substances and triggers.

Did You Know?

Students who are allergic to trees may complain of nasal congestion in the early spring, depending on when allergy season peaks. Those who are allergic to certain grasses tend to complain in late spring and early summer, and students with hay fever caused by weeds complain more in late summer through fall. Mold spores increase in the spring and peak in July in the warmer states and in October in states with cold weather. However, along the West Coast and the South, mold is found year-round. The most common cause of allergies in the fall is ragweed, which grows throughout the United States, but is especially widespread along the East Coast and in the Midwest (American College of Asthma, Allergies, & Immunology, 2017).

- Arrange for school accommodations (e.g., air conditioning) to avoid triggers.
- Common cold interventions include good hand hygiene and promoting fluids. Table surfaces, toys, and doorknobs should be routinely sanitized. Children with colds do not need to be excluded from the classroom unless they have other symptoms, such as fever or dyspnea.

Epistaxis

Epistaxis, or nosebleeds, are common in children. The nose has a rich blood supply from the internal and external carotid blood supply, centered at Kiesselbach's plexus located in the anterior inferior nasal septum (Rhoads & Petersen, 2021). Figure 16-1. Epistaxis can be triggered by nasal trauma, digital trauma (nose picking), inflammation, injury, forceful blowing, exposure to dry air, or rubbing the nose (Send et al., 2021). Students who have nosebleeds may have allergies, have a foreign body in the nose, be exposed to an environment with low humidity, or have an infection. Recurrent epistaxis can occur without an identified cause in children up to 16 years of age. Most cases are self-limiting and do not indicate underlying pathology; more severe recurrent cases need further evaluation by an ear, nose, throat (ENT) physician (Send et al., 2021). School nurses should develop an individualized healthcare plan (IHP) and an emergency action plan (EAP) for students with bleeding disorders who are at risk for epistaxis.

Focused History

- Onset of epistaxis, length of time, amount of bleeding
- Upper respiratory infection, trauma, nose picking, drug use, foreign body
- Triggers: heat, smoke, environmental
- History of allergies, asthma or eczema, bleeding disorder
- Family history of bleeding disorder, epistaxis

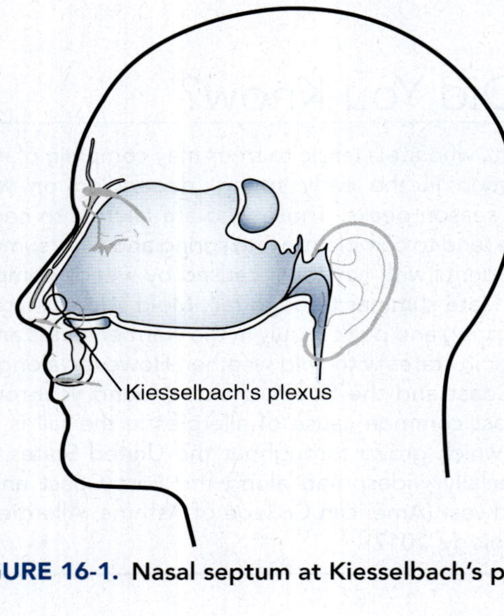

FIGURE 16-1. Nasal septum at Kiesselbach's plexus.

- History of tarry or black stools not associated with iron administration
- For girls, menstrual history of prolonged or excessive bleeding

Focused Assessment

- Examine the nares for crusting or clotting or foreign body.
- Inspect the skin on arms and legs for petechiae or bruises.
- Check vital signs.

Focused Interventions

- Compress the nares continuously with child upright and leaning slightly forward to prevent blood from draining back into the throat (Send et al., 2021).
- If direct pressure does not work, apply upward pressure to the labial artery by placing a cotton compress beneath the upper lip and putting upward pressure on it, while keeping pressure on the anterior nare.
- If bleeding is severe, the student may need to be transported for emergency care.
- Apply cool compresses to nasal bridge.
- Encourage the young child to breathe through the mouth.
- Teach students about the problems associated with nose-picking behavior and encourage keeping fingernails short.
- Educate student and family about humidification, nasal saline spray, and petroleum jelly to promote healing and prevent bleeding recurrence (Send et al., 2021).
- Inform a parent/guardian that the child may vomit a little blood or have a dark stool because of swallowed blood.
- Evaluate the classroom and school environment to identify irritating substances and ensure proper humidity levels.
- Work with physical education teachers and coaches regarding the importance of wearing protective face gear during contact sports.

FOREIGN BODY IN THE EYES, EARS, OR NOSE

It is not uncommon for children and adolescents to put small toy parts, beads, food, seeds, nuts, paper, cotton, foam, stones, or wads of tissue into their nose and ears. Similarly, other objects can get in the eyes, ears, and nose either by accident or on purpose. These may include environmental dust, dirt, sand, or insects. Students can present with a foreign body or a foreign body sensation in the eyes, ears, and nose. Allergy can also present with a foreign body sensation. It is important to determine whether there is any history of trauma.

A student who has a foreign body in the nose may present to the health office with other complaints, a foul odor around the face and nose, or have a visible purulent unilateral discharge. School-age students may be embarrassed to admit that they put an object in their nose or ear. Therefore the foreign body may be in the nose or ear for days before an odor or discharge is detected. Be advised that objects can also be inserted into the urethra, vagina, and rectum. If these are reported, the student must be seen by their primary care provider.

The student may be unaware of what is causing the problem, and it may be difficult to obtain a history. In these cases, phrase questions in an indirect way, such as "Sometimes students put things in their nose or ears; have you ever tried something like that?"

Focused History

- What happened right before the foreign body sensation? How long has sensation been present?
- Location: Was student playing in dirt or sand? Was it windy out?
- Type of object
- Trauma, bleeding, pain, discharge
- Change in vision or hearing; fluttering sensation in ear

Focused Assessment

Eye

- Inspect the eye to look for a foreign body.
- Inspect for any redness or localized area of irritation.
- Gently invert the upper lid to see if you observe a foreign object.
- Remove contact lenses if in place.

Nose

- Inspect the nasal openings.

Ear

- Inspect external ears, ear canals, and tympanic membranes. Use otoscope if available.

Focused Interventions

Eye Foreign Body

- Never remove a foreign body if the history indicates that a projectile object was possibly involved in the injury (Woo, 2020). Refer a parent/guardian to take the child directly to an eye specialist or emergency care.
- Shield the eye if there is any history of eye trauma with foreign body sensation. Have the student rest with the unshielded eye shut to decrease movement.
- Flush or remove foreign object *if nonpenetrating* (Table 16-3).
- Refer students continuing to complain of a foreign body sensation to a primary care provider or eye specialist.

Nasal Foreign Body

- If a foreign body is visualized, have child take a deep breath through the mouth and gently blow out the nose.
- If unsuccessful, child should be seen by primary care provider.

TABLE 16-3 Foreign Body in Eye

Type of Foreign Body	Intervention
Nonpenetrating—visualized	Flush with warm water—inner to outer part of eye.
Corner of eye	Remove with moistened cotton swab.
Upper eyelid—not visualized	Flush or gently invert upper lid using cotton-tipped applicator over the upper eyelid and pulling eyelid outward and up over the applicator.

Bryant (2024).

Foreign Body in the Ear

- Do not put any object into the ear to attempt removal as you may actually push the object farther into the canal.
- For an insect in the ear, take the student into a dark room and shine a bright light into the ear; the insect may come out on its own. With provider and parental approval, tilt the head so that the ear with the insect is upward and insert small amount of olive oil/mineral oil/vegetable oil. Insect may float out. Flush with warm water (DePietro, 2018).
- Blunt objects made of metal (iron, nickel, or cobalt) may be removed with a magnet.
- Disk batteries must be removed emergently; DO NOT irrigate the ear if the object is a disk battery or vegetable matter, or if the tympanic membrane is not intact.

MOUTH AND THROAT PROBLEMS

Tooth Pain

Many conditions can cause mouth and tooth pain. The origin of toothache complaints can include caries, infections, debris between the teeth, eruption of new teeth, movement of teeth due to braces, and trauma. Teeth and gums are sensitive and can cause significant pain. Within the United States, there is significant disparity in oral health care resulting in a twofold increase in cavities among children from low-income families. Dental caries are the most common chronic disease of childhood (CDC, 2021). Despite frequent contact with members of the healthcare team, students with special healthcare needs do not always get their dental care needs met and often have increased dental health needs (Cameron & Widmer, 2022). Treatment and preventive dental care for students are affected by economics, accessibility, past experiences, phobias, and cultural beliefs.

Young children have 20 primary or deciduous teeth. They begin falling out around age 5, followed by permanent teeth beginning to erupt around age 6. Adults have 32 permanent teeth, the last of which (the third molars or wisdom teeth) erupt around age 18 (see Chapter 9, Fig. 9-1).

Focused History

- Onset and location of tooth pain
- Duration and quality of pain (rate); radiating to head, neck, or ear
- Sensitivity to cold or heat
- Last dental visit; number of caries, fillings, crowns, braces, spacers
- Oral hygiene: brushing habits, frequency, flossing
- Recent trauma to face and/or teeth, tongue, or oral piercings

Focused Assessment

- Vital signs, especially temperature, to rule out dental abscess
- Inspect for caries; broken, loose, or missing teeth; lodged food between teeth.
- Inspect gum line for any swelling, pus, or redness. Excess fluoride use results in mottling of the teeth; oral iron intake may cause black staining if administered undiluted.
- Inspect jaw and neck lymph nodes for any enlargement.
- Note halitosis.

Focused Interventions

- Offer cool compresses to jaw for 20 minutes. Use warm water or saline rinses to clean inside of the mouth and teeth.
- Provide floss and help the student use it if absence of severe pain permits.
- Administer analgesic if medical orders are in place.
- Refer student for dental care.
- Provide parent/guardian with a list of community resources for preventive and emergent dental care, which may include dental schools or clinics, as well as local dentists in the area willing to work with families on payment plans.
- Review proper teeth brushing and flossing skills.

Oral Lesions

Children and adolescents can have oral lesions due to trauma, infections, immunodeficiency, cancer, celiac disease, Crohn's disease, poor dental care, or use of smokeless tobacco (Cameron & Widmer, 2022). Oral lesions such as canker sores or benign mouth ulcers are painful and cause distress for the student, interfering with learning. Some oral lesions are recurrent, such as aphthous ulcers/stomatitis (canker sores), gingivostomatitis (from herpes simplex virus), and herpangina (Cameron & Widmer, 2022). Aphthous ulcers are painful, shallow, pseudomembranous depressions with an erythematous halo. They can vary in size and number and can appear anywhere on the oral mucosa or lips. They can be caused by trauma (including dental work), vitamin deficiency, celiac disease, and Crohn's disease (Cameron & Widmer, 2022). Gingivostomatitis (fever blisters) are vesicular lesions on an erythematous base anywhere in the oral cavity, but generally on the outer lips and surrounding area. Herpangina is caused by an enterovirus (such as Coxsackie); they appear as bright-red ulcers generally in the posterior oral cavity (Cameron & Widmer, 2022). These may be treated with over-the-counter (OTC) products containing carbamide peroxide, such as Gly-Oxide.

Oral candidiasis (thrush) can occur in children who are immunocompromised, who have been on courses of antibiotics, or use dry powder inhalers for asthma (AAP, 2021). These white lesions are not common in well school-age students and appear on an erythematous base that bleeds when gently scraped. Candidiasis can be treated with medicated oral rinses, drops, and lozenges.

Focused History

- Onset and location of oral lesion
- Duration and quality of pain (rate), fever
- Trauma, allergy
- History of lesions; any family members with the lesions
- Recent dental work
- History of chewing smokeless tobacco, eating acidic foods, oral sex, biting one's tongue or cheek, mouth piercing
- Teeth brushing habits (the lesions may be caused by strenuous brushing) and last time toothbrush was replaced
- Any systemic complaints, such as joint pain, diarrhea, abdominal pain, sore throat, or dysphagia
- Health history of risk factors: immune deficiency, cancer chemotherapy treatment, stress, celiac disease, Crohn's disease

Focused Assessment

Temperature

- Assess size, depth, shape, color, amount, drainage
- Inspect lips, gums, under the tongue, tonsils, inner cheeks, neck, and glands
- Inspect hands and feet for vesicles caused by Coxsackie virus

Focused Interventions

- Notify a parent/guardian about lesions and refer to primary care provider or dentist.
- Healthcare provider may recommend OTC topical anesthetics or equal parts of diphenhydramine elixir (Benadryl) and aluminum and magnesium hydroxide (Maalox) that are ordered as "swish and spit" (Hockenberry, 2024).
- Recommend avoidance of carbonated beverages, citrus juices, and spicy foods, which can cause stinging and pain.
- Teach infection control measures: hand washing, disposable bathroom cups, separating toothbrushes.
- Advise a parent/guardian to replace student's toothbrush once lesions have resolved.

Throat Pain

Sore throat or pain on swallowing is a common complaint in the pediatric population. The onset of throat pain can be acute or gradual. Students with viral pharyngitis tend to have a history of rhinorrhea, cough, or diarrhea with gradual onset of throat pain. Symptoms with viral pharyngitis may also include hoarseness and conjunctivitis. In younger school-age children, a characteristic viral enanthem and/or exanthem may be present (Pelucchi et al., 2012).

In contrast, students with streptococcal infections tend to have rapid-onset throat pain, fever, and the absence of cough. Headache and abdominal pain with vomiting may accompany streptococcal infections (Shulman et al., 2012). Acute group A beta-streptococcal infections may present with any of the following: tonsillopharyngeal erythema and exudates, anterior cervical lymph node enlargement, soft palate petechiae, beefy red edematous uvula, strawberry tongue, and a scarlatiniform sandpaper-like rash. When accompanied by rash, streptococcal pharyngitis is called scarlet fever. Group A streptococcal pharyngitis is treated to prevent complications of rheumatic fever (Shulman et al., 2012). See Chapter 24 for more information on rheumatic fever and rheumatic heart disease.

Most sore throats are caused by viruses; only 15% to 30% of infections are caused by group A streptococcus (Shulman et al., 2012). A history of close contact with group A streptococcus and a high prevalence rate in the community can be a significant history point (Shulman et al., 2012). Other causes of sore throat include overuse of the voice, persistent cough, allergies, mouth breathing, dust, and dry weather.

Focused History

- Onset location and duration of throat pain: has it increased or decreased?
- Did the student choke or swallow something that got stuck in the throat?
- Length of time, quality of pain (rate), radiating to ear, fever, difficulty swallowing
- Triggers: second-hand smoke, forced hot air
- History of allergies, recreational drug use, oral sex, postnasal drip
- Other symptoms: headache, fever, cough

Focused Assessment

- Vital signs, including oximetry; pain scale
- Respiratory assessment: breath sounds, nose, lips, mouth, throat and lymph nodes, nailbeds
- Inspect for lesions/white patches noted on pharynx, including swollen tonsils.
- Inspect buccal mucosa for ulcerative lesions.
- Inspect teeth for dental caries or gum inflammation.
- Head tilt due to cervical node enlargement
- Inspect tonsils for erythema, swelling, exudate, odor, symmetry, position. A tonsil displaced anteriorly is of concern for peritonsillar abscess requiring further medical evaluation.

Focused Interventions

- Administer analgesic if medical orders are in place.
- Offer fluids to thin secretions and soothe throat if no vomiting or abdominal pain.
- Refer to primary care provider if pain persists and other symptoms exist.
- Teach student to gargle with warm salt water for relief of throat irritations and promote healing (¼ tsp salt in 8 oz water).
- Collaborate with school staff and family to identify and remove irritants from school/home environment (fumes, hairspray, perfumes, smoke, fragrant cleaning products).
- Advise to replace toothbrush and toothpaste when symptoms resolve.
- *Epiglottitis is a medical emergency:* Drooling or muffled voice, changes in vocal quality, an inability to swallow, drooling, and an ill-appearing child may indicate a retropharyngeal abscess or epiglottitis. Do not attempt to visualize the throat; call 911. Attempting to open the mouth to visualize the throat can result in occlusion of the airway and respiratory arrest.

NECK PROBLEMS

Torticollis

Torticollis occurs when a person laterally tilts their head to one side combined with a rotation of the head to the opposite side (Sargent et al., 2019). Torticollis is a physical sign that can result from trauma, inflammation, or neurological problems; it can be divided into congenital or acquired. Torticollis may be the manifestation of cervical muscle spasm or injury, vertebral subluxation, cervical fractures, or dislocations (Herman & Wolf, 2013).

The onset of cervical dystonia after a traumatic event may occur immediately or up to 12 months after an injury (Herman & Wolf, 2013). Torticollis can also result from inflammation due to cervical adenitis, retropharyngeal abscess, upper lobe pneumonia, cervical osteomyelitis, rheumatoid arthritis, or an infection of the head and/or neck (Rhoads & Petersen, 2021). Inflammatory torticollis may be due to infections in

Did You Know?

Tonsil size is best measured using the Brodsky scale:

Size 0 = Tonsils are absent or have been removed.
Size 1 = Barely visible (normal)
Size 2 = Tongue tissue is not beyond the tonsillar pillar. Also normal size
Size 3 = Up to 75% of the airway is taken up by tonsil.
Size 4 = More than 75% of airway is taken up by tonsil (often tonsils are touching).

Brodsky (1989); Kumar et al. (2014).

the upper respiratory tract (e.g., pharyngitis, tonsillitis, epiglottitis, sinusitis, otitis media, and mastoiditis) or soft tissue (e.g., retropharyngeal abscess) (Herman & Wolf, 2013). Neurologically, torticollis can be the manifestation of a posterior fossa tumor, cervical cord tumor, visual disturbance, dystonic drug reaction, or syringomyelia (Herman & Wolf, 2013). Torticollis can be confused with nuchal rigidity or stiff neck.

Focused History

- Onset, duration, and location of neck pain or muscle spasm
- History of head tilt, viral infection, trauma, vision issue
- Some genetic conditions may predispose students to subluxation (e.g., Down syndrome, dwarfism syndromes, or bone dysplasias)
- Some prescribed neuroleptic medications (e.g., antipsychotics such as phenothiazines and haloperidol) can cause acute, painful dystonic reactions

Focused Assessment

- Take vital signs (temperature).
- Identify history of trauma.
- Evaluate for extraocular movement: strabismus, nystagmus, and other eye deviations that may cause student to tilt head to avoid double vision; perform vision testing if indicated.
- Assess throat and cervical lymph nodes.
- Inspect passive and active neck range of motion; do not force neck movement that elicits pain.

Focused Interventions

- Activate emergency medical services (EMS) for acute trauma.
- Allow the student to rest in a position of comfort.
- Apply warm compress (wet or dry) to the neck muscle.
- Apply gentle massage on the posterior sternocleidomastoid muscle.
- Administer analgesics according to medical orders.
- Refer to primary care provider as indicated.

Neck Pain

Neck pain can overlap with torticollis but can present as an isolated complaint. This section discusses the child with neck pain without a history of trauma. The student with neck pain after a trauma is an emergency discussed in Chapter 17. When the student presents with neck pain, the nurse needs to determine whether the child is systemically ill, has a trauma with neurological symptoms, is asymptomatic neurologically, or is in a high-risk category for atlantoaxial dislocation (Rhoads & Petersen, 2021). Pain may be related to heavy or improperly worn backpacks or positioning during sleep, class, or playing video games.

Focused History

- Onset, duration, and location of neck pain or muscle spasm: Does it radiate down arm or back? Is there any pain during chewing or jaw movement?
- Precipitating factors: screen time, heavy backpack, trauma (whiplash)
- History of fever, scoliosis, or excessive time in front of a computer, mobile device, or playing video games
- Medications taken for pain or fever

Focused Assessment

- Assess vital signs and level of consciousness.
- Evaluate hand and arm strength/weakness bilaterally.
- Palpate cervical lymph nodes, evaluate for enlargement.
- Inspect skin for signs of injury.
- Palpate cervical spine for point tenderness.
- Gently inspect range of motion of the neck.
- Assess for scoliosis (see Chapter 12) and differences in the height of one shoulder, hip, or rib.

Focused Interventions

- Activate EMS for acute trauma.
- Allow the student to rest in a position of comfort; use a folded towel under the neck to support it while lying down and keep the neck in alignment.
- Apply warm compress (wet or dry) to the neck muscle.
- Administer analgesics if medical orders are in place.
- Refer for medical evaluation as indicated.

CHEST-RELATED PROBLEMS

Cough

Cough can result from a number of different causes, such as environmental irritants; infection; allergies; asthma; foreign bodies, aspiration; congenital or acquired disorders; cardiac disease; and extrinsic or intrinsic mechanical factors (Rhoads & Petersen, 2021). Pediatric cough can be acute or chronic (longer than 4 weeks), can be moist or dry, or can have identifiable underlying causative factors (Rhoads & Petersen, 2021).

Cough is a symptom that results from a reflex phenomenon in the cough receptors in the airways of the lung, pharynx, paranasal sinuses, and external auditory canal and is controlled by the cough center in the medulla. However, cough may be absent even in the presence of a foreign body in the airway because there is not a uniform stimulus threshold in the respiratory tree. Cough can be productive (where mucus is expectorated or swallowed) or dry and nonproductive. Children with a productive cough usually swallow their mucus, often resulting in nausea.

Acute respiratory infections such as bronchitis or pneumonia are the most common cause of an acute cough. Cough and tachypnea are common symptoms in children with pneumonia. *Pneumonia* is defined by fever, acute respiratory distress, and the presence of infiltrates on chest radiograph (World Health Organization, 2022). Tachypnea is defined as a respiratory rate greater than 40 in a child older than 1 year. Common organisms causing pneumonia in school-age children are *Mycoplasma pneumoniae, Chlamydia pneumoniae, Streptococcus pneumoniae,* and respiratory viruses (Krafft & Christy, 2020).

Pertussis, commonly called whooping cough, is an acute respiratory infection with a unique cough (CDC, 2022b). Pertussis presents as a paroxysmal cough in more than 72% of those affected, accompanied by post-tussive (i.e., after coughing spell) vomiting in 50% to 70%, and a whoop after spasms of coughing in 30% to 50% of infected children. The cough can persist for more than 3 months and is known as the "100-day cough." Antibiotic treatment for pertussis does not help the cough but decreases the spread of the infection (CDC, 2022b).

Focused History

- Onset and duration of cough; when is it worse: daytime or nighttime?
- Nature of the cough: dry versus wet, painful
- Expectorant: color, consistency, and amount; is it swallowed or expectorated?
- Triggers: place, food, exposure to smoking, inhalants, fumes
- Is cough related to eating a large meal? Are there complaints of heartburn?
- Current medications
- Up-to-date immunizations: diphtheria, pertussis, influenza
- Change in appetite, energy, exercise tolerance, or weight
- History of respiratory illness/asthma, allergy, cystic fibrosis
- Family history of respiratory illness
- Does student smoke or vape?
- Adult in the house with a history of a cough or current cough
- Is there sore throat, fever, rhinorrhea, or hemoptysis?

Focused Assessment

- Vital signs, including oximetry
- Overall appearance: flushed, pale, anxious, agitated, lethargic, cyanosis/dusky color
- Cough quality (dry, congested, productive or not, paroxysmal [multiple coughs in rapid succession without a breath between them, which may indicate pertussis]), use of accessory muscles
- Respiratory: breath sounds, nose, lips, mouth, throat and lymph nodes, nailbeds; assess for respiratory distress (see Box 16-2 and Table 16-4)
- Signs of allergy: allergic shiners, mouth breathing, allergic crease across the nose, cobblestone appearance in the back of the throat
- Inspect nose for dryness, crusting, congestion; inspect throat for redness.

BOX 16-2

Signs and Symptoms of Respiratory Distress in Children

- Inspiratory stridor
- Expiratory grunting
- Nasal flaring
- Increased heart rate and respiratory rate in absence of fever or drug/medication use
- Retractions: intercostal, subcostal, suprasternal/substernal
- Significantly decreased breath sounds unilaterally or bilaterally
- Difficulty talking and breathing
- Seated tripod position
- Sweating
- Restlessness; irritability
- Cyanosis: circumoral, nailbeds, or generalized
- Pulse oximetry less than 95% on room air

TABLE 16-4 Breath Sounds, Noisy Breathing, and Possible Problems

Sound	What You Hear	Location of the Problem
Polyphonic wheezing	High-pitched musical squeaking sounds; may occur during inspiration and expiration	Indicates problem with the small airways (asthma, cystic fibrosis, bronchiectasis, viral-induced wheeze)
Monophonic wheezing	Low-pitched, snoring sounds on expiration	Indicates problems with the intrathoracic trachea and upper airway (tracheomalacia, foreign body, obstruction of upper airway)
Coarse crackles (rhonchi)	Low-pitched bubbling gurgling sounds early on inspiration	Indicates secretions in large airways (pulmonary edema)
Fine crackles (rales)	Intermittent, high-pitched, short crackling popping sounds	Indicates problems with bronchioles (pneumonia, bronchitis, asthma)
Stridor	High-pitched inspiratory, loudest in neck	Upper airway obstruction due to swelling or foreign body, sign of severe distress (croup, epiglottitis, foreign body obstruction)
Grunt	Expiratory grunt occurs with extensive alveolar pathology	Child's attempt to improve oxygenation during severe respiratory distress (pneumonia)

Adapted from Jarvis (2020).

Focused Interventions

- Administer medications as ordered.
- Encourage student to maintain a position of comfort (e.g., sitting upright or leaning forward) until respiratory distress resolves or a parent/guardian arrives.
- Provide emotional support during an acute episode; keep student calm.
- Encourage warm liquids to help soothe the throat. Do not give anything by mouth if the danger of choking exists or if the student is experiencing dyspnea or tachypnea.
- Encourage evaluation by primary care provider if pertussis is suspected or cough lasts over 4 weeks (Weinberger & Hurvitz, 2020).

Chest Pain

Chest pain occurs in students of all ages. Causes of chest pain in children can be divided into cardiac and noncardiac (Rhoads & Petersen, 2021). The younger the student with chest pain, the more likely there is an organic cause for the pain. Males and females are equally affected. Chest pain can be from local sources, from structures within the thorax, or referred from visceral organs. The most common cause of chest pain in children and adolescents is musculoskeletal. Musculoskeletal chest pain can be caused by strained intercostal or pectoralis muscles, costochondritis, rib fracture, direct trauma to the ribs, or sternal trauma. Other causes of chest pain include infectious, gastrointestinal, psychogenic, pulmonary, cardiac, idiopathic, or miscellaneous disorders such as Marfan syndrome, sickle cell crisis, or shingles (Rhoads & Petersen, 2021).

Chest pain with a pulmonary cause can be due to severe cough, asthma, bronchitis, pneumonia, pleurisy, pulmonary embolism, or pneumothorax (Yeh & Yeh, 2015). Chest pain related to gastrointestinal problems can be caused by esophagitis, gastroenteritis, gastroesophageal reflux, or gastric ulcer disease. Adolescents with eating disorders who purge vomit are predisposed to esophageal ulcers, tears, ruptures, pneumomediastinum, and cardiac arrhythmias (Hornberger et al., 2021).

Psychogenic chest pain is particularly common in adolescents and is often related to anxiety. Psychosocial factors, especially depression, mental distress, and somatic complaints, have an influence on the development of upper-quadrant musculoskeletal pain in children and adolescents (Turk & Gatchel, 2018).

Cardiac causative factors of chest pain in children are uncommon. Cardiac chest pain may be related to hypertrophic cardiomyopathy, anomalous coronary artery, premature atherosclerotic coronary artery disease secondary to diabetes, Kawasaki disease, pericarditis, myocarditis, paroxysmal atrial arrhythmias, cocaine abuse, or ventricular arrhythmias (Rhoads & Petersen, 2021). Symptoms of cardiac rhythm disturbance in children and adolescents may include palpitations or the sensation of a rapid heartbeat, chest discomfort, syncope, or presyncope.

Adolescent girls taking oral contraceptives may be at a greater risk for venous thrombosis, pulmonary embolism, and myocardial infarction. Chest pain during exercise is a red flag for organic disease. Students with chest pain accompanied by fever should be immediately referred for medical evaluation to rule out a serious organic cause, such as myocarditis or pneumonia (Rhoads & Petersen, 2021).

Focused History

- Onset, duration, and location of chest pain and whether pain is reproducible by touch or deep breaths
- Quality of pain (rate), radiating, palpitations; cough, vomiting, fever
- History of dizziness, light-headedness, palpitations
- Triggers: position, stress, anxiety, medication, exercise, spicy or fatty foods (e.g., indigestion)
- History of sickle cell disease—acute chest syndrome is a serious complication and a cause of mortality in sickle cell disease (Kato et al., 2018); eating disorder; reflux; heart disorders; syncope; recreational drug use
- History of strenuous physical activity: dancing, gymnastics, contact sports, weightlifting
- History of blunt trauma musculoskeletal injury
- Family history of chest pain/cardiac disease
- The student's concerns about the chest pain
- Use of birth control pills and smoking; acute onset of sudden severe chest pain may indicate a pulmonary embolus
- Vesicular rash present on one side of chest; rule out shingles (Saguil et al., 2017)
- Recent breast development or breast tenderness

Focused Assessment

- Vital signs, including oximetry, pain scale
- Overall appearance: perspiration, pallor, bruising
- Respiratory assessment: breath sounds, nose, lips, mouth, throat and lymph nodes, nailbeds
- Cardiac assessment: heart sounds, rib/thorax tenderness, bilateral pulses
- Assess skin for petechiae of nearby muscles related to increased strenuous use.

Focused Interventions

- Observe student until stable or pain subsides.
- Initiate EMS for signs/symptoms of respiratory or cardiac compromise.
- Reassure the student if the history and assessment are normal.
- Encourage student to avoid activities that reproduce musculoskeletal pain.
- Suggest student keep a chest pain diary.
- Refer student with chest pain with exercise to primary care provider for evaluation and clearance to participate in physical education and sports.
- Share relaxation techniques to address anxiety-related chest pain.

INFECTIOUS MONONUCLEOSIS

Infectious mononucleosis (IM) is an acute, self-limiting, mildly contagious infection usually spread by saliva through kissing or sharing food and drink. The virus can live outside the body for hours (Sanderson & Gaylord, 2020). It presents with clinical symptoms ranging from a simple pharyngitis and fatigue to exudative pharyngotonsillitis with fever, hepatosplenomegaly, and lymphadenopathy (especially posterior cervical). Jaundice is seen in about 4% of those affected, and a skin rash may be present on the trunk in up to 15% (Heymann, 2022). The incubation period is 4 to 6 weeks. IM is most commonly seen in adolescents; younger children may have a more subclinical course (Sanderson & Gaylord, 2020).

Ninety percent of IM in adolescents is caused by the Epstein-Barr virus (EBV) (Sanderson & Gaylord, 2020). EBV is related to the herpesviruses and infects B-lymphocytes. Diagnosis is usually confirmed by the monospot blood test. Other causative organisms need to be considered if testing for EBV is negative.

Recovery from IM can take weeks to months (Heymann, 2022). The treatment of IM is supportive because there is no treatment to shorten the course of illness. Splenic rupture, although rare, can occur up to 28 days after symptomatic illness and has significant implications for the school nurse (Sanderson & Gaylord, 2020). *The student's activities, especially contact sports, should be limited while splenic enlargement exists;* the student must be asymptomatic without an enlarged spleen before gradual return to play. Return to full activity needs to be paced and is dependent on the severity of the illness; fatigue and weakness may persist for months (Sanderson & Gaylord, 2020).

Focused History

- When did illness begin? Are symptoms improving or worsening?
- What is the student's history of dating, kissing, sharing straws or utensils?
- What is the severity of associated fatigue? How many hours does the student sleep, including naps, per day?
- Is sore throat, myalgia, fever present?
- Is abdominal pain, which can indicate spleen or liver enlargement, present?

Focused Assessment

- Monitor vital signs.
- Palpate for enlarged cervical lymph nodes.
- Inspect tonsils for enlargement or exudate.
- Inspect for periorbital edema (present in 25% of patients with EBV).
- Palpate for liver and spleen enlargement.

Focused Interventions

- If fever, tonsillitis, or rash is present, send the student home with a parent/guardian and recommend physician follow-up.
- Educate family about variable severity of IM and lack of specific treatment.
- Discuss fever-reducing measures with parents/guardians.
- *Inform child and family about possible splenic enlargement and that contact play should be avoided, including physical education classes. Make sure the child has a clearance note from the healthcare provider before returning to any contact sports.*
- Discuss the importance of hydration.
- Educate family that the child may need to nap or sleep longer during the recovery period, including possible partial days or rest periods in the health office on return to school.
- Avoid kissing on the lips or sharing saliva; do not share toothbrushes, cups, or eating utensils.
- Clean and sanitize common surfaces, toys, and utensils after use.

GASTROINTESTINAL PROBLEMS

Abdominal Pain

Gastrointestinal (GI) problems can be acute, chronic, recurrent, or episodic. Acute abdominal pain is discussed in Chapter 17. Inflammatory bowel disease is discussed in Chapter 24. Abdominal pain, often generally referred to as *stomachache,* is among the most common complaint for which students visit the health office. Essentially, all children experience abdominal pain at some point. Recurrent abdominal pain can be somatic, subacute, and transient, or symptomatic of a more serious chronic GI problem or an evolving emergency. Therefore, it is imperative that all students with abdominal pain be taken seriously and evaluated each time. The school nurse should document each visit for abdominal pain and watch for changes and patterns indicating the need for further medical evaluation.

Biological, psychological, and social factors in the presence of altered intestinal motility and heightened sensation from the GI tract are thought to be modulated by the central nervous system and can result in pain. The Rome criteria for chronic or functional GI disorders in children include (1) pain once a week for 2 months that is either episodic or continuous; (2) symptoms that do not fit the criteria for another functional disorder; and (3) no evidence of any inflammatory, anatomical, metabolic, or neoplastic process to explain the symptoms (Friesen et al., 2021). The most common GI complaints are constipation, encopresis, and diarrhea.

GI concerns may have either a physiological or psychological origin (Rajindrajith et al., 2018). Students who have functional bowel disorders have physiological abnormalities in their gut motility and abnormal visceral perception. Psychological stress can also alter GI motility and cause abdominal pain.

Focused History

- Time and quantity of last food intake or meal
- Content of recent food intake: spiciness, food intolerance, sensitivity, or allergy
- Nutritional status: eating habits, consumption of foods of minimal nutritional value (i.e., junk food)
- Hydration status: water and fluid consumption habits and recent drinking intake (or lack thereof)
- Typical stooling pattern
- Last bowel movement: time, frequency, quantity, characteristics (hard, soft, loose, color, float, or sink)
- Psychological or social issues regarding going to the bathroom at school (e.g., lack of privacy, fear of bullying, lack of toilet paper)
- Associated pain and symptoms (onset, general or localized, severity); abdominal cramping, nausea, vomiting, dyspepsia, heartburn, belching or flatulence, pain while stooling
- Reproductive-age females: menstrual cycle symptoms or changes; pregnancy; sexually transmitted diseases
- Recent weight loss or gain
- The student's perceived stress level; recent changes in the student's life (divorce, parent/guardian away from the home, new baby)

Focused Assessment

- Assess whether weight loss, fever, anorexia, nausea, vomiting, or abdominal distention is present.
- Assess for altered nutritional status.
- Assess hydration status and skin integrity (e.g., tenting, edema).
- Assess level of activity: altered gait (slowed, shuffling, or bent over), fetal positioning, abdominal guarding, restlessness, or anxiety (generalized or associated with cramping or pain).
- Auscultate abdomen for bowel sounds in all four quadrants before palpation.
- Palpate away from the area of pain. Have the child flex at the knees to decrease tension from abdominal muscles. Determine whether pain is localized or diffuse or if there is rebound tenderness.
- Determine whether mouth ulcers (associated with inflammatory bowel disease) are present.
- Healthy students may have pain if palpated deeply in the left lower quadrant in the area of the descending colon with large amounts of stool palpable.
- Students with appendicitis may have pain on hopping.

Focused Interventions

- Have the student lie down in a comfortable position.
- Monitor for worsening or improving pain and fever.
- Explore stressors that cause abdominal pain.
- Teach relaxation exercise and imagery to manage pain and stress.

Constipation

Constipation is common, accounting for 3% of pediatric primary care office visits and 15% of pediatric gastroenterology specialty visits (Nurko & Zimmerman, 2014). *Constipation* is defined as a delay or difficulty in defecation for 2 or more weeks. School-age children should have approximately one stool per day, but not having a stool does not necessarily indicate constipation. It is the consistency and size of the stool that causes the problem. After passage of large or hard stools, the anus may be stretched, resulting in pain and development of anal fissures, which can result in withholding of stool. As a result, the rectum becomes larger and may fail to alert the student to the need to defecate. Students with constipation can have pain or discomfort, feelings of distention or fullness, rectal bleeding, and soiling from liquid stool leaking around impacted stool. The younger the student, the more difficult it is in the school setting to obtain a history of bowel habits (Ho & How, 2020).

Students with constipation need to eat a well-balanced diet that includes whole grains, fruits, and vegetables, as well as adequate fluid for mild constipation. The school nurse may need to advise the family to seek further medical evaluation and treatment, nutritional counseling, and behavioral management for a student with severe or chronic constipation (Ho & How, 2020). Underlying medical conditions that can cause constipation may need to be ruled out by a medical provider or gastroenterologist. It is important to reassure and support the student, while allowing the student to use a designated bathroom for privacy and time for defecation.

Focused History

- Student's toileting habits and schedule at home: color, size, frequency, ease, and consistency of bowel movement
- Medications with constipation as a side effect (e.g., vitamins, iron, calcium)
- Laxatives/enemas used/abused at home
- History of recent or chronic vomiting, diarrhea, constipation; withholding of stool, rectal bleeding, soiling, pain with defecation
- Student's self-image and view about defecation
- Dietary pattern: intake of fiber, fruits, vegetables, fluids, fats, dairy; processed or fast food, or prepared at home
- Accessibility of a toilet during school hours: psychological factors from restricted use/lack of privacy with toileting

Focused Assessment

- Palpate left lower quadrant for consolidated sausage-shaped stools.
- Indications of thyroid dysfunction (e.g., weight gain with fatigue; new onset of hair loss; sensitivity to cold; eye puffiness; or dry, rough skin)

- Indications of neuromuscular dysfunction (e.g., neurogenic bowel or bladder, myelomeningocele, cerebral palsy, Hirschprung's disease): unsteady or clumsy gait, lack of feeling or voluntary control of rectal muscles

Focused Interventions

- Educate the student and family about measures to promote regular bowel movements:
  - The importance of high-fiber foods (e.g., bran, graham crackers, oatmeal, popcorn, brown rice)
  - Constipating foods to avoid (e.g., white rice, bananas, low-carbohydrate foods that are low in fiber)
- Encourage fruits and vegetables; including apple, pear, cherry, grape, and prune juices; citrus juices are not helpful for constipation (Ho & How, 2020).
- Educate about the dangers of chronic laxative use and enemas.
- Encourage increased activity level.
- Promote the importance of adequate water and fluid intake for age. Allow student to have water bottle in class.
- Allow private time for defecation at school.
- Work with school administration to make sure bathrooms are safe, clean, and monitored for privacy and security with ample toilet paper and soap.
- Educate staff about sensitivity of subject and potential adverse effects of asking invasive questions.

Encopresis

Encopresis, also known as functional fecal incontinence, is defined as voluntary or involuntary repeated passage of normal or near-normal stool into places other than a toilet by a child who is older than 4 years of age chronologically and developmentally (Fisher, 2024; Sood et al., 2023). Encopresis is often associated with chronic constipation and withholding of stool (Ho & How, 2020). As stool is withheld in the rectum, the rectal muscle stretches; the urge to defecate can be diminished or lost. Retention of stool, whether voluntary or involuntary, is often followed by pain on defecation. A cycle of pain-retention-pain often develops, exacerbating the constipation. Stool stalled in the rectum becomes hard, which can lead to impaction and leaking of loose or small amounts of stool around the impaction. Large, hardened stools are painful to pass, which furthers the cycle.

Encopresis may be associated with other GI conditions or abnormalities in the bowel that cause chronic constipation. In some cases, encopresis may be associated with emotional distress (i.e., psychogenic encopresis) (Fisher, 2024). It is essential to distinguish encopresis from delayed toilet training, where the child never mastered the ability to stool independently into the toilet.

Treatment for encopresis begins with bowel cleansing and removal of impaction with laxatives or enemas, followed by dietary modifications (e.g., high-fiber diet) and bowel lubricants such as mineral oil. It may be followed by behavior modification. The school nurse must be alert to signs of encopresis such as staining of a student's underwear and fecal smell. This is usually an embarrassing issue for school-age children; the student may hide underwear to avoid shame or punishment and/or may lack friends and be teased or bullied by other students due to the foul smell. The school nurse should develop an individualized healthcare plan for a student with encopresis to ensure a comprehensive and therapeutic approach (LeLeiko et al., 2020). Section 504 plan accommodations in the learning environment may be indicated.

Focused History

- History/pattern of pain with defecation, abdominal pain, distention, or bloating
- Details of current bowel patterns: stooling pattern in toilet, soiling accidents, diarrhea, stool size, color, amount, consistency, urge to defecate; pain with defecation
- Withholding behaviors witnessed by parents/guardians or teachers: crossing the legs, tightening the anal sphincter to avoid defecating, squatting (LeLeiko et al., 2020)
- Altered bowel function and toilet training, diagnostic testing, surgeries, and treatments
- Systemic diseases or abnormalities in the GI tract that cause constipation (e.g., Hirschsprung's disease typically presents with difficulty in evacuation from birth due to lack of nerve innervation in the intestine, which results in recurrent abdominal distention, constipation, and leaking of liquid stood around the impaction) (Fisher, 2024)
- Family history of GI disorders or rectal bleeding
- Medications: misperception of diarrhea and treating of firm stool
- Associated rectal bleeding or anorectal lesions
- Dietary history; changes or decrease in appetite
- Social difficulties, bullying, or lack of friends

Focused Assessment

- Determine growth parameters: height, weight, and BMI.
- Look for abdominal distention.
- Auscultate bowel sounds in all four quadrants; hypoactive or absent bowel sounds may indicate acute constipation or obstruction.
- Palpate abdomen for tenderness or masses.

Focused Interventions

- Institute Section 504 plan if indicated.
- Maintain daily toileting diary and reward system (i.e., praise, stickers) for successful bowel movements.
- Schedule routine times for the student to sit on the toilet in a private low-traffic bathroom facility in the school, if possible (beginning of the day, after lunch).
- Teach the student to bear down using technique of blowing on a balloon while sitting on toilet and using foot support.

- Arrange for increased fiber in diet at school.
- Encourage student to drink water throughout the day; allow water bottle in class.
- Arrange for bathroom privileges and privacy any time needed.
- Establish private cleanup procedure for soiling episodes: provide soap, towels, and cleansing wipes, and change of clothes as needed in a private, accessible place.
- Refer the student to school counselor for individual counseling to support positive self-esteem and social interactions with peer group issues.
- Encourage participation in school activities and provide support and reassurance to reduce negative associations around toileting (LeLeiko et al., 2020).

Diarrhea

Diarrhea is an acute or chronic increase in frequency, volume, and loose consistency of stool. Acute diarrhea results from GI infections, including viruses, bacteria, and parasites, as well as medications such as antibiotics (Rodgers & Wilson, 2017). Chronic diarrhea lasts more than 2 weeks and can be caused by malabsorption syndromes, endocrine disorders, tumors, psychological issues, diet, or infections. Acute episodes of diarrhea can be related to oral-fecal contamination through direct/indirect contact or ingestion of contaminated foods or beverages, infections, medications, or allergic diseases. Dehydration and underlying causes related to diarrhea can be serious and require medical evaluation and treatment. Management of diarrhea includes reestablishment of fluid and electrolyte status, treatment of underlying cause, and adequate nutrition (Rodgers & Wilson, 2017). Clinical research demonstrates some improvement of diarrhea with the use of probiotics for children; however, further research is needed (Guo et al., 2019).

Focused History

- Onset, frequency, and consistency of recent stools (24 to 48 hours)
- Complaint of localized pain
- Members of the family or close contacts with recent illness
- Incontinence
- Use of OTC medications for diarrhea
- Recent travel to remote areas (e.g., camping) or out of the country
- Potential exposure to infectious causes (i.e., viral, bacterial, parasites)
- Fluid status: intake and urinary output in last 24 to 48 hours; thirst
- Food intolerances, sensitivities, or allergies
- Excessive ingestion of caffeine, sorbitol (artificial sweetener), or high-fructose corn syrup in food, juice, gum, or candy
- Recent history of weight loss or changed percentiles on the growth chart

Focused Assessment

- Presence of blood, mucus, or pus in the stool
- Abdominal pain, cramping, distention, nausea and vomiting
- Signs of dehydration such as increased pulse rate, dry skin, flushing of skin, tacky saliva, sunken orbits, delayed capillary refill, quiet behavior with lack of interest in surroundings, light-headed (Rhoads & Petersen, 2021)
- Signs of systemic disease (e.g., fever, jaundice of sclera)

Focused Interventions

- Refer for medical evaluation and treatment in the presence of fever, dehydration, abdominal pain, or protracted diarrhea.
- Provide privacy and easy access to a well-equipped restroom.
- Discourage use of OTC antidiarrhea medications unless discussed with the primary care provider.
- Encourage clear fluid intake and salty snacks to prevent dehydration.
- Encourage rehydration with commercially available oral rehydration solution.
- Educate about foods and fluids that can affect diarrhea.

Nausea and Vomiting

Nausea and vomiting can be acute or chronic and can be presenting symptoms of many conditions and diseases. Causes include side effect of medications, anatomical problems, foreign body obstruction in the gut, neurological problems, infectious diseases, endocrine disorders, respiratory problems, allergies, and other causes, including pregnancy and eating disorders. Nausea and vomiting may be the first indication of a migraine or simply the result of swallowing increased mucus secondary to postnasal drip or spinning on playground equipment. In older children, vomiting (emesis) occurs most often because of acute gastroenteritis accompanied by fever and diarrhea. Nausea and vomiting can also be a presenting symptom of viral and bacterial meningitis (Ingle & Gibbs, 2024). In students with diabetes, nausea and vomiting requires urgent medical evaluation and treatment. Protracted or chronic recurrent vomiting clearly needs evaluation by the primary care provider.

Focused History

- Onset, duration, and time of day that nausea and vomiting occurs
- Quantity, frequency, and consistency and appearance (e.g., undigested or digested food, bilious, red-tinged)
- Nature of vomiting: abrupt, forceful, dry heaves
- Complaint of localized pain
- Any sick members of the family or close contacts

- Potential exposure to infectious causes (viral, bacterial, parasites)
- Fluid status: intake and urinary output in last 24 to 48 hours; thirst
- Food intake, intolerances, sensitivities, or allergies; when was the last time the student ate?
- Possibility of pregnancy in childbearing age females
- Ingestion of nonfood products (pica or foreign body obstruction)
- Epigastric or abdominal discomfort
- Presence of other symptoms: sore throat, cough, headache, rash, abdominal pain, dizziness, postnasal drip
- Self-induced or related to body image

Focused Assessment

- Assess vital signs; weigh student to identify weight loss.
- Inspect characteristics of emesis.
- Inspect for signs of dehydration; for example, increased pulse rate; dry, flushing of skin; sticky saliva; sunken orbits; delayed capillary refill; quiet behavior with lack of interest in surroundings (Rhoads & Petersen, 2021); light-headedness; dry heaves.
- Inspect skin for color change—observe for jaundice in sclera, mucous membranes, and skin; check chest for rash.
- Auscultate bowel sounds and palpate for localized area of tenderness, especially in the right lower quadrant (may indicate appendicitis).
- Palpate for abdominal masses.
- Assess neck for pain and stiffness (may indicate meningitis).
- Inspect for thinning hair, sallow color, dental erosions, palatal scratches, or callus on the knuckles (Russell's sign, which may indicate an eating disorder) (Hornberger et al., 2021).
- Auscultate chest for adventitious sounds or respiratory distress.
- Assess orientation/level of consciousness to rule out encephalitis or drug overdose.

Focused Interventions

- Allow student to rest in a well-ventilated, quiet room.
- Allow student to rinse out mouth (swish and spit) after vomiting.
- Maintain nothing-by-mouth (NPO) status for approximately 1 hour; then begin rehydration with ice pops or Gatorade—1 tsp every 5 minutes.
- Students who are actively vomiting should be sent home from school with instructions to the parent/guardian on care and parameters of when to contact a healthcare provider for medical evaluation and possible treatment.
- Students should rehydrate and avoid dairy products; caffeine; carbonated drinks; and spicy, greasy foods until they return to normal.
- Encourage slow, deep breaths to help alleviate nausea.

Pinworms

Pinworms or thread worms (i.e., Enterobius vermicularis) are small (8 to 13 mm), thin, white or light gray roundworms that live in the colon and rectum of humans. While the infested person sleeps, female pinworms exit the anus and deposits eggs on the perineum (CDC, Division of Parasitic Diseases, 2020). Symptoms include perianal itching, difficulty sleeping, and restlessness. It is the most common worm infection in the United States, occurring most commonly among school-age and preschool-age children. Pinworm infections can affect all ages and socioeconomic status.

Pinworms are spread by the fecal-oral route, either directly by hand or indirectly through fomites such as contaminated clothing, bedding, food, or other articles (CDC, Division of Parasitic Diseases, 2020). Pinworm eggs can survive for 2 to 3 weeks on fomites. People become infected by ingesting infective pinworm eggs on fingers, under fingernails, or on clothing, bedding, and other contaminated objects and surfaces. The child is infectious as long as the female pinworm is laying eggs on the perineum.

The most common symptom of pinworms is nighttime perianal itching (Rodgers & Wilson, 2017). Other symptoms may include general irritability, poor sleep, bed wetting, perianal excoriation, or dermatitis from scratching. Pinworms can migrate to the vagina and urethra causing secondary infections.

Students suspected of having pinworms need medical evaluation for treatment. The diagnosis is made by a history of nighttime perianal itching or using the tape test. This involves pressing cellophane tape with the sticky side against the skin across the anus at night to capture the eggs. The tape is removed in the morning and put on a slide or on a commercially prepared product and examined microscopically. Pinworm eggs rarely are found in routine stool or urine samples (CDC, Division of Parasitic Diseases, 2020).

Medication to treat pinworms is given in a single dose and repeated in 2 weeks (AAP, 2021). All household contacts and caretakers of the infected person should be treated due to the high rate of reinfection. Students may return to school after taking one dose of medication, bathing, and trimming fingernails (AAP, 2021). Strict hand hygiene to prevent the spread of pinworms is essential, including proper hand washing; maintaining clean, short fingernails; avoiding nail biting; and avoiding scratching the perianal area. It is also important *not* to shake out the linen and underwear of children with pinworm infection because the ova can be spread into the air and respiratory transmission is possible (AAP, 2021).

Focused History

- Close contact with others with the same symptoms
- Differentiate from other causes of anal itching (e.g., sexual abuse and/or sexually transmitted disease, contact dermatitis, or allergy to new lotions or creams)

- Difficulty sleeping, irritability, distractibility, enuresis (Rodgers & Wilson, 2017)
- Urinary frequency from related urinary tract infections (UTIs)

Focused Assessment

- Observe the student for signs of discomfort and scratching anus.
- School nurses do not typically assess or inspect areas beneath the underwear.

Focused Interventions

- Reassure student and family by demystifying the shame and blame associated with pinworm infestation.
- If the healthcare provider has instructed the parent/guardian how to examine the perianal area and perform the "tape test," the school nurse can reinforce and clarify the directions.
- Encourage medication compliance for child and household contacts.
- Educate that careful handling and frequent laundering in hot water of underclothing, night pajamas, towels, and bedding can help reduce infection, reinfection, and environmental contamination with pinworm eggs (CDC, Division of Parasitic Diseases, 2020).
- Educate parents/guardians to shower rather than bathe child each morning to remove a large portion of eggs.

GENITOURINARY/ GYNECOLOGICAL PROBLEMS

Genital Discharge/Itch

The most common gynecological complaint in school-age females is vaginal discharge or itch (Emans & Laufer, 2019). A student who presents with this complaint needs a professional and sensitive school nurse for emotional support, guidance, and confidentiality of what is being said. This complaint may be the result of an overgrowth of bacteria from obesity, poor hygiene, tight clothing, or nonabsorbent underwear. Vaginal discharge is generally the result of a Candida fungal infection. Candida infections may result from antibiotic use, vaginal dryness, or diabetes in prepubescent students. Occasionally, students may contract group A streptococcal infections in the perianal and genital region from an untreated strep throat. A vaginal foreign body or a retained tampon may also lead to bacterial overgrowth and result in itch, discharge, and foul odor.

Pubertal girls may become concerned when they note a discharge on their underwear. Vaginal discharge that is clear or white and generally is odorless is relatively normal. Genital itch from sand, tight pants, pantyhose, tight-fitting underwear, wet bathing suits, bubble baths, soap, or detergent can lead to both vaginal irritation and urinary tract infections. Older students who are sexually active may have a sexually transmitted infection with presentation of vaginal discharge. Students on birth control pills may experience vaginal drying, which sets the stage for the growth of yeast infections (Galan, 2017). Young students who have been sexually abused may not know how to explain their complaint of vaginal itching and discharge. Emotional support is needed to guide the student with this complaint. If sexual abuse is reported or suspected, police and child protective agencies need to be contacted.

Focused History

- Onset, duration, and location of discomfort
- Burning on urination, itching, sores, rash
- Discharge: amount, color, consistency (may be clear or cloudy, thin or thick, curd-like)
- Triggers: tight-fitting or damp clothes, sand, bath products, vaginal douches
- Medications/birth control pills
- Sexual activity
- Onset of menarche and the relationship of the itching to the menstrual cycle

Focused Assessment

- Vital signs
- Physical assessment of the genital region is not usually performed in the school setting.
- Focused interventions
- Refer student for evaluation and treatment; confidential treatment can be provided to students beginning at the age indicated by state law.
- Educate student about proper hygiene, avoidance of irritants, tight and damp clothing, bubble baths. Teach females to wipe front to back, wear cotton-lined underpants, and remove them before sleeping.
- Counsel sexually active students on consistent use of condoms and to abstain from sexual activity until infection is cleared.
- Discuss avoidance of feminine hygiene cleansers and timely changing of tampons.

Dysmenorrhea and Menorrhagia

Dysmenorrhea is defined as painful menstruation during the onset and first few days of the menstrual period. Dysmenorrhea is differentiated as primary or secondary. Primary dysmenorrhea is most common in girls 1 to 3 years after menarche begins and is one of the leading causes of short-term school absenteeism (DeSanctis et al., 2015). In primary dysmenorrhea, lower abdominal cramping is the most common symptom; other symptoms include dizziness, nausea, vomiting, anorexia, headache, leg pain, abdominal pain, flushing, sleeplessness, depression, and irritability (Dharmapuri, 2019). It does not accompany any pelvic pathology, whereas secondary dysmenorrhea is usually due to a pathological condition. Secondary dysmenorrhea may be caused by tumors, complications of pregnancy, pelvic inflammatory disease, cysts on the ovaries, or endometriosis.

Menorrhagia is abnormally heavy bleeding at menstruation. The most common time for menorrhagia is the first 2 years after menarche. The blood loss during the entire cycle should be approximately 30 to 50 mL, with a high normal amount of 80 mL (Kabra & Fisher, 2022). During the initiation of menstruation, the cycle may be anovulatory, leading to disruption of the normal menstrual buildup of the endometrium. This lack of maturity of the hypothalamic-pituitary axis is the most common reason for menorrhagia. However, miscarriage, hematological bleeding disorders, thyroid disorders, infections, pathology within the reproductive tract, genital trauma, medications that inhibit platelets, and eating disorders can also cause excessive bleeding (Emans & Laufer, 2019). Menorrhagia can present with short, frequent cycles of heavy bleeding or long periods of bleeding.

The focused assessment and interventions for both dysmenorrhea and menorrhagia in the health office are similar, with emphasis on supporting the student and encouraging follow-up with a primary care provider.

Focused History

- Age of onset of menses and when this period started
- Length of time between cycles (The longer the time between the onset of menses and the onset of excessive bleeding, the less likely it is related to anovulatory cycles.)
- Presenting symptoms: pain, nausea/vomiting, diarrhea, heavy bleeding (refer)
- Sexual history: rule out pregnancy/miscarriage and sexually transmitted infection
- Medications and alternative treatments used to relieve cramps
- Number of pads used (heavy menstrual bleeding/menorrhagia is more than 8 pads or 12 tampons/day [Emans & Laufer, 2019]); clots or flooding through pads or tampons
- Bowel habits: rule out GI causes, such as constipation
- History of bruising or bleeding easily
- Energy level (to assess for anemia)

Focused Assessment

- Vital signs, pain scale
- Overall appearance: ambulatory or doubled up clutching abdomen
- GI assessment: bowel sounds, rebound tenderness

Focused Interventions

- Allow student to rest in a position of comfort until cramping subsides or until student needs to go home.
- Provide supportive measures: nonsteroidal anti-inflammatory medications as ordered; heating pad on low setting for 20 minutes to the abdomen or back (if allowed by protocol), pads (Emans & Laufer, 2019).
- Encourage follow-up with primary care provider.
- Educate about normal menstruation; provide emotional support and reassurance.

Enuresis

Enuresis refers to the continued incontinence of urine past the age of toilet training (Wilson & Gupta, 2022). Diurnal enuresis is daytime loss of urinary control; nocturnal enuresis refers to involuntary passage of urine during sleep. Nocturnal enuresis is further classified as primary (no prior period of sustained dryness) or secondary (recurrence of nighttime wetting after 6 months or longer of dryness) (Wilson & Gupta, 2022).

Occasional daytime wetting or dribbling of urine is not a cause for concern, but frequent daytime wetting is disconcerting for both the child and the parent/guardian (Walle et al., 2017). Nocturnal enuresis is common in early childhood. There is a slight male predominance for nocturnal enuresis; these children are typically deep sleepers (Collier et al., 2020). Nocturnal enuresis is not considered a healthcare problem until the child is 6 years old. Although there is a high rate of spontaneous remission, the social, emotional, and psychological costs to the children can be great.

In some children, enuresis may be related to a physical disorder, such as diabetes mellitus or diabetes insipidus, sickle cell disease, or urethral obstruction (Wilson & Gupta, 2022). Other causes common to both diurnal and nocturnal enuresis include a urine-concentrating defect, urinary tract infection, constipation, and emotional distress (Wilson & Gupta, 2022). Nocturnal enuresis can be related to either a high fluid intake or a high caffeine intake before bedtime, obstructive sleep apnea, or a family history of enuresis (Walker, 2019).

Focused History

- Access to a bathroom
- Recent fluid intake
- Voiding: pain, difficulty, color, odor, hematuria, urine-holding behaviors (squatting, dancing, or staring)
- Recent disruption in the family or other emotional stressors
- Toilet training history (for young children)
- Medications taken
- Bowel patterns, specifically constipation (Children with enuresis often have problems with constipation that must be resolved first before treating the enuresis.)

Focused Assessment

- Observe the student's general appearance.
- Palpate the bladder to check for distention, as indicated; palpate for stool.
- Take blood pressure.

Focused Interventions

- Schedule voiding times during the day at approximately 2-hour intervals.
- Educate family on importance of avoiding bladder irritants, such as chocolate, carbonated beverages, citrus, and caffeine (Rhoads & Petersen, 2019).
- Collaborate with family and teacher to develop a plan for regular voiding.

- Provide support and reassurance if student is incontinent.
- Assist student to maintain voiding diary as needed.
- Store change of clothing at school or in backpack.

Urinary Frequency

Urinary frequency is a symptom of several commonly encountered clinical pediatric problems such as UTIs, urethritis, vulvovaginitis, diabetes mellitus, drug side effects (e.g., caffeine, theophylline, and diuretics), daytime frequency syndrome of childhood (i.e., pollakiuria), and psychogenic stress (Fuentes et al., 2019).

Urinary frequency is defined as an increase in the number of voids per day. In the school-age population, urinary frequency is often described as voiding more than once every 2 hours. Urinary frequency may be caused by reduced bladder capacity or psychological stress (Austin et al., 2016). Teachers may tell the school nurse their concern about students who visit the lavatory frequently. The nurse has an important role in educating school personnel about problems of urinary frequency so that support for students can be provided.

Students with UTIs can present with frequency and burning while urinating. Urinary frequency is distinctly different from polyuria (excretion of excessive amounts of urine), although the two symptoms can be related (Austin et al., 2016). Frequency should also be differentiated from enuresis.

Urethral syndrome is a term used to describe the sudden onset of urinary frequency in adolescent girls; it is associated with dysuria with insignificant bacteria counts (Austin et al., 2016). Common causes of urethral syndrome are vaginitis, chlamydia, and gonorrhea. Urinary frequency can be attributed to vulvovaginitis or urethral trauma (related to straddle injuries, catheterization, masturbation, or sexual abuse) (Burgers et al., 2013). Taking a thorough history is the best way to try to differentiate the cause of urinary frequency.

Young children between the ages of 4 and 6 years can have an abrupt onset of urinary frequency every 15 to 30 minutes without any physiological cause, but it may be related to emotional stress. The school nurse needs to refer the student for medical evaluation to rule out a UTI. Classically, these students sleep through the night without episodes of voiding. Occasionally pinworms can cause urinary frequency. In general, nonpathological excessive daytime urinary frequency usually improves in 2 to 3 months (CDC, Division of Parasitic Diseases, 2020).

Focused History

- Onset: illness, fever, weight loss
- Voiding: pain, difficulty, color, odor, frequency, urgency, hematuria
- Hydration: fluid intake, thirst, 24-hour fluid intake history
- Rule out: pregnancy, sexually transmitted disease, GI disturbance, sexual abuse
- New stressors in the child's life: sadness, bullying, home stressors

Focused Assessment

- Vital signs, pain scale
- Observe the student's general appearance, signs of dehydration
- Presenting symptoms: chills, nausea/vomiting, flank pain
- Signs of acanthosis nigricans (i.e., darkening at the back of the neck and axilla that may be associated with type 2 diabetes)
- Palpate the bladder to check for distention, as indicated

Focused Interventions

- Ensure adequate access to the bathroom until the problem is resolved.
- Encourage follow-up with primary care provider.
- Notify child protective services about any suspicion of sexual abuse.

NEUROLOGICAL PROBLEMS

Headache

Headache is a common childhood complaint, and the incidence increases during adolescence (Klein & Koch, 2020). There are two main kinds of headaches in pediatric patients: tension and migraine.

Tension-type headaches are the most common and are believed to have a neurobiological basis. Central pain mechanisms are involved in frequent tension-type headaches; peripheral pain mechanisms are likely to be the cause of infrequent tension-type headaches (Oskoui et al., 2019). The student with tension-type headaches will complain of an equally distributed tightening feeling as though someone is putting a band around the head (Patel et al., 2022). Although the student may complain of photophobia or phonophobia, there is no nausea or vomiting. Activity does not make a tension-type headache worse.

The three subtypes of tension-type headaches are infrequent (headache less than 1 day a month), frequent (headache 1 to 14 days a month), or chronic (headache more than 15 days a month). Because children may not be able to describe headache symptoms with the same skill as an adult, it can be difficult to distinguish between migraine and tension headaches in students (Oskoui et al., 2019). Cluster headaches are rare and present with unilateral burning pain, more commonly around the eye and orbits on the affected side with a frequency of one to eight times per day (Patel et al., 2022).

The onset of *migraine headaches* typically begins during the early school-age years. The prevalence in females is twice that of males. The clinical presentation is a bilateral, frontotemporal headache with associated symptoms of nausea, vomiting, photophobia, or phonophobia. Migraines with an aura in males peak at 5 years between ages 12 and 13 in females (Oskoui et al., 2019). Headaches can be associated with menses as fluid is retained in the body, hypertension, and increased intracranial pressure. Headaches can also be related to depression (Patel et al., 2022).

Focused History

- History of head trauma, concussion, or recent accidental injury
- History of recent illness (e.g., fever, sinus infection, vision or dental issues)
- Recent food and fluid intake: hunger; dehydration; food allergies, sensitivities, and intolerances
- Sources of social and emotional stress, changes in the home or school situation, adverse childhood experiences
- Onset, frequency, time of day (when pain starts, increases, decreases), and duration of headache. Is it worse in the morning? Is it worse with activity or coughing?
- Warning signs: Auras that are persistently unilateral need medical evaluation (Oskoui et al., 2019).
- Characteristics of pain: intensity, duration, location, sharp, dull, squeezing, throbbing
- Bitemporal frontal headaches are common in migraines. Younger children describe migraines as pressing or heavy rather than throbbing.
- Tension headaches feel like a band around the head (Oskoui et al., 2019).
- Associated symptoms: fever, nausea, vomiting, numbness, weakness, imbalance, purulent nasal discharge
- Dizziness, unsteadiness, or vertigo may be associated with vestibular or cerebellar pathology. Throbbing headache accompanied by dizziness and vertigo at the onset may be a more complex form of migraine.
- Disruption of daily living: changes or disturbances in sleep, appetite, thirst, behavior, mood, affect, activity levels, school engagement and performance, loss of instructional time (i.e., absences, tardiness, health office utilization), withdrawal from caffeine
- Children with migraines have increased sleep disturbances (Oskoui et al., 2019).
- Precipitating factors: medications (e.g., prescription, OTC, or alternative) taken for headaches or other health issues, side effects, drug or alcohol use, oral contraceptives
- Exacerbating factors: increase or decrease in pain with activity, light, noise, smell, coughing, bending over, in specific social circumstances, or after consuming a particular food, drink, or caffeine
- Alleviating factors: nonpharmacological and pharmacological interventions:
  - Effectiveness of comfort measures the student seeks or has tried
  - Effectiveness of medications (prescription, OTC, alternative) that the student takes or has tried

Focused Assessment

- Vital signs: especially blood pressure changes and fever
- Conduct neurological assessment: changes in mental status, level of consciousness, behavior, visual disturbances or changes (e.g., blurred, or double vision, nystagmus, pupil changes), speech, balance, coordination, strength, sensation, gait, and motor symmetry
- Variants of migraines include visual migraines where the eyelid flutters in spasms but there is no pain; the student may also describe vision changes of wavy lines in their field of vision.
- Employ developmentally appropriate pediatric pain scale.
- Screen or rescreen vision.
- Inspect the nasal cavity for drainage, teeth for decay, tympanic membrane for signs of infection, and neck for stiffness, rigidity, spasms, or abnormality.
- Inspect chest and extremities for purpura or other rashes.

Focused Interventions

- Have the student rest in a dark, quiet room for a short period unless the student appears acutely ill with a change in mentation.
- Activate the EMS system if headache is associated with significant head trauma, change of level of consciousness, orientation, vital signs, or presence of nuchal rigidity with photophobia, and fever.
- Offer a snack and drink of water/fluid if the student indicates they are hungry, thirsty, or have not eaten or drunk sufficiently.
- Educate the parent/guardian and student about the need to maintain a headache diary to help the primary care provider in headache evaluation.
- Apply cool compresses over the eyes or forehead for 20 minutes.
- Explore with student and family how to eliminate possible triggers (including nutritional triggers) and how to institute a healthy lifestyle including adequate sleep, fluid, and diet, as well as starting pain medication at the onset of the headache.
- Administer analgesics if medical orders are in place.

Dizziness

Dizziness is classified into four categories: vertigo, presyncope, disequilibrium, and nonspecific complaints. *Vertigo* is a feeling that one is moving when still or the room is moving in circles or linearly. The student may have impaired balance, pallor, nausea, vomiting, or perspiration with the vertigo. Students may complain of dizziness by saying they feel like they are on a merry-go-round or that their head and/or body is spinning. Vertigo can indicate inner-ear disease or another neurological problem. The most common diagnosis related to vertigo in children is childhood paroxysmal vertigo related to migraines, which accounts for 25% of vertigo in children ages 2 to 12 years, and is associated with headache, nausea and vomiting, and occasionally photophobia (Fancello et al., 2021). Vertigo may be associated with psychological stress and inadequate sleep.

Neurological signs can also be associated with vertigo in the form of drug intoxication, encephalitis, paraneoplastic syndromes, and neuroblastomas (Fancello et al., 2021). In this case, equilibrium is more the issue than true vertigo. Rarely, vertigo may be the only presenting sign of chronic otitis media. Syncope can be related to cardiac arrhythmias, vagal and other reflexes, and, in some cases, is psychogenic. Cardiac arrhythmias and conditions related to syncope include bradyarrhythmias such as atrioventricular block, supraventricular tachycardia, and long QT syndrome (Fancello et al., 2021). Table 16-5 differentiates types of presentation of dizziness.

Students also use the term *dizziness* to describe lightheadedness from hyperventilation, dehydration, hypoglycemia, or comorbid cardiac conditions. Students may have different terms for dizziness or may not be able to accurately describe what they are feeling. Similar to headache, school nursing assessment of complaints of dizziness includes a careful assessment of precipitating and alleviating factors and careful neurological assessment. Exposure to inhaled drugs or solvents (sniffing or huffing), gases (carbon monoxide), or chemicals (gasoline) also needs to be assessed. Nursing interventions depend on underlying causes with a focus on safety and fall prevention. Students with dizziness or vertigo should be referred for medical evaluation.

Syncope

A syncopal episode, or fainting, causes significant anxiety for the family, playmates/peers, and school personnel. *Syncope* is a reversible, temporary, and acute loss of consciousness and postural tone (Li et al., 2021). The decrease in blood flow to the brain causes the cortical centers to release inhibiting influences on the reticular formation. The causes of syncope include dehydration, abnormalities of the autonomic nervous system, cardiac disease, neurological problems, medications, metabolic disorders, and psychogenic problems (Li et al., 2021). A syncopal episode may actually be temporal lobe epilepsy.

Neurally mediated syncope includes vasovagal and neurocardiogenic syncope (Villafane et al., 2021). Vasovagal syncope is commonly caused in the upright position with rapid gravitationally mediated venous pooling in the lower extremities (Villafane et al., 2021). This leads to transient hypovolemia causing a decrease in venous return and stroke volume. Emotional stress, physical stress, or a reflex mechanism (i.e., voiding or swallowing) can cause an increase in sympathetic output. The resulting hypotension causes a decrease in cerebral perfusion pressure causing a syncopal episode. A prodromal period of a few seconds to 1 to 2 minutes that consists of nausea, epigastric distress, diaphoresis, pallor, dizziness, and weakness is suggestive of vasovagal, neurocardiogenic, or a simple "faint" (Villafane et al., 2021).

Syncope can occur when adolescents or preadolescents have been in a warm place, have not eaten, have had limited fluid intake, or stand up too quickly. Situational syncope is common with this age group, especially when seeing blood or after receiving immunizations.

Cardiac syncope is associated with little or no prodrome and occurs suddenly even when the student is lying down. Students with syncope during exercise, with complaints of palpitations, or with chest pain during exercise need emergent medical evaluation. Students younger than 6 years with syncope are more worrisome unless there is a situational explanation such as fear, anxiety, pain, hunger, crowding, fatigue, injection, or the sight of blood.

Another cause of syncope is *postural orthostatic tachycardia syndrome* (POTS). The clinical presentation of POTS is excessive tachycardia, which leads to decreasing blood pressure and symptoms of orthostatic intolerance, followed by a simple postural faint (Fancello et al., 2021). Most definitions of POTS include a sustained increase in heart rate greater than or equal to 30 beats/min more than the child's normal pulse rate or greater than 120 beats/min within 10 minutes of orthostatic changes. The clinical features can be rapid or have an insidious progression. Other associated symptoms of POTS include weakness,

TABLE 16-5 Understanding Different Presentations of Dizziness

Term	Clinical Presentation	Nursing Intervention
Presyncope	Student will feel light-headed and may feel as though they are going to faint.	• Lay the student down. • Take vital signs. • Offer fluids with sodium and glucose.
Vertigo	Student complains of spinning of the body or that the room around the student is spinning.	• Lay the student down. • Get adequate history about recent illness. • Examine ears. • Ask about medications and illicit drug use. • Refer to primary care provider for further management.
Disequilibrium	Student feels off balance and has postural instability.	• Has the student fallen recently? • Are there signs of muscle weakness? • Is there any numbness, tingling reported?

palpitations, hyperhidrosis (i.e., excessive sweating), chest pain, vomiting, diarrhea, fatigue, and sleep disturbance (Fancello et al., 2021).

POTS is estimated to be quite prevalent in the United States, with the highest rates in females between 15 and 50 years of age (Fancello et al., 2021). The prevalence in females may be related to differences in sympathetic nerve discharge characteristics. The pathophysiology may include neuropathic dysfunction, hyperadrenergic response, genetic mutation, state of hypovolemia, and impaired cerebral autoregulation.

Pharmacological and nonpharmacological therapies are useful in the treatment of POTS. Making sure that the student consumes adequate amounts of water and salt together with regular aerobic exercise is an evidence-based intervention. For older adolescents, elastic support hosiery is also suggested to improve venous return.

Focused History

- Determine what preceded the episode. Was the student sitting or standing when the episode occurred?
- Determine past history and frequency of syncopal episodes.
- Inquire about the student's recollection of how they felt, saw, or heard (aura) before the syncopal episode: dizziness, palpitation, chest pain, tunnel vision, headache, belching, yawning, weakness, cold hands, sweating, or nausea.
- Note whether there are neurological deficits after a syncopal event, the length of time for recovery, and sequelae.
- Obtain a history of the event from witnesses: length of episode, student's appearance, cyanosis, incontinence, eye or limb movements, or sounds made by the student during the episode.
- Ascertain the precipitating factors: medications (prescription, OTC, or alternative) taken with headache side effects; drug or alcohol use (especially huffing/sniffing toxic fumes); breath holding; comorbid conditions (e.g., seizures, diabetes, cardiac conditions, familial history of sudden cardiac death); recent illness or stressful occurrences; adequate fluid/food intake, especially with sun exposure and after exercise.
- Determine whether there is history of trauma to the temporal bone region.

Focused Assessment

- Assess for airway patency. If the student is still unconscious after 2 minutes, call EMS.
- Assess for injuries if student fell as a result of syncope.
- Perform a neurological assessment: assess for blurred vision, tinnitus (ringing in the ears), decrease in hearing, sweating, extraocular eye movements, balance (Romberg test: stand with feet together and arms at sides; close eyes and hold position for 20 seconds; may sway slightly but should maintain balance [Jarvis, 2020]).
- Perform cardiac assessment, including checking for postural hypotension (positive orthostatic changes are changes of 20 mm Hg or more when moving from supine to standing position; take BP lying down, sitting, and standing).
- Check for hypoglycemia in students with known diabetes.

Focused Interventions

- Allow the student to lie down with the feet elevated (without a pillow under the head) for at least 10 to 20 minutes to increase blood flow to the brain. Monitor closely. A cool compress to the forehead may help if diaphoretic.
- Treat underlying cause, if known, according to medical orders. Provide fluid replacement (e.g., carbohydrates, fruit juice), ensure proper ventilation, decrease stimuli in the environment.
- Refer for further evaluation if indicated.

Weakness

To evaluate a student who complains of weakness, the school nurse should use a systematic approach to evaluate the musculoskeletal system for muscle atrophy, motor function, and strength (Rhoads & Petersen, 2019). Weakness can also be caused by a host of health conditions such as sleep deprivation; dehydration; poor nutrition; infectious diseases; and endocrine, cardiac, pulmonary, hematological (anemia), rheumatic, and neurological system disorders; as well as exposure to toxic substances. Activity levels, fine and gross motor function, gait, and the ability to rise independently from a seated or supine position are important indicators of the severity of weakness and potential underlying pathology. The focused history and assessment will guide appropriate nursing interventions and referral for medical evaluation and treatment if indicated. Note whether the recent weakness is affecting the student's academic performance.

MINOR WOUNDS

Many students present to the school health office with minor wounds that can be treated with first aid. Wounds can be classified as abrasions, lacerations, burns, punctures, and bites. Hemostasis is the primary concern with most wounds. Superficial wounds, such as abrasions and scrapes, require no suture closure. Injuries that penetrate into or beyond the dermis, such as deep or gaping lacerations, may require medical intervention (Bultas & Oldenburg, 2023). When subcutaneous fat is visible, the injured student needs to be seen by a healthcare provider to evaluate the need for wound closure (i.e., sutures, staples, surgical glue). A thorough history of the mechanism of trauma should be taken to elicit the possibility of deep injury (crush injury, blunt trauma), contamination from environmental substances (soil, manure, animal or human saliva), or retained foreign bodies (gravel, wood or metal splinters). Many abrasions and minor lacerations may appear to have significant ongoing blood loss, but this is usually an oozing type of bleeding (Bultas & Oldenburg, 2023).

Wound cleansing and débridement are the most important aspects of preventing secondary infections. Cleansing is performed best with mild soap and water or normal saline under mild pressure (Bultas & Oldenburg, 2023). It is important to remove dirt and gravel to reduce the risk for infection. Tap water should *not* be used in cases where a full-thickness injury has been sustained and tendons, blood vessels, or bones have been exposed (Bultas & Oldenburg, 2023). Antibiotic creams and other topical medications should be used only if standing orders specifically allow it and the child has no known allergies to the products.

Puncture wounds can be superficial or deep. Puncture wounds are reported to have the highest infection rate after animal bites because of the deposition of bacteria deep in the skin (Bultas & Oldenburg, 2023). Infection rates are also high if a nail punctures tennis shoes before entering the skin. Wounds that involve the chest, abdomen, neck, hand, and eye are considered serious penetrating trauma. See Chapter 17 for more information on students with acute traumatic wounds.

Focused History

- Mechanism, time, location of injury, and potential contaminants. What was the wounding agent (e.g., metal, glass, wood, plants, playground asphalt, dirt, pencil graphite, knife, etc.)?
- History of medical conditions or medications that interfere with blood clotting or wound healing, such as immunosuppression or the use of steroids
- Immunization history (e.g., tetanus)
- Wound character, size, shape, and depth
- Pain severity and character, amount of bleeding, associated symptoms, other body trauma

Focused Assessment

- Extent of bleeding, redness, swelling
- Underlying injury, bleeding, bruising, point tenderness, presence of foreign bodies
- Limitations in movement or function associated with injury

Focused Interventions

Scrapes and Cuts

- Clean the wound away from the area of injury, going from inside to outside. Never bring dirt toward the wound.
- Thoroughly irrigate the wound with a physiological solution, such as normal saline. If normal saline is not available, use tap water.
- Do not use agents that are cytotoxic to human fibroblasts and inhibit collagen tissue, such as povidone-iodine 10%, acetic acid, hydrogen peroxide, and benzalkonium chloride (Greener, 2016). The stronger the cleanser, the more toxic it is to cells.
- Apply topicals if allowed by school protocol. Silver sulfadiazine RX (Silvadene) and topical antibiotics have been shown to reduce the bacterial counts of wounds. Topicals do not sterilize the wound but rather control bacterial growth; they promote wound reepithelialization.
- Notify the parent/guardian of the scrape and how it was treated and when student was returned to the classroom.
- Document appearance of the wound and treatment: location, size, shape, depth, length, causative agent.
- Complete an incident/accident report in accordance with school policy and procedures.

Splinters

- Remove splinters, if possible, before they become hidden by swollen tissue or embedded in tissue. Deep, embedded, large splinters will need to be removed by the primary care provider.
- Superficial splinters may be washed off; some can be removed by using sticky tape or sterilized tweezers to pull out at the same angle it went in.
- Wash with soap and water; apply antibiotic ointment if appropriate, and apply a clean adhesive bandage or gauze dressing.
- Notify a parent/guardian and instruct on wound care at home.

Puncture Wounds

- Clean and irrigate the wound.
- Refer any student who stepped on a nail to their primary care provider for further evaluation and treatment.
- Document appearance of the wound and treatment as specifically as possible: location, size, shape, depth, length, treatment.
- Complete incident/accident report if injury occurred on school grounds, in accordance with school policy and procedures.

JOINT AND BONE PAIN

Joint pain is often referred pain from other sites, so it is important to examine above and below the area of complaint. Joint pain can be the result of musculoskeletal injury, but may also reflect systemic conditions such as leukemia, rheumatological disease, inflammatory bowel disease, or, rarely, tumors. Knee pain is more common in students who are extremely active, possibly related to overuse.

Knee pain in the younger adolescent can result from *Osgood-Schlatter syndrome* (i.e., aseptic necrosis of the tibial tuberosity), which causes a partial separation of the patella tendon from the anterior tibial tuberosity leading to pain (Ladenhauf et al., 2020). Because bone grows faster than muscle, the quadriceps muscle pulls across the apophysis of the tibial tubercle during activity causing a chronic avulsion of the tibial tuberosity ossification center. As the cartilage pulls away, there is ossification and subsequent enlargement of the anterior tibial tuberosity. Due to earlier onset of puberty in girls, the symptom of anterior tibial tuberosity pain more often occurs in girls from 8 to 12 years and in boys from 12 to 15 years of age (Ladenhauf et al., 2020). Initially, the pain is intermittent and mild; but during the acute phase the pain is more continuous and severe and is exacerbated by physical activity, especially involving bending or kneeling. Pain from Osgood-Schlatter syndrome usually resolves over time with the rest of the knee.

Patellofemoral pain syndrome presents as anterior knee pain involving the patella and surrounding soft tissues. It is a common knee problem among adolescents, particularly female athletes. Pain tends to get worse with climbing stairs, squatting, prolonged sitting, and running. However, there is usually no effusion present within the knee. Pain will present on palpation of the patellar tendon and surrounding structures (Sweeney et al., 2020).

Focused History

- Mechanism of injury (if known)
- Sports and activities that cause the knee or joint to hurt
- Quality and quantity of pain: precipitating and alleviating factors
- Functional impairment
- Comorbid conditions (e.g., inflammatory bowel disease, juvenile idiopathic arthritis, Lyme disease, lupus)

Focused Assessment

- Assess pain level on a developmentally appropriate pain scale.
- Inspect for swelling and/or bruising.
- Check range of motion above and below the joint or bone.
- Check for symmetry with joint/bone on opposite side of the body.
- Check for reproducible pain with extension of the knee against resistance of the examiner's hand; this is consistent with Osgood-Schlatter syndrome (Sweeney et al., 2020).
- Check for crepitus during joint movement.
- Determine whether student can get up and walk without difficulty.
- Assess hip flexion and extension, abduction and adduction, and internal and external rotation. It is not uncommon for hip pathology to be perceived as knee pain and vice versa.

Focused Interventions

- Elevate and ice painful or injured area as tolerated.
- Splint or immobilize suspected fractures.
- Encourage student to rest the injured part and not to try to "work through the pain."
- Avoid activities where student is on their knees.

CONCLUSION

This chapter has reviewed common student health complaints and problems that can present to the school nurse. Most students who visit the health office are able to return to class after the school nurse assesses the student and implements basic nursing interventions. Students with common health complaints require astute assessment by the school nurse because common complaints and presentations may herald more significant mental or physical health issues that require medical evaluation and a careful and coordinated follow-up plan of care. An organized approach to common complaints communicated to the parent/guardian and healthcare providers allows the school nurse the opportunity to have a positive impact on the health of students and reduces loss of instructional time in the classroom.

The Editors gratefully acknowledge the work of the previous chapter authors, Tami Jakubowski and Tracy Perron.

References

Adam, H. (2020). Fever. Quick references. *Pediatric Care Online.* https://doi.org/10.1542/aap.ppcqr.396073

Aggarwal, B. B. (2021). Acute abdominal pain in paediatrics. *Pedia Flash, 7*(1). https://wbhf.walterbushnell.com/docs/2021/pedia-flash/article-1.pdf

American Academy of Ophthalmology. (2023, June 14). *What is the difference between a stye and a chalazion? Causes, symptoms, treatment.* https://www.aao.org/eye-health/diseases/what-are-chalazia-styes

American Academy of Pediatrics. (2021). *Red book: 2021–2024 report of the Committee on Infectious Diseases* (32nd ed.). American Academy of Pediatrics.

American Academy of Pediatrics. (2022). *Bright futures tools and resource kit: Developmental, behavioral, psychosocial, screening, and assessment forms* (2nd ed.). Author. https://www.aap.org/en/practice-management/bright-futures/bright-futures-materials-and-tools/bright-futures-tool-and-resource-kit/bright-futures-developmental-behavioral-psychosocial-screening-and-assessment-forms/

American College of Asthma, Allergies, & Immunology. (2017). *Seasonal allergies.* https://acaai.org/allergies/seasonal-allergies

Armitage, R. (2021). Bullying in children: Impact on child health. *British Medical Journal Paediatrics Open, 5*(1), e000939. https://doi.org/10.1136/bmjpo-2020-000939

Austin, P. F., Bauer, S. B., Bower, W., Chase, J., Franco, I., Hoebeke, P., Rittig, S., Vande Walle, J., von Gontard, A., Wright, A., Yang, S., & Neveus, T. (2016). The standardization of terminology of lower urinary tract function in children and adolescents: Update report from the standardization committee of the International Children's Continence Society. *Neurourology and Urodynamics, 35*(4), 471–481. https://doi.org/10.1002/nau.22751

Barbi, E., Marzuillo, P., Neri, E., Naviglio, S., & Krauss, B. S. (2017). Fever in children: Pearls and pitfalls. *Children (Basel, Switzerland), 4*(9), 81. https://doi.org/10.3390/children4090081

Bielory, L., Delgado, L., Katelaris, C. H., Leonardi, A., Rosario, N., & Vichyanoud, P. (2020). ICON: Diagnosis and management of allergic conjunctivitis. *Annals of Allergy, Asthma & Immunology: Official Publication of the American College of Allergy, Asthma, & Immunology, 124*(2), 118–134. https://doi.org/10.1016/j.anai.2019.11.014

Boerner, K. E., Green, K., Chapman, A., Stanford, E., Newlove, T., Edwards, K., & Dhariwal, A. (2020). Making sense of "somatization": A systematic review of its relationship to pediatric pain. *Journal of Pediatric Psychology, 45*(2), 156–169. https://doi.org/10.1093/jpepsy/jsz102

Brodsky, L. (1989). Modern assessment of tonsils and adenoids. *Pediatric Clinics of North America, 36*(6), 1551–1569. doi:10.1016/S0031-3955(16)36806-7

Bryant, R. (2024). Impact of cognitive or sensory impairment on the child and family. In M. J. Hockenberry, E. A. Duffy, & K. D. Gibbs (Eds.), *Wong's nursing care of infants and children* (12th ed., pp. 621–647). Elsevier.

Bultas, M. W., & Oldenburg, A. P. (2023). Minor skin injuries at school: The role of the school nurse. *NASN School Nurse, 38*(2), 79–83. https://doi-org.ezproxy.tcnj.edu/10.1177/1942602X221144304

Burgers, R. E., Mugie, S. M., Chase, J., Cooper, C. S., von Gontard, A., Rittig, C. S., Homsy, Y., Bauer, S. B., & Benninga, M. A. (2013). Management of functional constipation in children with lower urinary tract symptoms: Report from the standardization committee of the International Children's Continence Society. *The Journal of Urology, 190*(1), 29–36.

Cameron, A. C., & Widmer, R. P. (2022). *Handbook of pediatric dentistry* (5th ed.). Elsevier Health Sciences.

Centers for Disease Control and Prevention. (2021). Oral health surveillance report, 2019: *Trends in dental caries and sealants, tooth retention, and endentulism, United States 1999–2004 to 2011–2016*. https://www.cdc.gov/oralhealth/publications/OHSR-2019-index.html

Centers for Disease Control and Prevention. (2022a). *Handwashing: Clean hands save lives*. https://www.cdc.gov/handwashing/index.html

Centers for Disease Control and Prevention. (2022b). *Pertussis (whooping cough)*. https://www.cdc.gov/pertussis/index.html

Centers for Disease Control and Prevention. (2023). *Data and statistics about hearing loss in children*. https://www.cdc.gov/hearing-loss-children/data/?CDC_AAref_Val=https://www.cdc.gov/ncbddd/hearingloss/data.html

Centers for Disease Control and Prevention, Division of Parasitic Diseases. (2020). Parasites: Erterobiasis (also known as pinworm infection). https://www.cdc.gov/parasites/pinworm/

Collier, E., Varon, C., Van Huffel, S., & Bogaert, G. (2020). Enuretic children have a higher variability in REM sleep when comparing their sleep parameters with nonenuretic control children using a wearable sleep tracker at home. *Neurourology and Urodynamics, 39*(1), 367–375. https://doi.org/10.1002/nau.24215

Danishyar, A., & Ashurst, J. V. (2022, December 11). Acute otitis media. *StatPearls* [Internet]. https://www.ncbi.nlm.nih.gov/books/NBK470332/

Das, J. (2018). *Trauma in otolaryngology*. Gateway East, Singapore: Springer Nature.

DeGeorge, K. C., Ring, D. J., & Dalrymple, S. N. (2019). Treatment of the common cold. *American Family Physician, 100*(5), 281–289.

DePietro, M. (2018). How to get a bug out of your ear. *Medical News Today*. https://www.medicalnewstoday.com/articles/322064.php

DeSanctis, V., Soliman, A., Bernasconi, S., Bianchin, L., Bona, G., Bozzola, M., Buzi, F., de Sanctis, C., Tonini, G., Rigon, F., & Perissinotto, E. (2015). Primary dysmenorrhea in adolescents: Prevalence, impact and recent knowledge. *Pediatric Endocrinology Reviews, 13*(2), 512–520.

Dharmapuri, S. (2019). Dysmenorrhea in adolescents. *Pediatric Medicine 2019, 2*(34), 1–9. https://doi.org/10.21037/pm.20

Earwood, J. S., Rogers, T. S., & Rathjen, N. A. (2018). Ear pain: Diagnosing common and uncommon causes. *American Family Physician, 97*(1), 20–27.

Elliott, D. B. (2020). *Clinical procedures in primary eye care* (5th ed.). Elsevier Health Sciences.

Emans, S. J., & Laufer, M. R. (2019). *Goldstein's pediatric and adolescent gynecology* (7th ed.). Lippincott Williams & Wilkins.

Fancello, V., Palma, S., Monzani, D., Pelucchi, S., Genovese, E., & Ciorba, A. (2021). Vertigo and dizziness in children: An update. *Children, 8*(11), 1025. https://doi.org/10.3390/children8111025

Fisher, B. (2024). Health problems of the school-age child. In M. Hockenberry, D. Wilson, & C. Rodgers, *Wong's nursing care of infants and children* (12th ed., pp. 483–509). Elsevier.

Friesen, C., Colombo, J. M., Deacy, A., & Schurman, J. V. (2021). An update on the assessment and management of pediatric abdominal pain. *Pediatric Health, Medicine and Therapeutics, 12*, 373–393. https://doi.org/10.2147/PHMT.S287719

Fuentes, M., Magalhães J., & Barroso, U., Jr. (2019). Diagnosis and management of bladder dysfunction in neurologically normal children. *Frontiers in Pediatrics, 7*, 298. https://doi.org/10.3389/fped.2019.00298

Galan, N. (2017). Birth control and yeast infections: What's the link? *Medical News Today*. https://www.medicalnewstoday.com/articles/319568.php

Greener, M. (2016). Wound care: Treating small wounds in the school setting. *British Journal of School Nursing*, 11(8), 376–378.

Guo, Q., Goldenberg, J. Z., Humphrey, C., El Dib, R., & Johnston, B. C. (2019). Probiotics for the prevention of pediatric antibiotic-associated diarrhea. *The Cochrane Database of Systematic Reviews, 4*(4), CD004827. https://doi.org/10.1002/14651858.CD004827.pub5

Herman, M. J., & Wolf, M. (2013). Torticollis in children. *Current Orthopaedic Practice, 24*(6), 598–603.

Heymann, D. (2022). *Control of communicable diseases manual* (21st ed.). American Public Health Association.

Ho, J. M., & How, C. H. (2020). Chronic constipation in infants and children. *Singapore Medical Journal, 61*(2), 63–68. https://doi.org/10.11622/smedj.2020014

Hockenberry, M. J. (2024). Childhood communicable and infectious diseases. In M. J. Hockenberry, E. A. Duffy, & K. V. Gibbs (Eds.), *Wong's nursing care of infants and children* (12th ed., pp. 167–195). Elsevier.

Hoersting, A., & Mullen, J. (2017). Traumatic brain injury. In C. Cartwright & D. Wallace, *Nursing care of the pediatric neurosurgery patient*. Springer International Publishing. doi:10.1007/978-3-319-49319-0_8

Hornberger, L. L., Lane, M. A., & Committee on Adolescence. (2021). Identification and management of eating disorders in children and adolescents. *Pediatrics, 147*(1), e2020040279. https://doi.org/10.1542/peds.2020-040279

Illinois Emergency Medical Services for Children & OSF HealthCare Children's Hospital of Illinois. (2022). *Guidelines for the nurse in the school setting* (4th ed.). https://www.osfhealthcare.org/media/filer_public/94/9a/949ae3b2-8927-416c-b009-a53ed47c4cc0/school_nurse_guidelines_osf_202forthosenotregistered.pdf

Ingle, T., & Gibbs, K. D. (2024). The child with cerebral dysfunction. In M. J. Hockenberry, E. A. Duffy, & K. D. Gibbs (Eds.). *Wong's nursing care of infants and children* (12th ed., pp. 1111–1171). Elsevier.

Jarvis, C. (2020). *Physical examination and health assessment* (8th ed.). Elsevier Health Sciences.

Jefferson, T., Dooley, L., Ferroni, E., Al-Ansary, L. A., van Driel, M. L., Bawazeer, G. A., Jones, M. A., Hoffmann, T. C., Clark, J., Beller, E. M., Glasziou, P. P., & Conly, J. M. (2023). Physical interventions to interrupt or reduce the spread of respiratory viruses. *Cochrane Database of Systematic Reviews*. https://doi.10.1002/14651858.CD006207.pub6

Johnson, D., Liu, D., & Simel, D. (2022). Does this patient with acute infectious conjunctivitis have a bacterial infection? The rational clinical examination systematic review. *JAMA, 327*(22), 2231–2237. https://doi.org/10.1001/jama.2022.7687

Kabra, R., & Fisher, M. (2022). Abnormal uterine bleeding in adolescents. *Current Problems in Pediatric and Adolescent Health Care, 52*(5), 101185. https://doi.org/10.1016/j.cppeds.2022.101185

Kasbekar, R., Naz, A., Marcos, L., Liu, Y., Hendrickson, K., Gorsich, J. C., & Baun, M. (2021). Threshold for defining fever varies with age, especially in children: A multi-site diagnostic accuracy study. *Nursing Open, 8*(5), 2705–2721. https://doi.org/10.1002/nop2.831

Kato, G. J., Piel, F. B, Reid, C. D., Gaston, M. H., Ohene-Frempong, K., Krishnamurti, L., Smith, W. R., Panepinto, J. A., Weatherall, D. J., Costa, F. F., & Vichinsky, E. P. (2018). Sickle cell disease. *Nature Reviews. Disease Primers, 4*, 18010. https://doi.org/10.1038/nrdp.2018.10

Klein, J., & Koch, T. (2020). Headache in children. *Pediatrics in Review, 41*(4), 159–171. https://doi.org/10.1542/pir.2017-0012

Krafft, C., & Christy, C. (2020). Mycoplasma pneumonia in children and adolescents. *Pediatrics in Review, 41*(1), 12–19. https://doi.org/10.1542/pir.2018-0016

Kumar, D. J., Valenzuela, D., Kozak, F. K., Ludemann, J. P., Moxham, J. P., Lea, J., & Chadha, N. K. (2014). The reliability of clinical tonsil size grading in children. *Journal of the American Medical Association Otolaryngology–Head & Neck Surgery, 140*(11), 1034–1037. https://doi.org/10.1001/jamaoto.2014.2338

Ladenhauf, H. N., Seitlinger, G., & Green, D. W. (2020). Osgood-Schlatter disease: A 2020 update of a common knee condition in children. *Current Opinion in Pediatrics, 32*(1), 107–112. https://doi.org/10.1097/MOP.0000000000000842

LeLeiko, N. S., Mayer-Brown, S., Cerezo, C., & Plante, W. (2020). Constipation. *Pediatrics in Review, 41*(8), 379–392. https://doi.org/10.1542/pir.2018-0334

Li, H. X., Gao, L., & Yuan, Y. (2021). Advance in the understanding of vasovagal syncope in children and adolescents. *World Journal of Pediatrics, 17*(1), 58–62. https://doi.org/10.1007/s12519-020-00367-z

Lieberthal, A. S., Carroll, A. E., Chonmaitree, T., Ganiats, T., Hoberman, A., Jackson, M. A., Joffe, M. D., Miller, D. T., Rosenfeld, R. M., Sevilla, X. D., Schwartz, R. H., Thomas, P. A., & Tunkel, D. E. (2013). The diagnosis and management of acute otitis media. *Pediatrics, 131,* e964–e999. https://doi.org/10.1542/peds.2012–3488

MedlinePlus. (2022). Fever. *MedlinePlus.* https://medlineplus.gov/ency/article/003090.htm

National Association of School Nurses. (2024). A contemporary framework update for today's school nursing landscape: Introducing the School Nursing Practice Framework. *NASN School Nurse, 39*(3), 140–147. https://www.doi.org/10.1177/1942602X241241092

Nurko, S., & Zimmerman, L. A. (2014). Evaluation and treatment of constipation in children and adolescents. *American Family Physician, 90*(2), 82–90.

Oskoui, M., Pringsheim, T., Holler-Managan, Y., Potrebic, S., Billinghurst, L., Gloss, D., Hershey, A. D., Licking, N., Sowell, M., Victorio, M. C., Gersz, E. M., Leininger, E., Zanitsch, H., Yonker, M., & Mack, K. (2019). Practice guideline update summary: Acute treatment of migraine in children and adolescents: Report of the guideline development, dissemination, and implementation subcommittee of the American Academy of Neurology and the American Headache Society. *Neurology, 93*(11), 487–499. https://doi.org/10.1212/WNL.0000000000008095

Patel, V. A., Liaw, J., Saadi, R. A., Isildak, H., Kalmar, C. L., & Polster, S. P. (2022). Headache diagnosis in children and adolescents. *Otolaryngologic Clinics of North America, 55*(3), 633–647. https://doi.org/10.1016/j.otc.2022.02.007

Paul, C. R., & Moreno, M. (2020). Acute otitis media. *JAMA Pediatrics, 174*(3), 308. https://doi.10.1001/jamapediatrics.2019.5664

Pelucchi, C., Grigoryan, L., Galeone, C., Esposito, S., Huovinen, P., Little, P., & Verheij, T. (2012). Guideline for the management of acute sore throat. *Clinical Microbiology and Infection, 18*(Suppl 1), 1–28.

Rajindrajith, S., Zeevenhooven, J., Devanarayana, N. M., Perera, B. J., & Benninga, M. A. (2018). Functional abdominal pain disorders in children. *Expert Review of Gastroenterology & Hepatology, 12*(4), 369–390. https://doi.org/10.1080/17474124.2018.1438188

Reinauer, C., Platzbecker, A. L., Viermann, R., Domhardt, M., Baumeister, H., Foertsch, K., Linderskamp, H., Krassuski, L., Staab, D., Minden, K., Kilian, R., Holl, R. W., Warschburger, P., & Meißner, T. (2021). Efficacy of motivational interviewing to improve utilization of mental health services among youths with chronic medical conditions: A cluster randomized clinical trial. *JAMA Network Open, 4*(10), e2127622. https://doi.org/10.1001/jamanetworkopen.2021.27622

Rhoads, J., & Petersen, S. W. (2021). *Advanced health assessment and diagnostic reasoning* (4th ed.). Jones & Bartlett Learning.

Rodgers, C. C., & Wilson, K. D. (2017). The child with gastrointestinal dysfunction. In M. J. Hockenberry, D. Wilson, & C. C. Rodgers (Eds.), *Wong's essentials of pediatric nursing* (10th ed., pp. 689–737). Elsevier.

Saguil, A., Kane, S., Mercado, M., & Lauters, R. (2017). Herpes zoster and postherpetic neuralgia: Prevention and management. *American Family Physician, 96*(10), 656–663.

Sanderson, S. K., & Gaylord, N. M. (2020). Infectious diseases. In D. Maaks, N. Starr, M. Brady, N. Gaylord, M. Driessnack, & K. Duderstadt (Eds.), *Burns' pediatric primary care* (pp. 456–510). Elsevier.

Sargent, B., Kaplan, S. L., Coulter, C., & Baker, C. (2019). Congenital muscular torticollis: Bridging the gap between research and clinical practice. *Pediatrics, 144*(2), e20190582. https://doi.org/10.1542/peds.2019-0582

Send, T., Bertlich, M., Eichhorn, K. W., Ganschow, R., Schafigh, D., Horlbeck, F., Bootz, F., & Jakob, M. (2021). Etiology, management, and outcome of pediatric epistaxis. *Pediatric Emergency Care, 37*(9), 466–470. https://doi-org.ezproxy.tcnj.edu/10.1097/PEC.0000000000001698

Shojaei, E., Jafari, Z., & Gholami, M. (2016). Effect of early intervention on language development in hearing-impaired children. *Iranian Journal of Otorhinolaryngology, 28*(84), 13–21.

Shulman, S. T., Bisno, A. L., Clegg, H. W., Gerber, M. A., Kaplan, E. L., Lee, G., Martin, J. M., & VanBeneden, C. (2012). Clinical practice guideline for the diagnosis and management of group A streptococcal pharyngitis: 2012 update by the Infectious Diseases Society of America. *Clinical Infectious Diseases,* 55(10), e86–e102. https://doi.org10.1093/cid/cis629

Sliwinska-Kowalska, M., & Davis, A. (2012). Noise-induced hearing loss. *Noise and Health, 14*(61), 274.

Sood, M. R., Li, B. U., & Hoppin, A. G. (2023). Chronic functional constipation and fecal incontinence in infants, children, and adolescents: Treatment. *UptoDate.* https://www.uptodate.com/contents/chronic-functional-constipation-and-fecal-incontinence-in-infants-children-and-adolescents-treatment/print?search=dyfunctional%20elemination&source=search_result&selectedTitle=5~150&usage_type=default&display_rank=5

Sweeney, E., Rodenberg, R., & MacDonald, J. (2020). Overuse knee pain in the pediatric and adolescent athlete. *Current Sports Medicine Reports, 19*(11), 479–485. https://doi.org/10.1249/JSR.0000000000000773

Tarhun, Y. M. (2020). The effect of passive smoking on the etiology of serous otitis media in children. *American Journal of Otolaryngology, 41*(3), 102398. https://doi.org/10.1016/j.amjoto.2020.102398

Thomas, M., & Bomar, P. A. (2022, June 27). Upper respiratory tract infection. In: *StatPearls* [Internet]. StatPearls Publishing. https://www.ncbi.nlm.nih.gov/books/NBK532961/

Turk, D. C., & Gatchel, R. J. (Eds.). (2018). *Psychological approaches to pain management: A practitioner's handbook* (3rd ed.). Guilford Publications.

Vallerand, A. H., & Sanoski, C. A. (2020). *Davis's drug guide for nurses* (17th ed.). F.A. Davis.

Varu, D. M., Rhee, M. K., Akpek, E. K., Amescua, G., Farid, M., Garcia-Ferrer, F. J., Lin, A., Musch, D. G., Mah, F. S., & Dunn, S. P. (2019). Conjunctivitis preferred practice pattern. *Ophthalmology, 126*(1), P94–P169. https://doi-org.ezproxy.tcnj.edu/10.1016/j.ophtha.2018.10.020

Villafane, J., Miller, J. R., Glickstein, J., Johnson, J. N., Wagner, J., Snyder, C. S., Filina, T., Pomeroy, S. L., Sexson-Tejtel, S. K., Haxel, C., Gottlieb, J., Eghtesady, P., & Chowdhury, D. (2021). Loss of consciousness in the young child. *Pediatric Cardiology, 42*(2), 234–254. https://doi.org/10.1007/s00246-020-02498-6

Walker, R. A. (2019). Nocturnal eneuresis. *Primary Care: Clinics in Office Practice, 46*(2), 243–248. doi.org/10.1016/j.pop.2019.02.005

Walle, J. V., Rittig, S., Tekgul, S., Austin, P., Yang, S. S., Lopez, P. J., & Van Herzeele, C. (2017). Enuresis: Practical guidelines for primary care. *British Journal of General Practice, 67*(660), 328–329. https://doi.org/10.3399/bjgp17X691337

Weinberger, M., & Hurvitz, M. (2020). Diagnosis and management of chronic cough: Similarities and differences between children and adults. *F1000Research, 9*, F1000 Faculty Rev-757. https://doi.org/10.12688/f1000research.25468.1

Wilson, M., & Gupta, V. (2022). Enuresis. *StatPearls.* https://www.ncbi.nlm.nih.gov/books/NBK560565/#_NBK560565_pubdet_

Woo, T. (2020). Eye disorders. In C. Burns, A. Dunn, M. Brady, N. Starr, C. Blosser, & D. Garzon (Eds.), *Pediatric primary care* (pp. 616–646). Elsevier.

World Health Organization. (2022). Pneumonia in children. https://www.who.int/news-room/fact-sheets/detail/pneumonia

Yeh, T. K., & Yeh, J. (2015). Chest pain in pediatrics. *Pediatric Annals, 44*(12), e274–e278. https://doi.org/10.3928/00904481-20151110-01

Zavdy, O., Viner, I., London, N., Menzely, T., Hod, R., Raveh, E., & Gilony, D. (2021). Intranasal foreign bodies: A 10-year analysis of a large cohort, in a tertiary medical center. *American Journal of Emergency Medicine, 50*, 356–359. https://doi-org.ezproxy.tcnj.edu/10.1016/j.ajem.2021.08.045

Chapter 17

Students With Acute Illness and Injury

Vicki L. Brzoza ▪ Mariann F. Cosby ▪ Christina Silva

CHAPTER OUTLINE

School nursing practice includes first-responder elements of emergency nursing in the educational setting (Cosby, 2023). Therefore, the school nurse must be prepared to respond to unexpected urgent or emergent health emergencies involving students, staff, and school visitors both at school and during school-related activities. An *emergency* is commonly regarded as an unanticipated circumstance that calls for immediate action.

Unintentional injury is a leading cause of death for children and young adults. Injury accounts for almost 42% of adolescent deaths (Centers for Disease Control and Prevention [CDC], 2022a). Adolescents are much more likely to die of injuries sustained from motor vehicle traffic crashes and firearms than are younger children (Panchal, 2022). From 2019 to 2021, firearm deaths rose to 3.6 deaths per 100,000 children, an increase of almost 50% (Panchal, 2022). Nonfatal injuries are important causes of child morbidity, disability, and reduced quality of life. For children younger than 14, the leading cause of nonfatal injury is falls (CDC, 2022f). For adolescents, nonfatal injury often results from violence, sports-related activities, or motor vehicle traffic crashes (CDC, 2022f). From 2010 to 2020, almost 180,000 school injuries resulted in a visit to an emergency department (ED) (SafeHome.org, 2022). Additionally, complications or exacerbations of many chronic conditions in children can present as emergencies during the school day.

These statistics highlight that emergencies are common reasons that students, staff, and visitors require nursing care in schools. Districts should have emergency policies, protocols, and procedures in place and train unlicensed staff to respond accordingly. A school's failure to provide adequate employee training in emergency care may result in unintended harm to students and place a school at risk for liability.

During a health emergency, the primary objectives for the school nurse are to triage, prevent further harm, stabilize, and expedite transport of the ill or injured individual(s) to a healthcare facility, such as an ED, that can perform a complete evaluation and provide medical treatment. The purpose of this chapter is to outline the school nurse's response to emergencies involving students, though the principles are applicable to staff members and visitors, and incidents involving multiple people. See Chapter 15 for discussion of school preparedness and response for emergencies and disasters involving multiple casualties.

THE SCHOOL NURSE'S ROLE IN HEALTH EMERGENCIES

School nurses advocate for student safety by preparing for a wide range of potential emergencies that might occur at school (National Association of School Nurses [NASN], 2022). As the leader on the school health services team, the school nurse must be knowledgeable about urgent and emergent healthcare issues and current evidence-based practice guidelines. The school nurse is responsible for mounting a confident response to acute situations at school that are urgent, emergent, or potentially life-threatening. The nursing standard of care includes clinical assessment, diagnosis, and professional interventions beyond those of simple first aid.

In every emergency situation, the school nurse completes a focused problem-based assessment of the student to manage the condition until the parent/guardian or emergency medical services (EMS) arrives and accepts responsibility for care. The nurse must be able to competently perform quick assessments to

- Recognize impending or actual emergencies and triage the severity of an illness or injury
- Triage to determine whether imminent referral to outside resources is necessary, summon appropriate EMS, or coordinate other nonemergent transport arrangements
- Provide initial emergency care, stabilizing the affected individual
- Communicate the assessment and interventions to EMS personnel
- Follow up with the healthcare provider and parent/guardian or legally responsible person

The school nurse may not always be available to respond at the time of the emergency due to competing job demands. In many school districts, school nurses cover more than one building. Therefore the school nurse should provide leadership and expertise in training the appropriate school staff to assist in emergency first response. The exact level of accountability in a specific urgent or emergent situation depends on the state's nurse practice act, relevant national and state standards, the school nurse's job description and assignments, and the district's health services policies, protocols, and procedures. The nurse should be familiar with these mandates, especially those related to delegation of healthcare tasks to unlicensed assistive personnel. See Chapters 30 and 31 for more information about delegation in the school setting.

Regardless of the availability of a school nurse, school districts are responsible for developing health emergency response programs to protect the safety of the population they serve. Districts should also develop prevention programs to mitigate injury to students, staff, and visitors to the school grounds. As the school's healthcare expert, the school nurse should be involved in the development and implementation of the school emergency preparedness response plan. Communication and coordination among the school nurse, parents/guardians, school administration, EMS, the local hospital ED, and primary care providers are recommended to optimize the plan and the availability of emergency care in schools.

THE HEALTH EMERGENCY RESPONSE PLAN

Health emergency response plans are part of more global school emergency preparedness. Planning to respond to health emergencies should include the following:

1. Developing a planning team of stakeholders, such as school administrators, staff members, school nurse, school district physician or medical advisor (as applicable), local EMS representatives, and area hospital representatives
2. Performing an emergency readiness assessment of the school and surrounding community
3. Developing a medical emergency response plan that includes written care protocols for when a nurse is available and not available
4. Identifying emergency response team members, including staff led by the school nurse, who will respond to an emergency health event
5. Outlining the process for activating this team
6. Developing a training program for the emergency response team that includes their role, scene safety, first aid, cardiopulmonary resuscitation (CPR) and automated external defibrillator (AED) use, and protocols for care, including how to respond when a student or staff experiences a sudden cardiopulmonary arrest
7. Training the emergency response team
8. Reviewing the plan and training methods at least annually or when reevaluation or changes are warranted
9. Identifying and obtaining equipment and supplies that would be needed during health emergencies and ensuring they are stored in a readily accessible area

All schools should have a cardiac emergency response plan in place to quickly activate the emergency response team, access the AED, and call 911 to increase survival rates of students or staff who suffer a sudden cardiopulmonary arrest (American Heart Association [AHA], 2016a, 2022a; Rose et al., 2016). This is especially important due to the increased numbers of children with chronic conditions in the schools. Two in five children ages 6 to 17 have chronic health conditions (CDC, 2022a). The American Heart Association recommends that CPR training be a high school graduation requirement. Currently, almost 40 states have this recommendation in place (AHA, 2022b).

Roles and Responsibilities

A delayed response by the school nurse or other members of the emergency response team may lead to serious complications or result in death. The health emergency response plan should stipulate the roles for teachers, physical education teachers, coaches/trainers, and other staff members. Understandably, many staff members express anxiety about accepting responsibility for what is perceived to be a medical rather than an educational issue, especially when they have received little to no emergency response education or training. The school nurse takes the lead in educating staff to ensure they have the lay first responder and communication skills, and the practice needed for an effective coordinated response. The school administrator or principal is typically responsible for designating the staff members involved in emergency response.

Employees who are responsible for covering the health office (e.g., staff nurses, licensed practical nurses/vocational nurses, health office assistants) have primary roles during an emergency at school. The school office and ancillary staff have important supportive roles in communication, notifying the family, and managing the scene and school environment. Student support team members, such as the school social worker or counselor, provide needed emotional support to students and staff during and following a frightening or traumatic emergency event. Local police, fire, EMS, health departments, and hospital EDs should be key partners in planning, training, and responding to health emergencies at school. Such partners are typically eager to provide first responder skills training with mannequins, equipment, and drills for school staff.

Written Emergency Guidelines and Protocols

Emergency guidelines and protocols are valuable resources for both school nurses and emergency response team members to address common urgent health presentations, high-risk conditions, and life-threatening events. Frequently cited in this chapter are the *Guidelines for the Nurse in the School Setting* (Illinois Emergency Medical Services for Children [IEMSC] & OSF HealthCare Children's Hospital of Illinois [OSF HCHI], 2022). This resource contains individual protocols for commonly encountered injuries and health problems of students that school nurses can apply to practice. Depicted as algorithms, these guidelines outline the assessment and triage processes that guide interventions for urgent and emergent health situations.

State and local guidelines may also provide guidance for basic or specialized healthcare procedures. Often, state school nurse consultants or state departments of health and/or education can direct the school nurse to these specific resources to ensure congruence with the district or site-specific plan. Keep in mind that protocols do not supplant nursing judgment. Many examples from the *Guidelines for the Nurse in the School Setting, 4th ed.*, (IEMSC & OSF HCHI, 2022) are used throughout this chapter.

> *The Illinois Emergency Medical Services for Children School Nurse Committee has exercised extreme caution that all information presented is accurate and in accordance with professional standards in effect at the time of publication. The information does not serve as a substitute for the professional advice of a physician/advanced practice nurse, does not dictate an exclusive course of treatment, and should not be construed as excluding other acceptable methods of treatment. It is recommended that care must be based on the student's clinical presentation and authorized policies. (p. V)*

Emergency Supplies

The availability of essential emergency supplies is an integral component of being able to render appropriate management of the emergency condition and should be incorporated into the health emergency plan. There is no nationally recommended list of minimal emergency equipment or supplies for schools; first-aid supply lists vary contingent on the local needs of the enrolled students and the local school community.

Meeting at least the minimal supply standard ensures that every student has the same opportunity for effective management and stabilization of likely emergencies. Backboards, evacuation chairs, blankets, and tourniquets may save lives in an emergency. A pulse oximeter can augment respiratory assessment. A generator for backup power for students dependent on electrically powered equipment may avert emergencies during power outages. An emergency *Go Bag* with emergency supplies should be ready for the school nurse to grab when responding to incidents outside of the school health office. See Online Material OM17-1 for NASN's *Emergency Resources, Equipment, and Supplies List for Schools*. Campus supply lists may have additional content based on the unique needs and ages of the student population. For instance, high schools may need a childbirth kit for pregnant teens or stock naloxone if the opioid epidemic is affecting the community.

Activating Emergency Medical Services or Public Safety Resources

The school plan for a health emergency response should include protocols and criteria for activating EMS and other public safety resources (e.g., police and fire departments) that should be summoned and the information that should be conveyed. Protocols or guidelines should contain information on when to activate EMS for unexpected urgent or emergent problems. Students with chronic conditions should have an individualized healthcare plan (IHP) and may have either a Section 504 plan or an individualized education program (IEP), depending on their unique needs. For students with life-threatening conditions, the school nurse should have developed an emergency action plan (EAP), detailing what lay staff should do when they see signs of an impending, urgent, or emergent situation, including when EMS should be activated. Note that the term emergency *action* plan is preferred over emergency *care* plan because lay school personnel take action as outlined in the plan, whereas nurses provide care under their professional licenses. The school nurse needs to train the appropriate staff and make sure that all plans are kept current and are readily accessible. See Chapter 8 for more information about student health and education plans.

In many regions, calling 911 activates EMS and dispatches an ambulance with paramedics and/or emergency medical technicians to the scene. In other areas, there are local numbers to call for EMS. In most jurisdictions, once EMS is called, a dispatcher follows protocols to determine the level of response. In many instances, firefighters and police officers or other public safety agencies may also respond, depending on the nature of the emergency and proximity to the event. For the purposes of this chapter, the terms "activate EMS" or "call 911" will be used interchangeably.

If there is a question as to the seriousness of an injury, it is always better to err on the side of safety and have the student transported to a medical facility for evaluation and treatment. The responsibility for care is transferred to EMS at the scene after the vital health information is exchanged. The health emergency response plan should designate the school staff member who accompanies the student to the ED and stays with the student until the parent/guardian arrives. Students should not be left unattended. The designee should have some experience in providing emotional support to the student while they are acutely ill or injured. Whether or not the nurse accompanies the child to the ED depends on how the health needs of the school campus will be met while the nurse is off campus.

Key staff members should be trained to activate EMS and not hang up the phone until instructed by the EMS dispatcher. The person who activates EMS should be prepared to provide the following information:

- The correct address of the school and a call-back number
- The exact location of the injured/ill person(s) and the best place to enter the building
- The type of incident or resources needed (e.g., EMS, law enforcement, fire department, hazardous materials team)
- The type of injury/illness, including pertinent medical history
- What care is being provided and by what level of responder

At the time of the emergency, a staff member should be directed to meet EMS at the school access point to guide EMS personnel to the scene. In the absence of a nurse, the school first responder should provide a brief report to the EMS crew, keeping in mind that confidential information can be shared on a need-to-know basis if it is pertinent to the safe transport and treatment of the individual. When a registered nurse (RN) is on the scene, an accurate report can be given to EMS using a systematic format such as *SBAR:* situation, background, assessment, recommendation (Blom et al., 2015; Institute for Healthcare Improvement, 2017). If the student has a known medical condition, the EAP should be copied and sent with EMS to the ED (Gereige et al., 2022). The following key data should be included, if available:

- Name
- Sex
- Age
- Chief complaint and precipitating factors
- Significant medical history, including allergies
- ABCDE (airway, breathing, circulation, disability, exposure) assessment findings, including vital signs

- Medications
- Interventions performed
- Primary care provider contact information
- Parent/guardian contact information

When time allows, the school nurse can call ahead to the ED to report the information for timely evaluation and treatment. The school administrator and parent/guardian should also be notified as soon as possible.

The health emergency response plan also needs to designate a staff member to contact the student's family or legal guardian or emergency contact immediately or as soon as safely possible. Emergency information is generally available on the student's health information card, in the school electronic records system, or on an EAP. Emergency information usually contains identifying data, critical parent/guardian contacts, and relevant health conditions. In the event of interruptions in power, Internet, or during an emergency building evacuation, contact and emergency care information should be easily accessible and portable. The school nurse should update vital health information at least annually or as changes in the student's health condition warrant. As part of this process, it is essential that parents/guardians be informed of the importance of communicating major changes in the health status of their child so that emergency response is appropriate and accurate.

Additionally, the health emergency response plan includes a mechanism to communicate with other parents/guardians and community members who may contact the school for information about the emergency. An administrator should be in charge of handling responses to information requests from the news media that reflect only objective information and respect the family's wishes and privacy.

After the Emergency

When the emergency incident is over, the school nurse should follow up with parents/guardians as soon as possible. Follow-up with healthcare providers may also be necessary, especially when changes in school medical orders are indicated. If the emergency illness is contagious, the school nurse must follow mandated communicable disease reporting to the local or state health department as required by state regulations. The health emergency response protocol should also include procedures to document the event, such as by incident reports. The school administrator and school nurse should debrief with the response team and staff involved about the incident and opportunities for improvement.

Unfortunately, some emergency events at school are extremely difficult and emotionally traumatic for students, staff, and community members. The school should communicate closely with the affected students and staff to provide needed information and support. Developmentally appropriate information needs to be shared with the students as agreed on by the ill or injured individual's family with respect to the privacy and dignity of the individual. For example, if an elementary student is transported via ambulance to the hospital for an asthma attack, the school nurse can visit the classroom to allay anxiety among classmates that they might "catch asthma" and let them know that they will be able to welcome the student back to class soon. If a student contracts bacterial meningitis, public health and school officials and the school nurse could hold a forum at school in the evening to address the fears of the school community. The school nurse can assist school administrators to craft appropriate media messages to post on the school Web site or for press releases, if needed.

Whether witnessed or not, emergencies that involve multiple individuals, trauma, blood loss, violence, critical illness, or death can have an immediate and lasting impact on the social and emotional health of the school community. Social workers and counselors should provide extra emotional support and teach coping skills. In the event of a tragic consequence or death of a student or staff member, grief counseling should be offered. An opportunity for the school community to come together can help begin the healing process and foster a return to learning as soon as possible.

SCHOOL NURSING EMERGENCY ASSESSMENT AND TRIAGE

The school nurse uses the nursing process and a systematic approach to assess and triage a student in an urgent or emergency situation. The four components of a systematic approach in an emergency are *scene safety assessment, across-the-room assessment, primary assessment,* and *secondary assessment.* The school nurse serves as a role model and remains calm and in control during an emergency. Although primary actions in an emergency must be directed toward care of the victim, crowd control is crucial to allow first responders to do their work without distraction, to protect the privacy and dignity of the injured or ill individual, and to prevent psychological trauma to bystanders. For these reasons, staff should be directed to remove bystanders and students to another location. Staff should be ready to assist with other aspects of care, such as applying pressure to a bleeding wound, reassuring the student, or communicating with the school office or EMS.

Scene Safety Assessment

Any time a nurse responds to an emergency situation, there is risk involved. It is important to remember that the emergency response team members' personal safety comes before the victim's; responders cannot help another person if they become a victim too. In the event of an emergency, whether in the health office, outside on the school grounds, or in the school community, the school nurse should first and foremost ensure that the emergency scene is safe. Before rendering aid, the school nurse should perform a quick mental determination of the situation and identify potential dangers for the responders, bystanders, or victim. In addition to potential environmental hazards, a responder is also at risk for exposure to communicable disease. Responders should wear basic personal protective equipment, such as gloves, and have masks and eye shields readily available to be used as needed.

Scene hazards include the following:

- Environmental dangers: unstable structures, fires, electrical hazards, gas leaks, traffic or other potential mechanisms of injury
- Situational dangers: potential for violence—armed perpetrator, hostages, and weapons
- Substances: blood or other body fluids, noxious fumes, toxic chemicals

If hazards are evident, the scene is not safe and should not be approached. **Activate EMS and wait until the risks are reduced before proceeding with care.**

Across-the-Room Assessment

The general appearance or across-the-room assessment begins as the school nurse approaches the ill or injured student/individual. In less than a minute, the school nurse should perform a hands-off, sensory assessment of the student and determine whether the student has physiological instability and the urgency of interventions that need to be implemented. The school nurse uses the *pediatric assessment triangle,* using **ABC** as a memory jog. The nurse looks, listens, and smells while assessing the physiological parameters that reflect the severity of illness or injury:

- General Appearance
- Work of Breathing
- Circulation to the skin (AHA, 2020b; Powers-Jarvis, 2023)

Use the mnemonic **TICLS—**Tone, Interactiveness, Consolability, Look, and Speech—to remember what to look for when assessing general appearance. Each of these parameters can convey the student's overall condition (Powers-Jarvis, 2023).

Based on this rapid initial assessment, the school nurse should compare the findings to the student's baseline and determine whether the student (a) appears sick or unstable and needs immediate action or (b) does not appear sick or unstable and requires no immediate action. In addition, the nurse should be alert for any unusual smells that may be suggestive of a disease process, such as diabetes or exposure to chemicals (AHA, 2020a; IEMSC & OSF HCHI, 2022; Powers-Jarvis, 2023). If a life-threatening condition is identified at any time, activate EMS immediately and proceed with the primary assessment and life-saving intervention.

Primary Assessment

Next, a more focused physical examination is done in two stages: a primary assessment followed by a more detailed secondary assessment. The goal of the primary rapid assessment is to provide the school nurse with a basis for identifying whether a life- or limb-threatening emergency exists and initiating treatment immediately, potentially decreasing morbidity and mortality. Experienced nurses find that they can conduct the physical assessment while simultaneously gathering information for the history and providing necessary interventions. When the need becomes apparent, both triage determination and EMS activation should occur (IEMSC & OSF HCHI 2022).

The primary assessment identifies and treats problems that threaten life, limb, or vision. The primary assessment follows the **C-ABCDE** format: Control hemorrhage/perform CPR, Airway (and simultaneous spinal motion restriction), Breathing, Circulation, Disability, and Exposure (IEMSC & OSF HCHI, 2022; Jamerson, 2023).

To assess the level of consciousness or disability, use the **AVPU** mnemonic: Alert, Verbal, Painful, Unresponsive (Table 17-1) (IEMSC & OSF HCHI, 2022; Jamerson, 2023). The *Pediatric Glasgow Coma Scale* (PGCS) is commonly used in acute care settings to assess level of consciousness. The PGCS scores range from 3 to 15. A score of 8 or lower can indicate a severe head injury (Waunch & Zaky, 2020). However, the PGCS is more complex to rate and document; therefore an accurate and objective description of level of consciousness may be more practical in the school setting.

If uncontrolled bleeding is identified at any time during the assessment process, interventions must be taken to control the hemorrhage. Direct pressure, pressure dressings, and tourniquets may be needed in order to control the bleeding. The U.S. Department of Homeland Security (2022) has a *Stop the Bleed Campaign* that provides lay person awareness and training on appropriate interventions to control bleeding. The American College of Surgeons' Stop the Bleed course also teaches the lay public how to control external bleeding by direct pressure, wound packing, and tourniquets, in that order (Jamerson, 2023). Schools should have protocols for both the school nurse and nonmedical staff who participate on the emergency response team that outline hemorrhage control measures, including the use of tourniquets (Erdman et al., 2019).

TABLE 17-1 AVPU Scale

Meaning	Associated Findings
A *Alert*	The student is awake and able to speak or interact spontaneously.
V *Verbal* (responds to verbal stimulus)	A verbal stimulus elicits some response; for example, the student's eyes may open when you call loudly, or agitation may lessen in response to a command.
P *Painful* (responds to painful stimulus)	The student responds to a painful stimulus by moaning, crying, or withdrawing from pain.
U *Unresponsive*	The student shows no response to verbal or painful stimuli.

Illinois Emergency Medical Services for Children & OSF HealthCare Children's Hospital of Illinois. (2022). *Guidelines for the nurse in the school setting* (4th ed.), with permission.

Secondary Assessment

The goal of secondary assessment is to gather additional information on the ill or injured student to assist with clinical decision making, interventions, and triage decisions. The secondary assessment obtains data following the **FGHI** mnemonic: a **F**ull set of vital signs and a pain assessment; **G**iving comfort measures; a **H**ealth history and head-to-toe or focused physical examination (inspect, palpate, auscultate); and **I**njuries, **I**nspect back, and provide additional **I**nterventions (IEMSC & OSF HCHI, 2022). To emphasize the need to continue to do reassessments, the letter J for **J**ust keep evaluating is the latest addition to the mnemonic. Reassessment for evolving signs and symptoms should be completed and include ongoing evaluation of the vital signs, identified abnormalities and effectiveness of interventions, primary survey, and pain (Cosby, 2023; Jamerson, 2023). See Box 17-1 for an overview of systematic assessment and immediate care of emergency situations.

Vital Signs and Pain Assessment

Establishing baseline vital signs is essential for ongoing reassessment and should be obtained during the physical examination. Abnormal vital signs may indicate significant pathophysiology, physical trauma, pain, or emotional distress. Normal vital signs can vary with a student's age and presenting condition (see Chapter 9). In the absence of a table of normal blood pressure values per age range, the following formula may be used to approximate the *lowest* acceptable limit for systolic blood pressure (BP): BP $70 + (2 \times \text{age in years})$. Do not rely solely on blood pressure to indicate the severity of the student's condition. Note that children can lose up 30% of their circulating blood volume and still be normotensive; beyond that point, decompensated shock sets in rapidly (AHA, 2020a).

The following are guidelines related to interpreting vital signs:

- Tachycardia and tachypnea are compensatory mechanisms for shock. The heart rate and respiratory rate can also increase in the presence of fear, anxiety, fever, hypoxia, or certain medications; these elements must be factored into the evaluation.
- Hypothermia and certain medications can cause bradycardia.
- Bradycardia, slow respirations, cyanosis, and hypotension are signs of decompensated shock in a critically ill or injured child (AHA, 2020a).

Another important element of the secondary assessment is focused pain assessment. Pain can be thought of as the fifth vital sign. The cause of pain should be taken into consideration. The **PQRST** (**P**roblem, **P**rovoking and **P**alliative factors; **Q**uality of the pain; **R**egion and **R**adiation of the pain; **S**everity, **S**igns, and **S**ymptoms; and

BOX 17-1

Systematic Assessment/Immediate Care

NOTE: Triage determination and EMS activation should occur as soon as the need becomes apparent.

SCENE SAFETY ASSESSMENT

Call for assistance as indicated before proceeding.

ACROSS-THE-ROOM ASSESSMENT

Use the Pediatric Assessment Triangle (PAT)

- Appearance: Mental status; muscle tone; and body position
- Breathing: Work of breathing (nasal flaring and retractions); abnormal airway sounds
- Circulation: Visible skin color

PRIMARY (C-ABCDE) ASSESSMENT/IMMEDIATE INTERVENTIONS

- Standard precautions
- Restrict motion of cervical spine
- Control obvious hemorrhage as applicable
- CPR as applicable
- Airway, positioning
- Breathing, O_2, mouth-to-mask
- Circulation, control bleeding
- CPR/AED
- Disability, AVPU, pupil check
- Exposure, brief inspection

SECONDARY (FGHI) ASSESSMENT

Full set of vital signs, temperature, weight, and blood glucose

Give comfort measures/pain assessment

- PQRST pain assessment
- Numerical pain scale
- FACES visual pain scale

History and head-to-toe/focused physical examination

- SAMPLE history: Symptoms, Allergies, Medications, Past health history, Last food/drink, Events
- Complete or limited physical examination: Inspect, Auscultate, Percuss, Palpate

Injuries, Inspect the back, and Additional Interventions

- Assess injuries; Inspect posterior surfaces; perform additional interventions based on findings

TRIAGE (E–U–N)

- Emergent: Activate EMS
- Urgent: Determine need for EMS
- Nonurgent: Return to class or send home

Illinois Emergency Medical Services for Children & OSF HealthCare Children's Hospital of Illinois. (2022). *Guidelines for the nurse in the school setting* (4th ed.), with permission.

Timing and Triggers) mnemonic can be used to assess pain depending on the age and developmental capacities of the individual student (IEMSC & OSF HCHI, 2022).

Because pain is a unique individualized experience, the nurse must believe the student's self-report of pain intensity and take into consideration the student's age, culture, gender, cognition, emotions, and past experiences. Multiple types of pain scales are available to measure pain in children. At approximately age 8, children have the ability to understand the concept of small and large numbers and therefore can self-report their pain on the 1 to 10 scale. The nurse can ask, "If 0 is no pain and 10 is the worst pain, what is the pain now?" Faces-based pain scales such as the Wong-Baker FACES or the FACES Pain Scale–Revised are also useful for younger children and English-language learners (Lawson et al., 2021). The nurse should be aware that this clinical standard of self-report of pain is limited to verbal and cognitively typical children.

For children under 8 or who are developmentally delayed or communicatively challenged and unable to self-report, observational methods using pain behavior scales or checklists should be used. For nonverbal or developmentally challenged students, objective pain scales such as the rFLACC (revised Face, Legs, Activity, Cry, Consolability) scale can be used (MacKeil-White, 2023a).

School nurses should be mindful that students who experience chronic pain (e.g., sickle cell disease) may not act as though they are in the amount of pain they are experiencing (MacKeil-White, 2023b). A student in pain may compensate by engaging in a diversionary activity such as playing or sleeping, whereas another student may exhibit anger and irritability when in pain. Physiological changes can occur as a result of acute pain and can be assessed by monitoring vital signs. Alterations in vital signs may not be apparent in a student who experiences chronic pain. Although parents/guardians are often a good source of information regarding how their child tolerates and demonstrates pain, self-report of pain is preferable and not to be substituted by caregivers (Lawson et al., 2021).

Health History

When possible during an emergency, gathering health history information helps the school nurse form a plan of care. The nurse may already be familiar with the student's history from information supplied by the parent/guardian, primary healthcare provider, and school staff or from previous interactions with the student. However, two mnemonics can assist the nurse in gathering pertinent health history information. The mnemonic CIAMPEDS (pronounced *C I am peds*) is a common aid for remembering the elements of a complete history (Powers-Jarvis, 2023). **CIAMPEDS** stands for

- Chief Complaint
- Immunizations/need for Isolation
- Allergies
- Medications, routine and given for illness
- Past health history
- Events preceding the problem
- Diet/elimination (last meal, when, what)
- Symptoms associated with the illness/injury

An alternative method for conducting the history uses the mnemonic **SAMPLE**, which stands for Signs/Symptoms, Allergies, Medications, Past medical history, Last meal, Events leading (Powers-Jarvis, 2023). See Table 17-2.

Especially important in the focused history is the mechanism of injury. It makes a difference in the potential degree of injury whether the student was standing, jumping, or in motion. Gravity and speed add weight and can result in a more severe status. The focus of the head-to-toe examination depends on the circumstances of the illness/injury. For example, in the case of a student with sudden onset of high fever and respiratory distress, the school nurse would assess for infectious disease exposure and determine the need to implement isolation measures based on public health policy. Remember to observe body substance isolation precautions to prevent exposure to body fluids. Provide additional interventions based on the findings of the physical examination. At any time during the examination process, if the student cannot maintain airway patency, adequate breathing, or adequate perfusion, EMS should be called to provide rapid transport and treatment.

TRIAGE

Based on the systematic assessment, the school nurse determines the triage category that denotes the severity of the student's condition. The word *triage* comes from the military French word meaning "to sort out or choose." Triage is the process of sorting and classifying individuals according to the type and urgency of their conditions (IEMSC & OSF HCHI, 2022). The concept of triage applies to both individual students and mass casualty situations (see Chapter 15).

School nursing practice is unpredictable. The school nurse must respond to episodes of acute illness or injury to one or multiple ill/injured individuals in the health office or on the school campus. The school nurse must quickly establish priorities and determine who needs immediate intervention and who can wait. Treatment priorities are set according to the seriousness of the presenting illness or injury and are not based on the order of arrival or onset. Triage places those whose condition is most critical ahead of others.

The three major triage acuity levels used in school nursing practice are *emergent, urgent,* and *nonurgent.*

- *Emergent* means EMS must be activated without delay.
- *Urgent* denotes that medical intervention is required within 2 hours.
- *Nonurgent* signifies that the condition is not severe but may need follow-up medical care (IEMSC & OSF HCHI, 2022).

TABLE 17-2 Pediatric Health History: SAMPLE

	Mnemonic/Topic	Questions
S	**Symptoms** Ask the student to describe current symptoms, particularly pain.	• What problem brings the student to the health office? • How long has the problem persisted? • If an injury, how and when did it occur? • Does the student have pain, apprehension, or guarding? • What are the location, quality, and duration of pain? • Does repositioning make the pain better or worse? • What strategies make other symptoms better or worse? • What is the student's impression of their condition?
A	**Allergies**	• Does the student have any known allergies to food, medications, latex, other materials, or environmental elements such as bee stings?
M	**Medications** List medications the student takes regularly, including dosage regimen and time of the last dose.	• Is the student using any prescription, over-the-counter, home, herbal, or cultural remedies? For what reasons? When was the last dose taken? • Did the student take any medications before coming to the health office? What was the result? • Has the student used any illicit drugs? When?
P	**Past health history** Note preexisting physical or psychological disabilities, previous trauma, and chronic conditions. Check immunization status, including tetanus prophylaxis.	• Does the student have a chronic illness (e.g., asthma, diabetes, hemophilia, or seizure disorder)? • Does the student have special healthcare needs?* • Does the student rely on a medical device (e.g., oxygen, tracheostomy, nebulizer, central venous line, or gastrostomy tube)? • Are immunizations up to date? • Is isolation necessary (e.g., varicella exposure, or immunosuppression)? • If a student is of childbearing age or has experienced menarche, when was her last menstrual period? Is she pregnant, or is there a possibility of pregnancy?
L	**Last meal** Document when and what the student last ate or drank.	• Is the student able to eat? • When was the last meal? • Has there been any nausea, vomiting, or diarrhea? • Is bowel and bladder function normal?
E	**Events** Ask the student to describe the events that led up to the illness or injury.	• When did the problem begin? • Were there precipitating factors? • If an injury occurred, were there witnesses? What did they report?

*You may need to modify your evaluation of assessment findings for students with special needs, because their baseline findings may differ from accepted averages.

Illinois Emergency Medical Services for Children & OSF HealthCare Children's Hospital of Illinois. (2022). *Guidelines for the nurse in the school setting* (4th ed.), with permission.

See Box 17-2 for an overview of triage categories.

Once the triage category of emergent, urgent, or nonurgent is determined, the school nurse considers specific health condition protocols or guidelines, such as an asthma action plan, to rapidly begin focused interventions. Delegating tasks related to the primary assessment and triage determination is not recommended because nursing knowledge and expertise is required to quickly recognize and categorize ill and injured students.

Triage is not a one-time decision but rather a continuous dynamic process. The importance of ongoing monitoring and frequent reevaluations cannot be stressed enough (Cosby, 2023). Children's bodies may be able to compensate for a severe illness or injury for some time and then decompensate rapidly. Therefore it is better to "overtriage" than to "undertriage." Generally, triage categories should not be downgraded. The signs and symptoms of a significant illness/injury, such as a change in the level of consciousness, swelling, or internal bleeding, may not be apparent at first or may develop more slowly. For example, a student who has fallen from a distance of over two or three times their own height onto a hard service initially may be awake and alert but would be anticipated to deteriorate; this student would be triaged as emergent. The school nurse actualizes each step of the nursing process (assessment, nursing diagnoses, outcomes identification, planning, intervention, and evaluation) until the student improves or care is transferred to the parent/guardian or EMS.

The nurse's assessment, triage category, and interventions and the student's response and disposition should all be documented in the student's health record. When

BOX 17-2

Triage Categories, Examples, and Dispositions

CATEGORY	EXAMPLES	DISPOSITION
Emergent: Student requires *immediate* medical attention. Condition is acute and potentially threatens life, limb, or vision.	■ Cardiopulmonary arrest ■ Altered mental status ■ Burns, severe or major ■ Caustic chemical exposure ■ Childbirth, imminent ■ Head injury, history of loss of consciousness ■ Pain, severe or significant location (e.g., chest) ■ Poisoning or drug overdose ■ Respiratory distress (severe) or respiratory failure ■ Shock, any type ■ Spinal cord injury, suspected ■ Status epilepticus or first-time seizure ■ Threatens harm to self or others ■ Trauma, severe; trauma to limb, no distal pulse	■ Monitor* in health office ■ Transport to emergency care facility via EMS
Urgent: Student requires additional medical intervention within 2 hours. Condition is acute but not severe or life-threatening.	■ Burns, minor ■ Deformity or suspected closed fracture without circulatory compromise ■ Febrile illness (temperature exceeds 100°F/37.8°C) ■ GI symptoms (e.g., nausea, vomiting, or diarrhea) ■ Lacerations requiring sutures without excessive blood loss ■ Pain, moderate, after abdominal trauma ■ Seizure, atypical, in student with history of seizures ■ Wheezing	■ Monitor in health office ■ Transport to emergency care facility via EMS, parent/guardian, or other adult as appropriate
Nonurgent: Student may require referral for routine medical care. Minor or nonacute condition.	■ Essentially well; S/S of mild noncommunicable illness or URI ■ Headache without fever or abnormal findings ■ Injury, minor (e.g., abrasions, ecchymoses, muscle sprains, or muscle strains) ■ Pain, mild (e.g., abdominal or menstrual pain, headache or toothache)	■ Monitor in health office ■ Contact parent/ guardian ■ Return student to class or send home as indicated

*Monitoring should be performed by the school nurse.

EMS, Emergency medical services; *F,* Fahrenheit; *C,* centigrade; *GI,* gastrointestinal; *S/S,* signs/symptoms; *URI,* upper respiratory infection.

Illinois Emergency Medical Services for Children & OSF HealthCare Children's Hospital of Illinois. (2022). *Guidelines for the nurse in the school setting* (4th ed.), with permission.

the stability of the student and time allow, the school nurse should write a status report on a simple form that is given to the parent/guardian or EMS personnel and subsequently communicated to the provider or ED personnel. The form should be addressed in bold: **"To Emergency Department, Medical Doctor, Registered Nurse, or Physician's Associate"**—to ensure that the EMT or parent/guardian passes it on. If a student is returned to class after a period of observation in the health office, the teachers should be informed to be alert to changes in status and send the student immediately back to the school nurse with any concerns.

The nurse should follow up with the student's parent/guardian and, if needed, the primary healthcare provider. Two-way exchange of information in person or by phone is optimal. At a minimum, communication should include time, date, reason for the visit, action taken, and recommendations for follow-up. The nurse's name and contact information should be provided. Written notification should also be sent with the student or mailed when a parent/guardian is not immediately available to confirm details of the event. Document the outcome in the student's health record and complete an incident report, as indicated.

STUDENTS WITH SPECIAL HEALTHCARE NEEDS

Students with chronic medical and mental health conditions may be especially vulnerable to adverse health outcomes and at greater risk for medical emergencies. For example, a student with sickle cell disease could potentially have a vaso-occlusive crisis, acute chest syndrome, or stroke at school. A student with Paget's disease may break bones during routine classroom activities. To effectively serve these students, the school nurse should be familiar with the student's baseline status so that changes in status can be readily identified (MacKeil-White, 2023b).

Each student's medical and emergency needs should be reflected in their emergency action plan (EAP) (Cosby, 2024; Gereige et al., 2022). See Chapter 8 for more information about student health and education plans including developing EAPs.

Students with limited mobility whose classes are on floors above the ground level or who do not have access to an exit without special assistance need an evacuation plan in their EAP. In addition, slings, transfer training, and emergency supplies for these students need to be planned out in advance with staff, parents/guardians, and healthcare providers. Access to emergency supplies and the ability to transfer safely and quickly from any building level is vital to their safety.

During assessment and triage, it is important to remember that some students may appear to be at a similar stage of physical development as their peers, but they may function at a level inconsistent with their chronological age. The nurse must also consider that baseline vital signs for individuals with a chronic condition may be outside the range of their same-age peers who do not have special needs. The school nurse may see day-to-day variations and is often the first to notice changes in a student's condition. The nurse must remember to use developmentally appropriate language, gestures, and techniques when communicating with a student who has cognitive impairment or developmental delay. See Chapter 20 for detailed information on caring for students with special healthcare needs.

RESPIRATORY EMERGENCIES

The respiratory system is involved in exchanging oxygen and carbon dioxide. Any condition that impairs the normal pathway of air can precipitate a respiratory emergency. Respiratory emergencies can range from mild to severe and can be life-threatening, leading to respiratory failure and arrest. When managing respiratory emergencies, it is important to keep the student calm and in a position of comfort. Crying and anxiety will increase the need for oxygen usage and potentially worsen the student's respiratory status (Cleveland Clinic, 2020).

Causes

Respiratory distress, failure, and arrest are physiological responses to an imbalance between breathing requirements and the ability to meet them that leads to hypoxia. *Respiratory distress/respiratory failure* occurs when a person experiences insufficient oxygen delivery and/or removal of carbon dioxide. Although this can be life-threatening, if recognized and responded to promptly, most children recover with no long-lasting consequences. There are many causes that trigger respiratory distress and failure (ACLS Algorithms, 2022):

Upper airway obstruction
- Croup
- Epiglottitis
- Foreign body
- Retropharyngeal abscess
- Anaphylaxis

Lower airway obstruction
- Bronchiolitis
- Asthma

Lung tissue disease
- Pneumonia
- Pulmonary edema

Central nervous system or neuromuscular issues
- Overdose
- Muscular dystrophy

Assessment

The school nurse uses across-the-room assessment and the pediatric triangle assessment to evaluate the student's appearance, work of breathing, and circulation (Powers-Jarvis, 2023). A complaint of shortness of breath, outside an obvious cause such as the completion of strenuous physical activity, should always be taken seriously. Clinical presentation of respiratory distress may include the following (IEMSC & OSF HCHI, 2022):

- Increased respiratory rate
- Increase heart rate
- Color changes in the skin such as bluish color seen around the mouth
- Grunting or drooling
- Nose flaring
- Retractions of muscles between the ribs
- Sweating
- Wheezing
- Stridor
- Accessory muscle use
- Change in level of alertness

The nurse should observe the student's position and chest expansion to determine whether there are signs of respiratory compromise, such as tripod position, pursed lips, and tachypnea (Powers-Jarvis, 2023). Assessment should include the student's color and other indications of work of breathing, such as observing the rate, depth, symmetry, and pattern of breathing. Furthermore, the use of accessory muscles (intercostal, substernal, and supraclavicular retractions) and the presence of nasal flaring, head bobbing, or paradoxical/seesaw breathing are signs of increased respiratory effort to improve oxygenation, ventilation, or both. These signs should be used to assess the severity and urgency of the situation (Powers-Jarvis, 2023). Use a stethoscope to auscultate for abnormal breath sounds bilaterally. As respiratory distress progresses to respiratory failure, the resulting hypoxia will also cause changes in mental status. Ongoing assessment should include airway patency, level of consciousness and interaction with the environment, work of breathing, breath sounds, oxygen saturation, and vital signs (IEMSC & OSF HCHI, 2022).

A pulse oximeter is a noninvasive electronic device used to measure the saturation level of oxygen carried in red blood cells. Normal pulse oximetry readings on a child range from 95% to 100%. Any reading below normal range requires intervention, unless the child is known to have lower baseline oxygen saturation levels due to a past medical history of lung or cardiac disease. Pulse oximeters can be attached to the fingers, forehead, nose, foot, ears, or toes. Pulse oximetry can give false readings in students with poor circulation, thick skin, cold extremities, or opaque fingernail polish. A false reading might be suspected if a critically low value is obtained but the child appears in no distress; reposition the pulse oximetry probe or place in a different location. Assess the student's breathing and circulation and check for cyanosis around the lips and nailbeds. The pulse oximetry should be used as an adjunct tool in the comprehensive nursing assessment of a student's respiratory and cardiovascular status; it is not a replacement for careful assessment and diligent monitoring (American Lung Association, 2020). It is just one data point on which to base nursing judgment.

A past or current asthma diagnosis or significant respiratory condition should be indicated on the school record as part of the student's medical history, IHP, EAP, and/or Section 504 plan.

Interventions

Basic interventions include allowing the person to find a position of comfort, reassessing frequently, calling EMS if the student's condition worsens, and using basic life support skills. The sitting position is preferred because it most easily allows the chest to expand fully. A supine position increases the risk of aspiration and choking. A student with severe tachypnea should not have anything by mouth (Volerman et al., 2021). If the student has medical orders, a fast-acting bronchodilator should be used immediately and repeated as directed. Maintain an open airway. This can be accomplished by doing a head tilt/chin lift maneuver. Clear the airway of secretions if necessary. Monitor the oxygen saturation using pulse oximetry. For severe respiratory distress with ineffective tidal volumes use a bag-valve mask to deliver rescue breaths (AHA, 2020b).

Asthma

Emergency action plans should be in place for students with known asthma and allergies that are potentially life-threatening (Cosby, 2024). *Asthma* is a disease of the lungs characterized by inflammation, overactive airways, and periodic bronchospasm (asthma attack). In an asthma attack, the airways narrow (bronchoconstriction) and increase mucous production. Symptoms include wheezing, coughing, chest tightness, and shortness of breath. Asthma can be triggered by viral infections, allergies, chemical irritants, and exercise (Mayo Clinic, 2023). The severity of asthma varies widely among students, from mild intermittent asthma to severe persistent asthma. An asthma attack may spontaneously resolve or may require the use of medication or other measures. If not treated, asthma can become life-threatening. See Chapter 22 for more detailed information on asthma.

Anaphylaxis

Anaphylaxis is a severe, potentially life-threatening systemic allergic reaction. Students with asthma and allergies to certain foods, insect stings, medications, or chemical products are at highest risk for developing anaphylaxis (Brown & Turner, 2017). However, anaphylaxis can develop unexpectedly in anyone during any time across the life span. Signs and symptoms of anaphylaxis include the following:

- Shortness of breath, wheezing, or coughing
- Skin color is pale or has a bluish color
- Weak pulse
- Fainting or dizziness
- Tight or hoarse throat
- Trouble breathing or swallowing
- Swelling of lips or tongue that bother breathing
- Vomiting or diarrhea (if severe or combined with other symptoms)
- Many hives or redness over body
- Feeling of "doom," confusion, altered consciousness, or agitation (AAP, 2019, p. 1)

The most severe symptoms are restriction of breathing and blood circulation, which can lead to shock (AAP, 2021). Although not common, note that biphasic reactions may occur up to 72 hours after the initial reaction. Treatment for biphasic reactions is the same as for initial reactions (Schoessler & White, 2013; Shaker et al., 2020). It is imperative that school staff are trained to recognize and respond to anaphylaxis in the absence of a school nurse. Careful planning is required. School nurses can find a standardized *allergy and anaphylaxis emergency plan* (AAP, 2019) online at no cost.

In out-of-hospital settings, the treatment for anaphylaxis is intramuscular injection of epinephrine administered via an autoinjector device, commonly referred to as an "epi-pen." *Epinephrine is the only rescue medication effective in controlling an anaphylactic reaction* and should be used immediately upon the first appearance of symptoms. There are no absolute contraindications to administering epinephrine for anaphylaxis (Simons, 2016). Delayed administration of epinephrine is associated with complications and possibly death (Sicherer & Simons, 2017). Although symptoms may appear improved after epinephrine, EMS *must* be called.

Epinephrine is available in three doses: 0.1 mg for infants, 0.15 mg for a young child, and 0.3 mg for a larger child or teenager (greater than 55 to 66 lb) to be administered intramuscularly in the mid-outer thigh and held in place for 3 seconds (Mayo Clinic, 2022). The half-life of epinephrine is shorter than the duration of a typical anaphylactic episode; therefore the student can go into rebound anaphylaxis physiology as a first dose of epinephrine is metabolized. Epinephrine can be repeated in 5- to 15-minute intervals via autoinjector until EMS arrives or symptoms improve. It may take repeated doses over 30 to 60 minutes for symptoms to resolve (Brown & Turner, 2017). Report to EMS the dose of epinephrine given.

All 50 states and Washington, DC, either mandate or allow schools to carry, or "stock," quick-relief inhaled bronchodilators and epinephrine autoinjectors with standing medical orders for treatment of anyone in the school, whether or not they have a known history or medical orders on file (Volerman et al., 2021). Undesignated stock rescue medication protocols are critical to decreasing morbidity and mortality when the student or person does not have an individualized order or does not have an inhaler available at school. Many schools also have protocols for oxygen administration in case of emergency. See Chapter 21 for more detailed information on allergies and anaphylaxis. See Chapter 30 for more information about stocking undesignated rescue medications at school.

Foreign Body Upper Airway Obstruction

Foreign body aspiration continues to be one of the leading causes of death in children. There are many factors that increase the risk of aspiration. Child anatomy and developmental structures of a child factor into why children are at such a risk for aspiration. *Choking* is defined as an obstruction that leads to the inability to ventilate and oxygenate the blood (Cramer et al., 2022). Most common choking items include food, coins, balloons, and toys. When upper airway obstruction occurs, fast action is required to decrease long-lasting effects to the brain and morbidity and mortality (Cramer et al., 2022).

Sudden onset of coughing, choking, and shortness of breath are common symptoms of choking. The student may also exhibit anxious behavior, restlessness, and changes in color or grasp at their neck. In all cases of obstruction, activate EMS because a partial airway obstruction can rapidly progress to complete obstruction.

The difference between mild and severe foreign body obstruction determines the interventions. In mild foreign body obstruction, the child is coughing and making sounds. Coughing is the body's attempt to clear the airway. In severe obstruction, a child cannot make sounds because they cannot move air past the obstruction; abdominal thrusts are required until the object is expelled, or the child becomes unresponsive. If the child becomes unresponsive, start CPR according to current resuscitation protocols. Check for a foreign body each time the airway is opened to give breaths and remove a foreign body if visible. Do NOT perform blind finger sweeps. This may push the foreign body deeper into the throat (AHA, 2020a).

Epiglottitis

Acute epiglottitis is an abrupt onset of inflammation of the epiglottis and surrounding structures. Epiglottitis is an emergent condition that can rapidly progress to severe respiratory distress with occlusion and obstruction of the airway and death in a matter of hours. Since the routine use of the *Haemophilus influenzae* type b 9 (Hib) vaccine, there has been a sharp decline in the cases of epiglottitis in childhood. *Haemophilus influenzae type b* is still typically the responsible organism and remains an important etiological agent, primarily in unvaccinated or incompletely immunized children. In rare instances, epiglottitis may occur in fully immunized children (Reichert & Foley, 2024).

A student with epiglottitis has a fever, appears anxious, and exhibits the classic three *D*'s of epiglottitis: respiratory **d**istress, **d**rooling, and **d**ysphagia (trouble swallowing). The student typically insists on sitting upright, assuming the tripod pose with the neck extended forward to keep the airway open. The tongue may be protruding with the chin thrust out and mouth open. The school nurse may notice a thick or muffled-sounding, low-volume voice. On inspiration, a frog-like croaking sound (stridor) may be heard. However, the child is not hoarse. Stridor is a late finding and suggests near or threatening airway obstruction (Sweeney, 2023).

When a student is suspected of having acute epiglottitis, activate EMS. *No attempts to visualize the back of the throat should be made.* The priority is to keep the student calm and avoid unnecessary agitation that may worsen the airway obstruction and increase respiratory distress. Close observation with frequent reassessment is essential as progressive obstruction leads to decreased oxygenation, altered level of consciousness, complete obstruction, and death. Nothing should be administered by mouth because the student may require an emergency airway procedure such as intubation or tracheostomy. The risk of complete airway obstruction needs to be clearly communicated to the EMS personnel. Suggest that efforts be made to keep the student calm and delay invasive procedures that may cause aggravation, such as starting an intravenous line, until the airway is secured (Reichert & Foley, 2024).

Pneumonia

Pneumonia is a serious disease in children and can be fatal if left untreated. *Pneumonia* presents as an acute inflammatory reaction in the lung, which may include the airways, alveoli, pleura, connective tissue, and vascular structures. Pneumonia usually follows an upper respiratory infection that allows the invasion of bacteria, viruses, or other pathogens to produce inflammation of the lower respiratory tract. The air spaces of the lower respiratory tract then fill with white blood cells, fluid, and cellular debris leading to reduction of lung compliance and collapse of distal air spaces (Milici, 2024a).

The clinical manifestations and severity of pneumonia vary depending on the pathogen and health status of the host. Bacterial pneumonia is most commonly due to *Streptococcus pneumoniae* and causes abrupt onset of symptoms (Milici, 2024a; Reichert & Foley, 2024). Viral pneumonia onset is often more gradual, following an upper airway infection.

Clinical features of mild pneumonia include the following:

- Increased respiratory rate
- Mild or absent retractions
- No grunting
- No nasal flaring
- Mild shortness of breath
- Normal skin color
- Normal mental status
- Normal heart rate

Clinical features of severe pneumonia include the following:

- Difficulty breathing
- Tachypnea
- Tachycardia
- Grunting
- Nasal flaring
- Altered mental status
- Hypoxemia
- Cyanosis

For severe respiratory distress, activate EMS. The student should be allowed to maintain a position of comfort to facilitate breathing. Oral fluids may be offered if the student is not vomiting.

Pneumothorax and Hemothorax

Pneumothorax and *hemothorax* are potentially life-threatening emergencies requiring immediate intervention in an acute care setting. Though not common in children, pneumothorax and hemothorax usually result from blunt trauma to the chest causing intrathoracic injury but can also occur in the presence of chronic or acute lung disease (Davis, 2024a).

A ***pneumothorax***, also called a collapsed lung, occurs when air is pushed outside the lung into the pleural space between the lung tissue and the chest wall, thus restricting the ability for the lung to expand. The lung may collapse partially or totally. A pneumothorax can be caused by any blunt chest injury, penetrating trauma, or ruptured blebs (weak, thin-walled air cysts in the lungs). If a child has had a previous history of pneumothorax, they are at an increased risk of recurrence (Davis, 2024a; Mayo Clinic, 2021).

Tension pneumothorax is a severe complication of pneumothorax that occurs when a large amount of air accumulates in the pleural space. This results in markedly increased intrathoracic pressure that causes a shift in the mediastinal structures, a decrease in venous return, and a drop in cardiac output leading to obstructive shock and potentially cardiac arrest. Clinical manifestations include tachypnea, hypoxemia, respiratory distress, unilateral diminished breath sounds, paradoxical chest wall movements, hypotension, crepitus in neck/chest, and distended neck veins, and, in severe cases, tracheal deviation away from the affected lung (Davis, 2024a).

Communicating pneumothorax, or open pneumothorax, is caused by a penetrating chest wound in which air audibly enters and exits through the chest wall with respiration (Davis, 2024a). Sometimes referred to as a "sucking chest wound," communicating pneumothorax does not lead to tension pneumothorax because air will escape the pleural space when intrathoracic pressure exceeds atmospheric pressure. Nevertheless, if left untreated, open pneumothorax can progress to respiratory failure. If communicating pneumothorax is suspected, an occlusive dressing may be applied (Davis, 2024a).

A ***hemothorax*** is a collection of blood between the chest wall and lung, also due to chest trauma in children (Davis, 2024a). Breath sounds are typically diminished on the affected side in the setting of hemothorax.

To assess for pneumothorax or hemothorax, auscultate lung sounds in the midaxillary area and observe for symmetrical chest rise and fall. If breath sounds are diminished on one side or chest rise is asymmetrical, a pneumothorax or hemothorax should be suspected (Miller, 2023). Signs and symptoms may appear as respiratory distress, tachypnea, asymmetrical lung expansion, hyperresonance on percussion, and hypotension (Daley, 2022). If a pneumothorax or hemothorax is suspected, activate EMS and call the parent/guardian. Be prepared to provide supportive care and CPR if necessary until EMS arrives.

CIRCULATORY EMERGENCIES

The circulatory system is responsible for transporting oxygenated blood from the lungs throughout the body, regulating body temperature, and maintaining normal water and electrolyte balance. A circulatory emergency is the result of the body's inability to supply the cells with enough oxygenated blood to meet metabolic demands. Circulatory emergencies in children may result from abnormal cardiac function, as in heart failure; from an insufficient volume of blood, as occurs in hemorrhage; or from systemic vasodilation, as may occur in septicemia (Delaney et al., 2017).

The most common circulatory emergency that occurs in children is hypovolemic shock, although other types of shock (e.g., anaphylactic, neurogenic) can occur. Fluid volume deficit from nausea, vomiting, and diarrhea can occur quickly, especially in younger children. Blood loss from trauma can also quickly lead to hypovolemic shock, a life-threatening emergency.

Sickle cell disease can also cause circulatory emergencies (CDC, 2022e). See Chapter 24 for a detailed discussion of school nurse care of students with sickle cell disease.

Shock

Shock is not a disease, but rather the physiological result of ineffective circulation and inadequate delivery of oxygen to the organs and tissues. There are four broad categories of shock: *hypovolemic, cardiogenic, distributive* (i.e., septic, anaphylactic, and neurogenic causes), and *obstructive* (Table 17-3). Early recognition and management of the different types of shock are critical to reestablishing adequate tissue perfusion before permanent organ damage and cardiac arrest occur (Giordano, 2023; Milici, 2024b). The school nurse should be alert for pending shock from internal or external hemorrhage following severe trauma.

Shock progresses quickly if not recognized and responded to promptly. As shock advances, so does the likelihood of death. Mortality rates increase 10-fold in severe shock compared with early shock. When pending

TABLE 17-3 Types of Shock

Pathophysiology	Examples	Signs and Symptoms	Interventions
Hypovolemic Fluid and electrolyte loss leading to intravascular and interstitial volume depletion	Nonhemorrhagic dehydration (vomiting, diarrhea, diabetic ketoacidosis, burn injury) Hemorrhagic (trauma)	Poor skin turgor, sunken eyes, dry mucous membranes, cool skin, delayed capillary refill, altered mental status, decreased urine output, tachycardia, active bleeding, hypotension (late sign)	Prevent further fluid loss (e.g., control hemorrhage). Lay the student supine. Activate EMS. Keep the child warm.
Cardiogenic Cardiac dysfunction (pump failure); reduced cardiac output and inadequate tissue perfusion despite adequate intravascular volume	Congenital heart defects Cardiomyopathy Arrhythmias Toxic drug exposure	Decreased cardiac output; tachycardia; normal or low BP; cool, pale, moist skin; absent or weak pulses; increased respiratory effort (retractions, cyanosis); syncope; cardiac arrest; toxicity	Maintain an open airway. Follow emergency care plan. Activate EMS.
Distributive Loss of vascular tone and subsequent capillary leakage causes relative hypovolemia due to vasodilation, maldistribution of blood flow, and myocardial depression.	**Septic** Life-threatening response to an infection coupled with new organ dysfunction	Tachycardia, altered mental status, hyperthermia or hypothermia, hypotension (late sign)	Maintain an open airway. Initiate isolation precautions.
	Anaphylaxis	Angioedema, respiratory distress, wheezing, hives, hypotension, tachycardia, syncope, cardiopulmonary arrest	Maintain an open airway. Administer oxygen (if available). Administer epinephrine (if available). Activate EMS.
	Neurogenic	Bradycardia; hypotension; warm, dry and flushed skin; decreased deep tendon reflexes	Maintain an open airway. Stabilize spine if spinal cord injury suspected. Lay victim supine. Keep the victim warm. Activate EMS.
Obstructive Compression or mechanical obstruction of the great veins, pulmonary arteries, aorta or the heart, which prevents adequate circulating volume	Pericardial tamponade Pulmonary emboli Tension pneumothorax	Muffled heart tones (cardiac tamponade), distended neck veins, decreased breath sounds on affected side, asymmetrical chest rise and fall, respiratory distress (tension pneumothorax)	Maintain an open airway. Stabilize spine if spinal cord injury suspected. Position of comfort to improve respiratory effort. Administer oxygen (if available). Activate EMS.

Miley (2023).

shock is a concern, the school nurse closely monitors vital signs, skin perfusion, peripheral pulses, and mental status. Pulse oximetry can also be used. Skin perfusion parameters include color, temperature and moisture, and capillary refill checked at frequent intervals. A normal capillary refill time is brisk—about 2 seconds. A prolonged refill time of greater than 2 seconds may indicate poor perfusion in a normothermic child (AHA, 2020a; Giordano, 2023; Reichert & Foley, 2024).

Early signs of circulatory compromise include the following:

- Tachycardia
- Delayed capillary refill
- Decreased peripheral pulses
- Cool, mottled skin
- Restlessness, agitation, or lethargy
- Decreasing level of consciousness

Tachypnea may be present, depending on the type and state (compensated or decompensated) of shock (Milici, 2024b). Although a student's blood pressure might be within normal ranges, they could be on the verge of circulatory collapse. Children developing shock are able to maintain adequate cardiac output for a long period because of compensatory peripheral vasoconstriction (Giordano, 2023). Hypotension with hypovolemic shock does not occur in a child until the vascular volume has decreased by approximately 30% to 40%. Therefore blood pressure is one of the least sensitive indicators of adequate circulation in children (AHA, 2020a).

It is imperative that the school nurse quickly assess and intervene when shock is suspected because children can decompensate very quickly. The goal is to improve the balance between tissue perfusion and metabolic demand. EMS with advanced life support capabilities should be activated immediately. See Box 17-3 for the school nurse protocol for trauma.

Sudden Cardiopulmonary Arrest

Sudden cardiopulmonary arrest (SCA) is an abrupt and unanticipated malfunction of the electrical system of the heart resulting in ventricular fibrillation or asystole (Erickson et al., 2021). Cardiac output and breathing cease. Sudden cardiac death is described as an unexpected sudden death from a cardiac cause occurring in the community or in the ED usually within an hour of the onset of symptoms.

SCA in children and youth is rare, but always tragic. Widespread media coverage of cases among high school athletes makes SCA appear more common than it actually is. SCA affects boys more than girls, and the unexpected sudden death of an apparently healthy family member before age 50 increases the risk (May & Menon, 2021). Fortunately, out-of-hospital deaths due to SCA in youth are declining, perhaps due to the increased availability of AEDs and CPR training.

Sudden cardiopulmonary arrest is caused by disorders that affect the structure of the heart and/or cause life-threatening arrhythmias. The leading causes of SCA in children less than 18 years are congenital heart disease, followed by arrhythmias, cardiomyopathies, and myocarditis (May & Menon, 2021). Many of these contributing conditions will not be detected during routine screening for school physical examinations or sports activities, so SCA may be the first and only indication of the life-threatening problem (May & Menon, 2021). However, SCA may be potentially preventable in some cases if forewarned by signs and symptoms such as dizziness, syncope/near syncope, chest pain, dyspnea, palpitations, elevated blood pressure, and heart murmur. The American Academy of Pediatrics recommends that all children be screened for the risk of sudden cardiac arrest and sudden cardiac death regardless of their athletic status every 3 years by their primary care provider (Erickson et al., 2021, p. 9; Erickson & Salerno, 2021). Routine electrocardiograms on all athletes are not currently recommended, but further evaluation may be indicated if students are suspected to be at increased risk.

Although not directly related to a cardiovascular abnormality, *commotio cordis* deserves mention as a cause of SCA (Erickson et al., 2021). Literally meaning concussion of the heart, death from commotio cordis results from a fatal dysrhythmia caused by the impact of a nonpenetrating object striking the chest, such as a baseball or hockey puck. It is thought that the blow must occur at a certain phase of the cardiac cycle, specifically ventricular repolarization, to be fatal. Episodes of commotio cordis are rare, and the likelihood of successful resuscitation has increased over the last 15 years to greater than 89%, which can be attributed to increased awareness, decreased time between collapse and CPR and defibrillation, and increased availability of AEDs in the community (National Operating Committee on Standards for Athletic Equipment, 2021).

When a student or staff member collapses, the nurse, trained school staff, or bystander must complete a basic life support assessment of responsiveness, circulation, airway, and breathing. A person with SCA is unresponsive with a clear airway, no breathing or gasping respirations, and no palpable pulse (AHA, 2020a). SCA victims need CPR and an AED applied immediately. Unless cardiac function is restored, death is certain.

AEDs are designed to quickly treat ventricular fibrillation by delivering an electric shock to the heart. The availability and utilization of AEDs have been shown to increase survival rates following SCA. AEDs should be universally available in schools; however, not all states require schools to have AEDs on the premises (Avive, 2023; Sherrid et al., 2017).

Training laypersons to safely and effectively use an AED and do CPR on a child or an adult with SCA can save lives. Protocols and procedures must be in place before initiating use of AEDs in the school setting. AEDs can be used on

BOX 17-3

Determine Triage Category and Activate EMS as Soon as the Need Becomes Apparent!

EMERGENT

- Profuse hemorrhage
- Slow or fast respiratory rate, other signs/symptoms (S/S) of respiratory distress/failure
- Capillary refill exceeds 2 seconds, other S/S of shock
- Currently/previously unconscious
- Penetrating wound or significant blunt trauma to head, chest, or abdomen
- Open chest wound
- Suspected pelvic/femoral fracture
- Suspected spinal injury with paresthesia
- Amputation/crush injury
- S/S of intra-abdominal injury:
  - Hematuria
  - Grey Turner sign (bluish discoloration of flank/periumbilical area)
  - Abdominal asymmetry/distention
- Tenderness/guarding/pain on gentle palpation

INTERVENTIONS

- Control hemorrhage
- Activate EMS
- Support C-ABCDE
- Maintain spinal motion restriction
- Place supine or in shock position
- Keep student warm
- Give nothing by mouth
- Stabilize impaled object with dressings—do not remove
- Splint/elevate suspected fracture
- Control hemorrhage
- Directly/continuously observe student
- Frequently reassess vital signs/AVPU
- Contact parent/guardian
- Notify school administrator
- Follow-up

Amputation Management

- Wrap part in gauze slightly moistened with sterile saline
- Place in plastic bag, seal securely, and label
- Place bag on cold packs (not ice) for transport
- Follow-up

URGENT

- Stable vital signs
- No loss of consciousness
- Deformity/suspected closed fracture without neurovascular compromise
- Controllable bleeding
- Significant mechanism of injury without other significant abnormalities

INTERVENTIONS

- Support C-ABCDE
- Reassess vital signs
- Determine need for EMS
- Control bleeding
- Proceed with detailed physical examination
- Splint/immobilize suspected fractures, elevate extremity, and apply cold packs

Blunt Abdominal Injury

- Observe closely for 15 min for S/S of intra-abdominal injury
  - Hematuria
  - Grey Turner sign (bluish discoloration of flank/periumbilical area)
  - Abdominal asymmetry/distention
  - Tenderness/guarding/pain on gentle palpation
- Reassess in 1 hour or if S/S recur

In All Cases

- Contact parent/guardian to transport student to medical care or home
- Follow-up

NONURGENT

- Stable vital signs
- No deformity or suspicion of fracture
- Minor abrasions or lacerations
- Mild muscle strain or sprain

INTERVENTIONS

- Proceed with detailed physical examination
- Refer to appropriate protocol

Blunt Abdominal Injury

- Observe closely for 15 min for S/S of intra-abdominal injury
  - Hematuria
  - Grey Turner sign (bluish discoloration of flank/periumbilical area)
  - Abdominal asymmetry/distention
  - Tenderness/guarding/pain on gentle palpation
- Reassess in 1 hour or if S/S recur

In All Cases

- Contact parent/guardian
- Return student to class or send home as indicated
- Follow-up (as needed or per policy)

Illinois Emergency Medical Services for Children & OSF HealthCare Children's Hospital of Illinois. (2022). *Guidelines for the nurse in the school setting* (4th ed.), with permission.

children of all ages and adults. Some models are designed to be used for both children and adults but may require adaptations for use in children such as preprogramming, different cable and pads, or a pediatric dose-attenuator system. *The emergency response team member should use a pediatric dose-attenuator system and/or the child-specific cable and pads if available for those under age 8.* However, if these are not available, then a standard AED is acceptable to use on any age/size child (AHA, 2020b). School nurses should advocate for regular CPR/AED training for school staff.

NEUROLOGICAL EMERGENCIES

The nervous system includes the central nervous system, consisting of the brain and spinal cord, and the peripheral nervous system, which is a complex network of motor and sensory nerves, including the cranial nerves, spinal nerves, somatic nervous system, and autonomic nervous system. The nervous system monitors, coordinates, and controls virtually all of the body's activities, including voluntary and involuntary reflexes, internal organ function, and responses to changes in the external environment. The somatic nervous system regulates voluntary activities, which include almost all coordinated muscle actions. The autonomic nervous system regulates the body functions that occur without conscious effort, such as many of the body's vital organs (Costello, 2023).

Normal brain function requires a continuous supply of glucose and oxygen. Neurological emergencies can occur as a result of alterations in cerebral blood flow, increased intracranial pressure, metabolic imbalances, hypoxia, or infections. Neurological emergencies can also result from substance use or abuse, exposure to toxins, shock, stroke, and seizures, or from a direct traumatic insult (Foley, 2024b). When an alteration in the level of consciousness is detected, the **AEIOU-TIPS** mnemonic can be used to try to determine possible causes. Determining the underlying cause of an abnormality will guide interventions.

A—**A**lcohol (acute intoxication, withdrawal)
E—**E**pilepsy(or any seizure) and environmental conditions (hypothermia, heat stroke)
I—**I**nsulin (too much, too little)
O—**O**xygen (underdose or overdose)
U—**U**remia (or other metabolic disorders)
T—**T**rauma, toxicity, tumors, and thermoregulation
I—**I**nfection, ischemia
P—**P**sychiatric/**P**oisoning
S—**S**troke, syncope, or other neurological or cardiovascular causes (Foley, 2024b)

During the triage process, the school nurse should follow the ABCDE format to determine whether there is a life-threatening emergency. During the primary assessment, the AVPU (Awake, Verbal stimuli, Painful stimuli, and Unresponsive/unconscious) scale can be used to determine the student's mental status (see Table 17-1) and pupils should be assessed (IEMSC & OSF HCHI, 2022). Once life-threatening emergencies are ruled out, during the secondary assessment the school nurse conducts a focused neurological examination and determines whether there are any gross alterations in motor and/or sensory functions and level of consciousness; events leading up to the episode; whether there are any signs of trauma; and whether there was a total loss of consciousness and its duration.

The nurse can expect a student with altered mental status to exhibit personality or behavior changes that are inappropriate for their age or developmental level. Therefore, it is important for the nurse to be familiar with age-appropriate behavior of children and adolescents to determine whether there is any alteration in neurological function. The school nurse should observe the student closely and perform the assessment in a consistent sequence so the subtle changes are not overlooked. Do NOT move the student if head or spinal cord trauma is suspected (IEMSC & OSF HCHI, 2022).

Signs and symptoms of altered mental and neurological status include the following:

- Disorientation, confusion, temporary amnesia, inability to recognize familiar people, delayed responses, inability to focus attention
- Emotionally labile (agitation, irritability, listlessness)
- Vision and eye abnormalities (inability to track objects, nystagmus, ptosis, staring, loss of visual field, pupillary changes)
- Slurred or incoherent speech, repetition of phrases ("What happened? What happened?")
- Changes in gait; ataxia; purposeless activity; gross observable uncoordinated movements; decreased or asymmetrical strength, movement, and coordination; changes in reflexes (Costello, 2023; IEMSC & OSF HCHI, 2022)

Although pupils may be checked initially, the nurse should keep in mind that pupil dilation is a late sign of increasing intracranial pressure. The most important indicator of cerebral function is the person's level of consciousness (Costello, 2023; IEMSC & OSF HCHI, 2022).

The potential cause of the neurological emergency and the findings in the primary and secondary assessment will dictate what interventions are needed. The following section reviews several common neurological emergencies to which the school nurse may need to respond and appropriate interventions for each. The brain and spinal cord have limited ability to regenerate after injury, so immediate action must be taken to minimize long-term effects of traumatic brain damage (Sharma, 2022). Overall, if there was a loss of consciousness or any other abnormal findings, the school nurse should activate EMS and perform cervical motion restriction as indicated by the mechanism of injury. The student should be seen at the most appropriate level in the ED for evaluation by a physician.

While in the nurse's office, the student should rest while the nurse observes and reassesses vital signs and mental status until EMS arrives. The school nurse should assess and evaluate the student for signs of increasing intracranial pressure, such as headache, nausea, vomiting, or altered level of consciousness. Nothing should be given by mouth until medical evaluations have been completed and it is determined that the patient has been stabilized.

Traumatic Brain Injury

Traumatic brain injury (TBI) resulted in 16,070 pediatric (birth to 17 years old) hospitalizations in 2019 and 2,774 TBI-related deaths in 2020 (CDC, 2022d). The major causes of TBI in children are falls, motor vehicle crashes, and bicycle crashes. Blows to the head can also occur due to collisions, falls, or impact with equipment in contact sports. TBIs may also be the result of violence, such as being hit with a blunt object, being thrown to the ground, or suffering a penetrating wound, such as a gunshot. The major complications of head trauma are hemorrhage, infection, and cerebral edema.

The severity of TBI is related to the strength of the blow because the force of impact causes the brain to move inside the skull. Bruising inside the brain at the point of initial impact is called the *coup,* and the second contusion at the opposite side is called the *contrecoup.* This rapid, forceful back and forth movement results in contusions and significant distortion as the brain changes shape with the impact (Costello, 2023). Severe head injury can cause diffuse axonal injury from the acceleration and deceleration forces that damage or stress axons and cause diffuse, microscopic hemorrhagic lesions. Severe impacts to the head can also cause intracranial hemorrhage that can result in a subdural, epidural, or intracerebral hematoma that occupies space inside the brain, compressing other brain structures and impairing function (Costello, 2023). Edema and space-occupying bleeds elevate intracranial pressure inside the rigid confines of the skull. Severely elevated intracranial pressure is a neurosurgical emergency that can cause brain herniation through the tentorium and death.

Initial assessment of a child with a head injury includes a mental status evaluation (outlined previously) and neurological examination, including assessment of sensation, movement, and strength of extremities; assessment of pupillary symmetry in response to light; and observation for seizures. TBIs can be classified as mild, moderate, or severe based on the presenting symptoms. The grading generally depends on the presence or absence of loss of consciousness and its duration, length of postinjury memory loss, and persistence of symptoms (Foley, 2024a).

In addition to assessing for changes in neurological status and abnormal behavior, the school nurse should assess for abnormal physical findings related to the trauma (IEMSC & OSF HCHI, 2022) such as the following:

- Deformities, lacerations, abrasions, and edema of the head and skull
- Seizure activity
- Loss of/decreased movement or sensation in extremities
- Clear fluid draining from the eyes or nose indicative of cerebral spinal fluid (CSF). CSF will form a halo sign when dabbed on an absorbent surface (gauze) and test positive for glucose when tested with a glucometer.
- Blood or CSF from the ears
- Paresthesia (tingling, numbness, "pins and needles")

Nursing management goals in TBI are to address complications of head trauma and prevent further brain and spinal injury. The student should not be moved until the cervical spine is immobilized (IEMSC & OSF HCHI, 2022). If a neck brace is not available, the head and neck should be held in position by placing hands on both sides of the student's head and maintaining that position until EMS arrives. While awaiting EMS, a dressing can be applied to open wounds, and ice can help relieve pain and swelling.

Concussion

Concussions are functional injuries. "A concussion is a type of traumatic brain injury caused by a bump, blow, or jolt to the head or by a hit to the body that causes the head and brain to move quickly back and forth. This fast movement can cause the brain to bounce or twist within the skull, creating chemical changes in the brain and sometimes stretching and damaging brain cells" (CDC, 2019a, para. 1). Concussions most commonly are sustained at school from physical contact to the head during physical education, recess on the playground, or school-based sports; but students may also present at school with signs and symptoms from a concussion sustained outside of school (CDC, 2019a).

Concussions are sometimes characterized as "mild" TBIs. However, because each student presents uniquely, concussions cannot accurately be categorized as mild, moderate, or severe. Concussions can result in both temporary and long-term consequences and must be monitored closely. Most students recover from concussions within 1 month, but approximately one third of children experience symptoms lasting 4 weeks or longer, especially those who had more significant initial signs and symptoms (Davis et al., 2024). Concussions are generally not life-threatening and do not require evaluation or treatment in a hospital, but all concussions should be taken seriously. See Box 17-4 for common signs and symptoms of concussions.

NASN (2021) takes the position that the school nurse "provides leadership/care coordination in collaboration with the school-based team to manage student concussion. The school nurse has the healthcare knowledge and skills to provide concussion prevention education to parents/guardians, students, and school staff; identify suspected concussions; and help guide students as they return to academics/learning, physical activities, and sports" (para. 1).

The school nurse should carefully assess and closely monitor a student who receives a blow, bump, or jolt to the head using the CDC's (2019c) *Concussion Signs and Symptoms Checklist.* According to the CDC (2019a), the school nurse should do the following when a student is seen in the health office after an impact to the head or jolt to the body:

1. Observe the student for signs and symptoms of concussion for a minimum of 30 minutes.
2. Ask people who saw the injury occur about how the injury happened and any concussion signs they observed.
3. Complete the *Concussion Signs and Symptoms Checklist* (found at cdc.gov/headsup/schools/nurses.html).
4. Notify the student's parent(s) or guardian(s) that their child had a head injury.

If the student has concussion signs or symptoms:

- Tell the parent(s) or guardian(s) that the student needs to see a healthcare provider experienced in concussion management.

BOX 17-4
Signs and Symptoms of Concussion

OBSERVED SIGNS

- Appears dazed or stunned
- Is confused about events
- Repeats questions
- Answers questions slowly
- Can't recall events *before* the hit, bump, or fall
- Can't recall events *after* the hit, bump, or fall
- Loses consciousness (even briefly)
- Shows behavior or personality changes
- Forgets class schedule or assignments

COGNITIVE SYMPTOMS

- Difficulty thinking clearly
- Difficulty concentrating
- Difficulty remembering
- Feeling more slowed down than usual
- Feeling sluggish, hazy, foggy, or groggy

PHYSICAL SYMPTOMS

- Headache or "pressure" in head
- Nausea or vomiting
- Balance problems or dizziness
- Fatigue or feeling tired
- Blurry or double vision
- Sensitivity to light
- Sensitivity to noise
- Numbness or tingling
- Does not "feel right"

EMOTIONAL SYMPTOMS

- Irritable
- Sad
- More emotional than usual
- Nervous

CDC (2019c, p. 1).

- Give the parent(s) or guardian(s) a copy of the completed Concussion Signs and Symptoms Checklist for the healthcare provider to review.
- Ask for written guidance from the student's healthcare provider about when the student can return to school and to physical activity.

If the student does not have concussion signs or symptoms:

- Have the student return to class, but do not allow them to return to sports or recreational activities on the same day of the injury.
- Send a copy of the completed Concussion Signs and Symptoms Checklist home with the student for the parent(s) or guardian(s) to review. Ask the parent(s) or guardian(s) to continue to observe the student for any changes.
- Tell the parent(s) or guardian(s) that if concussion signs or symptoms appear, the student should be seen right away by a healthcare provider with experience in concussion management (CDC, 2019a, p. 3).

Each student with a concussion presents and recovers uniquely. Specific guidance from a qualified healthcare provider should inform the school team on accommodations at school regarding the student's safe return to learning and play. Generally, most students require no more than 2 to 3 days of rest before gradually returning as tolerated to school and nonsports activities (CDC, 2019a). Accommodations should be consistent throughout the instructional environment and adjusted or removed according to the student's needs until the student recovers to their preconcussion baseline. Students recovering from concussions might benefit from allowance for rest breaks, shortened school day, extended time on tests or assignments, reduced screen or reading time, and help with homework (CDC, 2019a). Evidence suggests that return to light physical (aerobic) activity helps facilitate recovery in children, but continued play in competitive sports immediately post-injury can prolong recovery. With symptom resolution, most students are able to return to playing sports within 1 month, though caution to avoid reinjury is advised (Davis et al., 2024). A graduated approach as tolerated to full participation is recommended. Students should not return to athletic play until cleared by a qualified physician or healthcare provider (CDC, 2019b).

Practice Connection

Although not common, increased intracranial pressure (brain swelling) can evolve over the first 24 to 48 hours after a concussion. Severe intracranial swelling can lead to permanent damage to the brain and even death. EMS should be activated immediately for transport to an ED for any of the following signs and symptoms:

- A headache that gets worse and does not go away
- Weakness, numbness, or decreased coordination
- Significant nausea or repeated vomiting
- Unusual behavior, increased confusion, restlessness, or agitation
- Drowsiness or inability to wake up
- Slurred speech, weakness, numbness, or decreased coordination
- Convulsions or seizures
- Loss of consciousness (passing out) (CDC, 2019a, p. 2)

Much more information on concussions for school nurses, parents/guardians, school personnel, and athletic trainers and coaches can be found on the Web site *CDC HEADS UP: Safer Brain, Stronger Future* (CDC, 2019b).

Spinal Cord Injury

Spinal cord injuries result most frequently in children from motor vehicle injuries, falls, and sports injuries (Children's Hospital of Philadelphia [CHOP], 2022; National Institute of Neurological Disorders and Stroke [NINDS], 2023). Other common causes include diving accidents, gunshot or stab wounds, trampoline, and birth injuries. Spinal cord injuries should always be assumed in the presence of these traumatic events. They can occur in the cervical, thoracic, lumbar, or sacral areas, with the cervical spine being most vulnerable in children. The spinal cord can be bruised, lacerated, or transected, and the blood vessels supplying the cord can also be injured. The injuries occur because of hyperextension, hyperflexion, vertical compression, and rotational forces (CHOP, 2022; NINDS, 2023).

A rapid primary assessment of the mechanism of injury should be performed while restricting the student's spinal motion to prevent further damage (IEMSC & OSF HCHI, 2022). The student should be asked whether there is any pain, tingling, or loss of sensation in any extremity. Use neurological assessment techniques to determine upper and lower extremity movement, strength, and symmetry by checking hand grip and dorsiflexion. High cervical spine injuries may paralyze the victim from the neck down, including the diaphragm, causing respiratory arrest.

Do not move the victim unless the scene poses an imminent danger. EMS must be called immediately. The school nurse continues to monitor ABCDE and maintains spinal motion restriction by applying a cervical collar, if available, or by using manual traction. If the airway is not patent, the team member must use the jaw thrust maneuver instead of the head-tilt, chin-lift method (AHA, 2020b). In high cervical spine injuries, ventilation using a bag-valve mask may be required even if the student is conscious.

Seizures

Although seizures are the main sign of epilepsy, these two terms are not interchangeable. A *seizure* is a single occurrence; provoked seizures have an underlying cause or trigger. *Epilepsy* is a neurological disease diagnosed once a child has two or more unprovoked seizures (Epilepsy Foundation, 2023b). A seizure occurs when multiple neurons in the brain misfire at the same time. The area of the brain in which the seizure originates will determine its clinical manifestation. Common symptoms include muscle twitching, spasms, altered level of consciousness, and/or changes in mood and behavior. Any seizure that lasts longer than 5 minutes is a medical emergency (Epilepsy Foundation, 2022). The cause of epilepsy is unknown in about half of people diagnosed; in other cases, epilepsy may be due to abnormality or injury in the brain structure or function, traumatic brain injuries, metabolic abnormalities, and brain tumors (Epilepsy Foundation, 2023b).

Febrile seizures in infants and young children are common and typically benign. They usually occur in children ages 6 months to 5 years old. Febrile seizures are not due to the fever but due to the quick rise in body temperature. They do not cause chronic seizure disorder or brain damage (Emergency Nurses Association, 2019).

When a student experiences a seizure, it is important to accurately observe and document the events before, during, and after the episode, including the time of onset, duration, and characteristics (i.e., behavior, movement, respiratory effort, and incontinence). The nurse should avoid labeling the type of seizure and document only what is observed. Observation should continue after the seizure, noting the duration of the postictal period, level of consciousness, orientation, arousability, motor function, speech, and the student's recollection of preseizure sensations (Epilepsy Foundation, 2022).

Interventions during an active seizure are similar, regardless of the cause. The student should be assisted to the ground. Protect the head from injury by placing a soft pillow or blanket under the head. Position the student on their side to prevent aspiration. Do not attempt to restrain the patient or place anything in the mouth. The student's privacy should be protected by isolating the student from the view of others (Matesanz & Giovine, 2020).

If the student has a known seizure disorder, an EAP written in advance in consultation with the family and physician should direct the seizure response and care in the absence of the nurse.

In its training guide for school nurses, the Epilepsy Foundation (2022) states that EMS should be called in the following situations:

- Student has no known seizure history.
- Seizure is a result of trauma.
- The child has difficulty ambulating or difficulty breathing.
- Seizure lasts longer than 5 minutes.
- The child is hurt during the seizure.
- Seizure is different from any seizure the student has had in the past.

Did You Know?

Fast-acting benzodiazepines are prescribed as emergency medications to treat prolonged seizure activity (Epilepsy Foundation, 2023a). Diazepam (Valium), lorazepam (Ativan), and midazolam (Versed) are the most commonly prescribed rescue medications for repetitive or clustered seizures for out-of-hospital use in the United States. The Food and Drug Administration (FDA) has approved the following for children: rectal diazepam for children age 2 and older, nasal diazepam for children age 6 and older, and nasal diazepam for children age 12 and older.

- Student has repeated seizures without regaining consciousness.
- Student has diabetes or is pregnant.
- Seizure occurs in water.

School nurses should access NASN's *School Nursing Evidence-Based Practice Clinical Guideline: Students With Seizures and Epilepsy* (2023b) for more information about school nursing care for students with seizures and epilepsy. See Chapter 27 for more detailed information on seizures.

Meningitis

Bacterial meningitis is a potentially life-threatening acute inflammation of the meninges that surround and protect the brain and spinal cord (CDC, 2021a). There are three layers of meninges, the dura mater, the arachnoid mater, and the pia mater, which are separated by the epidural, subdural, and subarachnoid spaces. When infected, the meninges become inflamed causing acute pressure on the brain and spinal cord. In bacterial meningitis, bacteria invade the subarachnoid space. Although there are many different viruses and bacteria that can cause meningitis, the most common pathogens are *Haemophilus influenzae, Streptococcus pneumoniae,* and *Neisseria meningitides* (Reichert & Foley, 2024), which are spread by coughing, by sneezing, or through exchange of saliva (CDC, 2021a). Bacterial meningitis can be prevented with meningococcal, pneumococcal, and *H. influenzae* serotype b (Hib) vaccines. The CDC (2023) recommends that all preteens and teens receive meningococcal vaccinations and boosters. The incidence of cases of meningitis caused by *H. influenzae* type b has decreased dramatically since 1990 after the introduction of the Hib vaccine (CDC, 2021a, 2023).

Acute bacterial meningitis is a medical emergency that requires early recognition and immediate treatment to prevent death or disability. The primary symptoms include severe headache, stiff neck, and fever associated with other symptoms such as nausea, vomiting, light sensitivity, and altered mental status. The student is also at risk for seizures, coma, or even death (CDC, 2021a).

Viral meningitis is the most common type of meningitis. While the symptoms are similar to bacterial meningitis, it is typically less serious and may resolve within 7 to 10 days. Common causes of viral meningitis include the following (CDC, 2021c):

- Nonpolio enterovirus
- Measles
- Mumps
- Influenza
- West Nile virus
- Herpes
- Epstein-Barr virus

There is no way for the school nurse to know what type of meningitis might be suspected; therefore the same actions and precautions are indicated for any student with acute presentation of symptoms. EMS should be activated immediately. Due to the infectious nature of the disease, isolation of the child is important when symptoms indicate possible infection. The nurse should wear personal protective equipment, such as gloves, gowns, and masks, while awaiting EMS. Management of ABCDEs is a priority, and vital signs should be monitored until EMS arrives.

If bacterial meningitis is confirmed, public health officials must be contacted to conduct contact tracing to identify close contacts of the ill student and provide interventions and follow-up, including notification and treatment of other students and staff.

Syncope

Syncope is caused by a sudden decline in blood flow to the brain leading to brief loss of consciousness and loss of muscle control. When an individual faints, or falls out, they fall over or to the ground. Blood flow to the brain is restored, and the person regains consciousness. Syncopal episodes occur suddenly, last only a few minutes, and may or may not be proceeded by a brief period of dizziness, light-headedness, sweating, pallor, nausea, blurred vision, or other symptoms. *Vasovagal syncope* is estimated to account for nearly half of all syncopal episodes. It is a physiological response that induces vasodilation and bradycardia. Vasovagal syncope occurs when the body is overstressed by triggers such as standing for a long time, heat, dehydration, anxiety, pain, hunger, or the sight of blood (AHA, 2022c). *Postural syncope* occurs when there is a sudden change in body position, such as moving from lying to standing, which causes postural hypotension (Sweet, 2020). Syncopal episodes are most often benign but should be evaluated to rule out more serious underlying cardiac, metabolic, or neurological problems. Cardiac syncope is caused by heart or vascular conditions such as an arrhythmia, congenital heart disease, heart failure, or aortic stenosis. Syncopal-like episodes can also be caused by conditions such as stroke, seizures, and migraines (AHA, 2022c).

When a student presents with syncope, the nurse should check vital signs, especially blood pressure and pulse, with the student lying, sitting, and standing (if safe) to assess for orthostatic hypotension (CDC, 2017; Sweet, 2020). The nurse should perform a thorough assessment, including a history of preceding events and recent medication, alcohol, or drug intake. Check to see when and what the student last ate and whether any signs of dehydration are present. Conduct a neurological status examination. If the student has diabetes, blood sugar should be checked and treated per protocol (IEMSC & OSF HCHI, 2022).

If the student feels "faint," have the student lie down. If there are any injuries from a fall, provide first aid as needed and assess the need for spinal motion restriction if head/spinal injury is suspected. Periodic reassessment of vital signs may be indicated. It is good practice to call the parent/guardian and recommend consultation with the primary care provider. EMS should be activated if any of the following are present: sustained abnormal vital signs, acute change from baseline mental status, neurological deficit, head trauma, severe headache with altered mental status, or seizure activity (IEMSC & OSF HCHI, 2022).

EYE, EAR, NOSE, THROAT, AND DENTAL EMERGENCIES

Eye, ear, nose, throat, and dental medical problems involve multiple conditions that include infections, foreign bodies, thrombotic or embolic events, or trauma (Nolan-Kelley, 2020; Winter, 2020). Traumatic injuries involving the eyes, ears, nose, and throat are extremely painful and frightening for students. Such incidents include the following:

- Eye: Embedded foreign body, globe trauma/possible rupture, corneal ulcer, acute retinal detachment, central retinal artery occlusion, chemical burns, trauma around eye (blowout fracture), lacerations/abrasions
- Ear: Acute infections, ruptured tympanic membrane, burns, acute hearing loss, trauma with clear drainage (cerebral spinal fluid [CSF]), uncontrollable bleeding, piercing infection
- Nose: Uncontrolled nasal bleeding (epistaxis), trauma with suspected nasal fracture or CSF drainage, foreign body obstruction, piercing infection
- Throat: Tonsillar abscess/epiglottitis; tongue infection from piercing
- Dental: Trauma causing fractured tooth through the enamel and dentin, avulsed tooth (Nolan-Kelley, 2020; Waunch & Zaky, 2020; Winter, 2020)

Activate EMS for acute changes in vision, hearing, airway, breathing, swallowing, or mental status. Interventions for emergent eye injuries are outlined in Box 17-5. See Chapter 16 for more information on common complaints and injuries of the eye, ear, nose, and throat.

Impact injuries to the mouth at school commonly result in the avulsion of a tooth. Primary teeth should not be replaced. For an avulsed permanent tooth, students need to see a dentist within 60 minutes to increase the success of reimplantation. School staff should do the following:

- Handle the tooth by the crown (not the root).
- Rinse the dirty tooth in water or milk.
- Gently replace the tooth in the socket (do not force) *only* if the student is alert and able to cooperate. Instruct the student to keep pressure on the tooth by gently biting down on gauze.
- If unable to replace the tooth in the socket, place it in a protective container filled with pH-balanced solution for transport with the student to the ED or dentist. If pH-balanced solution is not available, use cold milk (or water if milk is not available) (IEMSC & OSF HCHI, 2022; Waunch & Zaky, 2020).

BOX 17-5

Emergent Triage Category for Eye Injuries in Students

EMERGENT

- Change in mental status
- Penetrating injury
- Chemical/thermal burn
- Unequal/irregular pupils
- Blunt injury (see Head/Spinal Cord protocol)
- Embedded foreign body
- Hyphema (haze or blood in iris)
- Reduced visual acuity/loss of vision
- Bilateral periorbital ecchymosis (raccoon eyes)

INTERVENTIONS

- Maintain spinal motion restriction as applicable
- Support C-ABCDE
- Activate EMS
- Protect eye from further injury

Chemical Burns

- Continue irrigation while awaiting EMS
- Send copy of SDS to ED

Penetrating Injuries

- Stabilize object with gauze pads
- Tape disposable drinking cup over dressing (do not allow it to contact object)

Thermal Burns

- Do not inspect eyes
- Apply loose, moist dressing

Radiation Burns

(From arc welder, sunlight, or sun lamp)

- Cover with eye patch

In All Cases

- Directly/continuously observe student
- Contact parent/guardian
- Notify school administrator
- Follow-up

SDS, Safety Data Sheet.

Illinois Emergency Medical Services for Children & OSF HealthCare Children's Hospital of Illinois. (2022). *Guidelines for the nurse in the school setting* (4th ed.), with permission.

ABDOMINAL EMERGENCIES

The abdominal organs and muscles include the digestive tract (stomach, small intestine, large intestine, cecum, and appendix), accessory organs (liver, gallbladder, and pancreas), urinary system (kidney and ureters), and other organs (spleen and reproductive organs). Abdominal trauma is the third most common type of trauma in children and is the most common site of missed injuries that result in death (Ernst, 2020; Miller, 2023). The large size of the organs in a relatively small space and the pliable rib cage predisposes children to have multiple organ injuries after blunt and penetrating kinetic forces. Blunt force is the most common cause of an abdominal injury in children (Waunch & Zaky, 2020). Subsequent internal bleeding is a common cause of death. The most commonly injured abdominal organ in blunt trauma is the spleen, followed by the liver, and then the kidney (Miller, 2023; Waunch & Zaky, 2020).

Causes

An abdominal emergency can be caused by infection, injury, obstruction, or inflammation of any of these organs. In the school setting, pain and discomfort are often the symptoms that precipitate a visit to the school health office. The school nurse must be able to differentiate between a serious emergency, such as appendicitis, from a less serious abdominal problem, such as constipation. Abdominal pain can occur during many acute and chronic illnesses and can be caused by many different conditions, even those originating from or referred from other parts of the body (Herrington, 2020). Abdominal pain, often described by children as a stomachache, may be a nonemergency caused by emotional distress, menstrual cramps, hunger, medications, or other minor causes. See Chapter 16 for discussion of less acute abdominal problems in children.

Assessment

The intensity of abdominal pain does not always reflect the seriousness of the condition. Severe abdominal pain can be caused by mild conditions, such as gas or cramping from viral gastroenteritis. Conversely, life-threatening conditions, such as early appendicitis, may present with relatively mild pain or no pain. The pain can be assessed using the PQRST mnemonic adapted for abdominal discomfort to determine the onset, location, frequency, and severity of the pain/tenderness or discomfort; time of the last bowel movement; presence of any urinary symptoms; and recent falls, blows, or other accidents, which are key assessment points (Dymond, 2023b; IEMSC & OSF HCHI, 2022). For adolescent females, the history should include onset of menarche, menstruation-related pain, and consideration of pregnancy. Students as young as 8 years old are at risk for ruptured ectopic pregnancy and hemorrhage. From the age of menarche until a negative pregnancy test has been confirmed, unilateral lower abdominal pain is considered an emergency (Dymond, 2023a). Ask the student to point with one finger to where the pain is greatest.

The nurse should perform a focused abdominal assessment including visual inspection, auscultation, and palpation (Dymond, 2023a; IEMSC & OSF HCHI, 2022). Following visual inspection, the nurse should listen in all four quadrants of the abdomen for bowel sounds. Gentle palpation of the nonpainful areas of the abdomen is done first and the painful area last. Assessment elements include rigidity of the abdominal muscles, rebound tenderness (increasing pain on release of pressure on the abdominal wall), distention, guarding, and positioning (maintaining a position of comfort). In a student with a recent fall or accident, the presence of *Kehr's sign* (referred left shoulder pain) suggests diaphragmatic irritation caused by an accumulation of blood in the peritoneal cavity indicative of possible splenic injury, leaking or ruptured ectopic pregnancy, or other internal bleeding in the abdominal cavity. Other related assessment elements can include hydration status with monitoring of vital signs, especially temperature for signs of fever. Diarrhea, vomiting, rectal bleeding, and jaundice are other significant indicators and should be documented if present (Waunch & Zaky, 2020).

The location of the pain may point to the pathology.

- Right upper quadrant pain could indicate problems in the liver, gallbladder, a duodenal ulcer, or right lower lobe pneumonia.
- Right lower quadrant pain could indicate involvement of the appendix, ovary, or fallopian tube.
- Left upper quadrant pain could be due to gastritis, left lower lobe pneumonia, or problems within the spleen, kidney, or pancreas.
- Left lower quadrant pain could be due to an ectopic pregnancy, ovarian problems, or diverticulitis.
- Flank pain could indicate renal problems, and lower abdominal pain could indicate pelvic inflammatory disease, ectopic pregnancy, ovarian or uterine problems, or a urinary tract infection (Waunch & Zaky, 2020).

Interventions

It is not advisable to give food or oral fluids until the cause of pain has been determined or the pain subsides. If mild or moderate pain persists after rest, contact the parent/guardian and recommend further evaluation by a medical provider. For severe abdominal pain (e.g., cannot walk or is constantly bent over), an abdominal mass, signs of shock, or when abdominal pain may indicate an ectopic pregnancy, EMS should be activated for transfer to the hospital for further evaluation and diagnostics (IEMSC & OSF HCHI, 2022).

Appendicitis

Appendicitis is the most common abdominal surgical emergency in children. The incidence is higher in males than females and peaks between ages 9 and 12 (Dymond, 2023b; Herrington, 2020). The appendix is a small pouch attached to the cecum, located near the transition from the small intestine to the colon in the lower right quadrant of the abdomen.

Appendicitis is the inflammation of the vermiform appendix or blind sac of the cecum and subsequent blockage of the lumen of the appendix. This blockage can be due to fecal debris or infection and results in an increase in pressure within the appendix and compression of the blood vessels. The resulting infection and edema can block blood flow to the area, causing ischemia and infarction. Bacterial overgrowth and pressure within the lumen can result in gangrene and rupture of the appendix. The release of toxins and bacteria causes inflammation of the lining of the abdominal cavity or peritonitis (Logee, 2020; Parsh & Jeffries, 2022).

Peritonitis is a high-risk complication if diagnosis is delayed. Peritonitis can progress to sepsis, intestinal obstruction, electrolyte imbalance, and hypovolemic shock (Herrington, 2020). Surgical intervention (i.e., appendectomy) or nonoperative approaches are the care options and are dependent on clinical status. Nonoperative intravenous antibiotic regimens and inpatient clinical observation may be used for low-risk patients (Dymond, 2023b). Early diagnosis is a challenge because appendicitis can be mistaken for other illnesses due in part to atypical presentations in children. Assessment for signs and symptoms of appendicitis should be a consideration of every abdominal pain presentation.

If appendicitis is suspected, the school nurse should contact the parent/guardian to take the student for urgent medical evaluation. The nurse should instruct the parent/guardian to refrain from applying heat or giving laxatives and enemas, as they stimulate bowel motility and may cause perforation of the appendix. If the appendix perforates, the temperature can be expected to increase to greater than 102.2°F (greater than 39°C), the respiratory rate increases, and the abdominal pain becomes less localized and more diffuse with rigid guarding (Dymond, 2023b; Logee, 2020). If perforation is suspected, the school nurse should activate EMS (IEMSC & OSF HCHI, 2022). Perforation of the appendix necessitates surgical intervention to avoid sepsis, shock, and potentially death. The student should not eat or drink anything because of the possibility of surgery. A follow-up contact with the parent/guardian should be made that evening or the next day to verify that the student was evaluated by a medical provider. If the student has not seen a medical provider, the potential risks should be emphasized and the parent/guardian encouraged to have the student evaluated.

Practice Connection

The early signs of appendicitis include mild fever with diffuse midabdominal or periumbilical pain, pain with coughing and walking, anorexia, nausea and/or vomiting, rebound tenderness, and abdominal rigidity. The student may prefer to lie still with legs flexed for pain relief. If pain can be elicited by hyperextension of the right hip while the child lays on the left side, appendicitis should be suspected. As appendicitis progresses, pain is localized to the right lower quadrant (McBurney's point between the iliac crest and the umbilicus), where the pain is most intense (Parsh & Jeffries, 2022).

GENITOURINARY EMERGENCIES

The term *genitourinary* (GU) refers to two different systems: urinary and reproductive. The reproductive system in females includes the ovaries, uterus, fallopian tubes, vagina, and cervix, and in males, the testes, seminal vesicles, prostate, seminal ducts, and penis. The urinary system is composed of the upper urinary tract, which includes the kidneys and the ureters, and the lower urinary tract, which includes the bladder and urethra (Baxter, 2020). GU emergencies in schools typically involve torsion of the testicle and blunt trauma to the genital area. The school nurse should gather a careful and objective history from the student and family regarding genital injuries sustained outside of school, such as blunt trauma and/or nonmenstrual vaginal or rectal bleeding, to rule out suspicions of physical or sexual abuse. It is not appropriate for school nurses to assess students beneath their underwear without consent of the parent/guardian and assent from the student; even then caution is advised. If a visual inspection is considered, a chaperone should be present with the school nurse to mitigate potential allegations of impropriety (Adimando, 2024; Zirkel, 2019).

Testicular Torsion

Testicular torsion is a surgical emergency (Logee, 2020). This painful condition is caused by twisting of the spermatic cord that causes a loss of blood flow to the testicle. The highest incidence of testicular torsion occurs during the neonatal period and puberty (Dymond, 2023a). Testicular torsion is characterized by acute onset of severe pain in one testicle accompanied by sudden swelling (Dymond, 2023a). Typically, the affected testicle is elevated. If there is a report of any asymmetry or enlargement, change in color, especially redness or darkening, or pain and discomfort, the nurse should refer the student emergently for medical attention. The student may also complain of nausea, vomiting, abdominal pain, and increase in pain when the testicle is elevated (Baxter, 2020; Dymond, 2023a).

Early diagnosis and treatment are key to avoiding testicular loss due to ischemia. All prepubertal and young adult males with a sudden onset of severe scrotal pain should be assumed to have testicular torsion until otherwise evaluated by a healthcare provider. Testicular swelling and pain must be evaluated promptly in an ED where there is access to surgical intervention if necessary. Although manual lateral rotation of the testes may be attempted in a medical setting, surgical intervention within 4 to 6 hours of onset is the treatment of choice (Baxter, 2020; Logee, 2020). If untreated for 24 hours, the testicle will likely become necrotic and be lost (Dymond, 2023a; Logee, 2020).

Genitourinary Trauma

Trauma to the GU system can result from physical force to organs such as the kidney, ureters, bladder, urethra, internal reproductive organs, or external genitalia. Injuries to the GU system can result from impacts such as motor vehicle collisions, sports activities, falls, all-terrain vehicle accidents, and so on. The kidney is the most commonly injured organ in the GU system, followed by injuries to the external genitalia, bladder/urethra, and ureter (Waunch & Zaky, 2020).

Although sports-related injuries and assaults account for the smallest number of GU system injuries seen in the ED, they are a common cause of GU injuries seen in the school setting. Common causes of female genitalia injuries are falls, straddle-type falls on monkey bars or chairs, and sexual abuse or assault. Male genitalia injuries include testicular trauma from straddle-type falls and direct force injuries to the penis such as from a zipper injury (Waunch & Zaky, 2020).

The evaluation and treatment of GU pain is difficult; different conditions may cause similar symptoms. School nurse interventions may include direct pressure to stop bleeding, application of ice to reduce swelling, and referral/transfer to an ED.

MUSCULOSKELETAL TRAUMA

Musculoskeletal injuries are common in children due to immature areas of the growing skeletal system. Many situations in school settings carry the risk for injuries to the musculoskeletal system such as recess, gym, sports, and training. Children have more porous and flexible bones compared with adults, so bone may bend before breaking, resulting in an incomplete (greenstick) fracture. As children grow, elongation of the long bones occurs at the epiphyseal plate (growth plate) at both ends of the long bones. Injury to this area may disrupt bone growth and result in long-term consequences. In some areas, the surrounding ligaments and tendons may be stronger than the skeletal system itself, making the bones more vulnerable. Skeletal injuries include dislocation of joints, fractured bones, amputations, or crush injuries (National Institute of Arthritis and Musculoskeletal and Skin Diseases, 2022).

Treatment of musculoskeletal injury depends on the type and degree of injury. Nonurgent injuries appear as mild soft tissue edema with mild pain and tenderness; the student is able to bear weight and will have normal neurovascular findings along with normal vital signs. Interventions for nonurgent injuries include icing and elevating the affected area. Contact the parent/guardian according to health office protocols.

A student with urgent musculoskeletal injuries may present with deformity, discoloration, moderate edema, and moderate pain; vital signs and neurovascular findings may be normal. The nurse evaluates the student for pain, pallor, pulselessness, pressure (tense feeling of the extremity on palpation—indication of compartment syndrome), paresthesia/paralysis, and poikilothermia (limb taking on the temperature of the surrounding environment) (Davis, 2024b). Interventions include applying ice packs, immobilizing, and elevating the extremity. Determine the need for EMS and reassess neurovascular status distal to the injury every 5 to 10 minutes. If EMS is not needed, contact the parent/guardian to transport the child to receive medical care.

When a student is emergently injured it is important to activate EMS immediately. Emergent injuries include, but are not limited to, open fractures, amputation, neurovascular compromise, severe edema, and hemorrhage. While waiting for EMS to arrive, the school nurse should immobilize the injured area, stop bleeding, monitor neurovascular status distal to the injured site, directly and continuously observe the student, and monitor airway, breathing, and circulation (ABC). In the event the student loses pulses distal to the injury, apply gentle traction until pulse is restored and reassess pulses every 5 to 10 minutes. Notify the guardian and follow school protocol for follow-up (IEMSC & OSF HCHI, 2022).

In the event of amputation, the severed body part should be wrapped in gauze slightly moistened with sterile saline, secured in a plastic bag, and placed on cold packs (not ice) to be transported via EMS with the student (IEMSC & OSF HCHI, 2022). For uncontrolled bleeding, apply pressure, and apply pressure dressings and a tourniquet if available and indicated. The school nurse should be trained in the proper use of tourniquets. Although painful to the victim, tourniquets should not be removed out of the hospital setting.

TOXICOLOGICAL EMERGENCIES

In 2020, over 2.1 million human exposures to toxic or poisonous substances occurred and telephone guidance to the poison control centers were made. The United States accounts for 91.45% of the world's poison control cases whereas international cases account for 8.55% (Poison Control, 2020). Although most exposures occur in the home, the school environment contains multiple poisonous substances, particularly in science laboratories. Children younger than 6 years old accounted for 39% of exposures and teens accounted for 8% (Poison Control, 2020). Poisoning for males is predominant in ages less than 13 and is more predominant in females during adolescence and adulthood. Adolescents are more likely to ingest harmful amounts of alcohol or recreational drugs. Prescription opioid misuse is one of the leading causes of unintentional death and injury in adolescents and young adults in the United States (Hudgins et al., 2019). In 2017, 2.2 million adolescents ages 12 to 17 were users of illicit drugs, adding it to the top five public health challenges (NASN, 2023a).

A *poison*, or toxin, is any substance that can cause harm to the body. Any substance can be poisonous depending on the amount ingested. A poisoning may be acute, as in an overdose of medication, or chronic, such as cirrhosis caused by alcohol. Poisonings are classified as either unintentional or intentional. Poisons enter the body through ingestion, inhalation, absorption, or injection. The reaction and signs and symptoms vary depending on the chemical and the quantity of the substance ingested (Poison Control, 2020).

A *toxidrome*, or toxicological syndrome, is a group of signs and symptoms constituting the basis for a diagnosis of poisoning. Toxidromes are helpful because they classify groups of drugs or chemicals according to the clinical findings typical in overdoses or poisonings. Knowledge of common toxidromes helps the school nurse make assessment and intervention decisions. See Box 17-6 for toxicological syndromes that the school nurse may encounter.

Causes

Many chemical substances are not toxic in appropriate amounts or levels. As is the case with prescription medications, many substances are beneficial at therapeutic doses but are dangerous, if not deadly, when taken in large amounts. For guidance on treatment of any poisoning, regardless of whether symptoms have developed, contact the National Poison Control Center at 1-800-222-1222 (Poison Control, 2024). The school nurse should request that another staff member contact the poison control center for guidance on management so as to not interrupt providing life-sustaining care to the student. For known toxins in the school, the school material safety data sheet (MSDS) should be obtained, copied, and given to EMS. Before initiating care, the nurse should determine whether personal protective equipment is needed to avoid becoming exposed to the poison. It is

BOX 17-6

Toxidromes

If assessment findings suggest a toxic ingestion and you do not know what substance is involved, it may be helpful to look for signs of identifiable toxic syndromes (toxidromes). Toxidromes involve a recognizable group of signs and symptoms that tend to occur consistently with particular toxins. The following table describes the four major toxidromes and provides mnemonics that can help you remember the associated findings. Examples of substances that can cause each toxidrome are included.

TOXIDROMES	CLINICAL FINDINGS	CAUSATIVE SUBSTANCES
Opioid	■ Constricted pupils ■ CNS depression ■ Respiratory depression	■ Heroin ■ Codeine ■ Fentanyl ■ Methadone
Sympathomimetic	■ Hypertension ■ Tachycardia ■ Hyperthermia ■ Diaphoresis ■ Dilated pupils	■ Epinephrine ■ OTC diet aids containing caffeine ■ Amphetamines ■ Oral decongestants (e.g., pseudoephedrine) ■ Bronchodilators
Anticholinergic (listed phrases may help you recall clinical findings)	■ Hyperthermia (hot as a hare) ■ Flushed skin (red as a beet) ■ Hypertension, dry skin (dry as a bone) ■ Delirium (mad as a hatter) ■ Dilated pupils (blind as a bat) ■ Urinary retention (full as a flask) ■ Tachycardia ■ Absent bowel sounds	■ Antihistamines ■ GI antispasmodics ■ Certain toxic plants (e.g., jimson weed, deadly nightshade, atropine) ■ Tricyclic antidepressants
Cholinergic	SLUDGE: ■ Salivation ■ Lacrimation ■ Urination ■ Diarrhea ■ Gastrointestinal distress ■ Emesis Other symptoms: ■ Miosis, muscle fasciculations ■ Bradycardia, bronchorrhea ■ Weakness	■ Organophosphate and carbamate insecticides ■ Physostigmine

Illinois Emergency Medical Services for Children & OSF HealthCare Children's Hospital of Illinois. (2022). *Guidelines for the nurse in the school setting* (4th ed.), with permission.

important to remove the offending irritant from the student as soon as possible.

Assessment

When a student presents to the nurse's office after a suspected exposure to a toxic substance or overdose, the nurse should act quickly. If the initial assessment reveals signs of distress or altered mental status, the substance is already causing a systemic reaction. In addition to vital signs, the school nurse should be alert for respiratory depression, skin and temperature changes, altered mental status and level of consciousness, unusual odors on the breath or skin, nausea, vomiting, and abdominal pain.

The school nurse conducts a focused history to ascertain the following:

- The type and amount of substance (get the container if available)
- Time and route of exposure (dermal, ocular, inhalation, or ingestion)
- The location where exposure occurred
- Whether any other students are involved
- Any history of allergies and underlying health problems (IEMSC & OSF HCHI, 2022)

The school nurse must be aware, however, that an alert and oriented and apparently stable student may have a lethal amount of poison in their system that has not yet had time to produce systemic reactions. The nurse must be vigilant with continued monitoring because the student's condition can change dramatically. Once initial life threats have been addressed, the nurse may complete a focused history and physical examination, including vital signs, and reassess the ABCDEs. The nurse should note any unusual odors or stains around the mouth or nose or on the clothes in addition to assessing the skin for areas of irritation.

Asking the appropriate questions to determine the type of poison will dictate the intervention. If the substance is known, the student (as developmentally appropriate), school staff, or witnesses should be questioned as to what time the exposure occurred, the amount and route of exposure, and whether any other students are known to have also been exposed. Quick recognition that a poisoning has occurred is key to effective treatment and recovery.

Interventions

Students suspected of ingesting a toxic substance or a toxic amount of drug should be transported immediately via EMS to the nearest medical facility. Monitoring and maintaining ABCDEs will be the primary focus until EMS arrives. If possible, identify the toxin for EMS and the ED so that appropriate treatment can begin without delay. The priority is to remove the victim from the toxin and prevent further exposure. Provide fresh air or oxygen for inhalation of hazardous substances. If ingestion of a toxin is suspected, do not induce vomiting. If possible, save the vomitus in a container to be transported with EMS. For topical exposure to chemical toxins, don personal protective equipment and remove contaminated clothing, brush off chemicals, and flush with water until EMS arrives. If a student is suspected of injecting an overdose of drugs, administer an opioid antagonist (naloxone) and be prepared to start CPR.

In response to the national crisis of opioid overdoses, states are increasingly allowing or mandating that naloxone be stocked as a rescue medication for suspected overdoses in schools. See Chapter 30 for more information on stock emergency medications. Due to the complicated issues related to this issue, the NASN (2023a) has developed the *Naloxone Education in Schools Toolkit* that provides resources to assist school nurses and school districts with developing a naloxone program and instituting campus protocols for emergency naloxone administration. Naloxone is an opioid antagonist that will temporarily reverse respiratory depression in opioid overdoses; it is available as an intramuscular injection or intranasal spray. This medication is useful in preventing opioid deaths and can be given every 2 to 3 minutes (NASN, 2023a). The half-life of naloxone is usually shorter than the drug ingested, therefore rebound overdose can occur. Monitor respiratory status continuously until EMS arrives and administer medications as needed. School nurses should be familiar with the legal implications in their state regarding this drug.

> **Did You Know?**
>
> An example of a highly toxic drug is fentanyl; it is 50 to 100 times more potent than morphine and is highly associated with drug overdoses. It is used in the medical field to treat patients with chronic pain or postsurgical patients; however, it can also be manufactured in a laboratory and sold illegally. Fentanyl is often added to illegal synthetic drugs, but the user may or may not know that it is an ingredient in the substance they are using. Fentanyl can cause serious life-threatening symptoms such as bradypnea, apnea, and hypoxia. If left untreated with an opioid antagonist (naloxone, discussed in the following paragraph), it will lead to death (U.S. Drug Enforcement Administration, 2022). See Chapter 29 for more information on students engaging in high-risk behaviors.

BITES AND STINGS

The school nurse should have knowledge of human bites and local animals, reptiles, insects, and arachnids (e.g., spiders, mites, ticks, and scorpions) in the school community that pose a risk of bites and stings. Although most bites and stings are relatively nonurgent and cause only minimal injury, others pose a significant risk. Protocols should be developed that outline care of common bites, scratches, and stings. See Table 17-4.

TABLE 17-4 General Interventions for Bites and Stings

Key Considerations	Assessment	Interventions
Human Bites • High risk for infection due to bacteria/viruses in the human mouth. • Signs of infection may occur 1–2 days after injury or later. • Identify whether the bite was accidental or intentional. • Assess for child abuse.	• Obtain thorough history. • Determine whether skin is broken or intact. • Look in and around the wound to determine the extent of injury. • Assess pain (complaints of pain in older bites may be a sign of infection). • Assess area for signs of infection and lymph nodes above the area for enlargement. • Assess immunization status of the biter and who was bitten (i.e., tetanus, hepatitis B).	• Treat as an open wound if unclear whether skin is broken. • Clean the wound with soap and water and apply clean bandage. • Apply pressure if the wound is actively bleeding. • Follow-up care with a primary doctor or in the ED is warranted if skin is broken. • Bites to the ear and nose need to be evaluated due to high risk of infection and complications. • Complete incident and/or accident report per policy. • Report suspected child abuse to authorities. • If a tetanus booster is needed, give within 48–72 hours of injury.

Animal Bites and Scratches
• Bites or scratches that produce an open wound are at risk for infection.
• Bites from potentially rabid sources (i.e., bats) need to be taken seriously.
• Claw wounds from cats should be treated the same as bite wounds.
• Some states require dog bites to be reported to the department of health and/or law enforcement.
	• Obtain thorough history.
	• Identify type of bite, location and time of bite, and number of bites or puncture wounds.
	• Assess area for swelling, discoloration, drainage, and any active bleeding.
	• Assess immunization status for need for tetanus booster.
	• For dog bites, if the owner is known, assess immunization status for the dog.
	• Assess for signs of infection in older bites.
		• If skin is not broken, apply ice indirectly to the skin for 20 minutes for pain relief.
		• Minor wounds (barely breaks the skin and no danger of rabies):
		  • Allow wound to bleed for 3–4 seconds then flush with running water.
		  • Wash/lightly scrub wound with soap and water.
		  • Apply bandage.
		• If skin is broken, seek medical evaluation and treatment.
		• Deep wounds (deep puncture, torn skin, active bleeding):
		  • Apply pressure with cloth or gauze to control bleeding.
		  • Activate EMS.
		• If rabies is suspected, activate EMS and call local animal control services.

• Snake bites may be venomous or nonvenomous, but most species of snakes are harmless, and bites are not life-threatening. • Children are at greater risk for death or serious complications from venomous snake bites.	• Obtain thorough history. • Identify type of snake, location and time of bite, and number of bites or puncture wounds. • Assess area for swelling, discoloration, drainage, fang marks, and active bleeding. • Assess for other possible symptoms depending on type of snake (blurred vision, burning of skin, convulsions, diarrhea, dizziness, excessive sweating, nausea, vomiting, loss of muscle coordination, numbness/tingling, skin discoloration, severe pain, weakness). • Assess immunization status for need for tetanus booster.	• Leave the area to prevent repeated bites or additional victims. • Do not hunt or try to capture the snake. • Activate EMS for rapid transport because antivenom may be needed. • Keep student calm and minimize movement. • Remove any rings or constrictive items. • If prolonged or delayed transport, wrap a loose splint on the affected area to restrict movement. • Monitor the student's vital signs. • Do not apply ice to the area. • Do not apply a tourniquet. • Do not allow student to eat or drink. • Do not raise the area of the bite above the level of their heart.
Insect Bites and Stings • Almost all spiders are venomous but may not be harmful to humans because of the inability of the spider's fangs to penetrate human skin or small amount of venom. • Brown recluse spiders and black widow spiders can cause problems in humans.	• Obtain thorough history. • Identify type of bite and location and time of bite. • Assess for symptoms of brown recluse or black widow spider bites: fever, nausea, vomiting, headache, joint pain or stiffness, malaise, rash, and muscle cramping. • Assess area for swelling, discoloration, drainage, blister formation, bull's-eye pattern to the area, fang marks. • Assess whether pain was delayed or sudden onset. • Assess immunization status for need for tetanus booster.	• Wash the area with soap and water. • Cover area with light dressing. • If a suspect bite is from brown recluse or black widow, immediate treatment is required (antivenom may be given for black widow and hospitalization may be needed following both types of bites). • Limit movement of affected area. • Contact the Poison Control Center for additional guidance. • If a tetanus booster is needed, give within 48–72 hours of injury.

Continued

TABLE 17-4 General Interventions for Bites and Stings—cont'd

Key Considerations	Assessment	Interventions
• Classified as venomous or nonvenomous • Some insects leave their stinger behind in the wound. • Risk for anaphylaxis • Examples of stinging or biting insects: wasps, hornets, yellow jackets, bees, fire ants, fleas, lice, scabies, ticks, mosquitos, chiggers, bedbugs	• Obtain thorough history. • Identify type of bite or sting and location and time of bite. • Assess area for swelling, discoloration, drainage. • Assess for signs of systemic reaction (hives, swelling to face or tongue, difficulty swallowing, fainting, wheezing). • Signs of infection may be present at least 24 hours after bite/sting. • Symptoms of a tick bite might only develop after the tick drops off or is removed (local redness, itching, burning, flu-like symptoms, fever, numbness, rash, weakness, joint pain, nausea, vomiting). • Assess immunization status for need for tetanus booster.	• Activate 911, activate care plan, and provide respiratory support for anaphylactic reactions. • If a stinger is present, brush it or scrape it to remove it using cardboard or credit card. • Do not squeeze the area. • Wash the area with soap and water. • Apply ice to the area for comfort. • Assess for systemic reactions such as flu-like symptoms. • Remove the tick using forceps or tweezers by pulling the tick straight out without twisting or turning (it is important to not break apart or only partially remove the tick). • Take care when removing stingers and ticks to prevent disease transmission. • Follow up with primary care or in the ED as indicated. • Educate parents/guardians regarding symptoms to watch. • If a tetanus booster is needed, give it within 48–72 hours of injury.

National Institute for Occupational Safety and Health (2018a, 2018b, 2021a, 2021b).

Bites

Bites can be from humans, animals, or insects. Human bites that break the skin should be treated seriously. Human bites should be meticulously cleaned to prevent infection. Human bites that break the skin pose a risk of infection and should be referred for medical evaluation and treatment (Barret & Brusch, 2021). Animal bites can be divided into categories of those that are wild and prone to rabies (e.g., bats, skunks, raccoons, foxes); small wild animals (e.g., rats, chipmunks, squirrels, prairie dogs, rabbits); and pets (e.g., indoor animals, horses, and farm animals). Although rare, *rabies* is a viral illness transmitted through the bites of infected animals. Rabies affects the brain and central nervous system in humans and can lead to death within days if not promptly and aggressively treated. Individuals bitten by wild animals should seek treatment in an ED without delay (CDC, 2022c). The local animal control unit should be contacted.

Snakes are more common in certain regions but are found across the United States. Snake bites can be venomous or nonvenomous. Rattlesnakes, copperheads, cottonmouths, water moccasins, and coral snakes are venomous (National Institute for Occupational Safety and Health [NIOSH], 2021b). Some nonvenomous snakes and venomous snakes resemble each other. If the type of snake is not seen or recognized, assume the bite to be from a venomous snake. The signs and symptoms of venomous snake bites include the following:

- Puncture marks at the wound
- Redness, swelling, bruising, bleeding, or blistering around the bite
- Severe pain and tenderness at the site of the bite
- Nausea, vomiting, or diarrhea
- Labored breathing (in extreme cases, breathing may stop altogether)
- Rapid heart rate, weak pulse, low blood pressure
- Disturbed vision
- Metallic, mint, or rubber taste in the mouth
- Increased salivation and sweating
- Numbness or tingling around the face and/or limbs
- Muscle twitching (NIOSH, 2021a, para. 1)

Victims should not wait for signs and symptoms to appear but seek immediate treatment in an ED. Immobilize the student and keep them calm.

Spiders are not inherently aggressive but may bite when unintentionally contacted. They are most commonly found around or under undisturbed places.

While most spiders are venomous, not all venomous spider bites are serious. Some nonvenomous spider bites (e.g., wolf spiders) may also cause severe reactions in some individuals. Symptoms of spider bites include the following:

- Itching or rash
- Pain radiating from the site of the bite
- Muscle pain or cramping
- Reddish to purplish color or blister
- Increased sweating
- Difficulty breathing
- Headache
- Nausea and vomiting
- Fever
- Chills

- Anxiety or restlessness
- High blood pressure (NIOSH, 2018c)

The most common species of venomous spiders in the United States are the black widow and the brown recluse, which may be found indoors and out. Black widow spiders, distinguished by a red hourglass shape on the abdomen, may bite when a human disturbs their web. The bite, distinguished by two fang marks, injects a venomous neurotoxin that causes pain as it spreads from the bite to the chest, abdomen, and across the body, requiring immediate medical attention (NIOSH, 2018c). Brown recluse spiders, sometimes called violin spiders, are found mostly in the Midwest and South. They bite when unintentionally trapped against the skin. The stinging and painful bite results in a white blister followed by localized skin necrosis, which requires medical attention (NIOSH, 2018c).

Immediate medical attention is needed for venomous spider bites or severe reactions to spider bites. First aid measures include washing the bite with soap and water and icing and elevating (if possible). No efforts to remove the venom from the site should be attempted. If possible, try to identify the type of spider so directed medical treatment can be initiated quickly (NIOSH, 2018c).

Ticks are found across the country in outside shaded areas in the warm weather months. Ticks feed on the blood of mammals (including humans), birds, reptiles, and amphibians. They can transmit a number of different pathogens between hosts that can cause disease in humans, such as Lyme disease, Rocky Mountain spotted fever, and tularemia, among others. If fever/chills, headache, fatigue, muscle aches, and/or joint pain develop within a few weeks, medical attention is needed (CDC, 2021b). See Chapter 18, Figure 18-6, for directions on tick removal.

Stings

School nurses must be aware that stings/bites of bees, wasps, hornets, yellow jackets, and fire ants may be life-threatening if the person is allergic to the stinging insect. Anaphylaxis is a severe allergic reaction that occurs after exposure to an allergen, which may result in death if untreated. Follow anaphylaxis protocols discussed earlier in this chapter. See Chapter 21 for more detailed information on anaphylaxis.

Mild reactions to stings include pain, redness, swelling, and itching at the site. Stingers should be removed by wiping with a gauze pad. Never pinch the stinger to remove, because this forces more venom through the stinger into the skin (American Academy of Allergy, Asthma, & Immunology, 2020). Wash the area with soap and water and apply ice.

Scorpions are found in the southern and southwestern parts of the country. They usually hide under rocks, wood, or anything lying on the ground during the day and become active at night (NIOSH, 2018a). A scorpion bite results in a stinging/burning sensation with little associated swelling or inflammation. The hallmark of a scorpion sting is a positive "tap test," which elicits extreme pain at the site when tapped by a finger. Immediate medical attention in an ED is needed. Symptoms include restlessness, convulsions, roving eyes, staggering gait, thick tongue sensation, slurred speech, drooling, muscle twitching, abdominal pain and cramps, and respiratory depression. Ice may be applied, but tourniquets should not. Treatment in a hospital is supportive; symptoms generally subside in 48 hours, though stings from the bark scorpion can be lethal (NIOSH, 2018a).

BURNS

A *burn injury* is defined as damage to the skin and underlying tissues that results from heat/thermal sources (i.e., exposure to flames, hot liquids, hot objects, and inhalation of heat or smoke), caustic chemicals, radiation, or electric current. Most burns affect only the epidermal and dermal layers of the skin. However, deeper tissues, such as muscle, bone, and blood vessels, may also be injured (American Burn Association [ABA], 2018). While fire-related deaths at school are rare, burns are not uncommon. Fire and safety burn prevention programs developed for community education can help educate families to mitigate fire and burn injuries and deaths (ABA, 2018).

Causes

Thermal burns result from the skin's exposure to hot temperatures. There are four types of thermal burns:

- Scalds: from hot liquids (water, oil, beverages, bath water) or steam
- Flame: from matches, lighters, house fires, cooking incidents, fireworks, wood stoves, or kerosene heaters
- Flash burns: caused by an explosion or ignition of gasoline fumes or electrical flash, furnace blast, or gasoline explosion
- Contact burns: from exposure to hot objects such as a radiator, iron, hot tar, or hot grease

The inhalation of smoke, superheated air, or burning toxic substances may lead to asphyxiation, carbon monoxide poisoning, and damage of the airways and lungs (Bidigare, 2023).

Chemical burns may be caused by the skin's exposure to a corrosive substance such as a strong acid or base. Common causes of chemical burns include cleaning agents, gasoline, paint removers, and battery acids. Damage from chemical burns may cause significant deep pathology that may not be immediately evident. Chemicals cause proteins to denature within the tissues or cause the desiccation of cells; therefore there may be only minimal cutaneous effects. More tissue damage is usually seen with alkali products than with acids (ABA, 2018).

Electrical burns are caused by an electrical shock or lightning. High-voltage electric shock occurs when the human body makes contact with any source of voltage high enough to cause sufficient current to damage the muscles, causing swelling of the fascia and interruption of blood flow (ABA, 2018). Because the electrical current passes through the body, there is an entrance and an exit wound, with damage occurring internally along the route of the current. The internal injuries of a high-voltage electrical burn may be disproportionate to the size of the burns seen; therefore the extent of the damage is not always obvious. If the path of the electricity is near or through the heart, the electrical conduction system of the heart can cause spontaneous ventricular fibrillation or other dysrhythmias. Nonfatal electrical injuries do occur, such as when children bite on electrical cords or place their fingers into electrical outlets. Adolescent risk-taking behaviors, such as climbing high-voltage transmission towers, may result in electrocution, a fatal injury.

Lightning strikes are a rare cause of electrical injuries in the United States. The southeastern states are most at risk. The odds of being struck by lightning in any year are less than 1 in 1 million. About one-third of lightning injuries occur indoors (CDC, 2022b).

Radiation burns are caused by exposure to electromagnetic or particulate ionizing radiation (ABA, 2018). Exposure to ultraviolet rays from the sun is the most common type of radiation burn. Other causes may be from extended exposure to radiation-producing machines or other radiation-producing devices. The school nurse is instrumental in developing sunburn prevention protocols (sunblock, hats, sunscreen) and monitoring compliance.

Assessment

The initial assessment of a burn victim focuses on whether the burning process is still occurring while simultaneously performing the systematic assessment of airway, breathing, and circulation. If there are still flames, smoke, or heat coming from the burned area, then the burning process is still occurring. Inspect the mouth, nose, and face for signs of burn injury or inhalation. The chest should be auscultated for any abnormal breath sounds, such as stridor or hoarseness. If injury is due to a flash explosion, be aware of the potential for serious inhalation injury. Assess the circulation by observing skin color, level of consciousness, capillary refill time (might not be reliable depending on the extent and location of the burn), heart rate, heart rhythm and quality, and the level of pain.

The burn location, depth, and extent are assessed to determine the severity of the burn injury. The location is important because burns in certain locations of the body indicate higher risk. Although final determination of the depth of the burn may not occur for several days, the school nurse should attempt to quantify this parameter to determine disposition and to communicate with others about the burn injury. According to the American Burn Association (2018), the following parameters are used to describe depth:

- A *superficial* burn involves only the epidermis, which is the outermost layer of the skin. It is characterized by erythema (redness), local pain, hypersensitivity, and no skin sloughing. These burns are not included as part of the total body surface area (TBSA) calculations of burned skin.
- A *superficial partial-thickness* burn involves both the epidermis and part of the dermis, which is directly beneath the epidermis. This type of burn generally produces erythema and blisters.
- A *deep partial-thickness* burn may appear white and dry, with locally reduced sensitivity to touch and pain but perceptive of pressure. This type of burn will not heal without intervention.
- A *full-thickness* burn is the destruction of the entire thickness of the dermis and epidermis. The burn has a tough brownish surface and a hard eschar. The area will be locally insensitive to touch or pain. This type of burn will not heal without intervention.
- *Fourth-degree* burn refers to wounds that penetrate into the subdermal fat below the skin. The burn may affect muscles and bones, with skin blackened or completely burned away. Due to the nerve damage, the person may not feel pain. The damage from this burn will not heal without intervention.

The extent of the injury is assessed by using formulas that estimate the percentage of the TBSA that has a partial- or full-thickness burn. A simple formula uses the size of the student's palm including fingers to represent 1% of the TBSA (ABA, 2018).

The extent of chemical burns is related to the chemical concentration and duration of exposure. Chemical burns may be deceiving as to their depth with an appearance similar in surface discoloration until the tissue begins to slough off days later. Therefore all chemical burns should be considered deep partial thickness or full thickness until proven otherwise. For electrical injuries that typically have only an entrance and exit burn wound, describing the injury anatomically is more important than calculating the percentage of TBSA burned (ABA, 2018).

Interventions

The emergency response interventions depend on the type and extent of the burn suffered. In all cases, the student should be removed from the source of the burn (Box 17-7).

Thermal Burns

The priority for a thermal burn is to stop the burning process. First, extinguish any flames by wrapping a blanket on the student or direct the student to stop, drop, and roll. Apply room temperature water to all types of thermal burns for 2 to 5 minutes or until heat cannot be felt coming from the site of burn injury. Too much cooling can quickly lead to hypothermia in a severe burn. Do NOT use ice on a burn injury because it will cause additional tissue injury. Remove burned clothing unless it is adhered to the burned skin area; cut around it but remove all loose areas. Quickly remove any jewelry from injured extremities before swelling occurs

BOX 17-7

Triage and Interventions for Burns

IMMEDIATE INTERVENTIONS

Even before you determine triage category, perform the following actions as indicated:

- Remove student from burn source (e.g., heat/electricity)
- Remove jewelry, rings, and constricting clothing (if possible)
- Do *not* remove clothing that has adhered to skin!
- Begin irrigation of chemical burns with cool water (clear off any chemical powders/dust before irrigation)
- Cool thermal burns if less than 20% of total body surface area (% TBSA) is involved

NOTE: Protect student from hypothermia; only immerse superficial or partial-thickness burns less than 5% TBSA

DETERMINE TRIAGE CATEGORY AND ADDITIONAL INTERVENTIONS

EMERGENT

- Apnea or pulseless
- Full-thickness burn (tough, brownish surface)
- Deep partial-thickness burn (charred/white)
- Burns involving face, hands, feet, eyes, ears, or genitalia (see Eye or Ear Emergencies protocols)
- Electrical burns
- Signs/symptoms of inhalation injury (singed nasal hair or carbonaceous sputum) or other complicating injuries
- Altered mental status
- Respiratory distress (see Respiratory Distress protocol)
- Suspected child maltreatment (see Child Maltreatment protocol after providing burn care)
- Severe pain

INTERVENTIONS

- Activate EMS
- Support C-ABCDE

Electrical burns

- Safely remove student from burn source
- Initiate CPR as needed/have AED ready
- Inspect for entrance and exit wounds

Chemical burns

- Continue copious irrigation of chemical burns with tepid running water for at least 20 min
- Consider contacting Poison Control Center (800-222-1222)
- Send burn agent and SDS to ED with student
- Do not apply cold packs

Thermal burns

- Cover with dry, sterile dressings or clean sheet in all cases
- Directly/continuously observe student
- Contact parent/guardian
- Notify school administrator
- Follow-up

URGENT

- Superficial partial-thickness burn without complicating factors
- Moderate pain
- Erythema/edema, wet/oozing blisters
- Too large to cover with adhesive bandage
- Signs of associated infection

INTERVENTIONS

- Determine need for EMS
- Flush copiously with tepid running water
- If unable to immerse, apply clean, wet, cool cloth
- Do not apply cold packs
- Do not break blisters
- Bandage loosely
- Observe student closely
- Contact parent/guardian to transport student to medical care or home
- Follow-up

NONURGENT

- Superficial burn (e.g., sunburn)
- Minor erythema
- Local, mild pain
- Student is alert

INTERVENTIONS

- Immerse area in tepid water 2–5 min
- Apply tepid cloths
- Bandage loosely
- Observe student
- Contact parent/guardian
- Return student to class or send home as indicated
- Follow-up (as needed or per policy)

Illinois Emergency Medical Services for Children & OSF HealthCare Children's Hospital of Illinois. (2022). *Guidelines for the nurse in the school setting* (4th ed.), with permission.

and to stop the burning process. Do not apply ointment or burn cream to any burn (ABA, 2018).

For minor, small, superficial burns, after cooling, wash the burned area with mild soap and water. Leave blisters intact and cover loosely with a clean dressing. The student can return to class with a small minor burn, although the parent/guardian should be notified.

For partial-thickness burns with redness, pain, swelling, and blisters, the burn location, depth, and an estimate of the TBSA that is burned can assist the nurse in determining whether EMS needs to be activated or whether the child can be released to the parent/guardian with instructions to follow up with their healthcare provider.

A full-thickness burn is always considered an emergency and EMS should be activated. The parent/guardian should be notified of any types of burns. Dry dressings should be applied to all burns. For burns that may have respiratory involvement, management of the airway is the priority. Assist respirations as needed using ventilation adjuncts if available, such as a pocket mask or bag-valve mask. Measure blood pressure in an unburned extremity when assessing circulation. Continue to monitor ABCDEs and consider covering the injured person with a sheet to maintain core body temperature.

Chemical Burns

For all chemical burns, the school nurse or responders should assess for scene safety and the need to use personal protective equipment to prevent exposure to the chemical. Removal of the contaminated clothes, shoes, jewelry, and belongings of the victim is critical to halting the burning process (ABA, 2018). If the chemical is dry, it can be brushed from the skin onto something under the patient that can be discarded properly before irrigating. Interventions should not be delayed while attempting to identify the causative agent (ABA, 2018). Review the safety data sheets, if available, for care recommendations. Chemical burns should be irrigated immediately with tap water for at least 20 to 30 minutes (ABA, 2018). After the wound is thoroughly irrigated, it is treated like a thermal burn.

If the burn is from an identified chemical, consider contacting the National Poison Control Center (Poison Control, 2024) for directions on management or locating the safety data sheet for recommended first-aid treatment (ABA, 2018). Chemical burns are considered emergent and EMS should be activated.

> **Practice Connection**
>
> The following are considered emergent burns that require immediate evaluation and treatment in an ED. Transfer to a regional burn center may be required.
>
> EMS should be activated for the following burns:
>
> - Partial-thickness burns that cover an area 10% or greater of the TBSA
> - Full-thickness burns
> - Burns involving the hands, feet, face, genitalia, perineum, or major joints
> - Chemical burns
> - Electrical burns, including lightning injury (ABA, 2018)

Electrical Burns

Electrical burns, including lightning strikes, are considered emergent and meet the criteria for transfer to a burn center, so EMS should be activated. The entrance and exit wounds should be located and cleansed with normal saline or sterile water and a light gauze dressing applied. Even though the tissue wounds may appear to be superficial, deep tissue injury should be suspected (ABA, 2018). The individual should be closely monitored until the arrival of EMS because of the risk of a cardiac arrhythmia (ABA, 2018).

Radiation Burns

The initial care for radiation burns (other than sunburn) should be the same as chemical burns with the caveat that the responder take appropriate precautions not to become the next victim from exposure (ABA, 2018).

HEAT-RELATED AND COLD-RELATED ILLNESS AND INJURY

Outside school activities or poor climate-controlled school environments in extreme weather conditions can be unsafe for students. The pace of climate change is increasing the frequency and duration of severe and prolonged hot weather. Heat-related illness (hyperthermia) and cold-related illness (hypothermia) can be prevented. School districts should implement clear policies and parameters for safe student activity and proper clothing in extreme temperatures based on the National Weather Service's heat index and wind chill charts (National Weather Service, n.d.a.; n.d.b.).

Hyperthermia

The *heat index* is defined as "what the temperature feels like to the human body when relative humidity is combined with the air temperature" (National Weather Service, n.d.a., para. 1). The body's response to heat is perspiration, which cools the body when sweat evaporates from the skin. High humidity decreases the body's ability to cool by decreasing the evaporation rate of sweat. The heat index chart displays the likelihood of heat disorders ranging across a continuum from caution to extreme danger.

Students may be exposed to extreme heat at school, increasing the risk of heat cramps, heat exhaustion, and heat stroke. Many school buildings lack air conditioning. The surface of playgrounds, tennis courts, and artificial turf playing fields can increase the environmental temperature. Many intense interscholastic and extracurricular sports are played under conditions that could potentially result in hyperthermia. For example, practicing football in full uniform and helmets in high heat can increase body temperature significantly. Athletes who do not take precautions to cool off and maintain adequate place are at risk for heat-related illness. School nurses, coaches, and athletic trainers must educate students about the signs and symptoms of heat-related illness. Coaches must also monitor students/athletes and provide additional breaks when the heat index rises.

Heat stroke is a medical emergency that can cause the body temperature to rise rapidly (10 to 15 minutes), potentially up 106°F or higher. Heat stroke is "when the body can no longer control its temperature: the body's temperature rises rapidly, the sweating mechanism fails, and the body is unable to cool down" (National Institute for Occupational Safety and Health [NIOSH], 2022, para.1). Extreme hyperthermia can cause permanent disability or death if not treated immediately in an acute care setting.

Heat exhaustion may result from dehydration associated with excessive sweating (NIOSH, 2022). *Heat cramps* can result from dehydration and low sodium levels in the muscles. Heat cramps are very painful and may also be a symptom of heat exhaustion. *Heat syncope* is an episode of fainting or dizziness in hot conditions associated with standing too long or standing up quickly after sitting or lying down for a prolonged period. See Table 17-5 for more information signs and symptoms and treatment of heat-related illnesses.

Hypothermia

Extremely cold temperatures can also be dangerous to students when the body loses heat faster than it can be generated. *Hypothermia* is a medical emergency (NIOSH, 2018b). Low body temperature will affect the brain's ability to think clearly. Early signs of hypothermia include shivering, fatigue, loss of coordination, confusion, and

TABLE 17-5 Heat-Related Illness

Heat-Related Illness	Signs & Symptoms	Interventions
Heat Stroke	• High body temperature (>103°F) • Hot, red, dry, or damp skin; or profuse sweating • Fast, strong pulse • Headache • Dizziness • Nausea • Altered mental status (confusion, disorientation, slurred speech) • Loss of consciousness • Seizures	• Heat stroke is a medical emergency: Activate EMS • Move the person to a shaded cool place • Apply wet cloths to the head, neck, armpits, or groin. Soak clothing in cool water • Do not give the person anything to drink
Heat Exhaustion	• Heavy sweating • Moderately elevated body temperature • Cold, pale, and clammy skin • Fast, weak pulse • Muscle cramps • Weakness or dizziness • Headache • Nausea/vomiting • Decreased/concentrated urine output	• Move to a shaded cool place • Loosen or remove unnecessary clothes • Apply cool, wet cloths • Sip cool water *Seek immediate medical attention if:* • Vomiting • Symptoms worsen • Symptoms last >1 hour
Heat Syncope	• Dizziness, tunnel vision • Brief fainting episode • Palor • Decreased heart rate	• Move to a shaded cool place • Apply cool, wet cloths • Encourage hydration
Heat Cramps	• Heavy sweating during intense exercise • Muscle pain or spasms	• Stop physical activity and move to a cool place • Encourage rehydration with cool water or a diluted electrolyte replacement drink if allowed by school protocol • Wait for cramps to go away before resuming physical activity *Seek immediate medical attention if:* • Cramps last ≥1 hour • History of other significant medical problems

Adapted from NIOSH (2022); IEMSC & OSF HCHI (2022); CDC (2024).

disorientation. Late symptoms of hypothermia include lack of shivering, blue skin, dilated pupils, slowed pulse and breathing, and loss of consciousness.

Immediate interventions include moving the person to a warm environment; removing wet clothing; and applying loose, dry layers of blankets (NIOSH, 2018b). If the person is alert, warm beverages can be given. If frostbite is suspected, the affected area will lose feeling and color due to decreased blood circulation. Until emergency personnel arrive, frostbitten parts should be immersed in warm (not hot) water. If possible, prevent the person from walking on frostbitten feet to avoid further tissue damage (NIOSH, 2018b). Do not rub or massage affected areas. During extremely cold weather, schools should ensure that students have appropriate winter clothing and limit outdoor exposure.

CONCLUSION

Preparing for health emergencies must be a priority for every school nurse every day. School nurses are often the first person to identify and respond to health emergencies at school. Whether the school nurse is on-site or available remotely, the school nurse serves as a leader on the school's emergency response team responsible for training others to quickly and effectively help an acutely ill/injured student, staff member, or school visitor. School emergency planning also involves emergency prevention.

Evaluation of current protocols and procedures and debriefing after an emergency event focuses efforts to improve the school's emergency response as a quality improvement imperative. Should protocols or guidelines be developed or changed to manage a situation like this in the future? Did the emergency plan work? Was the emergency quickly identified? Was the scene safe? Was help requested in a timely manner? Were the injuries identified? Was appropriate first-aid provided? Would it have been helpful to have had a particular piece of equipment? Was any information needed by the healthcare provider not available? Does the healthcare provider have any suggestions to improve emergency response? When school nurses are prepared for health emergencies at school, students, families, teachers, and the school community feel safer. School nurse emergency preparedness saves lives.

The Editors gratefully acknowledge the work of the previous chapter authors, Mariann F. Cosby, Evelyn Lyons, and Laura Prestidge.

References

ACLS Algorithms. (2022). *Pediatric advanced life support: Respiratory distress/failure/upper airway obstruction.* https://acls-algorithms.com/pediatric-advanced-life-support/respiratory-distress-failure/upper-airway-obstruction/

Adimando, A. (2024). Physical examination of children and adolescents in a school setting. In C. A. Resha & V. L Taliaferro (Eds.). *Legal resource for school health services* (2nd ed., pp. 377–385). SchoolNurse.com

American Academy of Allergy, Asthma & Immunology. (2020, September 28). *Stinging insect allergy.* https://www.aaaai.org/Tools-for-the-Public/Conditions-Library/Allergies/stinging-insect-allergy

American Academy of Pediatrics. (2019). *Allergy and anaphylaxis emergency plan.* https://downloads.aap.org/AAP/PDF/AAP_Allergy_and_Anaphylaxis_Emergency_Plan.pdf

American Academy of Pediatrics. (2021, January). *Anaphylaxis.* https://publications.aap.org/patiented/article-abstract/doi/10.1542/peo_document203/80176/Anaphylaxis?searchresult=1%3Fautologincheck

American Burn Association. (2018). *Advanced burn life support course: Provider manual 2018 update.* https://ameriburn.org/wp-content/uploads/2019/08/2018-abls-providermanual.pdf

American Heart Association. (2016a). *Cardiac emergency response planning for schools: A policy statement.* https://cpr.heart.org/-/media/CPR-Files/Training-Programs/Nation-of-Heartsavers/CERP/CERP-for-Schools-A-Policy-Statement.pdf

American Heart Association. (2020a). *Pediatric advanced life support (PALS) provider manual.* American Heart Association.

American Heart Association. (2020b). *Basic life support (BLS) provider manual.* American Heart Association.

American Heart Association. (2022a). *Cardiac emergency response plan.* https://cpr.heart.org/en/training-programs/cardiac-emergency-response-plan-cerp

American Heart Association. (2022b). *CPR in schools legislation map.* https://cpr.heart.org/en/training-programs/community-programs/cpr-in-schools/cpr-in-schools-legislation-map

American Heart Association. (2022c). *Syncope (Fainting).* https://www.heart.org/en/health-topics/arrhythmia/symptoms-diagnosis-monitoring-of-arrhythmia/syncope-fainting

American Lung Association. (2020, November 17). *Lung health & diseases.* https://www.lung.org/lung-health-diseases

Avive. (2023). *AED school law: A 2022 update.* https://avive.life/industry-guides/aed-school/aed-school-law/

Barret, J., & Brusch, J. L. (2021, March 4). Human bites treatment and management. *Medscape.* https://emedicine.medscape.com/article/218901-treatment

Baxter, C. S. (2020). Renal and genitourinary emergencies. In V. Sweet & A. Foley (Eds.), *Sheehy's emergency nursing: Principles and practice* (7th ed., pp 271–279). Elsevier.

Bidigare, C. (2023). Burns. In M. Harding, J. Kwong, D. Hagler, & C. Reinisch (Eds.), *Lewis's medical-surgical nursing: Assessment and management of clinical problems* (12th ed., pp. 494–511). Elsevier.

Blom, L., Peterson, P., Hagell, P., & Westergren, A. (2015). The situation, background, assessment, and recommendation (SBAR) model for communication between health care professionals: A clinical intervention pilot study. *International Journal of Caring Sciences* 8(3), 530–535. http://www.internationaljournalofcaringsciences.org/docs/2_2-Bloom_original_8_3.pdf

Brown, S., & Turner, P. (2017). Anaphylaxis. In D. Leung, S. Szefler, F. Bonilla, C. Akdis, & H. Sampson (Eds.). *Pediatric allergy: Principles and practice* (pp. 345–360). Elsevier.

Centers for Disease Control and Prevention. (2017). *Assessment: Measuring orthostatic blood pressure.* https://www.cdc.gov/steadi/pdf/Measuring_Orthostatic_Blood_Pressure-print.pdf

Centers for Disease Control and Prevention. (2019a). *CDC HEADS UP: A fact sheet for school nurses.* https://www.cdc.gov/headsup/pdfs/schools/TBI_factsheet_NURSE-508-a.pdf

Centers for Disease Control and Prevention. (2019b, February 12). *CDC HEADS UP: Safer brain. Stronger future.* https://www.cdc.gov/headsup/index.html

Centers for Disease Control and Prevention. (2019c, August). *Concussion signs and symptoms checklist.* https://www.cdc.gov/headsup/pdfs/schools/TBI_schools_checklist_508-a.pdf

Centers for Disease Control and Prevention. (2021a, July 15). *Bacterial meningitis.* Centers for Disease Control and Prevention. https://www.cdc.gov/meningitis/bacterial.html

Centers for Disease Control and Prevention. (2021b, November 3). *Tick bite: What to do.* https://www.cdc.gov/ticks/pdfs/FS_TickBite.pdf

Centers for Disease Control and Prevention. (2021c, May 25). *Viral meningitis.* https://www.cdc.gov/meningitis/viral.html

Centers for Disease Control and Prevention. (2022a). *Healthy schools.* https://www.cdc.gov/chronicdisease/resources/publications/factsheets/healthy-schools.htm

Centers for Disease Control and Prevention. (2022b). Lightning strike victim data. https://www.cdc.gov/disasters/lightning/victimdata.html

Centers for Disease Control and Prevention. (2022c, December 8). *Rabies.* Centers for Disease Control and Prevention. https://www.cdc.gov/rabies/index.html

Centers for Disease Control and Prevention. (2022d). *TBI data.* https://www.cdc.gov/traumaticbraininjury/data/index.html

Centers for Disease Control and Prevention. (2022e). *What is sickle cell disease?* https://www.cdc.gov/ncbddd/sicklecell/facts.html#:~:text=HbSS,severe%20form%20of%20the%20disease

Centers for Disease Control and Prevention. (2022f). Web-based injury statistics query and reporting system [online]. https://www.cdc.gov/injury/wisqars/nonfatal.html

Centers for Disease Control and Prevention. (2023, November 20). *Meningococcal vaccination.* https://www.cdc.gov/vaccines/vpd/mening/index.html

Centers for Disease Control and Prevention. (2024, February). *Symptoms of heat-related illness.* https://www.cdc.gov/extreme-heat/signs-symptoms/index.html

Children's Hospital of Philadelphia. (2022). *Acute spinal injury in children.* https://www.chop.edu/conditions-diseases/acute-spinal-cord-injury-children

Cleveland Clinic. (2020, January 24). *Respiratory system: Functions, facts, organs & anatomy.* https://my.clevelandclinic.org/health/articles/21205-respiratory-system

Cosby, M. F. (2023). Emergency nursing practice: Traditional and non-traditional settings and organizations. In P.W. Iyer (Ed.), *Medical record analysis: A guide for attorneys by LNCs* (pp. 11–18). The Pat Iyer Group.

Cosby, M. F. (2024). Life threatening emergencies: Anaphylaxis, asthma, and allergies. In C. A. Resha & V. L. Taliaferro (Eds.), *Legal resource for school health services* (2nd ed., pp. 413–427). SchoolNurse.com

Costello, K. J. (2023). Nervous system. In M. Harding, J. Kwong, D. Hagler, & C. Reinisch (Eds.), *Lewis's medical-surgical nursing: Assessment and management of clinical problems* (12th ed., pp. 1460–1463). Elsevier.

Cramer, N., Jabbour, N., Tavarez, M. M., & Taylor, R. S. (2022, August 1). *Foreign body aspiration.* https://www.ncbi.nlm.nih.gov/books/NBK531480/

Daley, J. B. (2022, May 9). *Pneumothorax clinical presentation.* History, physical examination. https://emedicine.medscape.com/article/424547-clinical#b3

Davis, G. A., Schneider, K. J., Anderson, V., Babl, F. E., Barlow, K. M., Blauwet, C. A., Bressnan, S., Broglio, S. P., Emery, C. A., Echemendia, R. J., Gagnon, I., Gioia, G. A., Giza, C. C., Leddy, J. J., Master, C. L., McCrea, M., McNamee, M. J., Meehan, W. P., ... Patricios, J. S. (2024). Pediatric sport-related concussion: Recommendations from the Amsterdam Consensus Statement 2023. *Pediatrics, 153*(1), e2023063489. https://doi.org/10.1542/peds.2023-063489

Davis, W. D. (2024a). Chest trauma. In A. Foley (Ed.), *Sheehy's manual of emergency care* (8th ed., pp.149–161). Elsevier.

Davis, W. D. (2024b). Musculoskeletal trauma. In A. Foley (Ed.), *Sheehy's manual of emergency care* (8th ed., pp.289–301). Elsevier.

Delaney, A., Baker, A. L., Bastardi, H., & O'Brien, P. (2017). The child with cardiovascular dysfunction. In M. J. Hockenberry, D. Wilson, & C. C. Rodgers (Eds.), *Wong's essentials of pediatric nursing* (10th ed., pp. 783–785). Mosby Elsevier.

Dymond, M. M. (2023a). The child with abdominal pain. In *Emergency Nurses Association: Emergency nursing pediatric course: Provider manual* (6th ed., pp.173–192). Jones & Bartlett Learning.

Dymond, M. M. (2023b). The child with vomiting. In *Emergency Nurses Association: Emergency nursing pediatric course: Provider manual* (6th ed., pp.157–172). Jones & Bartlett Learning.

Emergency Nurses Association. (2019). *Pediatric febrile seizure infographic.* https://enau.ena.org/Users/LearningActivity/LearningActivityDetail.aspx?LearningActivityID=fHMzWNzEmXzcWqhK9n7zKQ%3D%3D

Epilepsy Foundation. (2022). *Seizure training for school nurses: Using rescue therapies in epilepsy care—v2.0.* https://learn.epilepsy.com/courses/school-nurse-rescue-therapies-OD-v2

Epilepsy Foundation. (2023a). *Seizure rescue medications.* https://www.epilepsy.com/recognition/rescue-medications#:~:text=In%20the%20United%20States%2C%20nasal,acute%20repetitive%20seizures%20or%20clusters

Epilepsy Foundation. (2023b). *Understanding epilepsy.* https://www.epilepsy.com/

Erdman, M. O., Chardavoyne, P., & Olympia, R. P. (2019). School nurses on the front lines of medicine: The approach to a student with severe traumatic bleeding. *NASN School Nurse, 34*(5), 280–286. http://doi.org/10.1177/1942602X19837525

Erickson, C. C., & Salerno, J. C. (2021, June 21). *Policy: Incorporate cardiac risk screening for all youths at least every three years.* AAP News. https://publications.aap.org/aapnews/news/16505/Policy-Incorporate-cardiac-risk-screening-for-all?autologincheck=redirected

Erickson, C. C., Salerno, J. C., Berber, S., Campbell, R., Cannon, B., Christiansen, J., Moffatt, K., Pflaumer, A., Synder, C. S., Srinivasan, C., Valdes, S. O., Vetter, V. L., Zimmerman, F., & Section on Cardiology and Cardiac Surgery, Pediatric and Congenital Electrophysiology Society Task Force on Prevention of Sudden Death in the Young. (2021). Sudden death in the young: Information for the primary care provider. [Policy Statement, American Academy of Pediatrics.] *Pediatrics, 148*(1), e2021052044. https://doi.org/10.1542/peds.2021-052044

Ernst, G. (2020). Pediatric trauma. In J. E. Tintinalli , O. J. Ma, D. M. Yearly, G. D. Meckler, J. S. Stapczynski, D. M. Cline, & S. H. Thomas (Eds.), *Tintinalli's emergency medicine: A comprehensive study guide* (9th ed., pp. 789–797). McGraw Hill.

Foley, A. (2024a). Head, neck, and vertebral column trauma. In A. Foley (Ed.), *Sheehy's manual of emergency care* (8th ed., pp.189–206). Elsevier.

Foley, A. (2024b). Neurologic emergencies. In A. Foley (Ed.), *Sheehy's manual of emergency care* (8th ed., pp.173–188). Elsevier.Forum on Child and Family Statistics. (2021). *Adolescent injury and mortality.* https://www.childstats.gov/americaschildren21/phys8.asp

Gereige, R., Gross, T., & Jastaniah, E. (2022). Individual medical emergencies occurring at school. *Pediatrics, 150*(1), 1–16. https://doi.org/10.1542/peds.2022-057987

Giordano, D. (2023). The child in need of stabilization. In *Emergency Nurses Association: Emergency nursing pediatric course: Provider manual* (6th ed., pp. 94–115). Jones & Bartlett Learning.

Herrington, A. (2020). Gastrointestinal emergencies. In V. Sweet & A. Foley (Eds.), *Sheehy's emergency nursing: Principles and practice* (7th ed., pp. 260–270). Elsevier.

Hudgins, J. D., Porter, J. J., Monuteaux, M. C., & Bourgeois, F. T. (2019, November 5). Prescription opioid use and misuse among adolescents and young adults in the United States: A national survey study. *PLOS Medicine.* https://journals.plos.org/plosmedicine/article?id=10.1371%2Fjournal.pmed.1002922

Illinois Emergency Medical Services for Children & OSF HealthCare Children's Hospital of Illinois. (2022). *Guidelines for the nurse in the school setting* (4th ed.). https://www.osfhealthcare.org/media/filer_public/94/9a/949ae3b2-8927-416c-b009-a53ed47c4cc0/school_nurse_guidelines_osf_202forthosenotregistered.pdf

Institute for Healthcare Improvement. (2017). *SBAR tool: Situation-background-assessment-recommendation.* http://www.ihi.org/resources/Pages/Tools/SBARTechniqueforCommunicationASituationalBriefingModel.aspx

Jamerson, L. (2023). Initial assessment. In *Emergency Nurses Association: Emergency nursing pediatric course: Provider manual* (6th ed., pp. 69–82). Jones & Bartlett Learning.

Lawson, S., Hogg, M. M., Moore, C. A., Anderson, W. E., Osipoff, P. S., Runyon, M. S., & Reynolds, S. L. (2021, December). Pediatric pain assessment in the emergency department: Patient and caregiver agreement using the Wong-Baker FACES and the Faces Pain Scale–Revised. *Pediatric Emergency Care, 37*(12), e950–e954. http://doi.org/10.1097/PEC.0000000000001837

Logee, K. (2020). Pediatric emergencies. In V. Sweet & A. Foley (Eds.), *Sheehy's emergency nursing: Principles and practice* (7th ed., pp 556–575). Elsevier.

MacKeil-White, K. (2023a). Pediatric differences. In *Emergency Nurses Association: Emergency nursing pediatric course: Provider manual* (6th ed., pp. 29–46). Jones & Bartlett Learning

MacKeil-White, K. (2023b). The child with special healthcare needs. In *Emergency Nurses Association: Emergency nursing pediatric course: Provider manual* (6th ed., pp. 279–288). Jones & Bartlett Learning.

Matesanz, S., & Giovine, M. (2020, March 6). *Seizure first aid for children.* HealthyChildren.org. https://www.healthychildren.org/English/health-issues/conditions/seizures/Pages/Seizure-First-Aid-for-Children.aspx#%3a~%3atext=Lower%20the%20child%20to%20the%2c child%20still%20during%20the%20seizure

May, L., & Menon, S. (2021). *Sudden cardiac arrest in young people.* https://www.healthychildren.org/English/health-issues/injuries-emergencies/sports-injuries/Pages/Sudden-Cardiac-Death.aspx

Mayo Clinic. (2021, May 21). *Pneumothorax.* https://www.mayoclinic.org/diseases-conditions/pneumothorax/symptoms-causes/syc-20350367

Mayo Clinic. (2022). *Drugs and supplements: Epinephrine (injection route).* https://www.mayoclinic.org/drugs-supplements/epinephrine-injection-route/proper-use/drg20072429#:~:text=Push%20the%20needle%20end%20(orange,of%203%20seconds%20following%20activation

Mayo Clinic. (2023). *Asthma symptoms and causes.* https://www.mayoclinic.org/diseases-conditions/asthma/symptoms-causes/syc-20369653Merriam-Webster Dictionary. (n.d.). *Emergency.* https://www.merriam-webster.com/dictionary/emergency

Miley, H. (2023). Shock. In M. Harding, J. Kwong, D. Hagler, & C. Reinisch (Eds.), *Lewis's medical-surgical nursing: Assessment and management of clinical problems* (12th ed., pp. 961–985). Elsevier Inc.

Milici, J. J. (2024a). Respiratory emergencies. In A. Foley (Ed.), *Sheehy's manual of emergency care* (8th ed., pp.105–127). Elsevier.

Milici, J. J. (2024b). Shock emergencies. In A. Foley (Ed.), *Sheehy's manual of emergency care* (8th ed., pp.163–172). Elsevier.

Miller, S. (2023). The child with an injury. In *Emergency Nurses Association: Emergency nursing pediatric course: Provider manual* (6th ed., pp.129–145). Jones & Bartlett Learning.

National Association of School Nurses. (2021). Concussions: School based management [Position Statement]. https://www.nasn.org/nasn-resources/professional-practice-documents/position-statements/ps-concussions

National Association of School Nurses. (2022). *Framework for 21st century school nursing practice.* https://www.nasn.org/nasn-resources/framework

National Association of School Nurses. (2023a, September 9). *Naloxone education for school nurses toolkit.* https://learn.nasn.org/courses/58011#

National Association of School Nurses. (2023b). *School nursing evidence-based clinical guideline: Students with seizures and epilepsy.* https://learn.nasn.org/courses/63321#

National Institute for Occupational Safety and Health. (2018a). *Scorpions.* Centers for Disease Control and Prevention. https://www.cdc.gov/niosh/topics/insects/scorpions.html

National Institute for Occupational Safety and Health. (2018b). *Types of cold-related illness.* Centers for Disease Control and Prevention.

National Institute for Occupational Safety and Health. (2018c). *Venomous spiders.* Centers for Disease Control and Prevention. https://www.cdc.gov/niosh/topics/spiders/symptoms.html

National Institute for Occupational Safety and Health. (2021a, June 28). *Types of venomous snakes.* Centers for Disease Control and Prevention. https://www.cdc.gov/niosh/topics/snakes/types.html

National Institute for Occupational Safety and Health. (2021b, June 28). *Venomous snake bites: Symptoms & first aid.* https://www.cdc.gov/niosh/topics/snakes/symptoms.html

National Institute for Occupational Safety and Health. (2022). *Heat stress-Heat related illness: Types of heat-related illness.* https://www.cdc.gov/niosh/topics/heatstress/heatrelillness.html#:~:text=Heat%20stroke%20is%20the%20most,is%20unable%20to%20cool%20do

National Institute of Arthritis and Musculoskeletal and Skin Diseases. (2022, May 18). *Growth plate injuries.* U.S. Department of Health and Human Services. https://www.niams.nih.gov/health-topics/growth-plate-injuries

National Institute of Neurological Disorders and Stroke. (2023). *Spinal cord injury.* https://www.ninds.nih.gov/health-information/disorders/spinal-cord-injury

National Operating Committee on Standards for Athletic Equipment. (2021). *Performance standard to protect against commotio cordis.* https://nocsae.org/wp-content/uploads/2021/10/NOCSAE_Performance-Standard-to-Protect-Against-Commotio-Cordis-Fact-Sheet_October-11-2021.pdf

National Weather Service. (n.d.a.). *Understanding wind chill.* https://www.weather.gov/safety/cold-wind-chill-chart

National Weather Service. (n.d.b.). *What is the heat index?* https://www.weather.gov/ama/heatindex

Nolan-Kelley, L. (2020). Ocular emergencies. In V. Sweet & A. Foley (Eds.), *Sheehy's emergency nursing: Principles and practice* (7th ed., pp. 365–376). Elsevier.

Panchal, N. (2022). The impact of gun violence on children and adolescents. https://www.kff.org/other/issue-brief/the-impact-of-gun-violence-on-children-and-adolescents/#:~:text=From%202019%20to%202021%2C%20the,dying%20by%20firearm%20in%202021

Parsh, B., & Jeffries, D. (2022). Abdominal emergencies. In D. Jeffries & L. S. Visser (Eds.), *Rapid access guide for pediatric emergencies: Providing expert nursing care* (pp. 115–131). Springer Publishing.

Poison Control. (2020). *Poison statistics.* National Poison Control Center. https://www.poison.org/poison-statistics-national

Poison Control. (2024). *Get help online or by phone.* National Poison Control Center. https://www.poison.org/

Powers-Jarvis, R. (2023). Prioritization. In *Emergency Nurses Association: Emergency nursing pediatric course: Provider manual* (6th ed., pp 47–68). Jones & Bartlett Learning.

Reichert, G., & Foley, A. (2024). Pediatric emergency and trauma considerations. In A. Foley (Ed.), *Sheehy's manual of emergency care* (8th ed., pp. 453–475). Elsevier.

Rose, K., Martin Goble, M., Berger, S., Courson, R., Fosse, G., Gillary, R., Halowich, J., Indik, J., Konig, M., Lopez-Anderson, M., Murphy, M., Newman, M., Ranous, J., Sasson, C., Taras, H., & Thompson, A. (2016). Cardiac emergency response planning for schools: A policy statement. *NASN School Nurse, 31*(5), 263–270. https://doi.org/10.1177/1942602X16655839

SafeHome.org. (2022). 2021 school injury report. https://www.safehome.org/family-safety/school-injury-report/

Schoessler, S., & White, M. (2013). Recognition and treatment of anaphylaxis in the school setting: The essential role of the school nurse. *Journal of School Nursing, 29*(6), 407–415. https://doi.org/10.1177/1059840513506014

Shaker, M. S., Wallace, D. V., Golden, D. B., Oppenheimer, J., Bernstein, J. A., Campbell, R. L., Dinakar, C., Ellis, A., Greenhawt, M., Khan, D. A., Lang, D. M., Lang, E. S., Lieberman, J. A., Portnoy, J., Rank, M. A., Stukus, D. R., & Wang, J. (2020). Anaphylaxis—a 2020 practice parameter update, systematic review, and grading of recommendations, assessment, development and evaluation (GRADE) analysis. *Journal of Allergy and Clinical Immunology, 145*(4), 1082–1122. https://doi.org/10.1016/j.jaci.2020.01.017

Sharma, M. (2022). Treating, repairing the body's electrical system. https://www.mayoclinichealthsystem.org/hometown-health/speaking-of-health/treating-repairing-nervous-system

Sherrid, M. V., Aagaard, P., Serrato, S., Arajadjian, M. E., Lium, J. M., Lium, J. D., & Greenberg, H. M. (2017). State requirements for automated external defibrillators in American schools: Framing the debate about legislative action. *Journal of the American College of Cardiology, 69*(13), 1735–1743. https://doi: 10.1016/j.jacc.2017.01.033

Sicherer, S., & Simons, F. E. (2017). Epinephrine for first-aid management of anaphylaxis. *Pediatrics, 139*(3), e1–e9. https://doi.org/10.1542/peds.2016-4006

Simons, F. E. (2016). Anaphylaxis: Assessment and management. In D. Leung, S. Szefler, & F. Bonilla (Eds.). *Pediatric allergy: Principles and practice* (pp. 524–536). Elsevier.

Sweeney, A. (2023). The child with a cough. In *Emergency Nurses Association: Emergency nursing pediatric course: Provider manual* (6th ed., pp. 117–128). Jones & Bartlett Learning.

Sweet, V. (2020). Patient assessment. In V. Sweet & A. Foley (Eds.), *Sheehy's emergency nursing: Principles and practice* (7th ed., pp. 68–74). Elsevier.

U.S. Department of Homeland Security. (2022). *Stop the Bleed campaign.* https://www.dhs.gov/stopthebleed

U.S. Drug Enforcement Administration. (2022). *Drug fact sheet: Fentanyl.* U.S. Department of Justice. https://www.dea.gov/sites/default/files/2023-06/Fentanyl%202022%20Drug%20Fact%20Sheet-update.pdf

Volerman, A., Lowe, A. A., Pappalardo, A. A., Anderson, C. M. C., Blake, K. V., Bryant-Stephens, T., Carr, T., Carter, H., Cicutto, L., Gerald, J. K., Miller, T., Moore, N. S., Phan, H., Sadreameli, S. C., Tanner, A., Winders, T. A., & Gerald, L. B. (2021, September 1). Ensuring access to albuterol in schools: From policy to implementation: An official ATS/AANMA/ALA/NASN policy statement. *American Journal of Respiratory and Critical Care Medicine, 204*(5), 508–522. https://www.ncbi.nlm.nih.gov/pmc/articles/PMC8491259/

Waunch, A., & Zaky, K. (2020). Pediatric trauma. In V. Sweet & A. Foley (Eds.), *Sheehy's emergency nursing: Principles and practice* (7th ed., pp. 517–536). Elsevier.

Winter, J. L. (2020). Dental, ear, nose, throat, and facial emergencies. In V. Sweet & A. Foley (Eds.), *Sheehy's emergency nursing: Principles and practice* (7th ed., pp. 353–364). Elsevier.

Zirkel, P. A. (2019). Physical exams: Legal liability (versus professional norms). *NASN School Nurse, 34*(5), 270–273. http://doi.org/10.1177/1942602X19846641

Chapter 18

Students With Skin Conditions

Sarah Hallowell ▪ Melinda Jen

CHAPTER OUTLINE

The skin is the largest organ of the body (McCann et al., 2017). Skin conditions can cause alarm among teachers and peers, and cause embarrassment, stress, and concern for students and their families. The school nurse is in an ideal position to provide an accurate assessment of these problems and suggest treatment, referral, or exclusion from school when indicated. This chapter addresses the most common skin disorders seen in school-age children, including assessment, management, and relevant education for students and staff.

ASSESSMENT

Health History

The school nurse is often the first person who receives a report from a teacher, parent, or student regarding a dermatological concern. An organized approach to the evaluation of a rash or other skin finding simplifies the process of discerning potential causes.

A thorough and detailed history is the most important tool when assessing a skin finding. An accurate history can help the school nurse identify the problem for many presenting skin conditions. However, it may be challenging to obtain an accurate or complete history of the issue from students who are young or who have developmental delays; adult caregivers may need to be consulted. The first set of questions should relate to **onset and duration** of the skin finding.

- When did the presenting dermatological symptom start?
- Does it come and go, or has it persisted since the onset?
- Are any new lesions still forming?

The next questions relate to **location and distribution** of the lesions.

- What is the location of the current skin issue?
- Is there only one lesion or are there several lesions?
- Are the lesions isolated to one area of the body or more than one area of the body?
- Did the lesion begin in one spot or as one lesion, and has it spread to other areas?

The school nurse must next determine **characteristics** of the skin problem.

- Does the lesion itch, burn, or hurt?
- Has there been any bleeding or weeping from the lesion?

An **exposure history** is important to identify contact with any infected individuals, poisonous plants, or animals. Even gardening or visiting parks may place children at risk.

- Has there been potential exposure to poison ivy, insecticides, cleaning agents, or chemicals?
- What skin cleansers, makeup, and other skin products have been used recently?
- Has there been sun exposure or use of tanning booths? These may exacerbate skin lesions or cause photosensitive rashes.

Additional questions include **allergies** the child may have, any past history of dermatological conditions, and if anyone else at home has similar symptoms. Last, **alleviating and aggravating factors** need to be identified.

- What makes the skin condition worse and what makes it better?
- What treatments (including home remedies) have been used for the current skin condition?
- What over-the-counter, prescription (topical, oral, or injectable), and recreational medications does the student take?
- Are other symptoms present, such as fever, chills, or night sweats, that might indicate a systemic problem?

A helpful mnemonic for the school nurse to remember the components of a history is **OLDCARTS:** *Onset, Location, Duration, Characteristics, Aggravating factors, Relieving fractors, Time duration,* and *Severity.* Although this mnemonic does not entirely encompass how to obtain a thorough history, it may be helpful in time-sensitive situations (Buckley, 2021).

Physical Examination

A thorough physical assessment of the skin condition is the next step for the school nurse. School nurses should be familiar with their state guidelines and school's policy on the extent to which a school nurse is able to physically evaluate a student in the school setting. Gloves are indicated if you need to touch the student to view the lesion and perform the assessment, especially if bodily fluids present (Buckley, 2021).

Basic knowledge of primary and secondary lesions is necessary to determine whether the parent needs to be called, the student needs to be referred for follow-up, or if the student can return to class. Primary skin lesions appear at the onset of a disease (e.g., papule, nodule, or pustule), whereas secondary lesions result from disease progression, treatment, or manipulation of the lesion, such as picking or rubbing (Bland, 2020). To aid in the assessment, the school nurse should be able to describe the skin lesions. See Tables 18-1 and 18-2 for descriptions of commonly seen primary and secondary lesions. Since the school nurse may be the first-line healthcare provider, their description of skin findings is crucial when communicating with primary care or other healthcare providers. Additional assessments include the following:

- Is the distribution of lesions linear or circular (annular)? Are the lesions scattered or clustered, confluent (run together) or discrete, or limited to certain exposure sites? Is the location of the lesion directly related to contact with creams, jewelry, clothing, or the sun, or are the lesions primarily in areas of higher body heat (e.g., underarms, groin)? Are the lesions present in primarily exposed areas (e.g., face, neck, hands), which may be a sign of sensitivity to something in the environment?
- What color are the lesions? Skin-colored and erythematous rashes can be differentiated from honey-colored crusts.
- Describe the margins and center of the lesions. Are the borders well-demarcated or ill-defined? Are the colors different between the edges of the lesion compared with its center? Does it resemble a bullseye or other shape? Are scales present? If so, are they centrally or peripherally located?

Practice Connection

Children with painful rashes (possibly due to a spider bite) or signs of an infection at the site of the lesion (e.g., erythema, swelling, warmth) need to be seen by a primary care provider within a few hours of the identification of the skin problem.

TABLE 18-1 Primary Skin Lesions

Primary Lesion	Description
Macule	Flat, smooth, <1 cm. Examples: vitiligo or café-au-lait spots
Papule	Raised, <1 cm. Examples: acne, wart, or molluscum
Patch	Flat, nonpalpable, >1 cm. Examples: dermal melanocyte, café-au-lait spots
Plaque	Raised, >1 cm. Examples: eczema, psoriasis
Vesicle	Elevated, fluid filled, <1 cm. Examples: varicella (chickenpox), herpes simplex
Bulla	Elevated, fluid filled, >1 cm in diameter. Example: friction blister
Pustule	Elevated, filled with pus
Nodule	Elevated and extending into the dermis, >1 cm. Examples: neurofibroma, epidermal inclusion cyst, lipoma
Wheal/hives	Transient, firm edematous, elevated. Example: urticaria

Sources: Adapted from Bolognia et al. (2017); McCann et al. (2017).

TABLE 18-2 Secondary Lesions

Secondary Lesions	Description
Scales	Dry flakes of skin, silvery or white in color. Examples: seborrheic dermatitis, tinea corporis, xerosis
Crust	Dried exudate comprised of blood or pus. Example: impetigo
Fissure	Linear crack, break in skin. Example: athlete's foot
Erosion	Partial epidermal loss. Example: impetigo
Ulcer	Deep concave depression, loss of epidermis and dermis, irregular shape. Example: pressure or stasis ulcer
Lichenification	Thickening of the skin with accentuation of the skin lines. Example: chronic eczema

Sources: Adapted from Bolognia et al. (2017); McCann et al. (2017).

Full body or truncal rashes can be due to viral illness and be delayed in their onset. For example, 5 to 12 days after receiving the measles vaccine a child may break out in a fine pink maculopapular rash. The rash is benign and the student is not contagious (Paller & Mancini, 2022). Large areas with a macular rash could also be due to an allergic reaction to medication, including antibiotics and nonsteroidal anti-inflammatory drugs. These types of rashes can occur immediately or up to 6 weeks after the medication is discontinued (Bland, 2020).

Primary lesions should be described as clearly as possible. Palpate the lesion for induration (firmness) or warmth. Other signs of illness should be assessed. Signs of allergy and anaphylaxis require careful assessment of the respiratory system. If wheezing or severe respiratory difficulty is present, activate emergency medical services (see Chapter 21 on allergies). Fever, lethargy, and general discomfort should result in a multisystem assessment and referral to the student's healthcare provider. Acute onset of a rash manifested as purpura (large reddish-purple or gunmetal-gray areas that do not blanch) or petechiae (tiny red dots that do not blanch) associated with fever and not related to injury or friction indicates that the student needs to be transferred to an acute care setting immediately to rule out meningococcemia or bleeding disorders (Blosser et al., 2017).

Following the assessment, the school nurse should determine whether the student may return to class or if the lesion needs further assessment by a healthcare provider. The assessment and disposition should be documented on the student's health record. Parents/guardians should be contacted to determine whether they are aware of the skin condition, if the student is under the care of a healthcare provider, and to collaborate on a plan of care going forward. If the nurse suspects that the condition is contagious, the student should not return to class until the condition has been diagnosed and documentation provided.

When assessing skin in students of color, the school nurse should be aware that subtle skin changes might present differently than in students with pale or white skin. Erythema and purpura may be missed in students with darker pigmented skin, because erythema and purpura can present as hyperpigmentation (Poladian et al., 2019). Cyanosis may also not be as readily apparent in students of color. However, post-inflammatory skin changes may be more visible and bothersome for students of color. Knowing that school absence rates are higher in students of color with atopic dermatitis, the school nurse should be attentive to all visual and palpable changes in a student's skin (Poladian et al., 2019).

PRURITUS AND BASIC SKIN INTERVENTIONS

Pruritus (itching) is a very common, unpleasant sensation associated with many skin conditions, as well as many systemic diseases, such as renal failure and thyroid disorders, or the use of opiate drugs (Nicol & Huether, 2017). Pruritus often leads to a scratching or rubbing response that can disrupt the skin's integrity, causing inflammation, infection, cracking, lichenification (thickening), and scarring. Common causes of pruritus include direct irritation by an offending substance (e.g., wool and mohair fibers), histamine release from allergy, and dry skin (xerosis). The lesions of many infectious conditions (e.g., scabies and varicella [chicken pox]) are also extremely pruritic.

The school nurse should ask the student and/or consult with the parent/guardian about contact irritants, recent travel, and the use of new medications, soaps, moisturizers, or other skin products. Cold, dry weather may cause skin to become dry and present as slightly scaly with variable erythema and superficial fissuring, most commonly on the extremities.

A goal in the treatment of pruritus is to decrease the student's discomfort and prevent scratching by keeping the skin hydrated and lubricated with a plain, thick emollient. Moisturizing twice daily with a thick moisturizing cream or ointment can help strengthen the skin barrier. Moisturizers with fragrance or many additive ingredients can irritate the skin (Bland, 2020). The school nurse should consult with the parent regarding what care is provided at home and what support can be provided at school. Topical medications require a medical order to be administered at school. If moisturizers are to be kept at school, they should be labeled with the student's name. To provide cooling effect, moisturizers can also be placed in a refrigerator.

For new-onset pruritus, generalized suggestions can be made to students and parents for home care. If the cause can be identified, the obvious solution is to avoid the cause. A mild soap without fragrance and dye can be used to remove the irritant from the skin, but soap use should be limited until the situation resolves. Warm water can be used for cleansing. However, taking hot showers lasting longer than 10 minutes should be avoided, because heat dilates vessels and can exacerbate pruritus. Loofahs and exfoliators can allow irritants to invade the skin barrier and should be avoided (Habif, 2019). The student should pat dry after showering and apply the recommended moisturizers immediately while the skin is still moist. In the school setting, the simplest first aid for pruritus is to apply cool compresses for 10 to 20 minutes every 3 to 4 hours. If these approaches do not alleviate the problem, the student should be referred for further medical evaluation and treatment. See Box 18-1 for generalized care of skin problems.

ACNE

Acne is one of the most prevalent skin disorders among school-age students, often corresponding with the onset of puberty and lasting through adolescence. Increased androgen production during puberty stimulates the oil glands in the body to make more sebum (oil). Sebaceous glands are primarily on the face, upper chest, and upper back, which correspond to the locations where acne is often located (Nicol & Huether, 2017). Acne can cause embarrassment and anxiety in affected individuals.

Did You Know?

Ointments are the most potent topical formulation, followed by creams, lotions, and gels. Moreover, ointments burn the least when applied to skin, followed by creams, lotions, and gels. Absorption is enhanced in areas that are traumatized or broken down (Bland, 2020).

BOX 18-1

Generalized Care of Skin Problems

- Apply an ice pack or cool compress to an area of intense itching.
- Place emollients or other topical medications in the refrigerator for a cooling effect.
- Ensure that nails are short.
- Suggest limiting baths to no more than once a day, and preferably lasting less than 10 minutes. Use lukewarm water rather than hot water.
- Suggest keeping use of soap to a minimum. Use a mild, perfume-free soap (most liquid soaps contain fragrance, which can be irritating to the skin).
- Pat dry after showering and apply thick emollient to moist skin.
- If a steroid cream has been recommended by the healthcare provider, it should be applied as directed. It is important to closely follow the prescribed duration of treatment to prevent side effects.
- Oral antihistamines may be used but may cause sedation. Topical antihistamines, particularly diphenhydramine HCl, should be avoided due to increased findings of contact sensitization.
- Do not use bubble baths, loofahs, or exfoliators as they can be irritating.

Sources: Bland (2020); McInerny et al. (2017); Paller & Mancini (2022).

Assessment

The severity of acne can vary; influences include genetics, menses, stress, and use of facial and hair products that can occlude pores (Nicol & Huether, 2017; Tan et al., 2018). Other aggravating factors include sweating and friction, such as wearing protective helmets. Acne is not caused by foods, such as chocolate, nuts, or fried food, or sexual activity.

The lesions of acne (pimples) can be inflammatory or noninflammatory. Noninflammatory lesions are smaller than 5 mm and are known as *comedones;* they include blackheads (open comedones) and whiteheads (closed comedones). Blackheads do not contain dirt; they are black from oxidization of the comedone contents (Tan et al., 2018). Whiteheads (or closed comedones) are the precursor to inflammatory acne. Inflammatory lesions are often larger than 5 mm. Inflammatory lesions include papules, pustules, nodules, or cysts and can result in scarring (Nicol & Huether, 2017).

Impacted sebum and cellular debris leads to sebaceous gland swelling (pimples), preventing the normal shedding of follicular keratinocytes, obstructing the follicle. When the comedone ruptures, it spills sebum into the surrounding dermis and initiates the inflammatory process, forming pustules and cysts (McCann et al., 2017). Some of the lesions may be painful if touched.

Management

The goals of managing acne are to decrease the excess sebum and prevent or decrease scarring. Acne can take an emotional toll on adolescents. The school nurse can provide support and education. However, it is common for teens to follow the advice of their peers or trends on social media rather than those of the healthcare provider. Basic instructions on managing acne include the following:

- Wash the face twice a day with mild soap or cleansers; discourage excessive scrubbing with a loofah or washcloth. Moisturize once or twice a day with oil-free, noncomedogenic facial moisturizer, and use a facial moisturizer with sun protection factor (SPF) in the morning.
- Avoid picking or squeezing pimples; this can lead to skin damage and the spread of any infection. Picking or popping acne lesions also greatly increases the risk of scarring.
- Makeup used should be noncomedogenic (does not clog the pores); hair and face products should be oil-free and water-based. Makeup should be washed off the face every night.

- Identify aggravating factors, such as stress, menses, and activities (e.g., sports). The skin should be washed as soon as sweaty activity concludes. The longer the sweat remains on the skin, the more likely new acne will develop.

Acne treatment takes 2 to 3 months for improvement, so consistent skin care routines are critical to achieving desired outcomes. Many topical medications are available. Benzoyl peroxide is a safe, inexpensive agent effective against mild acne and is available over the counter as either a wash or topical gel. It is antibacterial but can cause dryness by decreasing free fatty acids, resulting in desquamation and peeling (Habif, 2019). Benzoyl peroxide is applied in a thin layer over the entire affected area; it is a bleaching agent and can stain clothing. If benzoyl peroxide is used within 30 minutes of tretinoin, these products inactivate each other.

Topical antibiotics (e.g., clindamycin or erythromycin) are effective in some acne cases. Topical antibiotics should always be combined with a second antimicrobial product, such as benzoyl peroxide, to prevent bacterial resistance to the antibiotic. Prescription products that combine benzoyl peroxide and topical antibiotics are available. If a student presents with acne that has a distribution particularly concentrated on the jawline, they may respond to a topical or oral preparation that can address the hormonal component of acne, such as oral contraceptives or spironolactone. For inflammatory or cystic acne, a student may be placed on oral antibiotics, such as doxycycline, for up to 6 months. Oral antibiotics can cause increased sun sensitivity and nausea if taken without food (Paller & Mancini, 2022).

The student may also be treated with a topical retinoid, such as tretinoin, or an oral retinoid, such as isotretinoin; both are derived from vitamin A. Retinoids are the mainstay of most acne treatment regimens. Topical retinoids are drying to the skin as well as photolabile; therefore, should only be used at night (Chen & Williams, 2017) . If a student presents with irritated skin and is currently using a topical retinoid, the nurse should encourage the student to pause use of the retinoid and use a gentle moisturizer for a few days until the inflammation subsides. It is unknown if topical retinoids are teratogenic; since some of the medication is absorbed through the skin, it is best to follow the same protocols as for oral retinoids.

Isotretinoin is used only after oral antibiotics have not been successful and is effective in treating severe acne. Close monitoring by the student's healthcare provider is required during treatment with isotretinoin. The most common side effects of isotretinoin are dry skin, dry eyes, dry nose, and dry lips. Isotretinoin also increases one's sensitivity to the sun, so attention to sun protection is important during treatment (Paller & Mancini, 2022). Because isotretinoin is a teratogen, its use is regulated by a monitoring system called *iPledge.* Additional monitoring may include liver function levels and triglycerides. Though no causative link has been proven, some individuals treated with isotretinoin report mood changes, such as depression and anxiety. The school nurse should be alert if a student taking isotretinoin displays a change in behavior, such as being withdrawn or erratic behavior, and the student's family should be alerted promptly. Students taking isotretinoin should also refrain from drinking protein shakes and energy drinks since there is an increased risk of elevated liver enzymes (Brzezinski et al., 2017).

ALLERGIC CONDITIONS

Urticaria

Urticaria, also known as hives, is the occurrence of an inflamed, edematous wheal and can be acute or chronic. Acute urticaria lasts 6 to 8 weeks. Approximately 15% of the American population will have at least one episode of hives, usually due to an immediate type I, IgE-driven allergic reaction (John & Brady, 2020; see Chapter 21). Hives can occur anywhere on the body. Individual lesions should resolve within 24 hours, though new lesions may appear. If an individual lesion is present for longer than 24 hours, then the diagnosis of urticaria is less likely (Habif, 2019). In rare instances, some individuals have chronic urticaria, which lasts longer than 6 to 8 weeks and can last up to 5 years (Paller & Mancini, 2022).

An allergic reaction occurs from within minutes to hours after contact. Urticaria can be caused by an altered response to cold, heat, exercise, sun, water, pressure, or vibration (John & Brady, 2020). *Aquagenic urticaria* is a reaction to immersion. *Cholinergic urticaria* is in response to an increase in one's core temperature for any number of reasons, including heat, cold, or stress (John & Brady, 2020). The most common cause of urticaria in the pediatric population is viral infection (Paller & Mancini, 2022). Urticaria may include *angioedema,* which is extravasation of fluid into deeper tissues that occurs gradually. Students with parasitic infections also may present with urticaria.

Assessment

Hives are transient pink, red, or flesh-colored plaques or wheals with sharp borders varying in size from 2 mm to 8 cm, sometimes with an annular or polycyclic appearance. See Fig. 18-1. The student with urticaria usually presents with intense itching (Nicol & Huether, 2017). The nurse should assess for respiratory involvement by asking about shortness of breath or any difficulty breathing in order to rule out anaphylaxis. Wheezing may also be present. Edema of the mouth and throat may compromise the airway and is a medical emergency.

Management

Most cases of urticaria are self-limited and resolve without treatment. The first intervention for urticaria is to remove the underlying cause. The school nurse should assist students with chronic urticaria to identify precipitating factors. Keeping a symptom diary that includes potential

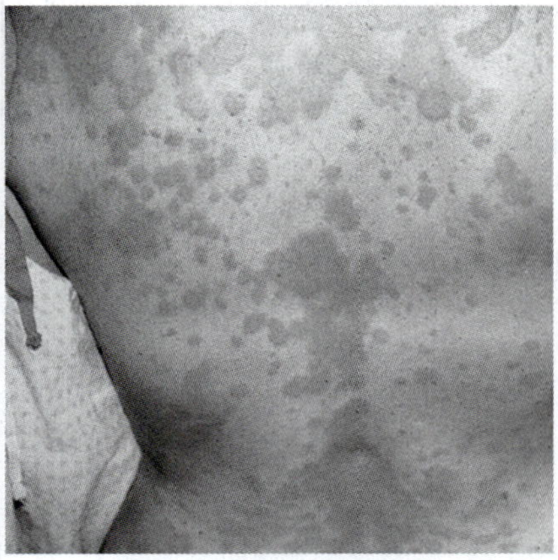

FIGURE 18-1. Urticaria.

triggers for urticaria and treatment efficacy may be helpful. However, many times it may not be possible to determine the etiology. These students may be placed on daily oral antihistamines to treat the urticaria (Bland, 2020).

Students with urticaria who present with signs of anaphylaxis (e.g., hypotension, tachycardia, respiratory distress, severe anxiety) need immediate administration of epinephrine and activation of emergency medical services for transport to the nearest emergency department. The administration of antihistamines (e.g., diphenhydramine) is not effective in reversing anaphylaxis and should not delay emergency treatment with epinephrine (Food Allergy Research and Education, 2022). The school nurse should ensure that students with a documented allergy have an epinephrine autoinjector (e.g., epi-pen) at school that is in an easily accessible location. The school nurse should periodically check expiration dates on all epinephrine autoinjectors. Students who present with hives and no indication of respiratory distress may be managed with over-the-counter or prescription antihistamines, if ordered. Cool compresses may also be helpful.

Atopic Dermatitis/Eczema

Atopic dermatitis, also known as eczema, is a common chronic, relapsing, and pruritic condition caused by two pathophysiological processes: impaired barrier function of the epidermis and altered immune function response to environmental factors (Nicol & Huether, 2017). Eczema is seen in 10% to 20% of children and 3% of adults in the United States; 85% to 95% are identified before the age of 5 years (Bland, 2020; McCann et al., 2017). Patients with atopic dermatitis may also have concurrent asthma and allergies, known as the allergic triad (Paller & Mancini, 2022). For more information on allergies and asthma, see Chapters 21 and 22.

Assessment

A thorough history includes a review of the student's allergies and current skin practices (Buckley, 2021). The student may complain of itching, one of the major criteria for a diagnosis of eczema. Examination of the involved skin areas will reveal erythema or hyperpigmentation, lichenification, and scaling. In some cases, tiny, clear, fluid-filled vesicles may weep and form crusts, which is concerning for eczema herpeticum (Habif, 2019). The most common sites are the antecubital and popliteal folds, thighs, neck, and hands. Younger children often have eczema on their cheeks and scalp. In chronic eczema, the dry skin is sensitive and easily irritated. Rubbing and scratching causes the skin to change over time, thickening and developing deeper skin lines. This lichenification (thickened skin) may present with hypopigmentation or hyperpigmentation (Poladian et al., 2019).

Management

Students with eczema should be under the care of a healthcare provider. The goal of eczema treatment is to optimize the student's skin maintenance plan (gentle soaps, moisturizers, and detergents) and break the inflammatory and itch-scratch cycles. In some students, eczema can be irritated by dog or cat dander. Avoiding fragrances is another key component to management of atopic dermatitis. The use of air fresheners, perfumes, cologne, essential oils, and other fragranced products should be avoided in the home (Bland, 2020). Treatment regimens include thick moisturizers, topical steroid ointments, topical immunomodulators, and the management of secondary infections (Poladian et al., 2019). Students with open erosions, vesicles, or pustules should be evaluated by their primary care provider for a skin culture and potential antibiotic therapy (Nicol & Huether, 2017).

The mainstay of treatment for eczema flares is topical steroids. Topical steroids are used only for the duration of time as outlined by the prescribing provider to prevent skin thinning associated with prolonged use. Oral corticosteroids are a temporary solution for eczema; usually when the oral steroid course is finished, eczema will flare again (Paller & Mancini, 2022). Dupilumab is a newer injectable medication that has greatly changed the landscape of atopic dermatitis therapy and improved quality of life for children with severe eczema who previously did not obtain relief from topical steroids. Dupilumab is an immunomodulator that suppresses one aspect of the immune system and greatly decreases pruritus. Since it is now approved for children as young as 6 months of age, school nurses may have students in their school who are being treated with dupilumab. The side effects of dupilumab include red, itchy eyes and injection site reactions (Siegfried et al., 2019).

Daily skin care that hydrates and lubricates is of primary importance for students with eczema. Families can be educated to avoid wool or other itch-provoking fabrics, avoid hot showers and baths lasting longer than 10 minutes, and to moisturize the skin with a thick cream or ointment twice a day. In the school setting, cool wet compresses to decrease itching and inflammation can be applied as often as needed for 30 minutes each. The school nurse can keep moisturizers and other topical medications in the refrigerator to provide a cooling effect to the skin. Emollients should be applied when the skin is moist for best results. Moisturizers should also be free of additives and fragrance (Bland, 2020).

POISON IVY, POISON OAK, AND POISON SUMAC

Reactions to poison ivy, oak, and sumac are caused by contact with the sap-like material (urushiol) from the *Rhus* genus of plants. Trauma to the leaves of these plants releases oils that are dragged across the skin or transferred by another vehicle, such as a pet. The urushiols bind rapidly to the skin, causing an extremely pruritic contact dermatitis. Approximately 85% of the population will develop a reaction after contact (American Academy of Dermatology [AAD], 2022b). The body's reaction to the plant is a delayed, cell-mediated hypersensitivity; the incubation period after the first exposure is 5 to 21 days, although reexposure can result in a reaction within 8 to 72 hours. Burning vines can release poison ivy particles into the air, which can also cause a respiratory reaction in sensitized individuals (Kim et al., 2019).

Assessment

The usual presentation of contact dermatitis due to poison ivy, oak, or sumac is linear or geometric erythematous, edematous to papulovesicular papules and plaques with intense itching. Vesicles drain serous fluid, and the skin surface becomes moist and crusted. The fluid from the vesicles does not spread the lesions and is not contagious (Kim et al., 2019).

Management

The development of lesions may be prevented if the skin is washed within 10 minutes after contact to any resin on the skin surface. After 10 minutes, only 50% of the urushiol can be removed, and more resin is absorbed as time increases (Habif, 2019). Lesions are not contagious to others. However, the student's clothing and anything else that has had contact with the plant resin, such as animal fur, can continue to transfer the sap. Therefore these items need to be removed and washed immediately. Once the lesions appear, treatment usually consists of cool soaks lasting 15 to 20 minutes multiple times a day; a thick emollient to assist in drying the lesions; antihistamines; and topical, oral, or injected steroids if necessary. The rash will resolve in 1 to 3 weeks (Kim et al., 2019).

INFECTIOUS SKIN CONDITIONS

Impetigo

Impetigo is a contagious, superficial bacterial infection of the skin seen commonly in children and caused by group A beta-hemolytic streptococcus (20%) and/or *Staphylococcus aureus* (80%; May et al., 2019). Exposed parts of the body, such as the face, extremities, hands, and neck, are commonly involved. Impetigo can be spread by direct or indirect contact with infected lesions (Nicol & Huether, 2017). The infection typically starts in an area of skin trauma or a skin lesion, including bug bites (Habif, 2019). Impetigo can spread to other areas of the body by scratching (autoinoculation). The incidence of impetigo is increased in warm humid weather and when students are in close physical contact with others, such as in contact sports like wrestling (Heymann, 2022).

Assessment

Impetigo begins as vesicles with a fragile covering, which rupture easily to form secondary lesions forming the classic honey-colored crust or scaling (Fig. 18-2). Lesions can be either bullous or nonbullous. Bullous lesions imply a staphylococcal cause. These thin-walled vesicles on an erythematous base expand laterally with the formation of satellite lesions. Regional lymphadenopathy and mild pruritus or soreness may be present (May et al., 2019). It should be noted that infections with other organisms, such as tinea capitis, can present a picture similar to impetigo. If impetigo is suspected, treat the lesions as contagious.

Management

Limited areas of impetigo may be effectively treated with an antibiotic preparation such as mupirocin (cream or ointment) two to three times a day (Habif, 2019). Soaking the lesions in warm water for 10 to 15 minutes three or four times a day to remove the crusts aids in the healing process, as crusts interfere with the function of antibacterial creams (May et al., 2019). Students with widespread infections or recurrent infections should be referred for systemic antibiotic treatment, such as with cephalexin or clindamycin. In students with recurrent bacterial infections, dilute bleach baths (a quarter of a cup of regular strength unscented bleach in a half bathtub of water) one to two times a week may help decrease further infections (Bland, 2020).

It is important to explain the contagious nature of impetigo to the parents/guardians. Good hand washing practices and isolation of the student's towels, washcloths, linens, and drinking glasses should be emphasized.

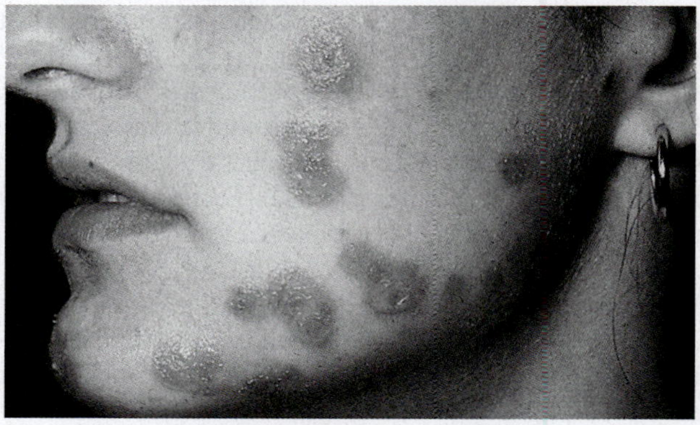

FIGURE 18-2. Impetigo.

Students with impetigo should be excluded from school until they have been treated for 24 hours to prevent the spread of infection (Kimberlin et al., 2021).

Methicillin-Resistant *Staphylococcus aureus*

Staphylococcus aureus is a common bacteria that is found in the external environment and in the anterior nares of 20% to 40% of adults. It can cause relatively mild infections of the skin and the soft tissue as well as life-threatening sepsis, pneumonia, and toxic shock syndrome (Guo et al., 2020). *S. aureus* is prone to develop resistance to methicillin and other beta-lactamase–resistant penicillins. As a result, two genetically and phenotypically distinct strains have developed: healthcare-associated/acquired methicillin-resistant *S. aureus* (HA-MRSA) and community-associated/acquired methicillin-resistant *S. aureus* (CA-MRSA). Most cases seen in the school setting are the less serious CA-MRSA. The incidence of MRSA is increasing, making it more difficult to treat (Kimberlin et al., 2021).

Staphylococcus aureus can be spread by direct skin-to-skin contact or by contact with objects and surfaces touched by those affected, including towels and used bandages. It is also spread by autoinfection (Heymann, 2022). It is not common for the infection to spread through the bloodstream to other organs beyond the skin, but it can occur, especially in those with weakened immune systems or central lines.

The first cases of CA-MRSA in the United States were in high school wrestlers in 1993 (Perloff, 2017). It is most commonly spread through open wounds, such as skin abrasions that occur when rubbing against a mat or turf or via skin-to-skin contact with an infected player. MRSA can also develop within infected skin, especially in students with eczema. Students presenting with open, punched-out lesions should be referred to their primary care provider for evaluation. A culture of the area is generally taken to determine the appropriate antibiotic course of treatment.

Assessment

CA-MRSA usually presents as boils (furuncles), folliculitis, abscesses, and infected lacerations (Heymann, 2022). The student may describe it as an "infected pimple" or an "insect bite" (Perloff, 2017). Examination may reveal a localized area of erythema, warmth, and swelling, sometimes associated with cellulitis. Pus may ooze from the lesion.

Management

The student can transmit the organism as long as the lesion continues to drain; therefore it is essential to keep the lesion covered (Heymann, 2022). Athletes should be removed from sports participation until 72 hours after starting on oral antimicrobial therapy and some demonstrated improvement is seen (Centers for Disease Control and Prevention [CDC], 2019a). Abscesses may need to be drained by the healthcare provider.

Education is essential to prevent spread, with hand washing being the initial intervention. Students should be instructed not to share towels, soaps, and sports-related items. Strict attention to policies that dictate cleaning and disinfection protocols for wrestling mats, locker room benches, floors, football equipment, and so forth is essential to prevent spread.

Hand, Foot, and Mouth Disease

Hand, foot, and mouth disease (HFMD) is caused by a coxsackievirus, a member of the enterovirus family. It is highly contagious and is a frequent cause of outbreaks in daycares and preschools. HFMD usually occurs in children less than 10 years of age. There are several strains of HFMD, so it is possible for student to contract HFMD more than once and for parents to develop HFMD even if they were exposed as a child. Although HFMD is benign, the skin lesions can be uncomfortable and visually distressing for students and families (Kimberlin et al., 2021).

Assessment

After contact with HFMD, students become symptomatic within 3 to 6 days. Typically, students will experience fatigue, fever (less than 102°F for 3 days or less), sore throat, and difficulty eating and drinking due to painful mouth sores that can develop in the back of the throat. This virus presents with small red papules and vesicles on the perioral skin, hands, feet, and buttocks and can occur with painful ulcers in the mouth (Bland, 2020). Over 7 to 10 days, the papules and vesicles will crust while the mouth ulcers should resolve within 7 days.

Management

Supportive treatment is the mainstay of therapy for HFMD. Due to potential painful mouth ulcers, staying hydrated is very important; cold drinks, smoothies, and a soft diet are helpful in maintaining hydration and nutrition. Spicy, citrus, or salty foods should be avoided. Acetaminophen and ibuprofen are appropriate supportive therapies (Nield, 2017). Students should not attend school while they are febrile or symptomatic. Temporary closure of daycare classes may be necessary to control the spread of HFMD (Kimberlin et al., 2021). Desquamation (peeling of fingers and toes) can occur 1 to 2 weeks after resolution of symptoms. Although this can be worrisome, it is benign and thick emollients should be applied to these areas at least twice a day. In 5% of severe cases, some fingernails and toenails can fall off weeks after infection. Reassurance should be provided to families that fingernails can take 3 to 6 months and toenails can take 6 to 12 months to grow back fully (Kimberlin et al., 2021).

Fifth Disease

Fifth Disease, *or erythema infectiosum*, is a viral disease caused by parvovirus B19 that primarily affects preschool and young school-age students. Parvovirus B19 infection is typically asymptomatic or causes only mild illness in healthy individuals (CDC, 2024). The peak incidence of this infection is usually late winter and early spring. It is slightly contagious and can appear randomly or in epidemics. The virus is spread by respiratory droplet, and children are most contagious before the rash appears. Asymptomatic infections are common. The incubation period is 13 to 18 days (Habif, 2016).

Assessment

The history associated with Fifth disease includes mild fever, headache, cough, sore throat, and joint pain. The hallmark sign is a diffuse, bright red patchy rash erupts on the cheeks, resembling "slapped cheeks." The rash is warm, nontender and may be itchy. It can last for 7 to 10 days and may come and go over several weeks (CDC, 2024). The student may also develop a lacy maculopapular reddened rash that begins on the trunk and then spreads peripherally to the extremities and buttocks.

Management

Students and parents can be assured that the rash will fade and no treatment is required. The concern is for the developing fetus of pregnant parents and staff; hydrops fetalis, an excessive fluid accumulation in the fetus that can result in fetal death, is remotely possible. Persons who have weakened immune systems or certain blood disorders (e.g., leukemia, organ transplant, HIV, sickle cell disease) may also be at risk for complications (CDC, 2024). *Pregnant and at risk students and staff should be referred to their healthcare provider for assessment.* Because the student is most contagious before the rash appears, health department policy should be followed as to whether to exclude the child from school until the rash subsides. Practical recommendations include having pregnant or immunocompromised staff maintain a reasonable physical distance from the infected person and practice good hand hygiene.

Warts

Verruca vulgaris, commonly known as warts, is a common cutaneous viral infection caused by human papillomavirus (HPV) infection of the skin. Warts are spread via contact and are common among school-age children and teenagers; about 30% of children have had a wart. (Silverberg, 2019). Untreated, their typical course lasts between 2 and 3 years; however, they can be stubborn and recalcitrant to treatment. In students with atopic dermatitis, warts can spread easily due to the impaired skin barrier and frequent itching. Autoinoculation is a common way that warts spread, so students should be counseled to avoid touching or scratching their warts (Chen & Willams, 2017).

Assessment

Warts are typically verrucous (rough), although warts can also be flat-topped, or filiform (protruding outwards). Common locations for warts are the knees, hands, feet, and elbows, although they can present in almost any location. Warts that are found on the feet can be painful, particularly if the student is involved in sports or other physical activities. Students should not share shoes, towels, pencils, or other personal items to prevent the spread of warts. Students should cover their warts with bandages or tape to prevent transmission while playing sports. Any student over 3 to 4 years of age with perianal or perineal warts should be referred to their primary care provider, as the transmission of these warts may have occurred though sexual abuse (Soenjoyo et al., 2020).

Management

Although warts are self-resolving, their appearance can be bothersome to students and cause psychosocial distress. Treatment approaches to warts include physical destruction of each lesion and stimulating the student's immune system to fight off the virus. Salicylic acid liquids and pads are widely available over the counter and can be applied nightly to each wart. It is important to emphasize that families must be diligent in applying treatment for the warts to resolve. A common side effect of salicylic acid is irritation of the surrounding normal skin, so the family should apply it just to the wart itself. Another common therapy that the school nurse may encounter is duct tape occlusion therapy (Silverberg, 2019). Salicylic acid and duct tape can also be used in combination to treat warts. Other topical prescription medications are available and can be trialed; however, rates of successful treatment for warts vary. Many offices offer cryotherapy, or liquid nitrogen treatment, for warts and serial treatments are needed. There have been reports of the HPV vaccine stimulating the immune system and helping resolve even common warts (Soenjoyo et al., 2020).

Molluscum Contagiosum

Molluscum contagiosum is another common skin infection caused by poxvirus infection, with an incubation period ranging from 1 week to 6 months (Heymann, 2022). Similar to warts, the virus enters through small openings in the skin. The infection is usually localized and self-limiting, resolving spontaneously in 6 to 24 months (Heymann, 2022). It can spread by direct and indirect contact via skin-to-skin contact or handling objects contaminated with the virus (e.g., towels, floor mats, swimming pool kickboards). Molluscum also frequently spreads via autoinoculation, so students should be advised to refrain from touching or scratching their lesions. Wrestlers and gymnasts are particularly susceptible to this skin infection (Habif, 2019).

Assessment

Lesions are often several months old when first reported. The number of lesions can vary from one to dozens of lesions and frequently involve the face, trunk, and proximal extremities. Involvement of the buttock and groin is common and usually not associated with sexual abuse. The palms, soles, and scalp are typically spared. Molluscum begin as small, almost shiny dome-shaped papules, 1 to 6 mm in diameter, that are flesh-colored, white, pink, or yellow and have a tiny dimple or umbilicated central area. Inflammation and redness may occur as a result of scratching or a hypersensitivity reaction, especially in students with a history of eczema (Bland, 2020). When students have both molluscum and atopic dermatitis, the molluscum lesions are often difficult to clear until the atopic dermatitis is under control. The student may complain of tenderness and itching associated with mild inflammation Due to the similarity with warts and herpes lesions, the student should be referred to their primary healthcare provider to make a definitive diagnosis (Chen & Willams, 2017).

Management

Molluscum lesions resolve spontaneously in 6 to 24 months in healthy individuals, and treatment is usually not necessary. The student is contagious as long as the lesions are present (Bland, 2020). The school nurse should teach those with the infection to avoid skin-to-skin contact to minimize transmission of the virus. If possible, students should keep the areas of infection covered with clothing or an adhesive bandage, but students should not be excluded from school because of molluscum infection (Kimberlin et al., 2021). Many of the treatment options lead to significant scarring, so treatment considerations should be individualized and directed by a healthcare provider. Treatments are aimed at destroying the lesion and virus by freezing it with liquid nitrogen, applying an irritating topical substance such as cantharone or a retinoid, or surgical removal (Habif, 2019). In addition to scarring, surgical removal can be painful. Reassurance and watchful waiting for natural resolution is often appropriate.

FUNGAL SKIN INFECTIONS

Superficial fungal infections of the skin are caused by various dermatophytes that infect the keratinized cutaneous tissues, including the skin, nails, and hair. The term *tinea* is used in conjunction with a specific part of the body infected with the fungus, by such additional terms as tinea capitis (head), tinea corporis or ringworm (trunk, legs, and arms, excluding the feet, hands, and groin), tinea cruris or jock itch (groin, pubic area, and thighs), and tinea pedis (athlete's foot). Technically, all could be considered ringworm—although that designation is usually limited to tinea corporis (Paller & Mancini, 2022).

Tinea Corporis

Tinea corporis, or ringworm, is a fungal (dermatophyte) infection with an incubation period of 4 to 10 days (Heymann, 2022) affecting the trunk and limbs. Tinea thrives on the top layer of dead skin. Tinea corporis may be transferred from other parts of the body affected with tinea, from household contacts, young kittens, puppies, and guinea pigs, or from contact during sports such as wrestling (Habif, 2019; Nicol & Huether, 2017).

Assessment

The student presenting with tinea corporis may have one or multiple lesions that spread peripherally. Physical findings usually include annular (ring-shaped), scaling, erythematous plaques with sharply demarcated, indurated, hyperkeratotic borders (Fig. 18-3) with a central clearing (Habif, 2019). The initial lesion may be a macule or a plaque, varying in size from less than a centimeter to greater than 8 cm. The student may be asymptomatic or complain of mild pruritus. The rash may be misdiagnosed as eczema or seborrheic dermatitis (Paller & Mancini, 2022). The student should be checked for dermatophyte infections involving other body areas.

Management

Children with tinea corporis are contagious as long as the lesions are present (Heymann, 2022). Prescription or over-the-counter topical antifungal medications (e.g., ketoconazole cream) may be used for treatment. A therapeutic response should occur after 2 weeks of treatment; therapy is continued for up to 4 weeks after the clinical symptoms have resolved (Habif, 2019). Students do not need to be excluded from school if lesions are covered and treatment has been initiated (Kimberlin et al., 2021).

Tinea Capitis

Tinea capitis has an incubation period of 10 to 14 days and most often occurs in children ages 2 to 10 years, with a decreasing incidence after puberty (Heymann, 2022). It is transmitted by personal contact and occasionally by pets, especially puppies, kittens, and guinea pigs. The infecting spores can remain viable for long periods of time and can be cultured from combs, brushes, blankets, hats, and theatre seats (Paller & Mancini, 2022). Tinea capitis is more common in crowded living conditions, and reinfection can occur (Habif, 2019).

Assessment

The student usually presents with patchy hair loss and/or scaling of the scalp, sometimes with cervical lymphadenopathy. The fungal organism can invade the hair shaft, causing it to break off 1 to 5 mm above the scalp (Nicol & Heuther, 2017); this may leave a circular area of hair breakage 1 to

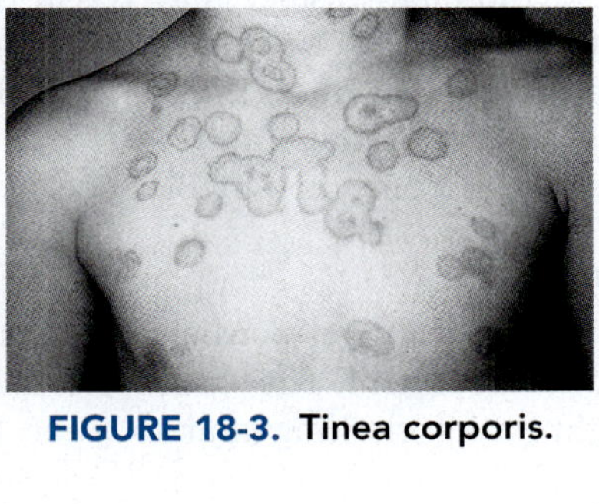

FIGURE 18-3. Tinea corporis.

5 cm in diameter with a "salt and pepper" appearing scalp. The assessment may reveal erythema, edema, and pustules. Weeping and gold-colored crusting can resemble impetigo. A kerion, or large crusting and potentially oozing area in the scalp, may appear if tinea capitis has been present for an extended amount of time (Paller & Mancini, 2022). If a kerion is present, the student needs to be promptly evaluated by their primary care provider.

Management

Management of tinea capitis requires oral antifungal medication (e.g., griseofulvin or terbinafine) for treatment. If oral griseofulvin is used, it is best taken with fatty foods for better absorption (Barnett, 2017). Topical shampoos (such as ketoconazole) may be used to decrease transmission. Students with suspected tinea capitis should be referred for medical evaluation and management. The student may return to school after treatment is started (Kimberlin et al., 2021). Parent/guardian and student education regarding the transmission and prevention of the infection is important. To prevent reinfection, it is important to scrupulously clean all possible objects contaminated by the child's head, including clothes, head coverings, hairclips, furniture, blankets, and sheets (Paller & Mancini, 2022).

Washing the hair with an over-the-counter shampoo with the active ingredient of selenium sulfide 1% or ketoconazole 1% can reduce the risk of shedding spores. All household contacts should be encouraged to shampoo with selenium sulfide, and siblings should be checked for similar scalp lesions. Students should be encouraged not to share hats to decrease the possibility of contracting tinea from those who are infected or asymptomatic carriers. Following treatment, normal hair growth will usually occur; however, in severe cases of tinea capitis and kerion, individuals may experience permanent alopecia (Habif, 2019).

Tinea Cruris

Tinea cruris, commonly referred to as jock itch, is a superficial infection that can occur in the crural folds of the groin and perianal region. It is more common in males and in individuals who are obese, have increased sweating, and/or experience chafing from tight clothing (Blosser et al., 2017).

Assessment

The student will usually complain of itching in the groin area, especially when sweating after vigorous exercise or during warm days. A thorough history may reveal the presence of another tinea infection elsewhere. Tinea cruris presents as well-defined scaling plaques, sometimes with a papular advancing edge extending out of the crural fold and onto the thigh, and may involve the scrotum (Blosser et al., 2017).

Management

Over-the-counter antifungal powders, creams, or lotions may be used for treatment. The student should be advised to avoid tight-fitting clothing and to wear loose-fitting underwear, and change their underwear frequently, especially after tasks that leave them hot and sweaty. Following a workout, the student should be taught to bathe or shower right away, dry well with a towel, and apply an antifungal preparation. Students should be encouraged to wash their hands after applying any medicinal preparation and avoid sharing towels (Paller & Mancini, 2022). The student should be taught to avoid storing damp clothing in a locker or gym bag, and to wash workout clothing after each wearing to avoid reinfection. The student with resistant infections should be referred for medical evaluation by their primary care provider and further treatment.

Tinea Pedis

Tinea pedis, commonly called athlete's foot, is frequently seen during puberty when the feet sweat and shoes provide a warm environment for the fungus to grow. It is usually acquired from the warm moist environment of a communal shower or locker room floor (Blosser et al., 2017).

Assessment

The student may present with itching, scaling, and/or burning pain between the toes (interdigital) or on other areas of the foot. In interdigital tinea pedis, the student may have fissures between the toes with underlying erythematous skin that may weep, often emitting a foul odor. Without proper treatment, tinea pedis can advance to cellulitis, osteomyelitis, and lymphangitis (Nigam, et al., 2023).

Management

All students, especially those with tinea pedis, should be instructed to wear shower shoes (flip-flops or plastic sandals) while showering in public facilities to try to decrease the spread of the fungus. They should dry their feet well after showering and wear cotton socks. Students may use an over-the-counter antifungal cream, powder, or spray applied beyond the borders of the rash until it is clear, which can take 3 to 6 weeks (Bland, 2020). Students may continue to participate in sports during treatment (Nigam, et al., 2023).

SKIN INFESTATIONS

Pediculosis

Pediculosis, or lice, is an infestation of a blood-obligate parasite. Pediculosis is distressing to students, parents, healthcare providers, and school personnel. There are three species of lice that infest humans: *Pediculus humanus capitis* (head louse), *Pediculus humanus corporis* (body louse [uncommon in children]), and *Pthirus pubis* (crab louse, pubic louse [a sexually transmitted infection]). Head lice are transmitted from person to person through direct contact and the environment but do not transmit any other disease (Kimberlin et al., 2021).

The Centers for Disease Control and Prevention (CDC, 2019b) estimates 6 to 12 million children between the ages of 3 and 11 have head lice infestation each year. Head lice affects children of all socioeconomic backgrounds, with females more susceptible than males (Habif, 2019).

The life cycle of adult lice is approximately 1 month. Head lice exist in one of three stages: the nit (or egg), the nymph (or small adult), and the adult lice. The female louse lays 6 to 10 eggs a day that attach firmly within 4 mm of the base of the hair shaft. The eggs hatch in 7 to 10 days and mature in an additional 9 to 12 days. The egg casings become more visible after the lice hatch. Eggs can survive 7 to 10 days without a host (Habif, 2019; Heymann, 2022).

Head lice do not jump or fly and are not transferred from person to person by pets. Lice are most likely spread from head to head by direct contact or from contact with objects containing the louse. For this reason, it is important to teach students not to share combs, brushes, headphones, scarves, hats, helmets, towels, pillowcases, toys, or stage props that fit on the head and not to have their hair touch another child's head. Within the past decade, increased transmission of lice has occurred due to children crowding around cell phones, computers, or other electronic devices, allowing lice the opportunity to spread from an infected student (Bragg & Wills, 2022).

Assessment

Most students with lice are asymptomatic. The student may complain of pruritus on the head, around the ears, at the hairline, or the base of the neck. The pruritus is likely caused by the lice saliva, which is injected as the lice feed on the skin. Cervical lymphadenopathy may result from scratching the skin. Although rare, staphylococcal infections associated with fever may result from abrasions in the skin caused by scratching (Habif, 2019).

In addition to attaching to the hair close to the scalp, head lice can also attach to the eyebrows and eyelashes. The definitive diagnosis of head lice is seeing the live louse on the head. Small eggs (nits) may look like dandruff or tiny pearls found near the hair root. Active lice will be moving on the scalp. Using a magnifying glass and a good light source may help identify infestation, as lice are small and difficult to see. Tiny eggs or nits are usually easier to identify on the scalp (Fig. 18-4). It is important not to confuse nits with dandruff, dried flaking hair product, hair spray, or other debris in the scalp. Nits will not release from the shaft if the hair is shaken (Bragg & Wills, 2022), whereas dandruff or other hair debris usually does not cling to the hair shaft. Nits may be easiest to identify at the nape of the neck. Head lice feed off human blood up to five times a day, and the nits must be close enough to the scalp for the louse to feed (Habif, 2019). Nits that are less than ¼ inch from the scalp are suggestive of a lice infestation; nits greater than ¼ inch from the scalp indicate that the infection is no longer active and does not need to be treated (Heymann, 2022).

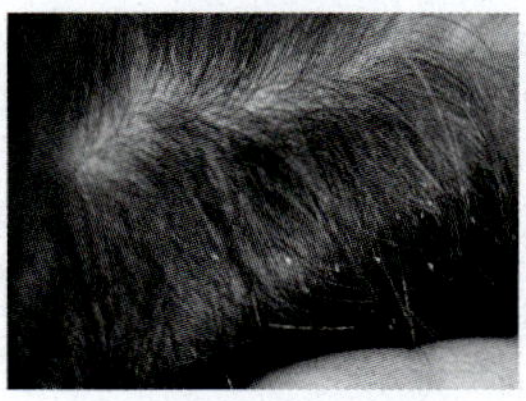

FIGURE 18-4. Nits.

Students found to have head lice do *not* need to be immediately excluded from school (Kimberlin et al., 2021). Parents/guardians should be notified of the infestation. A school form letter describing proper care and recommended treatments should be sent home with the child at the end of the school day. The letter informs parents/guardians that treatment needs to be done that evening so that the child is able to return to school the next day, although policies vary among schools. Once treatment has been applied, the student may return to school. All household members should be checked for lice and treated if lice are found. Everyone should be treated at the same time so the lice will not continue to spread (McInerny et al., 2017). Some parents may express anger at the diagnosis of lice; some may refuse treatment, but it is the duty of the school nurse to ensure that treatment is performed. For some, financial assistance is needed to access the pediculicide. It should be noted that the American Academy of Pediatrics (2022) and the National Association of School Nurses (2020) do not support "no nit" policies nor school exclusion due to pediculosis. No child should miss school time due to head lice (Kimberlin et al., 2021). The school nurse needs to reinforce that having lice has nothing to do with cleanliness.

Some schools notify the affected student's class while maintaining the student's privacy; others notify the entire school, although this is not recommended. A letter such as that in Figure 18-5 informs parents that treatment should not be given unless lice are present, but that they should assess their child to ensure that they are free of lice.

Management

There are several preparations that may be used to treat head lice. A pediculicide shampoo containing permethrin is the first-choice over-the-counter medication. Malathion is a prescription medication approved for those older than age 2. The American Academy of Pediatrics notes that malathion is the most pediculicidal and ovicidal agent with the best cure rate after just one application (Kimberlin et al., 2021). Benzyl alcohol 5% lotion is another approved product for the treatment of head lice (CDC, 2020; Habif, 2019). Other products include pyrethrums (should be avoided by those who are sensitive to ragweed), Spinosad, and ivermectin. All pediculicide products have specific guidelines for how they are to be applied (e.g., damp or dry hair) and a prescribed period of time to be left on before being washed with shampoo. A second treatment in 7 to 10 days is recommended for most products to ensure that any lice that may have hatched from the eggs are also killed (Bland, 2020).

PARENT BULLETIN

Head Lice

Date

A case of head lice (pediculosis) has been reported in your child's school. Lice are a common occurrence in schools. Head lice do not transmit disease.

When a child gets lice, it does not suggest that the child is not clean. It only indicates that the child has been near someone with lice. All families are being informed so that parents can examine their children's scalp and hair carefully each day for head lice.

Lice may cause itching and scratching of the scalp.

Head lice are insects the size and color of a sesame seed. They do not fly or jump but scamper on the scalp. Lice are spread by head-to-head contact or shared items.

Lice eggs (nits) are teardrop shaped and white or hair color. They are tightly attached to the hair shaft, usually behind the ears and at the back of the neck. Nits cannot be "flicked off."

If a head louse is found on your child, treatment is required before the child is permitted to return to school. All treatments need careful attention to directions to decrease any risk of side effects and to ensure elimination of the infestation. Use only treatments recommended for head lice, as products intended for animals or for other purposes will not be effective. Please contact your school nurse or healthcare provider for recommendations on treatment. The school nurse can also provide more information about head lice and school district policies.

____________________ School Nurse

FIGURE 18-5. Lice assessment letter. *(CDC, 2022b)*

Because pediculicides may kill the eggs but will not remove them, manual removal of nits is still recommended (Heymann, 2022). Removal of nits and lice with fine-tooth combs (supplied with most over-the-counter preparations) make the process easier. To remove nits from eyelashes, apply petroleum jelly to lashes twice a day for several days and gently wipe lashes clean. Vigilance and careful attention to product directions are imperative as lice are increasingly resistant to treatment. Objects in the school or home that have been in contact with the child's head (e.g., sheets, towels, and hats) should be washed in hot water and dried on high heat cycle. Items that cannot be washed should be placed in plastic trash bags and sealed for 3 weeks. All surfaces in the home should be vacuumed well, including carpets, floors, mattresses, and furniture (Kimberlin et al., 2021).

Parents who reject the use of recommended shampoos may try natural or home remedies. These products are not regulated by the U.S. Food and Drug Administration (USFDA), nor have they been demonstrated to be effective. Some of the common over-the-counter products that parents may massage into the hair in an attempt to smother the head lice are mayonnaise, olive oil, and petroleum jelly. The children sleep with the product on their hair (covered with a shower cap) and then wash it out the next day. The problem is that these products are *very* difficult to get out of the hair and often do not kill both live lice and eggs (CDC, 2020). Products such as dog shampoos for fleas, insect repellents, and kerosene are dangerous for children and should never be used to treat lice.

Screening for nits or live lice is not cost effective and does not have significant effect on decreasing the incidence of lice (Kimberlin et al., 2021). Assessing close contacts of persons who have head lice is appropriate. Successful care of students with head lice is a collaborative effort that includes open communication among the school nurse, family, and student. Care includes educating the student, family, and school staff about the myths around head lice, as well as having proper evidence-based school policies and procedures in place.

Scabies

Scabies is a mite infestation in the skin that causes intense itching. Scabies is usually contracted by close body contact with an infected individual who may be asymptomatic. Although rare, infection can occur by the use of contaminated towels, bed linen, and clothing. The mite burrows into the skin and deposits its eggs; once hatched over the next 2 weeks the mites mature and travel into the skin (May et al., 2019). The incubation period is 1 to 2 months in persons who have never been infected with scabies.

Focus on the Framework

Treatment of pediculosis (head lice) in the school community requires the school nurse to practice using all principles of the *School Nursing Practice Framework* (2024). The nurse uses the principle of **Care Coordination** in working with the parent/guardian to treat a student with lice. The principle of **Leadership** and **Standards of Practice** is demonstrated when ensuring that evidence-based "no nit" policies are in place. The principle of **Quality Improvement** is employed when school nurses evaluate the effectiveness of no-nit policies that increase instructional time. Finally, the school nurse practices within the principle of **Community/Public Health** when they dispel myths and teach families and school staff about pediculosis.

In persons who have previously had scabies, symptoms may occur in 1 to 4 days (Habif, 2019).

Assessment

A history of intense itching that is worse at night and visible burrows or tunnels under the skin may be reported; the pruritus is related to a reaction to the mite or feces of the mite. A rash that affects the hands, wrists, armpits, genital area, waist, buttocks, ankles, and areas around the knees and elbows is common; the face is not usually affected. More than one person in the household may have symptoms. Scratching destroys the burrows and is a possible source of spread of the mite (May et al., 2019). Skin lesions associated with scabies may include macules; papules; and linear, curved, or S-shaped erythematous or hyperpigmented lesions that represent the areas where the mite has burrowed (Paller & Mancini, 2022).

Management

Application of a prescription scabicide, such as topical permethrin, is curative. When treating the skin with topical permethrin, the skin below the neck should be covered with the lotion and left on the skin for 12 hours. A second treatment is recommended in 1 to 2 weeks (Heymann, 2022). Students should be excluded from school until the day after the initiation of treatment (Kimberlin et al., 2021). It is important to note that all household contacts should also be treated with permethrin in the same manner and the same time, regardless of symptoms (Kimberlin et al., 2021). Symptomatic treatment may include oral antihistamines as well as topical corticosteroids to help with the associated pruritus, which can last for weeks after successful treatment (Paller & Mancini, 2022).

Scabies is contagious. School nurses should advise teachers to watch for signs or symptoms of other students scratching, complaining of itching, and having a red or hyperpigmented rash on the arms, hands (between the fingers), and other areas of the body except the face. Persons who have had close contact with the infected student should be encouraged to wash their clothing and bedding using the hot cycle for both the washer and dryer. If there is a concern, articles that cannot be washed in hot water, such as mats, coats, and stuffed animals, can be placed in a dark plastic bag, sealed, and put aside for 3 weeks, although this is rarely done. If the mite does not have human contact, it will die in 10 to 18 days (McInerny et al., 2017).

TICK-TRANSMITTED DISEASES

Lyme Disease

Lyme disease occurs as a result of a bite from a deer tick infected with the spirochete *Borrelia burgdorferi*. Infestation was previously most common in the Northeast, Mid-Atlantic, and upper Midwest regions of the United States; however, over the past 20 years cases have expanded to the West coast and Southern states. Nationally, there are approximately 30,000 human cases of Lyme disease each year, but most cases are not reported (CDC, 2022). Symptoms usually occur during the spring and summer months and are present in 73% of patients (Schwartz et al., 2017).

Assessment

The onset of Lyme disease occurs 3 to 32 days after an infective tick bite, but it often presents as a localized inflamed, painless area that goes unnoticed (Heymann, 2022). It is important to educate parents to check for ticks on the body and in hair-bearing areas after being in wooded areas. The localized area presents as a bright red expanding eruption occurring at the site of the bite (Habif, 2019). The area of erythema (referred to as erythema migrans) begins as a small papule, slowly enlarges, but fades within 2 to 3 weeks, leaving a normal to light blue surface. The rash rarely itches, blisters, or swells; as the rash enlarges, the center may become clear, resulting in a bull's-eye appearance (Blosser et al., 2017). Not all individuals infected with Lyme disease develop the bull's-eye rash. Symptoms such as fatigue, headache, fever, chills, stiff neck, and muscle or joint pain may occur. Flu-like symptoms may occur in the absence of an identified rash.

If left untreated, Lyme infection can become systemic. In addition to erythema migrans, 27% of people infected with Lyme disease develop arthritis, and 1.5% develop carditis, primarily seen as atrioventricular block. Neurological symptoms are present in 12.5% of the cases, including facial palsy, radiculoneuropathy, lymphocytic meningitis, and encephalitis (Schwartz et al., 2017).

Management

Prevention of disease is the first line of defense, including teaching students to wear protective clothing, tucking pants into socks, and wearing closed-toed shoes when in areas infested with ticks. Permethrin can be sprayed

> **Practice Connection**
>
> Ticks should be removed as soon as detected using the following technique:
>
> 1. Use fine-tipped tweezers to grasp the tick as close to the skin as possible.
> 2. Pull upward with steady pressure to remove the tick. Don't twist or jerk the tick.
> 3. After removing the tick, clean the bite area and hands with rubbing alcohol or soap and water.
> 4. Dispose of the tick by flushing it down the toilet. If identification of the tick is recommended by a healthcare provider, place the tick in rubbing alcohol in a sealed bag or container.
> 5. For the next 30 days, watch for rash, fever, fatigue, headache, muscle pain, or joint swelling and pain.
>
> Adapted from the CDC (2021).

directly on clothing to ward off insects but should not be applied directly on the body. Insect repellent with 20% to 30% DEET or clothing impregnated with DEET can be used. Inspection of the skin and removal of ticks should be done as soon as possible when students have been in areas of potential exposure (Habif, 2019). Once infected, however, early Lyme disease is best treated with 2 to 4 weeks of antibiotics (Stagg & McCarthy, 2017).

Rocky Mountain Spotted Fever

Rocky Mountain spotted fever (RMSF) is caused by a *Rickettsia* species transmitted through a bite of an infected tick. The disease is seen throughout the United States, southern Canada, Mexico and Central America, and parts of South America. Although initially found in the Rocky Mountains, most cases of RMSF now occur between April and September in the southeastern and southcentral states, particularly Oklahoma, Arkansas, Tennessee, North Carolina, and South Carolina (McInerny et al., 2017). *Rickettsiae* affect the blood's ability to clot by reducing platelet function (Habif, 2019). This leads to increased vascular permeability and edema. In severe reactions, hypovolemia and shock can occur.

Assessment

The symptoms usually appear within 3 to 21 days of an infected American dog tick or Rocky Mountain wood tick bite and include abrupt onset of fever, rash, severe headache, muscle pain, and vomiting. The discrete, macular, skin rash that blanches with pressure most commonly occurs on the fourth day, starting on the wrists and ankles, and then moving to the palms and soles of the feet. The rash then becomes more petechial in nature (Bland, 2020); the fever and rash subside in 2 to 3 weeks (Habif, 2019). Note that the rash may be difficult to see in individuals with more darkly pigmented skin. Potential severe systemic symptoms of untreated RMSF include altered mental status, peripheral neuropathy, incontinence, cerebellar dysfunction, neck stiffness (suggestive of meningism), disseminated intravascular coagulation, necrosis of digits, and potentially coma (Kimberlin et al., 2021).

Management

The first line RMSF treatment for a child of any age is doxycycline (Habif, 2019). Treatment needs to be initiated within 5 days of the first symptoms in order to prevent possible systemic symptoms (Blosser et al., 2017). As with Lyme disease, RMSF is prevented by prevention of tick bites. Students should tuck their pants legs into their socks so that ticks cannot crawl up the inside of pant legs and apply DEET repellents to discourage tick attachment. Repellents containing permethrin can be sprayed on shoes and clothing and will last for several days. Check children for ticks, especially in the hair, when returning from potentially tick-infested areas. Ticks may also be carried into the household on clothing and pets and attach later.

SUN EXPOSURE ISSUES

Sun exposure prevention is a prime example of population health school nursing practice. Protecting the skin from excessive sun exposure is imperative to prevent sunburns and also prevent new melanocytic nevi (moles) from forming (Hallowell & Mehlmann, 2022). The sun emits two types of ultraviolet rays: ultraviolet A (UVA) and ultraviolet B (UVB). Both can damage the DNA of the skin, causing premature wrinkling and aging of the skin and increasing the risk of skin cancer. The incidence of skin cancer has been rapidly increasing worldwide for the last 2 to 3 decades. While UVA rays are responsible for the premature aging of the skin caused by the sun, the UVB rays are responsible for both the burning and tanning of the skin, as well as the development of new moles and potentially skin cancer (AAD, 2022a).

Children have varying sensitivities to the sun, usually due to the amount of melanin in the skin, with lighter skin tones more susceptible to sunburn than darker skin tones. Mild sunburn resembles a first-degree partial thickness burn, with symptoms of erythema and mild discomfort. Intense sun exposure can cause painful second-degree partial thickness burns that bister and cause more severe damage to the skin (AAD, 2022a). A number of medications can increase a child's sensitivity to the sun and therefore cause faster burning. These include doxycycline, nonsteroidal anti-inflammatory drugs, furosemide, antifungals, tretinoin, and isotretinoin (Young & Tewari, 2022).

It is not uncommon for students who have been burned by the sun to come to school when the discomfort is at its peak. In addition, 2 to 7 days after the burn, the burned skin layer begins to shed, and the student may experience a combination of itching and discomfort. Treatment in school may include cool water compresses or ice packs for edema. Ibuprofen or acetaminophen may be administered for discomfort according to school medication administration policies. Blisters should remain intact and can be covered with gauze until they heal, although the tape may be irritating to the surrounding burned skin. Gentle emollients are helpful in keeping the skin from drying. Although products containing aloe vera are commonly recommended, they can cause further irritation in students with sensitive skin or eczema. In addition, the child should stay hydrated (AAD, 2022a).

The American Academy of Dermatology (2022c) warns that even on overcast days, 80% of UV rays can pass through clouds. Limiting UV ray exposure is the best way to prevent skin damage and reduce skin cancer risk. There are two types of sunscreen to protect the skin—physical and chemical (Hallowell & Mehlmann, 2022). Physical (mineral) sunscreens block and reflect UV rays. They leave a white coating on the skin and are recommended for young children and persons with dry skin or eczema. Active ingredients in physical sunscreens include titanium dioxide or zinc oxide. Chemical sunscreens blend into the skin and absorb the UV rays. Active ingredients in chemical sunscreens include vobenzone, oxybenzone, octocrylene, homosalate, octisalate, and octinoxate.

Sunscreens have a sun protection factor (SPF), which is a "measure of how much solar energy (UV radiation) is required to produce sunburn on protected sun (i.e., in the presence of sunscreen) relative to the amount of solar energy required to produce sunburn on unprotected skin. As SPF value increases, sunburn protection increases" (USFDA, n.d., para. 1). A broad-spectrum sunscreen (protection against both UVA *and* UVB) with a minimum SPF of 30 is recommended for children. Sunscreen creams, sticks, gels, and foams are preferred over spray sunscreens (AAD, 2022c). Sunscreen should be applied 30 minutes before exposure to bind to the skin and reapplied at the water-resistant interval indicated on the sunscreen bottle when swimming, after showering, and during activity that results in excessive perspiration (Hallowell & Mehlmann, 2022).

Additional sun protection actions include wearing protective cotton clothing, hats with visors, and sunglasses with UV protection during hours of peak exposure. Since the sun's rays are strongest between 10 a.m. and 3 p.m., these are the times when the most protection is needed and when exposure should be limited, especially for younger children (CDC, 2023). Adolescents should also be discouraged from using tanning beds, which present risks similar to outdoor sun (see Chapter 29).

School nurses are in key positions to provide education and guidance regarding sun exposure risk to the greatest number of children and adolescents. Because students are often outside during recess, physical education, sports activities, and field trips, it is essential that school staff understand the importance of sun safety. There are a number of programs available to be used in educating children about sun safety. The Environmental Protection Agency's *Sunwise* program and SunSmart's "Slip, Slop, Slap, Seek and Slide" are two examples (AAD, 2022c). See Box 18-2 for the CDC's sun safety recommendations for schools.

BOX 18-2

CDC Recommendations for School Sun Safety

CDC's guidelines include seven recommendations for schools from prekindergarten through 12th grade and are meant to encourage skin cancer prevention on school property and elsewhere. The recommendations are as follows:

1. **Policy.** Establish policies that reduce exposure to UV radiation.
   - Encourage scheduling of outdoor activities during times when the sun is not at peak intensity, when possible.
   - Modify building and grounds codes to increase availability of shade in frequently used outdoor spaces.
   - Encourage or require students to wear protective clothing, hats, and sunglasses.
   - Establish sunscreen use routines before going outside.
   - Support health education activities needed for skin cancer prevention.
   - Disseminate skin cancer prevention information to families.
   - Develop guidance for allocation of resources for skin cancer prevention.
2. **Environment.** Provide and maintain physical and social environments that support sun safety and are consistent with the development of other healthy habits.
   - Consider sun protection in the design of new schools.
   - Identify opportunities to extend or create new shaded areas.
   - Work with community partners to facilitate provision of sunscreen at a reduced price or fee.
   - Use visual and audio messages to remind students to engage in sun-safe behaviors.
   - Encourage all adults to be sun-safe role models.
   - Have peer educators teach students about sun safety.
   - Recognize staff and students who practice sun safety.
3. **Education.** Provide health education to teach students the knowledge, attitudes, and behavioral skills they need to prevent skin cancer. This education should be age-appropriate and linked to opportunities for practicing sun-safe behaviors.
   - Include skin cancer prevention as part of a comprehensive health education curriculum.
   - Integrate skin cancer prevention into other subject areas as well.
   - Provide skin cancer education sequentially and reinforce key messages over time, from prekindergarten through 12th grade.
   - Deliver skin cancer education during times of the year when students have the most opportunities for sun exposure and sun protection.
4. **Families.** Involve family members in skin cancer prevention efforts.
   - Educate parents about the importance of sun-safe behaviors.
   - Inform parents about school initiatives and policies and obtain their input.
   - Encourage parents to advocate for sun-safe policies and practices in the school.
5. **Professional Development.** Include skin cancer prevention knowledge and skills in preservice and in-service education for school administrators, teachers, physical education teachers and

Continued

BOX 18-2
CDC Recommendations for School Sun Safety—cont'd

coaches, school nurses, and others who work with students.
- Integrate skin cancer prevention into existing professional development activities.
- Tailor professional development activities to the responsibilities of the audience.

6. **Health Services.** Complement and support skin cancer prevention with school health services.
   - Include parental permission for use of sunscreen in the health record.
   - Use sports participation checkups to educate students about skin cancer prevention.
   - Assess patients' sun exposure patterns and reinforce sun-protective behaviors.
   - Advocate for skin cancer prevention policies and practices.
7. **Evaluation.** Periodically evaluate whether schools are implementing the skin cancer prevention guidelines. They should be evaluated on policies, environment, education, family involvement, professional development, and health services.

CDC (2023), para. 6.

CONCLUSION

The school nurse is often the first person students seek when there is a dermatological issue. Parents and teachers will also consult the school nurse for guidance to address skin disorders. Acquiring a history using nonjudgmental therapeutic communication and performing a thorough physical assessment of the involved areas (as allowed) will help the school nurse determine the possible etiologies, make referrals for medical evaluation when needed, and initiate appropriate management of the presenting skin problem.

The Editors gratefully acknowledge the 3rd Edition authors of this chapter, Leatha Ross and Janice Selekman.

References

American Academy of Dermatology. (2022a). *How to treat sunburn.* https://www.aad.org/public/everyday-care/injured-skin/burns/treat-sunburn

American Academy of Dermatology. (2022b). Poison ivy, oak, and sumac. https://www.aad.org/public/diseases/itchy-skin/poison-ivy-oak-and-sumac#overview

American Academy of Dermatology (2022c). *Shade, clothing and sunscreen.* https://www.aad.org/public/everyday-care/sun-protection/shade-clothing-sunscreen

American Academy of Pediatrics. (2022). *American Academy of Pediatrics updates report on controlling and treating head lice in children, adolescents.* https://www.aap.org/en/news-room/news-releases/aap/2022/american-academy-of-pediatrics-updates-report-on-controlling-and-treating-head-lice-in-children-adolescents/

Barnett, N. K. (2017). Alopecia and hair shaft anomalies. In T. K. McInerny, H. A. Adam, D. E. Campbell, T. G. DeWitt, J. M. Foy, & D. Kamat, D. M. (Eds.), *American Academy of Pediatrics textbook of pediatric care* (2nd ed., pp. 1188–1194). American Academy of Pediatrics.

Bland, T. (2020). Dermatologic disorders. In D. Maaks, N. Starr, M. Brady, N. Gaylord, M. Driessnack, & J. Duderstadt (Eds.), *Burns' pediatric primary care* (7th ed., pp. 567–615). Elsevier.

Blosser, C., O'Keefe, C., & Sanderson, S. (2017). Infectious diseases and immunizations. In C. Burns, A. Dunn, M. Brady, N. Starr, C. Blosser, & D. Gatzone (Eds.), *Burns' pediatric primary care* (6th ed., pp. 474–548). Elsevier.

Bolognia, J., Schaffer, J., & Cerroni L. (2017). *Dermatology* (4th ed.). Elsevier.

Bragg, B. N., & Wills, C. (2022, August 8). Pediculosis. In *StatPearls* [Internet]. StatPearls Publishing. https://www.ncbi.nlm.nih.gov/books/NBK470343/

Brzezinski, P., Borowska, K., Chiriac, A., & Smigielski, J. (2017). Adverse effects of isotretinoin: A large, retrospective review. *Dermatologic Therapy, 30*(4). https://doi.org/10.1111/dth.12483

Buckley, D. (2021). History taking and examination. In D. Buckley & P. Pasquali (Eds.), *Textbook of primary care dermatology*. Springer. https://doi.org/10.1007/978-3-030-29101-3_2

Centers for Disease Control and Prevention. (2019a). *Methicillin-resistant* Staphylococcus aureus *(MRSA).* https://www.cdc.gov/mrsa/healthcare/outpatient.html

Centers for Disease Control and Prevention. (2019b). *Parasites: Lice.* https://www.cdc.gov/parasites/lice/head/treatment.html

Centers for Disease Control and Prevention. (2020). *Head lice: Frequently asked questions.* https://www.cdc.gov/parasites/lice/head/gen_info/faqs.html

Centers for Disease Control and Prevention. (2021). *Tick bite: What to do.* https://www.cdc.gov/ticks/pdfs/FS_TickBite-508.pdf

Centers for Disease Control and Prevention. (2022). *Lyme disease, data and statistics.* https://www.cdc.gov/lyme/stats/index.html

Centers for Disease Control and Prevention. (2023, April 18). *Guidelines for school programs to prevent skin cancer.* https://www.cdc.gov/cancer/skin/what_cdc_is_doing/guidelines.htm

Centers for Disease Control and Prevention. (2024). *About parvovirus B19.* https://www.cdc.gov/parvovirus-b19/about/index.html#:~:text=The%20clinical%20presentation%20most%20often,fever%20or%20flu%2Dlike%20symptoms

Chen, C., & Williams, J. V. (2017). Verrucae (Warts). In T. K. McInerny, H. A. Adam, D. E. Campbell, T. G. DeWitt, J. M. Foy, & D. Kamat, D. M. (Eds.), *American Academy of Pediatrics textbook of pediatric care* (2nd ed., pp. 2527–2563). American Academy of Pediatrics

Food Allergy Research and Education. (2022). *Food allergy & anaphylaxis emergency care plan.* https://www.foodallergy.org/living-food-allergies/food-allergy-essentials/food-allergy-anaphylaxis-emergency-care-plan

Guo, Y., Song, G., Sun, M., Wang, J., & Wang, Y. (2020). Prevalence and therapies of antibiotic-resistance in *Staphylococcus aureus. Frontiers in Cellular and Infection Microbiology, 10:107.* https://doi.org/10.3389/fcimb.2020.00107

Habif, T. (2019). *Clinical dermatology* (7th ed.). Elsevier.

Hallowell, S., & Mehlmann, S. (June 17, 2022). *Is sunscreen safe?* Children's Hospital of Philadelphia. https://www.chop.edu/news/health-tip/sunscreen-safe

Heymann, D. (2022). *Control of communicable diseases manual* (21st ed.). The American Public Health Association.

John, R. M., & Brady, M. (2020). Atopic, rheumatic and immunodeficiency disorders. In D. Maaks, N. Starr, M. Brady, N. Gaylord, M. Driessnack, & J. Duderstadt (Eds.), *Burns' pediatric primary care* (7th ed., pp. 520–566). Elsevier.

Kim, Y., Flamm, A., Elsohly, M., Kaplan, D., Hage, R. Hamann C., & Marks, J. (2019). Poison ivy, oak, and sumac dermatitis: What is known and what is new? *Dermatitis, 30*(3), 180–190. http://doi.org/10.1097/DER.0000000000000472

Kimberlin, D. W., Barnett, E. D., Lynfield, R., & Sawyer, M. H. (2021). *Red book: 2021–2024 report of the Committee on Infectious Diseases.* Committee on Infectious Diseases, American Academy of Pediatrics. https://doi.org/10.1542/9781610025782

May, P. J., Tong, S. Y., Steer, A. C., Currie, B. J., Andrews, R. M., Carapetis, J. R., & Bowen, A. C. (2019). Treatment, prevention and public health management of impetigo, scabies, crusted scabies and fungal skin infections in endemic populations: A systematic review. *Tropical Medicine & International Health, 24*(3), 280–293. https://doi.org/10.1111/tmi.13198

McCann, S., Nicol, N., & Huether, S. (2017). Structure, function, and disorders of the integument. In S. Huether, K. McCance, V. Brashers, & N. Rote (Eds.), *Understanding pathophysiology* (6th ed., pp. 1053–1083). Elsevier.

McInerny, T. K., Adam, H. A., Campbell, D. E., DeWitt, T. G., Foy, J. M., & Kamat, D. M. (2017). *American Academy of Pediatrics textbook of pediatric care* (2nd ed.). American Academy of Pediatrics.

National Association of School Nurses. (2020). *Head lice management in schools* (Position Statement). https://www.nasn.org/nasn-resources/professional-practice-documents/position-statements/ps-head-lice

National Association of School Nurses. (2024). A contemporary framework update for today's school nursing landscape: Introducing the School Nursing Practice Framework. NASN School Nurse, *39*(3), 140–147. https://www.doi.org/10.1177/1942602X241241092

Nicol, N., & Huether, S. (2017). Alterations of the integument in children. In S. Huether, K. McCance, V. Brashers, & N. Rote (Eds.), *Understanding pathophysiology* (6th ed., pp. 1084–1095). Elsevier.

Nield, L. S. (2017). Stomatitis. In T. K. McInerny, H. A. Adam, D. E. Campbell, T. G. DeWitt, J. M. Foy, & D. Kamat, D. M. (Eds.), *American Academy of Pediatrics textbook of pediatric care* (2nd ed., pp.2686–2689). American Academy of Pediatrics.

Nigam, P. K., Hasnain, A., & Saleh, D. (2023). *Tinea pedis.* StatPearls [Internet]. https://www.ncbi.nlm.nih.gov/books/NBK470421/#:~:text=Tinea%20pedis%2C%20also%20known%20as,and%20medial%20and%20lateral%20edges

Paller, A., & Mancini, A. (2022). *Hurwitz clinical pediatric dermatology* (6th ed.). Elsevier.

Perloff, S. (2017). MRSA skin infection in athletes. https://emedicine.medscape.com/article/108972-overview

Poladian, K., De Souza, B., & McMichael, A. (2019). Atopic dermatitis in adolescents with skin of color. *Cutis, 104*(3), 164–168.

Schwartz, A., Hinckley, A., Mead, P., Hook, S., & Kugeler, K. (2017). Surveillance of Lyme disease—United States, 2008–2015. *Morbidity and Mortality Weekly Report, 66*(22), 1–12. https://doi.org/10.15585/mmw.ss6622a1

Siegfried, E. C., Igelman, S., Jaworsk, J. C., Antaya, R. J., Cordoro, K. M., Eichenfield, L. F., & Paller, A. S. (2019). Use of dupilumab in pediatric atopic dermatitis: Access, dosing, and implications for managing severe atopic dermatitis. *Pediatric Dermatology, 36*(1), 172–176. https://doi.org/10.1111/pde.13707

Silverberg, N. B. (2019). Pediatric warts: Update on interventions. *Cutis, 103*(1), 26–27.

Soenjoyo, K. R., Chua, B. W. B., Wee, L. W. Y., Koh, M. J. A., & Ang, S. B. (2020). Treatment of cutaneous viral warts in children: A review. *Dermatologic Therapy, 33*(6). https://doi.org/10.1111/dth.14034

Stagg, D., & McCarthy, J. (2017). Lyme disease prevention and treatment: Education and early detection lead to the best outcomes. *American Nurse Today, 12*(6).

Tan, J. K., Gold, L. S., Alexis, A. F., & Harper, J. C. (2018). Current concepts in acne pathogenesis: Pathways to inflammation. *Seminars in Cutaneous Medicine & Surgery, 37*(3S), S60–S62.

U.S. Food and Drug Administration. (n.d.). *Sun protection factor (SPF).* https://www.fda.gov/about-fda/center-drug-evaluation-and-research-cder/sun-protection-factor-spf

Young, A., & Tewari, A. (2022). Sunburn. *UpToDate.* http://www.uptodate.com/contents/sunburn

part V

Caring for Students With Special Healthcare Needs

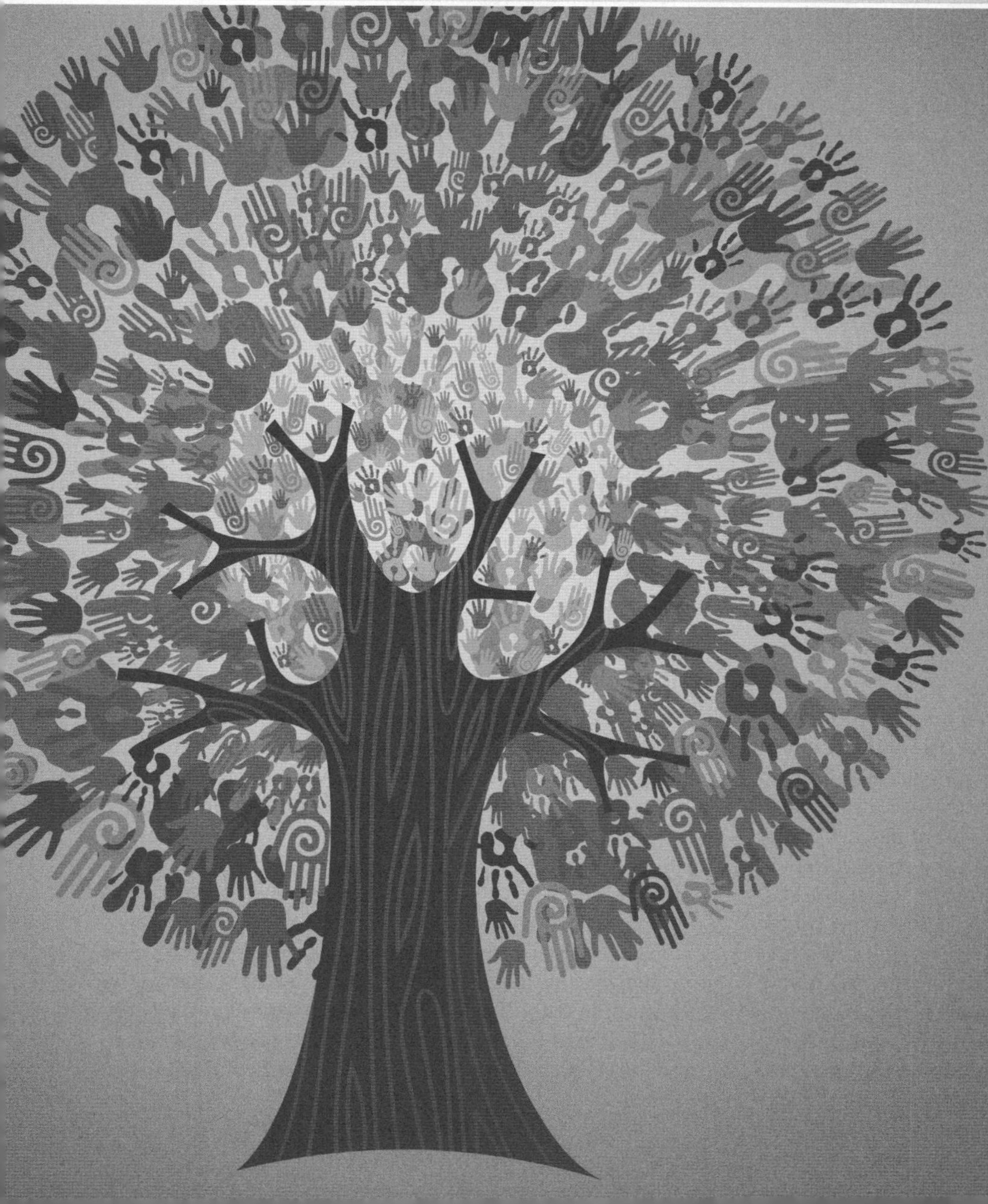

Chapter 19

Students Who Are Pregnant and Parenting

Sally Lemke ▪ Katherine L. Dato

CHAPTER OUTLINE

It is imperative that schools support pregnant students throughout the perinatal period. These students may have complex physical, social, and emotional needs requiring the assistance of the school nurse. Other interdisciplinary team members, such as counselors, school psychologists, and social workers, may also work with the student to help them successfully complete their education. Once the student learns of the pregnancy, they face many decisions. The student must decide if they desire to maintain the pregnancy and become a parent, maintain the pregnancy and develop an adoption plan, or terminate the pregnancy through abortion. The pregnancy, delivery, and postpartum recovery period can take a tremendous physical and emotional toll on the teen, their family, and the father of the baby. The purpose of this chapter is to discuss the implications of teen pregnancy and the school nurse's role in supporting students who are pregnant and parenting.

INCIDENCE AND PREVALENCE

When determining the incidence and prevalence of teen pregnancies, it is important to consider the ages used in the collection of data. Most statistics on pregnancy refer only to the 15- to 19-year age range, while others subdivide these into teens 15 to 17 and 18 to 19 years old. There are separate statistics for those 14 years of age and younger. There has been a steady decline in teen birth rates in the United States since 1991, with a continued decline for all races (Osterman et al., 2023). In 2021, there were 158,043 live births to mothers 15 to 19 years of age, a birth rate of 13.9 per 1,000 females 15 to 19 years of age. This was a 7% drop from 2020 and represents a record low for the United States (Osterman et al., 2023). See Figure 19-1.

Disparities exist in which teenagers experience pregnancy and birth. In 2021, the birth rate for Hispanic women ages 15 to 19 was 21.1 per 1,000 women, more than two times higher than their non-Hispanic white peers (9.4). The non-Hispanic black teen birth rate was 21.8 per 1,000. The highest birth rate was seen in American Indian or Alaska native women at 24.2 per 1,000 (Osterman et al., 2023). Teens in foster care or in the child welfare system are at a higher risk for pregnancy than others of their age; these teens are twice as likely to become pregnant compared with those not in foster care (Centers for Disease Control and Prevention [CDC], 2024b). State-specific variations in teen birth rates ranged from 5.4 per 1,000 teen births in New Hampshire for 15- to 19-year-olds, to 26.5 per 1,000 teen births in Arkansas. States in the southern United States have the highest teen birth rates, including Alabama, Arkansas, Mississippi, New Mexico, Oklahoma, and Texas. Connecticut, Massachusetts, New Hampshire, New Jersey, and Vermont were among those with the lowest rates (Osterman et al., 2023).

Some evidence suggests that the decline in teen birth rates may be a result of more teens abstaining from sexual activity, delaying the initiation of sexual activity, and using more birth control when sexually active, especially long-acting reversible contraceptives. Data on teen birth rates suggests a clear connection between social determinants of health and teen birth (World Health Organization [WHO], 2022); further decreases in teen birth rates could be attained by addressing the social and structural determinants of health that are "the conditions in which people are born, grow, work, live, and age and the wider set of forces and systems shaping the conditions of daily life" (WHO, 2023, para. 1).

Despite the decline in teen births, the rate of teen pregnancy in the United States continues to be higher than in most Western industrialized nations (Office of Population Affairs [OPA], n.d.). One factor that may be keeping the United States teen birth rate higher is income inequality. Reducing poverty rates and income inequalities while increasing investments in education are significant national policies that could reduce teen childbearing and their ability to afford to properly care for their child (CDC, 2024b).

The most recent examination of *repeat* birth rates studied trends between 2004 and 2015 (Dee et al., 2017). In 2025, the number of repeat births to women 15 to 19 years old declined significantly, but there were still 38,324 repeat births, which accounts for 16.7% of all teen births. This percentage varies from state to state with Vermont being the lowest at 10.6% to 21.4% in the District of Columbia. Repeat teen births were most prevalent in the Hispanic population (18.7%), followed by the non-Hispanic black population (17.9%), and then the non-Hispanic white population (14.3%). Despite the decline in repeat pregnancies in recent years, teens who are already parents present a unique opportunity for the school nurse related to health teaching and secondary pregnancy prevention (Dee et al., 2017).

According to the Guttmacher Institute (2019), teens have sex for the first time at about the age of 17, with most teens' first sexual partner (75% of females and 48% of males) being someone with whom they were in a relationship. Additionally, most teens report using contraceptives

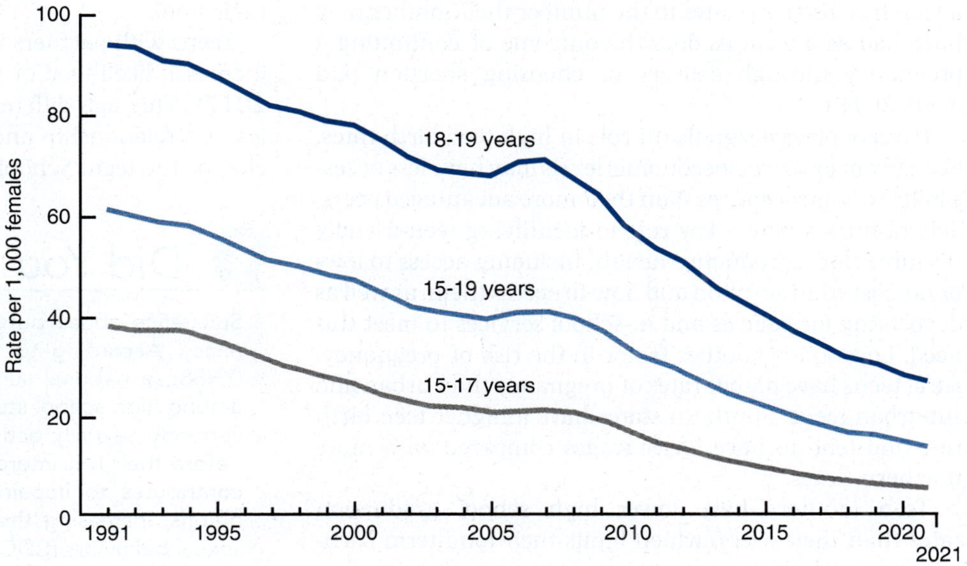

FIGURE 19-1. Birth rates for teenagers, by age of mother, United States, final (1991 to 2020) and provisional (2021). (Hamilton et al., 2022)

at both first sex and most recent penile-vaginal sex, with condoms being the contraceptive method most used.

In 2017, approximately 25% of pregnant 15-to 19-year-olds terminated their pregnancy, while nearly 60% of pregnancies in this age group resulted in birth (OPA, n.d.). Reasons given for the decision to have an abortion include concern about how their life would change and not feeling like they are mature enough to raise a child.

PREGNANCY RISK AND PROTECTIVE FACTORS

According to the CDC (2024b), nearly 75% of teen pregnancies are unplanned. These unintended pregnancies are associated with greater risk to the pregnant teen and baby. Pregnant teens are twice as likely not to seek prenatal care during the first trimester of pregnancy, which can lead to premature birth.

Risk Factors

There are many factors that put teens at risk for becoming pregnant. Some include the teen's cultural and family experiences, family patterns of early sexual experience, socioeconomic status, the community in which the teen lives, the educational attainment of the teen's parents, the teen's own attitudes about pregnancy, the lack of a sex education program in the schools, or living in a foster home, among others (Youth.gov, n.d.b). Daughters of teen mothers are two to three times more likely to become parents during their teen years; this phenomenon is referred to as the intergenerational cycle of teenage childbearing (Hendrick & Maslowsky, 2019). These teens are up to three times more likely to become mothers compared with those with mothers who were not teens when pregnancy first occurred (Black, 2018). The number of pregnancies a teen has also correlates to the number their mother may have had as a teen, as does the outcome of continuing a pregnancy through delivery or choosing abortion (Liu et al., 2018).

Poverty plays a significant role in high teen birth rates. Teens from lower socioeconomic levels may have less accessibility to contraceptives than their more advantaged peers. School nurses play a key role in identifying teen-friendly resources for reproductive health, including access to low- or no-cost contraception and how to access them, as well as advocating for policies and in-school services to meet this need. Location is another factor in the risk of pregnancy; rural teens have higher rates of pregnancy than urban and suburban teens. Southern states have a higher teen birth rate and tend to have lower wages compared with more northern states.

Teen mothers have lower high school graduation rates than their peers, which limits their long-term earning potential (Bullinger, 2017). However, even modest increases in the minimum wage may keep adolescents attached to the labor market, potentially increasing their future advancement opportunities, and thus provide a reason to delay childbearing or offer a chance to substitute work for leisure.

The number of families with both parents working outside of the home has increased due to shifting cultural norms and economic necessity. A decline in marriage rates and an increase in the number of single-parent families has resulted in children and teens frequently being unsupervised at home after school, placing young people at risk for involvement in early sexual activity. Adolescents with high levels of parental monitoring report less sexual activity, increased use of condoms, and fewer lifetime partners compared with their peers with lower levels of parental monitoring (Dittus et al., 2023). Providing more opportunities for after-school activities for teens might help these teens feel more connected to and supported by the school. School connectedness has been found to be a protective factor, especially in communities where teens experience hardship (Goetschius et al., 2023). A school that provides access to before- and after-school programming helps fill the gaps in adult supervision many teens experience.

A history of physical or sexual abuse is another risk factor for an unintended pregnancy. Youth who are involved with child protective services have higher rates of adolescent pregnancy even when controlling for race, ethnicity, and income level (Font et al., 2019; Garwood et al., 2015). One study demonstrated that teenagers with a history of childhood sexual abuse were 4.6 times more likely to present with pregnancy compared with teenagers without this history (Fortin-Langelier et al., 2019). School nurses should monitor for signs of abuse in all students but should pay particular attention to pregnant teens because the incidence of abuse for these students is disproportionately high. As mandated reporters, it is essential for the school nurse to understand the child abuse reporting process in their state.

Teens with partners who are 3 to 5 years older have an increased likelihood of becoming pregnant (Masho et al., 2017). This age difference can influence power dynamics in a relationship and increase the risk of sexual coercion of the teen. School nurses can talk with teens about

Did You Know?

Substance abuse puts students at risk for teen pregnancy. According to the Youth Risk Behavior Survey (YRBS), a national survey that assesses risk behaviors among high school students, 20.6% of teens who were currently sexually active drank alcohol or used drugs before their last intercourse. Use of alcohol and drugs contributes to impaired judgment and lowered inhibitions, increasing the likelihood of engaging in risky sexual behaviors (CDC, 2023b).

making informed choices when deciding who to date and talking about the characteristics of healthy relationships. School nurses can also be involved in efforts to educate and engage parents in their support of informed sexual decision making by their teens.

Another common risk factor is early pubertal development. Early puberty does not correlate with earlier brain maturation; consequently, young teens have mature bodies and immature decision-making abilities. Early puberty can have a significant impact both socially and psychologically on the teen and increase risk of depression, substance use, and early sexual activity (Mendle et al., 2019). School nurses need to support these young teens and preteens and recognize their unique developmental needs with targeted education.

School nurses should work with the school team to ensure that the school sexual health education curriculum includes evidence-based risk reduction strategies. The school nurse can participate in the development and delivery of this content. Today's teens have a substantial amount of exposure and easy access to adult-oriented sexual content from a broad range of media, including television and streaming services, Internet, music, social media, and games. These influence teen perceptions of the prevalence of sexual activity, encouraging earlier initiation of sex because of overestimation of sexual activity among their peers. Exposure to sexually explicit media at the beginning of adolescence relates to risky sexual behavior over the adolescent period (Lin et al., 2020). As a positive, the Internet and social media have also increased teen access to private, confidential sexual health services as well as accurate, teen-centric sexual health information. Honest discussions with teens about how sex is used and abused by the media and what constitutes positive online content are essential.

It is age-appropriate that teens are curious about sex and exploring their sexuality. Some teens feel the need to prove that they are "sexually normal" or "grown up"; others are rebelling against their families. Many who get pregnant describe peer pressure and the desire to belong to a group or be "loved" by someone. Adolescence is also a time when young people are actively exploring and questioning their sexual orientation and gender identity. The number of teens who identify as "nonheterosexual," or lesbian, gay, or bisexual, increased from 8.3% in 2015 to 25.8% in 2021 per the YRBS (CDC, 2023b). Many youths have embraced the term "queer" to express identity outside of straight and/or cisgender definitions. The school nurse should *not* assume that youth who are lesbian, gay, bisexual, transgender, queer, or identify otherwise along the sexual orientation and gender spectrum (LBGTQ+) are at decreased risk for pregnancy. LGBTQ+ youth report increased sexual risk-taking behavior and rates of sexual violence, increasing their risk for unintended pregnancy (Johns et al., 2019). School nurses should provide a safe and affirming environment for discussion of pregnancy-related issues for LGBTQ+ students.

Students With Disabilities

Adolescents with disabilities are as sexually curious as other adolescents and have many of the same desires to feel valued and desired in social relationships but routinely do not receive adequate sexual education and reproductive care (Houtrow et al., 2021). Teens with disabilities have the same sexuality and sexual health needs as other teens; they may also express interest in having a family and children. Studies indicate that teens with disabilities are more likely to have had sexual intercourse compared with their peers without disabilities (Horner-Johnson et al., 2021). There also appears to be a lower uptake of contraception in teens with disabilities than in their peers without disabilities (Senders & Horner-Johnson, 2022). However, teachers and parents may be reluctant to discuss sexuality with their teens due to a lack of knowing what to say. School nurses can share community resources and materials to assist parents/guardians and advocate for appropriate sexual education for students with and without disabilities (National Association of School Nurses [NASN], 2022).

Preventive/Protective Factors

Just as there are risk factors for teen pregnancy, there are protective factors that work to guard against teen pregnancy. Being enrolled and engaged in school can serve as a protective factor for the prevention of teen pregnancy. Participating in after-school activities, athletics, or clubs, having positive attitudes toward school, and performing well educationally reduce the likelihood of early sexual initiation (Office of Adolescent Health, n.d.b). Open communication with parents and guardians or other adult mentors about accurate contraception use and access is vital. Parents can also be a protective factor against teen pregnancy as those with open communication and parental support are less likely to experience teen pregnancy (Youth.gov, n.d.b). Teen pregnancy prevention programs should focus on the specific needs of the teens in the school's community, consider social and emotional learning needs, and be evidence-based (Office of Adolescent Health, n.d.a). Teens who received formal sex education before their first sexual experience report healthier sexual behaviors as they progress through their teen years. Teens who received sex education that included comprehensive information on abstinence and contraceptive choices were older at first sexual contact and were more likely to have used condoms or another form of contraception (Masho et al., 2017).

With a knowledge of prevention strategies and the consideration of the needs of those most at risk, the school nurse can work with the school team to develop targeted education programs for high-risk groups. Sex education for all students should be aimed at making informed choices about sexual activity and healthy relationships. When the school nurse develops trusting relationships with students, students may be more willing to come to the health office with questions and concerns.

> **Focus on the Framework**
>
> Within the National Association of School Nurses' *School Nursing Practice Framework* is guidance to provide student-centered care (NASN, 2024). When working with parenting teens, needs will vary and ebb and flow as they move through the experience of becoming parents. As the school nurse provides health education and works to coordinate and eliminate access to care barriers for the teen parent and child, the school nurse operates under the principles of **Care Coordination** and **Community/ Public Health.**

CONFIRMING PREGNANCY AND PARENTAL NOTIFICATION

Diagnosing Pregnancy

The school nurse is frequently the first adult the student, and sometimes a partner, contacts for advice or help when concerned about health issues for either a known or suspected pregnancy. Sometimes the student is unaware that the complaints being reported are those of potential pregnancy. The concerns may be worries over a missed period, breast tenderness, or nausea and vomiting. Based on the nurse's assessment of the student's chief complaint, it is within the scope of practice to ask about other signs and symptoms of pregnancy, sexual activity, use of contraceptives, and the date of the last period.

Some teens may have purchased a pregnancy test kit and will tell the nurse the results of the test. The early diagnosis of pregnancy has become revolutionized by the development of sensitive and highly specific over-the-counter tests for pregnancy, many of which are relatively inexpensive. These tests measure human chorionic gonadotropin and are about 99% accurate depending on how they are used, when they are used, and the brand of the test (Office of Women's Health, 2021). Students should be informed that results may vary based on the reliability of the test and encouraged to have a medical provider confirm the pregnancy.

Delayed confirmation of pregnancy can limit a teen's access to certain services, including early abortion services, or delay entry to prenatal care, resulting in increased risk to the pregnancy and child. The school nurse can assist the teen in getting timely medical confirmation of the pregnancy by finding an appropriate healthcare provider. Some school-based health clinics perform pregnancy testing, depending on state statutes and school district guidelines. Getting confirmation of the pregnancy from a healthcare provider with whom the student already has a relationship may be helpful (American Academy of Pediatrics [AAP], 2022a). In other instances, the teen may worry about a lack of confidentiality in speaking with an established healthcare provider and may benefit from referral to clinics and services designed to protect a minor's right to privacy for these circumstances.

For most teens, receiving a positive pregnancy result elicits many emotions. Initial reactions may be surprise, denial, fear, and confusion, which may affect the teen's ability to fully comprehend the diagnosis and its implications. The school nurse should affirm and normalize the range of emotions the teen may be feeling. The pregnant teen will likely need support for the emotional, moral, and financial challenges and discussions that will need to be faced. It is important that the teen be counseled in an environment of acceptance and confidentiality as early feelings about the pregnancy and decisions regarding the future are explored. The school nurse can provide the sensitivity and understanding needed to support a pregnant student in the next steps.

Studies show that pregnant teens feel varied levels of stigma because of their pregnancy. Teens have reported that when others stigmatize them due to their pregnancy they feel shame, fear, anger, resentment, and worthlessness. School nurses should be supportive but cautious about giving special attention, which can cause further stigmatization. Recommendations for providing support include creating a welcoming and safe environment in the health office and providing respectful care to all students (NASN, 2023; SmithBattle, 2020).

Informing Parents

The school nurse needs to balance the student's right to confidential health care with the need for support from parents or guardians. Receiving a diagnosis of pregnancy is a sensitive time for the teen, their partner, and each of their families. If the teen has confirmed the pregnancy but has not told their parent/guardian, the school nurse may offer to assist the teen in informing them. There is great benefit to having a supportive teen's parent/guardian or other trusted adult as an integral part of the care team. Often, the law and school policy and procedures do not clearly define when or if the school nurse should or must notify the parents/guardian about a possible pregnancy. Most states currently allow minors to consent for prenatal care, which includes medical visits and labor and delivery. However, in some states, the healthcare provider is at liberty to decide to inform the parents/guardians when they determine it is in the minor's best interest (Guttmacher Institute, 2023a). The school nurse must be aware of federal laws about parental notification, as well as any specific state regulations and school policies, and proceed accordingly. The school nurse should also inform the teen of their rights within the same scope.

If the teen decides to provide notification to their parents/guardians on their own, the school nurse can explore timing and methods with the teen, and practice language for the disclosure. If the teen consents to including the school nurse in parental/guardian notification, the nurse may contact the parent/guardian and request they attend a nurse/parent conference in the school nurse's office, or the nurse may go with the student to their home if this

Did You Know?

Many states explicitly permit all or some minors to obtain contraceptive, prenatal, and sexually transmitted infection (STI) services without parental involvement. Nearly every state permits minor parents to make important decisions on their own regarding their children. In sharp contrast, most states require parental involvement in a minor's abortion. Several states have no relevant policy or case law; in these states, medical providers commonly provide medical care without parental consent to minors they deem mature, particularly if the state allows minors to consent to related services. An overview of state-specific laws can be located at the Guttmacher Institutes Web site (Guttmacher Institute, 2023a).

practice is permitted by school policy. The advantage of hosting a meeting in the school environment is that help is more readily available if the parent/guardian becomes angry by the news of the pregnancy. For some, the advantage of making a home visit is that parents/guardians and the teen may feel more comfortable in the home setting. The teen's feelings about the anticipated reactions of the parents/guardians to the disclosure are a crucial factor to consider in determining where the discussions take place. It is wise to have another school support professional, such as the social worker, attend the home visit as well. It is important that the nurse document the home visit regarding informing the parent/guardian and any referrals made for counseling or prenatal care.

INITIAL COUNSELING AND DECISIONS IN EARLY PREGNANCY

Once the pregnancy is confirmed, it is important that the teen be counseled in an environment of acceptance and confidentiality as feelings about the pregnancy and decisions regarding the future are explored (AAP, 2022a). Comprehensive options counseling consists of a nondirectional, accurate discussion of (1) continuing the pregnancy and raising a child, (2) continuing the pregnancy and making plans for adoption, or (3) terminating the pregnancy through abortion.

Initial counseling of the pregnant teen by the school nurse about pregnancy options is important in establishing trust and reinforcing the school nurse as a source of support, information, and guidance, no matter the decision. State and/or school district policy may dictate to what extent school nurses can provide comprehensive options for counseling and referral services. School nurses must be aware of their own values and beliefs about teen pregnancy and pregnancy options to remain nonjudgmental and nondirectional. When the state and school district policy allows comprehensive options counseling, options should be presented accurately while taking into consideration the teen's personal, family, spiritual, and cultural beliefs (AAP, 2022a). When considered safe and desired by the teen, including the teen's parents/guardians in decision making can be a source of strength and support for the teen. If possible and appropriate, the baby's father and his family can also be included in discussions.

Regardless of whether the school district permits discussion of comprehensive pregnancy options, school nurses should be aware of community-based clinical and counseling resources that can be provided to the teen. The school nurse can work in collaboration with the school social worker or counselor to speak with representatives of various local agencies that provide these services before the need arises; it is important to know the agency's philosophy, the services they provide, and the associated costs to determine alignment with the teen's needs.

The school nurse should be prepared to assist the student with accessing pregnancy counseling and care services that provide information on all available options in a manner that is accurate, supportive, and adheres to confidentiality guidelines. Counseling should provide support for the teen's decisions and assist with any coping that is needed. If the student reports that providers at the counseling centers were judgmental, lacked knowledge, or provided biased or hurried counseling, the teen should be helped to find another source for services. It is imperative that the school nurse maintains continued communication with the teen to ensure follow-through and access to timely care needs.

Early and ongoing support for pregnancy-related counseling and decision making has significant positive effects on the student, their academics, the pregnancy, and any parenting outcomes. With the student's permission, the school nurse can consider sharing information with other school staff or in-school partners who have a legitimate need to know and who can be of support to the student as they move through their decision-making process and subsequent care. These staff may include the school counselor, social worker, teachers, or others that the student has identified as trusted adults. Many schools have community partners who provide in-school programming and support for pregnant and parenting youth. The school nurse should document what health information is shared with whom about the pregnant teen and assist in coordinating services as appropriate.

It will ultimately be up to the teen to decide between continuing the pregnancy and raising the child, continuing the pregnancy and making plans for adoption, or terminating the pregnancy through abortion. The school nurse should support the teen and provide accurate, up-to-date information on each option as school policy permits and/ or refer to community resources that can do the same. The school nurse should continue to provide supportive counseling to ensure that timely initiation of care that aligns with the decision is achieved.

The Option to Continue the Pregnancy to Delivery and Raise a Child

When the teen has made the decision to continue with the pregnancy to deliver the child, maintaining optimal health takes priority. Early initiation of care, regular prenatal care and checkups, eating healthy, staying active, and following instructions and guidance provided by the healthcare provider are some of the responsibilities a teen needs to fulfill to maintain good health throughout the pregnancy and deliver a baby at term. The nursing interventions offered by the school nurse and assistance from other key healthcare professionals in the school and community can affect the course of the pregnancy and the birth outcomes.

In most cases, the school nurse will have more opportunity for contact with the pregnant teen during the prenatal period than other healthcare providers. Establishing agreed-upon regular "check-ins" with the pregnant teen provides the necessary time for the nurse to establish a trusting relationship with the teen. The school nurse will often be the person to whom the teen will bring questions concerning the pregnancy and the health of the fetus. The school nurse may also help the pregnant teen determine when additional assessment is needed and help with referral to a healthcare provider. In the role of advocate, the school nurse serves as a source of encouragement to the teen to practice self-care during pregnancy and to continue educational aspirations.

Juggling roles and responsibilities associated with keeping up with academic work, the stressors of adolescence, and the responsibility of managing prenatal and self-care can be challenging. Compassionate school personnel can facilitate simple accommodations to help the student cope with these added stressors. The pregnant teen's needs may include more frequent restroom privileges, extra fluids, and snacks to relieve nausea in early pregnancy or meet pregnancy-related recommendations, help carrying heavy books or book bags, and a more comfortable chair/desk in the classroom. If students wear uniforms, an adjustment for the pregnant student should be made. Although physical exercise is important for pregnant teens, the type of physical education activities may need to be modified as the pregnancy continues (March of Dimes, 2020a). Pregnant students should be encouraged to share concerns regarding accommodations while in school with the school nurse, counselor, or other staff. The school nurse can be integral in working with the school team to ensure that the pregnant teen remains healthy, active, and safe throughout the pregnancy and that barriers to learning are addressed.

Individualized Healthcare Plans

The school nurse should develop an individualized healthcare plan (IHP) for the pregnant teen (see Chapter 8 for more information on IHPs). The IHP provides guidance on how the school nurse will assess, monitor, and advise the student during pregnancy and the postpartum period. The nurse should support the student in making and attending healthcare appointments. Routine school nurse office visits should be scheduled between prenatal or healthcare provider visits so that the school nurse can monitor weight, blood pressure, and general health status. This information should be documented in the student's electronic health record, and in a separate monitoring/counseling record that the student can share with healthcare providers.

The school nurse can help identify and connect the student to programs designed to educate and prepare the teen for successful childbirth and parenting. Many programs continue support after the birth of the child and are instrumental in keeping the student on track academically. The school nurse can also maintain contact with the teen father and monitor participation in teen father group activities as needed.

Some school personnel may express concern with the extra attention paid to pregnant teens for fear that attention provides reinforcement for being pregnant and that other teens may crave similar attention and see the pregnant teen as a role model. Accommodations should be made relative to the unique needs of the pregnant teen. Interactions should be kept professional, with the health of the teen and baby being the focus of the necessary extra attention.

The Option to Continue the Pregnancy to Delivery and Make an Adoption Plan

Adoption entails transferring the legal rights and responsibilities of parenthood from the birthing person to the adopting person. Adoptions can be open or semi-open, which allows for maintenance of certain types of contact, or closed, where ongoing contact between the parties ceases.

Fewer teens are choosing to place their babies for adoption. The National Survey for Family Growth is a source of data on family life, marriage and divorce, pregnancy, infertility, use of contraception, and men's and women's health in the United States, providing limited information about who relinquishes a child for adoption (CDC, 2024f). Voluntary relinquishment of infants for adoptions nationally has declined from 9% in the 1970s to less than 1% currently for never-married women (Jones & Placek, 2017).

The prevalence of teens choosing to relinquish their babies for adoption mirrors that of all never-married women. Teens who choose to relinquish their child for adoption are more likely to have a higher socioeconomic status, have educational aspirations, and live in suburban residences. If paternity has been established, both parents should have rights related to the decision to relinquish the baby (Education for Justice, 2021).

Nearly every state permits minor parents to make the decision to relinquish their infant for adoption. State policies in 40 states and the District of Columbia either make no distinction between adult or teen parents or are explicit that teen parents may place their child up for adoption. Ten states require parental involvement in a minor's decision to place an infant for adoption and five require legal counsel for the teen during the adoption process (Guttmacher Institute, 2023b).

School nurses can support teens exploring the option of adoption by informing them about the distinct types of adoption and making referrals to agencies that can help the teen learn more and navigate the next steps. Teens who choose adoption may feel guilt, loss, and grief because of their decision (AAP, 2022a). School nurses can provide ongoing support to the teen who relinquishes parenthood by ensuring the teen has adequate psychosocial support from school counselors and social workers or community-based services.

The Option to Terminate the Pregnancy Through Abortion

The abortion rate in the United States is 11.2 per 1,000 pregnant persons and 5.8 per 1,000 teens ages 15 to 19. As teen pregnancy rates have decreased, so have abortion rates. Adolescents up to 19 years old account for only 8.2% of all abortions, a decrease in the percentage of abortions for this age range (Kortsmit et al., 2022). Abortion rates for teens ages 15 to 19 are at their lowest since abortion was legalized in 1973 (Office of Adolescent Health, n.d.b). Birth rates still exceed abortion rates, which is indicative of more teens electing to continue their pregnancies (Kortsmit et al., 2022). When a teen chooses to have an abortion, the reasons frequently given are a concern for how a baby would change their life. Teens may feel they are not mature enough to have a child and may be concerned that they will be unable to afford a baby. Research shows teens who do choose to have an abortion tend to be from higher socioeconomic backgrounds, have greater educational aspirations, and have higher self-esteem than their peers who choose childbirth; it also shows that there are disparities in access to abortion for teens living in or near poverty, from racial and ethnic minority groups, living with disabilities, and for LGBTQ+ youth (AAP, 2022b).

In 2022, the U.S. Supreme Court overturned its decision formed in 1973 that the Constitution protects the right to abortion, giving individual states the full right to determine abortion regulation not protected by federal law. This ruling has resulted in rapidly changing state laws and policies on abortion ranging from various bans to significant restrictions in some states with other states moving to formally uphold the right to abortion. Most states have laws requiring some level of parental involvement in a minor's decision to have an abortion (Guttmacher Institute, 2023c). Variations in laws range from the strictest requirement of parental notification and consent of both parents to less restrictive with notification of only one parent. Some states will allow notification of a grandparent or other adult relative. Each state decides what constitutes notification; in some states 24-hour notice is sufficient. Some states also have a provision for a bypass law so that the teen can go to court to waive the parental notification requirement. The school nurse must know the state's laws governing pregnant adolescents seeking abortions, especially the rights of the teen's parents and the rights of the father. An up-to-date summary of state laws can be found online at the Guttmacher Institute Web site (2023c). The nonprofit organization Power to Decide (2023) maintains a Web site to assist individuals to find verified abortion care and support. It should be noted that the U.S. Supreme Court has stated that a parent cannot prohibit their teen's decision to have an abortion (Advocates for Youth, 2019).

Making the decision to continue or terminate a pregnancy is difficult; the adolescent should be allowed the necessary time to sort through all available information and be provided with additional information when necessary. Adolescents who decide to terminate their pregnancy should be encouraged to do so early in the pregnancy. While most abortions in teens occur early in pregnancy, some teens delay this decision until after 13 weeks of pregnancy when the medical and psychological risks and financial costs related to abortion are significantly greater. Over 18% of those under age 15 and 9.1% of those age 15 to 19 obtained an abortion after 13 weeks of gestation (Kortsmit et al., 2022). There are many reasons for these delays, including the timing of pregnancy diagnosis, understanding abortion procedures, the need for parental consent, and barriers related to cost and transportation (Assifi et al., 2020). There also may be pressure from the father of the baby, parents, and religious groups to maintain the pregnancy.

There are two main categories of abortion: medical and surgical. Medical abortion can be provided for pregnancies 11 weeks and under and entails taking medication to end a pregnancy. Surgical abortions involve a procedure to evacuate the uterus; state law dictates how late in the pregnancy surgical abortion can take place (American College of Obstetricians and Gynecologists [ACOG], 2022). Complications after abortion, although exceedingly rare, can include infection, intrauterine blood clots, cervical trauma, and bleeding. Having an abortion does not affect one's ability to conceive and deliver a healthy baby later in life, and there are rarely long-term physical consequences (National Academies of Sciences, Engineering, and Medicine, 2018).

HEALTH CARE AND HEALTH CONCERNS DURING PREGNANCY

Prenatal Care

Early, comprehensive prenatal care is a crucial factor in a healthy outcome for the pregnant person and newborn, regardless of the person's age. When the start of prenatal care is delayed, the consequences can include infant mortality, preterm birth, or having a low-birth-weight baby (Fairchild et al., 2022; Leftwich & Alves, 2017). Adolescents express many reasons for delayed or inadequate prenatal care, such as a fear of the reaction to news of the pregnancy by parents/guardians or significant others (including the baby's father), not recognizing the pregnancy, denial of the pregnancy until the second or third trimester, not understanding the importance of early prenatal care, confusion about available services, lack of transportation, and lack of health insurance or finances.

Other difficulties and concerns mentioned by some adolescents are negotiating paperwork, their perception of negative attitudes of community clinic clerical and nursing staff, fear of healthcare providers primarily because of their lack of previous contact with them, and the lack of availability of adolescent-only clinics (Leftwich & Alves, 2017). Through familiarity with local resources that are sensitive to the unique culture of the teen parent, the school nurse can provide support to pregnant teens in navigating these barriers.

Nutrition During Pregnancy

Nutritional habits of adolescents often do not meet daily dietary recommendations for their age group (Demory-Luce, 2022). Pregnant teens should be encouraged to eat nutritious, well-balanced meals using the MyPlate.gov pregnant and breastfeeding guidelines (U.S. Department of Agriculture, 2022). Pregnant teens should choose a variety of foods from each food group each day to help provide the vitamins and minerals needed to develop a healthy baby. Pregnant teens should limit foods with large amounts of sugar and fat to help limit unnecessary weight gain. Limiting caffeine, especially energy drinks, is also beneficial. Although vitamin and mineral supplements can never replace the benefits of a healthy diet, most healthcare providers recommend the addition of a prenatal vitamin supplement that contains folic acid and, often, iron, to assist in development of the fetus.

The prevalence of obesity in adolescents is 22.2% (CDC, 2023a). This means that some teens will have an unhealthy pre-pregnancy weight, potentially affecting the pregnancy and delivery outcomes. Obesity is associated with complications for the pregnant person and immediate, as well as long-term, risks for the infant. Gestational hypertension, gestational diabetes, and pre-eclampsia are among the risks to the obese teen. The fetal risks include birth defects, being large for gestational age, preterm birth, feeding difficulties, and the possibility of fetal death or stillbirth (Ramsey & Schenken, 2024).

There are risks later in life for the offspring as well. A relationship between greater pre-pregnancy weight and greater weight gain during gestation and adverse effects to the baby, including an increased risk of developing an autism spectrum disorder or having a developmental delay, has been postulated (Windham et al., 2019). The child is also at increased risk for poorer cardiovascular health throughout the course of its life (Kankowski et al., 2022).

Weight gain during pregnancy varies for each teen and depends on pre-pregnancy weight. Teens who have a healthy pre-pregnancy weight should gain 25 to 35 pounds. A teen who is overweight should gain 15 to 25 pounds, and an obese teen should gain 11 to 20 pounds; an underweight teen should gain 28 to 40 pounds (March of Dimes, 2020d).

Although dieting is usually not recommended during pregnancy, the school nurse can play a vital role in helping the teen understand the significance of making informed food choices to maintain a healthy weight. Helping the teen at this stage of life can affect lifelong health, as well as the health of the new family. The school nurse can reinforce the healthcare provider's instructions to the pregnant teen regarding food and nutrition. If a specific diet has been suggested or dietary supplements (e.g., vitamins, iron, folic acid) are prescribed, the nurse should inquire whether the student has obtained them, review the reasons for taking them, and encourage the teen to ask questions or help clarify information that is not understood.

When counseling a pregnant teen about nutrition and food choices, it is important to consider the student's ability to afford and access healthy foods, including fresh fruits and vegetables. The school nurse can assist the pregnant teen to obtain healthy food from school, community, or governmental resources.

Did You Know?

Iron deficiency anemia is a common medical disorder of pregnancy, occurring in almost one-half of all pregnancies. Female teens are one of the primary groups with the greatest need for iron. Pregnancy increases this need, doubling the requirement because of increased blood volume, placing the teen at risk for iron deficiency.

Symptoms of iron deficiency can include fatigue, headache, light-headedness, difficulty maintaining body temperature, and exercise intolerance. Iron deficiency anemia during pregnancy can cause low birth weight, premature birth, or even death of the baby at birth. The current minimum recommended supplementation for nonanemic women during pregnancy is 30 mg of ferrous sulfate, most of which can be obtained through prenatal vitamins (National Institutes of Health, 2023).

Preventing Neural Tube Defects

Neural tube defects occur within the first month of pregnancy when the neural tube does not close completely (March of Dimes, 2022a). Each year, about 3,000 pregnancies in the United States are affected by neural tube defects such as spina bifida. More than one-half of these defects could have been prevented with daily intake of at least 400 mcg of synthetic folic acid from supplements or fortified foods throughout the childbearing years (CDC, 2024a). Folic acid deficiency, together with the fact that the eating habits of many teens do not meet recommended standards, places the teen at risk for having a baby with neural tube defects. A major concern is that many teens' pregnancy diagnoses and prenatal care do not occur until after the neural tube is formed.

The U.S. Food and Drug Administration (USFDA) established standards for fortifying cereal and grain products (e.g., cereal, bread, rice, and pasta) with folic acid to better supply this important dietary supplement (USFDA, 2024). Naturally occurring sources of folic acid (vitamin B) include dark green leafy vegetables, beans, peas, lentils, broccoli, asparagus, oranges, and orange juice.

The link between adequate intake of folic acid and the incidence of neural tube defects, the devastating effects of iron deficiency anemia on the pregnant teen and fetus, and dietary choices of many adolescents make a compelling case for school nurse intervention with all adolescents to improve birth outcomes for all pregnancies. The school nurse can make presentations in the classroom and provide resources for health education and parenting teens. The school nurse has opportunities for spontaneous or planned teaching about nutrition and health to guide young people in making healthier choices regarding their nutrition.

Immunizations

The Advisory Committee on Immunization Practice (ACIP) of the CDC (2021) gives specific recommendations for vaccines that can and should be administered and those that are contraindicated during pregnancy. State laws often require immunizations for school attendance, including for adolescents. If a required vaccine is contraindicated for pregnancy, then it should be considered a medical exemption. Pregnant adolescents not currently protected should receive influenza (inactivated) and tetanus, diphtheria, and pertussis (Tdap) vaccinations (CDC, 2021). Those who are pregnant or were recently pregnant are at increased risk of complications from COVID-19, including severe illness and hospitalization (ACOG, 2023). Evidence shows that COVID-19 vaccination is safe in pregnancy and breastfeeding. It is recommended that pregnant and breastfeeding persons follow guidelines from health officials for COVID-19 vaccination and boosters (CDC, 2024c). Live virus vaccines are generally contraindicated during pregnancy because of the theoretical risk for transmission of the vaccine virus to the fetus; this includes influenza (live attenuated), measles, mumps, rubella, and varicella. Other vaccines are not usually required unless the pregnant teen is traveling to a specific location or there is an outbreak of the disease (CDC, 2021).

Medications During Pregnancy

The USFDA has assigned a pregnancy risk category to medications that are systemically absorbed based on available clinical and preclinical information. The five categories—A, B, C, D, and X—reflect a drug's potential to cause birth defects, with X being most likely to cause fetal anomalies; however, less than 10% of drugs approved by the USFDA have enough information to determine the risk factor to cause birth defects (CDC, 2024e). In 2018, new categories were initiated: affecting pregnancy (including labor and delivery), affecting lactation, and affecting females and males of reproductive potential (USFDA, 2021). Although all drugs are best avoided during pregnancy whenever possible, this new rating system permits an assessment of the risk/benefit ratio should a medication be required. The school nurse should advise pregnant teens not to stop any prescription medication until first speaking with their healthcare provider, who will be able to advise them on the benefits and risks of the medication to them and the baby.

Certain over-the-counter medications are known to cause problems in pregnancy, and teens should be specifically cautioned against taking anything over the counter without first speaking with their healthcare provider. These include nonsteroidal anti-inflammatory drugs and aspirin, including aspirin-containing products, as they may increase bleeding during pregnancy and at delivery, in addition to other more serious issues such as spontaneous abortion and renal impairment in the fetus (USFDA, 2020).

Herbal preparations are becoming increasingly popular and are easily accessible in health food, grocery, and drug stores. The FDA does not regulate these products for potency or content, nor does it study their claims of health benefits. Because they are advertised as "natural" and "traditional," some adolescents and adults do not consider them to be medications and do not realize they may be harmful to the pregnant person or developing fetus. Teens should also be cautioned against taking over-the-counter vitamins, because they may contain doses of vitamins and minerals that are too high and could harm the fetus. They should take only prenatal vitamins recommended by their healthcare provider to ensure that they are receiving adequate doses of iron and folic acid (March of Dimes, 2020c).

Smoking, Illegal Drugs, and Alcohol

Almost everything ingested in the body during pregnancy is passed on to the fetus (National Institute on Drug Abuse, 2020). Nicotine and other pollutants in cigarettes and vaporizers, alcohol, prescription medications, over-the-counter drugs, marijuana, illegal drugs, and many chemical products used for cleaning or as plant and insect killers may be dangerous to the pregnant person and to the fetus. Some of the consequences of exposure to these substances include miscarriage, preterm birth, low-birth-weight newborns, congenital anomalies, growth retardation, central nervous system abnormalities, and learning difficulties. Cigarette smoking is one of the major hazards of pregnancy, resulting in increased risk for spontaneous abortion, prenatal mortality, decreased fetal growth, and delayed childhood development. Parenting teens should not smoke because infants exposed to cigarette smoke are up to three times more likely to die of sudden infant death syndrome (SIDS). Secondhand smoke has many of the same effects as direct smoke inhalation (March of Dimes, 2019).

The 2021 YRBS found that 22.7% of high school students drank alcohol at least 1 day in the 30 days before the survey, while 10.5% reported binge drinking (CDC, 2023b). There is no safe time or amount of alcohol to drink during pregnancy (CDC, 2024d). High rates of unintended pregnancy among teens and delayed entry to prenatal care increase the likelihood of early fetal alcohol exposure. Alcohol consumption by pregnant teens can result in the development of fetal alcohol syndrome, which causes significant deficiencies in the child's cognitive development (see Chapter 26).

Marijuana is the most common illicit substance used by adolescents with 15.8% of adolescents reporting having used the substance at least once in the 30 days before completing the 2021 YRBS (CDC, 2023b). While more research is needed, marijuana has not been proven to be safe in pregnancy and may result in problems for a baby, including premature birth and problems with brain development (March of Dimes, 2020b).

While no state currently criminalizes the use of drugs during pregnancy, 24 states and the District of Columbia classify drug use during pregnancy as child abuse, and 25 states and the District of Columbia require healthcare providers to report suspected drug use during pregnancy (Guttmacher Institute, 2023d). Emphasis must be placed on drug treatment during pregnancy, as well as access to an inpatient drug treatment program, if necessary. Pregnant teens, in general, should be advised about the effects of alcohol and drugs during pregnancy and their impact on the health of the baby.

Spontaneous Abortion/Miscarriage

Miscarriage, or spontaneous abortion, is defined as pregnancy loss before 20 weeks of gestation and occurs in approximately 10% to 15% of all pregnancies. Spontaneous abortion is usually the result of abnormal chromosomes in the developing embryo or fetus (March of Dimes, 2023). Most miscarriages cannot be prevented, and some occur even before a person misses a period or has knowledge of a pregnancy. Ectopic or extrauterine pregnancy results when a pregnancy attaches to an area other than the uterus, such as a fallopian tube or ovary. Ectopic pregnancies always result in pregnancy loss. Without treatment, an ectopic pregnancy can progress to the point of rupturing the structure to which it is attached, causing serious complications, including death. Ectopic pregnancies occur in 1 out of every 50 pregnancies and are often the result of irregular fallopian tubes resulting from an STI or pelvic inflammatory disease (March of Dimes, 2017).

Bleeding, spotting, cramping, or low backaches are frequent complaints during pregnancy but are also symptoms of a potential miscarriage and ectopic pregnancy. School nurses should refer pregnant teens who report these symptoms to their healthcare provider for further diagnosis and care. Approximately one-half of those who bleed during early pregnancy do not go on to miscarry. However, if a miscarriage is inevitable, in process, or incomplete, a healthcare provider should be consulted to determine whether there is a need for medical or surgical intervention to remove pregnancy-related tissue from the uterus to prevent infection. This is necessary in about one-half of cases of miscarriage (American Pregnancy Association, n.d.b). If a teen receives medical or surgical treatment for a miscarriage, written permission from a healthcare provider may be necessary before resuming some activities.

No matter how early the pregnancy loss occurs, a powerful sense of bonding may have already occurred, and the loss can be accompanied by a range of emotions. The school nurse should acknowledge the pregnancy and loss and provide resources for support. It may also present an opportunity for the school nurse to talk to the teen about prevention and protection in future sexual encounters. The timing of this conversation is key. For others, there may be grief and an intense sense of loss or self-blame. Anger, disappointment, and grief may be misunderstood or misinterpreted by friends and family and may be vastly different from that of a partner (American Pregnancy Association, n.d.a). School nurses can help guide teens in need of emotional support after a pregnancy loss to appropriate school and community counseling resources.

Sexually Transmitted Infections

It is estimated that one-half of all new incidences of STIs are in young people ages 15 to 24; one in four sexually active females has an STI (CDC, 2024h). Adolescents are at increased risk for acquiring STIs, including human immunodeficiency virus (HIV), due to both physiological and behavioral reasons. The maturational stages of the adolescent cervix results in an increased susceptibility to STIs such as chlamydia and human papillomavirus (HPV; CDC, 2024h). Adolescents are also at a greater risk for acquiring STIs because they may be more likely to have multiple (sequential or concurrent) sexual partners rather than a single long-term relationship, and they may select partners at a greater risk for STIs (Miller et al., 2017). Adolescents also have rates of condom use at last intercourse of just a little over 50% (Szucs et al., 2020).

Screening for STIs in pregnancy is a routine part of adolescent prenatal care. STIs can result in pregnancy-related complications that include miscarriage, ectopic pregnancy, and premature birth. Some STIs can cause harm for the baby during and after birth (March of Dimes, 2022b). By supporting prompt access to prenatal care for pregnant teens, the school nurse can promote timely identification and treatment of STIs.

Adolescents often lack knowledge of the symptoms of STIs, and frequently experience barriers to quality STI prevention and treatment services, including lack of insurance or ability to pay, lack of transportation, discomfort with facilities and services designed for adults, and concerns about confidentiality (CDC, 2024h). A pregnant teen may also think there is no longer a reason to use condoms since protection from pregnancy is not a concern. School nurses can counsel pregnant teens on the continued need and measures to prevent STIs throughout pregnancy. This may be on a one-to-one basis or in health education or other classes.

State and local school policies and guidelines vary in what can be taught in the classroom about human growth and development and sexuality. School nurses should be well versed in the state laws and school board policies surrounding sexual health education before introducing resources or guest presenters. In one-on-one situations, school personnel may answer any questions a student may ask so it is important for information to be accurate and presented in an unbiased and nonjudgmental manner. School nurses can use their expertise and advocacy skills to pursue changes in regulations, policies, and guidelines that restrict information that might prevent harm to students (NASN, 2022). School nurses should always be willing to advocate for the best evidence-based practice that keeps students in school healthy and ready to learn.

Hypertensive Disorders

Hypertensive disorders are among the most common medical complications during pregnancy and contribute to pregnancy-related mortality. Uncontrolled preexisting hypertension and hypertension that develops during a pregnancy can result in serious complications for the pregnant teen, including fetal growth restriction, low birth weight, and preterm birth (March of Dimes, 2024a). These complications can damage kidneys and other organs and are a major contributor to pregnancy-related death (National Heart, Lung, and Blood Institute, 2022).

Hypertensive disorders that develop during pregnancy include gestational hypertension, pre-eclampsia, and HELLP (Hemolysis, Elevated Liver Enzymes, Lowered Platelets) syndrome (March of Dimes, 2024a). Of these, pre-eclampsia is more common in first pregnancies and teen pregnancies. Pre-eclampsia is new-onset hypertension with proteinuria that develops after the 20th week of pregnancy. It occurs in about 8% of pregnancies and results in mild to severe hypoperfusion to the placenta. Pre-eclampsia is the cause for about 15% of all premature deliveries in the United States (March of Dimes, 2024a). When pre-eclampsia progresses to eclampsia, it can cause life-threatening seizures and coma. The cure for eclampsia is the delivery of the baby. School nurses who work with pregnant teens should immediately refer them to their healthcare provider if the student presents with signs and symptoms of pre-eclampsia, including swelling of the hands and face, blurred vision, headache, and unusual belly pain (March of Dimes, 2024c).

The school nurse may monitor a pregnant teen's blood pressure, recording the results in the student's healthcare record. The use of proper blood pressure technique is imperative; any notable change should result in immediate referral to the student's healthcare provider.

Preterm Birth

Preterm and *premature birth* are the terms used to define infants who are born at less than 37 weeks' gestation (March of Dimes, 2021). Although risk factors for preterm labor and birth are largely unknown, research indicates that it may be due to a combination of factors. Certain lifestyle factors and medical conditions predispose a pregnant person for preterm labor, including being overweight or underweight before pregnancy, a history of a previous preterm birth, a multifetal pregnancy, infection, hypertension, multiple abortions (miscarriages or elective), anemia, poor nutrition, having late or no prenatal care, having less than 6 months between pregnancies, and use or abuse of tobacco, alcohol, or other substances (March of Dimes, 2024d). Medical and obstetrical complications that may lead to preterm birth include pre-eclampsia, fetal distress, fetal growth restriction, abruptio placentae, and fetal death. Demographically, the preterm labor rate is 50% higher in the non-Hispanic black population than in the white population, those younger than 17 years, and those of lower socioeconomic status (CDC, 2024g).

In 2022, the CDC reported that 1 in 10 babies were born prematurely, a rise to 10.5% from the 2020 rate of 10.1%, but still a decrease from previous years. Most of the decline is attributed to the decrease in teen pregnancies during the same period (CDC, 2024g). Preterm infants who survive are at greater risk for lifelong disability, including intellectual and developmental disabilities, cerebral palsy, behavior problems (including attention deficit disorders), asthma, and some respiratory and intestinal disorders compared with full-term births (March of Dimes, 2024b).

Low Birth Weight

Low birth weight describes infants weighing less than 5 pounds, eight ounces at birth; very low birth weight refers to infants weighing 3.3 pounds or less, and extremely low birth weight refers to infants weighing 2.2 pounds or less. Neonatal mortality rates are directly proportional to the infant's weight at delivery with preterm birth a primary cause of low birth weight (CDC, 2024g). Other risk factors for low birth weight or fetal growth restriction include insufficient weight gain, poor nutritional status, smoking, alcohol, or other substances of abuse, birth defects, ingestion of chemical teratogens, chronic conditions, placental and cord anomalies, and multiple fetuses (March of Dimes, 2021).

Many of the risk factors for low-birth-weight infants can be prevented or controlled before or during pregnancy. The school nurse plays a key role in educating the teen about risk factors for low birth weight and preterm labor. Teens should be able to recognize symptoms of preterm labor that may include low, dull back pain, cramps similar to those of a menstrual cycle, pelvic pressure, abdominal cramps with or without diarrhea, and a change in vaginal discharge. The pregnant teen should consult her healthcare provider whenever these symptoms persist (March of Dimes, 2021).

EMOTIONAL AND DEVELOPMENTAL ISSUES

Psychosocial Development of Adolescents

Pregnancy and parenting present additional areas of opportunity for school nurses to support social and emotional learning. *Social and emotional learning* (SEL) is a lifelong strengths-based process during which a person acquires knowledge, skills, and attitudes that result in emotional regulation, positive goal setting, establishment and maintenance of positive relationships, and healthy decision making (Weissberg, 2019). Many school districts have embedded the principles of SEL into various areas of teaching and services. During pregnancy and parenting, the SEL needs of the teen are intensified.

Pregnant and parenting teens often struggle with the dual challenges of meeting the normative developmental needs of adolescence and the demands associated with pregnancy and becoming a parent. Continuing school during pregnancy and returning to school following the birth of a child are not easy tasks. Although still a high school student, the teen parent must learn to cope with some very adult situations and is expected to make mature decisions regarding the child.

Many pregnant teens have not yet reached cognitive or psychosocial maturity. The developmental tasks of the pregnant adolescent are complicated by the developmental tasks of pregnancy and parenting. For instance, in normal development, teenagers are typically concerned with their body size, shape, and weight (CDC, 2024b). They may frequently compare themselves with other teens and feel uncertain about their attractiveness. The increase in size and weight that accompanies pregnancy may cause feelings of embarrassment and dissatisfaction.

Most young teens (ages 12 to 14) are interested in being with their peer group; they begin to show less affection to their parents, develop a stronger sense of right and wrong, and experience pubertal changes. Although they may have physically matured, their emotional maturity is still developing. They may show some degree of self-assurance, test parental and adult authority, have self-doubts, and be rebellious. Early adolescents are still moving in and out of the world of childhood, seeking guidance and support as they attempt to define a new status and become independent. Pregnancy complicates the accomplishment of many of these tasks.

Despite the challenges faced by pregnant and parenting teens, most report a commitment to staying on track academically and being good parents (SmithBattle, 2020). By understanding and supporting the additional social and emotional learning needs of the pregnant and parenting teen, school nurses can promote skill- and relationship-building that has lifelong impacts for the teen and their child. The school nurse, in collaboration with the social worker, guidance counselor, and other school personnel, can support pregnant and parenting teens in determining education and career goals as well as a plan to achieve them. School nurses can promote the inclusion of evidence-based programming and services as well as linkage to community-based services designed to support teens who are struggling to stay in school while successfully raising their children.

Postpartum Depression

It is common for those who have recently given birth to experience feeling stressed, sad, anxious, lonely, tired, and tearful; these feelings often resolve 2 to 6 weeks after delivery without treatment. However, one in eight of people with a recent birth will continue to feel these symptoms and will develop postpartum depression. Birthing teens are at increased risk for postpartum depression (CDC, 2024i). Studies show the prevalence of postpartum depression in adolescent mothers ranges anywhere from 14% to 53%, twice that of adult mothers (Dinwiddie et al., 2018). The impact of COVID-19 on the mental well-being of those with a recent birth increased the risk of postpartum depression, with recent research showing the prevalence ranging from 22% to 44% (Sangsawang & Sangsawang, 2023).

Symptoms of postpartum depression are more severe and last longer than the postdelivery "baby blues" (American Psychological Association [APA], 2022). Postpartum depression can manifest anytime within the first year after delivery. In postpartum depression, the teen may have thoughts of hurting the baby, have no interest in caring for the baby, or have thoughts of harming themselves. The teen may experience anxiety, racing or scary thoughts, guilt, sadness and crying, inability to sleep, or sleeping continuously. If any of these symptoms last longer than 2 weeks, treatment by a healthcare provider should be considered (APA, 2022). The Edinburgh Postnatal Depression Scale (Fig. 19-2A and Fig. 19-2B) is a common tool used to screen for postpartum depression and is appropriate for use with teenagers (Levis et al., 2020). While the exact cause of postpartum depression is unknown, it is suspected that fluctuations in hormones because of the pregnancy and delivery, as well as genetic risk, may trigger the depression. Additional risks include isolation or a lack of support, increased life stressors, and having a baby with special needs (APA, 2022). Although the teen may not be in school when postpartum depression begins, the school nurse who has developed a relationship with a pregnant student can maintain contact with the student or arrange a home visit during which depression can be assessed. If any signs of depression are noted, a referral to the teen's healthcare provider or a mental health specialist should be made. Teachers working with students in the home following delivery should also be familiar with the symptoms of postpartum depression and should share their observations with school nurses and mental health staff, and the family as appropriate.

Edinburgh Postnatal Depression Scale (EPDS)

Patient Label	Mother's OB or Doctor's Name: ______________
	Doctor's Phone #: ______________

Since you are either pregnant or have recently had a baby, we want to know how you feel. Please place a **CHECK MARK** (✔) on the blank by the answer that comes closest to how you have felt **IN THE PAST 7 DAYS**—*not just how you feel today.* Complete all 10 items and find your score by adding each number that appears in parentheses (#) by your checked answer. This is a screening test; not a medical diagnosis. If something doesn't seem right, *call your health care provider regardless of your score.*

Below is an example already completed.

I have felt happy:
Yes, all of the time ____ (0)
Yes, most of the time ✔ (1)
No, not very often ____ (2)
No, not at all ____ (3)

This would mean: "I have felt happy most of the time" in the past week. Please complete the other questions in the same way.

1. I have been able to laugh and see the funny side of things:
   As much as I always could ____ (0)
   Not quite so much now ____ (1)
   Definitely not so much now ____ (2)
   Not at all ____ (3)

2. I have looked forward with enjoyment to things:
   As much as I ever did ____ (0)
   Rather less than I used to ____ (1)
   Definitely less than I used to ____ (2)
   Hardly at all ____ (3)

3. I have blamed myself unnecessarily when things went wrong:
   Yes, most of the time ____ (3)
   Yes, some of the time ____ (2)
   Not very often ____ (1)
   No, never ____ (0)

4. I have been anxious or worried for no good reason:
   No, not at all ____ (0)
   Hardly ever ____ (1)
   Yes, sometimes ____ (2)
   Yes, very often ____ (3)

5. I have felt scared or panicky for no good reason:
   Yes, quite a lot ____ (3)
   Yes, sometimes ____ (2)
   No, not much ____ (1)
   No, not at all ____ (0)

6. Things have been getting to me:
   Yes, most of the time I haven't been able to cope at all ____ (3)
   Yes, sometimes I haven't been coping as well as usual ____ (2)
   No, most of the time I have coped quite well ____ (1)
   No, I have been coping as well as ever ____ (0)

7. I have been so unhappy that I have had difficulty sleeping:
   Yes, most of the time ____ (3)
   Yes, sometimes ____ (2)
   No, not very often ____ (1)
   No, not at all ____ (0)

8. I have felt sad or miserable:
   Yes, most of the time ____ (3)
   Yes, quite often ____ (2)
   Not very often ____ (1)
   No, not at all ____ (0)

9. I have been so unhappy that I have been crying:
   Yes, most of the time ____ (3)
   Yes, quite often ____ (2)
   Only occasionally ____ (1)
   No, never ____ (0)

10. The thought of harming myself has occurred to me:*
    Yes, quite often ____ (3)
    Sometimes ____ (2)
    Hardly ever ____ (1)
    Never ____ (0)

TOTAL YOUR SCORE HERE ▶ ____

Thank you for completing this survey. Your doctor will score this survey and discuss the results with you.

Verbal consent to contact above mentioned MD witnessed by: ______________

Edinburgh Postnatal Depression Scale (EPDS). Adapted from the *British Journal of Psychiatry*, June, 1987, vol. 150 by J.L. Cox, J.M. Holden, R. Segovsky.

FIGURE 19-2A. Edinburgh Postnatal Depression Scale, page 1.

Edinburgh Postnatal Depression Scale (EPDS) Scoring & Other Information

ABOUT THE EPDS

Studies show that postpartum depression (PPD) affects at least 10 percent of women and that many depressed mothers do not get proper treatment. These mothers might cope with their baby and with household tasks, but their enjoyment of life is seriously affected, and it is possible that there are long term effects on the family.

The Edinburgh Postnatal Depression Scale (EPDS) was developed to assist health professionals in detecting mothers suffering from PPD; a distressing disorder more prolonged than the "blues" (which can occur in the first week after delivery).

The scale consists of 10 short statements. A mother checks off one of four possible answers that is closest to how she has felt during the past week. Most mothers easily complete the scale in less than five minutes.

Responses are scored 0, 1, 2 and 3 based on the seriousness of the symptom. Items 3, 5 to 10 are reverse scored (i.e., 3, 2, 1, and 0). The total score is found by adding together the scores for each of the 10 items.

Mothers scoring above 12 or 13 are likely to be suffering from depression and should seek medical attention. A careful clinical evaluation by a health care professional is needed to confirm a diagnosis and establish a treatment plan. The scale indicates how the mother felt during the previous week, and it may be useful to repeat the scale after two weeks.

INSTRUCTIONS FOR USERS

1. The mother checks off the response that comes closest to how she has felt during the previous seven days.
2. All 10 items must be completed.
3. Care should be taken to avoid the possibility of the mother discussing her answers with others.
4. The mother should complete the scale herself, unless she has limited English or reading difficulties.
5. The scale can be used at six to eight weeks after birth or during pregnancy.

Please note: Users may reproduce this scale without further permission providing they respect the copyright (which remains with the *British Journal of Psychiatry*), quote the names of the authors and include the title and the source of the paper in all reproduced copies. Cox, J.L., Holden, J.M. and Sagovsky, R. (1987). Detection of postnatal depression: Development of the 10-item Edinburgh Postnatal Depression Scale. *British Journal of Psychiatry*, 150, 782-786.

FIGURE 19-2B. Edinburgh Postnatal Depression Scale, page 2.

Grieving for the Lost Child

Perinatal loss includes fetal death, stillbirth, premature birth resulting in death, loss of the infant after relinquishing it for adoption, and death caused by sudden unexplained infant death (SUID) and sudden infant death syndrome (SIDS), birth defects, disease, or unintentional injury. When perinatal loss occurs, the school nurse may be a strong support for the teen. Regardless of cultural background, the deep sense of loss and sorrow is nearly universal and can be overwhelming regardless of the length of the pregnancy or age of the infant.

Grief related to pregnancy or newborn loss may be complicated by the fact that the developmental tasks of adolescence may have been interrupted by the pregnancy. Developmentally, teens often look to others outside of their family for support. Following the loss of the baby, the teen may grieve differently than adults. Grief is a natural process experienced after death and loss; it will be unique to each individual teen and there is no "right or wrong" way to grieve (The Dougy Center, 2021).

Teens experiencing loss may not be able to concentrate, they may be emotionally unpredictable, and their emotions may be very intense. They may be unable to discuss their grief with parents or caregivers, may have thoughts of suicide or self-harm, or may experience a lack of appetite or be unable to sleep (The Dougy Center, 2021). Emotions may be further exacerbated by the reaction of one parent who is grieving the loss and the other who sees the event as a relief from the major changes that were about to take place in their lives.

The grief experience is a process that never ends. It will change over time, and likely, the intensity of the grief will decrease. Grief may be felt immediately by the teen, then dissipate and then return, especially on the anniversary of the child's birth, death, or adoption, including termination of the pregnancy. The school nurse can help teen parents by allowing them to ask questions, being open and honest with the teen, and just listening to them. If you do not have the answers to the questions they are asking, tell them you do not know and that you will find out and get back to them. If it is a question with no answer, let them know that too. Suggest support groups but allow them the choice to say no. Acknowledge their need for privacy; teens are struggling developmentally for independence and seeking privacy may be a way to express their independence (The Dougy Center, n.d.).

Adolescents who experience loss through adoption or foster care placement may not be able to understand or verbalize their feelings. The school nurse should continue to engage the adolescent in conversation privately and with sensitivity. The nurse needs to use compassionate inquiry to assess for signs and symptoms of grief and/or depression. In an adoption situation, the fact that the child is still alive and thriving may result in multiple types of feelings. In all cases of loss, a referral for professional counseling should be considered. The school nurse or social worker should maintain a comprehensive list of resources for referral for adolescents who are grieving and/or depressed before a need arises.

BECOMING A PARENT

As the pregnancy continues, the prospective parents need assistance with preparation for the parenting role. Many teens who progress to delivery choose to raise the infant themselves or within their families. When the choice is made to continue the pregnancy and become a parent, the school nurse and appropriate others in the school or community should focus on providing targeted education for the teen parent. The educational needs of a parenting teen are related to the medical, educational, psychological, and economic concerns that may arise from being pregnant, as well as the future demands of parenting at this stage in their life. Incorporating the principles of social and emotional learning, the school nurse should provide the following:

- Encouragement and linkage to resources to support completion of academic or vocational training
- Counseling and referrals to healthcare services to prevent subsequent unplanned pregnancies
- Guidance on how to use existing community resources that provide support and care to pregnant and parenting adolescents and their children

Several government benefits are available to pregnant and parenting adolescents, including Medicaid and other health insurance programs, Women, Infants, and Children (WIC) services, supplementary food programming, and financial assistance (Benefits.gov, 2019). Healthy Start, a federal government program, funds pregnancy and parenting education and support programs tailored to the needs of specific communities that operate in many cities and regions (Health Resources and Services Administration, 2024). Community-based organizations located in many communities deliver additional resources and support to pregnant and parenting adolescents. School nurses and other school support staff can assist students in accessing these programs.

The Father of the Baby

There is limited information on teen fathers, mostly because there is little information collected about fathers on birth certificates. It is estimated that about 8% of men became fathers before the age of 20 (SmithBattle et al., 2019). Most teen fathers are either 18 years old (27%) or 19 years old (39%). Almost one-half of teenage fathers are white; 29% are non-Hispanic black, and 19% are Hispanic (Scott et al., 2012). Risk factors for becoming a teen father include living at or below the poverty level, having parents who were teen parents, living in a single-parent home, ethnicity, early sexual activity, low self-esteem, use of drugs and alcohol, and conflict in the home (Youth.gov, n.d.b).

Teen fathers face many of the same challenges as teen mothers. The teen father who does assume parental responsibility is faced with socioeconomic, cultural, and educational factors that may complicate his successful negotiation of the developmental tasks of adolescence. Initially, he may be no more knowledgeable about assuming the parenting role than his pregnant partner. In addition, he may face negative responses from his family, from the family of the pregnant individual, from the pregnant individual, and from others in the school and community who know of the pregnancy. He may feel isolated and alone, at a time in his life when peer relationships are of great importance (National Responsible Fatherhood Clearinghouse, n.d.).

Teen fathers are less likely to remain involved in their child's life. Compared with men who become fathers later in life, 56% of teen fathers do not live with their child by the time they reach age 22 to 24 (Scott et al., 2012). Young fathers who want to be involved in their child's life often find it difficult to obtain the support necessary to do so (SmithBattle et al., 2019). When support that is designed to meet their unique needs is provided, a teen father's involvement in both the pregnancy and parenthood can greatly increase (National Responsible Fatherhood Clearinghouse, n.d.). School personnel aware of the teen's concerns can offer many of the same support services that the pregnant individual receives. School nurses can also advocate for inclusion of evidence-based school services that address his social and emotional learning.

The concerns of the teen father may be influenced by the amount of involvement he has with the pregnant individual and the relationship that continues or does not continue after the birth of the child. If he plans to be involved during the pregnancy and childbirth process, or if he plans to remain involved after the birth, the school nurse may encourage him to enroll in and complete childbirth classes. He may also be encouraged to participate in classes about child growth and development, parenting, and childcare. These classes may provide the opportunity for him to meet and learn with other young fathers.

Programs for young men, directed at teaching parenting skills to adolescent fathers as well as preparing those teens about to become fathers, have become increasingly prevalent in schools and community settings. The Office of Family Assistance (2024) has grants and programs for males that promote responsible fatherhood and provide temporary assistance for needy families. Federal law allows each state to establish paternity laws (Justia, 2021). Fathers are allowed to initiate paternity testing if they choose. State laws require that, before testing, both verbal

Did You Know?

Parenting skills are equally important to both parents, but research shows that when the father is engaged in the child's life there are benefits to the child, such as greater academic success, more positive social behavior, better self-esteem, fewer conduct issues, less depression, and fewer instances with the juvenile justice system (The Fatherhood Project, 2015).

The degree to which the adolescent father bonds with his new baby is often dependent on his relationship with the child's mother. Studies show that many teen fathers want an active relationship with their child, but barriers exist that make this difficult (The Fatherhood Project, 2016). In some cases, the relationship with the baby's other parent is problematic or there may be financial stress in the relationship. In many instances, these fathers feel alienated and judged harshly by their parents and peers at school (The Fatherhood Project, n.d.).

and written instruction on the consequences related to child support for a positive paternity test be provided. Child support can be an important source of income for families and is intended to reduce the number of families living in poverty and dependent on public assistance. School nurses can guide teen fathers to resources and current information on paternity-related laws in their state. School nurses should encourage teen fathers to seek more information through counseling services while deciding issues related to paternity. The decisions related to paternity will be lifelong and should not be entered into without understanding all the financial, social, and emotional implications associated with paternity.

SCHOOL-BASED AND COMMUNITY RESOURCES

After the baby's birth, most adolescents benefit from follow-up and intensive support; this may be required for several years to achieve both academic success and wellness. Without support, teens and their children face significant economic hardship and educational and socioeconomic challenges.

Preventing Unwanted Repeat Pregnancies

An area of impact for school nurses is supporting the prevention of unwanted pregnancy for the teen parent. Factors important in the prevention of repeat births to teen parents are distinctively different from and less well studied than primary pregnancy prevention. In primary prevention of a first birth, for example, there may be the issue of lack of knowledge about birth control and access to services or a lack of understanding of the demands of raising an infant and how it will change a teen's life. It is assumed that with second births, these issues would be less of a mystery for the teen. Despite this experience, 16.7% of births to 15- to 19-year-olds are repeat births (Dee et al., 2017). While this number continues to decline, there is still a need for more or improved counseling and contraception for newly parenting teens. While studies have shown that repeat pregnancies in teens do not result in more physical health complications, these teens often report more negative health behaviors, including lower use of prenatal care, smoking, inadequate weight gain, and sexually transmitted infections (Maslowsky et al., 2021).

No single factor has been found to be successful in reducing rapid repeat births among teens. Successful programs include those that establish a close, sustained relationship that begins during pregnancy, have effective and professionally trained personnel, provide childcare assistance, have a family planning emphasis, and encourage high school completion. A meta-analysis of programs aimed at preventing rapid repeat teen pregnancy in clinical settings found that immediate access to postpartum contraception as well as home visiting programs had impact on preventing rapid repeat pregnancy (Frederiksen et al., 2018). School nurses can play an active role in preventing repeat births to teens by encouraging decision making during the pregnancy about postdelivery contraception and linking teens to evidence-based support programs for pregnant and parenting teens. School nurses can also encourage policies and practices that provide appropriate access to health and informational resources at school, as well as in the community, for parenting teens.

Helping Teens Stay in School

Funding and implementation of supports that help teen parents stay in school have been limited and unequally distributed across states and school districts, yet they have impact on the future of the parents and child. The COVID-19 pandemic created increased strain on these students as they had to manage complications with school and childcare while also experiencing increased worry about the health of their children (Sadeghi et al., 2021). Many states and individual school districts have comprehensive programs for pregnant teens; some school districts have schools specific for pregnant and parenting teens. School-based health centers can play a key role in supporting all aspects of academic success. A comprehensive program to help keep pregnant teens in school can include the following components:

- Meaningful connection with school personnel who create a sense of belonging
- School setting dedicated to serving teen mothers (including breastfeeding support)
- Collaboration with outside community organizations
- On-site health care
- On-site childcare

- On-site counseling and mentoring
- On-site group therapy sessions (with referrals off-site as needed)
- Academic support services
- Career preparation services
- Case management services (U.S. Department of Education, Office for Civil Rights, 2013; Youth.gov, n.d.a)

School-based programs may struggle with community expectations that the school meets the needs of parenting students. Resources for competing educational dollars are becoming more difficult to access, and school-based programs frequently struggle to meet even the basic non-educational needs of this population. Many services and supports necessary for these young families are outside of the school's domain. School nurses and school social workers may facilitate collaboration between the school and existing community-based services to provide teens with a comprehensive system. This may include assisting the student to schedule appointments for themselves and their baby and finding transportation to those appointments.

Funding Services

State and local public health and social service agencies may have monies available for use in school programs for teen pregnancy and parenting. The Office of Adolescent Health administers the Teen Pregnancy Prevention program and funds many programs to help prevent teen pregnancy. The goal is to deliver evidence-based, medically accurate, and age-appropriate programming to decrease the number of pregnant teens nationwide (Office of Adolescent Health, n.d.a). In addition, over 40% of prenatal care provided in the United States is funded through Medicaid. Medicaid-covered pregnancy care includes prenatal vitamins and ultrasounds, deliveries, and care up to 60 days postpartum (Ranji et al., 2022). Some states are examining expansion of Medicaid coverage to include home visitation by nurses and care for up to a year for the mother.

School-based health centers, a healthcare delivery model that supports access to in-school health care and services, can play a key role in supporting academic achievement for pregnancy and parenting youth (School-Based Health Alliance, n.d.). These centers eliminate many barriers to care that adolescents may face in accessing health care. Governmental and foundation funding for this evidence-based healthcare delivery model has seen an increase; school nurses can find additional information on school-based health centers on the School-Based Health Alliance Web site (sbh4all.org).

Unstable and chaotic relationships can place teen families at risk for homelessness. Alternatives for safe housing are often limited for teens; however, the U.S. Department of Housing and Urban Development (HUD; 2018) has a funding program specifically designed for teen parents and their children called *Second Chance Housing.* School nurses should research whether this or similar programs are available in their area and provide referrals for students needing safe housing.

To prevent students who are at risk from dropping out of school, state and local education agencies may commit educational funds to develop alternative instruction methodologies and other innovative educational approaches in regular and alternative schools. Several states provide funds to local school districts through formulas based on the number of teen parents served. Funds may come to the district as a supplement to the average daily attendance dollars. The average daily attendance formula may generate additional funding for pregnant students when they are attending school and for a brief period following the infant's birth. Some states require the school to use this money for core services or other programs for pregnant and parenting students, whereas others do not stipulate a requirement, and the money may go to other programs.

School nurses who see the need for a school-based program should review and incorporate best practices and inclusive approaches in their program design. They may begin by forming work groups or committees, seeking funding, writing grants, and making proposals. These workgroups may be ultimately responsible for the initiation, ongoing development, and evaluation of the program, or for identifying the persons who can assume these responsibilities. In large school districts, personnel may include the program director of health services (if this individual is not a nurse, a nurse representative should also be selected), counseling services, and/or psychological/social services or other program administrators. A team approach that includes key stakeholders will contribute to the successful development of school-based programs.

> **Practice Connection**
>
> School nurses support lactating teens and other staff by advocating for their legal right to have safe, clean lactation spaces and unpenalized time to express breast milk at school. Federal law, such as Title IX, protects against discrimination, with state law and school district policies providing additional guidance. If no lactation *policy* exists for lactating students (and staff), the school nurse can work with the school board to draft one. If no lactation *space* is designated, the school nurse and building administrator can identify and prepare a private, clean, and comfortable space with available electrical outlets (U.S. Department of Education, Office for Civil Rights, 2013).

LEGAL IMPLICATIONS OF PARENTING

Education Law

Title IX of the Education Act of 1972 prohibits discrimination in educational institutions based on sex, marital, pregnancy, or parenting status. The teen mother and father have equal rights to an appropriate education (U.S. Department of Education, Office for Civil Rights, 2013). Title IX makes it clear that pregnant and parenting students must be allowed to choose either to continue to attend their regular school or classes, or to attend an alternative program or school. Alternative schools must have instructional programs that are equal to those of other educational programs. Special programs may be provided for pregnant or parenting students, but they must be voluntary. Female teen parents cannot be required to take parenting education unless male student parents are also required to take the course (National Women's Law Center, 2016).

Title IX requires that policies regarding absences and leave of absence are the same for both nonpregnant and parenting students. Schools may not require students to be absent for a specific number of days following the infant's birth. Schools must make the same requirements for making up assignments and for home instruction for pregnant students as for any student who may be absent frequently because of a diagnosed health issue. Students may not be penalized for absences because of childbirth. If the school has a policy regarding the maximum number of days a student may be absent and still pass and this policy is waived for students with medical conditions or temporary disabilities, the policy must also be waived for pregnant and parenting students (National Women's Law Center, 2016). In addition, no restrictions can be placed on pregnant or parenting students' participation in extracurricular activities. More information on the interpretation of Title IX and details of the information to be included in drafting a school policy are available from the National Women's Law Center in Washington, DC (www.nwlc.org).

Child Abandonment Law

During the postpartum period, some teens may feel that caring for a child is beyond their ability and that the child might have their needs better met by another family. These feelings may be amplified in mothers experiencing postpartum depression, putting the health and safety of newborns at risk. Increases in the prevalence of child abandonment have contributed to the need for measures to provide for a safe and confidential means of relinquishing an infant without threat of prosecution. Every state currently has provisions for relinquishing an infant, often termed *Infant Safe Haven* laws (Child Welfare Information Gateway, 2021).

The Infant Safe Haven laws vary from state to state, including limits on the infant's age and places or persons authorized to accept an infant. Individual state laws dictate "safe haven" sites, such as hospital emergency departments, fire stations, police stations, or adoption agencies (Child Welfare Information Gateway, 2021). Anticipatory support at school can reduce the likelihood of a teen parent relinquishing their infant. The school team can help teen parents and their families anticipate and prepare for the infant's needs before birth to try to lessen some of the overwhelming feelings that come with a newborn. Developing rapport with the pregnant teen before the birth and initiating a counseling referral for students who may be at risk for abandoning their infant can be instrumental in providing support for the teen family. However, supporting struggling/overwhelmed teens requires the school nurse to be well-versed in the options available for teen parents.

CONCLUSION

Despite declining rates of teen pregnancy and live births, teen pregnancy is often viewed as a "crisis" by the media, as well as by others. Although there is considerable evidence that teen parenting presents a unique set of challenges worthy of continued focus on pregnancy prevention efforts, the school nurse plays a key role in helping these teens move beyond pregnancy and toward the broader picture of young families as valued partners in decision making and primary caregivers for their children. The outcomes of successful school and community programs for pregnant and parenting teens include students who have a healthy pregnancy, have a healthy baby, complete high school, have no unintended repeat pregnancies, have adequate parenting skills, and provide a healthy start for their child.

The support and understanding of school personnel can assist the pregnant teen through this monumental time in their life and their partner's life. They will be successful and able to provide a successful life for their family with this support. School nurses can offer emotional support by fostering communication between the parent and pregnant or parenting student and connecting the pregnant student to resources within the community. These efforts by the nurse and school staff assist teen students to have a positive outcome of their pregnancy and parenting experience.

The Editors gratefully acknowledge the work of the previous chapter author, Valerie Beshears.

References

Advocates for Youth. (2019). *Abortion and parental involvement laws.* https://www.advocatesforyouth.org/wp-content/uploads/2013/12/Parental-Involvement-Policy-Brief-2019.pdf

American Academy of Pediatrics. (2022a). Options counseling for the pregnant adolescent patient. *Pediatrics, 150*(3), 1–5. https://publications.aap.org/pediatrics/article/150/3/e2022058781/188340/Options-Counseling-for-the-Pregnant-Adolescent

American Academy of Pediatrics. (2022b). The adolescent's right to confidential care when considering abortion. *Pediatrics, 150*(3), 1–11. https://publications.aap.org/pediatrics/article/150/3/e2022058780/188339/The-Adolescent-s-Right-to-Confidential-Care-When

American College of Obstetricians and Gynecologists. (2022). *Abortion care.* https://www.acog.org/womens-health/faqs/induced-abortion

American College of Obstetrics and Gynecology. (2023). *COVID-19, pregnancy, childbirth, and breastfeeding: Answers from OB-GYNs.* https://www.acog.org/womens-health/faqs/coronavirus-covid-19-pregnancy-and-breastfeeding

American Pregnancy Association. (n.d.a). *After a miscarriage: Surviving emotionally.* http://americanpregnancy.org/pregnancy-loss/miscarriage-surviving-emotionally/

American Pregnancy Association. (n.d.b). *D&C procedure after a miscarriage.* http://americanpregnancy.org/pregnancy-complications/d-and-c-procedure-after-miscarriage/
American Psychological Association. (2022). *Postpartum depression.* https://www.apa.org/topics/women-girls/postpartum-depression
Assifi, A. R., Kang, M., Sullivan, E. A., & Dawson, A. J. (2020). Abortion care pathways and service provision for adolescents in high-income countries: A qualitative synthesis of the evidence. *PloS One, 15*(11), e0242015. https://doi.org/10.1371/journal.pone.0242015
Benefits.gov. (2019). *Benefits for moms.* https://www.benefits.gov/news/article/369
Black, K. (2018). Intergenerational teen pregnancy and reproductive choices. *BJOG: An International Journal of Obstetrics and Gynaecology, 125*(13), 1775. https://doi.org/10.1111/1471-0528.15346
Bullinger, L. (2017). The effect of minimum wages on adolescent fertility: A nationwide analysis. *American Journal of Public Health, 107*(3), 447–452.
Centers for Disease Control and Prevention. (2021). *Pregnancy and vaccination.* https://www.cdc.gov/vaccines/pregnancy/index.html
Centers for Disease Control and Prevention. (2023a). *Obesity and overweight.* https://www.cdc.gov/nchs/fastats/obesity-overweight.htm
Centers for Disease Control and Prevention. (2023b). *Youth risk behavior survey data.* https://www.cdc.gov/healthyyouth/data/yrbs/index.htm
Centers for Disease Control and Prevention. (2024a). *About folic acid.* https://www.cdc.gov/folic-acid/about/index.html
Centers for Disease Control and Prevention. (2024b). *About teen pregnancy.* https://www.cdc.gov/reproductive-health/teen-pregnancy/?CDC_AAref_Val=https://www.cdc.gov/teenpregnancy/about/index.htm
Centers for Disease Control and Prevention. (2024c). *COVID-19 vaccines while pregnant or breastfeeding.* https://www.cdc.gov/coronavirus/2019-ncov/vaccines/recommendations/pregnancy.html
Centers for Disease Control and Prevention. (2024d). *Fetal alcohol spectrum disorders.* https://www.cdc.gov/fasd/about/index.html
Centers for Disease Control and Prevention. (2024e). *Medicine and pregnancy: An overview.* https://www.cdc.gov/medicine-and-pregnancy/about/index.html
Centers for Disease Control and Prevention. (2024f). *National survey for family growth.* https://www.cdc.gov/nchs/nsfg/index.htm
Centers for Disease Control and Prevention. (2024g). *Pre-term birth.* https://www.cdc.gov/maternal-infant-health/preterm-birth/?CDC_AAref_Val=https://www.cdc.gov/reproductivehealth/maternalinfant health/pretermbirth.htm
Centers for Disease Control and Prevention. (2024h). *Sexually transmitted diseases: Life stages and populations.* https://www.cdc.gov/sti/about/index.html
Centers for Disease Control and Prevention. (2024i). *Symptoms of depression among women.* https://www.cdc.gov/reproductive-health/depression/index.html#:~:text=Depression%20rates%20and%20risk%20factors,episode%20of%20recent%20major%20depression
Child Welfare Information Gateway. (2021). *Infant safe haven laws.* U.S. Department of Health & Human Services, Administration for Children and Families, Children's Bureau. https://www.childwelfare.gov/topics/systemwide/laws-policies/statutes/safehaven/
Dee, L., Pazol, K., Cox, S., Smith, R., Bower, K., & Kapaya, M. (2017). Trends in repeat births and use of postpartum contraception among teens—United States, 2004–2015. *Morbidity and Mortality Weekly Report, 66*(16), 422–426. https://dx.doi.org/10.15585/mmwr.mm6616a3
Demory-Luce, D. (2022). *Adolescent eating habits.* UpToDate. https://www.uptodate.com/contents/adolescent-eating-habits
Dinwiddie, K. J., Schillerstrom, T. L., & Schillerstrom, J. E. (2018). Postpartum depression in adolescent mothers. *Journal of Psychosomatic Obstetrics and Gynaecology, 39*(3), 168–175. https://doi.org/10.1080/0167482X.2017.1334051
Dittus, P. J., Li, J., Verlenden, J. V., Wilkins, N. J., Carman-McClanahan, M. N., Cavalier, Y., Mercado, M. C., Welder, L. E., Roehler, D. R., & Ethier, K. A. (2023). Parental monitoring and risk behaviors and experiences among high school students—Youth Risk Behavior Survey, United States, 2021. *Morbidity and Mortality Weekly Report. Supplement, 72*(1), 37–44. https://doi.org/10.15585/mmwr.su7201a5
The Dougy Center. (n.d.). *How to help a grieving teen.* The National Center for Grieving Children and Families. https://www.dougy.org/grief-resources/how-to-help-a-grieving-teen/
The Dougy Center. (2021). *Developmental responses to grief.* The National Center for Grieving Children and Families. https://www.dougy.org/assets/uploads/Developmental-Responses-to-Grief-ages-2-18.pdf
Education for Justice. (2021). *Fact sheet—The rights of teen parents.* http://www.lawhelpmn.org/files/1765CC5E-1EC9-4FC4-65EC-957272D8A04E/attachments/CBA92481-3E56-41B0-87B8-B1A2814C2C8E/y-09-rights-of-teen-parents.pdf
Fairchild, E., Kyle, S., Marion, S., Cheatham, A., Lecky, T., Harris, S., & Jensen, S. (2022). Prenatal considerations and outcomes for girls aged fourteen and under: Development of a multidisciplinary team in a large tertiary care facility. *Journal of Midwifery & Women's Health, 67*(4), 504–509. https://doi.org/10.1111/jmwh.13378
The Fatherhood Project. (n.d.). *Programs for dads: Teen dads.* Department of Psychiatry, Massachusetts General Hospital. http://www.thefatherhoodproject.org/programs/#teen-dads
The Fatherhood Project. (2015). *Ten facts about father engagement.* Department of Psychiatry, Massachusetts General Hospital. http://www.thefatherhoodproject.org/10-facts-about-father-engagement/
The Fatherhood Project. (2016). *Teen dads: the forgotten parent.* Department of Psychiatry, Massachusetts General Hospital. http://www.thefatherhoodproject.org/teen-dads-forgotten-parent/
Font, S. A., Cancian, M., & Berger, L. M. (2019). Prevalence and risk factors for early motherhood among low-income, maltreated, and foster youth. *Demography, 56*(1), 261–284. https://doi.org/10.1007/s13524-018-0744-x
Fortin-Langelier, E., Daigneault, I., Achim, J., Vézina-Gagnon, P., Guérin, V., & Frappier, J.-Y. (2019). A matched cohort study of the association between childhood sexual abuse and teenage pregnancy. *Journal of Adolescent Health, 65*(3), 384–389. https://doi.org/10.1016/j.jadohealth.2019.03.001
Frederiksen, B. N., Rivera, M. I., Ahrens K. A., Malcolm, N. M., Brittain, A. W., Rollison, J. M., & Moskosky, S. B. (2018). Clinic-based programs to prevent repeat teen pregnancy: A systematic review. *American Journal of Preventive Medicine, 55*(5), 736–746. https://doi.ogr/10.1016/j.amepre.2018.08.001
Garwood, S., Gerassi, L., Jonson-Reid, M., Plax, K., & Drake, B. (2015). More than poverty—Teen pregnancy risk and reports of child abuse reports and neglect. *Journal of Adolescent Health, 57*(2), 164–168. https://doi.org/10.1016/j.jadohealth.2015.05.004
Goetschius, L. G., McLoyd, V. C., Hein, T. C., Mitchell, C., Hyde, L. W., & Monk, C. S. (2023). School connectedness as a protective factor against childhood exposure to violence and social deprivation: A longitudinal study of adaptive and maladaptive outcomes. *Development and Psychopathology, 35*(3), 1219–1234. https://doi.org/10.1017/S0954579421001140
Guttmacher Institute. (2019). *Adolescent sexual and reproductive health in the United States: Fact sheet.* https://www.guttmacher.org/fact-sheet/american-teens-sexual-and-reproductive-health
Guttmacher Institute. (2023a). *An overview of minors' consent law.* https://www.guttmacher.org/state-policy/explore/overview-minors-consent-law
Guttmacher Institute. (2023b). *Minors' rights as parents.* https://www.guttmacher.org/state-policy/explore/minors-rights-parents
Guttmacher Institute. (2023c). *Parental involvement in minors' abortion.* https://www.guttmacher.org/state-policy/explore/parental-involvement-minors-abortions
Guttmacher Institute. (2023d). *Substance use during pregnancy.* https://www.guttmacher.org/state-policy/explore/substance-use-during-pregnancy
Hamilton, B. E., Martin, J. A., & Osterman, M. J. K. (2022). *Births: Provisional data for 2021.* NVSS Vital Statistics Rapid Release, Report No.20. Division of Vital Statistics, National Center for Health Statistics. https://www.cdc.gov/nchs/data/vsrr/vsrr020.pdf

Health Resources and Services Administration. (2024). *Healthy start.* Maternal and Child Health. https://mchb.hrsa.gov/programs-impact/healthy-start

Hendrick, C. E., & Maslowsky, J. (2019). Teen mothers' educational attainment and their children's risk for teenage childbearing. *Developmental Psychology, 55*(6), 1259–1273. https://doi.org/10.1037/dev0000705

Horner-Johnson, W., Senders, A., Higgins Tejera, C., & McGee, M. G. (2021). Sexual health experiences among high school students with disabilities. *Journal of Adolescent Health, 69*(2), 255–262. https://doi.org/10.1016/j.jadohealth.2021.03.001

Houtrow, A., Elias, E. R., Davis, B. E., Kuo, D. Z., Agrawal, R., Davidson, L. F., Ellerbeck, K. A., Foster, J. E. A., Fremion, E., O'Connor Leppert, M., Saunders, B., Stille, C., Vargus-Adams, J., Yin, L., Norwood, K., Coleman, C., Mann, M. Y., Simpser, E., Poon, J., & Yeargin-Allsopp, M. (2021). Promoting healthy sexuality for children and adolescents with disabilities. *Pediatrics, 148*(1),1098–4275. https://doi.org/10.1542/peds.2021-052043

Johns, M. M., Lowry, R., Andrzejewski, J., Barrios, L. C., Demissie, Z., McManus, T., Rasberry, C. N., Robin, L., & Underwood, M. (2019). Transgender identity and experiences of violence victimization, substance use, suicide risk, and sexual risk behaviors among high school students—19 states and large urban school districts, 2017. *Morbidity and Mortality Weekly Report, 68*, 67–71. http://dx.doi.org/10.15585/mmwr.mm6803a3

Jones, J., & Placek, P. (2017). *Adoption: By the numbers.* National Council for Adoption. http://www.adoptioncouncil.org/publications/2017/02/adoption-by-the-numbers

Justia. (2021). *Paternity laws and forms.* https://www.justia.com/family/child-custody-and-support/paternity-forms-50-state-resources/

Kankowski, L., Ardissino, M., McCracken, C., Lewandowski, A. J., Leeson, P., Neubauer, S., Harvey, N. C., Petersen, S. E., & Raisi-Estabragh, Z. (2022). The impact of maternal obesity on offspring cardiovascular health: A systematic literature review. *Frontiers in Endocrinology, 13*. https://doi.org/10.3389/fendo.2022.868441

Kortsmit, K., Nguyen, A. T., Mandel, M. G., Clark, E., Hollier, L. M., Rodenhizer, J., & Whiteman, M. K. (2022). Abortion surveillance—United States, 2020. *Morbidity and Mortality Weekly Report, 71*(10), 1–27. http://dx.doi.org/10.15585/mmwr.ss7110a1

Leftwich, H., & Alves, M., (2017). Adolescent pregnancy. *Pediatric Clinics of North America, 64*(2), 381–388. https://doi.org/10.1016/j.pcl.2016.11.007

Levis, B., Negeri, Z., Sun, Y., Benedetti, A., & Thombs, B. D. (2020). Accuracy of the Edinburgh Postnatal Depression Scale (EPDS) for screening to detect major depression among pregnant and postpartum women: Systematic review and meta-analysis of individual participant data. *BMJ, 371*, m4022. https://doi.org/10.1136/bmj.m4022

Lin, W. H., Liu, C. H., & Yi, C. C. (2020). Exposure to sexually explicit media in early adolescence is related to risky sexual behavior in emerging adulthood. *PloS One, 15*(4), e0230242. https://doi.org/10.1371/journal.pone.0230242

Liu, N., Vigod, S., Farrugia, M., Urquia, M., & Ray, J. (2018). Intergenerational teen pregnancy: A population-based cohort study. *BJOG: An International Journal of Obstetrics and Gynaecology, 125*(13), 1766–1774. https://doi.org/10.1111/1471-0528.15297

March of Dimes. (2017). *Ectopic pregnancy.* https://www.marchofdimes.org/find-support/topics/miscarriage-loss-grief/ectopic-pregnancy

March of Dimes. (2019). *Smoking during pregnancy.* http://www.marchofdimes.org/pregnancy/smoking-during-pregnancy.aspx

March of Dimes. (2020a). *Exercise during pregnancy.* https://www.marchofdimes.org/find-support/topics/pregnancy/exercise-during-pregnancy

March of Dimes. (2020b). *Marijuana and pregnancy.* https://www.marchofdimes.org/find-support/topics/pregnancy/marijuana-and-pregnancy

March of Dimes. (2020c). *Vitamins and other nutrients during pregnancy.* https://www.marchofdimes.org/find-support/topics/pregnancy/vitamins-and-other-nutrients-during-pregnancy

March of Dimes. (2020d). *Weight gain during pregnancy.* http://www.marchofdimes.org/pregnancy/weight-gain-during-pregnancy.aspx

March of Dimes. (2021). *Low birthweight.* http://www.marchofdimes.org/complications/low-birthweight.aspx

March of Dimes. (2022a). *Neural tube defects.* http://www.marchofdimes.org/complications/neural-tube-defects.aspx

March of Dimes. (2022b, June). *Sexually transmitted infections.* https://www.marchofdimes.org/find-support/topics/pregnancy/sexually-transmitted-infections

March of Dimes. (2023). *Miscarriage.* https://www.marchofdimes.org/find-support/topics/miscarriage-loss-grief/miscarriage

March of Dimes. (2024a). *High blood pressure during pregnancy.* https://www.marchofdimes.org/find-support/topics/pregnancy/high-blood-pressure-during-pregnancy

March of Dimes. (2024b). *Long-term health effects of premature birth.* http://www.marchofdimes.org/complications/long-term-health-effects-of-premature-birth.aspx

March of Dimes. (2024c). *Preeclampsia.* http://www.marchofdimes.org/complications/preeclampsia.aspx#

March of Dimes. (2024d). *Preterm labor and premature birth: Are you at risk?* http://www.marchofdimes.org/complications/preterm-labor-and-premature-birth-are-you-at-risk.aspx

Masho, S., Chambers, G., Wallenborn, J., & Ferrance, J. (2017). Associations of partner age gap as sexual debut with teenage parenthood and lifetime number of partners. *Perspectives on Sexual and Reproductive Health, 49*(2), 77–83. https://doi.org/10.1363/psrh.12022

Maslowsky, J., Stritzel, H., Al-Hamoodah, L., Hendrick, C. E., Powers, D., Barrientos-Gutierrez, T., & Santelli, J. (2021). Health behaviors and prenatal health conditions in repeat vs first-time teenage mothers in the United States: 2015–2018. *Journal of Pediatric and Adolescent Gynecology, 34*(1), 47–53. https://doi.org/10.1016/j.jpag.2020.08.003

Mendle, J., Ryan, R. M., & McKone, K. M. P. (2019). Early menarche and internalizing and externalizing in adulthood: Explaining the persistence of effects. *Journal of Adolescent Health, 65*(5), 599–606. https://doi.org/10.1016/j.jadohealth.2019.06.004

Miller, L., Pickett, M., & Reed, J. (2017). Adolescents at risk for sexually transmitted infection need more than the right medicine. *The Journal of Pediatrics, 189*, 23–25. http://dx.doi.org/10.1016/j.jpeds.2017.06.072

National Academies of Sciences, Engineering, and Medicine. (2018). *The safety and quality of abortion care in the United States.* National Academies Press. https://doi.org/10.17226/24950

National Association of School Nurses. (2022). *Comprehensive health education in schools* (Position Statement). Author.

National Association of School Nurses. (2023). *Safe, supportive, equitable schools* (Position Statement). Author.

National Association of School Nurses. (2024). A contemporary framework update for today's school nursing landscape: Introducing the School Nursing Practice Framework. *NASN School Nurse, 39*(3), 140–147. https://www.doi.org/10.1177/1942602X241241092

National Heart, Lung, and Blood Institute. (2022). *Pregnancy and high blood pressure.* National Institutes of Health, U.S. Department of Health & Human Services. https://www.nhlbi.nih.gov/health/high-blood-pressure/pregnancy

National Institute on Drug Abuse. (2020). *Substance use in women research report: Substance use while pregnant and breastfeeding.* National Institute of Health. U.S. Department of Health & Human Services. https://nida.nih.gov/publications/research-reports/substance-use-in-women/substance-use-while-pregnant-breastfeeding#:~:text=Recent%20research%20shows%20that%20smoking,triple%20the%20risk%20of%20stillbirth

National Institutes of Health. (2023). *Iron—supplement fact sheet.* U.S. Department of Health & Human Services. https://ods.od.nih.gov/factsheets/Iron-HealthProfessional/

National Responsible Fatherhood Clearinghouse. (n.d.) *Young fatherhood.* U.S. Department of Health & Human Services. https://www.fatherhood.gov/for-programs/young-fathers

National Women's Law Center. (2016). *Pregnant and parenting students' rights.* https://nwlc.org/resources/pregnant-and-parenting-students-rights-2/

Office of Adolescent Health. (n.d.a). *About the teen pregnancy prevention (TPP) program.* U.S. Department of Health & Human Services. https://www.hhs.gov/ash/oah/grant-programs/teen-pregnancy-prevention-program-tpp/about/index.html

Office of Adolescent Health. (n.d.b) *Trends in teen pregnancy and childbearing.* U.S. Department of Health & Human Services. https://opa.hhs.gov/adolescent-health/reproductive-health-and-teen-pregnancy/trends-teen-pregnancy-and-childbearing

Office of Family Assistance. (2024). *Responsible fatherhood.* An Office of the Administration for Children & Families, U.S. Department of Health & Human Services. https://www.acf.hhs.gov/ofa/programs/healthy-marriage/responsible-fatherhood

Office of Population Affairs. (n.d.). *Trends in teen pregnancy and childbearing.* U.S. Department of Health and Human Services. https://opa.hhs.gov/adolescent-health/reproductive-health-and-teen-pregnancy/trends-teen-pregnancy-and-childbearing

Office of Women's Health. (2021). *Pregnancy test.* U.S. Department of Health and Human Services. https://www.womenshealth.gov/a-z-topics/pregnancy-tests

Osterman, M., Hamilton, B., Martin, J. A., Driscoll, A. K., & Valenzuela, C. P. (2023). Births: Final data for 2021: National vital statistics reports. *National Center for Health Statistics, National Vital Statistics System Centers for Disease Control and Prevention, 72*(1), 1–53. https://www.cdc.gov/nchs/data/nvsr/nvsr72/nvsr72-01.pdf

Power to Decide. (2023). *Find verified abortion care and support.* https://www.abortionfinder.org/

Ramsey, P., & Schenken, R. (2024). *Obesity in pregnancy: Complications and maternal management.* UpToDate. https://www.uptodate.com/contents/obesity-in-pregnancy-complications-and-maternal-management

Ranji, U., Gomez, I., Salganicoff, A., Rosenzweig, C., Kellenberg, R., & Gifford, K. (2022). *Medicaid coverage of pregnancy-related services: Findings from a 2021 state survey.* Henry J. Kaiser Family Foundation. https://www.kff.org/report-section/medicaid-coverage-of-pregnancy-related-services-findings-from-a-2021-state-survey-report/

Sadeghi, N., Smiley, Y., & Chokshi, B. (2021). Supporting teen parents during COVID-19. *Journal of Adolescent Health, 68*(2S), S47. https://doi.org/10.1016/j.jadohealth.2020.12.097

Sangsawang, N., & Sangsawang, B. (2023). Postpartum depression, social support, and maternal self-efficacy between adolescent and adult mothers during the COVID-19 pandemic: A comparative cross-sectional study. *Journal of Advanced Nursing, 79,* 113–124. https://doi.org/10.1111/jan.15445

School-Based Health Alliance. (n.d.). *What we do.* https://www.sbh4all.org/what-we-do/

Scott, M., Steward-Streng, N., & Manlove, J. (2012). The characteristics and circumstances of teen fathers: At the birth of their first child and beyond. *Child Trends: Research Brief, 19,* 1–6. https://www.childtrends.org/wp-content/uploads/2013/03/Child_Trends-2012_06_01_B_TeenFathers.pdf

Senders, A., & Horner-Johnson, W. (2022). Contraceptive use among adolescents with and without disabilities. *Journal of Adolescent Health, 70*(1), 120–126. https://doi.org/10.1016/j.jadohealth.2021.06.028

SmithBattle, L. (2020). Walking on eggshells: An update on the stigmatizing of teen mothers. *The American Journal of Maternal/Child Nursing, 45*(6), 322–327. https://doi.org/10.1097/NMC.0000000000000655

SmithBattle, L., Phengnum, W., Shagavah, A. & Okawa, S. (2019). Fathering on tenuous ground. *The American Journal of Maternal/Child Nursing, 44*(4), 186–194. https://doi.org/10.1097/NMC.0000000000000536

Szucs, L. E., Lowry, R., Fasula, A. M., Pampati, S., Copen, C. E., Hussaini, K. S., Kachur, R. E., Koumans, E. H., & Steiner, R. J. (2020). Condom and contraceptive use among sexually active high school students—Youth Risk Behavior Survey, United States, 2019. *MMWR Supplements, 69*(1), 11–18. https://doi.org/10.15585/mmwr.su6901a2

U.S. Department of Agriculture. (2022). *Healthy eating for women who are pregnant or breastfeeding.* https://www.myplate.gov/life-stages/pregnancy-and-breastfeeding

U.S. Department of Education, Office for Civil Rights. (2013). *Supporting the academic success of pregnant and parenting students—Under Title IX of the education amendments of 1972.* https://www2.ed.gov/about/offices/list/ocr/docs/pregnancy.pdf

U.S. Department of Housing and Urban Development. (2018). *About second chance homes.* https://www.hud.gov/program_offices/public_indian_housing/other/sch/about

U.S. Food and Drug Administration. (2020). *Nonsteroidal anti-inflammatory drugs (NSAIDs): Drug safety communication—Avoid use of NSAIDs in pregnancy at 20 weeks or later.* https://www.fda.gov/safety/medical-product-safety-information/nonsteroidal-anti-inflammatory-drugs-nsaids-drug-safety-communication-avoid-use-nsaids-pregnancy-20

U.S. Food and Drug Administration. (2021). *Labeling information/Drug products: Pregnancy and lactation labeling (drugs) final rule.* https://www.fda.gov/drugs/labeling-information-drug-products/pregnancy-and-lactation-labeling-drugs-final-rule#:~:text=The%20PLLR%20requires%20changes%20to,need%20to%20take%20medication%2C%20thus

U.S. Food and Drug Administration. (2024). *Folate and folic acid on the nutrition and supplement facts labels.* https://www.fda.gov/food/new-nutrition-facts-label/folate-and-folic-acid-nutrition-and-supplement-facts-labels

Weissberg, R. P. (2019). Promoting the social and emotional learning of millions of school children. *Perspectives on Psychological Science, 14*(1) 65–69. https://doi.org/10.1177/1745691618817756

Windham, G. C., Anderson, M., Lyall, K., Daniels, J. L., Kral, T. V .E., Croen, L. A., Levy, S. E., Bradley, C. B., Cordero, C., Young, L., & Schieve L. A. (2019). Maternal pre-pregnancy body mass index and gestational weight gain in relation to autism spectrum disorder and other developmental disorders in offspring. *Autism Research, 12*(2), 316–327. https://doi.org/10.1002/aur.2057

World Health Organization. (2022). *Adolescent pregnancy.* https://www.who.int/news-room/fact-sheets/detail/adolescent-pregnancy#:~:text=Every%20year%2C%20an%20estimated%2021,per%201000%20women%20in%202021

World Health Organization. (2023). *Social determinants of health.* https://www.who.int/health-topics/social-determinants-of-health#tab=tab_

Youth.gov. (n.d.a). *Education and employment.* https://youth.gov/youth-topics/expectant-parenting-young-families/education-employment#_ftn1

Youth.gov. (n.d.b). *Risk and protective factors.* http://youth.gov/youth-topics/teen-pregnancy-prevention/risk-and-protective-factors

Chapter 20

Supporting Students With Special Healthcare Needs

Rachel McClanahan

CHAPTER OUTLINE

School nurses play a critical role in caring for students with special healthcare needs and chronic health conditions in the school setting by providing essential health assessments, administering medications and treatments, teaching self-care, and collaborating with other healthcare professionals to ensure the child's health and safety at school. As the health experts on the interdisciplinary school team, school nurses also provide education and support to parents/guardians and teachers and help to create and implement individualized healthcare plans that address the unique needs of each child. The National Association of School Nurses (NASN) identifies case management and chronic disease management as critical components of the *Care Coordination* principle of the *School Nursing Practice Framework* (NASN, 2024a). By providing this specialized care, school nurses help to ensure that children with special healthcare needs can attend school and participate in educational activities, promoting their overall health and well-being. The purpose of this chapter is to define the terms and describe the breadth of concepts and issues that affect students with special healthcare needs, their families, and the nursing care provided in the school setting.

STUDENTS WITH SPECIAL HEALTHCARE NEEDS

Children with special healthcare needs are defined as having at least one of the following lasting 12 months or longer:

- Need or use of prescription medication(s)
- Elevated need or use of medical care, mental health, or education services
- Functional limitation(s) (that limit daily activity)
- Need or use of special therapies (e.g., physical, occupational, or speech therapy)
- Emotional, developmental, or behavioral problem for which treatment or counseling is needed (Maternal and Child Health Bureau [MCHB], 2022, para. 1)

Students with special healthcare needs require services and support of a type and amount beyond what is typically needed by children (McPherson et al., 1998; MCHB, 2012). Students with special healthcare needs have or are at increased risk for chronic physical, developmental, emotional, and behavioral or mental health issues. Students with special healthcare needs may also have a broader range of healthcare needs that are not necessarily chronic. As a group, students with special healthcare needs are more prone to face challenges to their well-being than their peers without special healthcare needs. A small subset of children in this group is considered medically complex and require intensive services due to extensive health needs, functional limitations, and high resource utilization.

Chronic health conditions are medical conditions "that last one year or more and require ongoing medical attention or limit activities of daily living or both" (National Center for Chronic Disease Prevention and Health Promotion, 2022, para. 1). This chapter uses the terms *special healthcare needs* and *chronic health conditions* interchangeably. The school nursing care of students with select chronic health conditions or special healthcare needs is discussed in the upcoming chapters, including allergies; asthma and respiratory conditions; diabetes; cardiac, gastrointestinal, and blood disorders; epilepsy and seizures, cerebral palsy; meningomyelocele; hearing or visual impairments; neurodevelopmental disorders (e.g., attention deficit-hyperactivity disorder, autism spectrum disorder, congenital anomalies, etc.); mental health conditions; and others.

Chronic conditions can vary in severity, impact, and course over time. Chronic health conditions in children can exist in any organ or system in the body. Some chronic conditions involve only one organ system; others may affect multiple body systems, such as Down syndrome or cystic fibrosis. Some conditions are present at birth and may be treated before the student enters the school system; other conditions develop or become more evident during the school-age years. Many chronic conditions do not have a cure. While some chronic conditions can be managed or controlled with treatments and lifestyle changes, the underlying condition is still present and may require ongoing management. Some chronic conditions may have periods of remission and exacerbation, where symptoms come and go or fluctuate in intensity. There may be a pattern of decline, where the condition worsens over time, potentially leading to significant disability, complications, or death. However, the rate and extent of progression varies widely depending on the specific condition and the individual.

Management of multisystem conditions often involves a team of healthcare providers from multiple specialties working together to provide comprehensive care. Treatment may include a combination of medications, surgeries, therapies, and lifestyle changes to manage symptoms and prevent complications. School nurses must work closely with families and their healthcare providers to develop an individualized care plan that addresses their child's unique needs and optimizes learning. Students often move back and forth along the health continuum as they grow due to new stages of development, exacerbations, and remissions. Therefore the plan of care needs to be flexible to accommodate the changes in the student's health status.

Students with chronic health conditions may experience limitations in their activities, frequent pain or discomfort, abnormal growth and development, and an increased need for hospitalizations, outpatient visits, and medical treatments. For children with severe disabilities, there may be times when they are unable to participate in school and social activities with peers. How children respond to a chronic health condition can vary depending on the developmental stage at which the condition arises. The impact may differ for children who develop chronic conditions during infancy versus during their school-age years or adolescence. Adolescents may find it particularly difficult to cope with being viewed as different during a time when being similar to peers is important.

Prevalence

Prevalence refers to the proportion of individuals in a population with a particular health condition or disease at a specific time. It is calculated by dividing the number of cases of a particular disease or condition in a population by the total number of individuals in that population. Prevalence is an important concept as it provides a snapshot of the overall burden of a particular disease or condition in a population. It helps school nurses, administrators, researchers, and policymakers to understand the extent and distribution of health problems, and to identify populations that are particularly affected. This information is critical for planning and implementing effective health interventions.

According to the 2019 to 2020 *National Survey of Children's Health*, approximately 19% (14 million) of people under the age of 18 years in the United States have special healthcare needs (MCHB, 2022). In about 25% of U.S. households, there is at least one child with a special healthcare need. Furthermore, children with special healthcare needs are more likely to live in poverty, be non-Hispanic black, and have public insurance compared with households without children with special healthcare needs (MCHB, 2022).

Comorbidity is a term that describes the presence of more than one health condition in patients with a particular disease or disorder (Nasir et al., 2019). *Multimorbidity* is the co-occurrence of two or more chronic medical conditions in a single individual. These conditions can be physical and/or mental health conditions, and they may interact with each other, leading to a higher burden of illness and poorer health outcomes. Comorbidities and multimorbidity are more common among students with complex medical needs (Nasir et al., 2019).

With advances in medicine, more children are entering school who have survived complications of pregnancy, significant congenital anomalies, prematurity, and birth trauma or neonatal complications/severe illness. Surgical advances have resulted in the repair of many conditions in the early years of life. As children mature into adulthood, the potential for having more than one chronic condition increases. In addition, the student may be receiving medications for multiple conditions, resulting in the potential for drug reactions. The school nurse needs to be sure that individualized healthcare plans (IHPs) include all relevant components for each condition and are kept up to date.

Secondary effects, complications, or episodic illness may significantly affect the underlying chronic condition and require tertiary care. For example, a student with myelomeningocele that results in significant scoliosis may have more compromise with respiratory infections. A student with diabetes may become unstable if they experience gastroenteritis, which affects their food intake and insulin needs.

CAUSATIVE FACTORS

Chronic conditions in children can have various causes, including the following:

- Genes inherited from parents/guardians or caused by genetic mutations, such as Down syndrome, cystic fibrosis, and sickle cell disease
- Complications during gestation, maternal infection
- Risk factors of pregnancy: inadequate prenatal care, poor maternal nutrition, or maternal use of drugs, alcohol, or tobacco
- Preterm or with low birth weight

Did You Know?

Key Sources for Child Health and Education Data

- The National Survey of Children's Health (NSCH) is a household survey conducted annually by the U.S. Census Bureau that provides important national and state-level data on child health and well-being. These data are critical for understanding the health status and needs of children in communities across the country. The most up-to-date data can be found at the NSCH Web site.
- The National Center for Education Statistics (NCES) is the primary federal entity for collecting and analyzing data related to education. Current data can be found at the NCES Web site.
- Kids Count® is a source for data on children and families that looks at child well-being in the United States.
- The National Institute of Dental and Craniofacial Research (NIDCR) aims to advance fundamental knowledge about dental, oral, and craniofacial health and disease and translate findings into prevention, early detection, and treatment strategies that improve overall health for all individuals and communities across the life span.

- Traumatic experiences or physical injuries
- Exposure to certain environmental factors, such as pollution, toxins, or infectious agents, can lead to chronic conditions (e.g., lead poisoning)
- Immunological processes, such as allergy, asthma, or cancer
- Idiopathic, for which the cause is not known

Some chronic conditions have periods when symptoms are mild or absent (remission), followed by periods when symptoms are more severe (exacerbation). Examples of these conditions include multiple sclerosis, rheumatoid arthritis, lupus, inflammatory bowel disease, asthma, bipolar disorder, and psoriasis.

Some chronic conditions (e.g., type 1 diabetes, celiac disease, sickle cell disease) remain throughout life, although management requirements may change over time, and individuals may experience complications or acute episodes. Some chronic conditions result in a continual pattern of decline, such as cystic fibrosis, Duchenne muscular dystrophy, and chronic renal disease. In some cases, conditions improve or resolve as the child ages. For example, some children with asthma may see a reduction in symptoms or complete resolution of their condition as they age, and other children may outgrow allergies to foods, pet dander, or pollen.

IMPACT ON THE STUDENT AND FAMILY

Many parents/guardians are concerned when their child is diagnosed with a chronic condition, especially one involving mental health, fearing that the label of the condition will affect their child's academic and social opportunities. For a variety of reasons, students with chronic health conditions often feel different than their peers or feel like they don't fit in. The student may experience discomfort or embarrassment regarding the health-related technology or aspects of chronic health conditions. Students with chronic health conditions may struggle with disclosure challenges, such as who to tell, how much to reveal, and coping with peer reactions to the information. Classmates may be curious or fearful of the student's unexplained behaviors or of "catching" the disease or condition from the affected student. Students feeling different may feel isolated, lonely, or withdrawn and struggle with anger and frustration at not fitting in. When appropriate, and with parent/guardian permission, the school nurse and the classroom teacher can work together to provide information to the class regarding the specific condition and the technology and devices used.

Stigma

Stigma is a "set of negative and unfair beliefs that a society or group of people have about something" (Merriam-Webster Dictionary, 2023). Stigma is a social process in which an individual or group is socially devalued and labeled as deviant, undesirable, or inferior based on their characteristics, behavior, or status. When a person or group is stigmatized, it can result in negative attitudes, discrimination, and prejudice toward them (Phelan et al., 2014). This exclusion and marginalization can limit their opportunities in various areas of life, such as education, employment, health care, and social relationships. Such consequences can have a detrimental impact on the stigmatized person or group and can lead to a further perpetuation of stigmatization.

Stigma can harm an individual's physical and mental health, self-esteem, and well-being and contribute to broader societal issues, such as inequality and injustice. Stigmatization can result in discrimination and infringements on civil and human rights, inadequate healthcare access, and reduced treatment adherence, ultimately causing increased morbidity and mortality (Phelan et al., 2014).

Bullying

The stigma of being "different" physically, socially, or intellectually from more typical peers puts students with disabilities at increased risk of being bullied (Stopbullying.gov, 2020a). ***Bullying*** is unwanted, aggressive behavior among school-age children. It involves a real or perceived power imbalance, and the behavior is repeated or has the potential to be repeated over time. Both students who are bullied and students who bully others may have serious, lasting problems (Stopbullying.gov, 2020b.). Bullying can result in depression and anxiety, increased health complaints, decreased academic achievement, and increased days absent (Stopbullying.gov, 2020a). Severe bullying that creates a hostile school environment for the student is called *disability harassment*, which must be addressed or the school may be found in violation of the student's federal civil rights under Section 504 of the Rehabilitation Act of 1973 and Title II of the Americans With Disabilities Act of 1990. See Chapter 11 for more information on bullying.

Practice Connection

Peer support of students with disabilities reduces the risk of bullying. According to Stopbullying.gov (2020b), schools can take the following actions to increase peer support and a sense of belonging:

- Engaging students in developing high-interest activities in which everyone has a role to play in designing, executing, or participating in the activity
- Providing general up-front information to peers about the kinds of support children with special needs require, and have adults facilitate peer support
- Creating a buddy system for children with special needs
- Involving students in adaptive strategies in the classroom so that they participate in assisting and understanding the needs of others
- Conducting team-based learning activities and rotate student groupings
- Implementing social-emotional learning activities
- Rewarding positive, helpful, inclusive behavior (para. 10)

Person-First Language

When referring to students with special healthcare needs, *person-first language* must be used. Person-first language is a linguistic approach that emphasizes the person, rather than their condition or disability, by placing the person before the descriptor or diagnoses (Wooldridge, 2023). For example, the school nurse should say a "student with asthma" rather than an "asthmatic student." There is a greater risk of stigmatizing or treating students as "sick" if they are identified as having or being a disease; instead, they should be viewed as being in their normal state of health. When referring to students with chronic conditions, school nurses should model language that emphasizes health and wellness, such as "a healthy child with a seizure disorder." The goal of person-first language is to promote respect and dignity for individuals by emphasizing their humanity rather than reducing them to a single aspect of their identity. However, it is important to note that not all members of the disability community embrace person-first language. They may prefer *identity-first language* because they feel that the disability trait should not be viewed negatively because it is an essential part of who they are (Wooldridge, 2023). School nurses should simply ask what term students and families prefer.

School nurses should keep abreast of currently accepted terms. For example, Rosa's Law was signed into law by President Barack Obama in 2010. To promote respectful and accurate language, Rosa's Law amended several federal health, education, and labor statutes to replace the term "mental retardation" with *intellectual disability*. The law was named after Rosa Marcellino, a young girl with Down syndrome.

The term "handicapped" is considered outdated and offensive and should be avoided. Handicap generally refers to a disadvantage or limitation that prevents someone from fully participating in an activity or achieving a specific goal. Students with significant disabilities or who are dependent on technology may be labeled as *medically fragile* or *medically compromised students*. Identifying these children as "fragile" or compromised may underestimate their ability to participate in educational and social opportunities and their potential contribution to society. For students who have complex needs that often require support from medical technology, the student-first term that is preferred is students with medical fragility.

Yet another term used to describe some children with chronic conditions is *technology dependent*, which emphasizes technology rather than the child. Although this term is usually limited to those with respiratory and gastrointestinal technology, it is rarely applied to those who wear glasses or braces or use insulin pumps. Using phrases such as *students assisted or supported by medical technology* is preferable.

Impact on Growth and Development

Chronic conditions can often affect a child's growth and development. Chronic conditions such as asthma, diabetes, and obesity can affect a child's growth and development by causing disruptions in physiological processes and limiting physical activity (Consolini, 2022). Additionally, growth and development can affect medication absorption, metabolism, and elimination, which may affect the efficacy and safety of some treatments or interventions (van den Anker et al., 2018).

School nurses should recognize the complex interplay between chronic conditions and growth and development and provide children and adolescents with comprehensive care that addresses their medical and developmental needs.

Adolescents with chronic conditions who need assistance with activities of daily living, physical appearance, or cognitive delays may sometimes be treated like younger children, leading to frustration, isolation, and lack of independence (Russo, 2022). It is important to recognize that adolescents with chronic conditions are still developing and have unique developmental needs that may differ from those of younger children (Consolini, 2022).

Frequent absences from school due to hospital admissions, appointments with healthcare providers, therapy sessions, or illness may also cause students with chronic health conditions to fall behind academically, feel alienated from their peers, and experience a delay in their development. Disruptions to social development due to the inability to socialize with peers and participate in social activities can lead to feelings of isolation, anxiety, and depression, which may affect their social and emotional development. Some chronic conditions require medication that may have side effects, such as drowsiness, lethargy, and cognitive impairment, affecting the child's ability to focus and learn and hindering their academic progress and cognitive development. Many chronic conditions limit a child's ability to engage in physical activity, an important aspect of growth and development. Reduced physical activity can lead to decreased muscle strength, cardiovascular fitness, and bone density, which may affect a child's overall health and well-being. See Chapter 9 for more information on student growth and development.

Family Coping

Chronic illnesses in children can have a significant impact on families. The diagnosis of a chronic condition in a child can be emotionally overwhelming for parents/guardians and family members. Parents/guardians may experience feelings of guilt, sadness, anxiety, and stress. It may be expected that many parents/guardians experience *chronic sorrow;* they may worry about their child's future, grieve the expectations or dreams they had for their child, and feel helpless (Coughlin & Sethares, 2017). Children with chronic illnesses may require accommodations that can affect their educational progress, putting additional stress on parents/guardians as they advocate for their child's academic needs. Parents/guardians may displace increased levels of stress onto school staff. Nurses, teachers, and student support staff must be aware of the potential for family strife or unpredictable conditions in the home.

Caring for a child with a chronic illness can be expensive and put a strain on a family's finances, especially if the child requires frequent medical visits, hospitalizations, medications, or equipment. Financial burdens can further stress the family dynamics. The school nurse should be empathetic to how some parents/guardians rely on the school to provide care during work hours. School nurses can offer emotional support to families who may be struggling financially by listening to their concerns, offering encouragement, and providing resources to help them cope. School nurses can also assist by being well-informed and providing families with information about available financial resources, such as government health insurance, support programs, grants, and local nonprofit organizations.

Caring for a child with a chronic illness can be time-consuming. It can be physically and emotionally challenging for parents/guardians to meet work demands while meeting the care needs of their children. Parents/guardians may need to make significant adjustments to their daily routines, which can lead to changes in family dynamics, including a shift in roles and responsibilities. It may be hard for a parent/guardian to maintain employment when employers do not understand the stressors on the parent/guardian and the need to miss work to care for the child. Parents/guardians who are unemployed, work part-time, or hold low-wage jobs may not have adequate healthcare benefits or may not have any type of healthcare insurance. Families may need to plan for extended care as the student transitions out of school or if the parents/guardians can no longer provide the student's care.

Families of children with a chronic illness may experience social isolation as they limit their activities due to their child's health needs. Single-parent families may feel especially stressed if they lack strong support systems nearby to help. Having a child with a severe chronic condition may affect what the family can do as a unit. Some typical family activities are often out of the question or take considerable planning and assistance. Qualified babysitters may not be readily available to give parents/guardians time for themselves or quality time with the other children. Frequent adjustments in family life can cause siblings to have increased absences, less opportunity to participate in school activities, increased stress, and increased isolation. Healthy siblings may experience anger at not having their parent's/guardian's attention. They might also be either embarrassed by or overprotective of their sibling with a chronic condition.

Coping strategies depend on the type and severity of the condition and vary from child to child. For some children, the condition becomes a part of their identity. The degree of acceptance will be strongly influenced by parents' and caregivers' expectations of treatment and whether they have been treated as handicapped or dependent.

Coping by parents/guardians is a continual process; typical developmental milestones can be especially difficult for the families of students whose development is delayed. Support groups, counseling services, financial assistance programs, online forums, and peer networks can be excellent resources for finding support and connecting with others who can relate to what they are experiencing. School nurses should be able to identify and refer students and families to school- and community-based resources to help with coping issues.

There is no such thing as a vacation from a chronic condition; families can become exhausted, which further adds to stress. Some families of children with severe chronic conditions are candidates for respite care or short-term home health nursing services so the family can take a break and recharge. School nurses and social workers should be aware of the criteria to access and pay for local respite service or short-term in-home nursing services.

Rehabilitation and Habilitation

Rehabilitation is an interdisciplinary approach that involves specialized treatments, therapies, and exercises to help individuals who have experienced an illness, injury, or disability recover, regain their independence, and improve their physical, cognitive, and emotional functioning. Rehabilitation focuses on promoting the maximum level of functional ability and quality of life. The rehabilitative approach can involve various healthcare professionals, including school nurses, nurse practitioners, physicians, physical therapists, occupational therapists, speech therapists, and psychologists, who work collaboratively to develop and carry out an individualized care plan.

"The goal of the rehabilitation process is for infants, children, and adolescents, regardless of their disability or chronic illness, to function at maximum potential and become contributing members of both their families and society" (Association of Rehabilitation Nurses, 2018, para. 1). Developmental theory is the cornerstone of pediatric rehabilitation nursing. Pediatric rehabilitation nurses work with families and collaborate with the interdisciplinary team to support the child's growth and development. The school nurse's knowledge of rehabilitation and the role of pediatric rehabilitation nurses is essential. Understanding the rehabilitation process and the role of pediatric rehabilitation nurses can help the school nurse better support the student's rehabilitation needs, communicate effectively with other healthcare providers involved in the student's care, and facilitate a smooth transition back to school after hospitalization or rehabilitation. An in-depth understanding of the role of pediatric rehabilitation nurses can help the school nurse to identify appropriate resources and referrals for students who require specialized rehabilitation services beyond what is available at the school.

Unlike rehabilitation, which focuses on restoring lost function, ***habilitation*** aims to help individuals acquire new skills and behaviors necessary for their day-to-day functioning and overall well-being. The term *habilitation* often refers to functional training of children with congenital or developmental disabilities (American Psychological Association, 2023). For many children and adolescents, habilitation continues indefinitely. The focus of habilitation is often on the functional abilities of self-care (eating, grooming, bathing, dressing, and toileting), sphincter control for bowel and bladder, mobility, communication, speech, vision, and social cognition. Any habilitation program should be based on bringing that child to their highest level of functioning. At school, habilitation services are typically provided by physical, occupational, speech therapists and other related services as indicated by the student's unique needs. School therapy is aimed at optimizing the student's participation in the learning environment and therefore is often conducted in a group setting.

EDUCATION OF STUDENTS WITH SPECIAL HEALTHCARE NEEDS

Students with chronic conditions or special healthcare needs are protected against discrimination and afforded certain civil rights in public schools and private schools that receive federal funding. Under *Section 504 of the Rehabilitation Act of 1973*, if a student with a chronic health condition can learn in the general curriculum but needs *accommodations* to participate in the learning environment, then the school district should develop a Section 504 plan for the student.

Under the *Individuals With Disabilities Education Improvement Act* (IDEA, 2004), if a student requires special education and related services (i.e., *modifications* to the curriculum), then the school district is obligated to develop an individualized education program (IEP) for the student.

In some instances, parents/guardians may not want their student or the student themself may not want to be identified as having a disability; therefore they may choose to forgo the services available to them in an IEP or Section 504 plan. Refusing to acknowledge a diagnosis may result in failure to obtain needed services that may jeopardize the student's academic performance. Families must understand that the disability category label is legally mandated for the student to receive the necessary services or accommodations via an IEP. The school nurse can educate families that the services or accommodations a student receives are not solely based on the label but on the student's unique educational and functional needs at school.

For all students with special healthcare needs, the school nurse develops an individualized healthcare plan (IHP). The IHP is written by school nurses for nurses to capture the full breadth of nursing care provided for the student based on the current health status, medical orders, and healthcare needs at school. IHPs are an important method by which the school nurse documents that the student is receiving the expected standard of care.

See Chapter 7 for more information on the federal laws protecting students with disabilities. See Chapter 8 for a detailed discussion on the school nurse's role in developing IHPs, Section 504 plans, and IEPs for students with special healthcare needs.

Interdisciplinary Team Approach

The interdisciplinary team is responsible for implementing and evaluating the services and related supports for students with chronic conditions. In the school setting, interdisciplinary teams (i.e., student support teams, multidisciplinary teams, IEP teams) are comprised of general educators, special educators, the school nurse, social workers, physical therapists, occupational therapists, school psychologists, speech-language pathologists, and other professionals, such as mobility specialists, nutritionists, assistive technology specialists, and audiologists, to address the student's needs. The school nurse is a leader on the interdisciplinary team when medical and health issues must be addressed. Social workers may need to assist the family with financial issues related to healthcare costs and required equipment, food, housing, transportation, mental health issues, respite care, and family counseling. See the *Care Coordination* section later in this chapter.

Accommodations for Physical Education

Any restrictions for physical education (PE) activities should be individualized, specific, and regularly reevaluated, depending on the condition. Blanket restrictions should be avoided; student-specific needs and accommodations should be listed. Healthcare provider notes that are open-ended, such as "activity as tolerated," should be clarified and not accepted since student-specific guidance and parameters indicating the lack of tolerance are not indicated. Individuals with internally implanted medical hardware (e.g., ventriculoperitoneal shunts, pacemakers, or defibrillators) may be restricted from contact sports. Those activities considered contact sports should be specifically listed to minimize confusion about activities in this category. The student's IEP or 504 plan should include health-related PE accommodations.

Did You Know?

In 2020 to 2021, 7.2 million students ages 3 to 21 received special education services under the Individuals With Disabilities Education Act (IDEA), which accounted for 15% of all public school students (National Center for Education Statistics [NCES], 2022). Of these, specific learning disabilities (33%), speech and language impairments (19%), other health impaired (15%), and autism (12%) were the most common. This number represents just one segment of children with chronic conditions since not everyone with a chronic health condition qualifies for or receives special education services.

Adaptive PE is a related service included in a student's IEP. Usually, adaptive PE indicates a need to modify equipment, rules, or teaching modality (Wright's Law, 2018). For example, students in wheelchairs will need adaptive equipment to kick a soccer ball. Students with Down syndrome need to be evaluated for atlantoaxial instability of the neck before being allowed to do somersaults. The Section 504 plan for students with special healthcare needs should list PE modifications or accommodations. All PE modifications or accommodations should focus on physical fitness.

Sexual Health Education

Sexuality is a sensitive subject in schools. Even when sexuality content is provided, it rarely addresses the specific needs of students with special healthcare needs and/or disabilities. All children, including students with chronic conditions, are sexual beings and have the same dreams and aspirations as other children their age. As they mature, students with chronic conditions have questions about sex and sexuality and want to form relationships and experience sexual feelings. Acknowledging these needs and providing them with answers and support is important. Students need up-to-date information related to how chronic conditions may affect puberty.

Research indicates that individuals with disabilities are more vulnerable to sexual victimization and experience poorer sexual health outcomes compared with those who are developing typically (Michielsen & Brockschmidt, 2021). Females ages 17 to 34 with disabilities are more likely to report nonconsensual sex and higher rates of sexually transmitted infections than their peers without disabilities (Holdsworth et al., 2018). Teenagers with mild to moderate intellectual disabilities are more likely to engage in unsafe sexual practices, and women with similar disabilities are more likely to become pregnant by age 20, compared with their typically developing counterparts (Baines et al., 2018).

Comprehensive sex education can help students with disabilities to better understand their bodies, their rights, and their relationships, which can help them to make informed decisions and protect themselves from exploitation, abuse, and unintended consequences of sexual activity. It is important for educators and schools to provide comprehensive sex education that is tailored to the individual needs and abilities of students with disabilities and to ensure that students have access to appropriate resources and support. Providing appropriate education may involve working with parents/guardians, caregivers, and healthcare professionals to develop a comprehensive sexual health education plan appropriate for the student's needs and abilities. School nurses should work with the teachers responsible for sexuality content to ensure that the educational needs of children with chronic conditions are included.

Did You Know?

Content in sexual health education curriculum for intellectually and developmentally disabled (I/DD) students includes healthy relationships, anatomy, physiology, puberty, and adolescent development.

- I/DD students have difficulty initiating and maintaining friendships and sexual relationships, and they have decreased knowledge of sexual and reproductive health, puberty, and body part identification (Schmidt et al., 2020).

Curriculum should include information about pregnancy, sexually transmitted infections, HIV, and personal safety.

- Women who are I/DD have a higher probability of smoking during pregnancy, are less likely to receive inadequate prenatal care during the first trimester, and face a greater risk of adverse pregnancy outcomes (Schmidt et al., 2020).
- Individuals with I/DD and learning disability are more likely to have STIs and experience sexual abuse (Schmidt et al., 2020).

Students in early and middle adolescence showed improvements in sexual health knowledge; therefore sexual health education should start in early adolescence (Schmidt et al., 2020).

Transitioning

The term *transitioning* generally describes the process of preparing and supporting students with identified disabilities as they move from one educational stage or institution to another. Transitioning may include moves from early intervention to preschool, from elementary school to middle school, from high school to postsecondary education or employment, or from school to adult life. This process aims to ensure that students are adequately prepared for the changes ahead and can smoothly transition to the next stage of their education or life. Transitioning occurs at every stage of development and education and is a process, not an event. The process of transitioning involves a variety of activities and support measures, including developing individualized transition plans, providing career counseling and job exploration opportunities, offering training in independent living skills, connecting students with community resources and services, and ensuring students receive the necessary accommodations and support to succeed in their new environment. The aim of these measures is to help the students successfully navigate the transition and achieve their goals in the next stage of their education or life.

Students with chronic conditions benefit from increased attention to self-care needs and future responsibilities beyond high school. Students with complex care needs, such as those with type 1 diabetes, benefit from enhanced knowledge about their condition and independent management needs to ensure readiness for college transition (Klein et al., 2018). The school nurse is responsible for evaluating the student's understanding of self-management concepts and providing education on decision-making and self-management skills that promote their understanding and active involvement in managing and caring for their health needs (Charlucien-Koech et al., 2021).

Transition Plans

Educational teams should prepare for transitions for students with IEPs. If a child receives early intervention services (from birth to 3 years), their individualized family service plan (IFSP) is the initial point for an IEP outlining early childhood services. The next transition occurs when the preschool-age child enters kindergarten or first grade. To ensure a seamless transition, the kindergarten teacher must know the child's communication support, adaptive equipment, and health services requirements during preschool. A clear understanding of a child's adaptation needs and what works well can save time and money on assessments, reduce the need to experiment with various equipment, and minimize the student's lost class time. Planning for the next grade level should always be included in the annual review process for students with IEPs.

IDEA mandates a formal *transition plan* be developed for students with IEPs in secondary education; this process must begin no later than age 16 (earlier in some states) to prepare students for life beyond high school and adulthood. For these students, transition services must be

> *a results-oriented process that is focused on improving the academic and functional achievement of the child with a disability to facilitate the child's movement from school to post-school activities, including postsecondary education, vocational education, integrated employment (including supported employment), continuing and adult education, adult services, independent living, or community participation; [it must also be] based on the individual child's needs, taking into account the child's strengths, preferences, and interests. [IDEA, 2004, Sec 614(d)(1)(A)(VIII)]*

The plan should include "measurable postsecondary goals based on age-appropriate transition assessments related to training, education, employment, and, where appropriate, independent living skills" (IDEA, 2004). It must also include the courses the student will need to take to reach these goals. See Chapters 7 and 8 for more information on special education transition plans.

CORE TENETS OF CHRONIC CONDITION MANAGEMENT IN SCHOOLS

In 2021, the National Center for Chronic Disease Prevention and Health Promotion, Division of Population Health, Healthy Schools Branch (NCCDPHP) gathered representatives from several children's health-focused organizations (e.g., American Academy of Pediatrics Council on School Health, the Center for Health and Health Care in Schools, NASN, and others) to collaborate on the *Consensus Statement on the Core Tenets of Chronic Condition Management in Schools.* The consensus statement's purpose is to outline a framework of fundamental principles schools should follow when managing chronic health conditions in their students. The framework is made up of seven core tenets and three foundational supports. It aims to set a "universal standard for high-quality chronic condition management in schools that establishes accountability and promotes equity" (NCCDPHP, 2021, p. 3).

The tenets of the framework are derived from existing models, including the patient-centered medical home (American Academy of Pediatrics [AAP], 2022), Chronic Care Model (Center for Accelerating Care Transformation, n.d.), NASN's *Framework for 21st Century School Nursing Practice,* and the CDC's *Whole School, Whole Community, Whole Child Model* (CDC, 2023), among others. The tenets are designed to guide schools in providing a comprehensive and collaborative approach to caring for students with chronic health conditions, focusing on optimizing their health outcomes and educational success.

The core tenets incorporate developing a culture of health, promoting a comprehensive approach to care, ensuring communication and collaboration between all stakeholders, creating individualized care plans, providing ongoing professional development and training, addressing health disparities, utilizing data and evaluation to improve care, and promoting wellness and prevention (NCCDPHP, 2021). By adhering to these core tenets, schools can provide high-quality care to their students with chronic health conditions and help them achieve their full potential in school and beyond. See Box 20-1 for the core tenets of the *Consensus Statement on the Core Tenets of Chronic Condition Management in Schools.*

Operationalizing and sustaining the *foundational supports* for these tenets requires (1) supportive leadership and organizational culture, (2) information and communication systems, and (3) sustainable and equitable funding. See Online Materials OM20-1 for the full consensus statement.

Care Coordination and School Nurse–Led Case Management

Care Coordination is one of the five principles in NASN'S (2024a) *School Nursing Practice Framework* and Standard 5A of the *School Nursing Scope and Standards of Practice* (NASN, 2022). It is essential to promoting student health and well-being and can help ensure that students with chronic conditions receive the healthcare services they need to succeed in school. Care coordination is a process by which the school nurse works collaboratively with students, families, healthcare providers, and the school's multidisciplinary team to promote optimal student health outcomes. The school nurse assesses the student's health needs, provides education and guidance to students and families, and helps to ensure that appropriate healthcare services are provided. In addition to providing longitudinal care at school, school nursing care coordination includes the following activities:

- Connect student and family to available resources.
- Collaborate with families, school community, mental health team (including school counselors, social workers, and psychologists), and medical home.
- Develop and implement plans of care.
- Foster developmentally appropriate independence and self-advocacy.
- Provide evidence-based health counseling.
- Facilitate continuity of care with family during transitions (NASN, 2024b, para 1).

While the school nurse leads the process, care coordination involves multiple stakeholders collaborating as a cohesive team to promote students' health and academic achievements and ensure that policies and procedures are consistent with federal and state laws and regulations related to students with special healthcare needs. This team-based approach necessitates ongoing engagement and communication among the student, parents or caregivers, community-based providers, other individuals directly interacting with the student, and the school-based care team. The primary objective is to manage chronic health conditions and enable students to remain safely in school, prepared to learn.

Case management is a concept within the **Care Coordination principle** of the *School Nursing Practice Framework* (NASN, 2024a). ***School nurse–led case management*** (SNLCM) is a specialized form of case management that is provided within the school setting by a school nurse, involving assessing the health needs of individual students, developing and implementing healthcare plans, monitoring and evaluating the effectiveness of interventions, and coordinating with other healthcare providers and resources in the community (NASN, 2021). The school nurse works collaboratively with the student's personal and school health teams, including family members, healthcare providers, teachers, and instructional support personnel, to ensure that the student's healthcare needs are met. SNLCM may also involve addressing transportation, housing, and food security concerns, and promoting self-care and independence. The goal of SNLCM is to promote optimal health and academic outcomes for students with acute or chronic health conditions while ensuring a safe and healthy learning environment for all students. NASN's (2021) *A Model for School Nurse–Led Case Management* is a tool that provides guidance and resources for school nurses to implement a successful case management program for students with chronic health conditions. The SNLCM resources can be accessed from NASN's Learning Center.

Delegation

Delegation is often an important component of nursing practice, but one that often raises concerns for school nurses. The *National Guidelines for Nursing Delegation* developed by

BOX 20-1

Core Tenets of Chronic Condition Management in Schools

Effective, high-quality care for children with chronic conditions is accessible, comprehensive, coordinated, culturally effective, equitable, evidence-based, and child- and family-centered. The key elements of these tenets are further described in the following.

ACCESSIBLE

School stakeholders:

- Work to ensure that children with chronic conditions are able to receive the care they need, when and where they need it, including access to school nursing services, a primary care medical home, and specialty and dental care.
- Assist children with chronic conditions in navigating barriers to care such as cost, transportation, appointment times, language and literacy, technology, and physical accessibility.
- Minimize barriers to care within schools and partner organizations.

COMPREHENSIVE

School stakeholders:

- Advance a comprehensive system of care to meet the needs of children with chronic conditions.
- Apply a whole-child orientation with consideration of physical, emotional, social, cultural, and academic needs.
- Support children with chronic conditions across all school settings (including field trips, before- and after-school care, virtual learning, homebound, etc.) and during emergencies and disasters (e.g., pandemics, natural disasters, lockdowns).
- Provide care that follows children with chronic conditions seamlessly from pre-K through high school and from school to community-based care.

COORDINATED

School stakeholders:

- Implement team-based care for children with chronic conditions, with roles defined according to local circumstances.
- Actively share responsibility and decision making across the team.
- Establish mechanisms and agreements for sharing information among members of the child's care team.
- Support transitions in care for children with chronic conditions.
- Provide case management and care planning for children with chronic conditions when appropriate.

CULTURALLY EFFECTIVE

School stakeholders:

- Understand the cultures represented in their school and community.
- Consider and respect the beliefs, values, customs, and needs of all cultures.
- Develop and maintain awareness of how their own cultural framework impacts their interactions with children and families with chronic conditions.
- Use strategies such as motivational interviewing and active listening as a vehicle to understand and respond to the cultural beliefs and practices of the children and families they serve.

EQUITABLE

School stakeholders:

- Provide individualized care and resources for all children with chronic conditions according to their needs.
- Work to eliminate bias, discrimination, and inequity within their organizations and community.

EVIDENCE-BASED

School stakeholders:

- Implement evidence-based best practices and clinical guidelines for chronic condition management.
- Actively engage in performance and quality improvement activities to ensure the provision of high-quality, safe care for children with chronic conditions.
- Ensure that all children with life-threatening chronic conditions have an emergency action/care plan and access to life-saving medications and equipment at school.

CHILD- AND FAMILY-CENTERED

School stakeholders:

- Collaborate with children with chronic conditions and their families to identify needs and goals and engage in shared decision making.
- Use a strengths-based approach to develop a partnership with children and their families based on trust and respect.
- Provide self-management education and support that builds independence and confidence.
- Advocate for policies, programs, and services to meet the needs of children with chronic conditions and their families.
- Include children with chronic conditions and/or their families on advisory and decision-making bodies.

NCCDPHP (2021, pp. 4–5).

the National Council of State Boards of Nursing and the American Nurses Association (2019) provides important principles and concepts about best practices. In situations authorized by the state's nurse practice act and school regulations, delegating healthcare procedures and medication administration to unlicensed assistive personnel (UAP) may be appropriate for some students with chronic health conditions.

School nurses must know their state's nurse practice act, educational regulations, and school rules to determine whether delegation is permissible. Delegation is a nursing skill requiring critical thinking and nursing judgment.

The school nurse's decision to delegate takes into consideration each child, the child's condition and needs, and potential complications. Some states have clear delegation rules that help delineate what tasks can and cannot be delegated and under what circumstances. For instance, in many states when a student's condition is stable and predictable, it is acceptable to delegate routine daily care, such as oral medication administration. In some states, UAP can be trained to perform a higher level of care, such as colostomy care, gastrostomy tube feedings, and urethral catheterization. Therefore in addition to gaining the skills needed to care for these students, the school nurse is also responsible for training other school staff who may provide services to children with special healthcare needs during the school day.

The school nurse should use standardized processes or checklists to train, monitor, and evaluate UAP competence to perform delegated tasks and reduce delegation risks. A consistent and clear communication, monitoring, and evaluation method must be maintained between the nurse delegating the healthcare task or procedure and the person delegated to perform that procedure. See Chapters 6, 30, and 31 for more discussion of the principles of delegation.

Personal Nursing Services

Some students with medical complexity require continuous nursing assessment, judgment, and interventions for chronic and complex conditions at school. However, due to high caseloads and busy job demands, school nurses may not be continuously available to provide this level of care. In 1999, the Supreme Court of the United States determined that school districts must provide the nursing services that students need in order to access their free and appropriate public education (FAPE), including the right to personal nursing services (*Cedar Rapids Community School District v. Garret F.*, 1999), also called one-on-one or private duty nursing. For example, a student with a tracheostomy who is ventilator dependent needs personal nursing care for continuous monitoring, scheduled and as-needed medication administration, and suctioning during the school day, including during transportation to and from school.

In coordination with the family and healthcare provider, the school nurse is the expert team member to evaluate a student's health status, determine whether individual nursing care is necessary, and suggest the most suitable model for the specific circumstance (Tapper Strawhacker, 2023). The student's physician or licensed provider serves in an advisory capacity; however, the school district does not have to respect medical orders for personal nursing services if deemed not appropriate for the school setting (Lipkin & Okamoto, 2015). If the parent disagrees with the school district's decision, they have the right to due process under the law (see Chapter 7).

Decisions regarding the proper staffing model for students requiring personal nursing care at school should be coordinated with the family, the student's primary or specialty care provider, and school administration guided by the school nurse (Shannon & Minchella, 2015; Tapper Strawhacker, 2023). Staffing models depend on the student's needs and the needs of other students at school or in the district. A one-to-one nurse or a nurse who cares for more than one student in the class could be hired directly by the district or contracted by a nursing agency. A licensed practical or vocational nurse (LPN/LVN) may be able to care for students that have stable and predictable conditions under the supervision of a registered nurse (RN) according to the given state's nurse practice act. In contrast, an RN may be more appropriate to care for students with unstable or unpredictable health conditions. If appropriate to the job description and school policy, licensed nursing staff sometimes are hired to also serve as instructional or classroom paraeducators for their assigned student. Regardless of the chosen staffing model, the direct and indirect nursing services should be outlined in the student's IEP, including the number of nursing service minutes daily or weekly provided by the personal nurse for direct care and the school nurse for case management.

When contracting with an agency to provide nursing services within the school setting, it is necessary to consult with district human resources to ensure the completion of district onboarding mandated hiring processes beyond what the staffing agency requires for their employee. As their employer, the staffing agency is responsible for ensuring that the personal nurse has the necessary licensure, certification, or credentials as required by the state. Agency nurses must comply with federal and state education-related laws, rules, and regulations while practicing in the school setting. All school employees are responsible for reporting any problematic behavior or inadequate care the agency nurse provides. To ensure the safety and appropriateness of student care, it is crucial to clearly understand the roles, responsibilities, and relationships between school nurses, school staff, and agency nurses. Orientation of the personal nurse to school rules and protocols (e.g., school schedule and hours, cellphone use, breaks, privacy and confidentiality, emergency preparedness procedures) should be provided by school staff. See Box 20-2 and Online Materials 20-2 for a checklist that districts can use when contracting with agency personnel.

When a child also receives personal nursing services at home, the family may or may not prefer that the student be cared for at school by nurses from the same nursing agency (Shannon & Minchella, 2015). If the student's one-on-one nurse from home comes to school with the student, clear expectations must be delineated in terms of communication and confidentiality. If the student rides the bus, the agency nurse should be contracted to escort the child on the bus to and from school. Parents/guardians might also request that personal nursing services at school be covered by the Medicaid nursing hours or personal insurance, but they cannot be required to use their own health insurance coverage. Keep in mind that the school has the authority to make decisions whether or not to accept such requests (Tapper Strawhacker, 2023).

BOX 20-2

Example of a Checklist for Contracted (Agency) Personal Nurses at School

DISTRICT ADMINISTRATOR

- Develop policy and procedures for use of contracted personal nurses.
- Establish contracts and memorandum of understanding with contract agency.
- Obtain signatures.
- Meet with agency administrator if needed.

SCHOOL NURSE (WITH SUPPORT FROM DISTRICT ADMINISTRATOR)

- Meet with IEP team (including family); establish need for personal nurse; review procedures with team.
- Complete forms for release of information between family, agency, and a school.
- Participate in IEP and develop IHP including plan for personal nurse.
- Obtain doctor orders and parent/guardian authorization for medications, procedures, treatments, and equipment in school.
- Provide training for personal nurse about school health protocols and procedures, including the following:
  - Assessment of condition and equipment before coming to school
  - Responsibility to care for student at all times
  - Health procedure protocols in school (e.g., where procedures will be done)
  - Emergency procedures and response
  - Sharing IHP and agency care plans
  - Documentation system and requirements
- Provide training of school staff to assist as needed and roles in emergencies.
- Arrange training of personal nurse about protocols and responsibilities, including the following:
  - Chain of command
  - School schedule and hours
  - Campus emergency and disaster protocols
  - Transportation protocols (may need involvement of transportation staff)
  - Confidentiality (FERPA): Only teaching staff communicates educational information to family
  - Personal rules: No smoking, limit cellphone use, no leaving campus, no visitors, etc.
- Arrange meeting with teacher to clarify classroom role and responsibilities.
- Monitor and document student health status and personal nurse competency.
- Communicate regularly with personal nurse, family, and IEP team regarding student health status.

RESPONSIBILITIES OF CONTRACT AGENCY

- Provide documentation of personal nurse: credentials, licensure, CPR certification, insurance, criminal check, ID, tuberculosis test, immunizations.
- Provide contact information of agency supervisor.
- Train personal nurse on special procedures and medical equipment.
- Provide plan for personal nurse call off and substitute personal nurses.
- Share agency plan of care with school nurse (at least every 60 days).
- Supervise personal nurse competence and professionalism in the school setting.

RESPONSIBILITIES OF PERSONAL NURSE

- Provide ongoing assessment of the student and healthcare equipment maintenance at school.
- Provide competent student care at all times.
- Communicate condition updates and changes to the school nurse.
- Maintain confidentiality according to HIPAA and FERPA.
- Documentation of student health status, medications, treatments, procedures for school and agency
- Follow school personnel rules and procedures and demonstrate professional behavior.

Source: Shannon & Minchella (2015), with permission.

When a school district contracts with nursing agencies, assurances should be established that daily competent nursing coverage is guaranteed. Coverage for the absence of the primary nurse is expected to be completed by the agency (Shannon & Minchella, 2015). In the event that agency nursing is absent, contingency plans must be put in place by the district to identify a nurse substitute to cover the student's care on short notice. Families are responsible for providing the medical orders so that treatments, procedures, and medications can be administered correctly. Again, the school must cover all services outlined in the IEP; it is a denial of FAPE if the student is withheld from school or sent home due to lack of nursing care.

Although a personal nurse provides care for the student under their license, the school nurse should regularly assess the student, monitor the care provided, and communicate with the personal nurse, teacher, and family regarding the child's health status—just as the school nurse would be expected to do for any student in their school(s) (Shannon & Minchella, 2015). It is essential that the school nurse has up-to-date medical orders for the student's care. The school nurse should develop a system of regular communication with the agency, personal nurse, and parents/guardians.

SPECIAL CONSIDERATIONS

Students Supported by Assistive Technology

According to the Assistive Technology Act of 2004, Public Law 108-364, *assistive technology* for students with special healthcare needs refers to "any item, piece of equipment, or product system, whether acquired commercially off the shelf, modified, or customized, that is used to increase, maintain, or improve the functional capabilities of a child with a disability."

Students with physical, cognitive, or sensory impairments often require assistive technology to participate in daily activities, communicate with others, and access information and education. Assistive technology can help students with special healthcare needs improve their independence, socialization, quality of life, and achieving their full potential.

Specialized school professionals, such as physical therapists, occupational therapists, mobility specialists, and vision and hearing teachers, are responsible for the integration of assistive technology at school that students need to optimize participation in the learning environment. Assistive technology includes mobility apparatus, augmentive communication devices, hearing and vision aids, computer hardware and software, sensory integration equipment, prosthetics, adapted utensils, and so on. School nurses are responsible for the care and management of medical equipment and technology, such as respiratory equipment (tracheostomy tubes, oxygen delivery systems, ventilators); alternative feeding devices (nasogastric tubes, gastrostomy tubes, portable electronic feeding devices); alternative elimination devices (ostomies, catheters); and implanted devices for medication or therapy (e.g., peripherally inserted central catheter lines, inserted ports, pacemakers, shunts, and vagus nerve stimulators).

Consideration should be given to any modifications that might be needed in common areas of the school, such as bathrooms, the cafeteria, the physical education area, the playground, and art and music classes (such as ramps, lifting equipment, grab bars in bathrooms, and adaptive play equipment).

Students with special healthcare needs who require medical technology may have decreased opportunity to explore their environment, attend extracurricular activities, and freely socialize with other children their age. Some students are embarrassed by their dependence on technology and try to conceal it from teachers, school nurses, and their peers so that they will not appear different. These concerns can be particularly problematic in middle and high schools.

The presence of assistive technology adds additional strain on the family. Not only must they be attentive to their child's health needs, but they must also learn to manage complex technology. Because it is helpful, and in some cases essential, to have a set of equipment in the school building and home, there is the added expense of buying and maintaining additional equipment and potential financial strain.

School nurses lead or participate in the interdisciplinary team working with the family and healthcare provider to determine the child's specific needs and to identify any technology that will help support those needs in the school setting. When there is a device in the body, the school nurse must ensure that the student and device are protected from trauma and infection and anticipate emergency measures should it be dislodged.

School nurses should be educated in using specific technological devices that students use. Primary and specialty healthcare providers, device manufacturers, and vendors are excellent resources for providing literature, training, and hands-on training regarding the technology, its uses, and how to troubleshoot when problems arise. The school nurse is responsible for determining which school staff should be trained on the technology the student uses and ensuring their competence.

The school nurse should work with families to ensure that backup supplies are available in the health office (e.g., batteries, tubing), that any necessary or specialized cleaning agents are in stock, and that the equipment is serviced per manufacturer instructions. There should be a backup power source in case of a power outage or emergency evacuation.

As the liaison for communication among the student, family, educators, and healthcare providers related to assistive technology, the school nurse must be updated by parents/guardians and the primary care provider regarding changes in the child's prescribed technological interventions to ensure the school IHP is up to date. See Chapter 25 for more information on students who are supported by assistive technology.

Chronic Pain

Some chronic conditions are accompanied by pain (e.g., juvenile rheumatoid arthritis, sickle cell disease) or painful treatments (glucose-monitoring finger sticks for diabetes). Research has demonstrated that chronic pain, pain intensity, medication use, and stress associated with school attendance are predictors of absenteeism (Owiredua et al., 2023). Pain interferes with the ability to learn. The burden of pain and maladaptive coping increases with age; therefore early interventions to help children cope with pain should be implemented to prevent adverse outcomes.

Young children and students with intellectual disabilities often cannot express that they are in pain or indicate the nature or severity of their pain. Many school nurses are not confident in assessing pain in students with intellectual disabilities and identify the need for more training (Quinn & Smolinksy, 2018). Inadequate time and school nurse staffing also pose barriers to thorough assessment of pediatric pain in students with intellectual disabilities. It is imperative that school nurses take the time to gain the necessary skills and to complete pain assessments in students with disabilities.

Strategies to assess pain include the following:

- Asking caregivers (e.g., parents/guardians, teachers, other professionals) who know the student well how they suspect the student is in pain and what interventions appear to be effective. The Individualized Numeric Rating Scale may be a helpful pain assessment scale to gather caregiver input.

- Observe the student in the learning environment when they are not experiencing pain to determine "well" behaviors versus behavior when the student is apparently not feeling well or is in pain.
- If the student is not acting typically or displaying maladaptive behavior, then assume the student is in pain. Offer nonpharmacological interventions (e.g., rest, ice or heat pack, distraction) first. If appropriate, over-the-counter or prescribed analgesics may be administered if medical orders and parental permissions are in place (Thompson et al., 2020).

The school nurse should carefully assess the experience of pain in students with chronic conditions, including baseline status, pain triggers and relievers (pharmacological and comfort measures), and coping strategies. The school nurse should remain in close communication with parents/guardians, healthcare providers, and educational staff in developing and implementing an effective pain management plan to optimize the student's participation, minimize loss of instructional time during the school day, and prevent unnecessary absences due to pain.

Patient-Centered Medical Home

Children with chronic conditions are often managed by specialists for their particular condition. According to the American Academy of Pediatrics (2022), high-quality primary care is received by only 43% of students with special healthcare needs. Because healthcare visits are so common, the parents/guardians may forget to ensure that the primary care needs of the child are met, including dental care. School nurses can educate families about the importance of establishing a patient-centered medical home for their child.

A patient-centered medical home is a healthcare delivery model that provides comprehensive, coordinated, and patient-centered care to children and adolescents, with the aim of improving their health outcomes and overall well-being. In a medical home, a primary care provider is a central point of contact for families, overseeing and coordinating all aspects of a child's health care, including preventive care, acute and chronic care, and specialty care. The medical home model emphasizes the importance of family-centered care, continuity of care, cultural competence, and shared decision making among healthcare providers, patients, and families. It also incorporates health information technology, quality improvement, and population health management to optimize care delivery and outcomes (AAP, 2022).

Oral Health

Dental caries, or tooth decay, is a prevalent chronic condition among children; 23% of children ages 2 to 5 years and 52% of children ages 6 to 8 years have had dental caries in their primary teeth, and nearly 57% of adolescents ages 12 to 19 years have had dental caries in their permanent teeth from 2011 to 2016 (CDC, 2019). Children without special healthcare needs have higher rates of oral health problems (16%) than students without special healthcare needs (11%) (Lebrun-Harris et al., 2021). Oral health problems in students with special healthcare needs tend to be more advanced, such as decayed teeth, cavities, gingivitis, and periodontal disease. This disparity is associated with lack of access to dentists and dental staff specializing in students with special healthcare needs and risk factors such as use of sugar-containing medicines and dependence on caregivers for oral care. Students with special healthcare needs from disadvantaged households are even more likely to have oral health problems due to increased barriers to consistent dental care (Lebrun-Harris et al., 2021).

Students with dental caries or poor oral health may miss school or have difficulty concentrating in class due to pain or other health issues, affecting their academic performance and potentially their long-term educational outcomes. If left untreated, dental caries can lead to more severe dental problems and affect a child's overall health and well-being. Families may need to spend time and money on dental treatment for their children, which can be a significant burden, especially for those with limited financial resources. Preventive measures such as regular dental checkups, good oral hygiene, and healthy dietary habits can help to reduce the incidence and severity of dental caries.

The school nurse's role in working with children and families experiencing dental caries includes educating students and parents/guardians about proper dental hygiene and nutrition, performing dental screenings, referring children to dental professionals for treatment, and promoting community resources for dental care. School nurses may also help with preventive measures such as fluoride treatments and sealants and assist in managing children with dental emergencies or pain.

Do Not Attempt Resuscitation Orders

IDEA (2004) gives children with chronic conditions the right to attend school, including when they are in the terminal stage of a disease. An increasing number of students with life-threatening medical conditions are enrolled in schools. *Do Not Attempt Resuscitation* (DNAR) orders for terminally ill patients in hospitals and other healthcare settings are prevalent; yet DNAR orders in the school setting are rare and somewhat controversial (Weiler et al., 2022).

When a medical condition is too advanced to expect recovery and death is imminent, the family may make the difficult decision to request that a DNAR order be honored at school. These orders may also be referred to as *Do Not Resuscitate* (DNR), *Allow Natural Death* (AND), or *Physician* or *Medical Order for Life-Sustaining Treatment* (POLST or MOLST). DNAR orders instruct school staff not to perform cardiopulmonary resuscitation (CPR) in the event of cardiac or respiratory arrest. The purpose of the DNAR order is to provide the child with supportive and compassionate care without prolonging the process or discomfort of dying. When families choose this option, often with the child's assent, there is the possibility that the child will die in school, although this is a rare event. At any time, the parents/guardians can change their minds and rescind the order.

No family wants their child to die at school, but the student and their family may prefer the student to be actively engaged with their friends and enjoying school to the fullest extent possible through the end of life. Although teachers and other parents/guardians might be concerned about how the other students will react and the long-term impact the death may have, parents/guardians of terminally ill children support their child's right to attend school. Some people may argue that withholding CPR violates the nurse's duty to provide care and may cause emotional distress for the nurse and other school staff involved in the student's care. However, it is important to consider the student's quality of life and to note that the out-of-hospital CPR survival rate is poor (less than 10%) (Fink et al., 2016). It is ethically prudent to respect DNAR orders when the outcome of resuscitation will likely not prolong life, but if successful may cause further harm and suffering (Putman, 2024).

There is no federal guidance on DNAR orders in schools. Not all states allow schools to honor a DNAR order. In some states, schools are required by law to have policies in place regarding DNAR orders for students (Weiler et al., 2022). School officials must address complicated ethical, legal, and moral issues. School nurses should advocate that school policies and protocols be developed well in advance of the need to implement a school DNAR plan (Putman, 2024). A school board policy may need to be written or revised to address how DNAR orders are addressed. These policies typically outline the circumstances in which a DNAR order can be issued, the process for obtaining consent from the student's parents/guardians, and the school nurse's role in implementing the order. School nurses must be familiar with state laws and the school's policy regarding DNAR orders and understand their role in implementing them.

Planning to respect a student's DNAR is complex and dynamic. The primary goal of a DNAR order is to prevent unnecessary suffering and ensure a peaceful death. The school nurse is in an ideal position to explain the child's condition, advocate for the family's rights, and lead the development of a comprehensive DNAR plan at school. The school nurse should work with the student's healthcare provider and the student's parents/guardians, communicate with school staff regarding the student's medical condition, and ensure that the DNAR order is appropriately documented and easily accessible in the event of a life-ending event.

The medical orders should clearly define what is meant by DNAR. It is never okay for the order to be written to "do nothing" (Putman, 2024). At a minimum, a DNAR order means not providing CPR, allowing individuals to die naturally without emergency intervention. Provide palliative measures such as positioning for comfort, oxygen administration, mucus suctioning, and controlling bleeding and pain as outlined in the DNAR. Some refer to this plan as a "comfort care plan."

Practice Connection

The NASN (2023) *Position Statement on Do Not Attempt Resuscitation (Orders) in School* states the following:

> *It is the position of the National Association of School Nurses (NASN) that schools and districts should establish DNAR policies, protocols, and practices that enable each student to receive best practice care, as designated by clear and specific directives for the individual, throughout the entire course of their condition while they are in school. Each student with a Do Not Attempt Resuscitation (DNAR) order benefits from having an Individualized Healthcare Plan (IHP) and an Emergency Action Plan (EAP), developed by the registered professional school nurse (hereinafter referred to as school nurse). As professionals who bridge education and health and who advocate for students, school nurses work closely with school teams, families, and students' healthcare providers to appropriately meet the special healthcare needs of students with a DNAR.* (para. 1)

The DNAR order is just one part of the comprehensive interdisciplinary approach. The IHP and EAP written by the school nurse should be incorporated into the DNAR plan, specifically addressing how the death will be handled (NASN, 2023).

The frequency with which a school DNAR order should be reviewed may vary depending on the state and school district policies. However, as a general guideline, it is recommended that DNAR orders be reviewed at least annually or more frequently if there is a significant change in the student's medical condition, treatment plan, or family wishes.

Planning for allowing the natural death of a child at school is an emotional and complex endeavor for everyone involved. It is understandable that teachers and school staff may be scared that the student will die in their classroom. The school nurse can help to ease anxiety regarding the possibility of a child's death by helping the school team to understand what to expect and delineating the specific roles and responsibilities of the student support team members, teachers, administration, and other school staff. Preparation and practice drills may help alleviate anxiety.

School nurses and school staff must be prepared to respond appropriately in the event the student appears to be dying, which includes communicating with the family immediately; providing comfort, support, privacy, and dignity to the student and their family; and coordinating with emergency medical services. Staying with the child and providing psychosocial support to the child, family, and school personnel is essential. The emotional needs of the student's friends and classmates must be carefully considered by the student support team and mental health professionals at school such as the social workers, counselors, and psychologists. See DNAR planning guidance for school nurses and personnel in Box 20-3.

BOX 20-3

Do Not Attempt Resuscitation (DNAR): Planning for the Child in School

PRE-DNAR ORDER

- Hold team meeting, including family.
- Obtain assessment data.
- Obtain current medical summary.
- Acquire equipment.
- Order/obtain supplies.
- Determine schedule.

DNAR ORDER

- Obtain releases of information for emergency medical services (EMS) and appropriate agencies.
- Write DNAR plan congruent with state laws and district policies.
- Obtain DNAR (original order if required).
- Obtain out-of-hospital DNAR bracelet (if required).
- Note DNAR order expiration date.
- Obtain student permission for DNAR if 18 years old.
- Determine need for full-time or 1:1 nurse in school.
- Contact EMS.
- Contact medical examiner.
- Determine emergency contacts.
- Involve palliative care or hospice.
- Include Comfort Care orders, POLST/MOLST as appropriate.
- Determine protocol for calling in case of emergency: family, physician, prearranged EMS.
- Communicate plan between school nurse and
  - Palliative care team
  - Local EMS
  - Funeral director
  - Involved local agencies, others as needed
  - All members of student's healthcare team
- Develop a code that everyone will recognize.
- Determine which staff members should be informed and receive training/education.
- Train designated staff.
- Address staff: moral, cultural, and ethical issues.
- Conduct student population assessment for education and needs if DNAR is implemented.
- Plan transportation
  - To and from school
  - Field trips
  - After school activities
  - Door to door, curb to curb
  - Special bus (air conditioning, seating)
  - Bus aide (UAP, healthcare aide, RN)

IMMINENT DEATH

- Clarify end-of-life issues vs. acute issues.
- Designate an area for care to be delivered.
- Direct Comfort Care orders, POLST/MOLST if appropriate.
- Plan for comfort care, including
  - Holding
  - Positioning
  - Oxygen
  - Pain management
  - Bleeding control
- Outline what may and may not be performed by staff that requires treatment/management vs. comfort care.
- Determine plan if no risk of imminent death:
  - EMS consultation
  - Consultation with parent/guardian
  - Transport to hospital (hospital of choice vs. nearest hospital needs to be discussed)

Death

- Determine where student will be moved.
  - For serious distress event or death
  - To provide privacy for student and family
- Plan for other students and staff.
- Determine who can pronounce death (per state regulations).
  - Physician
  - Nurse practitioner
  - Physician assistant
- Determine when student will be moved from school.
  - EMS may not be able to move the body once death has occurred.

Transportation and Mortuary Arrangements

- Determine plans for
  - Funeral home
  - Type of vehicle and where it will be parked
  - How student will be transported (stretcher, etc.)
  - Who will clear the hallways
  - Which doors to use

ROLE OF THE CRISIS TEAM

- Utilize bereavement team for staff and students.
- Determine who will call parents/guardians).
- Determine a plan if sibling in same building.
- Review and update plan whenever student's condition changes, at least annually.

Source: Zacharski et al. (2013), with permission.

CONCLUSION

Perhaps the most important concept related to students with chronic health conditions is that they are children first. Each child is unique and should not be defined solely by their diagnoses or medical condition. School nurses are key in providing care coordination, case management, and direct care to students with special healthcare needs and chronic conditions. They are valuable members of an interdisciplinary team that works to optimize these students' health, safety, learning, and overall well-being while at school. School nurses utilize their full range of skills and knowledge, in accordance with their state's nurse practice act, to anticipate potential complications, provide appropriate interventions, treat exacerbations, offer anticipatory guidance, support independence, and evaluate the outcomes of the care provided (McCabe, 2020). As child health experts, school nurses coordinate care, provide case management, promote health education, facilitate quality improvement, and utilize critical thinking skills to benefit schools, families, the healthcare system, and—most important—the students with chronic health conditions that they serve.

The Editors gratefully acknowledge the work of the 3rd edition chapter authors, Janice Selekman and Michelle Ness.

References

American Academy of Pediatrics. (2022). *About the National Resource Center for Patient/Family-Centered Medical Home.* https://www.aap.org/en/practice-management/medical-home/about-the-national-resource-center-for-patientfamily-centered-medical-home/

American Psychological Association. (2023). *Habilitation: Definition.* https://dictionary.apa.org/habilitation

Assistive Technology Act. (2004). Public Law 108–364. https://www.ataporg.org/ATActSummary

Association of Rehabilitation Nurses. (2018). *What does the pediatric rehabilitation nurse do?* http://www.rehabnurse.org/pubs/role/Role-Pediatric-Rehab-Nurse.html

Baines, S., Emerson, E., Robertson, J., & Hatton, C. (2018). Sexual activity and sexual health among young adults with and without mild/moderate intellectual disability. *BMC Public Health, 18*(667), 1–12. https://doi.org/10.1186/s12889-018-5572-9

Cedar Rapids Community School District v. Garret F., 525 U.S. 66. (1999). https://supreme.justia.com/cases/federal/us/526/66/

Center for Accelerating Care Transformation. (n.d.). *The chronic care model.* American College of Physicians. https://www.act-center.org/application/files/1616/3511/6445/Model_Chronic_Care.pdf

Centers for Disease Control and Prevention. (2019). *Oral health surveillance report: Trends in dental caries and sealants, tooth retention, and edentulism, United States, 1999–2004 to 2011–2016.* https://www.cdc.gov/oralhealth/publications/OHSR-2019-index.html

Centers for Disease Control and Prevention. (2023). *Whole school, whole community, whole child.* https://www.cdc.gov/healthyschools/wscc/index.htm

Charlucien-Koech, R., Brady, J., Fryer, A., & Dias-Gonzalez de Ferris, M. E. (2021). School nurse practices promoting self-management and healthcare transition skills for adolescents with chronic conditions in urban public schools: A mixed methods study. *Journal of School Nursing.* https://doi.org/10.1177/10598405211053266

Consolini, D. M. (2022). *Children with chronic health conditions.* Merck Manual. https://www.merckmanuals.com/professional/pediatrics/caring-for-sick-children-and-their-families/children-with-chronic-health-conditions#:~:text=Children%20with%20chronic%20health%20conditions%20may%20have%20some%20activity%20limitations,in%20school%20and%20peer%20activities

Coughlin, M. B., & Sethares, K. A. (2017). Chronic sorrow in parents of children with a chronic illness or disability: An integrative literature review. *Journal of Pediatric Nursing, 37*, 108–116. https://doi.org/10.1016/j.pedn.2017.06.011

Fink, E. L., Prince, D. K., Kaltman, J. R., Atkins, D. L., Austin, M., Warden, C., Hutchison, J., Daya, M., Goldberg, S., Herren, H., Tijssen, J. A., Christenson, J., Vaillancourt, C., Miller, R., Schmicker, R. H., & Dallaway, D. W. (2016). Unchanged pediatric out-of-hospital cardiac arrest incidence and survival rates with regional variation in North America. Resuscitation Outcomes Consortium. *Resuscitation, 107*, 121–128. doi:10.1016/j.resuscitation.2016.07.244

Holdsworth, E., Trifonova, V., Tanton, C., Kuper, H., Datta, J., Macdowall, W., & Mercer, C. H. (2018). Sexual behaviours and sexual health outcomes among young adults with limiting disabilities: Findings from third British National Survey of Sexual Attitudes and Lifestyles (Natsal-3). *BMJ Open, 8*, 1–12. http://dx.doi.org/10.1136/bmjopen-2017-019219

Individuals With Disabilities Education Improvement Act of 2004, 20 U.S. C. § 1400 (2004). http://.ed.gov/download/statute.html

Klein, K., Wheeler, M., & Yonkaitis, C. F. (2018). College-bound: Transition planning strategies for students with type 1 diabetes. *NASN School Nurse, 34*(1), 17–20. https://doi.org/10.1177/1942602X18794891

Lebrun-Harris, L. A., Canto, M. T., Vodicka, P., Mann, M. Y., & Kinsman, S. B. (2021). Oral health among children and youth with special health care needs. *Pediatrics, 148*(2). Article 2020025700. https://doi.org/10.1542/peds.2020-025700

Lipkin, P. H., & Okamoto, J. (2015). The Individuals With Disabilities Education Act (IDEA) for children with special educational needs. *Pediatrics, 136*(6), e1650–e1662.

Maternal and Child Health Bureau. (2012). Data Resource Center for Child and Adolescent Health. *Who are children with special health care needs?* U.S. Department of Health and Human Services, Health Resources and Services Administration. https://www.childhealthdata.org/docs/nsch-docs/whoarecshcn_revised_07b-pdf.pdf

Maternal and Child Health Bureau. (2022). *Children and youth with special health care needs. NSCH Data Brief.* Health Resources and Services Administration, https://mchb.hrsa.gov/sites/default/files/mchb/programs-impact/nhsc-data-brief-children-youth-special-health-care-needs.pdf

McCabe, E. M. (2020). School nurses' role in self-management, anticipatory guidance, and advocacy for students with chronic illness. *NASN School Nurse, 35*(6), 338–343. https://doi.org/10.1177/1942602X20906534

McPherson, M., Arango, P., Fox, H., Lauver, C., McManus, M., Newacheck, W., Perrin, J. M., Shonkoff, J. P., & Strickland, B. (1998). A new definition of children with special health care needs. *Pediatrics, 102*(1 Pt 1), 137–140. https://doi.org/10.1542/peds.102.1.137

Merriam-Webster Dictionary. (2023). *Stigma: Definition.* https://www.merriam-webster.com/dictionary/stigma

Michielsen, K., & Brockschmidt, L. (2021) Barriers to sexuality education for children and young people with disabilities in the WHO European region: A scoping review. *Sex Education, 21*(6), 674–692. https://doi.org/10.1080/14681811.2020.1851181

Nasir, A., Nasir, L., Tarrell, A., Finken, D., Lacroix, A., Pinninti, S., Pitner, S., & McCarthy, M. (2019). Complexity in pediatric primary care. *Primary Health Care Research & Development, 20*(e59), 1–7. https://doi.org/10.1017/S146342361800035X

National Association of School Nurses. (2021). *A model for school nurse–led case management.* https://www.nasn.org/blogs/nasn-profile/2021/08/24/manual-a-model-for-school-nurse-led-case-mgmt

National Association of School Nurses. (2022). *School nursing: Scope and standards of practice* (4th ed.). Author.

National Association of School Nurses. (2023). *Do not attempt resuscitation (orders) in school.* (Position Statement). Author. https://www.nasn.org/nasn-resources/professional-practice-documents/position-statements/ps-dnar

National Association of School Nurses. (2024a). A contemporary framework update for today's school nursing landscape: Introducing the School Nursing Practice Framework. *NASN School Nurse, 39*(3), 140–147.

National Association of School Nurses. (2024b). *School Nursing Practice Framework: Handout.* https://www.nasn.org/nasn-resources/framework

National Center for Chronic Disease Prevention and Health Promotion. (2022). Centers for Disease Control and Prevention. *About chronic diseases.* https://www.cdc.gov/chronicdisease/about/index.htm

National Center for Chronic Disease Prevention and Health Promotion, Division of Population Health, Healthy Schools Branch. (2021, August). *Consensus statement on the core tenets of chronic condition management in schools.* Cooperative Agreement Number NU38OT000282. Centers for Disease Control and Prevention. https://downloads.aap.

org/AAP/PDF/Consensus%20Statement%20-%20Core%20Tenets%20of%20CCMS%20%202021-08%20.pdf?_ga=2.180171041.445658547.1676225993-38208536.1676225992

National Center for Education Statistics. (2022). Students with disabilities. *Condition of education*. U.S. Department of Education, Institute of Education Sciences. https://nces.ed.gov/programs/coe/indicator/cgg

National Council of State Boards of Nursing & American Nurses Association. (2019). *National guidelines for nursing delegation*. https://www.ncsbn.org/public-files/NGND-PosPaper_06.pdf

Owiredua, C., Flink, I., & Boersma, K. (2023). Prevalence and risk factors for pain-specific school absenteeism in adolescents with recurrent pain: A prospective population-based design. *European Journal of Pain, 27*, 390–400. https://doi.org/10.1002/ejp.2065

Phelan, J. C., Lucas J. W., Ridgeway, C. L., & Taylor, C. J. (2014). Stigma, status, and population health. *Social Science Medicine, 103*, 15–23. https://doi.org/10.1016/j.socscimed.2013.10.004

Putman, S. (2024). Do not attempt to resuscitate (DNAR) in the school setting. In C. A. Resha & V. L. Taliaferro (Eds.), *Legal resource for school health services* (pp. 277–287). SchoolNurse.com

Quinn, B. L., & Smolinski, M. (2018). Improving school nurse pain assessment practices for students with intellectual disabilities. *The Journal of School Nursing, 23*(6), 480–488. https://doi.org/10.1177/1059840517722591

Rehabilitation Act of 1973 (Pub. L. 93-112). https://www.gpo.gov/fdsys/pkg/STATUTE-107/pdf/STATUTE-107-Pg718.pdf

Rosa's Law: Public Law 111–256. (2010, October 5). https://www.govinfo.gov/content/pkg/PLAW-111publ256/pdf/PLAW-111publ256.pdf

Russo, K. (2022). Assessment and treatment of adolescents with chronic medical conditions. *Journal of Health Service Psychology, 48*(2), 69–78. https://doi.org/10.1007/s42843-022-00059-4

Schmidt, E. K., Brown, C., & Darragh, A. (2020). Scoping review of sexual health education interventions for adolescents and young adults with intellectual or developmental disabilities. *Sexuality and Disability, 38*, 439–453. https://doi.org/10.1007/s11195-019-09593-4

Shannon, R. A., & Minchella, L. (2015). Students requiring personal nursing care in school: Nursing care models and a checklist for school nurses. *NASN School Nurse, 30*(2), 76–80. https://doi.org/10.1177/1942602X15569781

Stopbullying.gov. (2020a, July 21). *Bullying and youth with disabilities and special health needs*. https://www.stopbullying.gov/bullying/special-needs

Stopbullying.gov. (2020b, July 21). *Bullying and youth with disabilities and special health needs: Tip sheet*. https://www.stopbullying.gov/sites/default/files/2017-09/bullyingtipsheet.pdf

Tapper Strawhacker, M. (2023). Legal issues 101: Students who require one-to-one nursing services. *NASN School Nurse, 38*(4), 178–181. https://doi.org/10.1177/1942602X231176568

Thompson, V. N., Morse, B. L., & Peters, A. B. (2020). Pain assessment approaches for students with intellectual disability. *NASN School Nurse, 35*(5), 250–253. https://doi.org/10.1177/1942602X20915819

van den Anker, J., Reed, M. D., Allegaert, K., & Kearns, G. L. (2018). Developmental changes in pharmacokinetics and pharmacodynamics. *Journal of Clinical Pharmacology, 58*(S10), S10–S25. https://doi.org/10.1002/jcph.1284

Weiler, S., Birnbaum, M., & Westbrook, P. (2022). An examination of state statutes and school district policies addressing minors with do not resuscitate orders. *Educational Policy*. Advance online publication. https://doi.org/10.1177/08959048221120278

Wooldridge, S. (2023, April 12). *Writing respectfully: Person-first and identity-first language*. National Institutes of Health. https://www.nih.gov/about-nih/what-we-do/science-health-public-trust/perspectives/writing-respectfully-person-first-identity-first-language

Wright's Law. (2018). *Physical education for students with disabilities*. http://www.wrightslaw.com/info/pe.index.htm

Zacharski, S., Minchella, L. Gomez, S., Grogan, S., Porter, S., & Robarge, D. (2013). Do not attempt resuscitation (DNAR) orders in school settings: Special needs school nurses review current research and issues. *NASN School Nurse, 28*(2), 71–75. https://doi.org/10.1177/1942602X12472540

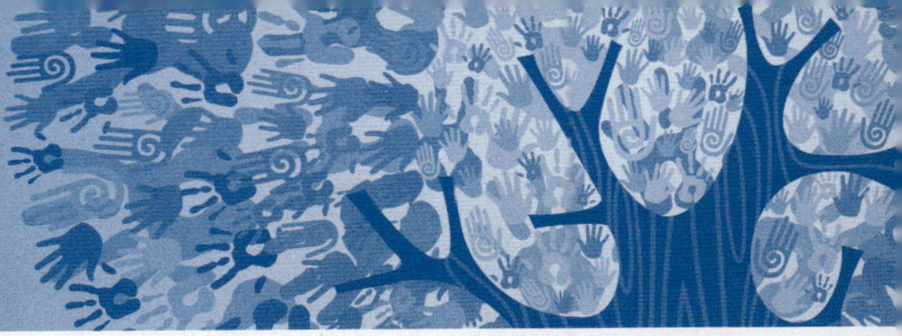

Chapter 21

Students With Allergies

Megan O. Lewis ▪ Jonathan M. Spergel

CHAPTER OUTLINE

The school nurse provides care coordination and case management for students with chronic health conditions in the school setting, including students with allergies. Students with allergies have a range of clinical presentations, from mild reactions such as sneezing, itching, and nasal congestion to severe reactions with urticaria, wheezing, vomiting, and anaphylaxis. School nurses are the health professionals that provide safe educational environments with allergen avoidance strategies and leadership when an emergency response is required.

Allergic disease is a high-impact worldwide health issue. Over 5.2 million children (7.2%) reported symptoms of allergic rhinitis in the past year (Centers for Disease Control and Prevention [CDC], 2022a). It is estimated that 8% of children in the United States have a food allergy, approximately two students per classroom (CDC, 2022c). These numbers illustrate that allergies have a profound impact on students and schools.

Allergy care in the school setting is a shared responsibility that incorporates both prevention and emergency response (Schoessler & White, 2013). The school nurse is integral to ensuring that all members of the school community understand the sources of common allergens, as well as how to provide life-saving treatment in the event of anaphylaxis. Policies and protocols should be in place to guide the school nurse in implementation of interventions aimed at environmental controls and emergency response.

CAUSATIVE FACTORS OF ALLERGIES

According to the American Academy of Allergy, Asthma, and Immunology (AAAAI; 2023), "An allergy is a chronic condition involving an abnormal reaction to an ordinarily harmless substance called an allergen. Allergens can include aeroallergens such as dust mite, mold, and tree weed and grass pollen, as well as food allergens such as milk, egg, soy, wheat, nut or fish proteins" (para. 1). A child is 75% more likely to have allergies when both parents are allergic and 50% more likely if one parent has allergies (Allergy & Asthma Network, 2023b). The tendency to be allergic and to produce higher quantities of immunoglobulin E (IgE) is passed to the child, not the type of allergy; therefore the child has a greater likelihood of developing some kind of allergy.

Allergic disease tends to progress from infancy to adulthood, which is often referred to as the *allergic march*. It often begins with an infant suffering from atopic dermatitis, or eczema, progressing to food allergies in later infancy and allergic rhinitis and asthma during the school-age years (Liu & Martinez, 2016). Research is exploring whether early exposure will decrease allergic diseases. Repeated environmental exposure can also influence allergies. For example, children with spina bifida who have daily exposure to latex in catheters are at higher risk for developing latex allergies (Bowman et al., 2001).

The cause of allergies in particular individuals is not completely understood. The hygiene theory speculates that allergy and asthma are more common in industrialized nations because of the lack of early exposure to dirt, germs, and allergic triggers and the overuse of antibacterial cleansers (Liu, 2015). Climate change is another proposed cause, including longer pollen seasons, mold growth following floods, and airborne irritants following wildfires (Collins, 2018). Evidence supports delaying the introduction of solid foods in infants until after 4 months of age can increase the risk for the development of allergy. Multiple clinical trials have demonstrated that certain foods, such as peanut and egg, when given around 6 months of life, can prevent food allergy. Consensus guidelines have been published about the importance of early introduction and food allergy (Fleischer et al., 2020).

PATHOPHYSIOLOGY OF ALLERGIES

An understanding of the interaction between the immune system and potential allergens provides the nurse with a basis for allergy care in the school setting. The immune system has three main functions: recognizing self from nonself, destroying invading pathogens, and getting rid of worn-out or damaged cells. When the immune system is functioning properly, pathogens are eradicated, and homeostasis is maintained. However, there are times when the immune system overperforms its functions and hyperreacts to products to which the body does not normally react. This is the basis for the allergic response.

Immune Cells

All cells have markers on their outside shell. These markers are highly specific. Some markers within one human being are the same so that the body can recognize itself. When a substance with a different set of markers enters the body, the immune system is stimulated to attack, neutralize, and eliminate that substance, with or without injury to the person's body. A foreign/nonself product is called an antigen, and antibodies are made in response. In allergy, the antigen is referred to as an allergen.

There are three main types of white blood cells: granulocytes (neutrophils, eosinophils, and basophils); monocytes; and lymphocytes (T and B). Neutrophils (also called polymorphonuclear leukocytes, polys, or segs) are the first cells that arrive at the site of trauma or invasion. They are the most numerous of the white blood cells (approximately 60%) but are short lived. They attack bacteria and fungi and function by phagocytosis. Once they leave the blood vessel, they stay in the general area of the trauma or invasion (Rote & McCance, 2017). Their presence at the site and the chemicals they release result in the *signs of inflammation*. Although not usually associated with allergy, the inflammatory process is always present after initiation of the allergic response and is the cause of many of the secondary symptoms of inflammation that are observed, especially edema.

Mast cells (in the tissues) and basophils (in the blood) have similar functions involved in the allergic reaction. Basophils circulate in the bloodstream and migrate into the tissue during the inflammatory process. Mast cells are found throughout the body but are more prevalent under the epithelial surface of the skin, in the mucosal linings of the nose and upper airways, in the conjunctival lining of the eyes, and along the gastrointestinal (GI) tract, all positioned to have direct contact with external environmental allergens. All of these sites are prime entry sites for antigens/allergens (Rote, 2017). Histamine and leukotrienes are the main products released when basophils and mast cells are stimulated and cause the symptoms of allergic reaction, including swelling, sneezing, runny nose, and, in severe cases, hypotension.

The primary focus of eosinophils is to release toxic granules. They stimulate inflammation, especially in response to mast cell degranulation, and therefore have an increased presence during an allergic attack that involves a histamine reaction. They are most abundant in tissues near mucosal linings, similar to mast cells (Schwartz et al., 2017).

Antibodies fall into five immunoglobulin classes: IgM, IgG, IgA, IgD, and IgE. Although most antibodies made to antigens are of the IgG family, the one with the most relevance to allergy is IgE; it is this class that stimulates the most common allergic reactions. Normally in a low concentration in the body, individuals with allergies have much higher concentration of IgE. Immunoglobulins are unique and they recognize specific antigen or allergens. Memory B cells can make immunoglobulin years after the initial exposure (Rote, 2017).

Immunology of Immediate Type I Immunoglobulin E–Mediated Allergic Reactions

Allergies are described in multiple ways, including the type of white blood cell involved, the timing of the allergic reaction (immediate or delayed), the organ system involved, and the route or source of the allergen. The most common allergic reaction is classified as an immediate type I hypersensitivity reaction or an IgE-mediated reaction. An IgE reaction may manifest as allergic rhinitis, atopic dermatitis, bronchial asthma, food allergy, or anaphylaxis.

A type I hypersensitivity reaction begins within 10 minutes of exposure to the allergen (Rote, 2017); thus it is called an *immediate* reaction. It can be delayed up to 2 hours if there is delayed absorption with a high-fat meal. The early phase of the response resolves within 1 to 3 hours. A secondary inflammatory response, or late phase response, occurs 6 to 12 hours later and can last for up to 24 hours as a result of the influx of other white blood cells and the inflammation (Oettgen, 2016). This concept is essential to understand the medications prescribed for allergy and asthma.

On first encounter with an allergen, whether by contact, ingestion, inhalation, or injection, the macrophages take the allergenic markers from the wall of the allergen and present them to B cells. With the signal from a particular type of CD4 T cell, the B cell makes IgE antibodies. All immunoglobulins are in the shape of the letter Y. The tail of the Y for IgE is perfectly suited to fit into receptor sites on basophils and mast cells, where it then sits waiting for the next exposure to the allergen (Rote, 2017). This process occurs the first time the individual is exposed to the antigen, yet the symptoms of an allergic reaction, including the possibility of anaphylaxis, are not always seen until the second and future exposures when the products of the mast cells (i.e., histamine, leukotrienes, and prostaglandins) are released. This concept can be an educational opportunity with parents and caregivers who may challenge the nurse's observation of allergy symptoms by reporting that the child had previously ingested or contacted the allergen and not experienced a reaction.

The Role of Histamine

The degree of severity of an allergic reaction is dependent on multiple factors, including the amount of IgE sitting on mast cells and the amount of allergen; an individual's overall health; and other exacerbating factors, including illness and exercise. The mediators include histamine, which dilates and increases the permeability of the blood vessels, providing a "doorway" for immune cells to exit the vessel and enter the tissues with resulting edema, erythema of the skin, and respiratory symptoms (sneezing, itching, congestion, and rhinorrhea). When this reaction occurs in the GI tract, the individual may experience cramps, bloating, diarrhea, and vomiting (Rote, 2017). In addition to increasing vessel permeability, histamine also causes constriction of bronchiolar and vascular smooth muscle (resulting in wheezing) and respiratory distress. The signs and symptoms of an individual's allergic reaction depend on the site of the histamine release in the body.

The symptoms commonly seen in a type I reaction are primarily due to the histamine released from the mast cells. Histamine is locally irritating and causes sneezing and an "itchy" sensation in the ears, on the skin, and in the back of the throat. As the permeability increases because of the histamine, fluid and substances are released from the vessels into the tissue, resulting in edema and erythema of tissues and hives.

Delayed Hypersensitivity Reactions

Delayed reactions are commonly discussed surrounding drug allergy. They have previously been classified as type II to IV delayed cell-mediated hypersensitivity reactions. Delayed hypersensitivity reactions can occur in a variety of forms. For instance, drug-induced hemolytic anemia may occur days to more than 72 hours after drug exposure. It is thought to be driven by an IgG and IgM cytotoxic reaction against the cell surface. Serum sickness reactions can occur 1 to 3 weeks after exposure to a drug and are thought to be driven by an immune complex reaction (Khan et al., 2022).

A type IV delayed cell-mediated hypersensitivity reaction does not involve IgE; it involves T lymphocytes. This results in a delay in symptoms by up to 48 hours after contact. Tuberculin skin testing is an example of a type IV reaction, as are many cases of contact dermatitis, such as poison ivy. In this type of delayed reaction, chemicals are released that can cause tissue destruction, but the reaction is rarely fatal and does not result in anaphylaxis (Rote, 2017).

PRESENTATION OF ALLERGY

When a student comes to the health office frequently with undiagnosed allergic symptoms, it is the responsibility of the school nurse to identify a pattern of the symptoms. It may be that symptoms occur in a particular classroom (such as one with rugs or pets), when the student is engaged in a particular activity (such as lunch or outdoor physical education), during a particular season, or when the student is with particular people (who may have pets or use perfumes). Identification of a family history of atopic (allergic) disease helps support the diagnosis. A mild allergic reaction may advance in severity and should be carefully observed. The school nurse can recommend to the parents that the student be evaluated by an allergist.

Allergic Rhinitis

Allergic rhinitis is sometimes inaccurately called "hay fever", even though fever is not associated with allergy. Allergic rhinitis usually develops around 9 to 10 years of age and peaks during mid- to late adolescence, although it can begin in preschool years. Students who have respiratory allergies are usually aware their symptoms are worse at certain times of the year, lasting 1 to 2 months at a time. It is important for school nurses to understand the pattern of pollination of their geographical region related to seasonal allergies. Ragweed is the biggest environmental allergen during the fall. Trees and grass are the most common allergens in the spring.

Allergic rhinitis can be characterized by inflammation of the nasal mucosa. The symptoms are IgE mediated; mast cells are activated in the nasal mucosa, conjunctiva, and the upper respiratory tract, resulting in histamine release and increased permeability. Clinical signs and symptoms include nasal congestion, watery rhinorrhea, sneezing, headache, and itching of the throat, nose, ears, and eyes (Allergy & Asthma Network, 2023a).

The nasal mucosa will have a pale, bluish hue; nasal discharge will be clear. Examination of the external portion of the nose often shows a transverse crease across the lower third of the nose. This crease is caused from pushing the nose up with the heel of the hand in an effort to relieve itching and nasal congestion, referred to as an "allergic salute" (Conlon & Wilson, 2015). As a result of chronic congestion, darkened areas under the eyes or "allergic shiners" are commonly seen in children with allergy. See Figure 21-1.

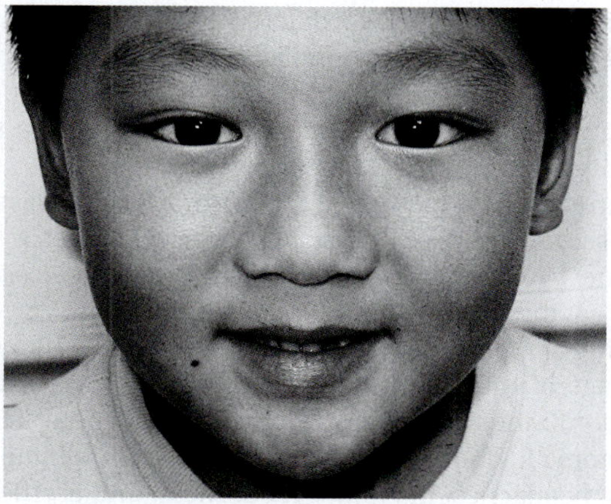

FIGURE 21-1. Allergic shiner and nasal crease.

The nose humidifies and warms inhaled air, provides the sense of smell, and contributes to the sense of taste. The nasal congestion of allergic rhinitis leads to mouth breathing, which results in altered smell and taste, a dry mouth, and can increase the chances of respiratory infection. Mouth breathing and nasal obstruction can also lead to sleep apnea with resultant daytime somnolence and decreased attentiveness (Allergy & Asthma Network, 2023a).

Rhinoviruses are the most prevalent cause of the "common cold" (CDC, 2023). Therefore it is often difficult to distinguish rhinosinusitis from allergic rhinitis. Rhinovirus infects the upper respiratory tract causing inflammation of the mucosa of the nose down to the bronchi. The symptoms of sneezing, coughing, nasal obstruction or congestion, rhinorrhea, malaise, low-grade to no fever, and watery or inflamed conjunctiva usually last 7 to 10 days. On nasal examination, it is noted that the nasal mucosa is erythematous and inflamed rather than pale to bluish as with allergic rhinitis. Seasonal allergies can last for weeks to months as cold viruses typically last significantly less. Establishing a differential diagnosis is essential because the symptoms of allergic rhinitis are similar to the common cold and other upper respiratory conditions, such as influenza (flu) or COVID-19. See Table 21-1 (CDC, 2023).

TABLE 21-1 Symptoms of Allergies, Colds, Flu, and COVID-19

Symptom	Allergy	Cold	Flu	COVID-19
Headache	Rare	Rare	Usually	Usually
Cough	Sometimes	Usually	Usually	Usually (dry)
Muscle aches	Never	Sometimes	Usually	Usually
Tiredness	Sometimes	Sometimes	Usually	Usually
Sneezing	Usually	Usually	Usually	Rarely
Sore throat	Rarely	Usually	Usually	Usually
Runny or stuffy nose	Usually (also itchy mouth, eyes, inner ear)	Usually	Usually	Usually
Fever	Never	Sometimes	Usually	Usually
Diarrhea	Never	Never	Sometimes (more common in children)	Sometimes
Nausea or vomiting	Never	Never	Sometimes (more common in children)	Sometimes
New loss of taste or smell	Sometimes	Sometimes (especially with stuffy nose)	Rarely	Usually (early—often without a runny or stuffy nose)
Shortness of breath	Sometimes (with asthma/reactive airway)	Rarely	Usually	Usually

Mayo Clinic (2023); Cleveland Clinic (2024); CDC (2023).

It is also important to differentiate allergy from substances, such as tobacco smoke, that are respiratory irritants but do not stimulate the allergic response. Certain strong odors, such as perfumes, also can irritate a hypersensitive airway.

Untreated allergies place a person at an increased risk for a secondary infection such as ear infection or sinusitis due to constant swelling of the nasal mucosa and sinus cavities, including persistent fluid in the ear canal. Swelling in the upper respiratory track prevents natural drainage of mucus, resulting in immobile secretions and infection. Sinusitis can last anywhere from 7 to 21 days. Symptoms include purulent drainage, fever, fatigue, body aches, headaches, maxillary tenderness, and erythema of the nasal mucosa and posterior pharynx. Pain between the eyes and forehead may also be present (Skoner, 2000). Children may also experience nausea from the constant swallowing of mucus.

Allergic conjunctivitis, an IgE-mediated immune response, is commonly seen with allergic rhinitis. Because it is rare to have ocular allergic symptoms without nasal symptoms, the combination of the two can be helpful in the diagnosis of allergic conjunctivitis. Clinical signs and symptoms include upper and lower eyelid swelling, watery clear discharge, intense itching of the eye, and redness of the conjunctiva and sclera. On physical examination, symptoms most often occur bilaterally, the cornea is usually not involved, and edema of the eyelid or conjunctiva may be present (Dupuis et al., 2020).

Complications of allergic conjunctivitis can be corneal abrasion secondary to intense scratching of the eye and infection resulting from frequent touching of the eye with dirty hands. Standard treatment for allergic conjunctivitis is ocular antihistamines for itching and swelling and ocular steroids for redness and swelling. Antibiotics are not needed for resolution unless underlying infection is suspected. It is important to carefully differentiate between allergic conjunctivitis and infectious conjunctivitis (viral or bacterial) (Dupuis et al., 2020). A thorough health history can help to differentiate the cause of symptoms and help the school nurse decide whether the student can stay in school, needs to go home, or needs medical evaluation. See Chapter 16 for more information on the types of conjunctivitis.

The school nurse can provide eye relief by using the eye wash station to rinse allergens from the sclera and conjunctiva. Cool compresses can provide some comfort but are not clinically indicated for treatment. If a child has repeat episodes of allergic ocular symptoms, refer the student for medical evaluation and possible orders for oral antihistamine or eye drops.

Urticaria and Angioedema

A dermal response to histamine release in a type I reaction is *urticaria*, commonly known as hives or wheals. Urticaria is an intensely itchy rash that appears as discrete, erythematous, raised, irregularly shaped lesions. The wheals have a blanched center surrounded by a red flare or halo of dilated vessels (Zuraw, 2016). It should be noted that hives can also occur due to nonimmunological causes, such as exposure to cold temperatures and emotional stress. Viral infection is another common cause of hives that is not allergic.

Angioedema is similar to urticaria but occurs at a deeper layer of the skin, therefore the swelling can cause pain or burning, rather than itching, yet the skin may appear normal. Depending on the location, angioedema can make it painful for a student to do simple things like hold a pencil or walk. Symptoms include swelling of the lips, tongue, eyes, face, or extremities (Zuraw, 2016). When any swelling compromises the airway, it should always be considered an emergency.

Atopic Dermatitis

Atopic dermatitis refers to either contact dermatitis or eczema. *Eczema* is an inflammatory skin condition producing pruritus that can be severe and presenting with a dry, inflamed, scaly rash on the cheeks, scalp, trunk, and extensor surfaces in infants. However, in older children, it appears in flexural areas, such as the antecubital and popliteal fossae, neck, wrists, ankles, and feet (Wilson, 2015). General signs and symptoms of dermatitis include skin dryness, pruritus, erythema, plaque eruption (weeping and crusting), and lichenification in severe cases. Lichenification is thickening of the skin due to repeated scratching. Genital areas are usually not affected. Children with atopic dermatitis often have interrupted sleep due to itching and can experience infected lesions created by scratching (American College of Allergy, Asthma, and Immunology [ACAAI], 2023a). Eczema is a major risk factor for developing food allergy, with studies showing varying rates of eczema and co-occurring food allergy. Evidence has shown that sensitization through a disrupted skin barrier can lead to food allergy (Johansson et al., 2017).

Atopic dermatitis is a chronic inflammatory skin disease that affects up to 20% of all children. The "atopic march" has been extensively studied; evidence suggests atopic dermatitis is the initial step in 30% to 50% of pediatric allergy (Davidson et al., 2019). Chronic eczema can be seen in older children. It may be exacerbated by inhalants, foods, cosmetics, fragrances, plants, metals, and several other natural and chemical compounds.

Treatment involves avoidance of the allergen, prevention of secondary infection from scratching, and comfort measures to decrease pruritus. Skin hydration measures and moisturizers are needed to repair and help maintain skin integrity. Certain fabrics, such as wool, rough fabrics, and furry stuffed animals, may irritate the skin condition. Perspiration associated with heat and high humidity may also increase itching (Wilson, 2015).

Home care recommendations include a warm daily bath followed by immediate application of a moisturizer (referred to as "soak and seal"). Hypoallergenic moisturizers can be used liberally throughout the day, but should not be applied over any topical medication. Vaseline is another inexpensive treatment option, but should only be applied to damp skin, as it is an occlusive agent (Boguniewicz et al., 2017).

Atopic dermatitis is a condition that can cause a high level of frustration and anxiety for students and their families. Sleep disturbances occur in 67% of children due to pruritus, and parents are likely to sleep less than 6 hours per night (Fishbein et al., 2021). Students with atopic dermatitis are more likely to be diagnosed with attention deficit-hyperactivity disorder and conduct disorders. Additionally, they are 2 to 6 times more likely to develop anxiety and depression. The care of a child with atopic dermatitis can be involved, and education regarding treatment has been shown to significantly improve the family's quality of life (National Eczema Association, 2023). For more information on atopic dermatitis, see Chapter 18.

ANAPHYLAXIS

Anaphylaxis is defined as an acute, potentially life-threatening hypersensitivity reaction involving the release of mediators from mast cells, basophils, and recruited inflammatory cells (Brown & Turner, 2017). Anaphylaxis is a severe allergic reaction typically caused by exposure to food, insect stings, medications, or latex. Massive histamine release results in bronchoconstriction and vasodilation and generalized vascular permeability affecting multiple systems in the body if left untreated, leading to anaphylactic shock. Symptoms may vary among individuals and can occur within minutes or up to 2 hours after exposure to a provoking agent; reactions may be mild, moderate, or severe (Brown & Turner, 2017). Symptoms and severity of anaphylaxis may also vary with each exposure to the allergen. See Figure 21-2 for signs, symptoms, and response to anaphylaxis.

There has been a significant increase in the number of emergency department visits and hospitalizations for anaphylaxis since the 1990s. Most fatalities from anaphylaxis occur outside the hospital setting and are due to a delay in epinephrine administration (Turner et al., 2020). Twenty percent of children experience their first anaphylactic episode in school. Food allergies are the most common trigger, followed by allergy to insect stings (Simons, 2016). Certain factors amplify anaphylaxis, including exercise, use of alcohol, use of nonsteroidal anti-inflammatory drugs, concurrent illness, and emotional stress.

Epinephrine

The prompt administration of epinephrine is critical because epinephrine is the only medication that can stop an anaphylactic reaction (Brown & Turner, 2017). Rapidly affecting alpha- and beta-adrenergic receptors, epinephrine works to reverse anaphylaxis by promoting vasoconstriction, decreasing vascular permeability, and relaxing the smooth muscle tissue of the lungs, gut, and bladder. Within 10 minutes, heart rate and blood pressure should increase. However, because epinephrine is quickly metabolized by the body, a second dose may be needed 10 to 15 minutes after the first administration.

The risk for complications and death from anaphylaxis is associated with a delay in the administration of epinephrine (Sicherer & Simons, 2017). *"There is no absolute contraindication to epinephrine treatment"* (Simons, 2016, p. 528). It rarely causes serious adverse events. Other ancillary medications, such as antihistamines, may also be ordered, but should not replace or delay the administration of epinephrine (Shaker et al., 2020). Emergency medical services (EMS) should *always* be called as soon as epinephrine is administered and the student should be transferred to the nearest emergency department (Mayo Clinic, 2022).

Epinephrine is injected intramuscularly in community settings such as home and school. Epinephrine is available in three doses: 0.1 mg for infants, 0.15 mg for a young child, and 0.3 mg for a larger child or teenager (greater than 55 to 66 lb) to be administered intramuscularly in the mid-outer thigh and held in place for 3 seconds (Mayo Clinic, 2022). The dose can be repeated in 5- to 15-minute intervals as needed to relieve symptoms (Sicherer & Simons, 2017). It may take 30 to 60 minutes for the anaphylactic reaction to begin to resolve (Brown & Turner, 2017). There are many different epinephrine delivery devices, most commonly autoinjectors. Administration directions can be found on autoinjector manufacturer Web sites. Clinical trials are underway evaluating other routes of epinephrine administration, such as intranasal or sublingual delivery options.

A secondary or biphasic reaction can occur following treatment for anaphylaxis within 72 hours of the initial event. Biphasic reactions are associated with more severe initial reactions and occur in less than 1% to 20% of all reactions (Shaker et al., 2020). Treatment for this secondary reaction remains the same; epinephrine is the treatment of choice. The school nurse needs to bring the possibility of a biphasic reaction to the caregiver's attention as it is important not to leave the child alone during the first few days following a reaction (Schoessler & White, 2013). It is equally important for the family to inform the school nurse when epinephrine had been administered at home.

Both the family and the school must ensure that they have sufficient epinephrine on hand should signs and symptoms of anaphylaxis recur. Self-injectable epinephrine is predominantly provided to the school by the student's family; two should be requested and medical orders should be secured. The student's epinephrine may be kept in the health office or the classroom, or the student may keep the epinephrine on their person during the day (self-carry) (Bingemann et al., 2021). However, approximately one quarter of events happen in persons who have not experienced anaphylaxis before. Consequently, schools are prudent to "stock" undesignated epinephrine that can be administered to anyone displaying signs and symptoms of anaphylaxis.

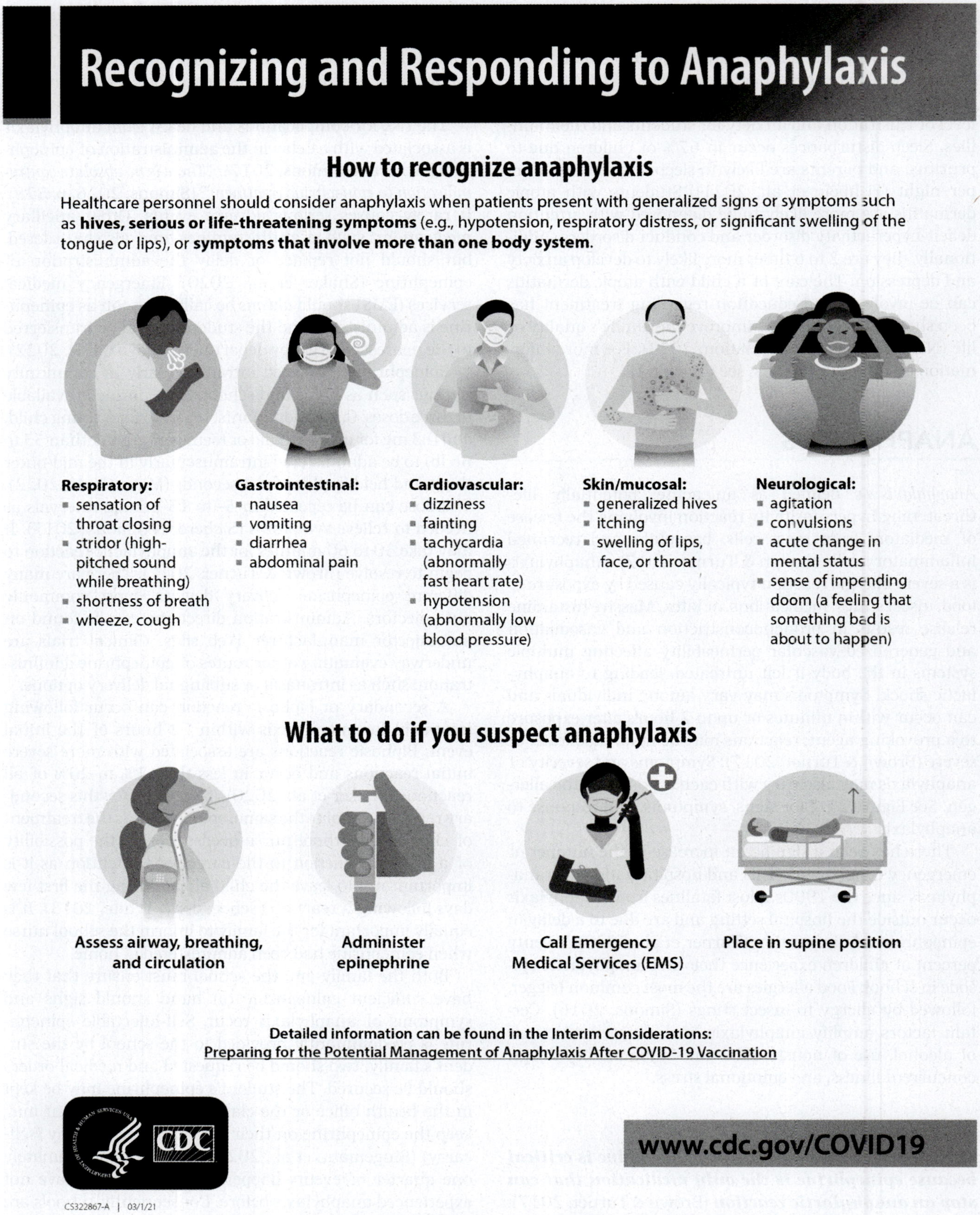

FIGURE 21-2. Recognizing and responding to anaphylaxis. *(CDC, 2021)*

> **Practice Connection**
>
> As of 2021, undesignated epinephrine in schools is allowed in all 50 states and Washington, DC, to treat anaphylactic reactions in students or adults without an individualized medical order. However, school policies, protocols, and procedures for using "stock" epinephrine vary widely between states. Only about one-third of states mandate schools to have stock epinephrine. Who is responsible for developing and implementing stock epinephrine protocols also varies widely between districts (Volerman et al., 2022). Finding cooperating licensed prescribers and funding for stock epinephrine can be challenging. School nurses are the most highly qualified professionals to advocate for, develop, and lead stock epinephrine policies and programs. School nurses can educate school boards, teachers, and families that the administration of undesignated stock epinephrine in an emergency is a safe investment that saves lives.

Regular training of parents and school personnel on the use of epinephrine autoinjectors is an essential part of allergy management. While training increases accuracy and speed, the skill is lost within a few months of training (Simons, 2016). Therefore retraining should occur once or twice each year and before sending a staff person with students on a field trip.

SOURCES OF ALLERGENS

An allergen is defined as a usually harmless substance capable of triggering a response that starts in the immune system and results in an allergic reaction (AAAAI, 2023). The most common allergens are environmental, food, latex, insect venom, and medications (Allergy & Asthma Network, 2023a). Environmental allergies can be divided into two major categories: outdoor allergens and indoor allergens.

Outdoor Allergens

Pollen consists of grains that are produced by trees, grasses, and weeds and can float through the air in spring, summer, and fall as it fertilizes plants. Exposure to pollen particles affects susceptible patients when the small particles enter the nasal passage, eyes, ear canal, and mouth (Allergy & Asthma Network, 2023a). Pollen particles are small and light and are often blown long distances by wind. Trees are the first plants to release their pollen in late winter and early spring, with grass pollen emerging in late spring and summer. Pollen from weeds, especially the potent ragweed, arrives in late summer and fall.

Pollen counts are measured daily and can be accessed online from the National Allergy Bureau. Many local allergists' offices post these counts daily on their Web sites, and local news stations may broadcast or post them for public information. Students with extreme sensitivity to certain pollens may need to stay in from recess on days when the pollen counts are excessively high. Allergy season varies in different parts of the country based on when trees, grasses, and weeds pollinate. During pollen seasons, levels are highest in the morning, during mildly windy conditions, and when grass is being mowed. Students allergic to pollen usually present with respiratory symptoms. Immunotherapy, or allergy shots, can often be used to relieve symptoms of pollen allergies by inducing tolerance of the allergen.

Outdoor mold is a fungus that grows in damp, dark places, often out of sight of those working to put environmental controls in place for allergy management. Mold is made up of microscopic spores, or reproductive seeds that become airborne when disturbed and cause an allergic reaction (Allergy & Asthma Network, 2023a). Mold digests whatever it lands on, including wood, paper, and compost piles. Students with mold allergies often present with nasal and sinus congestion, sore throat, and watery eyes, among other symptoms.

Indoor Allergens

Cats, dogs, and **other animals** are a common source of indoor allergens. The proteins found in the skin and dander (the sloughed epithelial skin cells) of animals with fur, as well as their saliva and urine, can cause allergic reactions. These tiny proteins can settle in furniture, rugs, and house dust that circulates throughout the home (Allergy & Asthma Network, 2023a). The severity of the reaction is directly proportional to the dose of the allergen. The risk associated with animal allergens should be considered before introducing classroom pets. School district policy on the topic should also be determined. Cat dander can be detected in schools without pets as it travels with students' clothes from home. Animal allergens can cause reactions when inhaled or when there is contact with eyes or skin. Reactions can happen within minutes or may be delayed for hours after exposure. They can be moderate to severe, including asthma-like symptoms such as wheezing and shortness of breath, hives, and itchy skin and eyes. There is no scientific evidence to support the existence of "hypoallergenic" pets (Sheehan & Phipatanakul, 2016). Early exposure of infants to cats, dogs, and farm animals is thought to be protective for asthma and other atopic conditions (Fall et al., 2015; Sheehan & Phipatanakul, 2016).

Dust mites can be found virtually everywhere—in carpeting, stuffed toys, mattresses, pillows, and upholstered furniture. They are tiny, microscopic insect-like pests that feed on human skin flakes. The feces, saliva, and body parts of dust mites can trigger asthma and allergic reactions in sensitive individuals. Dust mites are present year-round but are more of a problem during fall and winter when windows are closed, heating systems are in use, and students spend more time indoors. Warmth and humidity greater than 50% especially promote the growth of dust mites (Sheehan & Phipatanakul, 2016). Regular dust also contains dust mites. Routine dusting and vacuuming in the classroom can make a significant difference in reducing dust mites and other allergens. Symptoms include itchy eyes and scratchy throats, and the allergen is considered a potent trigger of asthma. There is good evidence about the importance of dust mite controls in the home, such as utilizing mattress/pillow covers, hot water washing of the bedding weekly, and limiting stuffed animals (Allergy & Asthma Network, 2023a).

Cockroaches are mostly nocturnal, scavenge at night for food and water, and leave behind trails of allergens that can cause symptoms on contact or when inhaled. Cockroach allergens are believed to consist of feces, saliva, and body parts. These pests hide in cracks and crevices in homes and schools and move freely from room to room or adjoining units via wall spaces, plumbing, and other utility installations. Cockroaches prefer a moist, warm habitat. Allergen levels are usually highest in kitchen or food service cabinets and floors, while moisture-laden bathrooms are secondary areas. Poorly contained food and garbage in kitchens is a well-known risk factor. Studies suggest that the bedroom is another prime location for cockroaches, particularly in heavily infested homes (Allergy & Asthma Network, 2023a). This has an impact for students who live in urban settings or for students in older school buildings. Cockroach allergens are known to affect the severity of asthma.

Indoor mold typically appears as brown/yellow or black/green splotches and often has a musty odor. It can grow on any organic substance, as long as moisture and oxygen are present, and often is present in areas of high humidity, especially basements, bathrooms, locker rooms, and kitchens. Mold can become a significant problem if it remains undiscovered or unaddressed. It will destroy anything on which it grows, and when inhaled, mold can cause allergy symptoms (Allergy & Asthma Network, 2023a). The U.S. Environmental Protection Agency (USEPA) recommends professional remediation to remove mold and preventive measures to prevent moisture problems in school buildings (USEPA, 2022). Indoor air quality should be addressed in the school setting. Resources from the EPA may be helpful for schools. See Chapter 13 for more on indoor air quality.

Food Allergies

Food Intolerance Versus Food Allergy

There is often confusion and misconception about the difference between food intolerance and food allergy (Table 21-2). *Food intolerance* involves a nonimmune system response in the digestive system that causes discomfort; it may include metabolic, pharmacological, or toxic mechanisms. Food intolerance may be due to an enzyme deficiency that prevents a food from being broken down in the intestines, leading to abdominal discomfort.

Lactose is the most common food intolerance; it is found in milk and other dairy products. Gluten is another product that is often misidentified as an allergen. Gluten intolerance or celiac disease is an inability to digest wheat, rye, barley, and oats, leading to GI discomfort. Celiac disease is an autoimmune process against ingested gluten that causes damage in the small intestines. The most common symptoms of celiac disease include bloating, diarrhea, constipation, and failure to thrive (Sables-Baus & Fidanza, 2017).

A *food allergy* is defined as "an adverse health effect arising from a specific immune response that *occurs reproducibly* on exposure to a given food" (Bock & Sampson, 2016, p. 371). Food allergies can be IgE mediated, non–IgE mediated, or mixed type, although IgE-mediated allergies are much more common and are generally caused by a combination of genetic and environmental factors. Food allergies are not typically associated with triggering asthma or chronic rhinitis in children (Sicherer et al., 2017).

Approximately 8% of U.S. children and 10% in the general population have food allergies (CDC, 2022c). Prevalence rates have increased over the last 2 to 3 decades (Sicherer & Sampson, 2018). There are nine food allergens that are responsible for 90% of all food allergy reactions in the United States: cow's milk, tree nuts, peanuts, eggs, fish, wheat, soybean, shellfish, and sesame (Nowak-Wegrzyn et al., 2017).

Some food allergies typically resolve during childhood, such as milk, egg, wheat, and soy; others, such as seeds and nuts, typically persist into adulthood. The symptoms of allergic reactions to food differ among individuals. One of the

TABLE 21-2 Food Intolerance Versus Food Allergy

	Food Intolerance	Food Allergy
Where reaction takes place	Digestive system	Immune system
Kind of reaction	Mild to moderate discomfort	Possible life-threatening reaction
Symptoms	Bloating, abdominal pain, diarrhea, vomiting	Multiple body systems (skin [rash, flushing, pruritus], respiratory [bronchoconstriction/dyspnea], cardiac [hypotension], and/or gastrointestinal [nausea, abdominal pain, diarrhea, vomiting])
Reaction time	May be delayed	Usually immediate
Action to take	See healthcare provider	Activate EMS

Adapted from Allergy and Asthma Network (2017).

Did You Know?

Students who have a history of egg allergy of any severity *can* receive influenza vaccination and measles, mumps, and rubella (MMR) vaccines without additional precautions beyond those recommended for any vaccine (CDC, 2013a, 2022b).

challenges of caring for students with allergies is that a student's reaction can be different from one episode to the next.

Diagnosis of food allergy is based on a thorough health history, a food diary, and allergy testing (Sicherer et al., 2017). The clinical history is the most important element in diagnosis (Sicherer & Sampson, 2018). Testing can produce false positives, thus the gold standard to diagnose a food allergy is a food challenge.

Oral allergy syndrome, also called pollen-food allergy syndrome, is often seen in individuals with hay fever or pollen allergies (especially to birch, ragweed, and mugwort pollens), who then react to certain plant proteins (Nowak-Wegrzyn et al., 2017). Symptoms are usually mild and limited to the mouth and throat and include itching and swelling of the lips, tongue, and throat. Oral allergy reactions occurs because the proteins in some fruits and vegetables are similar to those found in pollen, thus confusing the immune system. For instance, fresh apples can trigger mouth and throat pruritus, but applesauce may be tolerated without issue.

Peanut and Tree Nut Allergy

Peanuts are legumes. Aptly named, tree nuts (e.g., almonds, Brazil nuts, cashews, hazelnuts, pecans, pistachios, and walnuts) grow on trees. Both peanut and tree nut allergy typically persist throughout the lifespan and are major causes of anaphylaxis. Approximately 2% to 3% of U.S. children have peanut allergies (Soriano et al., 2021), with lower percentages estimated to have tree nut allergies (McWilliam et al., 2020). Many children with peanut allergy also have allergy to one or more tree nuts. Research has shown that early introduction of peanuts to infants significantly decreases the chance of developing peanut allergy (Logan et al., 2023; Soriano et al., 2021). Consensus guidelines resulting from the *Learning Early About Peanut Allergy (LEAP)* study state that peanuts (as well as eggs and other allergens) can be introduced around 6 months of age to prevent the future development of those allergies (Fleischer et al., 2020). To reduce the risk of choking, peanut butter can be mixed in pureed fruit or vegetables (Sicherer et al., 2017). The significant success of studies focusing on early introduction of peanuts may indicate that there will be a decrease in the number of students with peanut allergy in the future. Follow-up studies have found that even though peanut allergy may decrease with this intervention, rates of asthma or seasonal allergies were not affected (Du Toit et al., 2018).

Latex Allergy

Latex is a liquid produced by the brasiliensis tree that is used to make natural rubber. Latex allergy can be found in 1% to 7.6% of the general population. Students who have undergone repeated medical procedures as small children, especially those with spina bifida, are at higher risk for latex allergy (Parisi et al., 2021). Latex allergy symptoms may be mild at first with flushed cheeks, itchy eyes, or sneezing. Symptoms can quickly progress to a more systemic response including urticaria, wheezing, coughing, periorbital erythema and swelling, and even nausea and vomiting (Beierwaltes & Schoessler, 2017). Latex can be transmitted by direct contact and inhalation of latex particles in the air. While most latex allergies are IgE mediated, a type IV reaction (non-IgE delayed reaction) is usually limited to the skin and may develop 24 to 48 hours after exposure.

Creating a latex-safe environment at school can be difficult, but it is imperative for the student with a latex allergy. Products containing latex should be removed from school, including latex balloons, latex gloves (most commonly found in health and food service), and certain brands of erasers, rubber bands, and art supplies, as well as science, physical education, and sports equipment. Bicycle tires, swim goggles, gym mats, mouse pads, condoms, blood pressure cuffs, stethoscopes, and the rubber stoppers in vials may contain latex (Allergy & Asthma Network, 2023a).

Insect Allergies

Outside play and warm weather often lead to insect encounters. Recess, field day, outdoor physical education classes, and open windows (including on school buses) all place students allergic to insects at increased risk. Most insect sting reactions are mild, involving only a dermal reaction of swelling, pain, itching, or discomfort at the site. Insect sting allergy occurs in 0.4% to 3% of the general population. The incidence of anaphylaxis occurring from an insect sting in children is 0.3% to 1% (Elberink, 2016).

Biting insects (mosquitoes, flies, fleas, and bedbugs) inject saliva while feeding; this rarely causes anaphylaxis. Stinging insects (wasps, bees, and yellow jackets) inject venom that can be allergenic. Large local reactions peak in 24 to 48 hours and take 5 to 10 days to resolve. Systemic reactions can range from mild to life-threatening; symptoms usually start within 15 minutes of the sting and can progress quickly to anaphylaxis (Elberink, 2016). See Chapter 17 for more information on insect bites.

Did You Know?

Latex allergy is unique in that it can cross-react with foods that have similar proteins, especially fruits such as banana, avocado, chestnut, and kiwi. When eating these cross-reactive foods, some people with latex allergy may experience an allergic reaction (Allergy & Asthma Network, 2023a).

Treatment for large local reactions can include cold compresses, antihistamines to reduce itching, and nonsteroidal anti-inflammatory drugs (NSAIDs) to decrease pain. Keep the student calm to decrease the absorption of venom, raise the affected body part above the heart, and apply cold compresses. The school nurse should observe for symptoms of anaphylaxis. Treatment for insect venom anaphylaxis is no different from other anaphylactic reactions—injection of epinephrine.

If the stinger is still in the skin, it should be removed as soon as possible to prevent more venom from entering the body. Scrape the stinger off horizontally with a blunt edge of a knife, credit card, or fingernail; do not squeeze the stinger because this will increase the amount of venom released into the skin. The site can then be washed with soap and water.

In the case of fire ants, it is important to carefully brush off the fire ants and leave the site of the nest. The painful stings of the fire ants can cause blisters in the first 24 hours. These blisters will then appear cloudy and may become pustular. If the blisters are open, care must be taken to prevent secondary infections.

The following measures can be taken to decrease the chance of insect stings in the allergic student:

- Don't walk barefoot on grass; wear shoes.
- Avoid trash cans.
- Avoid strong scents and bright-colored clothing that can attract stinging insects.
- Avoid loose clothing or open shoes that can trap insects.
- Avoid being outdoors alone.
- If a nest is encountered, remain calm and slowly back away from the area.
- When eating outdoors, keep food and drinks covered; avoid drinking from cans or straws that may hide insects.
- When an area of stinging insects is located on school property, inform school personnel so that steps can be taken to get rid of the nests (Golden, 2017).

Medication Allergies

Medications can also be an allergen source for some students. Allergic reactions can occur within minutes of ingesting a medication or up to several hours later. The reaction can be immediate (IgE-driven reaction) or delayed and may not appear for 7 to 10 days after treatment has started (Hausmann, 2017). The most common clinical symptoms are maculopapular eruptions and urticaria.

The medications that most often cause an allergic reaction include the following:

- Antibiotics
- Aspirin and NSAIDs (e.g., ibuprofen)
- Drugs used in anesthesia
- Insulin (rarely)
- Topical medications: antibiotic ointments can cause a contact dermatitis (Allergy & Asthma Network, 2023a)

While many families report their child is allergic to penicillin, less than 10% of these children test positive and therefore are often given inappropriate or ineffective antibiotics to treat infections (Khan et al., 2022). In addition, many children with penicillin allergy during infancy lose their skin test positivity over time and are rarely tested again during childhood (Trubiano et al., 2017).

Other Sources of Allergies

There are other less common causes of allergies. Some children are allergic to particular wavelengths of the *sun*, resulting in a pruritic papular rash only on exposed areas of skin and only at certain times of the year (Harvard Health Publications, 2014). *Chemicals* such as formaldehyde and those used in cleaning products and pesticides can also result in an allergic response. Chemicals present in cosmetics and personal care products that can cause contact and respiratory symptoms include aerated scents from hairsprays, craft glues, permanent markers, and aromatherapy. The USEPA (2017) refers to these reactions as *multiple chemical sensitivities* or *idiopathic environmental intolerances*. Parental requests for the use of essential oils as a means of calming their child should be discouraged in the school setting, because the odor may trigger an allergic response in sensitized students and staff; there is little empirical support for this practice.

Contact dermatitis from chemicals, irritants, topical medications, metals, and fabrics (e.g., wool) results in a localized flare. If the nurse observes that the rash is localized, a detailed history of what has been in contact with the skin in that specific area can help identify the etiology and possible treatments. Nickel dermatitis is a common metal allergy that can manifest in various degrees from minor itching to blisters at the site of contact. Many products contain nickel, including fashion jewelry and piercings, watches, buttons, zippers, belts, silver wear, and electronic devices (Rishor-Olney & Gnugnoli, 2023).

Cold urticaria results in hives within 2 to 5 minutes of contact with cold temperatures or substances, including contact via cold weather, going into cold water, and eating and drinking cold food and drink. The cause of cold urticaria is not well understood (National Institutes of Health [NIH], 2015). *Stress* is another potential cause of hives due to unknown etiology.

ALLERGY TESTING AND MANAGEMENT

Testing

Parents/guardians may report an allergy, but it is vital to have medical confirmation of the diagnosis. Allergy testing has two key components: a detailed medical history and diagnostic tests to determine a patient's allergens (ACAAI, 2023b). While allergy testing should be done by a board-certified allergist in a medical setting, the school nurse should confirm that allergy testing has been completed and recognize the dermatological signs and symptoms resulting from the testing.

Allergy tests frequently used may include the following:

1. Skin prick test: A diluted extract of the allergen is placed on the patient's skin; then the skin is scratched with a prick device. A raised skin reaction (i.e., wheal) at the site of the prick indicates a possible allergy.
2. Blood tests for allergen-specific immunoglobulin E antibodies.
3. Oral food challenge tests are the gold standard for diagnosing food allergies. Oral food challenges should be performed by an allergist at a medical facility that has epinephrine, oxygen, IV fluids, and other treatments for potential anaphylactic reactions (Allergy & Asthma Network, 2023a).

Immunotherapy

Subcutaneous immunotherapy entails a series of injections of specific allergens administered in gradually increasing dosages over a defined period. The goal of immunotherapy is to desensitize the body to known allergens by forcing IgG to bind to receptors before IgE, thus preventing the allergic cascade. Once desensitized, the patient is able to better tolerate exposure with few or no symptoms. Immunotherapy is most effective for allergic rhinitis, stinging insects, and managing patients with allergic asthma; it is not indicated for atopic dermatitis, food allergy, chronic urticaria, or angioedema (Matsui & Eggleston, 2016).

The most common side effect of immunotherapy is a local reaction. Redness and itching at the site are common complaints. Antihistamines, topical steroid creams, and ice can minimize these adverse effects. Systemic reactions are rare, but not predictable based on local reactions. Most systemic reactions occur within 20 to 30 minutes after injection; therefore patients must wait in the medical office for 20 to 30 minutes after injection.

Sublingual immunotherapy is effective for seasonal allergic rhinitis, especially allergies to grasses and ragweed; side effects are usually oral or gastrointestinal (Matsui & Eggleston, 2016). Contraindications include uncontrolled asthma, eosinophilic esophagitis, or a previous reaction to this treatment. The first dose should always be administered in a medical setting.

Oral immunotherapy is a well-studied intervention to desensitize to food allergens. Oral immunotherapy works by giving the child small quantities of the allergen at home every day, then gradually increasing the amount under medical supervision. In many cases, daily ingestion can reduce a child's sensitivity to a food. Research trials demonstrate 60% to 80% effectiveness of oral immunotherapy and regular ingestion has proven to reduce the risk of accidental exposures. For instance, if a child who is allergic to peanuts can tolerate 300 mg of peanut (one very large peanut) daily for more than 6 months, they can likely tolerate exposure to 2 grams of peanut (seven peanuts). At the time of publication, there is one U.S. Food and Drug Administration–approved oral immunotherapy product for peanut allergy, called Palforzia®, which requires procedures to ensure the patient's safety, such as exercise restrictions for a period of time after taking the daily dose (Children's Hospital of Philadelphia, 2023).

Medications

The American Academy of Allergy, Asthma, and Immunology (2018) provides information on medication for allergies. The major categories are as follows:

- *Antihistamines* (pills, liquids, nasal sprays, eye drops) block histamine and relieve sneezing, rhinorrhea, itching of the eyes, and hives. (NOTE: Some over-the-counter antihistamines can be sedating.)
- *Decongestants* (pills, liquids, nasal sprays, eye drops) shrink the blood vessel lining of the nasal passage and reduce nasal congestion. Some nasal decongestants can cause rebound congestion when used for more than 3 days.
- *Corticosteroids* (nasal sprays and eye drops) relieve sneezing, nasal congestion, and itching of the eyes.
- *Leukotriene modifiers*, or leukotriene receptor antagonists (tablets or granules), such as montelukast, zafirlukast, and zileuton, relieve ocular and nasal symptoms.
- *Mast cell stabilizers* (nasal sprays and eye drops) prevent release of histamine and relieve sneezing, nasal congestion, postnasal drip, and itching of the eyes.
- *Saline sprays* (liquid and spray) flush nasal passages (Gentile et al., 2016).

Generalized Management Measures

The primary and most effective treatment for allergy is avoidance of the allergic trigger. The goal is to decrease the allergic load, or the amount of allergen in the environment. Multiple environmental control measures can be taken in both the home and school setting in this regard (Box 21-1). Implementing environmental control measures will benefit students and staff with allergies, decrease discomfort, minimize absences and lost instructional time, and perhaps reduce the amount of allergy medication needed. Avoidance can be almost impossible for children with outdoor and indoor allergens. Visiting another school or a field trip requires assessment and preparation based on the source of the allergies.

Maintaining good health via adequate sleep, exercise, and nutrition supports the immune system. Maintaining psychological health can also assist in maintaining immune health. Comorbid conditions such as diabetes or inflammatory bowel disease need to be well controlled; deficits in one condition could affect the ability to control allergy symptoms.

Home measures to decrease allergic symptoms include keeping windows closed and using air conditioning during

BOX 21-1

Allergen Avoidance and Control Measures for the Home and School

CLASSROOM AND HEALTH OFFICE MEASURES

- Remove carpeting from floors.
- Damp-dust often when the student is not in the immediate area.
- No curtains or blinds; window shades are preferable.
- No stuffed chairs (unless they can be wiped down).
- Decrease clutter; remove nonwashable dust collectors from classrooms, such as stuffed animals.
- Use plastic, metal, and wood toys that can be wiped down.
- No feather pillows or comforters; no wool blankets (cotton or synthetic only).
- Wash bed sheets weekly on the hot cycle ~130 degrees.

POLLENS AND OUTDOOR MOLDS

- Stay indoors when grass is being cut and close classroom windows.
- Use air conditioning with regular changing of filters to reduce indoor exposure to outdoor pollen.
- Reduce outdoor exposure during times of high pollen counts in season.
- Shower after outdoor activity to remove pollen from self.
- Do not hang clothes on a clothes line.
- Wipe the fur of outdoor animals before they come indoors to remove the pollen.
- Avoid outdoor gym class when the pollen or mold count is high.

INDOOR MOLD

- Clean visible mold growth in bathrooms, showers, locker rooms, concrete, or cement block walls (especially in basements) and damp wood surfaces with bleach-based agents.
- Clean showers and locker room daily; keep well ventilated with the appropriate-sized ventilation exhaust system.
- Repair indoor leaks and seepage (besides mold, cockroaches like humid moist areas).
- Reduce humidity in the school building below 50% to avoid excess humidity; in areas with high relative humidity, the use of dehumidifiers may be necessary.
- Classroom walls should have washable paint.

ANIMALS

- Remove pets from home if able or keep outdoors.
- Keep furry pets out of classroom (turtles and fish are OK).
- Ensure that rooms are swept daily and garbage is removed to prevent food from attracting cockroaches.
- Use a high efficiency particulate air (HEPA) filter (studies on the effects of air cleaners on clinical symptoms have been inconclusive).
- Keep cat allergen low by bathing cats twice a week.

IRRITANTS THAT MAY AFFECT STUDENTS

- Live flowers in the classroom
- Sprays, paints, cleaners, disinfectants, insecticides used while students are in the area
- Smoking in the school environment or at entryways
- Perfumes, incense, or other strong smells

periods of high pollen counts. Decrease clutter, rugs, curtains, stuffed toys, and anything that can accumulate dust. Damp dusting is more effective than just spreading the dust around with dry dusting. Dehumidifiers can be used in parts of the home that may be damp, especially basements and bathrooms. Smoking and the use of aerosol products should not occur in the home, because they act as respiratory irritants. In the school setting, chalk dust can also act as a respiratory irritant.

SCHOOL NURSING CARE FOR STUDENTS WITH ALLERGIES

In alignment with the nursing process, the first step in caring for students with allergies/anaphylaxis is a comprehensive assessment. Once a student with an allergy is identified, the school nurse should collect objective and subjective data from the student, parent/guardian, and healthcare provider regarding specific allergen(s), presentation of previous allergic reactions, treatments, and when the last allergic reaction occurred. The school nurse should assess the school environment (classrooms, cafeteria, school grounds, etc.) to identify and limit potential sources of exposure.

> **Focus on the Framework**
>
> School nurses should care for students with allergies and risk for anaphylaxis (National Association of School Nurses [NASN], 2021) according to the **Care Coordination** principle of NASN's *School Nursing Practice Framework* (NASN, 2024). School nurse–led case management of students with allergy/anaphylaxis is quite complicated and must be individualized to the student's health status, developmental stage, learning environment, cultural considerations, and family priorities.

School nurses are responsible for detailed planning for students with significant allergies and risk for anaphylaxis, beginning with the development of an individualized healthcare plan (IHP). Development and implementation of a Section 504 plan may be indicated to establish the accommodations the student needs to participate safely in learning and in school activities (U.S. Department of Education, Office for Civil Rights, 2016). If the student receives special education services, the required school health/school nursing services should be outlined in the student's individualized education program (IEP).

Healthcare providers should provide an allergy action plan including medication orders and emergency response for students at risk for anaphylaxis. See Figure 21-3 for the American Academy of Pediatrics (AAP) Allergy and Anaphylaxis Emergency Plan (AAP, 2019). See Online Materials OM21-1 for this plan in a customizable and fillable format. Food Allergy Research and Education (FARE; 2023) also has a sample *Food Allergy and Anaphylaxis Emergency Care Plan* available in English and Spanish, as well as other helpful resources for school management of anaphylaxis, on its Web site. If the medical emergency plan is overly complex or requires actions that cannot be delegated to lay staff, the school nurse should develop an emergency action plan (EAP) written in clear and simple terms for school staff that outlines how to identify and respond to an allergy emergency: "If you see this: ... Do this ..." See Chapter 20 for generalized information on caring for students with special healthcare needs. See Chapter 8 for more information about IHPs, Section 504 plans, IEPs, and EAPs for students with special healthcare needs.

Preventing Allergen Exposure

Throughout this process, it is important to develop a collaborative relationship with the family as well as the student. The school nurse should assure the parents/guardians that every reasonable precaution will be taken to create a safe school environment for their child; however, it cannot be guaranteed that a future allergic reaction will never happen at school.

The number one goal is to reduce the risk of allergen exposure. There are multiple routes of exposure that should be considered, depending on the student's specific allergies. In reality there is no way to ensure that a classroom or lunchroom table is "allergy safe" or "allergen-free" (e.g., "nut-free"). In a 5-year review of Massachusetts schools, there was no difference in the use of epinephrine in schools that banned peanuts versus those that allowed them (Bartnikas et al., 2017). Therefore many school districts prefer the term *allergy aware*.

Some strategies to prevent allergen exposure include the following:

- Read food labels to identify sources of allergens. Pay close attention to hidden ingredients and the possibility of cross-reactivity of foods.
- Be aware that nonfood items may pose a risk to students with allergies, including finger paint (wheat, milk, corn, oat), paste (wheat), crayons (soy), balloons (latex), and elastic bands (latex).
- Policies should be in place to prevent food sharing.
- Determine routine cleaning schedules for classrooms and lunchroom tables. Use fragrance-free hypoallergenic cleaning products.
- Develop classroom snack policies that are inclusive. Home-prepared foods should be prohibited.
- Use nonfood items for classroom incentives and celebrations.
- The school nurse should be aware of pollen counts and local pollen patterns.
- Involve food service managers in coordinating strategies for the daily management of food allergies for individual students:
  - Identify students with allergies while maintaining their right to confidentiality.
  - Identify appropriate food substitutions and accommodations; understand how to read food labels and share food information with parents/guardians as requested.
  - Clean cafeteria tables between lunch periods as indicated.
  - Prepare and respond to food allergy emergencies.
  - Participate in professional development on food allergies (CDC, 2020).

While many schools have identified nonfood alternatives for celebrations, the exclusion of all food in the classroom is debatable. Even when all foods are eliminated, the transmission of ingested allergens is still possible. Younger students often put objects or fingers in their mouths, potentially transmitting allergens through saliva on classroom objects. Older students may engage in risk-taking behaviors that pass allergens, such as kissing. Consider designating *food-free zones*, such as computer labs and buses, which are more difficult to clean. If meals are eaten in the classroom, washing desks with commercial cleaning products will remove the allergens (FARE, 2023). Multiple reports have highlighted the importance of considering the age of the students when developing school guidelines, as younger children need more supervision and have greater risk for sharing food. The school nurse should monitor the school environment periodically to reinforce prevention strategies and assess staff compliance with allergen avoidance policies.

Education and Training

The school nurse must remain abreast of best practices in allergy management and care to provide optimal education to school staff, students, and families. Using evidence-based allergy guidelines, the school nurse can lead the education effort for the school community. Parents and school staff may have been exposed to false information through the Internet or well-meaning friends and family; it is therefore important to assess baseline knowledge before beginning an educational session. Many states require mandatory staff training on allergies and anaphylaxis.

Education of all school staff, including substitutes and coaches, should include signs and symptoms of mild allergic reactions and anaphylaxis, prevention strategies, and initiation of an emergency response. All staff need to have access to information regarding the allergies and accommodations for the children who they supervise. It is vital that the school nurse remind staff about the student's rights to keep their health information confidential under the

Allergy and Anaphylaxis Emergency Plan

American Academy of Pediatrics
DEDICATED TO THE HEALTH OF ALL CHILDREN®

Attach child's photo

Child's name: ______________________ **Date of plan:** ____________

Date of birth: ___/___/___ **Age** _______ **Weight:** _______kg

Child has allergy to ______________________________

Child has asthma. ☐ Yes ☐ No (If yes, higher chance severe reaction)
Child has had anaphylaxis. ☐ Yes ☐ No
Child may carry medicine. ☐ Yes ☐ No
Child may give him/herself medicine. ☐ Yes ☐ No (If child refuses/is unable to self-treat, an adult must give medicine)

IMPORTANT REMINDER
Anaphylaxis is a potentially life-threating, severe allergic reaction. If in doubt, give epinephrine.

For Severe Allergy and Anaphylaxis **What to look for** ➡	**Give epinephrine!** **What to do**
If child has ANY of these severe symptoms after eating the food or having a sting, **give epinephrine**. • Shortness of breath, wheezing, or coughing • Skin color is pale or has a bluish color • Weak pulse • Fainting or dizziness • Tight or hoarse throat • Trouble breathing or swallowing • Swelling of lips or tongue that bother breathing • Vomiting or diarrhea (if severe or combined with other symptoms) • Many hives or redness over body • Feeling of "doom," confusion, altered consciousness, or agitation ☐ **SPECIAL SITUATION**: If this box is checked, child has an extremely severe allergy to an insect sting or the following food(s): ____________. Even if child has MILD symptoms after a sting or eating these foods, **give epinephrine**.	1. Give epinephrine right away! Note time when epinephrine was given. 2. Call 911. • Ask for ambulance with epinephrine. • Tell rescue squad when epinephrine was given. 3. Stay with child and: • Call parents and child's doctor. • Give a second dose of epinephrine, if symptoms get worse, continue, or do not get better in 5 minutes. • Keep child lying on back. If the child vomits or has trouble breathing, keep child lying on his or her side. 4. Give other medicine, if prescribed. Do not use other medicine in place of epinephrine. • Antihistamine • Inhaler/bronchodilator
For Mild Allergic Reaction **What to look for** ➡	**Monitor child** **What to do**
If child has had any mild symptoms, **monitor child.** Symptoms may include: • Itchy nose, sneezing, itchy mouth • A few hives • Mild stomach nausea or discomfort	Stay with child and: • Watch child closely. • Give antihistamine (if prescribed). • Call parents and child's doctor. • If more than 1 symptom or symptoms of severe allergy/anaphylaxis develop, use epinephrine. (See "For Severe Allergy and Anaphylaxis.")

Medicines/Doses
Epinephrine (list type): ______________ Intramuscular: ☐ 0.10 mg (7.5 kg to less than13 kg)*
☐ 0.15 mg (13 kg to less than 25 kg)
☐ 0.30 mg (25 kg or more)
(*Use 0.15 mg, if 0.10 mg is not available)
Intranasal: ☐ 2 mg (30 kg or more)
**If more than one epinephrine is selected, then either one can be usec

Antihistamine, by mouth (type and dose): ______________
Other (for example, inhaler/bronchodilator if child has asthma): ______________

______________ ______ ______________ ______
Parent/Guardian Authorization Signature **Date** **Physician/HCP Authorization Signature** **Date**

This information should not take the place of talking with your child's doctor. Page 1 of 2.

FIGURE 21-3. Allergy and anaphylaxis emergency plan. *(Copyright © 2019 by the American Academy of Pediatrics, with permission.)*

Family Educational Rights and Privacy Act of 1974 (FERPA). School staff also need to understand that Section 504 of the Rehabilitation Act of 1973 prohibits discrimination in the school setting related to a disability; life-threatening allergies may be classified as a disability (CDC, 2013b). The impact of staff training by the school nurse is immense. In one study (Tsuang et al., 2019), knowledge scores increased immediately after training sessions on food allergy and anaphylaxis management and persisted 24 months later.

Staff education needs to promote inclusion for the student in all school activities; therefore *all* staff need to be prepared in an emergency. Hands-on practice with epinephrine autoinjector trainers (available from pharmaceutical companies) should be included in regular training for school staff. All staff must be included in training, including coaches and after-school activity staff. For example, outdoor school activities or school trips may present risks for the child who has pollen or sting insect allergy. While no student may be excluded from an activity due to their disability, it is always helpful to consult with the parent or guardian before the child experiences a new environment where allergens may be present.

It is valuable to perform "tabletop drills" with school staff who need to respond if an emergent event occurs. Topics to consider as part of each school's drill include the following:

- Staff willingness to carry out an emergency action plan—ask a staff member to talk through how they would react in an emergency
- Knowledge about where a student's epinephrine is stored (self-carry or in health office)
- Demonstration of how to administer epinephrine using an autoinjector
- Location of school's stock epinephrine (in states that permit it)

Another issue that should be discussed with staff is the potential for bullying. Whole-school education may be needed to prevent students from putting their friends at risk. Bullying has occurred when students taunt their classmates with items that might cause anaphylaxis or pretending to put food triggers near them.

Education of students with allergies should be developmentally appropriate and include self-management skills, recognition of the signs and symptoms of anaphylaxis, use of an epinephrine autoinjector, and knowledge of when to notify an adult they need help. Younger children with allergies may need help knowing how to tell an adult they need assistance. Students who are developmentally able should carry their epinephrine with them (often considered around 12 years of age based on the individual). The school nurse should assess readiness and competency of students to autoinject and provide appropriate education to meet the student's needs. The nurse and parents of younger children who cannot yet self-carry may need to develop a strategy to safely ensure the epinephrine autoinjector stays with the child to and from school. One strategy is for the parent to hand a bag with the autoinjector to the bus driver who then hands it off to the teacher at school.

The school nurse can spearhead an effort to provide parent/guardian education at school, including nursing and food service personnel addressing relevant issues during school open house nights. Developing support groups can help to connect parents/guardians and promotes the acceptance of school policies and practices. Parents of students with multiple food allergies can experience a high level of anxiety, especially during transitions for their child, including a new school year, new teacher, and especially a new school.

School Policies and Protocols

School districts must have clear, concise, all-inclusive policies in place to address the management of allergies in the school setting. The school nurse must advocate for policies and protocols that are consistent with federal and state laws, nursing practice standards, and established safe practices in accordance with evidence-based information. Students benefit from well-developed school district allergy management policies and protocols that instruct staff about appropriate prevention strategies and emergency response. Policies and protocols protect school staff by providing them direction for action.

Each school district will have its own food and environmental allergy policies and protocols. NASN (2019) outlines the components of a comprehensive anaphylaxis school policy in Box 21-2.

The CDC (2013b) has extensive resources for schools to guide the development of plans, policies, and protocols specifically for food allergies, called the *Voluntary Guidelines for Managing Food Allergies in Schools and Early Care and Education Programs* (ECE). Developed by a panel of national experts, the guidelines "provide practical information, planning steps, and strategies for reducing allergic reactions and responding to life-threatening reactions in schools" (CDC, 2013b, p. 17). The CDC (2020) also offers a *Food Allergies in Schools Toolkit* with helpful tip sheets, presentations, and podcasts. These resources specifically outline recommendations and roles for school administrators, superintendents, health services directors, school nurses, teachers and paraeducators, nutrition professionals, mental health professionals, and transportation staff.

Putting Plans Into Action

Despite the best prevention strategies, exposures to allergens happen. School staff and nurses need to be ready in the event that anaphylaxis occurs. The school and/or district should have emergency response plans in place, and an allergic emergency should be included in those plans.

Staff need to be prepared to respond to and treat anaphylaxis without delay. With the leadership of the school nurse, specific roles should be assigned to identify trained staff members willing and confident to perform given tasks.

BOX 21-2

Comprehensive Anaphylaxis School Policy

School districts and schools need to prepare for school anaphylactic reactions in all children and youth—with or without a prior history of allergies considering state and local laws, policy, and protocols.

1. Individuals covered, including those with first-time anaphylaxis emergencies
2. School programs and environments covered
3. Epinephrine
   a. School prescription and standing order
   b. Stock locations, usually multiple
   c. Ensured secure access
   d. Stock supply dosages, number of doses
   e. Procurement—initial and periodic
   f. Disposal—after use and expiration
   g. Administration and documentation
   h. Reporting
4. Individuals authorized to administer
5. Emergency protocol for administration
6. Education, training, notification
   a. When to administer
   b. Who will be educated (every staff member needs to be trained to know the signs and symptoms of anaphylaxis and know how to initiate the emergency protocol)
   c. Levels of education to be provided
   d. Parent notification
7. Communication plan—district, school, parents, healthcare provider, EMS, community (a part of a school's all-hazard emergency plan)

Adapted from NASN (2014, p. 1; 2019).

Each school building has a unique layout and staffing pattern, so individual school plans should be reviewed. Potential roles for each staff member may include the following:

- School nurse—Directs emergency care, including administration of epinephrine, and has someone activate EMS (911). NOTE: In the absence of a school nurse, this person may be a trained staff or health office designee.
- School administrator—Provides support, directs students to appropriate location
- School counselor—Provides emotional support to witnesses, classmates
- School office staff—Calls parent, copies student's personal information for EMS responders (Allergy & Asthma Network, 2023c)

If stock epinephrine is available at the school, it should be stored in an unlocked, accessible location and have a mechanism in place to monitor the expiration dates of the medication. Nurses must remain current on state laws and regulations about who can give this medication.

Following an emergency, the school nurse should always lead a debriefing meeting with all involved in the incident. It allows nonmedical staff to express their feelings and concerns and helps to evaluate the incident and improve outcomes as you move forward.

School Nurse Leadership

School nursing care for students with allergies and risk for anaphylaxis is complex and can be anxiety producing. It requires strong school nursing leadership. Fortunately, NASN offers robust resources to support school nurses in caring for these students. NASN's *Evidence-Based Clinical Practice Guidelines: Students With Allergies and Risk for Anaphylaxis* (2023b) offers a systematic approach to care coordination according to the nursing process. According to NASN,

> *The purpose of this CPG is to provide best practice recommendations for implementation by school nurses to improve outcomes and provide quality care to students at risk for allergic reactions and anaphylaxis. The focus of this CPG is to provide safe and supportive school and classroom settings for the student to learn in a low risk environment. Students at risk for an allergic reaction should be able to participate fully in all academic, physical education, and extracurricular activities as outlined in the Office [for] Civil Rights (OCR) designation of a free and appropriate public education (FAPE) (U.S. Office for Civil Rights, 2020). This CPG includes practice recommendations and strategies to assist school nurses in their role of improving the health and safety of the school-age child at risk for an allergic reaction and anaphylaxis. Student goals resulting from successfully implementing the guidelines include:*
>
> - *improved management of allergen exposure and minimizing the risk for allergen exposure in school settings*
> - *decreased time spent out of the classroom*
> - *improved student academic success*
> - *full participation in all school activities*
> - *decreased allergic reactions and episodes of anaphylaxis*
> - *improved quality of life*
> - *improved mental well-being*
> - *decreased social isolation (NASN, 2023b, p. 7).*

To accompany this clinical practice guideline, NASN also developed an *Allergy and Anaphylaxis Toolkit* (2023a) as part of a cooperative agreement with the Healthy Schools branch of the CDC and in cooperation with the American Academy of Pediatrics. This toolkit incorporates evidence from over 60 references and is an essential free online resource for all school nurses. See Box 21-3 for the full list of available resources in the toolkit.

BOX 21-3

NASN's Allergy and Anaphylaxis Toolkit Table of Contents

Section A: Assessment (History, EAP/ECP, Self-Carry, Communication, Policy, Mental Health)

A-1 Types of Food Allergy Fact Sheet
A-2 Allergy and Anaphylaxis Latex Allergies Fact Sheet
A-3 Anaphylaxis Algorithm
A-4 Mild Allergic Reaction Versus Anaphylaxis and Biphasic Reactions
A-5 Sample School District Anaphylaxis Response Policy
A-6 Checklist to Initiate and Sustain Stock Epinephrine Programs
A-7 EpiPen Self-Administration Assessment
A-8 Language Considerations
A-9 Food Allergy and Anaphylaxis Family Mental Health Considerations/Resource

Section B: Diagnosis

B-1 Sample Allergy and Anaphylaxis Nursing Diagnoses

Section C: Planning (Outcomes)

C-1 Guidelines for Health Personnel Roles Managing Student Anaphylaxis/Allergy
C-2 Out of School Time (OST) Programs—Students With Allergies/Anaphylaxis Care Coordination Checklist
C-3 Field Trip Preparation Checklist

Section D: Implementation (IHP, Collaboration, Documentation, Education)

D-1 Sample Severe Allergy Health History Intake Form
D-2 School Nurse Consideration Checklist—Allergy and Anaphylaxis
D-3 Allergy and Anaphylaxis Program—Sample Development of the Student Healthcare Plans Checklist
D-4 Engaging Stakeholders to Support Students With Food Allergies Through a Coordinated Food Allergy Management Program Checklist
D-5 Allergy and Anaphylaxis Training for All School Staff Checklist
D-6 Sample Training PowerPoint Presentation for School Staff—Allergy and Anaphylaxis
D-7 Sample Notification Letter to Parents About Food Allergies in the Classroom

Section E: Evaluation (Data)

E-1 Allergy Clinical Practice Guide Data Points Table
E-2 Sample Allergy and Anaphylaxis Program Quality Improvement Checklist

NASN (2023a).

CONCLUSION

The school nurse is vitally important in management of student allergies at school. The school nurse functions in the role of care coordinator by overseeing that medical orders are followed, student care plans are developed and in place, and school staff are well educated in allergen avoidance and prepared to provide an emergency response. The school nurse, as a student advocate, should lead efforts to ensure evidence-based school allergy management policies are implemented. Effective management is maximized when the student is at the center of care, and the family home, educational home, and medical home strive to coordinate needed support for the student to fully access their educational program in the least restrictive environment.

The Editors gratefully acknowledge the work of the previous chapter authors, Sally Schoessler and Janice Selekman.

Resources

Allergy & Asthma Network. (2023). *Managing allergies at school: A guide for staff.* https://allergyasthmanetwork.org/allergies-and-asthma-at-school/managing-allergies-in-schools-a-guide-for-staff/

American Academy of Pediatrics. (2019, March). *Allergy and anaphylaxis emergency plan.* https://downloads.aap.org/HC/AAP_Allergy_and_Anaphylaxis_Emergency_Plan.pdf

Centers for Disease Control and Prevention. (2013b). *Voluntary guidelines for managing food allergies in schools and early care and education programs.* https://www.cdc.gov/healthyschools/foodallergies/pdf/20_316712-A_FA_guide_508tag.pdf

References

Allergy & Asthma Network. (2017). *Allergy & anaphylaxis: A practical guide for schools and families.* Vienna, VA: Author.

Allergy & Asthma Network. (2023a). *All about allergies.* https://allergyasthmanetwork.org/allergies/

Allergy & Asthma Network. (2023b). *Allergy statistics in the US.* https://allergyasthmanetwork.org/allergies/allergy-statistics/

Allergy & Asthma Network. (2023c). *Managing allergies at school: A guide for staff.* https://allergyasthmanetwork.org/allergies-and-asthma-at-school/managing-allergies-in-schools-a-guide-for-staff/

American Academy of Allergy, Asthma & Immunology. (2018). *AAAAI allergy & asthma medication guide.* https://www.aaaai.org/conditions-and-treatments/drug-guide/allergy

American Academy of Allergy, Asthma & Immunology. (2023). *Allergy defined.* https://www.aaaai.org/tools-for-the-public/allergy,-asthma-immunology-glossary/allergy-defined

American Academy of Pediatrics. (2019, March). *Allergy and anaphylaxis emergency plan.* https://downloads.aap.org/HC/AAP_Allergy_and_Anaphylaxis_Emergency_Plan.pdf

American College of Allergy, Asthma & Immunology. (2023a). *Eczema in children.* http://acaai.org/allergies/who-has-allergies/children-allergies/eczema

American College of Allergy, Asthma, & Immunology. (2023b). *Testing and diagnosis.* https://acaai.org/allergies/testing-diagnosis/

Bartnikas, L. M., Huffaker, M. F., Sheehan, W. J., Kanchongkittiphon, W., Petty, C. R., Leibowitz, R., Hauptman, M., Young, M. C., & Phipatanakul, W. (2017). Impact of school peanut-free policies on epinephrine administration. *Journal of Allergy and Clinical Immunology, 140*(2), 465–473. https://doi.org/10.1016/j.jaci.2017.01.040

Beierwaltes, P., & Schoessler, S. (2017). Latex-safe at school: A student-centered approach. *NASN School Nurse, 32*(6), 343–345. https://doi.org/10.1177/1942602X17715495

Bingemann, T. A., Nanda, A., & Russel, A. F. (2021). Pharmacology update: School nurse role and emergency medications for treatment of anaphylaxis. *NASN School Nurse, 35*(5), 264–270. https://doi.org/10.1177/1942602X211021902

Bock, S. A., & Sampson, H. (2016). Evaluation of food allergy. In D. Leung, S. Szefler, F. Bonilla, C. Akdis, & H. Sampson (Eds.). *Pediatric allergy: Principles and practice* (pp. 371–376). Elsevier.

Boguniewicz, M., Fonacier, L., Guttman-Yassky, E., Ong, P. Y., Silverberg, J., & Farrar, J. R. (2017). Atopic dermatitis yardstick: Practical recommendations for an evolving therapeutic landscape. *Annals of Allergy Asthma and Immunology, 120*, 10–22. https://doi.org/10.1016/j.anai.2017.10.039

Bowman, R. M., McLone, F. G., Grant, J. A., & Ito, J. A. (2001). Spina bifida outcome: A 25 year prospective. *Pediatric Neurosurgery, 34*, 114–120. https://doi.org/10.1159/000056005

Brown, S., & Turner, P. (2017). Anaphylaxis. In D. Leung, S. Szefler, F. Bonilla, C. Akdis, & H. Sampson (Eds.). *Pediatric allergy: Principles and practice* (pp. 345–360). Elsevier.

Centers for Disease Control and Prevention. (2013a). Prevention of measles, rubella, congenital rubella syndrome and mumps, 2013: Summary recommendations of the Advisory Committee on Immunization Practices (ACIP). *Morbidity and Mortality Weekly Report, 62*(4), 1–34. https://www.cdc.gov/mmwr/pdf/rr/rr6204.pdf

Centers for Disease Control and Prevention (CDC). (2013b). *Voluntary guidelines for managing food allergies in schools and early care and education programs*. https://www.cdc.gov/healthyschools/foodallergies/pdf/20_316712-A_FA_guide_508tag.pdf

Centers for Disease Control and Prevention. (2020). *Food allergies in schools toolkit*. https://www.cdc.gov/healthyschools/foodallergies/toolkit.htm

Centers for Disease Control and Prevention. (2021). *Recognizing and responding to anaphylaxis*. https://www.cdc.gov/vaccines/covid-19/downloads/recognizing-responding-to-anaphylaxis-508.pdf

Centers for Disease Control and Prevention. (2022a). *Allergies and hay fever*. https://www.cdc.gov/nchs/fastats/allergies.htm

Centers for Disease Control and Prevention. (2022b). *Flu vaccine and people with egg allergies*. https://www.cdc.gov/flu/prevent/egg-allergies.htm#print

Centers for Disease Control and Prevention. (2022c). *Food allergies*. https://www.cdc.gov/healthyschools/foodallergies/index.htm

Centers for Disease Control and Prevention. (2023, March 8). *Rhinoviruses*. https://www.cdc.gov/ncird/rhinoviruses-common-cold.html

Children's Hospital of Philadelphia. (2023). *Oral immunotherapy*. https://www.chop.edu/centers-programs/oral-immunotherapy-oit-program?-callsource=ctm&insitesid=1399&gclid=CjwKCAiAuOieBhAIEiwAgjCvcghZAFIJviCCQTIEdnM5MPwMGZXxlxr7l1nOCd_FHG3reWA1L5BtzRoC5qsQAvD_BwE

Cleveland Clinic. (2024). *How to know if it's COVID-19, a cold or allergies*. https://health.clevelandclinic.org/is-it-covid-19-a-cold-or-seasonal-allergies

Collins, T. (2018). Climate change is worsening allergies, expert says. *Pediatric News*. https://www.mdedge.com/pediatricnews/article/160418/pulmonology/climate-change-worsening-allergies-expert-says/page/0/1

Conlon, P., & Wilson, D. (2015). The child with respiratory dysfunction. In M. Hockenberry & D. Wilson (Eds.). *Wong's nursing care of infants and children* (pp. 1164–1250). Elsevier.

Davidson, W. F., Leung, D. Y. M., Beck, L. A., Berin, C. M., Boguniewicz, M., Busse, W. W., Chatila, T. A., Geha, R. S., Gern, J. E., Guttman-Yassky, E., Irvine, A. D., Kim, B. S., Hong, H. H., Lack, G., Nadeau, K. C., Schwaniger, J., Simpson, A., Simpson, E. L., Spergel, J. M., ... & Plaut, M. (2019). Report from the National Institute of Allergy and Infectious Diseases workshop on "Atopic dermatitis and the atopic march: Mechanisms and interventions." *Journal of Allergy and Clinical Immunology, 143*(3), 894–913. https://doi.org/10.1016/j.jaci.2019.01.003

Dupuis, P., Prokopich, C. L., Hynes, A., & Kim, H. (2020). A contemporary look at allergic conjunctivitis. *Allergy, Asthma & Clinical Immunology, 16*(5), 1–18. https://doi.org/10.1186/s13223-020-0403-9

Du Toit, G., Sampson, H. A., Plaut, M., Burks, A. W., Akdis, C., & Lack, G. (2018). Food allergy: Update on prevention and tolerance. *Journal of Allergy and Clinical Immunology, 141*(1), 30–40. https://doi.org/10.1016/j.jaci.2017.11.010

Elberink, H. (2016). Insect sting allergy. In D. Leung, S. Szefler, F. Bonilla, C. Akdis, & H. Sampson (Eds.). *Pediatric allergy: Principles and practice* (pp. 513–523). Elsevier.

Fall, T., Lundholm, C., Ortqvist, A., Fall, K., Fang, F., Hedhammar, A., Kampe, O., Ingelsson, E., & Almqvist, C. (2015). Early exposure to dogs and farm animals and the risk of childhood asthma. *JAMA Pediatrics, 169*(11), e153219. doi:10.1001/jamapediatrics.2015.3219

Family Educational Rights and Privacy Act of 1974 (FERPA), (20 U.S.C. § 1232g; 34 CFR Part 99). https://www.law.cornell.edu/uscode/text/20/1232g

Fishbein, A. B., Cheng, B. T., Tiley, C. C., Smith Begolka, W., Carle, A. C., Forrest, C. B., Zee, P. C., Paller, A. S., & Griffith, J. W. (2021). Sleep disturbances in school-aged children with atopic dermatitis: Prevalence and severity in a cross-sectional sample. *Journal of Allergy and Clinical Immunology: In Practice, 9*(8), 3120–3129. https://doi.org/10.1016/j.jaip.2021.04.064

Fleischer, D. M., Chan, E. S., Venter, C., Spergel, J. M., Abrams, E. M., Stukus, D., Groetch, M., Shaker, M., & Greenhawt, M. (2020). A consensus approach to the primary prevention of food allergy through nutrition: Guidance from the American Academy of Allergy, Asthma and Immunology; American College of Allergy, Asthma and Immunology; and The Canadian Society for Allergy and Clinical Immunology. *Journal of Allergy and Clinical Immunology: In Practice, 9*(1), 22–43e4. https://doi.org/10.1016/j.jaip.2020.11.002

Food Allergy Research & Education. (2023, January). *Food allergy and anaphylaxis emergency care plan*. https://www.foodallergy.org/living-food-allergies/food-allergy-essentials/food-allergy-anaphylaxis-emergency-care-plan

Gentile, D., Pleskovic, N., & Bartholow, A. (2016). Allergic rhinitis. In D. Leung, S. Szefler, F. Bonilla, C. Akdis, & H. Sampson (Eds.). *Pediatric allergy: Principles and practice* (pp. 210–218). Elsevier.

Golden, D. (2017). Insect allergy. In R. O'Hehir, S. Holgate, & A. Sheikh (Eds.). *Middleton's allergy essentials* (pp. 377–393). Elsevier.

Harvard Health Publications. (2014). *Sun allergy (photosensitivity)*. https://www.health.harvard.edu/allergies/sun-allergy-photosensitivity

Hausmann, D. (2017). Drug allergy. In R. O'Hehir, S. Holgate, & A. Sheikh (Eds.). *Middleton's allergy essentials* (pp. 225–248). Elsevier.

Johansson, E. K., Bergstrom, A., Kull, I., Lind, T., Soderhall, C., van Hage, M., Wickman, M., Ballardini, N., & Wahlgren, C. F. (2017). IgE sensitization in relation to preschool eczema and filaggrin mutation. *Journal of Allergy and Clinical Immunology, 140*(6), 1572.

Khan, D. A., Banerji, A., Blumenthal, K. G., Phillips, E. J., Solensky, R., White, A. A., Bernstein, J. A., Chu, D. K., Ellis, A. K., Golden, D. B. K., Greenhawt, M. J., Horner, C. C., Ledford, D., Lieberman, J. A., Oppenheimer, J., Rank, M. A., Shaker, M. S., Stukus, D. R., ... & Wang, J. (2022). Drug allergy: A 2022 practice parameter update. *Journal of Allergy and Clinical Immunology, 150*(6), 1333–1392. https://doi.org/10.1016/j.jaci.2022.08.028

Liu, A. H. (2015). Revisiting the hygiene hypothesis for allergy and asthma. *Journal of Allergy and Clinical Immunology, 136*(4), 860–865. https://doi.org/10.1016/j.jaci.2015.08.012

Liu, A., & Martinez, F. (2016). Natural history of allergic diseases and asthma. In D. Leung, S. Szefler, F. Bonilla, C. Akdis, & H. Sampson (Eds.). *Pediatric allergy: Principles and practice* (pp. 7–17). Elsevier.

Logan, K., Bahnson, H. T., Ylescupidez, A., Beyer, K., Bellach, J., Campbell, D. E., Craven, J., Du Toit, G., Clare Mills, E. N., Perkin, M. R., Roberts, G., van Ree, R., & Lack, G. (2023). Early introduction of peanut reduces peanut allergy across risk groups in pooled and causal inference analyses. *Allergy, 78*(5), 1307–1318. https://doi.org/10.1111/all.15597

Matsui, E., & Eggleston, P. (2016). Immunotherapy for allergic disease. In D. Leung, S. Szefler, F. Bonilla, C. Akdis, & H. Sampson (Eds.). *Pediatric allergy: Principles and practice* (pp. 203–209). Elsevier

Mayo Clinic. (2022). *Drugs and supplements: Epinephrine (injection route)*. https://www.mayoclinic.org/drugs-supplements/epinephrine-injection-route/proper-use/drg20072429#:~:text=Push%20the%20 needle%20end%20(orange,of%203%20seconds%20following%20activation

Mayo Clinic. (2023, November 3). *COVID-19, cold, allergies and the flu: What are the differences?* https://www.mayoclinic.org/diseases-conditions/coronavirus/in-depth/covid-19-cold-flu-and-allergies-differences/art-20503981

McWilliam, V.L., Perrett, K.P., Dang, T., & Peters, R.L. (2020). Prevalence and natural history of tree nut allergy. *Annals of Allergy, Asthma & Immunology, 124*(5), 466–472. https://doi.org/10.1016/j.anai.2020.01.024

National Association of School Nurses. (2014). Epinephrine policies and protocols. https://higherlogicdownload.s3.amazonaws.com/NASN/8575d1b7-94ad-45ab-808e-d45019cc5c08/UploadedImages/PDFs/Epinephrine%20Policies%20Protocols%20and%20Reporting/Comprehensive_Anaphylaxis_School_Policy.pdf

National Association of School Nurses. (2019). *Practice topics: Allergies and anaphylaxis.* https://www.nasn.org/nasn-resources/practice-topics/allergies-anaphylaxis

National Association of School Nurses. (2021). *A model for school nurse–led case management.* https://learn.nasn.org/courses/33713

National Association of School Nurses. (2023a). *Allergy and anaphylaxis toolkit.* (Lead author: Newman, L.). https://learn.nasn.org/courses/58035

National Association of School Nurses. (2023b). *Evidence-based clinical practice guidelines: Students with allergies and risk for anaphylaxis.* https://learn.nasn.org/courses/58496

National Association of School Nurses. (2024). A contemporary framework update for today's school nursing landscape: Introducing the School Nursing Practice Framework. *NASN School Nurse, 39*(3), 140–147. https://www.doi.org/10.1177/1942602X241241092

National Eczema Association. (2023). *Eczema stats.* https://nationaleczema.org/research/eczema-facts/

National Institutes of Health. (2015). *Cold urticaria.* https://rarediseases.info.nih.gov/diseases/6131/cold-urticaria

Nowak-Wegrzyn, A., Burks, W., & Sampson, H. (2017). Food allergy and gastrointestinal syndromes. In R. O'Hehir, S. Holgate, & A. Sheikh (Eds.). *Middleton's allergy essentials* (pp. 301–344). Elsevier.

Oettgen, H. (2016). Regulation and biology of immunoglobulin E. In D. Leung, S. Szefler, & F. Bonilla (Eds.). *Pediatric allergy: Principles and practice* (pp. 31–40). Elsevier.

Parisi, C. A., Kelly, K. J., Ansotegui, I. J., Gonzalez-Diaz, S. N., Bilo, M. B., Cardona, V., Park, H. S., Braschi, M. C., Macias-Weinmann, A., Piga, M. A., Acuna-Ortega, N., Sanchez-Borges, M., & Yanez, A. (2021). Update on latex allergy: New insights into an old problem. *World Allergy Organization, 14*(8), 1–15. https://doi.org/10.1016/j.waojou.2021.100569

Rishor-Olney, C. R., & Gnugnoli, D. M. (2023, July 22). *Nickel allergy.* In StatPearls [Internet]. https://www.ncbi.nlm.nih.gov/books/NBK557638/

Rote, N. (2017). Innate immunity: Inflammation and wound healing. In K. McCance & S. Huether (Eds.). *Understanding pathophysiology* (pp. 134–157). Elsevier.

Rote, N., & McCance, K. (2017). Structure and function of the hematologic system. In K. McCance & S. Huether (Eds.). *Understanding pathophysiology* (pp. 490–512). Elsevier.

Sables-Baus, S., & Fidanza, S. (2017). Alteration of digestive function in children. In K. McCance & S. Huether (Eds.). *Understanding pathophysiology* (pp. 950–967). Elsevier.

Schoessler, S., & White, M. (2013). Recognition and treatment of anaphylaxis in the school setting: The essential role of the school nurse. *Journal of School Nursing, 29*(6), 407–415. https://doi.org/10.1177/1059840513506014

Schwartz, A., McCance, K., & Rote, N. (2017). Alterations of hematologic function. In K. McCance & S. Huether (Eds.). *Understanding pathophysiology* (pp. 513–553). Elsevier.

Shaker, M. S., Wallace, D. V., Golden, D. B., Oppenheimer, J., Bernstein, J. A., Campbell, R. L., Dinakar, C., Ellis, A., Greenhawt, M., Khan, D. A., Lang, D. M., Lang, E. S., Lieberman, J. A., Portnoy, J., Rank, M. A., Stukus, D. R., & Wang, J. (2020). Anaphylaxis—a 2020 practice parameter update, systematic review, and grading of recommendations, assessment, development and evaluation (GRADE) analysis. *Journal of Allergy and Clinical Immunology, 145*(4), 1082–1122. https://doi.org/10.1016/j.jaci.2020.01.017

Sheehan, W., & Phipatanakul, W. (2016). Indoor allergens. In D. Leung, S. Szefler, & F. Bonilla (Eds.). *Pediatric allergy: Principles and practice* (pp. 191–195). Elsevier.

Sicherer, S., Allen, K., Lack, G., Taylor, S., Donovan, S., & Oria, M. (2017). Critical issues in food allergy: A National Academies Consensus Report. *Pediatrics, 140*(2), 1–8. https://doi.org/10.1542/peds.2017-0194

Sicherer, S., Sampson, H., Eichenfield, L., & Rotrosen, D. (2017). The benefits of new guidelines to prevent peanut allergy. *Pediatrics, 139*(6), 1–4. https://doi.org/10.1542/peds.2016-4293

Sicherer, S., & Simons, F. E. (2017). Epinephrine for first-aid management of anaphylaxis. *Pediatrics, 139*(3), e1–e9. https://doi.org/10.1542/peds.2016-4006

Sicherer S. H., & Sampson, H. A. (2018). Food allergy: A review and update on epidemiology, pathogenesis, diagnosis, prevention and management. *Journal of Allergy and Clinical Immunology, 141*(1), 41–58. https://doi.org/10.1016/j.jaci.2017.11.003

Simons, F. E. (2016). Anaphylaxis: Assessment and management. In D. Leung, S. Szefler, & F. Bonilla (Eds.). *Pediatric allergy: Principles and practice* (pp. 524–536). Elsevier.

Skoner, D. P. (2000). Complications of allergic rhinitis. *Journal of Allergy and Clinical Immunology, 105*(6), S605–S609. https://doi.org/10.1067/mai.2000.106150

Soriano, V., Peters, R., Ponsonby, A., Perrett, K., Dharmage, S., Gurrin, L., & Koplin, J. (2021). Has the prevalence of peanut allergy changed following the introduction of peanut? The EarlyNuts study. *Journal of Allergy and Clinical Immunology, 147*(2), supplement. https://doi.org/10.1016/j.jaci.2020.12.009

Trubiano, J., Adkinson, M. F., & Phillips, E. (2017). Penicillin allergy is not necessarily forever. *JAMA, 318*(1), 82–83. doi:10.1001/jama.2017.6510

Tsuang, A., Atal, Z., Demain, H., Patrick, K., Pistiner, M., & Wang, J. (2019). Benefits of school nurse training sessions for food allergy and anaphylaxis management. *Journal of Allergy and Clinical Immunology: In Practice, 7*(1), 309–311.

Turner P., Campbell D., Motosue M., & Campbell R. (2020). Global trends in anaphylaxis epidemiology and clinical implications. *Journal of Allergy and Clinical Immunology, 8*, 1169–1176. https://doi.org/10.1016/j.jaip.2018.05.015

U.S. Department of Education, Office for Civil Rights. (2016). *Parent and educator resource guide to section 504 in public elementary and secondary schools.* https://www2.ed.gov/about/offices/list/ocr/docs/504-resource-guide-201612.pdf

U.S. Environmental Protection Agency. (2017). *Indoor air pollution: An introduction for health professionals.* https:www.epa.gov/sites/production/files/2015-01/documents/indoor_air_pollution.pdf

U.S. Environmental Protection Agency. (2022). *Mold remediation in schools and commercial buildings guide.* https://www.epa.gov/mold/mold-remediation-schools-and-commercial-buildings-guide

U.S. Office for Civil Rights. (2020). *Disability discrimination. Protecting students.* https://www2.ed.gov/about/offices/list/ocr/frontpage/pro-students/ disability-pr.html

Volerman, A., Brindley, C., Amerson, N., Pressley, T., & Woolverton, N. (2022). A national review of state laws for stock epinephrine in schools. *Journal of School Health, 92*(2), 209–222. https://doi.org/10.1111/josh.13119

Wilson, D. (2015). Health problems of the infant. In M. Hockenberry & D. Wilson (Eds.). *Wong's nursing care of infants and children* (pp. 452–487). Elsevier.

Zuraw, B. (2016). Urticaria and angioedema. In D. Leung, S. Szefler, & F. Bonilla (Eds.). *Pediatric allergy: Principles and practice* (pp. 458–466). Elsevier.

Chapter 22

Students With Asthma and Cystic Fibrosis

Marciarose Winston ▪ Mary Bridget Kastl ▪ Robin Adair Shannon

CHAPTER OUTLINE

School nurses often care for students with asthma and cystic fibrosis. Students with these chronic conditions require long-term medications, management, and additional therapeutic interventions during times of exacerbation. The school nurse has the unique role of school-based case management, assisting students with their daily care regimens and intervening when medical attention is needed to treat symptoms, prevent complications, and elevate care when necessary. The school nurse can use their knowledge of the disease process to partner with students, families, and local care providers to coordinate care. Timely intervention facilitates an optimal learning environment by minimizing health-related barriers to education for the student with asthma and cystic fibrosis.

ASTHMA

School nurses in all settings, from preschool to high school and in urban, suburban, and rural schools, are responsible for caring for students with asthma. Despite its prevalence, asthma is often misdiagnosed, undertreated, and not well controlled, placing children at risk. This can affect students' ability to attend school, learn, and fully participate in school activities. Asthma is the leading medical cause of school absenteeism (Centers for Disease Control and Prevention [CDC], 2022). Due to the amount of time students are in school, school nurses can play an indispensable role in helping them manage their asthma.

Pathophysiology and Epidemiology

Asthma is a condition of chronic airway inflammation that is present even in the absence of symptoms. When a student is asymptomatic, their asthma is under control. Episodic asthma symptoms are the result of airway hypersensitivity to triggers. Symptoms result from a combination of three factors that reduce the capacity of small airways: increased edema, mucus production, and smooth muscle constriction. See Figure 22-1. Chronic inflammation leads to remodeling of the airways (Liu et al., 2025). The etiology of asthma development is not completely understood, but arises from a combination of genetic, immunological, and environmental factors (American Academy of Allergy, Asthma, and Immunology [AAAAI], 2024a).

Asthma is the most prevalent chronic illness in school-age children in the United States. In 2021, asthma affected 6.5% of children under age 18 years representing almost 4.7 million children. The prevalence is higher in boys (7.3%) than girls (5.6%) (CDC, 2023). There are also differences in asthma prevalence in children by race and ethnicity: 11.6% among black/non-Hispanic, 9.2% among American Indian/Alaska Native, 5.9% among Hispanic, 5.5% among white/non-Hispanic, and 3.3% among Asian populations (CDC, 2023). The prevalence of asthma among U.S. children also varies between states and territories, from 7.6% in Nebraska to 18.0% in Puerto Rico, and it often affects children living in conditions of poverty at greater rates.

While asthma is most commonly a condition with waxing and waning symptoms, asthma exacerbations can be fatal, even in children. Students with controlled asthma should be able to safely attend school and avoid excessive absences. The factors that increase the risk of death related to asthma include the following:

- A history of near fatal asthma requiring intubation and mechanical ventilation
- Hospitalization or treatment in the emergency department for asthma in the last year
- Currently and recently on an oral corticosteroid
- Not using inhaled corticosteroid (ICS), poor adherence to ICS
- Overuse of short-acting beta-2 agonist (SABA) (use of more than one albuterol metered-dose inhaler [MDI] that contains 120 puffs monthly)
- History of psychiatric disease or psychosocial problems

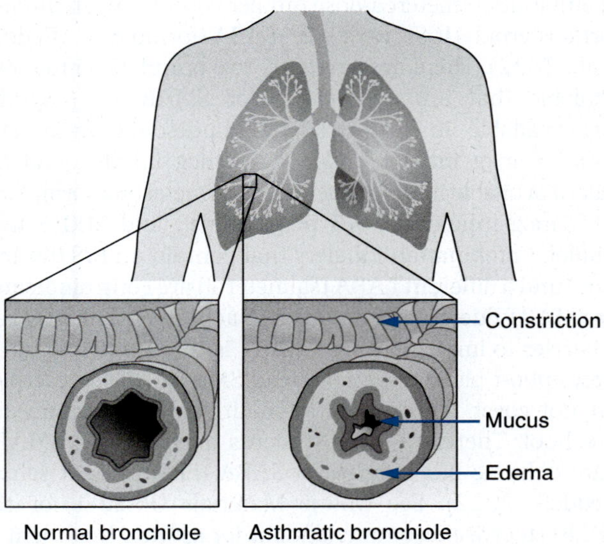

FIGURE 22-1. Asthma episode.

- History of food allergy
- Comorbidities (e.g., obesity, chronic sinusitis, gastroesophageal reflux, sleep apnea) (Global Initiative for Asthma [GINA], 2023)

School nurses should review the medical history of their students with asthma, assess current status and monitor students who are at high risk (National Association of School Nurses [NASN], 2024b).

The Global Initiative for Asthma began in 1993 as a partnership between the National Heart, Lung, and Blood Institute, the National Institutes of Health, and the World Health Organization. GINA strives to improve the lives of people affected with asthma globally by providing evidence-based asthma resources to reduce asthma morbidity, mortality, and prevalence and increasing awareness of asthma through World Asthma Day (GINA, 2023).

Signs and Symptoms

The symptoms of asthma are cough, wheeze, dyspnea, and chest discomfort, including tightness and pain (AAAAI, 2024a). Symptom presentation varies and can change over time. The most common asthma symptom is cough; either dry, hacking, barky, brassy, seal-like, croupy, or like a smoker's cough (Jarvis & Eckhardt, 2024). Wheezing in asthma is typically high pitched or whistling and sounds differently throughout the lung fields (Corjulo & Schoessler, 2016). Some students with asthma only present with cough; not all students with asthma wheeze, or wheezing may only be appreciated on auscultation (GINA, 2023). When auscultating breath sounds, instruct the student to take deep

Focus on the Framework

Standards of Practice

The National Association of School Nurses sponsored subject matter experts to develop the *School Nursing Evidence-Based Clinical Practice Guideline: Students with Asthma* (2024b) according to a standardized and rigorous process.

> *The purpose of this Clinical Practice Guideline (CPG) is to provide best practice recommendations for implementation by school nurses to improve student health and educational outcomes and provide high quality care to students with asthma. The focus of this CPG is to provide safe and supportive school and classroom settings for the students to learn. (NASN, 2024b, p. 6)*

The practice recommendations of this CPG set the standard of practice for safe and effective school nursing care of students with asthma, referenced throughout this chapter. ***Standards of Practice*** is an enveloping principle of NASN's *School Nursing Practice Framework* (2024a) that encompasses all dimensions of the specialty. School nurses will recognize that NASN's asthma CPG follows the nursing process in alignment with NASN's *School Nursing: Scope and Standards of Practice* (2022).

breaths in and out. If the school nurse only auscultates the chest during tidal breathing, then abnormal breath sounds (wheeze, crackles, rhonchi) may be missed. Place the diaphragm of the stethoscope chest piece directly on the student's skin; do not auscultate breath sounds through clothing. It is important to differentiate wheeze from stridor, which could indicate upper airway obstruction.

Diagnosis

Students with complaints of cough, wheeze, dyspnea, and chest discomfort should be evaluated for asthma. Clinical findings include the pattern of symptoms (seasonal, frequency, day, night, duration (aids in determination of level of severity), triggers, history of prior episodes, treatments, and response to treatments (Jarvis & Eckhardt, 2024). Diagnostic testing for asthma includes spirometry and bronchodilator responsiveness testing. Fractional exhaled nitric oxide measurement may be of value as adjunct diagnostic data for some children (National Institutes of Health, National Heart, Lung and Blood Institute [NHLBI], 2020). The school nurse can contribute to the diagnostic picture by sharing objective and subjective assessment data with the student's healthcare provider (NASN, 2024b).

A student's asthma can be more difficult to control if comorbid health conditions are not properly addressed, such as allergies, allergic rhinitis/sinusitis, gastroesophageal reflux, obesity, obstructive sleep apnea, and depression and/or anxiety (GINA, 2023). Differential diagnoses for students being evaluated for asthma include chronic upper airway cough syndrome (postnasal drip), inhaled foreign body, bronchopulmonary dysplasia, primary ciliary dyskinesia, cystic fibrosis, congenital heart disease, immune deficiency with recurrent respiratory infections, and vocal cord dysfunction (GINA, 2023; Kavanaugh et al., 2019).

ASTHMA CLASSIFICATION AND MANAGEMENT

According to the National Institutes of Health's National Heart, Lung and Blood Institute (2012), asthma in children is categorized by four levels of severity: *intermittent, mild persistent, moderate persistent,* and *severe persistent.* Asthma medications are generally divided into two categories: quick-relief or "rescue" medications, and long-term control medications. Quick-relief medications are inhaled short-acting beta-agonists (SABAs), a class of bronchodilators that work primarily by relaxing the bronchial smooth muscles and secondarily by inhibiting immediate hypersensitivity mediator release from mast cells. Long-term control medications include inhaled corticosteroids, long-acting beta-agonists (LABAs), long-acting muscarinic antagonists (LAMAs), leukotriene receptor antagonists (LTRAs), and biological/immunological therapies (Chu & Bajaj, 2024; NHLBI, 2020).

Treatment Recommendations

Based on the frequency of symptoms and levels of severity, treatment recommendations are stepwise and categorized based on three age groups: 0 to 4 years of age, 5 to 11 years of age, and 12 years of age and older. See Figure 22-2.

- ***Intermittent asthma:*** Students have symptoms 1 or 2 days a week and wake during the night with symptoms one or two times per month. Intermittent asthma is usually treated with a short-acting beta-agonist (SABA), most commonly albuterol, on an as-needed basis (prn). Although students with intermittent asthma have infrequent symptoms, they can still have exacerbations requiring acute treatment and are still at risk for a fatal exacerbation.
- ***Mild persistent asthma:*** Students have symptoms at least twice a week and wake at night no more than once a week with symptoms. Mild persistent asthma is usually managed with one asthma control medication such as an inhaled corticosteroid (ICS) and a quick-relief medication (SABA) to treat symptoms.
- ***Moderate persistent asthma:*** Students have symptoms daily and wake approximately once a week on average with symptoms. They require more than one control medication (ICS) and a long-acting beta agonist (LABA) in addition to quick-relief medication.
- ***Severe persistent asthma:*** Students have frequent daily symptoms and wake often at night with symptoms. Severe persistent asthma requires treatment with multiple control medications, possibly including systemic corticosteroids and biological therapy (NHLBI, 2012, 2020).

The NHLBI *2020 Focused Updates to the Asthma Management Guidelines* describe a new strategy called SMART, which stands for *Single Maintenance and Reliever Therapy.* SMART can simplify the treatment plan for students 5 years of age and older with persistent asthma. SMART is a combination metered-dose inhaler containing an inhaled corticosteroid (ICS) with the LABA formoterol (Reddell et al., 2022). There are currently two brands/formulations available that are appropriate for SMART: (1) Symbicort available in two strengths: budesonide/formoterol 160/4.5 mcg inhaler and 80/4.5 mcg inhaler, and (2) Dulera available in three strengths: mometasone/formoterol 50/5 mcg inhaler, 100/5 mcg inhaler, and 200/5 mcg inhaler. Combination inhalers that contain an ICS (fluticasone) and a different LABA (salmeterol) are contraindicated for SMART due to a slower onset of action (NHLBI, 2021a). A barrier to implementing SMART is that some insurance prescription plans may cover the SMART MDI prescribed but not cover the cost of the additional inhalers needed at school. Therefore some students may be on a SMART plan at home but only use a SABA (albuterol) at school (Reddell, 2022). See Online Materials OM22-1 for the NHLBI stepwise recommendations for asthma treatment in children and adolescents.

Components of Severity	Intermittent			Persistent								
				Mild			Moderate			Severe		
	Ages 0–4 years	Ages 5–11 years	Ages ≥12 years	Ages 0–4 years	Ages 5–11 years	Ages ≥12 years	Ages 0–4 years	Ages 5–11 years	Ages ≥12 years	Ages 0–4 years	Ages 5–11 years	Ages ≥12 years
Symptoms	≤ 2 days/week			>2 days/week but not daily			Daily			Throughout the day		
Nighttime awakenings	0	≤ 2x/month		1–2x/month	3–4x/month		3–4x/month	>1x/week but not nightly		>1x/week	Often 7x/week	
SABA* use for symptom control (not to prevent EIB*)	≤ 2 days/week			>2 days/week but not daily	>2 days/week but not daily and not more than once on any day		Daily			Several times per day		
Interference with normal activity	None			Minor limitation			Some limitation			Extremely limited		

FIGURE 22-2. Pediatric classification of asthma severity. *(National Heart, Lung, and Blood Institute, 2012, p. 6)*

Medication Delivery Devices and Techniques

Adherence to medication orders at home and at school promotes effective asthma management. Generally, asthma control medications are given at home, not at school. Many control medications are delivered in the form of dry powder inhalers. Quick-relief medications are often given at school to treat an asthma episode and are typically delivered via a metered-dose inhaler (MDI). However, many students have not been properly taught or have not mastered MDI techniques; therefore school nurses should teach and reinforce proper techniques to improve asthma medication response.

For effective medication delivery, an MDI should be attached to a spacer or valved holding chamber that has either a face mask or mouthpiece (American Lung Association [ALA], 2024). Both devices are plastic tubes that create a "space" between the mouth and the MDI to trap and suspend the medication so it can move more easily and deeply into the lungs. Cardboard disposable spacers are also available. A valved holding chamber is a type of spacer that has a one-way valve at the mouthpiece to prevent the medication from being inadvertently exhaled into the atmosphere.

Spacers make the administration of an MDI easier to time. Students as young as infants can be given asthma medications via an MDI with a holding chamber that has a face mask; the medication is pumped into the spacer and the mask is held on the face while the child does tidal breathing for at least six breaths (ALA, 2023). Masks are available in sizes for infants, young children, and adolescents/adults. Developmentally capable school-age children can generally master MDI technique with a spacer that has a mouthpiece, instead of a mask (Jarvis & Eckhardt, 2024). Students should be instructed to exhale fully; then the asthma medication is pumped into the holding chamber and the student should take a slow, deep inhalation and hold their breath for as long as they can, ideally 10 seconds. Students who cannot coordinate this technique or are too dyspneic to breath hold can perform tidal breathing for at least 6 breaths (ALA, 2023). See Figure 22-3.

Despite the ease of use and portability of MDIs with spacers, barriers to their consistent use exist for students. Traditional plastic valved holding chambers require a prescription for a pharmacy to dispense, and health insurance may not cover the cost of a second spacer for school. Additionally, spacers are bulky and inconvenient to carry on one's person (Volerman et al., 2021). This may be especially problematic for socially conscious adolescents.

Asthma MDIs require priming, maintenance, and cleaning in order to function properly, especially if unused for more than a few weeks. If the plastic actuator is not cleaned and the MDI is not primed properly, a complete dose of medication may not be delivered even though the activated MDI appears to spray out a dose. School nurses should consult the manufacturers' instructions for details on how and when to properly clean and prime specific MDIs.

Did You Know?

The Case for Metered-Dose Inhalers and Spacers

MDI administration without a spacer requires synchronized inhalation and breath holding, which is difficult to perform, even for adults. MDIs can spray as fast as 60 miles per hour, which can cause the medication to impact on the tongue, the roof of the mouth, or the back of the throat if a spacer is not used (ALA, 2024). Systemic absorption of a SABA in the mucosa of the mouth and throat can amplify side effects such as increased heart rate, headache, dizziness, and/or feeling nervous and excitable. Similarly, systemic absorption of inhaled corticosteroids can lead to systemic/extrapulmonary corticosteroid effects.

Extensive research has demonstrated that the administration of a SABA via MDI is as effective as by nebulizer treatment (Mitselou et al., 2016; Roncada et al., 2018; Snider et al., 2018; Volerman et al., 2021). Given that nebulizer equipment is expensive and treatments are administered over 15 to 20 minutes, MDIs are generally easier, more portable, more cost effective, and result in less missed instructional time at school.

Preventing Triggers

An equally important component of asthma management is the identification and avoidance of environmental asthma triggers in all settings. There can be many triggers

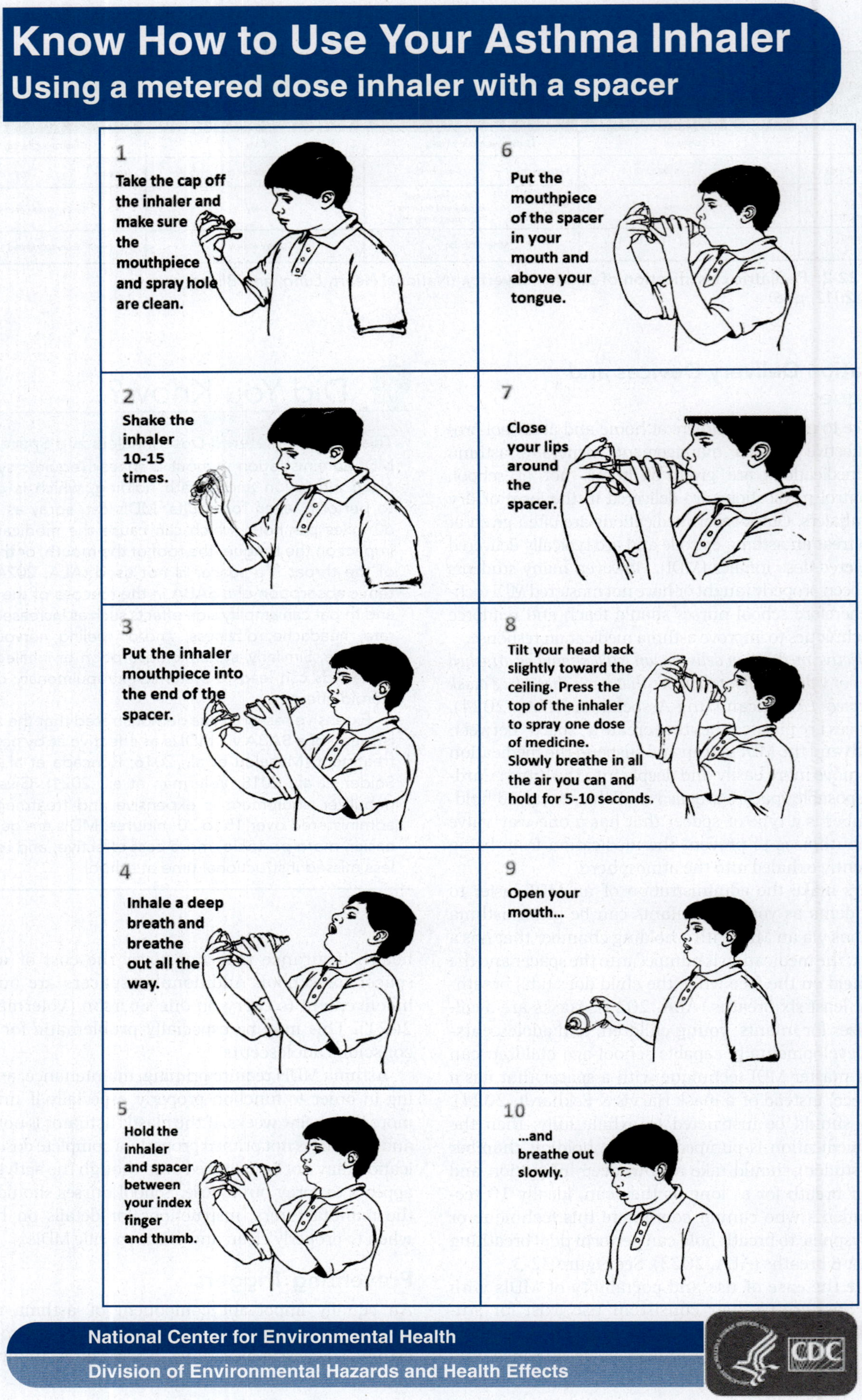

FIGURE 22-3. Metered-dose inhaler technique. *(CDC, n.d.)*

in the school environment whether the school is in an urban, suburban, or rural setting, or an old or new building. Asthma episodes are highly associated with allergen exposure in the environment. Students can also be exposed to any number of respiratory irritants such as chemicals, odors, fumes, and poor indoor and outdoor air quality from high ozone levels or pollution. When assessing the symptoms of a student with asthma, the school nurse should inquire about allergies, triggers, and the pattern of occurrence both at home and school (NASN, 2024b). Common triggers include the following:

- Viral upper respiratory tract infection
- Smoke (all types, including second- and third-hand tobacco smoke, incense, candles, fireplace)
- Pets (furry animals)
- Cleaners, chemicals, strong air fresheners, paint
- Dust mites
- Mold, humidity
- Pests (cockroaches, rodents)
- Cold/extreme weather, season/weather changes
- Air quality issues; smoke (tobacco, fires), vehicle exhaust, sprays, odors
- Physical activity
- Emotions: stress, anxiety, laughing, crying (Jakobowski & Perron, 2019; Jarvis & Eckhardt, 2024)

Air Quality

Fine particulate matter in poor quality indoor or outdoor air can trigger asthma. School nurses should advocate that cleaning, painting, insecticide or pesticide spraying, or mowing grass should be scheduled during times when students are not present. Additionally, exposures can be the result of outside air pollution from vehicle, bus, and train idling, roadway exhaust, nearby industries, or fires. Indoor air quality can be diminished by mold, dust, pests (e.g., cockroaches and rodents), and poorly cleaned ventilation systems (Jakubowski & Perron, 2019). School nurses can monitor AirNow.gov (n.d.) for the local air quality index to help decide if children with asthma should stay inside. The air quality index (AQI) is a "color-coded index designed to communicate whether air quality is healthy or unhealthy" (AirNow.gov, n.d., para. 2). Many school nurses have been instrumental in their districts in implementing policies to prohibit or restrict vehicle idling (buses and cars) outside of their school buildings.

Upper Respiratory Tract Infections

Upper respiratory tract infections, most commonly from cough and respiratory viruses, are common asthma triggers, especially for young children. An asthma cough is often worse at night and persistent beyond the expected course of a cough associated with viral upper respiratory tract infection. When asthma is controlled, students should have minimal symptoms and be able to tolerate viral upper respiratory tract infections, sleep through the night, and play with normal exercise tolerance and endurance. Students with controlled asthma should not need treatment with oral corticosteroids in the emergency department or hospitalization (Conlon, 2017).

Physical Activity

Physical activity is a common asthma trigger for *exercise-induced bronchospasm* in students, sometimes referred to as "exercise-induced asthma." Parents/guardians and school personnel may sometimes unnecessarily restrict students with asthma from participating in physical activities such as recess, physical education class, and sports. However, exercise-induced bronchospasm is not a problem for all children with asthma. Students with well-controlled asthma should be able to participate in all school activities (NHLBI, 2012).

Students with exercise-induced bronchospasm commonly have orders to take a SABA before physical education class, recess, or sports activities. However, exercise-induced bronchospasm can indicate inadequate management of persistent asthma with control medications (NHLBI, 2012). In other cases, students may have orders for a SABA before routine physical activity during which they may not otherwise experience symptoms, resulting in unnecessary medication use. The school nurse should carefully monitor the student's symptoms during exercise and communicate with the student, family, and healthcare provider so that the most effective medication management can be prescribed for school. Participation in outdoor activities may need to be adjusted in severely cold or hot weather.

Students with asthma should be taught to notify their teacher or a supervising adult if they are experiencing asthma symptoms so they can be assessed and treated while at school. School nurses should educate school staff and teachers, including physical education teachers, recess monitors, and coaches, about asthma. The nurse should identify students with asthma and inform staff about their symptoms, the plan for treatment, and any special accommodations that need to be in the student's asthma action plan (discussed later in this chapter).

Asthma Versus Vocal Cord Dysfunction

School nurses must be aware that *vocal cord dysfunction* (VCD) is a relatively common condition in school-age children that causes shortness of breath. The symptoms and triggers of VCD can mimic asthma, but they differ in several important ways (Corjulo & Schoessler, 2016). Asthma is a result of chronic inflammation and constriction of the bronchioles of the lungs that relaxes when treated with bronchodilators. Contrastingly, VCD occurs above the lungs, involving constriction of the vocal cords, and does not respond to asthma quick-relief medications (AAAAI, 2024c). Therefore VCD should be considered in students whose symptoms do not respond to bronchodilators. Yet the presentation can be complex because some students with VCD are misdiagnosed as having asthma, and some students with asthma also have VCD.

Symptoms of VCD include difficulty breathing, coughing, wheezing, throat tightness, hoarseness, and voice changes. Students with asthma complain of chest tightness, whereas students with VCD often complain of throat tightness. Asthma typically causes more difficulty on exhalation, whereas VCD causes more difficulty on inhalation. The triggers of VCD include exercise, lung irritants, upper respiratory tract infections, and gastrointestinal reflux (AAAAI, 2024b). Wheezing in VCD originates in the upper airway and has a harsh quality that typically resonates throughout the chest and sounds distant on auscultation (Corjullo & Schoessler, 2016). The school nurse should activate emergency medical services (EMS) for students with respiratory distress that is unresponsive to asthma quick-relief medications. Careful objective and subjective assessment data should be communicated to the family, EMS, and healthcare providers to aid in accurate diagnosis and treatment of VCD.

Assessing Asthma Control

National and global asthma guidelines divide asthma control into two domains considered simultaneously: risk and control (GINA, 2023; NHLBI, 2021a). Risk reduction focuses on preventing an asthma exacerbation that requires treatment with oral corticosteroids, treatment in the emergency department, and hospitalization. Assessment of risk for asthma exacerbations includes triggers, comorbid conditions, social/emotional well-being, stress factors, and focused history (NASN, 2024b). The school nurse should also collect data regarding access to healthcare, medical home, and insurance coverage. In addition to a general health history, the school nurse should determine the student's pattern of asthma episodes, emergency department visits, hospitalizations, specialized care, and school absences. Family factors are important such as the student's and family's understanding of the disease, how the student's asthma is treated at home, cultural preferences and practices, use of alternative and complementary treatments, appropriateness of over-the-counter medications (e.g., Primatene Mist), and coping mechanisms. The student's baseline activity levels at home and school should be outlined (NASN, 2024b).

The school nurse should manage a student who presents with symptoms by taking a baseline assessment of how well the student's asthma is controlled. A commonly used validated tool to measure asthma control is the *Asthma Control Test* (NHLBI, 2021b). There are two age-specific versions available online or from the student's healthcare provider:

- *Child-Asthma Control Test©* (C-ACT): Seven items for children ages 4 to 11; answered by both child and parent/guardian.
- *Asthma Control Test™:* Five items for children ages 12 and older (adult version); can be answered alone by the child or with assistance (Asthma Control Test, 2023).

The Asthma Control Test is simple to administer and takes only a few minutes. The results are given as score that determines whether the student is within the range of *well-controlled asthma, poorly controlled asthma,* or *very poorly controlled asthma* (see Resources). The school nurse can share results with a parent/guardian and the student's healthcare practitioner if the student has medical orders for asthma treatment at school or with consent of the parent/guardian. Other validated tools to assess asthma control are also available and should be honored if preferred by the family or provider (NHLBI, 2021b).

Another important aspect of assessing control is monitoring the frequency of SABA use. If a student is taking albuterol more than twice a week to treat symptoms (not including pre–physical activity treatment), their asthma is not under control (Allergy and Asthma Network, 2024a). The student should be evaluated and their treatment plan reviewed to determine whether a step up in treatment is indicated. The National Heart, Lung, and Blood Institute (2012) recommends that before initiating a step increase in treatment, a review of inhaler technique, compliance with prescribed regimen, and environmental control is needed.

Peak expiratory flow rate (PEFR), commonly called "peak flow", "measures the maximum flow of air (in liters per minute) that can be forcefully exhaled in 1 second using a peak expiratory flow meter" (Conlon, 2017, p. 656). Peak flow monitoring can be useful when recommended by a healthcare provider as an adjunct assessment tool to provide data regarding a student's asthma control and status during an episode. Accurate monitoring of peak flow rates can assist in school nurse case management of a student's asthma and care coordination with the family and healthcare provider by developing an asthma action plan, deciding on medication adjustments, identifying triggers, determining when to seek emergency care, and promoting self-care (Asthma and Allergy Foundation of America, 2017). It can also help the school nurse to collect referral data for students who have symptoms but do not have an asthma diagnosis.

Peak flow meters are portable, affordable, and easy to use hand-held nonelectronic devices. See Figure 22-4. Small children should use a low range peak flow meter,

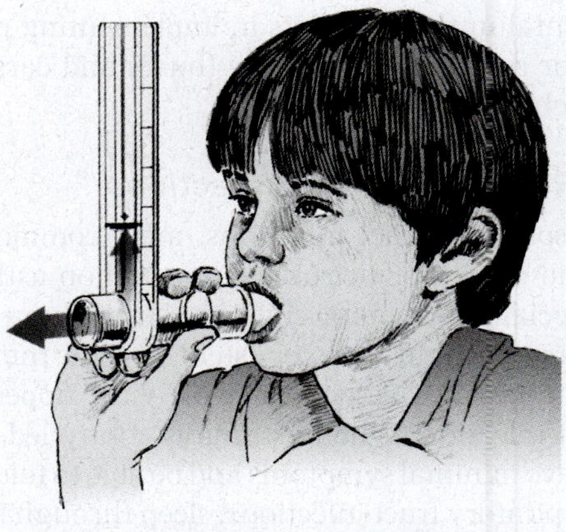

FIGURE 22-4. Peak flow meter.

whereas older children and youth can use a standard peak flow meter for adults (ALA, 2024). Peak flow readings are compared with the student's "personal best" reading, which should be established by multiple readings over a 2- to 3-week period when the student is without symptoms (Conlon, 2017). See Box 22-1 for guidance on how to instruct a student to use a peak flow meter. Peak flow readings are normed by age, height, and gender. Generally, peak flow rates are interpreted and categorized into green, yellow, and red zones that correspond to the zones of an asthma action plan (discussed later in this chapter).

- *Green zone:* Peak flow rate is 80% to 100% of personal best, indicating that the student is predominantly symptom free and under control with routine management.
- *Yellow zone:* Peak flow rate is 50% to 79% of personal best, indicating caution; the student is not well controlled and is having symptoms. The student's asthma practitioner should be contacted to adjust treatment.
- *Red zone:* Peak flow rate is less than 50% of the student's personal best, indicating an acute episode and possible emergency if there is no relief and no improvement in peak flow from the rescue medication (ALA, 2024).

BOX 22-1

Teaching Students to Use a Peak Flow Meter

How to Use Your Peak Flow Meter

Follow these steps:

1. Put the sliding marker or arrow at the bottom of the numbered scale. Use personal mouthpiece or disposable mouthpiece if using the health office peak flow meter. Make sure that there is nothing in your mouth (gum, food).
2. Stand up straight.
3. Take as deep a breath as possible. Put the mouthpiece of the peak flow meter into your mouth and close your lips tightly around the mouthpiece. Keep your tongue away from the mouthpiece.
4. In one action, blow out as hard and as fast as possible until you have emptied almost all of the air from your lungs.
5. Write down the number where the marker is.
6. Repeat steps 1 to 5 two more times and write down the numbers you get. You know that you are doing it correctly if the numbers are close together.
7. Record the highest reading (*not* the average of the three).
8. The number can then be compared with your personal best peak flow rate:
   a. Green zone if it is 80% to 100% of your personal best.
   b. Yellow zone if it is 50% to 79% of your personal best.
   c. Red zone if it is less than 50% of your personal best.
9. Check your Asthma Action Plan as to the action that should be taken based on your results.

However, peak flow parameters should be individualized by the healthcare provider for each student and categorized into green, yellow, and red zones that correspond to the zones of an asthma action plan, discussed in the following section (Asthma Control Test, 2023). Some practitioners prefer more conservative parameters such as green zone of 90% to 100% (ALA, 2024). Note that the reliability of peak flow monitoring in pediatrics is debated because its accuracy depends on a student's ability to understand the directions and the consistency of their technique and expiratory effort. Therefore peak flow monitoring is not universally recommended, especially for small children or children with developmental disabilities (NHLBI, 2021b).

Asthma Action Plans

Every student with asthma needs a written asthma action plan for school (Lemanske et al., 2016). An *asthma action plan* is an "asthma-specific treatment plan completed by the healthcare provider and outlining student-specific symptoms and treatment related to asthma and emergency contact information" (NASN, 2024b, p. 9). An asthma action plan is divided into three sections designated by colors similar to a traffic light: green, yellow, and red (ALA, 2022).

- The green section specifies the student's control medication or medications taken daily, even when asymptomatic, as well as instructions for pretreatment before physical activity.
- The yellow section provides instructions to begin at the onset of a student's symptoms. Prompt identification and treatment of symptoms when they start can prevent the student's condition from worsening.
- The red section specifies the child's emergency plan. A student's asthma action plan should include emergency contact information for their parent/guardian, the child's primary care provider, and/or the child's asthma specialist.

There are many different available forms of asthma action plans such as a school-specific, state-wide, or hospital system/healthcare provider asthma action plan. Asthma action plans are offered by professional organizations (ALA, American Academy of Pediatrics) and government health Web sites. See Figure 22-5 for an asthma action plan from the National Heart, Lung, and Blood Institute. School nurses should review all asthma action plans and medical orders submitted for students annually and when updated as changes in status indicate.

Asthma action plans should be shared with school personnel who are expected to initiate the plan in the absence of the school nurse, where delegation is allowed and appropriate. However, asthma action plans contain protected health information; the school nurse should carefully consider with whom an asthma action plan should be shared. Therefore the school nurse also develops an emergency action plan (EAP) for students with asthma that can be shared with school personnel who have supervision of

ASTHMA ACTION PLAN

For: ______________ Doctor: ______________ Date: ______________

Doctor's Phone Number: ______________ Hospital/Emergency Department Phone Number: ______________

GREEN ZONE

DOING WELL

- No cough, wheeze, chest tightness, or shortness of breath during the day or night
- Can do usual activities

And, if a peak flow meter is used,

Peak flow: more than ______ (80 percent or more of my best peak flow)

My best peak flow is: ______

Daily Medications

Medicine	**How much to take**	**When to take it**

Before exercise ☐ ______ ☐ 2 or ☐ 4 puffs 5 minutes before exercise

YELLOW ZONE

ASTHMA IS GETTING WORSE

- Cough, wheeze, chest tightness, or shortness of breath, or
- Waking at night due to asthma, or
- Can do some, but not all, usual activities

–Or–

Peak flow : ______ to ______ (50 to 79 percent of my best peak flow)

1st **Add: quick-relief medicine—and keep taking your GREEN ZONE medicine.**

______ (quick-relief medicine) Number of puffs ______ or ☐ Nebulizer, once Can repeat every ______ minutes up to maximum of ______ doses

2nd **If your symptoms (and peak flow, if used) return to GREEN ZONE after 1 hour of above treatment:**

☐ Continue monitoring to be sure you stay in the green zone.

–Or–

If your symptoms (and peak flow, if used) do not return to GREEN ZONE after 1 hour of above treatment:

☐ Take: ______ (quick-relief medicine) ______ Number of puffs or ☐ Nebulizer

☐ Add: ______ (oral steroid) mg per day For ______ (3–10) days

☐ Call the doctor ☐ before/ ☐ within ______ hours after taking the oral steroid.

RED ZONE

MEDICAL ALERT!

- Very short of breath, or
- Quick-relief medicines have not helped,
- Cannot do usual activities, or
- Symptoms are same or get worse after 24 hours in Yellow Zone

–Or–

Peak flow : less than ______ (50 percent of my best peak flow)

Take this medicine:

☐ ______ (quick-relief medicine) ______ Number of puffs or ☐ Nebulizer

☐ ______ (oral steroid) mg

Then call your doctor NOW. Go to the hospital or call an ambulance if:

- You are still in the red zone after 15 minutes AND
- You have not reached your doctor.

DANGER SIGNS

- **Trouble walking and talking due to shortness of breath**
- **Lips or fingernails are blue**

- **Take ______ puffs of ______ (quick relief medicine) AND**
- **Go to the hospital or call for an ambulance ______ (phone) NOW!**

FIGURE 22-5. National Heart, Lung, Blood Institute *Asthma Action Plan.* (NHLBI, 2021a).

the student during the school day and school-sponsored activities. An EAP is a very simple and brief plan for lay personnel that has the following format: IF YOU SEE THIS (asthma signs/symptoms)—then DO THIS (how to respond and get help). See Chapter 8 for more discussion of EAPs.

Asthma Episode Management

All schools need an emergency protocol that can be implemented if a student presents with an asthma episode or is not responding to treatment (Allergy and Asthma Network, 2024a; NASN, 2024b). The school nurse must be proficient in rapid assessment of students presenting to the health office with signs and symptoms of asthma. When a student presents with acute symptoms (cough, wheeze, dyspnea, complaints of chest pain or chest tightness), school nurses should assess the student and implement the yellow zone of the action plan by administering the prescribed quick-relief inhaler (SABA, i.e., albuterol) via an MDI with spacer or combination SMART therapy (SABA plus ICS-LABA). Notify a parent/guardian.

The school nurse conducts a focused history to identify what triggered the symptoms, the onset and duration, and activities before the onset of symptoms. The students' symptoms may have just started at school or been present for some time. Did the student treat the symptoms at home? Are they taking their control medication? Are they anxious or afraid?

School nurse physical assessment of students experiencing an asthma episode include the following:

- Quality of speech: ability to finish a sentence without taking breaths, increased voice pitch or decreased volume.
- Auscultate breath sounds anteriorly, posteriorly, and laterally to identify adventitious lung sounds. Listen for wheezing to identify pitch, timing in the breath cycle (inspiratory, expiratory, or both), generalized or localized. Assess for air movement throughout all lung fields (present, diminished, or absent).
- Assess respiratory rate for increased work of breathing/distress; cough (character and frequency), use of

accessory muscles, nasal flaring, leaning forward to breathe (Jakubowski & Perron, 2019).

- Heart rate, pulse oximetry (SaO_2), and temperature (rule out fever).
- Peak flow rate can be assessed if tolerated but should not delay treatment.

The student should be evaluated to be sure the correct technique is being used to administer quick-relief medications. Students should be reassessed and breath sounds auscultated after treatment. Notify the parent/guardian and continue monitoring and treatment (yellow zone). If the student does not respond and remains in respiratory distress, initiate red zone instructions and activate EMS to transport the student to the emergency department. Continue to treat and support the student until EMS arrives. Administer oxygen if ordered or allowed by school policy. See Chapter 17 for more discussion of students in respiratory distress.

SCHOOL NURSING CONSIDERATIONS

School nurses can increase self-efficacy and confidence in caring for students with asthma by engaging in evidence-based clinical practice and continuing education resources (McCabe et al., 2019; NASN, 2024b). Although most school nurses feel prepared to care for students with asthma episodes, significant barriers to best practices remain such as lack of student access to medications, absence of or inadequate school asthma policies and protocols, discomfort and/or variances in state nurse practice acts regarding delegation of asthma care to unlicensed assistive personnel (UAP), and legislative gaps in supporting undesignated (i.e., stock) quick-relief asthma medication (Gibson-Young et al., 2022).

School nurses are the most accessible healthcare provider for many students. Therefore school nurses are often in a position to identify students who may have undiagnosed asthma. Undiagnosed students may present to the nurse with persistent cough, breathing difficulties with physical activity, or observation of difficulty breathing by a physical education teacher, coach, or recess monitor. The school nurse may also be alerted because an undiagnosed student has excessive absences. The parent should be notified and the student referred for evaluation by their healthcare provider.

Asthma Education

School nurses are responsible for asthma education for students, families, and school staff. The parents/guardians of students with asthma may not be aware of the importance of controlling exacerbations, or the rationale for adherence to the control medications of the asthma action plan when the student is asymptomatic. Some parents may not fully understand their child's medications, how to administer them properly, how to implement the asthma action plan, or what can be developmentally expected of their child's engagement in their own care. Based on their readiness and health literacy level, the school nurse helps educate parents/guardians on care concepts and reinforces that asthma is a chronic condition that requires preventive medication when the child is asymptomatic and identification of and avoidance of asthma triggers. The school nurse can begin teaching students about self-care at their learning level as soon as they are diagnosed.

School nurses should facilitate tiered training of school personnel from individual teachers with students with asthma action plans to general training of all school staff. Individual training should be done face-to-face; general staff training can be done virtually. Many states require mandatory staff training on specific chronic conditions of childhood that are conducted via purchased online modules. The school nurse can also enlist the expertise of qualified health professionals from local health systems or certified asthma educators (NASN, 2024b). School nurses are also responsible for training UAP to implement the student's asthma action plan when the nurse is not immediately available or during after-school activities or field trips, as allowed by the state nurse practice act. See Chapters 6, 30, and 31 for more information on school nurse delegation. See Chapter 4 for detailed discussion of the school nurse's role as educator.

Fortunately, robust resources are available to support school nurses and their schools when caring for students with asthma, such as the following:

- American Academy of Allergy, Asthma, and Immunology. (2024b). *The School-Based Allergy, Asthma and Anaphylaxis Management Program®: Comprehensive Asthma Educational Resources* (SA³MPRO™).
- American Lung Association. (2024). *Asthma Friendly Schools Initiative Toolkit.*
- U.S. Department of Health and Human Services, National Institutes of Health, National Heart, Lung, and Blood Institute. (2014). *Managing asthma: A guide for schools.*

See Resources for links.

Health and Education Plans

Students with asthma should be able to participate to the full extent of their abilities in all academic, physical education, and extracurricular activities as outlined in the U.S. Office for Civil Rights (USOCR) designation of free and appropriate public education (FAPE) (NASN, 2024a, p. 6; USOCR, 2020). The school nurse develops an individualized healthcare plan (IHP) for students with asthma that outlines the full range of health services beyond just health office visits and medication administration. See Online Materials OM22-2 for a sample IHP for a student with asthma. Students with asthma may need Section 504 plans to ensure that the student does not face discrimination at school due to their asthma and that accommodations for academic success are respected. Examples of Section 504 accommodations include the right to self-carry their quick-relief medication, the right to use a cellphone, access to a trained asthma UAP, access to the elevator, extended time on assignments or standardized testing, no penalties for late assignments due to asthma absences, and guarantee of full participation in school-sponsored activities and field trips (NASN, 2024b). Students who receive special education services should have these safeguards incorporated in their individualized education programs (IEPs). See Chapter 8 for more information on Section 504 plans.

Self-Carry of Quick-Relief Inhalers

Students often have asthma episodes at school when a school nurse or trained personnel are not readily available to assist them with taking their asthma medications. School nurses should promote self-care for students with asthma. To that end, all 50 states have enacted legislation that protects a student's right to self-carry and self-administer their quick-relief asthma medication (Allergy and Asthma Network, 2024b). However, only about 25% of students who self-carry their quick-relief asthma inhalers are ready to do so upon objective measurement of their knowledge and skills. Students who are older than 11 years, in higher grade levels, and have parents/guardians who are more familiar with asthma policies are more likely to demonstrate higher levels or readiness to self-carry their asthma medications. Parents/guardians tend to overestimate a student's competence to self-carry. In contrast, school nurses are often hesitant to allow students to self-carry (Volerman et al., 2019). Although not stipulated legally, the licensed prescriber can indicate on the medication order form whether they deem the student has the capacity to self-carry their medication. Therefore careful assessment and education by providers and school nurses on the asthma action plan and proper inhaler techniques support the student's ability to self-manage their asthma at school.

School nurses can meet with students known to self-carry to assess their knowledge, technique, and competence to administer their medications independently. To demonstrate a student's readiness and willingness to accept responsibility can be outlined in a written agreement with the school. See Chapter 30 for more information on best practices in self-carry medications and a sample student medication self-carry contract.

Stock Quick-Relief Inhalers

As of 2024, twenty-three states and the District of Columbia have laws or guidelines that permit schools to stock quick-relief (albuterol) inhalers with orders from a licensed prescriber. This allows schools to keep a supply of undesignated quick-relief inhalers to administer to any student whether or not they are known to have asthma or have a personal medical order on file. In 2021, federal legislation, called the *School-Based Allergies and Asthma Management Program Act*, was enacted to encourage more states and schools to implement comprehensive asthma management programs such as having policies allowing undesignated quick-relief asthma medication (Allergy and Asthma Network, 2024b). The goal of stock albuterol in schools is to save students' lives.

As a component of part of SA³MPRO™, the American Academy of Allergy, Asthma, and Immunology developed a *Stock Inhaler Toolkit* (2023) in collaboration with the American Academy of Pediatrics, NASN, the American Lung Association, and other professional organizations. This toolkit is a compendium of resources to support schools in instituting stock quick-relief asthma inhaler programs, including the following:

- Why stock inhalers are important to you and your students
- How to recognize respiratory distress
- How to find and understand your state's law pertaining to stock medication
- Using stock medication and what follow-up care is needed
- Ways to get your staff trained to be prepared for asthma emergencies
- What policies, protocols, and processes you need to have in place before using the medication on campus
- Examples of the documents you may need to get medication and implement the program (AAAAI, 2023, p. 6)

See Resources at the end of this chapter for a link to the *Stock Inhaler Toolkit.*

Evaluation

School nurses can demonstrate their effectiveness as case managers, care coordinators, and leaders in school asthma care by collecting school- or district-wide data on their interventions. Such data can be shared with district decision makers, educators, families, and community partners to advocate for needed school health services and programming related to asthma. See Box 22-2.

CYSTIC FIBROSIS

Cystic fibrosis (CF) is a chronic, genetic condition that affects a protein in the body that affects mucus, sweat, and digestive enzymes. Mutations to the cystic fibrosis transmembrane conductance regulator (CFTR) gene lead to a dysfunctional CFTR protein. This makes mucus thick and sticky thereby causing progressive damage to the respiratory tract and chronic gastrointestinal symptoms along with other organ complications. People with CF can experience complications to their lungs, sinuses, pancreas, liver, intestines, reproductive tracts, and sweat glands (CDC, 2024).

BOX 22-2

School Nurse Data Collection Related to Asthma

NASN's *School Nursing Evidence-Based Clinical Practice Guideline: Students With Asthma* states the following:

In addition to regular evaluation of student progress to adjust individual student's care plans (e.g., IHP, EAP/ECP, 504 plan, IEP) needed to meet goals, the school nurse will collect the following information to track progress and evaluate efforts:

- *Effectiveness of school nurse interventions*
  - *Number of students diagnosed with asthma*
  - *Number of students using asthma reliever inhalers*
  - *Number of students within target range (TIR) of peak flow meter reading (if available)*
  - *Number of students who have an asthma action plan (completed by HCP)*
  - *Number of students who have an IHP, EAP/ECP, 504 plan, and/or IEP to address asthma-related needs in the school setting*
  - *Number of students receiving care from UAP*
  - *Number of health office visits of students with asthma*
  - *Number of students who experience an asthma exacerbation in the school setting*
  - *Number of students with impaired respiratory status*
  - *Number of students who are allowed to self-carry their asthma reliever inhalers*
  - *Number of school staff educated and trained for asthma response*

NASN (2024b, p. 22).

According to the 2022 Cystic Fibrosis Foundation (CFF) registry, there were over 32,000 people living with CF in the United States (CFF, 2023). CF can affect individuals of any race or ethnicity, though it is most common in populations of European descent. The incidence of CF is estimated to be between 1 in 3,000 and 1 in 6,000 live births (Scotet et al., 2020). The predicted median survival is 53 years old, increased from 35 years old in 2005. Currently more than half of people with CF are adult age due to improved therapeutic options (CFF, 2023). There is no cure for CF, but airway clearance regimens, medications, and nutritional optimization are helping people with CF better manage their disease.

Genetics

Mutations to the cystic fibrosis transmembrane conductance regulator (CFTR) gene, located on chromosome 7, lead to a dysfunctional CFTR protein. More than 1,700 mutations have been found in the CFTR gene; the most common mutation is delta F508 (F508del) and almost 90% of individuals in the CFF registry have at least one copy of this variant (CFF, n.d.a). CF is an autosomal recessive disease, meaning a person with CF has inherited one CFTR mutation from each parent. An individual who has inherited only one CFTR mutation does not have CF but is carrier for the mutation. About 10 million people in the United States are CF carriers (CFF, n.d.c).

In CF, secretory cells of the sweat glands, airway, gastrointestinal tract, pancreas, and reproductive tract have either not enough or malfunctioning CFTR protein. Suboptimal amount and function of CFTR protein impedes the passage of chloride from the cell's interior to exterior; this subsequently affects the balance of chloride, bicarbonate, sodium, and water throughout the body (Cabrini et al., 2022).

Diagnosis

All 50 states screen for CF through state newborn screening programs. CF newborn screening tests the level of immunoreactive trypsinogen, which is elevated in people with CF, although false positive results can occur due to prematurity (CFF, 2007). Quantitative pilocarpine iontophoresis, or a "sweat test," is the gold standard for CF diagnosis; a sweat chloride concentration of 60 mmol/L or higher meets diagnostic criteria for CF. Genotyping or genetic testing allows for identification of an individual's CFTR mutations (CFF, n.d.b).

Respiratory Management

In the respiratory tract, the defective CFTR protein leads to thick, dehydrated mucus, which is difficult to clear and can lead to both upper and lower airway complications. Students with CF can experience chronic rhinosinusitis and nasal polyps. Symptoms can be flared by allergens, environmental irritants, or viral triggers. Nasal or sinus complications may present with worsening nasal congestion, sinus pressure or pain, headaches, or fever. Students with CF may require regular sinus rinses or nasal spray to manage upper airway symptoms; chronic symptoms may warrant surgical intervention (CFF, 2023). Thick mucus causes airway obstruction and bacterial growth in the lungs, which can subsequently lead to inflammation, infections, bronchiectasis, and progressive lung damage. Treatment is focused on controlling infection, reducing airway obstruction, and decreasing inflammation of the airway. Respiratory cultures are performed at outpatient specialty appointments to determine whether bacterial growth is present in the respiratory tract. Careful antibiotic selection is required during times of illness or CF exacerbations. Students with CF may be treated with antibiotics administered orally, by inhalation, or intravenously through a centrally inserted catheter (CFF, 2023).

Mucolytics, such as hypertonic saline and dornase alpha, assist by thinning mucus, making it easier to mobilize with CPT therapies. Small portable positive expiratory pressure (PEP) devices, known by their name brands of Flutter®, Acapella®, AerobikA®, and RC-Cornet®, are recommended by CF care teams for additional CPT options.

Practice Connection

Reducing airway obstruction and inflammation in the lungs is achieved through medications and airway clearance techniques. Bronchodilators are given before airway clearance techniques to help dilate and relax the smooth muscles lining the airway. Chest physiotherapy (CPT) is used in addition to mucolytics to hydrate and mobilize thick, heavy mucus. CPT techniques consist of manual percussion over the five lobes of the lungs, performed in conjunction with postural drainage to optimize mucus draining from the lungs. High-frequency chest wall oscillation (HFCWO) is a machine that enables a wearable vest to inflate and deflate rapidly causing clapping-like pressure over the five lobes of the lung. The vibration created both loosens and moves mucus, which can then be mobilized with huffing and coughing maneuvers (CFF, n.d.c). See Chapter 25, Figure 25-9.

Students with CF perform airway clearance techniques on a routine basis, usually twice daily when they are feeling well. During times of illness, it is recommended students increase their airway clearance regimens, which may occur during school hours (CFF, n.d.a). Finally, regular exercise and good physical fitness are important factors for airway clearance, better lung function, and overall health in people with CF.

CFTR modulator therapies are the newest therapeutic option for many people with CF and are designed to correct the malfunctioning CFTR protein. Only people with specific mutations can take modulator therapies since different mutations lead to varying defects in the CFTR protein. There are four CFTR modulator therapies available, all taken orally: Kalydeco® (ivacaftor), Orkambi® (lumacaftor/ivacaftor), Symdeko® (tezacaftor/ivacaftor), and Trikafta® (elexacaftor/tezacaftor/ivacaftor) (CFF, n.d.d). All modulators help the CFTR protein function more effectively, though not perfectly, so chronic airway clearance therapies and medications are often continued.

There are several important respiratory considerations for school nurse–led case management at school:

- Students with CF tend to cough more than students without CF. Students should never be made to feel self-conscious about coughing or try to suppress it; coughing is the body's way of clearing secretions. Students with CF should have a box of tissues to cough into with a trashcan for disposal followed by hand hygiene. They also need to stay well hydrated and should be allowed to carry a water bottle and encouraged to drink often.
- It is not necessary for the student to be referred to the school nurse for coughing, unless the student is having difficulty controlling their cough or has signs of respiratory distress.
- Students with CF should never be given any medications to suppress coughing or to dry up secretions, as both are counterproductive in keeping mucus moist and easy to expectorate.
- Signs of respiratory distress that need immediate medical attention are uncontrolled coughing, dyspnea, tachypnea, exercise intolerance, wheezing, retractions, a dusky appearance, and hypoxemia, as observed and measured by pulse oximetry. Intervention may include administration of bronchodilators and airway clearance regimens. School nurses can receive instruction from the student's parent or local CF care center on use of airway clearance equipment and direction on manual CPT techniques.
- Students with CF are not contagious to classmates. However, students with CF can easily transmit bacteria and respiratory illness to other students with CF. Therefore it is recommended to place children with CF in different classrooms. ***To minimize the spread of bacteria and viruses, if there is more than one student with CF in the school (and they are not siblings), it is essential to maintain at least 6 feet of separation.*** They should never sit next to each other in class, lunch, or on the bus, and water bottles or personal items should never be shared; lockers and common areas should also be as far away as possible.
- In general, students with CF do not have physical restrictions, unless designated by their CF care team. Student with CF benefit from routine activity and exercise.
- Routine childhood immunizations and an annual seasonal influenza vaccine are recommended.
- The school nurse develops an IHP for a student with CF. The school nurse is integral in outlining respiratory considerations and academic accommodations in the student's IEP or Section 504 plan.
- Close communication with the student's parents/guardians and the CF center care team is important in managing aspects of both acute and chronic care (CFF, n.d.e).

Gastrointestinal and Nutritional Management

Approximately 84% of individuals with CF are pancreatic insufficient and require pancreatic enzyme replacement therapy (PERT) (CFF, n.d.f). Pancreatic enzymes allow for the digestion of fat and subsequent absorption of calories, nutrients, and vitamins. People with pancreatic-insufficient CF require lifelong pancreatic enzyme replacement therapy and fat-soluble vitamin supplementation with vitamins A, D, E, and K. Pancreatic enzyme replacement therapy preparations are porcine-derived capsules that are administered before any foods containing fat (Shteinberg et al., 2021a). The capsules can be opened, and enteric-coated beads can be sprinkled on an acidic soft food and administered by spoon for young children or individuals unable to swallow pills. Pancreatic enzyme replacement therapy capsules should be stored only at room temperature; cold and warm temperatures can degrade effectiveness of the medication. The amount or number of pancreatic enzyme replacement therapy capsules is calculated by the student's CF care team and is based on the individual's weight and typical amount of food eaten for meals and snacks. Poor weight gain or symptoms such as steatorrhea, flatulence, abdominal discomfort, and abdominal distention are signs of fat malabsorption and possibly related to inadequate pancreatic enzyme replacement therapy dosing.

School-age children and adolescents are recommended to maintain a body mass index at or above the 50th percentile on the CDC growth chart. Good nutritional status has been shown to lead to better pulmonary function and outcomes (CFF, 2023). Individuals with CF often need up to twice the daily calories to adequately gain weight as similarly aged people without CF. In some instances, enteral feeds are used to boost daily calorie and nutrient intake.

Conversely, now that highly effective CFTR modulator medications are available for many individuals with CF, some people are starting to gain weight excessively given improved fat and nutrient absorption in the gastrointestinal tract. It is suspected that excessive weight gain may have a negative impact on the health of individuals with CF, as it does with the general population (Gabel et al., 2022).

Students with CF are prone to constipation because fat malabsorption and faulty CFTR proteins in the GI tract limit intestinal fluid and cause thick mucus. Constipation can present as decreased stooling frequency and volume as well as hard, difficult to pass stools with straining, abdominal discomfort, loss of appetite, and early satiety. Constipation can be treated with daily or as-needed medication, most commonly osmotic laxatives, which help draw in fluid to soften hard stool. In severe cases, constipation can lead to distal intestinal obstruction syndrome where stool blocks the junction of the small intestines with the large intestines, requiring treatment at a hospital. Symptoms of distal intestinal obstruction syndrome often consist of severe abdominal pain, nausea with vomiting, hematochezia, or fever unexplained by lung disease (CFF, 2023).

Individuals with CF can be prone to gastroesophageal reflux disease (GERD), or refluxing of stomach acid into the esophagus, which can be exacerbated with coughing. Treatment to suppress stomach acid can be achieved with proton pump inhibitors or histamine H2-receptor antagonists (Borowitz et al., 2002).

Cystic fibrosis–related diabetes is the most common comorbidity in CF, affecting up to 20% of adolescents and 50% of adults (CFF, 2023). This complication is a result of pancreatic damage when the exocrine tissue of the pancreas is damaged or destroyed by fibrosis and fat. Management recommendations focus on insulin therapy and optimizing glycemic control (Weber, 2025). Screening for hyperglycemia begins at 10 years old and is facilitated by CF care centers.

The CFTR protein in sweat glands ineffectively reabsorbs sodium, therefore individuals with CF have higher rates of salt and water loss through their sweat. Replenishment with a high-salt diet and liberal hydration with water and electrolyte drinks is important in avoiding hyponatremia and dehydration, especially on warm or active days.

There are several important considerations for school nurse–led case management at school:

- The school nurse should ensure that students with pancreatic-insufficient CF take their pancreatic enzymes immediately before a meal. Enzyme capsules must not be crushed or chewed. If swallowing a capsule is difficult, the capsule may be opened and the contents sprinkled on a small amount of acidic food, such as applesauce or a pureed fruit, then swallowed. If sprinkled, the enzyme beads should be swallowed immediately, rather than prepared in advance. Enzymes should be stored at room temperature. Foods that do not require enzymes include fat-free foods and beverages; this includes fruits, most vegetables, electrolyte drinks, and some candies or snacks.
- Students with CF should be allowed unlimited bathroom privileges outlined in their Section 504 plan or IEP. Some students may prefer to use a noncommunal bathroom due to flatulence or stool characteristics.
- Constipation is manageable through daily or as-needed bowel regimens, often osmotic laxatives. Signs of distal intestinal obstruction syndrome indicate an emergency that must be addressed in a hospital setting.
- Students with CF often follow a high-fat, high-calorie, and high-salt diet to optimize nutritional status and replenish salt wasted through sweating. Some students on CFTR protein modulators do not require a high-fat diet if experiencing excessive weight gain.
- Some students may obtain caloric enhancement through enteral tube feeds via gastrostomy, nasogastric, or jejunostomy tubes to promote weight gain and nutritional status.
- Access to an air-conditioned room, electrolyte-rich fluids, and salt may be necessary if a student is overheated or showing signs of dehydration.
- Students with CF-related diabetes often require blood glucose monitoring before meals or if symptomatic for hypoglycemia or hyperglycemia. Insulin is generally used to facilitate glycemic control. The school nurse may be responsible for administering or supervising the student's self-administration of insulin (CFF, n.d.f).

Mental Health

Managing a chronic health condition can put students with CF at a higher risk for mental health concerns such as depression and anxiety. In addition, highly effective modulator therapies have been shown to affect the mental health of people with CF (Dagenais et al., 2020). The school nurse needs to be aware of students with CF who are struggling with mental health concerns. The Cystic

Fibrosis Foundation recommends an annual screening for depression and anxiety starting at 12 years of age through the *Patient Health Questionnaire–9* (PHQ-9) and the *Generalized Anxiety Disorder–7* (GAD-7). It is recommended that children 7 to 10 years old be assessed for depression and anxiety if the child is exhibiting symptoms of anxiety or depression or a caregiver is concerned (Quittner et al., 2016). The school nurse should partner with the student's family and CF center to be aware of any mental health concerns and treatment regimens such as counseling or medications.

Fertility

Fertility and pregnancy are subjects to be addressed in the adolescent and young adult population; 95% of males with CF are infertile secondary to congenital bilateral absence of the vas deferens. Although there is functioning sperm in the testes, most men with CF lack the ability to transport sperm (Shteinberg et al., 2021b). Some females with CF may experience decreased fertility secondary to thick cervical secretions, ovulation irregularity, malnutrition, and additional factors. However, given improved treatments and improved health outcomes, the number of pregnancies in women with CF has markedly increased since the 2000s. According to the 2022 CFF Registry (2023), there were over 600 pregnancies in women with CF in 2020 compared with 222 pregnancies in 2010. Unplanned pregnancy rates of women with CF are elevated, estimated up to 50% (Godfrey et al., 2020). School nurses should be knowledgeable with information regarding fertility, pregnancy, and available resources.

Inpatient Care

Students with CF may have acute pulmonary or gastrointestinal complications that require hospitalization. Hospitalizations may be lengthy with weeks of school missed. The school nurse is the liaison between the school and healthcare providers; this can be instrumental in promoting continuity of care as the student transitions back to school. Hospital home-bound services may be indicated to support the student's ongoing academic progress.

School Nursing Considerations

School nursing care of students with CF requires case management and care coordination skills. Evidence-based care requires not only that the school nurse has knowledge of the most current and relevant scientifically derived practice recommendations, but that they also consider the student's and family's cultural contexts and healthcare priorities. As with all students with special healthcare needs, the school nurse develops an IHP that outlines the comprehensive nature of care at school according to the nursing process. An EAP may also be indicated so that school personnel can respond quickly and appropriately in case of emergency when the school nurse is not immediately available. Students with CF need their school health services and educational accommodations/modifications stipulated on their Section 504 plan or IEP to help protect their right to a free and appropriate public education (FAPE). See Chapter 20 for further discussion on supporting students with special healthcare needs.

CONCLUSION

School nurses need to remain current on evidence-based treatment recommendations of students with asthma and CF. The treatment and overall management of these conditions are constantly evolving. School nurses should include asthma and CF in their own learning/continuing education plans, focusing on understanding assessment, current medications, and emerging treatment strategies for different asthma phenotypes. Partnering with students, families, and local healthcare providers allows for a collaborative approach in helping a student manage their asthma or CF both during times of wellness and episodes of escalated care. Through collaboration and education, school nurses are in positions of advocacy to ensure the health requirements of students with chronic conditions are met. This in turn gives the student the opportunity to focus on their educational priorities and optimization of learning and growth.

The Editors gratefully acknowledge the work of previous chapter authors, Melinda Barrett & Carol Murphy Moore.

Resources

Allergy and Asthma Network. (2024). *School health resources.* https://allergyasthmanetwork.org/wp-content/uploads/2020/05/asthma-action-plan.pdf

American Academy of Allergy, Asthma, and Immunology. (2023). *School-based asthma, allergy, anaphylaxis Management PROgram®. Stock inhaler toolkit.* https://www.aaaai.org/Aaaai/media/Media-Library-PDFs/Tools%20for%20the%20Public/School%20Tools/Stock-Inhaler-Toolkit-for-Schools.pdf

American Academy of Allergy, Asthma, and Immunology. (2024). *The school-based allergy, asthma and anaphylaxis management program: Comprehensive asthma educational resources (SA³MPRO™).* https://www.aaaai.org/tools-for-the-public/school-tools/sampro

American Lung Association. (2024). *Asthma friendly schools initiative toolkit.* https://www.lung.org/lung-health-diseases/lung-disease-lookup/asthma/health-professionals-educators/asthma-friendly-schools-initiative/toolkit

Asthma Control Test. 2023. *Welcome to the asthma control test.* https://www.asthmacontroltest.com/welcome/

National Association of School Nurses. (2024). *School nursing evidence-based clinical practice guideline: Students With asthma.* Author.

National Heart, Lung and Blood Institute. (2021). *Asthma action plan.* https://www.nhlbi.nih.gov/sites/default/files/publications/Asthma-Action-Plan-2020_rev_508.pdf

Respiratory Health Association & Illinois Department of Public Health. (2020). *Implementation guidance for quick-relief stock asthma medication.* https://resphealth.org/wp-content/uploads/2021/10/Stock-Albuterol-Schools-Toolkit.pdf

U.S. Department of Health and Human Services, National Institutes of Health, National Heart, Lung, and Blood Institute. (2014). *Managing asthma: A guide for schools* (NIH Publication No. 14-2650). https://www.nhlbi.nih.gov/sites/default/files/publications/14-2650%20NACI_ManagingAsthma-508%20FINAL.pdf

References

AirNow.gov. (n.d.). *About AirNow.* https://www.airnow.gov/about-airnow/

Allergy and Asthma Network. (2024a). *School health resources.* https://allergyasthmanetwork.org/wp-content/uploads/2020/05/asthma-action-plan.pdf

Allergy and Asthma Network. (2024b). *State laws.* https://advocacy.allergyasthmanetwork.org/laws-to-protect-those-with-allergies-and-asthma/state-laws/

American Academy of Allergy, Asthma, and Immunology. (2024a). *Asthma overview.* https://www.aaaai.org/conditions-treatments/asthma/asthma-overview

American Academy of Allergy, Asthma, and Immunology. (2024b). *The school-based allergy, asthma and anaphylaxis management program: Comprehensive asthma educational resources (SA³MPRO™).* https://www.aaaai.org/tools-for-the-public/school-tools/sampro

American Academy of Allergy, Asthma, and Immunology. (2024c). *Vocal cord dysfunction: Overview.* https://www.aaaai.org/conditions-treatments/related-conditions/vocal-cord-dysfunction

American Academy of Allergy, Asthma, and Immunology & School-Based Asthma, Allergy, Anaphylaxis Management PROgram®. (2023). *Stock inhaler toolkit.* https://www.aaaai.org/Aaaai/media/Media-Library-PDFs/Tools%20for%20the%20Public/School%20Tools/Stock-Inhaler-Toolkit-for-Schools.pdf

American Lung Association. (2022). *My asthma action plan for home and school.* https://www.lung.org/getmedia/aa8ce6f5-667e-4726-b4ab-8ac8d5d448e4/FY22-ALA-Asthma-Action-Plan_Home_School-with-QR-codes.pdf

American Lung Association. (2023, December 4). *Valved holding chambers and spacers.* https://www.lung.org/lung-health-diseases/lung-disease-lookup/asthma/treatment/devices/chambers-spacers

American Lung Association. (2024). *Measuring your peak flow rate.* https://www.lung.org/lung-health-diseases/lung-disease-lookup/asthma/treatment/devices/peak-flow

Asthma and Allergy Foundation of America. (2017, December). *Peak flow meters.* https://aafa.org/asthma/asthma-diagnosis/lung-function-tests-diagnose-asthma/peak-flow-meters/

Asthma Control Test. (2023). *Welcome to the asthma control test.* https://www.asthmacontroltest.com/welcome/

Borowitz, D., Baker, R. D., & Stallings, V. (2002). Consensus report on nutrition for pediatric patients with cystic fibrosis. *Journal of Pediatric Gastroenterology and Nutrition, 35*(3), 246–259. https://doi.org/10.1097/00005176-200209000-00004

Cabrini, G., Rimessi, A., Borgatti, M., Pinton, P., & Gambari, R. (2022). Overview of CF lung pathophysiology. *Current Opinion in Pharmacology, 64.* https://doi.org/10.1016/j.coph.2022.102214

Centers for Disease Control and Prevention. (n.d.). *Know how to use your metered dose inhaler.* https://www.cdc.gov/asthma/pdfs/Inhaler_Spacer_FactSheet.pdf

Centers for Disease Control and Prevention. (2022). *CDC's national asthma control program.* https://www.cdc.gov/asthma/nacp.htm

Centers for Disease Control and Prevention. (2023, May 10). *Most recent asthma data. 2019–2021 National Health Interview Survey.* https://www.cdc.gov/asthma/most_recent_national_asthma_data.htm

Centers for Disease Control and Prevention. (2024, May 15). *About cystic fibrosis.* https://www.cdc.gov/cystic-fibrosis/about/index.html

Chu, R., & Bajaj, P. (2024, July). *Asthma medication in children.* StatPearls [Internet]. https://www.ncbi.nlm.nih.gov/books/NBK441823/

Conlon, P. M. (2017). The child with respiratory dysfunction. In M. L. Hockenberry, D. Wilson, & C. C. Rodgers (Eds.), *Wong's essentials of pediatric nursing* (10th ed., pp. 636–688). Elsevier.

Corjulo, M., & Schoessler, S. (2016). Asthma and vocal cord dysfunction: Can you tell the difference? *NASN School Nurse, 31*(6), 325–327. doi:10.1177/1942602X16659350

Cystic Fibrosis Foundation. (n.d.a). *Airway clearance.* https://www.cff.org/managing-cf-/airway-clearance

Cystic Fibrosis Foundation. (n.d.b). *Basics of the CFTR protein.* https://www.cff.org/research-clinical-trials/basics-cftr-protein#:~:text=Summary,protein%20called%20an%20ion%20channel

Cystic Fibrosis Foundation. (n.d.c). *CF genetics: The basics.* https://www.cff.org/intro-cf/cf-genetics-basics

Cystic Fibrosis Foundation. (n.d.d). *CFTR modulator therapies.* https://www.cff.org/managing-cf/cftr-modulator-therapies

Cystic Fibrosis Foundation. (n.d.e). *A teachers guide to cystic fibrosis.* https://www.cff.org/intro-cf/teachers-guide-cystic-fibrosis

Cystic Fibrosis Foundation. (n.d.f). *Use the right gastrointestinal medications.* https://www.cff.org/managing-cf/use-right-gastrointestinal-medications

Cystic Fibrosis Foundation. (2007). *Newborn screening clinical care guidelines.* https://www.cff.org/medical-professionals/newborn-screening-clinical-care-guidelines

Cystic Fibrosis Foundation. (2023). *2022 Patient registry annual data report.* https://www.cff.org/medical-professionals/patient-registry

Dagenais, R. V., Su, V. C., & Quon, B. S. (2020). Real world safety of CFTR modulators in the treatment of cystic fibrosis: A systematic review. *Journal of Clinical Medicine, 10*(1), 23. https://doi.org/10.3390/jcm10010023

Gabel, M. E., Fox, C. K., Grimes, R. A., Lowman, J. D., McDonald, C. M., Stallings, V. A., & Michel, S. H. (2022). Overweight and cystic fibrosis: An unexpected challenge. *Pediatric Pulmonology, 57*(S1), S40–S49. https://doi.org/10.1002/ppul.25748

Gibson-Young., L, Waldrop, J., Lindahl, B., & Buckner, E. (2022). School nurses perceptions on managing asthma in Alabama schools. *The Journal of School Nursing, 38*(2), 194–202. https://doi.org/10.1177/1059840520924455

Global Initiative for Asthma. (2023). *Global strategy for asthma management and prevention.* https://ginasthma.org/wp-content/uploads/2023/07/GINA-2023-Full-report-23_07_06-WMS.pdf

Godfrey, E. M., Mody, S., Schwartz, M. R., Heltshe, S. L., Taylor-Cousar, J. L., Jain, R., Sufian, S., Josephy, T., & Aitken, M. L. (2020). Contraceptive use among women with cystic fibrosis: A pilot study linking reproductive health questions to the Cystic Fibrosis Foundation National Patient Registry. *Contraception, 101*(6), 420–426. https://doi.org/10.1016/j.contraception.2020.02.006

Jakubowski, T., & Perron, T. (2019). Asthma assessment in the school health office: Can they stay or should they go? *NASN School Nurse, 34*(1), 37–43. https://doi.org/10.1177/1942602X18803336

Jarvis, C., & Eckhardt, A. (2024). *Physical examination and health assessment* (9th ed.). Elsevier.

Kavanaugh, J., Jackson, D., & Kent, B. (2019). Over and under-diagnosis in asthma. *Breathe, 15,* e20–e27. https://doi.org/10.1183/20734735.0362-2018

Lemanske, R. F., Jr., Kakumanu, S., Shanovich, K., Antos, N., Cloutier, M. M., Mazyck, D., Phipatanakul, W., Schantz, S., Szefzer. S., Vandlik, R., & Williams, P. (2016). Creation and implementation of SAMPRO™: A school-based asthma management program. *Journal of Allergy and Clinical Immunology, 138*(3), 711–723. https://doi.org/10.1016/j.jaci.2016.06.015

Liu, A. H., Bacharier, L. B., Fitzpatrick, A. M., & Sicherer, S. H. (2025). Childhood asthma. In R. M. Kliegman, J. W. St. Geme, N. J. Blum, R. C. Tasker, K. M. Wilson, A. M. Schuh, & C. L. Mack (Eds.). *Nelson textbook of pediatrics* (22nd ed., pp. 1385–1410.e.1). Elsevier.

McCabe, E. M., McDonald, C., Connolly, C., & Lipman, T. H. (2019). A review of school nurses' self-efficacy in asthma care. *The Journal of School Nursing, 35*(1), 15–26. https://doi.org/10.1177/1059840518808886

Mitselou, N., Hedlin, G., & Hederos, C. A. (2016). Spacers versus nebulizers in treatment of acute asthma—a prospective randomized study in preschool children. *Journal of Asthma, 53*(10), 1059–1062. https://doi.org/10.1080/02770903.2016.1185114

National Association of School Nurses. (2022). *School nursing: Scope and standards of practice* (4th ed.). Author.

National Association of School Nurses. (2024a). A contemporary framework update for today's school nursing landscape: Introducing the School Nursing Practice Framework. *NASN School Nurse, 39*(3), 140–147. https://www.doi.org/10.1177/1942602X241241092

National Association of School Nurses. (2024b). *School nursing evidence-based clinical practice guideline: Students with asthma*. Author.

National Heart, Lung and Blood Institute. (2012). *Asthma care quick reference: Diagnosing and managing asthma guidelines* (NIH Publication No. 12-5075). National Asthma Education and Prevention Program Expert Panel Report, National Institutes of Health. https://www.nhlbi.nih.gov/files/docs/guidelines/asthma_qrg.pdf

National Heart, Lung and Blood Institute. (2020). The 2020 focused updates to the asthma management guidelines: A report from the National Asthma Education and Prevention Program Coordinating Committee Expert Panel. *Journal of Allergy and Clinical Immunology, 146* (6), 1217–1270. doi:10.1016/j.jaci.2020.10.003

National Heart, Lung and Blood Institute. (2021a). *Asthma action plan.* https://www.nhlbi.nih.gov/sites/default/files/publications/Asthma-Action-Plan-2020_rev_508.pdf

National Heart, Lung and Blood Institute. (2021b). *Asthma management guidelines: Focused updates 2020.* (NIH Publication No. 20-HL-8140). U.S. Department of Health and Human Services, National Institutes of Health. https://www.nhlbi.nih.gov/health-topics/asthma-management-guidelines-2020-updates

Quittner, A. L., Abbott, J., Georgiopoulos, A. M., Goldbeck, L., Smith, B., Hempstead, S. E., Marshall, B., Sabadosa, K. A., & Elborn, S. (2016). International committee on mental health in cystic fibrosis: Cystic Fibrosis Foundation and European Cystic Fibrosis Society consensus statements for screening and treating depression and anxiety. *Thorax, 71*(1), 26–34. https://doi.org/10.1136/thoraxjnl-2015-207488

Reddel, H. K., Bateman, E. D., Schatz, M., Krishnan, J. A., & Cloutier, M. M. (2022). A practical guide to implementing SMART in asthma management. *The Journal of Allergy and Clinical Immunology in Practice, 10*(1S), S31–S38. https://doi.org/10.1016/j.jaip.2021.10.011

Roncada, C., Andrade, J., Bischoff, L. C., & Pitrez, P. M. (2018). Comparison of two inhalational techniques for bronchodilator administration in children and adolescents with acute asthma crisis: A meta-analysis. *Revista Paulista de Pediatria, 36*, 364–371.

Scotet, V., L'Hostis, C., & Férec, C. (2020). The changing epidemiology of cystic fibrosis: Incidence, survival and impact of the CFTR gene discovery. *Genes, 11*(6), 589. https://doi.org/10.3390/genes11060589

Shteinberg, M., Haq, I. J., Polineni, D., & Davies, J. C. (2021a). Cystic fibrosis. *Lancet, 397*(10290), 2195–2211. https://doi.org/10.1016/S0140-6736(20)32542-3

Shteinberg, M., Taylor-Cousar, J. L., Durieu, I., & Cohen-Cymberknoh, M. (2021b). Fertility and pregnancy in cystic fibrosis. *Chest, 160*(6), 2051–2060. https://doi.org/10.1016/j.chest.2021.07.024

Snider, M. A., Wan, J. Y., Jacobs, J., Kink, R., Gilmore, B., Arnold, S. R. (2018). A randomized trial comparing metered dose inhalers and breath actuated nebulizers. *The Journal of Emergency Medicine, 55*(1), 7–14. https://doi.org/10.1016/j.jemermed.2018.03.002

U.S. Department of Health and Human Services, National Institutes of Health, National Heart, Lung, and Blood Institute. (2014). *Managing asthma: A guide for schools* (NIH Publication No. 14-2650). https://www.nhlbi.nih.gov/sites/default/files/publications/14-2650%20NACI_ManagingAsthma-508%20FINAL.pdf

U.S. Office for Civil Rights. (2020). *Free appropriate public education (FAPE). Protecting students.* https://www2.ed.gov/about/offices/list/ocr/frontpage/pro-students/issues/dis-issue03.html

Volerman, A., Kan, K., Carpenter, D., & Press, V. G. (2021) Strategies for improving inhalation technique in children: A narrative review. *Patient Preference and Adherence, 15*, 665–675. https://doi.org/10.2147/PPA.S267053

Volerman, A., Toups, M., Hull, A., Dennin, M., Kim, T. Y., Ignoffo, S., Sharp, L. K., & Press, V. G. (2019). Assessing children's readiness to carry and use quick-relief inhalers. *The Journal of Allergy and Clinical Immunology: In Practice, 7*(5), 1673–1675.e2. https://doi.org/10.1016/j.jaip.2018.11.040

Weber, D. R. (2025). Diabetes mellitus. In R. M. Kliegman, J. W. St. Geme, N. J. Blum, R. C. Tasker, K. M. Wilson, A. M. Schuh, & C. L. Mack (Eds.), *Nelson textbook of pediatrics* (22nd ed., pp. 3515–3549.e.4). Elsevier.

Chapter 23

Students With Diabetes

Jennifer Saylor ▪ Joya Kabel

CHAPTER OUTLINE

INTRODUCTION

Diabetes is one of the oldest conditions known to humans, having been identified circa 1500 B.C. It was almost always fatal until the discovery of insulin by Banting and Best in 1921. Advancements in care continue to inform and improve the management of diabetes, including the development of human insulin made with recombinant DNA in the 1980s, the 1993 Diabetes Control and Complications Trial (DCCT), the ongoing Epidemiology of Diabetes Interventions and Complications (EDIC) study, new glucose monitoring and insulin delivery systems, and the growing use of telehealth. We now know that intensive treatment and tight control of blood sugar results in dramatic decreases in long-term vascular complications from diabetes, especially with type 1 diabetes (ElSayed et al., 2023a; Nathan, 2021; Vanderniet et al., 2022). Self-management coupled with a supportive home and school community is integral to achieving positive outcomes.

GLUCOSE METABOLISM: THE FUNCTION OF INSULIN

Blood glucose (BG) levels are influenced by three factors: absorption of glucose in the circulatory system from external sources, glucose production from the breakdown of stored glucose in the liver and skeletal muscle (glycogenolysis), and production of glucose by the liver (gluconeogenesis; Kapoor & Mittal, 2023; Ojo et al., 2023). Excess glucose not needed for energy is stored as glycogen in the liver or metabolized to generate fat stores. Insulin is the hormone that functions as a chemical messenger, allowing glucose to enter cells where it can be utilized. It is secreted by beta cells in the islets of Langerhans inside the pancreas in response to elevated BG; it cannot be produced by any other cell in the body. Notably, the liver, kidney, and brain cells take up glucose by diffusion and do not require insulin.

It was once thought that normal glucose metabolism was dependent on insulin alone, given that the secretion of insulin is mainly influenced by BG levels. However, the hormones amylin, glucagon-like peptide-1 (GLP-1), glucose-dependent insulinotropic peptide (GIP), and glucagon also play important roles in glucose metabolism (Kapoor & Mittal, 2023). GIP functions as a synergistic partner to insulin and is cosecreted with insulin from pancreatic beta cells in response to food intake. GLP-1 and GIP are endogenous incretin (metabolic) hormones that are secreted within minutes of nutrient ingestion. Their role is to facilitate the rapid disposal of ingested nutrients, promote satiety and reduction of appetite, and reduce hepatic glucose output, as well as enhance insulin secretion, thus inhibiting the production of glucagon. Glucagon is produced in the alpha cells of the pancreas and is secreted in response to decreases in BG levels, stimulating the release of stored glucose (glycogen) from the liver. As these stores become depleted, glucagon then encourages the liver to synthesize additional glucose by gluconeogenesis. Glucagon secretion is inhibited by insulin (Kapoor & Mittal, 2023; Ojo et al., 2023).

TYPES OF DIABETES

Diabetes is a condition governed by insulin and the body's ability to utilize it. In addition to conditions involving the pancreas, hyperglycemia can also occur due to use of corticosteroids. There are three main types of diabetes: type 1 diabetes (T1D), type 2 diabetes (T2D), and gestational diabetes. In addition, there are numerous subcategories of diabetes (Nandhini et al., 2023), including cystic fibrosis–related diabetes (CFRD) and maturity-onset diabetes of the young (MODY). In the school environment, most students with diabetes will have either T1D or T2D. The approach used in the treatment, care, and instruction of the individual varies by the type of diabetes (Libman et al., 2022).

Type 1 Diabetes

Incidence and Prevalence

T1D predominates among the 283,000 youth diagnosed with diabetes, accounting for over 85% of all cases (Centers for Disease Control and Prevention, 2024). This translates into about 244,000 individuals under the age of 20 with T1D. The incidence of T1D for youth in the United States is increasing. A study of diabetes among youth in five centers across the United States found a 10.2% increase in T1D over an 8-year period (Lawrence et al., 2021). Incidence is highest in non-Hispanic whites.

There are a variety of risk factors associated with the development of T1D. Genetics significantly increases the risk for the development of T1D in first-degree relatives (Miranda Lora et al., 2023). Environmental factors implicated in the development of T1D in youth include infant diet and viruses. Enteroviruses such as congenital rubella and coxsackie B4 have been associated with the development of islet autoimmunity, which may take months or years before symptoms begin. Other possible environmental triggers include foreign antigens in an infant's diet, such as casein, bovine insulin, root vegetables, and cereals. Human breast milk, vitamin D, and vitamin E have been shown to have some protective properties against these antigens. Additionally, there is a seasonal component to the diagnosis with the highest incidence being in the fall and winter.

Pathophysiology

T1D is an autoimmune condition in which the destruction of beta cells of the pancreas results in the cessation of insulin production and the need for exogenous insulin (ElSayed et al., 2023a; Gomez-Diaz, 2023; Ojo et al., 2023). In T1D, autoantibodies are made against one's own antigenic markers on the beta cells (also known as islet cells) in the pancreas, causing their deactivation. This immunological response may happen before the onset of clinical symptoms (ElSayed et al., 2023a; Gomez-Diaz, 2023). The presence of one or more autoantibodies classifies T1D. Those that have been identified and associated with T1D include glutamic acid decarboxylase (GAD), IA-2, IA-2B, and zinc transporter 8 (ZnT8) (ElSayed et al., 2023a; Wojciechowska et al., 2023). Additionally, there is an association of human leukocyte antigens with ties to DQA and DQB genes in T1D that can be protective or predisposing in nature (ElSayed et al., 2023a; Gomez-Diaz, 2023).

Diagnostic Criteria

Specific criteria for the diagnosis of diabetes established by the American Diabetes Association (ADA; ElSayed et al., 2023a) include (1) hemoglobin A1C (average glucose over 2 to 3 months) greater than or equal to 6.5% (using certified and standardized assay); or (2) a fasting plasma glucose level greater than or equal to 126 mg/dL; or (3) a 2-hour plasma glucose level greater than or equal to 200 mg/dL using the 75-g oral glucose tolerance test; or (4) a random plasma glucose level greater than or equal to 200 mg/dL in an individual with classic symptoms of hyperglycemia. According to the SEARCH for Diabetes Study, 38.5% of T1D youth are diagnosed with diabetes as a result of diabetic ketoacidosis (DKA) presentation (Jensen et al., 2021). Unless the patient is clearly in a hyperglycemic crisis or displays classic hyperglycemia symptoms, the abnormal screening test should be repeated using either the same sample or a different sample. In either case, the repeat test for confirmation may occur on the same day; there should be no delay in confirming the diagnosis. A glucometer should not be used to make a diabetes diagnosis (Libman et al., 2022).

Some youth who are newly diagnosed with T1D may experience a *honeymoon phase* within days or weeks of initial diagnosis. The honeymoon phase occurs only once and is very individualized, lasting from a few weeks to 2 years (Cengiz et al., 2022; Libman et al., 2022; Miranda Lora et al., 2023). During this phase, the pancreas begins producing insulin on its own again, allowing approximately 80% of youth to decrease the amount of insulin they are taking. Intensive insulin therapy may sustain beta-cell function initially and this preservation of beta-cell function can decrease the possibility of severe hypoglycemia and vascular complications (Cengiz et al., 2022; Miranda Lora et al., 2023). The honeymoon phase can be misinterpreted by some as either having been misdiagnosed or being cured, resulting in decreased adherence to the food regimen or to BG monitoring. It must be reinforced to families that the student still has a diabetes diagnosis, that symptoms will reappear, and that their vigilance is essential. This vigilance extends to the school nurse.

Early identification of T1D is critical because the autoimmune attack on the insulin-secreting beta cells happens before symptoms become evident (Gomez-Diaz, 2023). Clinical guidelines provide for the presymptomatic staging of those children who have a family history of T1D (Table 23-1). The presence of two or more autoantibodies is a good predictor of T1D. The number of antibodies, antibody specificity, and titer relate to the speed of T1D development (ElSayed et al., 2023a). The school nurse may be aware of students who have positive autoantibodies (e.g., siblings with T1D), but have not yet developed T1D. In these cases, the nurse can support early detection through monitoring for diabetes symptoms.

Presentation

Classic symptoms at onset of T1D include polyuria, polydipsia, nocturia, weight loss, blurry vision, polyphagia, and significant hyperglycemia (ElSayed et al., 2023a; Libman et al., 2022; Nandhini et al., 2023). Fatigue, behavior changes, and decreased attention span may also be indicators of hyperglycemia. Symptom onset typically occurs within a short time frame. Predispositions include being Caucasian, slender, around pubertal age, and having a family history of T1D or other autoimmune conditions. Those diagnosed with T1D are susceptible to developing other autoimmune conditions, including thyroid and celiac conditions, as well as other rare comorbidities such as adrenal insufficiency, autoimmune hepatitis, vitiligo, pernicious anemia, and myasthenia gravis (ElSayed et al., 2023a; Nandhini et al., 2023).

The peak ages at which T1D occurs is 5 to 14, both globally and nationally. According to the search data, the annual T1D incidence increased by 2.02% per year from 2002 to 2018 (Magliano et al., 2021). T1D appears to have a seasonal peak in the month of January, which may be due to an increase in viral infections. As the incidence of T1D has increased, the age of onset has decreased (Pasi & Ravi, 2022). Thus T1D can occur at any age, which is why the term "juvenile diabetes" is no longer accurate.

Type 2 Diabetes

Incidence and Prevalence

Type 2 diabetes, once known as adult-onset diabetes, now accounts for 20% to 50% of all new cases among youth ages 10 to 19 in the United States. Incidence is rising at a higher rate than T1D, increasing by 45% between the years 2009 and 2017 (Lawrence et al., 2021). This incidence is higher among Native Americans, African Americans, Hispanics, and Asian Pacific Islanders (Lawrence et al., 2021; Shah et al., 2022). Similar trends are observed globally (Shah et al., 2022). Projections indicate that the prevalence of T2D in youth will quadruple in the United States by 2050 (Perng et al., 2023).

Pathophysiology

T2D in youth is caused by a combination of genetic, metabolic, and environmental factors. It is the result of insulin resistance and a relative (not absolute) insulin deficiency,

Did You Know?

When BG levels exceed approximately 180 mg/dL, the kidneys stop absorbing excess glucose; the excess spills into the urine (glycosuria). Glucose acts as a diuretic, causing fluid and electrolyte loss, increased urination (polyuria), and increased thirst (polydipsia) (ElSayed et al., 2023a). Glucose-starved cells trigger hunger and increased food intake (polyphagia). Protein and fat break down to satisfy unmet fuel needs. At the same time, the liver tries to help by converting its limited supply of triglycerides to fatty acids to use as energy; these transform into ketone bodies, which are excreted via the kidneys. The large amounts of free hydrogen ions in the ketones build up, leading to diabetic ketoacidosis (DKA), a medical emergency.

TABLE 23-1 Presymptomatic/Symptomatic Staging of Type 1 Diabetes

Stage 1	Stage 2	Stage 3	Stage 4
• Normoglycemia • Presymptomatic • Multiple autoantibodies • No IGT or IFG	• Dysglycemia: IFG and/or IGT • FBG 100–125 mg/dL • Usually presymptomatic • Multiple autoantibodies • 2-hr BG 140–199 mg/dL	• FBG >126 mg/dL • 2-hr BG >200 mg/dL • Symptomatic • Multiple autoantibodies • Meets standard diabetes diagnostic criteria	• Established T1D

BG, Plasma glucose; *FBG*, fasting plasma glucose; *IFG*, impaired fasting glucose; *IGT*, impaired glucose tolerance.
(Besser et al., 2022)

both of which are associated with inflammation and metabolic stress (ElSayed et al., 2023a; Miranda Lora et al., 2023; Nandhini et al., 2023; Shah et al., 2022). In fact, insulin levels in T2D may be normal or elevated but still insufficient, which is indicative of defective glucose-stimulated insulin secretion. In youth, unique properties of T2D include rapid development of beta-cell dysfunction and diabetes complications. T2D is unlikely in youth under 10 years of age; incidence begins to rise at puberty. Since T2D may develop slowly, it commonly is undetected. While the T2D symptoms are less severe, up to 25% may present with DKA at diagnosis (Miranda Lora et al., 2023; Shah et al., 2022).

Diagnostic Criteria

The diagnostic criteria for T2D are the same as it is for T1D with the addition of a negative test for islet autoantibodies (Miranda Lora et al., 2023; Shah et al., 2022). Individuals with diabetes symptoms and elevated laboratory values who do not meet the criteria are diagnosed with prediabetes (ElSayed et al., 2023a). The diagnostic criteria for prediabetes are impaired fasting glucose (100 to 125 mg/dL) or an impaired glucose tolerance test (140 to 199 mg/dL) or A1C between 5.7% and 6.4%. Risk factors for prediabetes include familial history of T2D, obesity, dyslipidemia/high triglycerides, low high-density lipoprotein (HDL) cholesterol, and high blood pressure (ElSayed et al., 2023a; Miranda Lora et al., 2023). These individuals have an increased risk for future development of diabetes and cardiovascular conditions. Students with prediabetes would benefit from education regarding specific nutrition and physical activity interventions that can prevent or delay the onset of T2D or gestational diabetes.

Presentation

Symptoms at onset of T2D are similar to those seen in T1D: polyuria, polydipsia, nocturia, and unexplained weight loss; however, T2D develops slower with less severe symptoms and is commonly undetected. Obesity and family history are primary risk factors for T2D in youth. Seventy-five percent of families with children diagnosed with T2D will have experience with the disease (Miranda Lora et al., 2023; Shah et al., 2022). Youth-specific risk factors include fetal exposure to maternal factors (obesity, diabetes, and increased weight gain during pregnancy) and high infant birth weight. Breastfeeding may be a protective factor (Shah et al., 2022). Other non–youth-specific risk factors include low socioeconomic status, limited education, physical inactivity, and a diet high in fat and refined carbohydrates. Additionally, in girls, the mean age of onset is earlier than in boys. Adolescent females also have a greater risk of developing T2D than adolescent males, which may be related to the earlier onset of pubertal insulin resistance, greater adiposity, and decreased sensitivity to insulin and physical activity. T2D is associated with other metabolic disorders, including dyslipidemia, hypertension, and polycystic ovary syndrome.

Other Types

Gestational

Like T2D, gestational diabetes mellitus is characterized by insulin resistance and relative insulin deficiency that occurs in the second or third trimester of pregnancy among individuals without a previous history of diabetes (ElSayed et al., 2023a; Garcia Argueta et al., 2023; Sweeting et al., 2022). Typically, glucose metabolism is affected as the pregnancy progresses, with the highest effect in the third trimester due to increased insulin resistance. Worldwide, gestational diabetes is estimated to complicate 6% to 7% of pregnancies (Garcia Argueta et al., 2023). Risk increases with factors such as gestational diabetes mellitus in a previous pregnancy, maternal age, maternal overweight or obesity, polycystic ovary disease, and race/ethnicity. Individuals with gestational diabetes are up to 10 times more likely to develop T2D (ElSayed et al., 2023b; Vounzoulaki et al., 2020). Sustained weight loss and a healthy lifestyle can prevent or delay disease onset. Persons with gestational diabetes should be screened for persistent diabetes 4 to 12 weeks postpartum; lifelong screenings should continue every 3 years (ElSayed et al., 2023a; Garcia Argueta et al., 2023).

Infants of mothers with gestational diabetes are at risk for macrosomia (excessive fetal growth) and neonatal hypoglycemia (Garcia Argueta et al., 2023; Sweeting et al., 2022). As children, they are more likely to develop impaired glucose tolerance, metabolic complications, obesity, and diabetes. Positive health outcomes for mother and baby are optimized through an individualized treatment plan that includes glucose monitoring and goal glucose ranges that may differ from those for students with T1D or T2D.

Cystic Fibrosis

Cystic fibrosis–related diabetes (CFRD) is the most frequent comorbidity for those with cystic fibrosis (Ode et al., 2022). The loss of pancreatic cells and insulin insufficiency is the main contributing factor (ElSayed et al., 2023a; Ode et al., 2022). Youth with cystic fibrosis are routinely assessed for CFRD, as the occurrence of diabetes increases with age in this population. Diagnosis is based on persistent elevated glucose levels. Nutrition in CFRD includes a diet high in calories, fat, and salt. Monitoring of blood glucose levels is important and should be encouraged. Glycemic goals are the same as in T1D, and insulin therapy with continuous glucose monitoring (CGM) is the preferred treatment (Ode et al., 2022).

Maturity-Onset Diabetes

Maturity-onset diabetes of the young (MODY) is a monogenetic condition in which gene mutations disrupt the availability of insulin by decreasing either beta-cell function or insulin release. Although there are approximately 40 different types of monogenetic diabetes, it represents only 1% to 6% of all cases of diabetes in the pediatric population (Greeley et al., 2022; Libman et al., 2022). The determination of a MODY diagnosis is related to family history,

Practice Connection

School nurses incorporate screening for acanthosis nigricans, a thickening and hyperpigmentation of the skin at the neck and flexural areas, which typically signifies insulin resistance (Miranda Lora et al., 2023; Shah et al., 2022). Skin affected by acanthosis nigricans may have a velvety appearance or look like dirty, dark patches around the neck and axilla (ADA, 2022a). Screening tools, coupled with waist circumference measurement, are useful for identifying and staging this condition (Scott & Hall, 2012) providing important information that can assist families in seeking follow-up healthcare services.

genetic testing, lack of islet autoantibodies, impaired insulin secretion, age of onset less than 25 years old, C-peptide levels, and absence of T2D. Youth with MODY may have only mild fasting hyperglycemia and generally have fewer diabetes-related complications. They may require daily insulin and/or oral hypoglycemic medication for control.

DIABETES CARE MANAGEMENT

Youth with all types of diabetes struggle as they transition through the developmental stages and their diabetes-related self-care increases. The goals for children and youth with diabetes are no different than those for their unaffected peers: to promote normal growth and development, good quality of life, optimal learning, safety from short-term complications, prevention of long-term complications, and planned reproduction (de Wit et al., 2022; Lawrence et al., 2022).

Diabetes management requires an individualized approach to maintain normal blood glucose levels (Fig. 23-1). Variables that affect the medical treatment plan include the type of diabetes, student's age, developmental level, diabetes-related technology, family support, and support from the student's pediatric diabetes care team (ADA, 2022a; ElSayed et al., 2023c; Lawrence et al., 2022). Challenges in managing diabetes in school-age youth include the need for lifestyle modification, medical treatment, the possibility of socioeconomic and psychosocial issues, and the potential for limited availability of disease management resources (ADA, 2022a; de Wit et al., 2022). Adolescent perceptions regarding health and their lack of concern for long-term complications may increase risk. Peer pressure is a major factor that can inhibit adolescents from following through on the prescribed plan of care.

Reducing glycemic variability is critical for optimal diabetes management and includes a multipronged approach that includes nutrition, physical activity, pharmacotherapy, and technology. A comprehensive diabetes management plan may include the following:

- Planned/spaced meals and snacks
- Carbohydrate counting

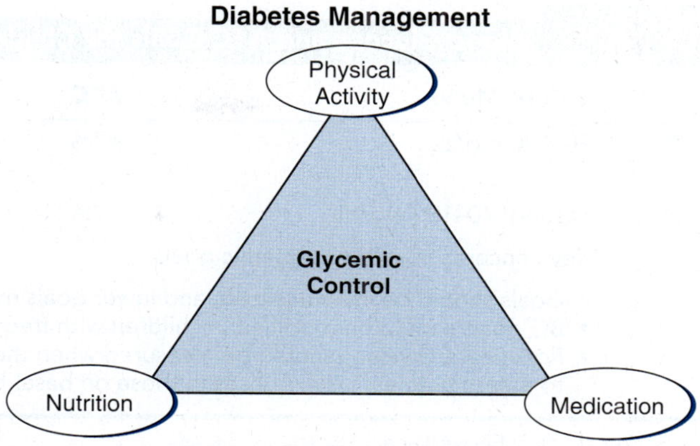

FIGURE 23-1. Diabetes management.

- Regular physical activity
- Glucose-lowering medications
- Use of an insulin pump or syringe pen
- Premeal/snack glucose monitoring (de Bock et al., 2022; ElSayed et al., 2023d)

Glycated hemoglobin (HbA_{1c} or A1C) testing remains the gold standard in measuring overall glycemic control (Besser et al., 2022). A1C levels reflect average BG levels over a 3-month period, providing a glimpse into the immediate past history of BG control (Table 23-2). The A1C goal for children with T1D is less than 7.0% (ElSayed et al., 2023c); however, healthcare providers may increase the A1C goal to less than 7.5% for younger children or youth who experience moderate to severe hypoglycemia. For children with T2D, the target is 7% and, in most cases, it can be less than 6.5% (de Bock et al., 2022; Table 23-3). Elevated A1C levels are linked to increased diabetes-related complications. Data from the Type 1 Diabetes Exchange clinic registry indicate that the A1C levels of the majority of youth with diabetes are above the recommended range of less than 7.5%, and that A1C actually increased in the last data collection period from 2016

TABLE 23-2 A1C to Average Blood Glucose Level Conversion

A1C Value (%)	Average BG (mg/dL)
6	126
6.5	140
7	154
7.5	169
8	183
8.5	197
9	212
9.5	226
10	240

(ADA, 2023)

TABLE 23-3 Blood Glucose and A1C Goals for Children and Adolescents With T1D and T2D

	Before Meals	A1C	Notes
T1D	90–130 mg/dL	<7%	A higher goal of <7.5% is reasonable for young children or youth experiencing moderate-to-severe hypoglycemia.
T2D	Fasting: 70–130 mg/dL	<7%	In most cases, a lower goal of <6.5 is appropriate.

Key concepts in setting glycemic goals:

- Goals should be individualized, and lower goals may be reasonable based on a benefit-risk assessment.
- BG goals should be modified in children with frequent hypoglycemia or hypoglycemia unawareness.
- Postmeal BG values should be measured when there is a discrepancy between premeal BG values and A1C levels and to assess premeal insulin doses in those on basal-bolus or pump regimens.

(de Bocket al, 2022; ElSayed et al., 2023c)

to 2018 (Demeterco-Berggren et al., 2023). This reflects a need for improving interventions to advance glycemic outcomes. Postprandial monitoring may provide additional helpful information when evaluating the effectiveness of different insulin regimens or in gestational or T2D. If postprandial testing is needed, peak BG should be obtained 2 to 3 hours after food intake. The goal for a postprandial BG level is less than 180 mg/dL (ElSayed et al., 2023d). Recent interventions such as the improved rapid- and long-acting insulins, advances in technology (e.g., CGM and better pump algorithms), and a focus on self-monitoring of BG have made achieving A1C targets, as well as decreasing episodes of hypoglycemia, a realistic goal (Abraham et al., 2022; ElSayed et al., 2023a).

Focus on the Framework
Care Coordination

The school nurse supports the student by providing direct care, as well as leading the school health services team through supervision, education, and stakeholder collaboration (National Association of School Nurses [NASN], 2020a, 2024a). Diabetes self-management is encouraged through school nurse supervision of BG monitoring, insulin injections, activity, and diet. These interventions improve BG control significantly and mitigate diabetes-related complications. The school nurse develops the student's individualized healthcare plan (IHP) and emergency action plan (EAP) based on the diabetes medical management plan (DMMP) supplied by the student's home diabetes care team (ADA, 2022a; NASN, 2020b). A sample DMMP is shown in Online Materials OM23-1. The IHP and the EAP direct diabetes management at school. Participation in school team meetings to develop and implement a 504 plan or an individualized education program (IEP); educating staff on the signs, symptoms, and appropriate response to hypoglycemia/hyperglycemia; providing feedback to the home diabetes care team; and generating/supporting research in pediatric diabetes care are also key elements of the care coordination role of the school nurse role (NASN, 2020a).

Pharmacological Management

Pharmacotherapy for treating diabetes in youth is determined by diabetes type, symptoms, BG levels, and the presence of DKA (ElSayed et al., 2023c).

Non-Insulin Agents

ORAL. Most oral diabetes medications work to increase insulin sensitivity at the cellular level or to influence receptor proteins in the pancreas. They are used in combination with physical activity and healthy nutrition to improve glycemic control. In youth, oral agents are only typically used in the treatment of T2D (ElSayed et al., 2023e; Shah et al., 2022), although the school nurse should be aware that a student with newly diagnosed T2D may also require insulin for a period of time. Metformin (Glucophage) is frequently the first medication to be prescribed for a new T2D diagnosis when the A1C is less than 8.5% (Berman et al., 2023; Shah et al., 2022). It belongs to the biguanide class of drugs, which decreases glucose production in the liver while increasing insulin sensitivity in liver and muscle cells. Metformin does not have a direct effect on insulin-producing cells and therefore does not cause hypoglycemia. It is approved for use in ages 10 and up. The usual starting dosage is 250 to 500 mg twice a day with meals; the dosage may increase by 500 mg every 1 to 2 weeks, up to a maximum of 2,000 mg daily (Shah et al., 2022). The DMMP for students receiving metformin may or may not include routine BG checks at school.

Empagliflozin (Jardiance®) was approved in 2023 for treatment of T2D in youth more than 10 years old. It works by increasing urinary glucose excretion via inhibition of sodium glucose cotransporter 2 (SLGT-2), leading to improved glycemic control and metabolism, reduced glucotoxicity, and reduced insulin resistance. Synjardy® is a proprietary combination of empagliflozin *and* metformin and is also approved for use in youth older than 10 years of age. Compared with metformin alone, both medications carry a higher risk of hypoglycemia, regardless of concurrent T2D therapies. Rosiglitazone and pioglitazone (Avandia® and Actos®, respectively) belong to the thiazolidinediones class. These drugs reduce insulin resistance and increase insulin sensitivity (Xu et al., 2022). While not approved by the U.S. Food and Drug Administration (USFDA) for use in youth, they have been prescribed off-label with some success to treat T2D in young people, especially when used in combination with metformin (Shah et al., 2022; Xu et al., 2022). Due to linkage with cardiovascular adverse events in adults, both drugs carry boxed warnings.

INJECTABLE. Two injectable medications are approved for use in youth over 10 years old: liraglutide (Victoza®) and its extended-release formulation, exenatide (Bydureon®). These fall under the GLP-1 receptor agonist class, and they improve BG levels by stimulating pancreatic receptors that control insulin release while simultaneously reducing glucagon release (Berman et al., 2023; Nauck et al., 2021). Both medications carry a low risk for hypoglycemia.

Did You Know?

Metformin may cause abdominal discomfort. This can be minimized by educating the student about foods that create gas so that they can be avoided.

Presently, pharmacological management of T2D in youth is rapidly changing. Advances in pediatric diabetes research will likely yield new pharmacological classes of medications in the coming years. New combinations of oral agents are also emerging. Thus it is imperative that the school nurse continually update their pharmacology knowledge to ensure their practice keeps pace with advancements.

Insulin Agents

TYPES OF INSULIN. Table 23-4 provides an overview of several different types of insulin classified according to the onset, peak, and duration of action (ADA, 2024). When developing the IHP, the school nurse must be aware of the type of insulin the student uses for their diabetes. Rapid-acting, or short-acting, insulin is known simply as regular, or R insulin; intermediate-acting insulin is also known as NPH; and peakless long-acting or basal insulin analogs include glargine and detemir (Cengiz et al., 2022). Regardless of the insulin type, storage guidelines must be followed to ensure potency and efficacy (Box 23-1).

TABLE 23-4 Insulin Preparations for Subcutaneous Injection

Type of Insulin	Time to First Effects	Peak Time	Duration	Generic Name (Brand Name Examples)
Rapid-Acting Insulin	*Range:*	*Range:*	*Range:*	Insulin aspart (Fiasp, NovoLog)
	5–30 min	30 min–3 hr	3–5 hr	Insulin gulisine (Apidra)
	Usually in 10–15 min	Usually in 30–90 min	Usually in 4 hr	Insulin lispro (Admelog, Humalog)
Regular or Short-Acting Insulin	30–60 min	2–4 hr	6–9 hr	Regular insulin (Humulin R, Novolin R, Velosulin R)
Intermediate-Acting Insulin	2–4 hr	4–12 hr	12–18 hr	NPH insulin (Humulin N, Novolin N, ReliOn)
Long-Acting Insulin	Several hours after injection		18–34 hr	Insulin degludec (Tesiba)
				Insulin detemir (Levemir)
				Insulin glargine (Basaglar Lantus)
Ultra Long-Acting Insulin	6 hr	Does not peak	36 hr	Insulin glargine u-300 (Toujeo)

(ADA, 2024)

BOX 23-1
Insulin Storage

- Keep sealed vials, disposable pens, and cartridges refrigerated.
- Most opened insulin can be kept at room temperature (below 86°F); consult manufacturer's guidelines regarding the recommended window for use after opening and for expiration questions.
- Write the date insulin was opened on the label and note in the log.
- Visually inspect insulin for sediment each time a dose is to be given.
- Discard if sediment is present, regardless of expiration date.

(ADA, 2022a)

INSULIN DOSING. There are generally two types of insulin dosing regimens: basal-bolus dosing and fixed dosing (Cengiz et al., 2022; ElSayed et al., 2023e). The selection is based on many individual factors, including age, length of diagnosis, lifestyle, and health literacy. The meal planning approach used (consistent carbohydrate or carbohydrate counting) is determined by the selected type of insulin dosing regimen. Among individuals newly diagnosed with T1D, initial insulin dosing is based on weight and then titrated based on BG levels (ElSayed et al., 2023e). A basal-bolus regimen consists of a long-acting insulin given 1 to 2 times per day to control high resting BG levels combined with doses of rapid-acting insulin given at meals and/or for correcting high blood sugars occurring outside of meals (Fig. 23-2). The number of grams of carbohydrate consumed at a given meal determines the bolus dose. Basal-bolus dosing is most often prescribed for students with T1D because it is flexible and mimics the insulin action of the pancreas. In fixed-dosing insulin therapy, the student takes fixed doses of either rapid-, short-, intermediate-, or long-acting insulin. The consistent carbohydrate meal planning approach is used with fixed-dosing therapy, as it provides predictability in BG rise (ADA, 2022a; Cengiz et al., 2022).

Each student with diabetes will have a target BG level that is individually determined by the pediatric diabetes care team and should be included in the student's IHP. Parameters for adjusting insulin doses at school need to be clearly outlined in the student's IHP in accordance with the diabetes medical management plan. Insulin orders in the DMMP need to include the following information:

- Insulin brand and type
- Administration times
- Insulin administration device: syringe pen, pump, or pod
- Insulin dose, either:
  - Standard dose based on a preset amount of insulin (e.g., Humalog insulin, 3 units each day before lunch)
  - Variable based on insulin/carbohydrate (I:C) ratio (e.g., 1 unit Novolog insulin for every 15 g carbohydrate consumed or 1 unit Humalog for each carbohydrate choice at lunch (e.g., 4 carbohydrate choices = 4 units Humalog)
  - Sliding scale insulin dose based on BG results—example:
    - Before lunch and every 3 hours if needed for hyperglycemia
    - BG 100 to 150 mg/dL, give 0 units Humalog insulin
    - BG 151 to 200 mg/dL, give 1 unit Humalog insulin
    - BG 201 to 250 mg/dL, give 2 units Humalog insulin

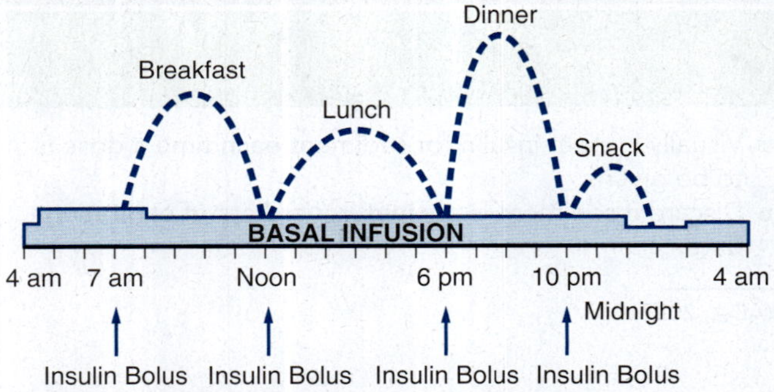

FIGURE 23-2. Basal infusion plus bolus.

A correction dose of insulin (also called insulin sensitivity factor) may be given with a meal dose and during episodes of hyperglycemia not associated with a meal as ordered by the healthcare provider in the DMMP. The target BG and specific BG correction calculation instructions are found in the student's individual DMMP. Care should be taken to avoid "stacking" insulin by considering any insulin on board that is still working in the body at the time of correction (ADA, 2022a).

- Correction dose example: In addition to meal dose, give 1 unit Humalog for every 50 points of BG greater than 150 mg/dL. If the student's lunchtime BG is 250, the calculation would be as follows:
  - BG (250) minus target BG (150) = correction factor (100)
  - Correction factor (100) divided by 50 = 2; therefore correction dose = 2 units
  - NOTE: The correction dose is added to any standing mealtime dose.

The correction dose for hypoglycemia or increased activity may be in the DMMP or agreed upon by the school nurse and parent as needed. The healthcare provider may provide further guidance for values that are fractions of units based on whether the student is going to the gym or taking an examination or is more prone to having episodes of hypoglycemia (ADA, 2022a; Frohnert & Chase, 2022). Insulin's absorption rate can be influenced by age, adiposity, insulin dose, exercise, insulin concentration, overuse of an injection site, and body temperature. For example, if a student injects insulin in their leg and exercises soon after, their insulin absorption may be enhanced (Cengiz et al., 2022; ElSayed et al., 2023e).

INSULIN ADMINISTRATION. The task of administering multiple insulin injections can be overwhelming for many students and families. Pens, pumps, and pods help by increasing dose accuracy, convenience, and adherence to the prescribed regimen (ElSayed et al., 2023e). Insulin pumps will be discussed in the Technological Management section of this chapter. Disposable insulin syringe pens come prefilled with insulin, whereas reusable pens require an insulin cartridge. The prescribed dose is simply dialed-in, and a small needle is screwed on the end of the device, which is removed and discarded after each use. Insulin syringe pens, whether disposable or reusable, are for individual student use only; they cannot be shared between students. See Online Materials for the injection procedure using a syringe (OM23-2) and an insulin pen (OM23-3).

State law may allow school nurses to delegate insulin administration in the school setting; the use of an insulin syringe pen may improve ease of training nonnursing staff. When correction doses are to be administered by someone other than a registered nurse (in states that allow delegation per the state's nurse practice act), the school nurse should review the student's status and approve the correction dose before administration. The correction dose should be indicated on the IHP (ADA, 2022a).

Technological Management

Intermittent Blood Glucose Monitoring

Meters that check BG are compact, give rapid results, and require just a small sample of blood from a fingerstick. Many BG meters (and all continuous glucose meters, discussed later in this chapter) interface with computers, cellphones, smart watches, tablets, and/or insulin infusion systems. Monitoring BG levels provides feedback on how nutritional intake, physical activity, and medications are affecting the student's diabetes (de Bock et al., 2022; ElSayed et al., 2023d). The memory within these devices can be downloaded for analysis of trends in BG levels. Retractable lancets and wicking test strips have greatly minimized the risk for blood exposures. However, the school nurse should establish a lancet disposal plan with the student that complies with standard precautions and local community sharps disposal laws. Many students, especially young children or newly diagnosed youth, will require assistance with BG monitoring (BGM) or with interpreting the results (ADA, 2022a).

The accuracy of BG readings can be affected by soiled hands, poor test strip storage practices, or a meter/test strip mismatch. Before using a BG meter ensure that

- The test site is dry and without food residue, dirt, or chemicals
- The test strips have been stored properly and are not expired
- The BG meter is programmed with the correct test strip code (usually 1 or 2 digits)

The DMMP will indicate how often the student should perform glucose monitoring. BG should be checked as often as is necessary to optimize the student's BG control (Tauschmann et al., 2022). BG level is typically checked before meals, before snacks, and at bedtime. The DMMP will indicate how often the student should perform glucose monitoring and the IHP should include when and where BG levels will be obtained, who will interpret them, and with whom this information will be shared. Additional monitoring may be needed before or after physical activity, before academic testing, at the end of the day (before boarding the bus, walking, biking, or driving home), when feeling sick, or when experiencing symptoms of hyperglycemia or hypoglycemia (ElSayed et al., 2023d; Tauschmann et al., 2022). Studies have shown that greater frequency of glucose monitoring can have a favorable impact on A1C levels and decrease acute complications (ElSayed et al., 2023f; Tauschmann et al., 2022). Recording and regular communication of BG results to parents/guardians and/or the healthcare provider is an important aspect of the school nurse's role in facilitating effective diabetes management (ADA, 2022a).

> **Practice Connection**
>
> Proper needle disposal is a nursing concern. A sharps container should be available for those students seen in the nursing office. Students who self-manage their insulin should be helped to develop a plan for safe and appropriate administration and needle disposal outside the nurse's office.

Self-Monitoring of Blood Glucose

Self-monitoring of BG is a necessary skill that all individuals with diabetes must possess. School nurses support students in mastering this self-care skill, increasing the student's level of self-care as their knowledge and developmental level allow (ADA, 2022a; ElSayed et al., 2023d). Students who have demonstrated correct BG monitoring technique and know how to respond to the results should be allowed to monitor and treat their BG whenever and wherever needed, including in the classroom (ADA, 2022a; Frohnert & Chase, 2022; Lawrence et al., 2022). When hypoglycemia is suspected, the student's BG should be checked immediately on-site (Abraham et al., 2022); *symptomatic students who need to go to the health office should always be escorted.* Alternatively, the school nurse can be called to the classroom. The location for the student's routine BG monitoring should be a collaborative decision among the school nurse, parent/guardian, student, healthcare provider, and school administrator. Student safety (i.e., preventing treatment delays), assistance needs, student preference, respect for privacy, and decreased time out of the classroom should be considered (ADA, 2022a). The school nurse should become familiar with their BG monitoring equipment used by the students under their care, even for those who self-monitor in case of emergency. If a student becomes incapacitated (i.e., severely hypoglycemic), the nurse will need to be able to measure BG in order to intervene appropriately. Information on how to use the glucose monitoring device can come from the family, through the manufacturer's toll-free number or Web site, or from the pediatric diabetes care team.

Continuous Glucose Monitoring

Continuous glucose monitors (CGMs) provide data regarding an individual's current glucose level and trends in the BG levels around the clock. Their use is associated with improved glycemic control (Laffel et al., 2020). CGMs are increasing in popularity; only 7% of persons with diabetes used a CGM in 2010 to 2012 compared with 47% in 2016 to 2018 (Sawyer et al., 2022). A number of CGM systems

Did You Know?

In addition to traditional fingersticks, many BG monitors and lancing devices can be used for alternate site monitoring (i.e., forearm). Results from alternate sites differ from fingerstick results when glucose levels are changing rapidly, such as after a meal, after taking insulin, during exercise, or when ill or under stress. Readings obtained from alternate sites lag 15 minutes behind fingerstick results. Always obtain a fingerstick sample if hypoglycemia is suspected.

have been authorized by the U.S. Food and Drug Administration for use in youth with diabetes, and most of them are approved for use in nonadjunctive insulin dosing (ElSayed et al., 2023h; Tauschmann et al., 2022). CGM glucose values are used for insulin dosing decisions without needing fingerstick BG verification. It is critical, however, that students using a CGM have access to a BG meter at all times so that they may perform a fingerstick BG measurement whenever necessary for instance if symptoms do not correlate with CGM reading, a CGM error message, or with rapidly changing BG levels (ElSayed et al., 2023f).

The CGM system consists of a sensor worn on the skin and a receiver (a smartphone or separate device). The sensor uses a small plastic filament into the subcutaneous tissue to sample glucose from interstitial fluid every 1 to 5 minutes. Glucose values are sent to the receiver wirelessly. Sensors are changed every 7 to 14 days, depending on the brand, and may require calibration with a BG meter. The receiver can be set to alarm for high and low glucose readings (ADA, 2022b; ElSayed et al., 2023f; Tauschmann et al., 2022). Sharing digital CGM data with the school nurse and/or parents requires access to a cellular data plan or the school's wireless network (ADA, 2022a). Expectations about how CGM readings will be used should be incorporated into the student's IHP and Section 504 plan.

The benefits of CGMs include the ability to predict impending hypoglycemia, availability of trend data for dose adjustments, identification of undetected hypoglycemia or hyperglycemia, increased BG time spent in-range, decreased fingersticks, and remote monitoring capabilities, including while away from parent at school or other events and when asleep (Abraham et al., 2022; Frohnert & Chase, 2022; Lin et al., 2023). Barriers to CGM use are related to the cost and insurance coverage of the CGM system and the aversion to wearing a device. Teens may have mixed feelings about using CGM. They may not appreciate being continuously reminded about their diabetes or their parents having remote monitoring capability. They may, however, appreciate fewer fingersticks and the ability to easily check BG levels during physical activity (Divan et al., 2022).

The school nurse may be asked to observe the sensor insertion site or assist the student with record-keeping (ADA, 2022a). As with any medical device, the nurse should be familiar with the specific alarms and nonadjunctive dosing requirements. CGMs should be set to alarm only when an action is required in order to avoid both frequent disruptions in the learning setting and calling attention to the student with the CGM. The DMMP should indicate specific actions to take for alarms that may alert the student to impending hypoglycemia or hyperglycemia. Alarms may be set for treating a low blood sugar (i.e., less than 80 mg or below target range), for treating a high BG (as determined by the care team), or for special circumstances (e.g., severe hypoglycemic unawareness). The school nurse should educate parents about CGM safety measures and collaborate with them to ensure they are followed (Box 23-2). Trending arrows are a feature of CGMs that provide projections regarding the rising and falling movement of BG levels (ADA, 2022a; Tauschmann et al., 2022), enabling more exact treatment. Safe use of the trend arrows for treatment is a concern. The school nurse who is considering using trend arrows for the treatment of hypoglycemia/hyperglycemia must have the knowledge base to carry out the task, understand the limitations of trend arrows/CGM data, and use a recommended method for the pediatric and young adult population. For the school nurse considering delegation (in states that allow delegation per their nurse practice act), the complexity of the task and the knowledge required to implement it properly must be considered in determining whether this task can be delegated. The use of trend arrows in the school setting is not best practice as this may increase the student's stress level (ADA, 2022b).

Ketone Monitoring

Ketone monitoring is a critical tool for caring for a child with hyperglycemia, illness, or both and is performed per the DMMP, typically when BG levels are greater than 250 or 300 mg/dL, or when the student is experiencing nausea, vomiting, abdominal pain, drowsiness, or rapid breathing

BOX 23-2
Safety Measures for Continuous Glucose Monitor

- Calibrate (if required) per manufacturer's instructions.
- Avoid use of acetaminophen, salicylic acid, and vitamin C (may cause incorrect high readings).
- Assess when sensor was inserted (some systems may be less accurate the first day).
- Confirm BG with fingerstick when readings are erratic or if symptoms do not match CGM reading.
- Ensure display shows both the glucose level and the directional arrow.
- Consider the rate of change and lag time if glucose levels are changing quickly.
- Assess insulin on board to avoid overdosing.
- Collaborate with parents to ensure that safety measures are being followed.

(ADA, 2022a)

(ADA, 2022a; Lawrence et al., 2022). Causes of elevated ketone levels include the following:

- Illness
- Inadequate or no insulin
- Cloudy or expired insulin
- Continuous insulin infusion site failure
- Traumatic stress (e.g., surgery, injury)
- Food regimen (e.g., low-carbohydrate diet)
- Prolonged exercise
- Pregnancy
- Alcohol intoxication

The IHP should include when to check for ketones, who will perform the testing, and what actions are to be taken when moderate to large amounts of ketones are detected (ADA, 2022a). Ketone levels can be checked using urine or blood, depending on the supplies and equipment available (Lawrence et al., 2022). Urine ketone monitoring is performed using a test strip that is dipped into a urine specimen (ADA, 2022a). The resulting color change of the strip is then compared with the chart on the package to determine the amount of ketones present. Brands of test strips may vary with regard to when the color should be read (timing), or to colors themselves and their corresponding ketone levels. The test strip container should be dated when opened and discarded in 6 months. Individually wrapped strips are preferred. Some BG meters have the ability to also monitor blood ketones using specialized strips. If moderate to large amounts of ketones are present, the parent/guardian should be notified and the plan for the management of ketones and/or illness should be initiated per the DMMP (Lawrence et al., 2022). Additional insulin is often required, and fluid replacement (water or noncaloric fluids) is important. The student should not participate in exercise, such as gym class or recess, if ketone levels are moderate to large or greater because this may increase the BG level and worsen the ketosis.

Administration Technology

Smart Insulin Pens. Diabetes management and insulin administration is driven by data, including BG, carbohydrates being consumed, time of day, activity, insulin on board, and so on (Ilkowitz et al., 2022). These data are tracked and used to assist in small incremental amounts of safe dosing of insulin using insulin pump therapy. However, smart insulin pens are another option for students who find insulin pumps challenging, prefer not to have a device attached to them, struggle when their insulin pump malfunctions, or want a "break" from their insulin pump. Though the literature is limited in the pediatric population, healthcare providers may prescribe a smart insulin pen that calculates an insulin dose based on BG, carbohydrates consuming, and insulin on board (active insulin). Although insurance and out-of-pocket costs remain a barrier, smart insulin pens have many benefits, including no charging needed for 1 year, dosing reminders, monitors insulin temperature, integration with some CGM and Bluetooth glucose meters, automatically logs doses, and shareable reports with time-based meal analysis. Currently the smart pen calculator rounds down to the half-unit, only automatically tracks rapid-acting insulin doses so long-acting insulin must be entered, no real-time remote monitoring, and reports must be retrieved from the app. As with any diabetes technology, frequent reminders and ongoing education about performing manual calculations in the event of app and/or managing device failure are critical.

Insulin Pumps. Insulin pump therapy, also called continuous subcutaneous insulin infusion, is an automated insulin delivery system that delivers programmed doses of rapid-acting insulin steadily around the clock, supplemented with additional insulin doses for food intake and correcting hyperglycemia (ElSayed et al., 2023f; Sherr et al., 2022). The healthcare provider determines pump settings and dosing parameters; any adjustments are the responsibility of the parent and provider (ADA, 2022a; Lawrence et al., 2022).

Advantages of insulin pump therapy include the following:

- Reduced glucose variability
- Precise insulin dose to 1/100th of a unit, which is critical for small children
- Diminished insulin absorption differences (compared with the use of various sites)
- Improved insulin absorption (due to continuous delivery)
- Easier management of the *dawn phenomenon* (early morning increase in BG levels) and *dusk phenomenon* (late afternoon increase in blood sugar levels)
- Lower incidence of nocturnal hypoglycemia
- Easier illness adjustments
- Enhanced lifestyle flexibility, including more customized meal/snack schedules

Limitations of insulin pump therapy include the following:

- Successful adaptation may take weeks to months.
- Technical failure can happen.
- Forgetting or neglecting to bolus for meals/snacks
- Increased risk for ketosis (when only fast-acting insulin is used)
- Rapid ketone development if insulin delivery is interrupted
- Potential for added expense for the pump and supplies
- Potential for weight gain due to increased food consumption and insulin use
- Potential for skin infection or irritation (ElSayed et al., 2023f; Frohnert & Chase, 2022; Sherr et al., 2022)

Continuous subcutaneous insulin therapy is administered via a system consisting of an insulin pump or an insulin pod. Pumps deliver insulin using a small mechanical pump and thin tubing (called an *infusion set*) that connects to a subcutaneous cannula in the student's abdomen, upper buttocks, posterior upper arm, or upper thigh. The cannula is routinely changed every 2 to 3 days, or when BG levels are persistently above target or when ketones are present (Sherr et al., 2022). A disconnect mechanism allows students to remove the pump from the cannula while leaving the catheter in place so they can swim, bathe, or engage in sports (ADA, 2022a). An insulin pod is similar to a pump, but much smaller and without tubing. It attaches directly to the skin's surface and uses a very tiny cannula that automatically inserts itself into the skin. Insulin pods are refillable and can be programmed for continuous insulin delivery using a handheld controller or via a smartphone app (ADA, 2022a; Frohnert & Chase, 2022). Like the pump infusion cannula, the pod site must be changed every 2 to 3 days. The advantage of the insulin pod system is that it is tubeless and affords more movement for the wearer. Both infusion systems can deliver both bolus and basal rate doses. Pumps offer additional bolus options that can be set to accommodate special situations. One example, called *extended bolus*, is used for eating over a period of time (e.g., popcorn at a movie). Another bolus, called a *dual wave bolus*, allows the individual to give a fraction of the insulin dose immediately and then deliver the other fraction over a set time that may be advantageous during a high-carbohydrate/high-fat meal such as pizza (Frohnert & Chase, 2022). Additionally, temporary basal patterns can be preset for short-term events (e.g., football practice).

Insulin pump technology is rapidly improving with sensor-augmented pump therapy and hybrid closed-loop pump systems (Sherr et al., 2022). Sensor-augmented pumps allow the BG data to be displayed and used by the pump. The CGM takes BG measurements every 5 minutes and relays this to the pump computer. Studies have shown that using sensor-augmented pumps has improved A1C levels, increased treatment satisfaction, and reduced glucose variability if worn more than 60% of the time. Hybrid closed-loop pump systems are approved for children as young as 2 years of age (USFDA, 2020). These devices automatically calculate basal insulin dosing using a control algorithm and CGM values, with the target goal of 120 mg/dL. A temporary target of 150 mg/dL can be set as needed (e.g., for exercise). The pump will automatically adjust or suspend basal insulin based on the CGM data. The user must put in the number of carbohydrates and manually bolus for mealtime insulin dosing. Trial studies have shown the safety and efficacy in improving glycemic control with the hybrid closed-loop system (Bergenstal et al., 2021; Kariyawasam et al., 2022; Sherr et al., 2022).

Smart phone apps that connect students and their families to the pump and CGM data are available for many insulin infusion systems. These apps provide remote monitoring capabilities and provide real-time trending of BG data. This information can be useful to the school nurse and access should be discussed with the parent and student (ADA, 2022a).

More complex insulin pumps that use CGM data and advanced pump algorithms to prevent hypoglycemia are becoming available (ElSayed et al., 2023f; Sherr et al., 2022). These pumps use the CGM data to either suspend the pump at the preset hypoglycemic BG level (minimum of 60 mg/dL) or suspend before a predictive hypoglycemia event occurs using prediction algorithms. Studies have shown that the pumps with hypoglycemia reduction capabilities do reduce hypoglycemia in the pediatric population with no increase in incidence of DKA.

> **Practice Connection**
>
> Consideration must be given to the number of students under the school nurse's care who are using remote glucose monitoring (ADA, 2022a). The type and amount of remote glucose monitoring the school nurse is expected to provide need to be clearly outlined in the IHP, IEP, or 504 plan, and all parties (including school administration) need to be in agreement. The Rehabilitation Act of 1973 ensures every student's right to attend school. This may mean that school nurse building assignments may need to be altered to provide the proper coverage as outlined in a 504 plan or IEP. If a school nurse monitors the student's blood sugar from another school, the parents should be made aware of this, and the plan for who will intervene to support the student with their BGM, insulin dosing, and treatment of hypoglycemia and hyperglycemia or other issues such as dislodged pumps or sensors should be outlined. The school cannot require the parent to be present during the school day to address their child's needs. If competing responsibilities limit the nurse's ability to monitor all students' device data continuously, then additional nurses or, if allowed by state law, unlicensed assistive personnel may need to be hired.

Nutrition Management

Food Regimen

A registered dietitian should take the lead in nutritional care, collaborating with the family and school nurse who supports its implementation (Annan et al., 2022). The school nurse may be involved in helping students make menu choices, count carbohydrates, and plan for special events while at school. Nutrition therapy to improve glycemic control is focused on being flexible and accommodating appetite, eating behaviors, and schedules while meeting the child's nutritional requirements (ADA, 2022a; Annan et al., 2022). Consideration of environmental, physiological, cultural, and social factors improves nutritional outcomes.

Families of children and youth with all types of diabetes should engage in individualized meal planning focused on healthy eating, achieving and maintaining a healthy weight, and physical activity (Annan et al., 2022; ElSayed et al., 2023g). For children with diabetes, nutrition focuses on nutritionally balanced amounts of carbohydrate, protein, and fat with specific emphasis on a consistent eating pattern of food intake for those with T1D. The student's DMMP should include the timing, amount, and type of foods to be eaten (ADA, 2022a). This individualized nutritional planning is an especially important component of the DMMP for student athletes engaged in intense physical activity, serving to prevent hypoglycemic and hyperglycemic episodes during and after the activity (Adolfsson et al., 2022; Annan et al., 2022). Table 23-5 provides carbohydrate intake suggestions and actions to be taken before engaging in physical activity. Multiple barriers to assisting the student in following their individualized meal plan exist. They include rotating class schedules (resulting in lunch breaks as early as 10:30 a.m.), parents packing inappropriate foods, student trading foods with friends, access to high-carbohydrate foods for purchase, and variations in school physical education programs. The nurse may need to assist administrators and teachers to adjust lunch or physical education (PE) schedules or allow extra time between classes for BG monitoring. Every effort should be made to keep students with diabetes from feeling singled out (e.g., placing them on a different schedule than their same peers), as this can negatively affect the student's willingness to participate in diabetes care management (ADA, 2022a; Lawrence et al., 2022).

Celiac disease is a comorbidity in up to 16% of children with T1D (Frohlich-Reiterer et al., 2022; Taczanowska et al., 2021), resulting in the inability to absorb gluten (wheat, rye, oats, and barley), thus increasing the nutritional planning complexity (Annan et al., 2022). Celiac disease causes variable absorption of carbohydrates that leads to BG fluctuations and an increased risk for hypoglycemia. Symptoms may include chronic diarrhea, failure to thrive, abdominal pain, stomach pain, and hypoglycemia (Frohlich-Reiterer et al., 2022). However, some youth may be asymptomatic or exhibit only mild symptoms (Imran et al., 2021; Taczanowska et al., 2021). A celiac disease diagnosis may follow a T1D diagnosis at any time, therefore ongoing screening is important (Flores Monar et al., 2022; Frohlich-Reiterer et al., 2022).

Principles for Meal Planning

A balance of carbohydrates (40% to 50%), protein (15% to 25%), and fat (30% to 40%) is needed for optimal nutrition planning (Annan et al., 2022). Because all carbohydrates consumed are converted into BG, monitoring carbohydrate intake is a key strategy in achieving glycemic control (Bonsembiante et al., 2021). Carbohydrate

TABLE 23-5 Carb Intake to Cover Moderate Exercise*†

Blood Glucose	Before Exercise	During Exercise	After Exercise
<90 mg/dL	**Aerobic and anaerobic exercise** • Eat 10–20 g of carbs before starting. • Wait until BG is >90 to start exercise.	**Aerobic exercise** • Eat 10–20 g of carbs per hour of activity. **Anaerobic exercise** • Extra carbs not typically needed	Eat meal or 10–15 g carb snack within 1 hr of exercise. Drink fluids with meal/snack. Before sleep, may eat additional bedtime snack (especially with prolonged or intense activity).
90–125 mg/dL	**Aerobic exercise** • Eat 10–20 g of carbs before starting. **Anaerobic exercise** • No carbs, start exercise.	**For all activity** • Drink fluids (water sports drink or other fluids before or during the exercise to avoid dehydration).	
126–180 mg/dL	**Aerobic and anaerobic exercise** • No carbs, start exercise.		
181–250 mg/dL	**Aerobic and anaerobic exercise** • No carbs, start exercise.	**Aerobic exercise** • Follow trend; when dropping below 180, give 10–20 g of carbs per hour of activity. **Anaerobic exercise** • Extra carbs typically not needed **For all activity** • Drink fluids (water, sports drink, or other fluids before and during the exercise to avoid dehydration).	
>250 mg/dL	**Aerobic and anaerobic exercise** • No carbs • Check ketones. No exercise if ketones are detected (blood: >0.6; urine: small, moderate, or large).		

carb, Carbohydrate.
*Moderate exercise (i.e., walking, leisurely cycling, lawn mowing). With strenuous exercise (i.e., jogging, bicycle racing, playing basketball, or digging in the garden), additional food may be required.
†The amount of carbohydrate varies based on exercise intensity and insulin on board during activity. Younger children may need fewer carbs than older teens and young adults; some may need up to 60 g/hr of carbs with intense exercise or a significant amount of insulin on board. If no insulin is on board, carbohydrates may not be needed in the first hour of exercise.
(Frohnert & Chase, 2022)

restriction is not recommended in children and adolescents; instead, meal planning should focus on the carbohydrate content of food choices. Dietary sources of carbohydrate are fruit, milk, yogurt, breads, cereal, grains, sweets, and starchy vegetables, such as corn and peas. Hidden sources of carbohydrates include condiments such as low-fat salad dressings, barbecue sauce, pasta sauce, and ketchup. Even sugar-free and sugar-substitute foods may contain carbohydrates.

Large quantities of dietary fat and protein increase postprandial (after meal) glucose levels and should be avoided when planning meals (Annan et al., 2022). Saturated and trans fatty acids should be limited to reduce the risk of cardiovascular disease. Additionally, dietary supplements (herbal and nonherbal) are not recommended as there is no strong evidence to support use by those with diabetes unless there is an identified deficit (ElSayed et al., 2023h). The general principles for meal planning include the following:

- *Eat a well-balanced diet.*
- *Be aware of insulin action times and time meals and snacks accordingly.* Mealtimes or PE class times that change throughout the school year may require an adjustment in meal planning to prevent hypoglycemia.
- *Use snacks to prevent hypoglycemia* (e.g., 15 grapes, ½ banana, apple, or orange juice).
- *Balance carbohydrate intake and insulin carefully.* The rise in postprandial BG is dependent on the total amount of carbohydrates eaten, not the form of carbohydrate. For a young child who is a picky eater, the mealtime insulin may be calculated after the meal based on the actual amount of carbohydrate consumed.
- *Avoid overtreating low BG.* This can be difficult because of the powerful response of feeling ravenously hungry that often occurs with hypoglycemia.
- *Reduce cholesterol and saturated fat intake.* If BG levels are too high, then blood cholesterol and triglyceride levels can also be elevated, which can lead to cardiovascular complications.
- *Monitor height and weight.*
- *Avoid foods high in sodium* (Abraham et al., 2022; Annan et al., 2022).

CONSISTENT CARBOHYDRATE MEAL PLAN. In a *consistent carbohydrate meal plan,* there is a set amount of carbohydrate grams or carbohydrate choices for each meal and snack, and the dose of insulin is not adjusted (ADA, 2022a; Annan et al., 2022). Although the type of carbohydrate can vary, consistency in the number of choices and grams of carbohydrate is important. *One carbohydrate choice, or serving, is 15 g of carbohydrate.* More carbohydrates (i.e., a snack) may be needed for increased activity (Adolfsson et al., 2022; Frohnert & Chase, 2022). This method of meal planning is often used by students who receive a preset amount of rapid-acting or short-acting insulin at lunch or who take intermediate-acting insulin in the morning (ADA, 2022a; Annan et al., 2022; Frohnert & Chase, 2022).

COUNTING CARBOHYDRATE MEAL PLAN. The *counting carbohydrate meal plan* involves counting carbohydrate grams and giving an adjusted dose of insulin based on the amount of carbohydrate in the meal or snack (ADA, 2022a; Annan et al., 2022). The insulin-to-carbohydrate (I:C) ratio determines the number of units of insulin to be given for the number of grams of carbohydrate eaten. The I:C ratio is very individualized and changes frequently based on BG levels 3 to 4 hours postprandial. Different ratios may be prescribed for meals, snacks, before exercise, and/or at bedtime (Frohnert & Chase, 2022).

This type of meal plan emphasizes carbohydrate intake while keeping protein and fat intake relatively constant. The variability of carbohydrate intake and insulin provides more flexibility and reduces the risk for hypoglycemia (Frohnert & Chase, 2022). This meal planning is used by students who are on multiple daily injections of rapid-acting insulin and basal or peakless insulin, or students receiving rapid-acting insulin through an insulin pump or pod.

Physical Activity Management

Regardless of diabetes type, regular physical activity (aerobic, anaerobic, and interval training) is an important component of diabetes management to improve glycemic control, decrease total daily insulin requirements, decrease cardiovascular risk factors, help with weight loss, and improve overall health (Adolfsson et al., 2022; ElSayed et al., 2023h). Additional factors are related to glycemic response during exercise at the site of insulin delivery, amount of circulating insulin, BG levels before exercise, and the ingredients of the last meal before exercise.

Hypoglycemia is one of the main concerns for those who receive insulin and are physically active, particularly if it occurs at a peak time of insulin action or before a meal or snack. The student's BG must be monitored before, during, and after exercise (ADA, 2022a; Adolfsson et al., 2022). The risk of hypoglycemia is increased during and after exercise and can last up to 24 hours; therefore the most pronounced risk for hypoglycemia occurs in the nighttime following afternoon activity.

Exercise intensity and duration recommendations for youth with diabetes are the same as those for all youth: at least 60 minutes of moderate to vigorous daily physical activity, along with muscle and bone strength activities at least 3 days per week (Adolfsson et al., 2022; ElSayed et al., 2023c). Unfortunately, schools vary in the amount of physical activity that is incorporated into the curricula; this will require planning and accommodations, such as adjusting the student's schedule, snacks, and/or insulin dosing. To ensure safe physical activity, school staff supervising activities such as PE classes, recess, and sporting events must be able to identify a hypoglycemic emergency and call for assistance.

To avoid hypoglycemia due to physical activity, the student's DMMP may include insulin adjustment via injection or pump (reduced basal or bolus insulin) and/or additional

Focus on the Framework

Care Coordination: Collaborative Communication

The school nurse should collaborate with school administrators, teachers, parents, and the student to encourage participation in physical activity and ensure safety. The student's emergency supplies (emergency action plan, quick-acting source of glucose, BGM, and water) should be readily available on site where the physical activity is occurring to provide for immediate treatment of low BG (ADA, 2022a).

carbohydrates before the activity. Students using an insulin pump may suspend or not wear their pump during physical activity, yet the time limit a pump should be suspended or not worn should not exceed 2 hours to avoid complications, such as DKA (Adolfsson et al., 2022; Frohnert & Chase, 2022). General guidelines for physical activity include providing an extra carbohydrate before exercise when the BG is less than 90 mg/dL and when exercise is expected to last longer than 30 minutes. Students with a BG greater than 270 mg/dL with moderate to large ketonemia/ketonuria (less than 1.5 mmol/L) not attributable to insulin deficiency and/or carbohydrate excess should not exercise (Adolfsson et al., 2022).

EMERGENCIES AND COMPLICATIONS

Hypoglycemia

Hypoglycemia represents the greatest immediate danger to the student with diabetes, especially for those with T1D. Hypoglycemia can occur from excessive physical exercise, too much insulin, and/or altered amount or food intake. Classifications for hypoglycemia have been defined by the International Hypoglycemia Study Group (2017; Abraham et al., 2022). A BG less than 54 mg/dL is considered serious and *always* requires immediate treatment. BG values greater than or equal to 70 mg/dL are classified as alert values that *may* cause symptoms and require treatment. Alert values often indicate the need for insulin dose adjustment. It should be understood, however, that the severity of a hypoglycemic episode is defined not by an absolute glucose value but by cognitive impairment requiring external assistance for recovery (Abraham et al., 2022).

The symptoms of hypoglycemia can vary from person to person. The BG level at which the symptoms are felt can also be different. Hypoglycemia symptoms include appearing pale, feeling shaky, weak, tired, and hungry, sweating, and exhibiting behavioral changes or confusion. These can progress to loss of consciousness and/or seizures (Abraham et al., 2022; Faradji et al., 2023). The symptoms of hunger, paleness, weakness, and shakiness are related to the effects of adrenaline, and the progressing symptoms are related to a lack of glucose to the brain (Frohnert & Chase, 2022). The school nurse should speak with the parent/guardian and the student to identify each student's symptoms of hypoglycemia and the treatment used. Some young children may only say, "I have an itchy nose," or "I am hungry," when they are feeling a low BG level. Individuals with diabetes can often identify the symptoms they experience when their BG level is mildly decreased, moderately decreased, and severely decreased (Table 23-6).

The student's DMMP will include orders for the treatment of hypoglycemia, including glucagon. These orders, along with symptoms and treatment procedures, should be written into the student's IHP and EAP. The EAP should be distributed to all school and transportation staff who have responsibility for the student (ADA, 2022a; NASN, 2020b). During an acute hypoglycemic episode, even an independent student may not be able to self-manage because of impaired cognitive and motor function. Urgent treatment on the spot is necessary to prevent worsening of symptoms.

Hypoglycemia unawareness is a phenomenon characterized by an individual's inability to sense that their BG level has dropped until it reaches a dangerously low level (Abraham et al., 2022; Faradji et al., 2023). The phenomenon is believed to be caused by changes in hormonal counterregulation systems, especially a decrease in the hormonal response of epinephrine. To counter hypoglycemia unawareness, the pediatric diabetes care team may increase BG target ranges for several weeks in an effort to reverse this phenomenon (de Bock et al., 2022; ElSayed et al., 2023d). The use of CGMs has been found to be helpful for children who experience hypoglycemia unawareness (Abraham et al., 2022; Faradji et al., 2023). Special considerations may be necessary for these students to prevent episodes of hypoglycemia.

TABLE 23-6 Reported Symptoms for Hypoglycemia

Mild Hypoglycemia	Moderate Hypoglycemia	Severe Hypoglycemia
• Hunger • Irritability • Shakiness • Weakness • Sweaty • Anxious • Dizziness • Headache • Unable to concentrate • Not feeling well • Feeling "funny" • Heart racing • Tingling in extremities	All symptoms of mild hypoglycemia, plus: • Sleepiness • Erratic behavior • Poor coordination • Confusion • Slurred speech • Slow thinking • Numbness • Combative	• Unable to swallow • Unresponsive • Unconscious • Seizures

(Abraham et al., 2022; Frohnert & Chase, 2022)

Hypoglycemia Treatment

Hypoglycemia treatment is individualized and based on the student's BG target ranges and history. It is important to know treatment for symptoms a student experiences with low BG episodes should begin at the first indication, even if a glucose meter is unavailable to verify a low BG result (Abraham et al., 2022; ADA, 2022a; Frohnert & Chase, 2022; Lawrence et al., 2022). Confirmed low BG readings in an asymptomatic student also need to be treated promptly.

A supply of fast-acting carbohydrates should always be accessible to students and staff (Abraham et al., 2022; ADA, 2022a; Lawrence et al., 2022). A supply of glucose tablets, gels, candy, or similar items should be kept in various places (e.g., the student's backpack, in the classroom, and the nurse's office). Once hypoglycemia is recognized, the student should consume *15 g of a carbohydrate*, which will raise the BG level approximately 54 to 72 mg/dL in a child who weighs 110 lb (50 kg). Glucose in a pure form is the ideal treatment because it is most rapidly absorbed. Examples of 15 g of carbohydrates include 4 oz of fruit juice; 4 to 6 oz (half a can) of regular (not low-calorie or reduced sugar) soda; four glucose tablets; one tube of glucose gel; three to four Starburst candies; 15 Skittles candies; or 3 tsp of sugar, syrup, jelly, or honey (Abraham et al., 2022; ADA, 2022a; Lawrence et al., 2022). Note that a student who is having hypoglycemia should never be left unattended or sent anywhere alone in case the BG declines to a dangerously low level and the student loses consciousness.

Fifteen minutes after the treatment, the student or school personnel must retest the student's BG. If the BG is still less than 70 mg/dL (or lower than target range specified in the DMMP), the student should repeat treatment with another 15 g of carbohydrate (Abraham et al., 2022; ADA, 2022a). The parents/guardians should be contacted at this point. Once BG returns to normal, it should be checked again 1 hour later. To avoid a recurrent episode of hypoglycemia, *after the student's BG level has returned to target range, the student should eat their typical meal or snack if it is due. If a meal/snack is not due, the student should eat 15g of a slower-acting carbohydrate (e.g., fruit, whole grain/graham crackers, yogurt, granola bar)*. Note that a meal or snack may not always be necessary, especially if an insulin pump is in use.

To prevent hypoglycemia, students should check their BG before, during, and after physical activity, especially when they are newly diagnosed and exercising and/or engaging in a new type of physical activity. Students who have a BG less than 90 mg/dL should not engage in physical activity until BG is between 100 and 200 mg/dL. Some students will require a snack (15 to 30 g of carbohydrates) before activities such as gym class or recess, depending on their BG result. A student experiencing severe hypoglycemia with BG results of less than 40 mg/dL and cognitive and motor dysfunction may not return to normal for more than an hour.

When BG is low, blood glucose monitoring is important to avoid overtreatment (ADA, 2022a). Although it is usually not necessary to send a child home for a mild to moderate hypoglycemic episode, a parent or guardian should be notified. It is also important to discuss the episode with the student so that they can learn about the symptoms of low BG and help problem-solve to prevent episodes in the future. Frequent mild hypoglycemia can deplete glycogen stores and put students at increased risk for prolonged or severe hypoglycemia in the future.

When a student has a severe hypoglycemia episode resulting in a decreased level of consciousness or inability to swallow, *do not attempt to give anything by mouth*. Activate the emergency medical system (EMS) immediately and administer glucagon per the DMMP (ADA, 2022a). Glucagon is a hormone that increases the BG level within 5 to 15 minutes by releasing glucose that has been stored in the liver as glycogen (Abraham et al., 2022). The emergency glucagon kit may consist of either a powdered intranasal spray (Lowe & Trujillo, 2020), a vial of powdered glucagon plus a saline-filled syringe for reconstitution and injection, or a prefilled, premixed pen for injection (ADA, 2022a). The glucagon kit must be accessible at all times; if it is in the health office, it should be stored in an *unlocked* cabinet or drawer. The location of the glucagon should be noted in the student's EAP. *Once glucagon is administered, the student should be placed in a side-lying position to protect the airway, as vomiting is a common side effect* (Abraham et al., 2022; ADA, 2022a). The parent/guardian and pediatric diabetes care team should always be notified immediately of a severe hypoglycemic episode.

The use of glucagon to address severe hypoglycemia is a standard part of a DMMP (ADA, 2022a). However, not every student will have glucagon at school. This can be related to a number of barriers that parents face, including affordability for families to have doses at home and school, lack of concern that a hypoglycemic event will occur, and family priorities that supersede filling the prescription or transporting it to school. The school nurse should work with the family to address barriers so that each student at risk for severe hypoglycemia has glucagon available (Yonkaitis & Jacobs, 2022). In addition, states such as Illinois, Ohio, and Oklahoma have passed laws allowing schools to stock undesignated glucagon, similar to the state laws that allow undesignated epinephrine in schools across the country (Abdelshehed & Clothier, 2023). In states that allow undesignated glucagon, the school nurse can work with school administration, state health and education departments, and pharmaceutical companies to provide undesignated glucagon in their schools. School nurses working in states that do not allow stock glucagon in schools can advocate for changes to their state laws (Yonkaitis & Jacobs, 2022).

Hyperglycemia

Hyperglycemia is defined as a BG level above 180 mg/dL and/or in excess of the individualized target range (ElSayed et al., 2023d; Sundberg et al., 2022). Hyperglycemia can occur gradually or rapidly (e.g., due to an insulin pump malfunction). A major benefit of BGM is the ability to monitor trends to prevent dangerously high BG levels. Symptoms of high BG include frequent urination, excessive thirst, blurred vision, fatigue, hunger, weight loss, abdominal pain, lack of concentration, headache, numbness in extremities, the development of sweet fruity breath, and a change in the respiratory status. Extended periods of hyperglycemia can lead to microvascular and macrovascular damage affecting major organs in the body, such as the circulatory system, eyes, kidneys, and nervous system (Bjornstad et al., 2022; ElSayed et al., 2023d). Most children are not concerned about the long-term effects of high BG and often do not appreciate that hyperglycemia, if unaddressed, can progress to a medical emergency.

Hyperglycemia can be caused by anything that results in insufficient insulin, such as missed insulin doses, not taking enough insulin because of eating more food than planned, or eating foods that are higher in carbohydrate content than anticipated (Glaser et al., 2022; Nandhini et al., 2023). In addition, some medications, illness and infection, growth spurts, menses in girls, stress, and decreased activity may lead to hyperglycemia. Medications associated with hyperglycemia include corticosteroids, diuretics, beta blockers, and antipsychotics. Students receiving insulin via an insulin pump are at increased risk for hyperglycemia because of infusion site failure or malfunction and may require insulin by injection to avoid ketoacidosis.

Hyperglycemia Treatment

Hyperglycemia is considered an immediate emergency medical situation when symptoms of diabetic ketoacidosis (DKA; see diabetic ketoacidosis section later in this chapter) are present (ADA, 2022a; Glaser et al., 2022). Overreaction to hyperglycemia should be avoided in the absence of DKA symptoms. Treatment for hyperglycemia is largely determined by the level of ketones in the blood or urine. A check for ketones should be performed per the DMMP, typically when the BG level is greater than 300 mg/dL (greater than 250 mg/dL if insulin pump is in use) or when the student is ill (ADA, 2022a). While both urine and blood ketone testing are considered reliable, urine ketone levels may be affected by how long the urine has been in the bladder (Frohnert & Chase, 2022). Correction of the elevated BG levels with insulin is necessary (Miranda Lora et al., 2023) and will be specified in the DMMP orders. Students who are experiencing hyperglycemia may remain at school unless they have moderate to large amounts of ketone. Should symptoms indicative of DKA, such as nausea, vomiting, stomachache, labored breathing, or lethargy, be present, EMS should be activated (ADA, 2022a). If insulin is given for hyperglycemia, the BG and ketone levels should be monitored per the DMMP.

Additional interventions for hyperglycemia include drinking extra water or noncaloric beverages and exercising moderately if no ketones are present (ADA, 2022a; Miranda Lora et al., 2023). If asymptomatic, the student can return to the classroom with access to fluids and unrestricted bathroom privileges and should be encouraged to return to the health office if symptoms reoccur. It may be helpful to discuss with the student what may have caused the glucose to be elevated. Problem-solving may also extend to a discussion with the parent or guardian. If hyperglycemic episodes persist, the school nurse should suggest that the parent/guardian contact the healthcare provider to alert them to the situation and clarify whether adjusting the insulin dosing is necessary in order to keep the student's BG levels within the target range while at school. Additionally, the needs of the student with recurrent hyperglycemia may need to be addressed in the IHP.

Recognition and early intervention for hyperglycemia are of special concern for students receiving insulin via insulin infusion systems (ElSayed et al., 2023f; Glaser et al., 2022; Sherr et al., 2022). DKA can occur rapidly because the student is not receiving any long-acting insulin. Problems with infusion sets, such as tube kinking or site failure, can result in DKA in as few as 3 to 6 hours. A student using an infusion system who experiences hyperglycemia in the presence of ketones should have the infusion site changed immediately and receive insulin by injection as per the DMMP (Frohnert & Chase, 2022; Miranda Lora et al., 2023).

Diabetic Ketoacidosis

Diabetic ketoacidosis (DKA) is one of the most serious outcomes of poorly controlled diabetes; it primarily occurs in T1D but can also occur in children with T2D. Ketoacidosis is usually caused by profound insulin deficiency and can lead to coma as the result of dehydration, electrolyte imbalance, and acidosis (Glaser et al., 2022). It develops over hours to days as hyperglycemia triggers the release of stored fats and proteins for energy, leading to the formation of ketones that result in acidosis. Ketone formation begins after 3 to 4 hours without insulin (ADA, 2022a; Frohnert & Chase, 2022). The biochemical diagnostic criteria for DKA are a BG level greater than 200 mg/dL, venous blood pH less than 7.3, or bicarbonate less than 15 mEq/L, and with ketonemia (blood beta-hydroxybutyrate 3 mmol/L or higher) and/or moderate to large ketonuria (Glaser et al., 2022). Symptoms include severe abdominal pain, nausea, vomiting, dry mouth and extreme thirst, fruity breath, blurry vision, heavy breathing and/or shortness of breath, chest pain, increased lethargy, weakness, and/or a change in the level of consciousness (ADA, 2022a; Frohnert & Chase, 2022). *DKA is considered a medical emergency. EMS should be activated for any student with diabetes for whom DKA is suspected.* For children who have several DKA episodes in a year, ongoing supervision, reeducation, support, and possible referral are appropriate.

Complications

Microvascular and macrovascular complications begin to develop around puberty and/or with 5 years of disease duration for youth with T1D diabetes (ElSayed et al., 2023c) and are the result of elevated glucose levels in the bloodstream. For young people with T2D, evidence exists that they may develop complications earlier than those with T1D (Barrett et al., 2020; Bjornstad et al., 2022). Students with any type of diabetes should be screened regularly, based on age and diagnosis duration for factors that increase the risk for diabetes-related complications (ElSayed et al., 2023c). Appropriate screens include those for hypertension, dyslipidemia, urine albumin excretion, and retinopathy. A landmark 10-year study demonstrates that early glycemic control in youth, with particular emphasis on reducing glycemic variability, has lasting effects on reducing complications (National Institute of Diabetes and Digestive and Kidney Diseases [NIDDK], 2017).

TABLE 23-7 American Diabetes Association Levels of Staff Training

Level	Topics	Audience
Level 1 Training	Basics of diabetes care, including recognizing and responding to an emergency	All school staff
Level 2 Training	Level 1 training, plus additional training based on roles/ responsibilities	School staff who have responsibility for students with diabetes (e.g., classroom teachers)
Level 3 Training	Specifics of diabetes care tasks, equipment, and comprehensive training on the DMMP, IHP, and EAP	School staff who assist the student with diabetes care tasks as permitted by local and state law

(ADA, 2022a)

CONSIDERATIONS IN THE SCHOOL ENVIRONMENT

Staff Training and Delegation

Some state nurse practice acts allow delegation of diabetes care in the school setting. Other states mandate that schools train care aides to assist the student in the absence of a school nurse. When delegating diabetes care tasks, the school nurse must take into consideration that the complexity of insulin action and timing requires the expertise of a school nurse (ADA, 2022a). The nurse should maintain close communication with the parents and provide adequate preparation of school personnel to ensure student safety during school or when participating in extracurricular activities. Staff training *must* include the recognition and treatment of hypoglycemia as per the student's EAP. Additionally, all school personnel who have responsibility for the student should have a copy of the EAP and know how to respond in an emergency (ADA, 2022a). The DMMP should never be substituted as an emergency action plan as it is too complicated for use in emergent situations and is meant as a communication tool between healthcare providers and the parents/guardians. The 2022 ADA *Guide for School Personnel* outlines three levels of staff training (Table 23-7).

Eating at School

Collaboration with school nutrition services on meal planning should take place as a part of IHP development for a student with diabetes (ADA, 2022a; Annan et al., 2022). Access to nutritional information, including the carbohydrate content of school menu items, is essential to ensure a proper insulin dose. Close collaboration between the school cafeteria and the nurse enables accurate collection of meal carbohydrate counts and may also provide an opportunity to educate the cafeteria staff on nutritionally sound meal preparation for students with diabetes. When school meals are provided by a contracted company, a daily calendar or other resource that outlines the carbohydrate content for each meal or food item should be available. The popularity of à la carte choices (e.g., vending machines and grab-and-go windows) in upper grades offers a wide variety of food options but creates an additional challenge as carbohydrate information may not be readily available on these items. Resources such as smart phone apps and calorie-counting Web sites such as CalorieKing (see Resources at the end of this chapter) can provide extra support to students in accessing accurate carbohydrate information.

Class Parties

Students with diabetes should participate fully in class parties and special events, as they are an important aspect of the overall school experience. Planning for these events in the IHP is the best way to identify possible food options (ADA, 2022a; Annan et al., 2022). School wellness policies may delineate that class parties only include healthy alternatives to high-calorie, low-nutrition choices. These may include extra recess time or nonfood treats (e.g., pencils). The school nurse should involve the family and pediatric diabetes care team in problem-solving for both planned and unplanned scenarios to guide the school nurse in insulin dosing changes that may be needed. Some options to accommodate increased carbohydrate consumption at class parties include the following:

- The student will eat the treat and may or may not receive an extra dose of insulin to cover the extra carbohydrate intake.
- Parent/guardian will provide a replacement treat alternative.
- Treat will be placed in a bag and sent home to be eaten as part of a scheduled snack.

Field Trips

Field trips are also an important part of the school experience and planning for them needs to include the school nurse (ADA, 2022a). Access to a field trip cannot be denied because of a student's diabetes (NASN, 2023); many students have a Section 504 plan that addresses necessary accommodations. It is the school's responsibility to make sure that trained staff are available to provide for these specified accommodations. At the beginning of each school year, the school nurse should remind staff that advanced notification of field trips is required to facilitate proper planning for the needs of all students with chronic health concerns.

The extent of care accommodations for a field trip may vary (ADA, 2022a). Students who are in elementary grades or newly diagnosed may require more assistance or direct care from school staff. For intensely active field trips, the parent/guardian should send extra snacks to be eaten during increased activity and may elect to obtain medical orders to reduce the insulin dose to prevent hypoglycemia. Field trips that involve a meal or snack being consumed away from school involve additional planning to maintain a balance between the nutritional intake and the insulin dosing.

Some field trips encompass only a few hours, whereas older students may have an opportunity for extended, even overnight field trips. The school nurse in collaboration with parents should assess and plan for the necessary diabetes care on field trips and school-sponsored extracurricular activities that occur off campus (ADA, 2022a). If neither a parent/guardian nor a school nurse can attend, the school will need to hire another registered nurse or trained school staff (if permitted by the state nurse practice act and delegation law) to accompany the student (NASN, 2023). School-sponsored field trips that occur out of state or country require special planning. The school nurse may need to seek licensure from the host state's board of nursing or contact the country's consulate for permission to practice nursing outside the United States (see Chapter 6).

The following supplies are needed for extended field trips:

- Copies of the EAP, including emergency contact information and phone numbers
- Blood glucose monitor and supplies (including extra battery)
- Ketone monitoring supplies
- Insulin and supplies for administration
- Pump supplies (including extra battery and charging cord)
- Appropriate insulin storage
- Meal and snack foods
- Fast-acting carbohydrate to treat hypoglycemia
- Glucagon (subcutaneous or inhalable) emergency kit (ADA, 2022a)

School-Sponsored Events and Extracurricular Activities

School-sponsored events and extracurricular activities also require planning so that hypoglycemic emergencies are avoided. Students with diabetes must have testing supplies and a fast-acting carbohydrate supply plus glucagon readily available in the event of low BG. Coaches, teachers, and other school staff involved in after-school activities need to be educated about diabetes and how to prevent, identify, and respond to symptoms of hypoglycemia and hyperglycemia as outlined in the student's EAP and IHP. The EAPs should be in a place easily accessible for staff (ADA, 2022a).

Insulin Pumps at School

Advance notification by the parents that a student with an insulin pump will be attending school ensures that the school nurse is able to work with the family to develop a DMMP-based individual healthcare plan (NASN, 2020b). A Section 504 plan is also typically indicated (see the Academic and Social Impact of Diabetes on Students section). Students often wear the pump on the waist of their pants, belt, or in a pocket. To the untrained eye, an insulin pump might look like a cellphone or other contraband. The school nurse is responsible for educating school staff about the nature of insulin pumps and, with parental permission (documented in the IHP or 504 plan), alerting staff when a student uses one of these devices. Doing so avoids confusion and potential student embarrassment that could result from being questioned by well-meaning but uninformed staff.

Many students using an insulin infusion system will be proficient in its use. Young children or students new to the infusion system, however, may need more assistance and supervision (ADA, 2022a). The student, school nurse, or other trained adult (if allowed by state law) may increase, decrease, or stop insulin delivery as the situation requires per the DMMP. It is the responsibility of the family to make routine infusion set changes; this is usually completed at home. Nonetheless, supplies should be available at school so that, in the event an unplanned set change needs to be made, the time a student is without insulin is minimized.

The following continuous subcutaneous insulin infusion system supplies should be kept at school:

- Extra pump supplies: infusion set, reservoir, inserter, skin prepping solution, batteries
- Insulin syringe pen and needles in case of system failure
- Urine or blood ketone strips

Practice Connection

The school nurse must be able to administer a bolus, suspend and stop a pump, recognize and troubleshoot alarms, and know who to call for technical help (ADA, 2022a). Manuals and online instructions are usually available on the manufacturer's Web site. The infusion system model and manufacturer's helpline phone number should be readily available (e.g., on the IHP) for any urgent problems that occur. In-person training by a manufacturer's representative is sometimes available. *Insulin infusion system alarms, including low battery, low cartridge, and occlusion, should never be silenced or ignored. These alarms require immediate attention to prevent interruption in the delivery of insulin.*

- BG meter, strips, and batteries
- Glucose tabs, gel, and glucagon emergency kit (ADA, 2022a)

ACADEMIC AND SOCIAL IMPACT OF DIABETES ON STUDENTS

Learning

The school team needs to take the student's diagnosis of diabetes into account when evaluating them for learning accommodations and special education services. T1D can have both short- and long-term consequences on student cognition and learning (de Wit et al., 2022; Oakley et al., 2020; Shapiro et al., 2023). Hyperglycemia and glycemic variability have been shown to affect the central nervous system in very young children with diabetes (ElSayed et al., 2023c; Jaser & Jordan, 2021; Mauras et al., 2021; Sundberg et al., 2022). Severe hypoglycemia is associated with negative effects on verbal intelligence and memory (Shapiro et al., 2023). Age of diabetes onset (less than 5 or 6 years old) is a significant risk factor for experiencing adverse effects (ElSayed et al., 2023c).

A student newly diagnosed with diabetes may still be experiencing the transient physiological effects of hyperglycemia, such as blurred vision and decreased memory and concentration, as their BG levels are brought under control. They can have difficulty concentrating and may miss out on learning opportunities, especially if they need to leave the classroom frequently to use the restroom or must go home because of symptoms and/or ketones (ADA, 2022a; Lawrence et al., 2022). These students will need extra support, hence the importance of educating teachers and school administration not only on the signs and symptoms of hyperglycemia, but also on the consequences.

The school nurse can support both the teacher and student by discussing the student's self-management ability and by visiting the classroom to observe and support the student and address any questions the teacher might have (ADA, 2022a). When a student has experienced an episode of hypoglycemia or hyperglycemia, nurse-teacher communication enables the teacher to assess the student's need to repeat lessons that were taught right before or right after the episode. When students are hypoglycemic or hyperglycemic, they may experience cognitive impairment; adolescents taking lengthy examinations should check their blood sugars at the beginning of the examination and approximately halfway through to maintain glucose levels in their target range. Poor glycemic control can also affect school attendance (ElSayed et al., 2023c). When a student is struggling in school and/or demonstrates frequent school absences, it may be beneficial to review the student's BG control to rule out fluctuations as a possible cause. Students who receive school nurse support should be considered for a Section 504 plan or an IEP evaluation.

> **Did You Know?**
>
> Learning and behavior can be affected by the short-term effects of hypoglycemia and hyperglycemia due to autonomic nervous system activation and lack of glucose to the brain (de Wit et al., 2022; ElSayed et al., 2023c; Shapiro et al., 2023). Symptoms related to the brain's lack of glucose include decreased concentration, blurred vision, difficulty hearing, poor judgment, impaired short-term memory, confusion, and other behavioral changes such as agitation, crying, and irritability (Abraham et al., 2022). Fine motor speed and coordination may also be affected in the hypoglycemic state (Sundberg et al., 2022).

Efforts to maintain the student's BG levels in their target range should be balanced with the student's quality of life. Accommodations (documented in the Section 504 plan and/or IHP) ensure equal access to school and school-sponsored events (ADA, 2022a). The school nurse is an active participant in the development of the Section 504 plan, working collaboratively with the parents and school staff to identify necessary and appropriate accommodations. These may include adjusting the student's school schedule and routine diabetes care (e g., BGM, insulin administration) to avoid disruption to class time, lunch, recess, or other school events. Since the student with diabetes may have frequent medical appointments for diabetes management, accommodations to keep the student from being penalized for these absences are appropriate.

If diabetes significantly affects a student's ability to learn, the school nurse should consider if an evaluation for special education services is appropriate under the Individuals With Disabilities Education Improvement Act (IDEA; 2004). Students with diabetes may qualify for services under the Other Health Impairment (OHI) category. Federal law mandates a free and appropriate public education for all students regardless of disability (U.S. Department of Education, Office for Civil Rights, 2023). It is the responsibility of the school and/or prekindergarten program to identify students with disabilities (IDEA, 2004). If a request is made by the family, teachers, or school nurse for evaluation of special education services, the school nurse conducts an initial evaluation to identify concerns related to the student's diabetes that affect learning (see Chapter 8). For example, a student with uncontrolled diabetes who has frequent episodes of hypoglycemia and hyperglycemia that affect their ability to focus and concentrate at school may qualify for IEP services. These services may include supplemental aid and/or education modifications (ADA, 2022a). If the student does not qualify for IEP services, then most often the student's needs can be met by accommodations identified in a Section 504 plan.

Psychosocial Well-Being

Successful diabetes management requires a significant investment of effort, time, attention, and vigilance—students and their families don't get a "day off" from blood sugar checks and medication doses. The student with diabetes must incorporate nutrition guidelines, physical activity, medications, and BGM into their daily routine and may grieve the loss of their previous lifestyle. This added responsibility places students with diabetes at greater risk of experiencing psychosocial issues related to depression, low self-esteem, and anxiety (de Wit et al., 2022; Gregory et al., 2022).

Depression or depressive symptoms are more likely in individuals with diabetes. It is estimated that 30% of youth with T1D have depression (Gregory et al., 2022). Youth with diabetes and their families may also experience *diabetes distress*. This term describes the range of emotional responses that children and their families may experience because of the day-to-day demands of living with diabetes, not to mention fears of hypoglycemia or hyperglycemia, injections/infusions, or concerns over meeting glycemic goals (de Wit et al., 2022; Morrissey et al., 2020). Diabetes distress is distinct from depression, although both can be present, and both can interfere with glycemic control and self-management. In adolescents, approximately one-third will have diabetes distress.

Eating disorders occur more frequently among individuals with diabetes compared with their peers without diabetes (de Wit et al., 2022). In school, the desire to be like one's friends may motivate the student to disregard their routine care. Diabetes management becomes more challenging during preadolescence and adolescence because of the perceived stigma of diabetes combined with the developmental tasks facing youth during these stages. Experimentation with alcohol, drugs (both illicit and prescription), tobacco, and cannabis is not unusual among youth as they move toward their teen years; use of these substances carries added risk for students with diabetes because of the potential effects on BG. Other psychosocial issues arise when the student with diabetes is overprotected and not allowed similar privileges and independence as their peers. They may feel helpless and lacking control or may become overly dependent on the assistance of others, particularly during episodes of hypoglycemia.

Family support is critical to the students' ability to manage their diabetes at school and must be considered when assessing for psychosocial concerns (de Wit et al., 2022). Factors contributing to poor diabetes management include functional issues (e.g., literacy), knowledge deficit related to diabetes care, lack of routine, psychological and emotional issues, absence of support, and erroneous beliefs or misinformation (Virmani et al., 2022). Maintaining parental support and guidance supports success in BG control (de Wit et al., 2022). As teenagers become more independent in managing their diabetes, parent/guardian guidance can—and should—wane. Positive outcomes result when parents can find a balance between parental involvement and allowing independence with self-care. Achieving this balance requires that parents pivot toward an attitude of partnership with their teen. This independence may also mean the student spends less time in the health office, often managing their diabetes independently with trips to see the nurse only when there are issues with equipment or significant BG issues. School nurses can assist families and students by referring them to available resources, including their local Juvenile Diabetes Research Foundation or ADA support groups, diabetes camps, and school-based support groups (see the Resource section).

Assessment for psychosocial concerns is vitally important for students with diabetes (ADA, 2022a; de Wit et al., 2022). Communication with the student's pediatric diabetes care team and school health team is imperative (ADA, 2022a). The school nurse may need to make referrals for counseling or mental health support. Early identification of psychological concerns can lead to appropriate treatment and decrease negative outcomes. Studies have shown that school nurses can have a positive impact on students' health behaviors using motivational interviewing, which is a patient-centered, respectful method of counseling (ElSayed et al., 2023h; Lindholm Olinder et al., 2022). Assisting the student in identifying strengths that are unrelated to the diabetes diagnosis can also help mitigate psychosocial concerns.

Applying cultural competence to diabetes care in the school setting may enhance the promotion of health and decrease health disparities (Flores-Luevano et al., 2020; Limbert et al., 2022). The school nurse is well-positioned to identify cultural factors such as language, education, literacy, economic concerns, and religious, health, and illness beliefs. For example, diet and food choices may vary among ethnicities and cultures. A school nurse's sensitivity to the student's cultural differences increases the nurse's ability to promote and sustain quality diabetes care (see Chapter 10). The school nurse can work with families to build upon the student's preferred traditional meal choices to support glycemic control and growth and development. Helping parents and students to set diabetes care goals at school that reflect cultural awareness establishes concordance or harmony and may improve diabetes outcomes (ADA, 2022a; Annan et al., 2022). Diabetes education that considers these cultural issues has improved results (Association of Diabetes Care and Education Specialists, 2019; Flores-Luevano et al., 2020).

Self-Care

The rate at which students learn diabetes self-care varies depending on their psychomotor and intellectual development, experience with diabetes, and motivation to provide self-care. Figure 23-3 provides general guidelines for expectations related to participating in and performing self-care diabetes activities. School staff, including administration, and parents may find it beneficial to have information on the student's developmental level relative to diabetes.

The student transitioning from middle school to high school or high school to emerging adulthood (i.e., college, work) will need assistance in identifying and developing skills to make the transition a success (ADA, 2022a; ElSayed et al., 2023c; Gregory et al., 2022; NASN, 2024b). Assessment and planning are integral to promoting readiness and should begin before the transition occurs. For the student transitioning to college, families must decide to either

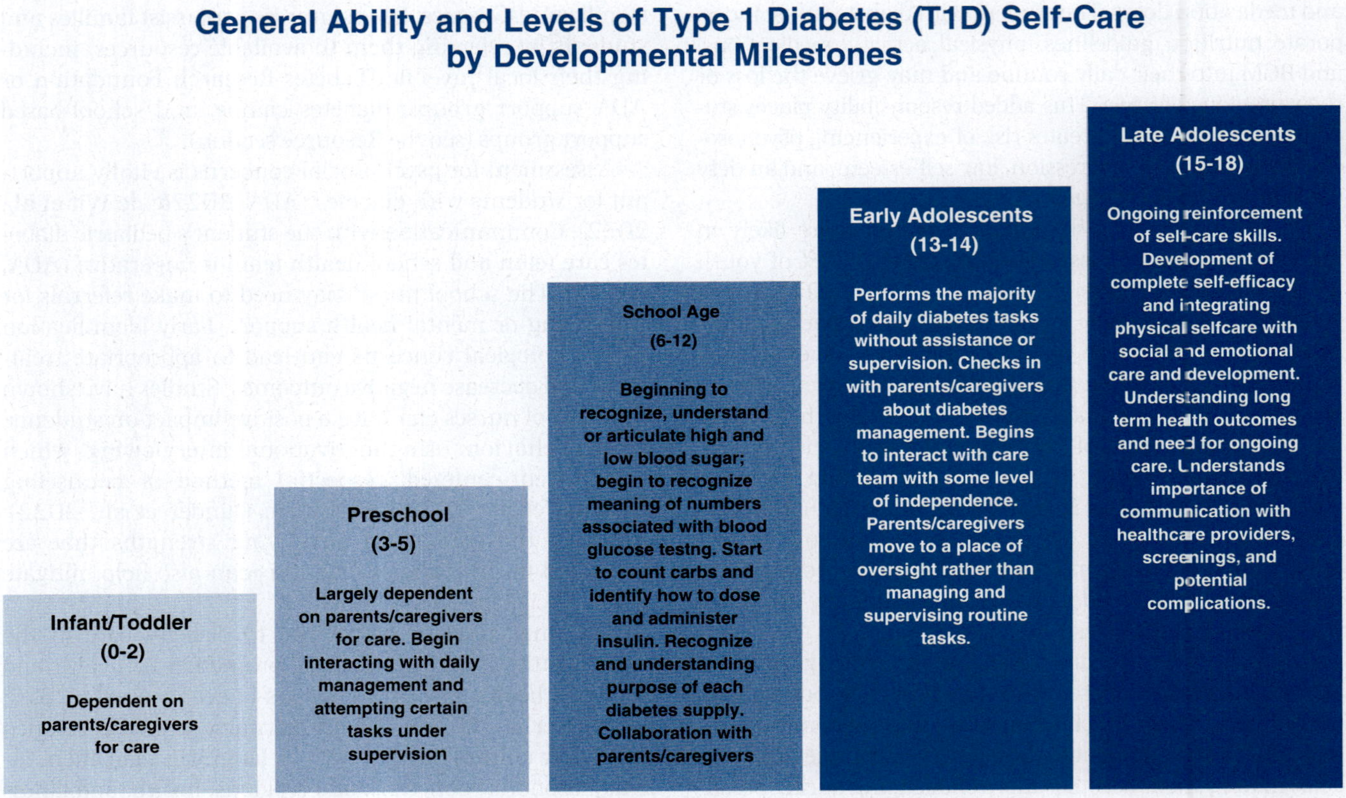

FIGURE 23-3. **Promoting self-care and independence: developmental considerations.** *(NASN, 2021a)*

identify and transfer diabetes care to a new healthcare provider closer to the college campus or remain with a current healthcare provider if they are able and willing to provide care virtually. Furthermore, families will need to begin the transition from pediatric to adult healthcare provider for the student's endocrinology care. The school nurse should review daily diabetes management skills with the student to assist in readiness (Klein et al., 2019). The ADA's position statement recommends that a transitional process to support the adolescent's move toward adulthood should begin at least 1 year in advance (Peters et al., 2011). Additionally, The Diabetes Link (n.d.), formerly known as the College Diabetes Network, helps youth with diabetes make the transition to college.

CONCLUSION

Effective diabetes management in school is necessary for the safety and long-term health of students with diabetes. It maximizes their readiness for learning and participation in school activities and minimizes the possibility of hypoglycemic and hyperglycemic emergencies during school hours, as well as when participating in extracurricular activities. Additional benefits for the student include better attendance and improved alertness and physical stamina. School nurses are the key school staff members to coordinate healthcare services for a student with diabetes at school and school-related activities (ADA, 2022a; NASN, 2021b). School nurses work with parents, students, the pediatric diabetes care team, and the community in a comprehensive and coordinated approach to ensure that students with diabetes have the same educational opportunities as other students.

The Editors gratefully acknowledge the work of the previous chapter author, Leah Wycoff.

Resources

This list of links is also available as Online Materials OM23-4.

A1C to Average BG Calculator: https://professional.diabetes.org/diapro/glucose_calc

Association of Diabetes Care and Education Specialists: https://www.diabeteseducator.org/

American Diabetes Association: http://www.diabetes.org

ADA Consumer Guide to Insulin: https://consumerguide.diabetes.org/collections/insulin

American Diabetes Association Safe at School: https://www2.diabetes.org/tools-support/know-your-rights/safe-at-school-state-laws/training-resources-school-staff/diabetes-care-tasks-school

American Dietetic Association: http://www.eatright.org

CalorieKing: https://www.calorieking.com/us/en/

CDC, Diabetes: https://www.cdc.gov/diabetes/index.html

Children With Diabetes: https://childrenwithdiabetes.com/

Colorado Diabetes Care and Prevention Collaboration: www.coloradokidswithdiabetes.org

Cultural Consideration in Diabetes Education: https://www.diabeteseducator.org/docs/default-source/practice/educator-tools/cultural-considerations.pdf?sfvrsn=2

Diabetes Exercise and Sports Association: http://www.diabetes-exercise.org

Individualized Health Care Plans for the School Nurse: http://www.schoolnursesupplyinc.com/Individualized-Health-Care-Plans-for-the-School-Nurse_p_8547.html

Indian Health Service IHS National Diabetes Program: https://www.ihs.gov/diabetes/

Joslin Diabetes Center: https://www.joslin.org

Juvenile Diabetes Research Foundation (JDRF): http://www.jdrf.org

National Diabetes Education Program (NDEP): http://www.yourdiabetesinfo.org

National Diabetes Information Clearinghouse: https://www.niddk.nih.gov/health-information/diabetes

National Institute of Diabetes and Digestive and Kidney Diseases (NIDDK): http://www.niddk.nih.gov

Link to sample DMMP: https://www.niddk.nih.gov/-/media/Files/Health-Information/Health-Professionals/Diabetes/health-care-professionals/Diabetes_Medical_Management_Plan.docx

The Diabetes Link (formerly known as the College Diabetes Network): https://thediabeteslink.org/

References

Abdelshehed, S., & Clothier, D. (2023). *Expanding health care access: Undesignated glucagon in schools.* The Council of State Governments. https://www.csg.org/2023/01/23/expanding-healthcare-access-undesignated-glucagon-in-schools/

Abraham, M. B., Karges, B., Dovc, K., Naranjo, D., Arbelaez, A. M., Mbogo, J., Javelikar, G., Jones, T. W., & Mahmud, F. H. (2022). ISPAD clinical practice consensus guidelines 2022: Assessment and management of hypoglycemia in children and adolescents with diabetes. *Pediatric Diabetes, 23*(8), 1322–1340. https://doi.org/10.1111/pedi.13443

Adolfsson, P., Taplin, C. E., Zaharieva, D. P., Pemberton, J., Davis, E. A., Riddell, M. C., McGavock, J., Moser, O., Szadkowska, A., Lopez, P., Santiprabhob, J., Frattolin, E., Griffiths, G., & DiMeglio, L. A. (2022). ISPAD clinical practice consensus guidelines 2022: Exercise in children and adolescents with diabetes. *Pediatric Diabetes, 23*(8), 1341–1372. https://doi.org/10.1111/pedi.13452

American Diabetes Association. (2022a). *Helping the student with diabetes succeed: A guide for school personnel.* https://diabetes.org/sites/default/files/2023-10/School-guide-final-11-16-22.pdf

American Diabetes Association. (2022b). *Safe at school®: Guidelines for the use of continuous glucose monitoring in the school setting.* https://diabetes.org/sites/default/files/2022-10/CGMguidance10-26-22final.pdf

American Diabetes Association. (2023). *eAG/A1C conversion calculator.* https://professional.diabetes.org/diapro/glucose_calc

American Diabetes Association. (2024). *Medication: Insulin basics.* https://diabetes.org/health-wellness/medication/insulin-basics

Annan, S. F., Higgins, L. A., Jelleryd, E., Hannon, T., Rose, S., Salis, S., Baptista, J., Chinchilla, P., & Marcovecchio, M. L. (2022). ISPAD clinical practice consensus guidelines 2022: Nutritional management in children and adolescents with diabetes. *Pediatric Diabetes, 23*(8), 1297–1321. https://doi.org/10.1111/pedi.13429

Association of Diabetes Care and Education Specialists. (2019). *Cultural and health literacy considerations with diabetes* [Practice paper]. Author. https://www.adces.org/docs/default-source/practice/practice-documents/practice-papers/adces-cultural-and-health-literacy-considerations-with-diabetes-final-4-1-20.pdf

Barrett, T., Jalaludin, M. Y., Turan, S., Hafez, M., Shehadeh, N., on behalf of the Novo Nordisk Pediatric Type 2 Diabetes Global Expert Panel. (2020). Rapid progression of type 2 diabetes and related complications in children and young people—A literature review. *Pediatric Diabetes, 21*(2), 158–172. https://doi.org/10.1111/pedi.12953

Bergenstal, R. M., Nimri, R., Beck, R. W., Criego, A., Laffel, L., Schatz, D., Battelino, T., Danne, T., Weinzimer, S. A., Sibayan, J., Johnson, M. L., Bailey, R. J., Calhoun, P., Carlson, A., Isganaitis, E., Bello, R., Albanese-O'Neill, A., Dovc, K., Biester, T., . . . FLAIR Study Group. (2021). A comparison of two hybrid closed-loop systems in adolescents and young adults with type 1 diabetes (FLAIR): A multicentre, randomised, crossover trial. *Lancet, 397*(10270), 208–219. https://doi.org/10.1016/S0140-6736(20)32514-9

Berman, C., Vidmar, A. P., & Chao, L. C. (2023). Glucagon-like peptide-1 receptor agonists for the treatment of type 2 diabetes in youth. *TouchREVIEWS in Endocrinology, 19*(1), 38–45. https://doi.org/10.17925/EE.2023.19.1.38

Besser, R. E., Bell, K. J., Couper, J. J., Ziegler, A. G., Wherrett, D. K., Knip, M., Speake, C., Casteels, K., Driscoll, K. A., Jacobsen, L., Craig, M. E., & Haller, M. J. (2022). ISPAD Clinical Practice Consensus Guidelines 2022: Stages of type 1 diabetes in children and adolescents. *Pediatric Diabetes, 23*(8), 1175–1187. https://doi.org/10.1111/pedi.13410

Bjornstad, P., Dart, A., Donaghue, K. C., Dost, A., Feldman, E. L., Tan, G. S., Wadwa, R. P., Zabeen, B., & Marcovecchio, M. L. (2022). ISPAD clinical practice consensus guidelines 2022: Microvascular and macrovascular complications in children and adolescents with diabetes. *Pediatric Diabetes, 23*(8), 1432–1450. https://doi.org/10.1111/pedi.13444

Bonsembiante, L., Targher, G., & Maffeis, C. (2021). Type 2 diabetes and dietary carbohydrate intake of adolescents and young adults: What is the impact of different choices? *Nutrients, 13*(10). https://doi.org/10.3390/nu13103344

Cengiz, E., Danne, T., Ahmad, T., Ayyavoo, A., Beran, D., Ehtisham, S., Fairchild, J., Jarosz-Chobot, P., Ng, S. M., Paterson, M., & Codner, E. (2022). ISPAD clinical practice consensus guidelines 2022: Insulin treatment in children and adolescents with diabetes. *Pediatric Diabetes, 23*(8), 1277–1296. https://doi.org/10.1111/pedi.13442

Centers for Disease Control and Prevention. (2024). *National diabetes statistics report.* https://www.cdc.gov/diabetes/php/data-research/

de Bock, M., Codner, E., Craig, M. E., Huynh, T., Maahs, D. M., Mahmud, F. H., Marcovecchio, L., & DiMeglio, L. A. (2022). ISPAD clinical practice consensus guidelines 2022: Glycemic targets and glucose monitoring for children, adolescents, and young people with diabetes. *Pediatric Diabetes, 23*(8), 1270–1276. https://doi.org/10.1111/pedi.13455

de Wit, M., Gajewska, K. A., Goethals, E. R., McDarby, V., Zhao, X., Hapunda, G., Delamater, A. M., & DiMeglio, L. A. (2022). ISPAD clinical practice consensus guidelines 2022: Psychological care of children, adolescents and young adults with diabetes. *Pediatric Diabetes, 23*(8), 1373–1389. https://doi.org/10.1111/pedi.13428

Demeterco-Berggren, C., Ebekozien, O., Noor, N., Rompicherla, S., Majidi, S., Jones, N. Y., McDonough, R., Odugbesan, O., Kim, A., Izquierdo, R., Kamboj, M. K., & Jacobsen, L. M. (2023). Factors associated with achieving target A1C in children and adolescents with type 1 diabetes: Findings from the T1D exchange quality improvement collaborative. *Clinical Diabetes, 41*(1), 68–75. https://doi.org/10.2337/cd22-0073

Diabetes Control and Complications Trial Research Group. (1993). The effect of intensive treatment of diabetes on the development and progression of long-term complications in insulin-dependent diabetes mellitus: Diabetes Control and Complications Trial. *New England Journal of Medicine, 329*(14), 977–986.

The Diabetes Link. (n.d.). *All things college*. https://thediabeteslink.org/all-things-college/

Divan, V., Greenfield, M., Morley, C. P., & Weinstock, R. S. (2022). Perceived burdens and benefits associated with continuous glucose monitor use in type 1 diabetes across the lifespan. *Journal of Diabetes Science and Technology, 16*(1), 88–96. https://doi.org/10.1177/1932296820978769

ElSayed, N. A., Aleppo, G., Aroda, V. R., Bannuru, R. R., Brown, F. M., Bruemmer, D., Collins, B. S., Gaglia, J. L., Hilliard, M. E., Isaacs, D., Johnson, E. L., Kahan, S., Khunti, K., Leon, J., Lyons, S. K., Perry, M. L., Prahalad, P., Pratley, R. E., Seley, J. J., ... Gabbay, R. A., on behalf of the American Diabetes Association. (2023a). 2. Classification and diagnosis of diabetes: Standards of care in diabetes—2023. *Diabetes Care, 46*(Suppl. 1), S19–S40. https://doi.org/10.2337/dc23-S002

ElSayed, N. A., Aleppo, G., Aroda, V. R., Bannuru, R. R., Brown, F. M., Bruemmer, D., Collins, B. S., Hilliard, M. E., Isaacs, D., Johnson, E. L., Kahan, S., Khunti, K., Leon, J., Lyons, S. K., Perry, M. L., Prahalad, P., Pratley, R. E., Jeffrie Seley, J., Stanton, R. C., & Gabbay, R. A., on behalf of the American Diabetes Association. (2023b). 15. Management of diabetes in pregnancy: Standards of care in diabetes—2023. *Diabetes Care, 46*(Suppl. 1), S254–S266. https://doi.org/10.2337/dc23-S015

ElSayed, N. A., Aleppo, G., Aroda, V. R., Bannuru, R. R., Brown, F. M., Bruemmer, D., Collins, B. S., Hilliard, M. E., Isaacs, D., Johnson, E. L., Kahan, S., Khunti, K., Leon, J., Lyons, S. K., Perry, M. L., Prahalad, P., Pratley, R. E., Seley, J. J., Stanton, R. C., & Gabbay, R. A., on behalf of the American Diabetes Association. (2023c). 14. Children and adolescents: Standards of care in diabetes—2023. *Diabetes Care, 46*(Suppl. 1), S230–S253. https://doi.org/10.2337/dc23-S014

ElSayed, N. A., Aleppo, G., Aroda, V. R., Bannuru, R. R., Brown, F. M., Bruemmer, D., Collins, B. S., Hilliard, M. E., Isaacs, D., Johnson, E. L., Kahan, S., Khunti, K., Leon, J., Lyons, S. K., Perry, M. L., Prahalad, P., Pratley, R. E., Seley, J. J., Stanton, R. C., & Gabbay, R. A., on behalf of the American Diabetes Association. (2023d). 6. Glycemic targets: Standards of care in diabetes—2023. *Diabetes Care, 46*(Suppl. 1), S97–S110. https://doi.org/10.2337/dc23-S006

ElSayed, N. A., Aleppo, G., Aroda, V. R., Bannuru, R. R., Brown, F. M., Bruemmer, D., Collins, B. S., Hilliard, M. E., Isaacs, D., Johnson, E. L., Kahan, S., Khunti, K., Leon, J., Lyons, S. K., Perry, M. L., Prahalad, P., Pratley, R. E., Seley, J. J., Stanton, R. C., & Gabbay, R. A., on behalf of the American Diabetes Association. (2023e). 9. Pharmacologic approaches to glycemic treatment: Standards of care in diabetes—2023. *Diabetes Care, 46*(Suppl. 1), S140–S157. https://doi.org/10.2337/dc23-S009

ElSayed, N. A., Aleppo, G., Aroda, V. R., Bannuru, R. R., Brown, F. M., Bruemmer, D., Collins, B. S., Hilliard, M. E., Isaacs, D., Johnson, E. L., Kahan, S., Khunti, K., Leon, J., Lyons, S. K., Perry, M. L., Prahalad, P., Pratley, R. E., Seley, J. J., Stanton, R. C., & Gabbay, R. A., on behalf of the American Diabetes Association. (2023f). 7. Diabetes technology: Standards of care in diabetes—2023. *Diabetes Care, 46*(Suppl. 1), S111–S127. https://doi.org/10.2337/dc23-S007

ElSayed, N. A., Aleppo, G., Aroda, V. R., Bannuru, R. R., Brown, F. M., Bruemmer, D., Collins, B. S., Hilliard, M. E., Isaacs, D., Johnson, E. L., Kahan, S., Khunti, K., Leon, J., Lyons, S. K., Perry, M. L., Prahalad, P., Pratley, R. E., Seley, J. J., Stanton, R. C., & Gabbay, R. A., on behalf of the American Diabetes Association. (2023g). 8. Obesity and weight management for the prevention and treatment of type 2 diabetes: Standards of care in diabetes—2023. *Diabetes Care, 46*(Suppl. 1), S128–S139. https://doi.org/10.2337/dc23-S008

ElSayed, N. A., Aleppo, G., Aroda, V. R., Bannuru, R. R., Brown, F. M., Bruemmer, D., Collins, B. S., Hilliard, M. E., Isaacs, D., Johnson, E. L., Kahan, S., Khunti, K., Leon, J., Lyons, S. K., Perry, M. L., Prahalad, P., Pratley, R. E., Seley, J. J., Stanton, R. C., . . . Gabbay, R. A., on behalf of the American Diabetes Association. (2023h). 5. Facilitating positive health behaviors and well-being to improve health outcomes: Standards of care in diabetes—2023. *Diabetes Care, 46*(Supple 1.), S68–S96. https://doi.org/10.2337/dc23-S005

Faradji, R. N., Urive-Weichers, A. C., & Sainz de la Maza, E. (2023). Hypoglycemia: Diagnosis, management, and prevention. In J. Rodriguez-Saldana (Ed.), *The diabetes textbook: Clinical principles, patient management and public health issues* (2nd ed., pp. 711–738). Springer International Publishing. https://doi.org/10.1007/978-3-031-25519-9

Flores-Luevano, S., Pacheco, M., Shokar, G. S., Dwivedi, A. K., & Shokar, N. K. (2020). Impact of a culturally tailored diabetes education and empowerment program in a Mexican American population along the US/Mexico border: A pragmatic study. *Journal of Clinical Medicine Research, 12*(8), 517–529. https://doi.org/10.14740/jocmr4273

Flores Monar, G. V., Islam, H., Puttagunta, S. M., Islam, R., Kundu, S., Jha, S. B., Rivera, A. P., & Sange, I. (2022). Association between type 1 diabetes mellitus and celiac disease: Autoimmune disorders with a shared genetic background. *Cureus, 14*(3), e22912. https://doi.org/10.7759/cureus.22912

Frohlich-Reiterer, E., Elbarbary, N. S., Simmons, K., Buckingham, B., Humayun, K. N., Johannsen, J., Holl, R. W., Betz, S., & Mahmud, F. H. (2022). ISPAD clinical practice consensus guidelines 2022: Other complications and associated conditions in children and adolescents with type 1 diabetes. *Pediatric Diabetes, 23*(8), 1451–1467. https://doi.org/10.1111/pedi.13445

Frohnert, B. I., & Chase, H. P. (2022). *Understanding diabetes* (15th ed.). The Pink Panther book. Children's Diabetes Foundation.

Garcia Argueta, M. I., Gonzalez Espejel, M., & Rodriguez-Saldana, J. (2023). Pregnancy: Pregestational and gestational management. In J. Rodriguez-Saldana (Ed.), *The diabetes textbook: Clinical principles, patient management and public health issues* (2nd ed., pp. 1095–1104). Springer International Publishing. https://doi.org/10.1007/978-3-031-25519-9

Glaser, N., Fritsch, M., Priyambada, L., Rewers, A., Cherubini, V., Estrada, S., Wolfsdorf, J. I., & Codner, E. (2022). ISPAD clinical practice consensus guidelines 2022: Diabetic ketoacidosis and hyperglycemic hyperosmolar state. *Pediatric Diabetes, 23*(7), 835–856. https://doi.org/10.1111/pedi.13406

Gomez-Diaz, R. (2023). Pathophysiology of type 1 diabetes. In J. Rodriguez-Saldana (Ed.), *The diabetes textbook: Clinical principles, patient management and public health issues* (2nd ed., pp. 115–126). Springer International Publishing. https://doi.org/10.1007/978-3-031-25519-9

Greeley, S. A. W., Polak, M., Njolstad, P. R., Barbetti, F., Williams, R., Castano, L., Raile, K., Chi, D. V., Habeb, A., Hattersley, A. T., & Codner, E. (2022). ISPAD clinical practice consensus guidelines 2022: The diagnosis and management of monogenic diabetes in children and adolescents. *Pediatric Diabetes, 23*(8), 1188–1211. https://doi.org/10.1111/pedi.13426

Gregory, J. W., Cameron, F. J., Joshi, K., Eiswirth, M., Garrett, C., Garvey, K., Agarwal, S., & Codner, E. (2022). ISPAD clinical practice consensus guidelines 2022: Diabetes in adolescence. *Pediatric Diabetes, 23*(7), 857–871. https://doi.org/10.1111/pedi.13408

Ilkowitz, J., Wissing, V., & Gallagher, M. P. (2022). Pediatric smart insulin pen use: The next best thing. *Journal of Diabetes Science and Technology, 16*(3), 635–640. https://doi.org/10.1177/19322968211041362

Imran, Cheema, H. A., Alvi, M. A., Rehman, M. U., Ali, M., & Sarwar, H. A. (2021). Spectrum of clinical presentation of celiac disease in pediatric population. *Cureus, 13*(6), e15582. https://doi.org/10.7759/cureus.15582

Individuals With Disabilities Education Improvement Act of 2004 (Pub. L. 108-446). https://www.gpo.gov/fdsys/pkg/PLAW-108publ446/content-detail.html

International Hypoglycemia Study Group. (2017). Glucose concentrations of less than 3.0 mmol/L (54 mg/dL) should be reported in clinical trials: A joint position statement of the American Diabetes Association and the European Association for the Study of Diabetes. *Diabetes Care, 40*(1), 155–157. https://doi.org/10.2337/dc16-2215

Jaser, S. S., & Jordan, L. C. (2021). Brain health in children with type 1 diabetes: Risk and protective factors. *Current Diabetes Reports, 21,* 1–10. https://doi.org/10.1007/s11892-021-01380-w

Jensen, E. T., Stafford, J. M., Saydah, S., D'Agostino, R. B., Dolan, L. M., Lawrence, J. M., Marcovina, S., Mayer-Davis, E. J., Pihoker, C., Rewers, A., & Dabelea, D. (2021). Increase in prevalence of diabetic ketoacidosis at diagnosis among youth with type 1 diabetes: The SEARCH for Diabetes in Youth study. *Diabetes Care, 44*(7), 1573–1578. https://doi.org/10.2337/dc20-0389

Kapoor, N., & Mittal, M. (2023). Homeostasis of glucose and intermediate metabolism: From the lens of a clinician. In J. Rodriguez-Saldana (Ed.), *The diabetes textbook: Clinical principles, patient management and public health issues* (2nd ed., pp. 104–114). Springer International Publishing. https://doi.org/10.1007/978-3-031-25519-9

Kariyawasam, D., Morin, C., Casteels, K., Le Tallec, C., Sfez, A., Godot, C., Huneker, E., Garrec, N., Benhamou, P. Y., Polak, M., Charpentier, G., Franc, S., & Beltrand, J. (2022). Hybrid closed-loop insulin delivery versus sensor-augmented pump therapy in children aged 6–12 years: A randomised, controlled, cross-over, non-inferiority trial. *Lancet Digital Health, 4*(3), e158–e168. https://doi.org/10.1016/S2589-7500(21)00271-5

Klein, K., Wheeler, M., & Yonkaitis, C. F. (2019). College-bound: Transition planning strategies for students with type 1 diabetes. *NASN School Nurse, 34*(1), 17–20. https://doi.org/10.1177/1942602X18794891

Laffel, L. M., Kanapka, L. G., Beck, R. W., Bergamo, K., Clements, M. A., Criego, A., DeSalvo, D. J., Goland, R., Hood, K., Liljenquist, D., Messer, L. H., Monzavi, R., Mouse, T. J., Prahalad, P., Sherr, J., Simmons, J. H., Wadwa, R. P., Weinstock, R. S., Willi, S. M., & Miller, K. M., for the CGM Intervention in Teens and Young Adults with T1D (CITY) Study Group. (2020). Effect of continuous glucose monitoring on glycemic control in adolescents and young adults with type 1 diabetes: A randomized clinical trial. *JAMA, 323*(23), 2388–2396. https://doi.org/10.1001/jama.2020.6940

Lawrence, J. M., Divers, J., Isom, S., Saydah, S., Imperatore, G., Pihoker, C., Marcovina, S. M., Mayer-Davis, E. J., Hamman, R. F., Dolan, L., Dabelea, D., Pettitt, D. J., Liese, A. D., for the SEARCH for Diabetes in Youth Study Group. (2021). Trends in prevalence of type 1 and type 2 diabetes in children and adolescents in the US, 2001–2017. *JAMA, 326*(8), 717–727. https://doi.org/10.1001/jama.2021.11165

Lawrence, S. E., Albanese-O'Neill, A., Besancon, S., Black, T., Bratina, N., Chaney, D., Cogen, F. R., Cummings, E. A., Moreau, E., Pierce, J. S., Richmond, E., & Mahmud, F. H. (2022). ISPAD clinical practice consensus guidelines 2022: Management and support of children and adolescents with diabetes in school. *Pediatric Diabetes, 23*(8), 1478–1495. https://doi.org/10.1111/pedi.13432

Libman, I., Haynes, A., Lyons, S., Pradeep, P., Rwagasor, E., Tung, J. Y., Jefferies, C. A., Oram, R. A., Dabelea, D., & Craig, M. E. (2022). ISPAD clinical practice consensus guidelines 2022: Definition, epidemiology, and classification of diabetes in children and adolescents. *Pediatric Diabetes, 23*(8), 1160–1174. https://doi.org/10.1111/pedi.13454

Limbert, C., Tinti, D., Malik, F., Kosteria, I., Messer, L., Jalaludin, M. Y., Benitez-Aguirre, P., Biester, S., Corathers, S., von Sengbusch, S., & Marcovecchio, M. L. (2022). ISPAD clinical practice consensus guidelines 2022: The delivery of ambulatory diabetes care to children and adolescents with diabetes. *Pediatric Diabetes, 23*(8), 1243–1269. https://doi.org/10.1111/pedi.13417

Lin, T., Manfredo, J. A., Illesca, N., Abiola, K., Hwang, N., Salsberg, S., Akhtar, Y., Mathioudakis, N., Brown, E. A., & Wolf, R. M. (2023). Improving continuous glucose monitoring uptake in underserved youth with type 1 diabetes: The IMPACT study. *Diabetes Technology & Therapeutics, 25*(1), 13–19. https://doi.org/10.1089/dia.2022.0347

Lindholm Olinder, A., DeAbreu, M., Greene, S., Haugstvedt, A., Lange, K., Majaliwa, E. S., Pais, V., Pelicand, J., Town, M., & Mahmud, F. H. (2022). ISPAD clinical practice consensus guidelines 2022: Diabetes education in children and adolescents. *Pediatric Diabetes, 23*(8), 1229–1242. https://doi.org/10.1111/pedi.13418

Lowe, R. N., & Trujillo, J. M. (2020). Intranasal glucagon: A new way to treat hypoglycemic emergencies. *Annals of Pharmacotherapy, 54*(8), 780–787. https://doi.org/10.1177/1060028020905846

Magliano, D. J., Chen, L., Islam, R. M., Carstensen, B., Gregg, E. W., Pavkov, M. E., Andes, L. J., Balicer, R., Baviera, M., Boersma-van Dam, E., Booth, G. L., Chan, J. C. N., Chua, Y. X., Fosse-Edorh, S., Fuentes, S., Gulseth, H. L., Gurevicius, R., Kyoung, H. H., Hird, T. R., Jermendy, G., ... Shaw, J. E. (2021). Trends in the incidence of diagnosed diabetes: A multi-country analysis of aggregate data from 22 million diagnoses in high-income and middle-income settings. *The Lancet: Diabetes & Endocrinology, 9*(4), 203–211. https://doi.org/10.1016/S2213-8587(20)30402-2

Mauras, N., Buckingham, B., White, N. H., Tsalikian, E., Weinzimer, S. A., Jo, B., Cato, A., Fox, L. A., Aye, T., Arbelaez, A. M., Hershey, T., Tansey, M., Tamborlane, W., Foland-Ross, L. C., Shen, H., Englert, K., Mazaika, P., Marzelli, M., & Reiss, A. L., for the Diabetes Research in Children (DirecNet). (2021). Impact of type 1 diabetes in the developing brain in children: A longitudinal study. *Diabetes Care, 44*(4), 983–992. https://doi.org/10.2337/dc20-2125

Miranda Lora, A. L., Espinosa Espíndola, M., Beauregard Paz, M., Molina Díaz, J. M., & Klünder Klünder, M. (2023). Diabetes in children and adolescents. In J. Rodriguez-Saldana (Ed.), *The diabetes textbook: Clinical principles, patient management and public health issues* (2nd ed., pp. 1063–1094). Springer International Publishing. https://doi.org/10.1007/978-3-031-25519-9

Morrissey, E. C., Casey, B., Dinneen, S. F., Lowry, M., & Byrne, M. (2020). Diabetes distress in adolescents and young adults living with type 1 diabetes. *Canadian Journal of Diabetes, 44*(6), 537–540. https://doi.org/10.1016/j.jcjd.2020.03.001

Nandhini, L. P., Kamalanathan, S., & Sahoo, J. (2023). Definition, diagnostic criteria, screening, diagnosis, and classification of diabetes and categories of glucose intolerance: An update. In J. Rodriguez-Saldana (Ed.), *The diabetes textbook: Clinical principles, patient management and public health issues* (2nd ed., pp. 89–104). Springer International Publishing. https://doi.org/10.1007/978-3-031-25519-9

Nathan, D. M. (2021). Realising the long-term promise of insulin therapy: The DCCT/EDIC study. *Diabetologia, 64,* 1049–1058. https://doi.org/10.1007/s00125-021-05397-4

National Association of School Nurses. (2020a). *The school health services team: Supporting student outcomes* (Position statement). Author.

National Association of School Nurses. (2020b). *Use of individualized healthcare plans to support school health services* (Position statement). Author.

National Association of School Nurses. (2021a). *School nursing evidence-based clinical practice guideline: Students with type 1 diabetes: Type 1 toolkit.* https://learn.nasn.org/courses/44058

National Association of School Nurses. (2021b). *School nursing evidence-based clinical practice guideline: Students with type 1 diabetes.* https://learn.nasn.org/courses/37660

National Association of School Nurses. (2023). *School-sponsored before, after, and extended school year/out of school time programs* (Position statement). Author.

National Association of School Nurses. (2024a). A contemporary framework update for today's school nursing landscape: Introducing the School Nursing Practice Framework. *NASN School Nurse, 39*(3), 140–147. https://www.doi.org/10.1177/1942602X241241092

National Association of School Nurses. (2024b). *Transition planning for students with healthcare needs* (Position statement). Author.

National Institute of Diabetes and Digestive and Kidney Diseases. (2017). *Recent advances & emerging opportunities: Diabetes, endocrinology, and metabolic diseases.* https://www.niddk.nih.gov/about-niddk/strategic-plans-reports/Pages/niddk-recent-advances-emerging-opportunities-2017.aspx

Nauck, M. A., Quast, D. R., Wefers, J., & Meier, J. J. (2021). GLP-1 receptor agonists in the treatment of type 2 diabetes—state-of-the-art. *Molecular Metabolism, 46,* 101102. https://doi.org/10.1016/j.molmet.2020.101102

Oakley, N. J., Kneale, D., Mann, M., Hilliar, M., Dayan, C., Gregory, J. W., & French, R. (2020). Type 1 diabetes mellitus and educational attainment in childhood: A systematic review. *BMJ Open, 10*(1), e033215. https://doi.org/10.1136/bmjopen-2019-033215

Ode, K. L., Ballman, M., Battezzati, A., Brennan, A., Chan, C. L., Hameed, S., Ismail, H. M., Kelly, A., Moran, A. M., Rabasa-Lhoret, R., Saxby, N. A., & Craig, M. E. (2022). ISPAD clinical practice consensus guidelines 2022: Management of cystic fibrosis–related diabetes in children and adolescents. *Pediatric Diabetes, 23*(8), 1212–1228. https://doi.org/10.1111/pedi.13453

Ojo, O. A., Ibrahim, H. S., Rotimi, D. E., Ogunlakin, A. D., & Ojo, A. B. (2023). Diabetes mellitus: From molecular mechanism to pathophysiology and pharmacology. *Medicine in Novel Technology and Devices, 19*. https://doi.org/10.1016/j.medntd.2023.100247

Pasi, R., & Ravi, K. S. (2022). Type 1 diabetes mellitus in pediatric age group: A rising endemic. *Journal of Family Medicine and Primary Care, 11*(1), 27–31. https://doi.org/10.4103/jfmpc.jfmpc_975_21

Perng, W., Conway, R., Mayer-Davis, E., & Dabelea, D. (2023). Youth-onset type 2 diabetes: The epidemiology of an awakening epidemic. *Diabetes Care, 46*(3), 490–499. https://doi.org/10.2337/dci22-0046

Peters, A., Laffel, L., & the American Diabetes Association Transitions Working Group. (2011). Diabetes care for emerging adults: Recommendations for transition from pediatric to adult diabetes care systems: A position statement of the American Diabetes Association, with representation by the American College of Osteopathic Family Physicians, the American Academy of Pediatrics, the American Association of Clinical Endocrinologists, the American Osteopathic Association, the Centers for Disease Control and Prevention, Children With Diabetes, The Endocrine Society, the International Society. *Diabetes Care, 34*(11), 2477–2485. https://doi.org/10.2337/dc11-1723

Sawyer, A., Sobczak, M., Forlenza, G. P., & Alonso, G. T. (2022). Glycemic control in relation to technology use in a single-center cohort of children with type 1 diabetes. *Diabetes Technology and Therapeutics, 24*(6), 409–415. https://doi.org/10.1089/dia.2021.0471

Scott, L., & Hall, L. (2012). Reliability and validity of the acanthosis nigricans screening tool for use in elementary school-age children by school nurses. *The Journal of School Nursing, 28*(6), 442–447. https://doi.org/10.1177/1059840512455364

Shah, A. S., Zeitler, P. S., Wong, J., Pena, A. S., Wicklow, B., Arslanian, S., Chang, N., Fu, J., Dabadghao, P., Pinhas-Hamiel, O., Urakami, T., & Craig, M. E. (2022). ISPAD clinical practice consensus guidelines 2022: Type 2 diabetes in children and adolescents. *Pediatric Diabetes, 23*(7), 872–902. https://doi.org/10.1111/pedi.13409

Shapiro, A. L. B., Bellatorre, A., Dabelea, D., Stafford, J. M., D'Agostino, R., Shah, A. S., Urbina, E. M., Barrett, C. E., Pihoker, C., Marcovina, S., Liese, A. D., Mottl, A. K., Jensen, E. T., & Wilkening, G. (2023). Diabetes complications and cognitive function in young adults with youth-onset type 1 or type 2 diabetes: The SEARCH for diabetes in youth study. *Pediatric Diabetes, 2023*, 1–10. https://doi.org/10.1155/2023/4860831

Sherr, J. L., Schoelwer, M., Dos Santos, T. J., Reddy, L., Biester, T., Galderisi, A., van Dyk, J. C., Hilliard, M. E., Berget, C., & DiMeglio, L. A. (2022). ISPAD clinical practice consensus guidelines 2022: Diabetes technologies: Insulin delivery. *Pediatric Diabetes, 23*(8), 1406–1431. https://doi.org/10.1111/pedi.13421

Sundberg, F., deBeaufort, C., Krogvold, L., Patton, S., Piloya, T., Smart, C., Van Name, M., Weissberg-Benchell, J., Silva, J., & diMeglio, L. A. (2022). ISPAD clinical practice consensus guidelines 2022: Managing diabetes in preschoolers. *Pediatric Diabetes, 23*(8), 1496–1511. https://doi.org/10.1111/pedi.13427

Sweeting, A., Wong, J., Murphy, H. R., & Ross, G. P. (2022). A clinical update on gestational diabetes mellitus. *Endocrine Reviews, 43*(5), 763–793. https://doi.org/10.1210/endrev/bnac003

Taczanowska, A., Schwandt, A., Amed, S., Toth-Heyn, P., Kanaka-Gantenbein, C., Volsky, S. K., Svensson, J., & Szypowska, A. (2021). Celiac disease in children with type 1 diabetes varies around the world: An international, cross-sectional study of 57.375 patients from the SWEET registry. *Journal of Diabetes, 13*(6), 448–457. https://doi.org/10.1111/1753-0407.13126

Tauschmann, M., Forlenza, G., Hood, K., Cardona-Hernandez, R., Giani, E., Hendrieckx, C., DeSalvo, D. J., Laffel, L. M., Saboo B., Wheeler, B. J., Laptev, D. N., Yarhere, I., & DiMeglio, L. A. (2022) ISPAD clinical practice consensus guidelines 2022: Diabetes technologies: Glucose monitoring. *Pediatric Diabetes, 23*(8), 1390–1405. https://doi.org/10.1111/pedi.13451

U.S. Department of Education, Office for Civil Rights. (2023, July). *Free appropriate public education for students with disabilities: Requirements under section 504 of the Rehabilitation Act of 1973.* https://www2.ed.gov/about/offices/list/ocr/docs/edlite-FAPE504.html

U.S. Food and Drug Administration. (2020, August). *FDA approves first-of-its-kind automated insulin delivery and monitoring system for use in young pediatric patients.* https://www.fda.gov/news-events/press-announcements/fda-approves-first-its-kind-automated-insulin-delivery-and-monitoring-system-use-young-pediatric

Vanderniet, J. A., Jenkins, A. J., & Donaghue, K. C. (2022). Epidemiology of type 1 diabetes. *Current Cardiology Reports, 24*(10), 1455–1465. https://doi.org/10.1007/s11886-022-01762-w

Virmani, A., Brink, S. J., Middlehurst, A., Mohsin, F., Giraudo, F., Sarda, A., Ajmal, S., von Oettingen, J. E., Pillay, K., Likitmaskul, S., Calliari, L. E., & Craig, M. E. (2022). ISPAD clinical practice consensus guidelines 2022: Management of the child, adolescent, and young adult with diabetes in limited resource settings. *Pediatric Diabetes, 23*(8), 1529–1551. https://doi.org/10.1111/pedi.13456

Vounzoulaki, E., Khunti, K., Abner, S. C., Tan, B. K., Davies, M. J., & Gillies, C. L. (2020). Progression to type 2 diabetes in women with a known history of gestational diabetes: Systematic review and meta-analysis. *BMJ, 369*, m1361. https://doi.org/10.1136/bmj.m1361

Wojciechowska, J., Krajewski, W., Zatoński, T., & Rodriguez-Saldana, J. (2023). Diabetes and cancer. In J. Rodriguez-Saldana (Ed.), *The diabetes textbook: Clinical principles, patient management and public health issues* (2nd ed., pp. 1041–1060). Springer International Publishing. https://doi.org/10.1007/978-3-031-25519-9

Xu, B., Xing, A., & Li, S. (2022). The forgotten type 2 diabetes mellitus medicine: Rosiglitazone. *Diabetology International, 13*(1), 49–65. https://doi.org/10.1007/s13340-021-00519-0

Yonkaitis, C. F., & Jacobs, J. (2022). Undesignated glucagon in Illinois: An issue of access and equity. *NASN School Nurse, 37*(6), 331–336. https://doi.org/10.1177/1942602X221120820

Chapter 24

Students With Select Chronic Conditions

Margaret W. Bultas

CHAPTER OUTLINE

Although there is no one single definition of a chronic condition in childhood in the United States, approximately 20% of children and youth have a special healthcare need lasting at least 1 year (Maternal and Child Health Bureau, 2022). Today, school nurses are managing increasingly complex health conditions in the school setting because all children have the right to attend school (Individuals With Disabilities Education Improvement Act [IDEA] of 2004; Section 504 of the Rehabilitation Act of 1973). The purpose of this chapter is to discuss less prevalent chronic health conditions of childhood not discussed elsewhere in this text. Organized according to bodily systems, this chapter presents a synopsis of less common chronic conditions experienced by students and provides suggested nursing interventions to allow the student to maximize learning.

Chronic conditions can originate in any organ system and the impact of these conditions on the student may increase or decrease over time. Chronic conditions diagnosed during the school-age and adolescent years may be identified by the school nurse during health office encounters, be identified outside of the school system, or the child may have had the condition since birth. The school nurse should remember that students may present with more than one condition, which may complicate care. Examples of individualized healthcare plans (IHPs), 504 accommodation plans, and emergency action plans (EAPs) are included throughout in different formats, because there is no standard prototype. See Chapter 8 for more information on student health and education plans. Health and education-related concepts common to many students with chronic conditions are discussed in Chapter 20.

ALTERATIONS IN CARDIOVASCULAR HEALTH

In children, cardiovascular alterations include congenital heart defects and acquired heart conditions such as hypertension, rheumatic heart disease, cardiomyopathy, and Kawasaki disease. Congenital heart anomalies and defects are one of the most common birth defects, occurring in 6 to 10 per 1,000 live births (Chu et al., 2017) and are due to an interaction of environmental and genetic factors (Scott & Neal, 2021). Chronic heart defects are commonly associated with genetic syndromes such as trisomy 21, Turner syndrome, DiGeorge syndrome, Noonan syndrome, and Marfan syndrome, among others. Congenital heart defects involve structural defects of the septum, valves, or major blood vessels that may alter the flow and pressure of blood through the heart, often resulting in symptoms of hypoxemia and/or congestive heart failure. Many congenital heart defects require corrective surgery before the child enters the school system and no further interventions are necessary; other cardiac conditions require ongoing care by a cardiologist. Due to advances in medications and interventions, the mortality rate for congenital heart defects has decreased significantly; there are more than 2.4 million adults in the United States who are survivors of congenital heart disease (Zimmerman et al., 2020). However, children with a history of a congenital heart defect are more likely to miss days in school, have challenges participating in sports or physical activities, and have been found to have more difficulty with learning and focusing (Farr et al., 2018).

Hypertension

Rates of hypertension in the pediatric population have increased significantly over the last decade; this trend is attributed to the increase in childhood obesity (Fox, 2021). Students with body mass index (BMI) greater than 95% have significantly increased risk of developing hypertension (Bell et al., 2019). Blood pressure categories and parameters are different for children less than 13 years of age and for those over 13 years of age. For children less than 13 years of age, the categorical ranges are developed based on sex, age, and height (considering normal weight percentiles). For children 13 years and older, the categories interface with the adult categories as shown in Table 24-1.

Hypertension is further classified as either primary (idiopathic) or secondary, which is attributed to another disease process such as kidney failure. Risk factors for development of primary hypertension include genetics, obesity, insulin resistance, low birth weight, sleep disorders, and a maternal history of smoking (Fox, 2021). Lifestyle choices, including sedentary activity level, diet, smoking, and stress, are also implicated in primary hypertension. Common causes of secondary hypertension include congenital heart disease, renal disorders, endocrine disorders, and autoimmune diseases.

Childhood hypertension is associated with increased risk of adult hypertension and other comorbidities (Fox, 2021). Additionally, long-term hypertension causes damage to the heart and vasculature. Hypertrophy of the left ventricle, increased thickness of the carotid artery, and calcification of the coronary arteries can lead to cardiac compromise in early adulthood and an early death.

All children over the age of 3 years should be screened regularly for hypertension, especially those who are obese or have a known risk factor for the development (Flynn et al., 2017). Important aspects of screening include the use of the appropriate-size blood pressure cuff and obtaining a manual blood pressure reading as these provide a more accurate measure (Fox, 2021). Before taking the reading, it is important to allow the student to rest in a normal seated position with uncrossed legs for a few minutes to gain an accurate reading. Blood pressure screening by the school nurse is an important way to identify hypertension as most children exhibit no other symptoms. Students with elevated blood pressure should be referred to their healthcare provider for further evaluation. Children who present with increased blood pressure along with symptoms of headache, dizziness, or visual changes warrant immediate evaluation by a healthcare provider (Fox, 2021).

TABLE 24-1 Blood Pressure Categories in Children ≥13 Years

Blood Pressure Category	Children ≥ 13 years
Normal BP	<120/< 80 mm Hg
Elevated BP	120/<80 to 129/<80 mm Hg
Stage 1 Hypertension	130/80 to 139/89 mm Hg
Stage 2 Hypertension	≥140/90 mm Hg

Flynn et al. (2017).

Did You Know?

Students with stage 2 hypertension should not be cleared to participate in sports until further evaluation. Additionally, these athletes should avoid heavy intensity static exercises such as powerlifting and bodybuilding (Fox, 2021).

Initial interventions for children with elevated blood pressure include lifestyle modifications such as physical activity, decreased sodium intake, weight control, healthy eating habits/nutritional consultation, and promoting healthy sleep habits (Fox, 2021). Once lifestyle modifications have been maximized or if the blood pressure is remaining in the stage 2 category, oral antihypertensives may be indicated. However, many antihypertensives are considered off-label use in children.

Congestive Heart Failure and Hypoxemia

Congestive heart failure (CHF) may occur as a result of a congenital heart defect, as a consequence of an acquired heart condition, or secondary to a chronic respiratory condition such as cystic fibrosis or chronic asthma. CHF is often a final outcome of significant heart conditions (Price, 2019). Some acquired conditions resulting in CHF are rheumatic fever, hypertension, myocarditis/endocarditis, radiation and chemotherapy for cancer, arrhythmias, and sickle cell disease.

CHF results from increased pressure or volume that strains the myocardium, leading to reduced cardiac output and a backup of blood in the cardiac circulation. Impaired ventricular contractility and increased systemic blood pressure also strain the myocardium, causing it to weaken and lead to CHF. Failure in one chamber usually causes a change in another chamber. As the heart muscle becomes damaged, it is unable to maintain adequate cardiac output to meet the body's oxygen demands and needs (Watanabe & Shih, 2020). This decreased cardiac output leads to decreased blood flow to the kidneys and stimulates sodium and water reabsorption, fluid volume overload, and an increase in systemic blood pressure (Watanabe & Shih, 2020). The additional fluid increases the workload of the heart leading to pulmonary congestion and peripheral edema.

The decreased cardiac output from CHF may present in children as tachypnea and tachycardia at rest, dyspnea, activity intolerance, cool extremities with delayed capillary refill, and chest pain (Price, 2019). The peripheral effects from CHF are less commonly seen in children but may present as lung congestion, murmur, weight gain caused by fluid retention, edema, and hepatomegaly (Price, 2019). Decreased food intake because of decreased energy to eat is a classic sign of CHF, especially in young children.

Students with CHF may experience hypoxemia, an arterial oxygen saturation below normal limits, which may result in cyanosis of the skin, especially around the mouth (circumoral cyanosis) and mucous membranes caused by deoxygenated hemoglobin. The school nurse can use pulse oximetry as a helpful tool to assess hypoxemia; however, oximetry often overestimates oxygen saturation in readings below 90% (Kim et al., 2019). The nurse should consult with the student's healthcare provider to determine the student's normal oxygen saturation at rest and when intervention is needed. The nurse should also note that chronic hypoxemia can result in polycythemia (increased numbers of red blood cells [RBCs] associated with hypoxemia) and clubbing of the digits. Polycythemia places the student at risk for thrombosis. Many students with cardiovascular alterations are on anticoagulant and antiplatelet medications (Abdelghani et al., 2021).

Chronic hypoxia places the child at risk for developmental delays and neurological complications of stroke. Children with hypoxemia may have difficulty concentrating and learning difficulty in the academic setting (Liamlahi & Latal, 2019), qualifying them for special education and an individualized education program (IEP). Modifications for physical education may be necessary and healthcare provider clearance should be obtained for sports. Contact sports should be avoided for students with pacemakers or those taking anticoagulants.

The treatment goals for CHF and hypoxemia include decreasing cardiac demands to improve cardiac function, removing accumulated fluid and sodium when indicated, supporting nutritional requirements, and managing symptoms (Price, 2019). Control of CHF is usually achieved using diuretics, inotropes (e.g., digitalis, dopamine), and afterload reducers (e.g., hydralazine, nitroprussides, and captopril). Dietary restriction of sodium and fluids may be recommended for some children to help decrease fluid retention (Price, 2019). Students with CHF in distress need to rest, may need oxygen, and may be more comfortable in a seated position rather than lying flat. Oxygen is a medication and requires a medical order from a licensed prescriber. Additionally, students with CHF have increased metabolic needs, which may result in poor growth if additional nutritional requirements are not met (Rohit & Budakoty, 2020). Students with arrhythmias should avoid caffeine-containing foods and drinks.

Rheumatic Fever and Rheumatic Heart Disease

Rheumatic fever refers to the body's autoimmune inflammatory response to upper airway infections caused by group A beta-hemolytic *Streptococcus* (group A strep), typically pharyngitis (Delaney et al., 2017). Rheumatic fever can affect the joints, skin, brain, and heart (de Loizaga & Beaton, 2021). It most often occurs in children ages 5 to 15 years as they are most frequently affected with repeated streptococcal infections (de Loizaga & Beaton, 2021). Prevalence of rheumatic fever in the United States is low; however, globally rheumatic fever contributes significantly to cardiovascular morbidity and mortality (Arvind & Ramakrishnan, 2020). Therefore, students who immigrate may have higher rates of rheumatic fever–related complications.

Signs and symptoms of rheumatic fever vary widely for subclinical to acute. Common presentations include fever, throat pain, headaches, and chills (Chowdhury et al., 2023). Gastrointestinal symptoms such as abdominal pain, nausea, and vomiting may be present. Migrating joint pain resembling arthritis occurs in 60% to 80% of cases manifested typically by erythema, swelling, and tenderness in the large joints such as the knees, ankles, or wrists. Carditis is the most serious concern in rheumatic fever which can affect the pericardium, layers of the heart wall, heart valves, and most commonly the mitral valve.

Rheumatic fever is preventable with appropriate and timely antibiotic treatment of group A strep infections. The primary goal of treatment for rheumatic fever includes prevention of permanent cardiac damage and recurrences of rheumatic fever. Recurrence of rheumatic fever can be as high as 50% (Watkins et al., 2018). Penicillin is the drug of choice, with erythromycin as a substitute in penicillin-sensitive children. The recommendation is to receive prophylactic antibiotics until age 21 years whether or not carditis was present; prophylaxis may extend beyond 21 years of age if there is an increased risk of recurrent group A strep infection after age 21 (de Loizaga & Beaton, 2021). Joint pain usually resolves in a few weeks and is commonly treated with nonsteroidal anti-inflammatory drugs (NSAIDs). School nurses play an important role in rheumatic fever reduction by referring students to a healthcare provider when they suspect group A strep pharyngitis.

Rheumatic heart disease is an acquired cardiac connective tissue disorder following a single or repeated group A strep infections damaging the cardiac valves. Clinical manifestations, presence of group A strep antibodies, and echocardiography confirm a diagnosis of rheumatic heart disease (Delaney et al., 2017). The mitral valve is affected in almost all cases of rheumatic heart disease. Mitral regurgitation is the most common problem in children; a murmur is heard on auscultation. Mitral regurgitation is generally mild to moderate in severity and typically well tolerated without medical intervention. Mitral stenosis may also be present less commonly.

Rheumatic heart disease may affect more than one cardiac valve. The aortic valve is involved in 20% to 30% of cases resulting in aortic regurgitation and sometimes aortic stenosis. The tricuspid valve is affected in 15% to 40% of cases. The pulmonary valve is rarely affected (Sika-Pautonu et al., 2017). Significant cases of rheumatic heart disease can be progressive and lead to CHF. Long-term cardiac follow-up may be necessary for individuals who develop valvular heart disease or CHF. Activity restrictions or modifications at school may be indicated for students with advanced rheumatic heart disease.

Cardiomyopathy

Pediatric *cardiomyopathy* denotes disease of the myocardium, or heart muscle (National Organization for Rare Disorders [NORD], 2023). The incidence of cardiomyopathy in the pediatric population is approximately 1 in 100,000 children in both males and females equivalently. The prevalence is thought to be higher due to an unknown number of children who are asymptomatic and therefore undiagnosed. Cardiomyopathy is often progressive and associated with significant mortality and morbidity. It is the most common reason for heart transplants in children over 1 year of age (Lipshultz et al., 2019).

Causes of pediatric cardiomyopathy may be inherited or acquired, including genetic abnormalities, bacterial or viral myocarditis, or excessive exposure to toxins such as heavy metals or alcohol. However, the etiology is unknown in approximately 79% of cases (NORD, 2023). Cardiomyopathy may be present at birth or occur at any time during life; however, children are 10 times more likely to develop cardiomyopathy in the first year of life than between the ages of 2 and 18 years.

According to NORD (2023), there are several different categories and subtypes of cardiomyopathy:

- ***Ischemic cardiomyopathy*** refers to a lack of blood flow and oxygen (ischemia) to the heart and in pediatrics is due to a congenital abnormality of the blood vessels that supply the heart (coronary arteries).
- ***Nonischemic cardiomyopathy*** refers to structural damage or malfunction of the heart muscle due to causes other than coronary artery abnormalities (para. 2).

Almost all pediatric cases are nonischemic cardiomyopathy, mostly affecting the left ventricle and less commonly involving the right ventricle and atria (NORD, 2023). The most common subtypes of cardiomyopathy are dilated cardiomyopathy and hypertrophic cardiomyopathy.

- ***Dilated cardiomyopathy*** may be inherited or acquired. It primarily affects the left ventricle wherein the walls of the heart muscle are stretched and thinned, resulting in decreased strength of contractions and reduced cardiac output leading to CHF (NORD, 2023).
- ***Hypertrophic cardiomyopathy*** is an inherited autosomal dominant condition in over 50% of cases. It decreases cardiac output as a result of abnormal thickening and stiffening of the heart wall (National Center for Chronic Disease Prevention and Health Promotion, 2017). Hypertrophic cardiomyopathy is a common cause of sudden cardiac death in adolescents and young adults; symptoms include anginal chest pain, dysrhythmias, and syncope (Choudhry et al., 2019).

Treatments for cardiomyopathy are supportive and include lifestyle changes, medications, surgery, implanted pacemakers to correct arrhythmias, or a heart transplant (NORD, 2023). The school nurse should work with the student's family and healthcare provider regarding accommodations at school and physical activity levels. Children should be allowed to self-restrict and stop activity to rest when they feel symptomatic. Contact sports are generally restricted, especially if the child has a pacemaker or takes medication that interferes with clotting.

An emergency action plan (EAP) should be developed in conjunction with the healthcare provider and family because students with cardiomyopathy are at risk for sudden cardiac arrest. Staff should have cardiopulmonary resuscitation (CPR) training and an automated external defibrillator (AED) should be on site. Students who demonstrate the following signs and symptoms should be referred for immediate medical attention: dizziness or fainting, shortness of breath, rapid or irregular heartbeat, chest pain or pressure, disorientation, or new-onset exercise intolerance (Garcia & Peddy, 2018). The school nurse should be alert for signs of infection, especially for post–heart transplant students who are immunocompromised. Students with advanced cardiomyopathy may have orders for *Do Not Attempt Resuscitation* (DNAR) or *Practitioner (or Physician, Provider, or Medical) Order for Life Sustaining Treatment* (POLST or MOLST), which should be honored at school (see Chapter 20).

Kawasaki Disease

Kawasaki disease is a febrile illness that causes inflammation of blood vessels and can result in cardiovascular and coronary artery complications. The etiology is unknown but is suspected to be linked to a preceding viral illness (Rowley, 2020). Kawasaki disease is a common cause of acquired heart disease primarily affecting children younger than 5 years of age. The incidence is highest in Japan; incidence in the United States is estimated to affect between 9% and 20% of children under 5 years of age (Centers for Disease Control and Prevention [CDC], 2020). Typical manifestations of Kawasaki disease include fever for more than 5 days, bilateral conjunctival inflammation without exudate, erythema of the lips and a "strawberry" tongue, polymorphous rash, cervical lymphadenopathy, and peeling of skin on the hands and feet (Diorio et al., 2020). Inflammation of the vessels can damage the coronary arteries and may lead to aneurysms. Diagnosis is based on clinical findings and is time sensitive to prevent cardiovascular damage.

Without treatment, about 20% of children with Kawasaki disease will develop a coronary artery aneurysm placing them at risk for rupture (Diorio et al., 2020). The child is at greatest risk for aneurysm development during the subacute phase, which occurs after the fever resolves and lasts about 3 weeks. Aneurysm rupture can lead to myocardial infarction and sudden death. Symptoms of acute myocardial infarction in children may include abdominal pain, vomiting, restlessness, inconsolable crying, pallor, and shock (McCrindle et al., 2017). In the initial acute period, treatment of Kawasaki disease includes high-dose IV gamma globulin and salicylate therapy. Low-dose aspirin is continued in children without evidence of coronary abnormalities until the platelet count has returned to normal, which is usually 6 to 8 weeks. Most children recover completely with no special adaptations needed.

Multisystem Inflammatory Syndrome in Children

Multisystem inflammatory syndrome in children, also referred to as MIS-C, is a cluster of symptoms that appears in children post infection with SARS-Co-V-2 (COVID-19) infection. Multisystem inflammatory syndrome in children is an emerging disorder that produces a range of clinical symptoms appearing about 4 to 6 weeks after a COVID-19 infection (Soma et al., 2021). Multisystem inflammatory syndrome in children is thought to be caused by an ongoing inflammatory response from an inefficient or altered immune response to a COVID-19 infection; most children recover fully but some become severely ill (Soma et al., 2021).

The signs and symptoms may vary, but common presentations include the following:

- Kawasaki disease–like features: conjunctivitis, red eyes; red or swollen hands and feet; rash; red, cracked lips; swollen glands. In some children, coronary artery enlargement and/or aneurysms have been described. Some children presenting with Kawasaki disease–like syndrome have been noted to have a broader age range and present with more gastrointestinal (abdominal pain or diarrhea) and neurological (headaches/meningitis) manifestations.
- Gastrointestinal symptoms such as abdominal pain, diarrhea, nausea/vomiting (patients have presented with colitis, hepatitis, and questionable appendicitis)
- Toxic shock syndrome–like features with hemodynamic instability and poor heart function
- Cytokine storm/macrophage activation or hyperinflammatory features
- Thrombosis or acute kidney injury
- Shortness of breath suggestive of congestive heart failure or pulmonary embolism
- Respiratory symptoms typically reported in adults with COVID-19 may or may not be present in pediatric patients with MIS-C (American Academy of Pediatrics [AAP], 2023, para. 4).

MIS-C is potentially life-threatening. Children with acute MIS-C require hospitalization, often intensive care (AAP, 2023). Treatment depends on the severity of presenting symptoms. School nurses may be the first to identify symptoms of MIS-C in students who present with new complaints of activity intolerance, changes in neurological status, or gastrointestinal symptoms 4 to 6 weeks after a COVID-19 infection or exposure (Bultas & Fuller, 2021). Students should be referred to tertiary care without delay.

Care of Students With Cardiovascular Alteration

For children with a history of cardiovascular alteration, it is important to have baseline information including vital signs, respiratory effort, color, weight, presence of murmur, and activity level, including any activity restrictions. The school nurse should monitor for changes in vital signs (including pulse oximetry); respiratory effort, including changes with exertion; weight gain, which could be an indicator of fluid retention; complaints of chest pain; and syncope (Garcia & Peddy, 2018). Accurate records on height, weight, and body mass index (BMI) are also important as they help monitor proper growth, development, and obesity, which may be a risk for children who have activity restrictions.

The school nurse should have a current list of medications the student is taking. These may include medications that alter blood pressure and heart rate and prolong bleeding, which can increase risk of bruising, petechiae, and bleeding. Many cardiovascular medications have the potential for serious interactions with foods, supplements, vitamins, and other medications. For example, NSAIDs can decrease the effectiveness of beta blockers and angiotensin-converting enzyme inhibitors. If the student is taking a digoxin preparation, it is important to know that vomiting and anorexia may occur secondary to digoxin toxicity. Also, grapefruit is known to interact with many medications, including those taken for blood pressure control, lowering of cholesterol, transplant rejection, antiarrhythmics, and antianxiety medications (U.S. Food and Drug Administration, 2021).

The student with cardiac conditions that present a potential risk should wear a medical alert bracelet for emergency situations. Parents and school staff should be trained in CPR and an AED should be on site. Care should be taken to monitor exposure to infectious diseases and early identification of illness as these can exacerbate the student's condition by increasing metabolic rate and oxygen demands. Last, some students may need modified meals or have dietary and fluid restrictions. These may require the school nurse to work with classroom teachers and cafeteria personnel to ensure nutritious meals.

A plan should be developed to account for missed school due to hospitalizations, recuperation from surgery, and healthcare provider visits. The student may qualify for a Section 504 plan or may need home or in-hospital schooling for prolonged absences. The student should be allowed to participate in activity as allowed and tolerated (Scott & Neal, 2021); students should not be placed in a situation where they cannot rest or are pushed beyond fatigue. Psychosocially, children could have body image concerns related to scars, small stature, or exercise intolerance. IHPs may be necessary to address learning delays and developmental disabilities, which are not uncommon in children with chronic cardiovascular disease (Liamlahi & Latal, 2019). See Box 24-1 for an EAP and Online Materials OM-1 for IHP for a student with cardiovascular disease.

Practice Connection

Individualized healthcare plans (IHPs) for students with special healthcare needs are nursing care plans written by school nurses for nurses. IHPs are written in nursing language to communicate the plan of care consistently between nurses. IHPs are important to document that the student is receiving comprehensive school health services. IHPs are confidential because they contain more protected health information than lay personnel usually need to know. Generally, IHPs should *not* be shared with educational staff.

Emergency actions plans (EAPs) are written by school nurses in lay language for "need to know" school staff. EAPs outline how nonnurses should identify and respond to a health emergency in the absence of a nurse or until a nurse or emergency medical services arrive and assume care. EAPs are confidential but should be shared with the school staff who may need to respond.

ALTERATIONS IN GASTROINTESTINAL HEALTH

Chronic gastrointestinal (GI) system conditions can affect students in the school setting and frequently lead to complaints of pain, constipation, diarrhea, upset stomach, bloating, and missed school days. Some of the most common conditions seen in the school setting include gastroesophageal reflux, inflammatory bowel disease, celiac disease, and GI symptoms associated with cystic fibrosis. The school nurse should be aware that foods the student eats during the day may either exacerbate or reduce symptoms.

Cystic Fibrosis

Cystic fibrosis (CF) is a disorder that affects many organ systems, most significantly the GI and respiratory systems. See Chapter 22 for information on the respiratory manifestations of CF. CF affects all parts of the GI system including the intestines, pancreas, and liver. Almost all students with CF report some degree of gastroesophageal reflux, which is thought to be related to prolonged gastric emptying and increased abdominal pressure from frequent coughing (Konrad et al., 2022). A high-fat diet is recommended for energy and weight gain. Approximately 85% of children with CF will be affected by pancreatic insufficiency from thick mucus obstructing the pancreatic duct. Pancreatic insufficiency leads to alteration in food and nutrient absorption in the gut, altered stools, and pancreatitis in some cases. Students with CF take oral pancreatic enzymes with each snack and meal to aid the breakdown and digestion of food. CF can also affect the liver causing abnormally thick bile and lead to hepatic fibrosis, gallbladder disease, and biliary cirrhosis. In addition, students with CF may experience intestinal obstruction, constipation, altered microbiome of the intestine, rectal prolapse, and a significant increase in risk of GI cancers (Konrad et al., 2022).

Gastroesophageal Reflux

Gastroesophageal reflux (GER) in children can cause pain, regurgitation, coughing, and respiratory complications such as recurrent pneumonias (Rosen, 2022). GER is

BOX 24-1

Emergency Action Plan for Student With Heart Disease

Student: ______________________________

Grade/Teacher: ______________________________

Parents: ______________________________

Home: ______________ Cell: ______________ Work: ______________

IF YOU SEE THIS:	**DO THIS:**
■ Extremely tired ■ Telling you they feel tired, weak, or dizzy ■ Struggling to keep up their normal pace ■ Irritable ■ Restless ■ Worried or uneasy expression	■ Call nurse ■ Have student sit quietly ■ Encourage slow deep breathing ■ Stay with student ■ Remain calm ■ Call student's emergency contact
■ Difficulty breathing ■ Unable to speak in sentences ■ Flaring nostrils ■ Rubbing or clutching chest ■ Blue- or gray-colored lips ■ Blue- or gray-colored fingernails ■ Becomes UNRESPONSIVE	■ CALL 911 ■ GET AED ■ DO CPR IF INDICATED ■ Call student's emergency contact

Staff members trained in CPR and AED in building:

______________________________ ______________________________

Hospital Preference: ______________________________

Emergency Department # ______________________________

Physician: ______________________________ Contact # ______________

Emergency contact #2 ______________________________

Home: ______________ Cell: ______________ Work: ______________

The parent/guardian agrees with this emergency action plan that will be shared confidentially with appropriate school staff in the best interest of the student.

Copy to: __ Principal __ Secretary __ Parent __ Teachers __ Substitute __ Cafeteria __ Ed Aid __ Phys Ed Teacher __ Playground Monitor __Other

Prepared by: ______________________________ *(School Nurse)* Date: ______________

Contact the school nurse with any questions/concerns.

caused by the relaxation of the lower esophageal sphincter allowing food to reflux back to the esophagus. The acids in refluxed food cause irritation and inflammation of the esophagus leading to classic symptoms of epigastric pain, that is, heartburn. In addition to numerous physiological causes, GER can also be caused by obesity and overeating, which increases abdominal pressure on the lower esophageal sphincter. Other conditions that have similar clinical features as GER include eosinophilic esophagitis, food allergy, achalasia, cyclic vomiting syndrome, pill esophagitis, infectious esophagitis, and rumination syndrome. Diagnosis is made by measuring the esophageal pH or by treating symptoms empirically with acid suppression medications. The mainstay of medication treatment involves acid suppression using H-2 receptor agonists and proton pump inhibitors. More recently, medications to increase GI motility are being used to increase the rate of gastric emptying resulting in a more rapid clearance of acid and food in the stomach (Rosen, 2022). There is a lack of evidence on dietary restriction to relieve symptoms, and restricting food may lead to eating disorders in adolescents. When required, thickening of enteral nutrition may be beneficial for students.

Inflammatory Bowel Disease

Inflammatory bowel disease (IBD) refers to two forms of chronic intestinal inflammation: Crohn's disease and ulcerative colitis. Rates of IBD have increased dramatically, especially in industrialized countries, with the United States having one of the highest rates globally. These increased rates have affected the pediatric population, including children under the age of 6 years (Subedi et al., 2022). About one-third of cases of IBD are diagnosed during childhood or adolescence (GBD 2017 Inflammatory Bowel Disease Collaborators, 2020).

The cause of IBD is not completely understood but is thought to be related to a multitude of factors including genetics, immune dysregulation, and environmental factors (Kleinhenz & Wagner, 2022). Researchers speculate IBD results from defects in the innate and adaptive immune system in genetically susceptible individuals (Subedi et al., 2022). Environmental factors, including reduced enteric pathogen exposures, are implicated in altering the gut microbiome, which has been found to be less diverse in industrialized nations (Subedi et al., 2022). Several environmental triggers have also been implicated in IBD including smoking, diet, stress, sleep, physical activity, gut infections, medication use, and vitamin D ultraviolet light exposure deficiency (Ananthakrishnan, 2015; Zhang & Li, 2014).

Crohn's disease is characterized by inflammation of the full thickness of the bowel. This inflammation involves any part of the GI tract from the mouth to the anus, although it most commonly affects the small intestine and colon (Kleinhenz & Wagner, 2022). Unique to Crohn's disease is the development of "skip lesions" where some parts of the bowel wall are affected while others are not. Common symptoms include abdominal pain, diarrhea, mucus and blood in the stool, fatigue, decreased appetite, and overall malabsorption of nutrients, which can result in weight loss. Fever from the inflammatory response, growth delay due to malabsorption, and delayed sexual development are also seen (Kleinhenz & Wagner, 2022). Chronic inflammation can result in bowel strictures and adhesions from the development of scar tissue, as well as the formation of fistulas and abscesses, which may require surgical intestinal resection (Kleinhenz & Wagner, 2022).

In contrast, ***ulcerative colitis*** involves inflammation of only the mucosal layer of the bowel and is limited to the area of the colon and rectum. Ulcers form on the surface of the bowel lining causing bleeding and tenesmus (urgency to stool) (Subedi et al., 2022). Students with ulcerative colitis usually experience crampy diarrhea, rectal bleeding, blood and mucus in the stool, and abdominal pain. Loss of appetite, weight loss, and fatigue are also common. In cases of severe GI blood loss, anemia may occur. The inflammatory process in the bowel results in decreased absorption because bowel mobility is accelerated. A serious and emergent complication is toxic megacolon. Toxic megacolon is an acute form of colonic distention where gas accumulates and can lead to bowel rupture and enterocolitis (Subedi et al., 2022).

Some individuals with IBD experience symptoms in areas other than the intestines. These include pain in the joints, mouth sores, skin complications such as rashes, and even kidney and liver complications (Crohn's and Colitis Foundation, 2022). These are thought to be related to the altered immune response and inflammation related to IBD. Because the symptoms of Crohn's disease and ulcerative colitis are so similar and children with Crohn's disease have more colon involvement, it is sometimes difficult to establish the diagnosis (Subedi et al., 2022).

The goals of treatment for both forms of IBD include controlling symptoms to achieve remission, healing the mucosa, minimizing the adverse effects of medications and immunosuppression, and optimizing quality of life (Subedi et al., 2022). Treatment involves the use of biological therapies, immunomodulators, nutritional therapies, and surgery. Biological therapies include monoclonal antibodies, which promote mucosal healing and remission by decreasing inflammatory cytokine tumor necrosis factor–alpha (TNF-α). These treatments have been found to reduce the need for surgical intervention; however, they pose risks of immunosuppression and infusion reactions. Immunomodulators are typically used as maintenance therapy as they are effective in inducing remission; however, they lead to an increased risk of infection due to immunosuppression (Subedi et al., 2022).

School nurses should be alert to the increased risk of infection of students with IBD who take immunosuppressive medications. The student's immunization schedule of live-attenuated vaccines (e.g., measles, mumps, rubella [MMR]; varicella, rotavirus, and intranasal influenza) may be altered while receiving immunomodulators and/or biologicals (see discussion later in this chapter) (Subedi et al., 2022). Students receiving methotrexate, a known teratogen, should receive education about contraception. Side effects of long-term corticosteroid therapy, often a part of treatment, include decreased bone density, growth suppression, immunosuppression, and weight gain. Adolescents being treated with metronidazole should be informed that alcohol should be avoided and may result in severe nausea and vomiting. Due to the medications needed to manage IBD, the school nurse should coordinate medication administration to optimize adherence and minimize loss of instructional time.

Adequate nutritional support is important to reduce symptoms and inflammation, correct nutritional deficits, provide adequate energy for healing, and promote normal growth. Exclusive enteral nutrition entails a complete liquid diet with a specific formula, usually for a limited time period (e.g., 6 to 12 weeks). Exclusive enteral nutrition has been found to enhance gut microbiome, decrease inflammation, and improve intestinal wall health with fewer side effects than many of medications (Rehman et al., 2022). The use of partial enteral therapy has been found to be helpful, although less robust of a treatment. Other dietary options can include specific diet therapies that may limit amount and types of carbohydrates or exclude specific foods (e.g., meats, dairy, gluten), as well as anti-inflammatory diets (Rehman et al., 2022).

Surgery may be indicated in IBD when medical treatments are insufficient or intestinal complications develop. Surgical procedures include intestinal resection including the formation of an ileostomy or colostomy. In IBD, the development of fistulas, abscesses, strictures, or perforation often requires surgery. Early and aggressive use of biological agents has reduced the need for surgical intervention (Subedi et al., 2022).

Psychosocially, students with IBD have a higher risk of anxiety and depression related to adjusting to their chronic illness, medication regimen, and dietary restrictions (Subedi et al., 2022). The cosmetic side effects of corticosteroids may be disturbing to the school-age child, overwhelming to the adolescent, and can lead to poor medication adherence. Unwelcome side effects include excessive weight gain, hair growth, and acne. Fortunately, these are temporary conditions that disappear when the dose is lowered or discontinued. If the disease is severe enough to require long-term therapy, alternate-day steroids lessen the impact on growth. Dietary restrictions or the use of enteral nutritional therapies can be challenging for children in school and the school nurse may need to work with the cafeteria staff or the classroom teacher to ensure the student's nutritional needs are met during the school day. Support groups are a helpful resource for some who are having difficulty coping with their illness (Subedi et al., 2022).

Disease symptoms, which often include diarrhea, pain, or gas, may make students fearful of being in school. Section 504 plan accommodations allow students with IBD to leave the classroom quickly without attracting unnecessary attention for bathroom visits. Students may prefer to use the bathroom in the health office; it is a good idea to have extra change of underwear and clothing at school. Teachers need to be educated on the student's health needs. Height and weight for age and BMI are important growth parameters to monitor (Rehman et al., 2022). Vision screening by an eye specialist may be warranted as IBD increases the risk of developing uveitis (Crohn's and Colitis Foundation, 2022). School nurses need to be sensitive to the psychosocial needs of the student and assist them to participate in school activities to the fullest extent possible. Students with IBS benefit from school nurse–led case management as outlined in the IHP. See Box 24-2 for an example of an IHP for a student with inflammatory bowel disease. See Chapter 8, Online Materials OM8-3, for a sample Section 504 plan for a student with inflammatory bowel disease.

Celiac Disease

Celiac disease, also known as celiac sprue or gluten-induced immune-mediated enteropathy, is a chronic disorder. In celiac disease, ingestion of gluten and gluten-related proteins found in wheat, rye, barley, and oats trigger an inappropriate immune response in genetically predisposed individuals. This autoimmune response causes damage to the villi of the small intestine and leads to malabsorption issues (Cheung et al., 2022). Untreated celiac disease is associated with the development of other autoimmune diseases (multiple sclerosis and type 1 diabetes), anemia, and skin rashes, as well as increased risk of intestinal cancer and lymphoma (Celiac Disease Foundation, 2022).

It is difficult to identify the prevalence of celiac disease; it is estimated only about 30% of those with celiac disease are properly diagnosed (Celiac Disease Foundation, 2022). Serological testing can be used to screen for celiac disease; however, a small bowel biopsy of the villi will confirm the diagnosis (Williams et al., 2022). Clinical manifestations are often insidious and chronic. Classic symptoms may not appear for several months after the ingestion of gluten in the diet. In children, manifestations typically include impaired growth, chronic diarrhea, abdominal pain and distention, poor appetite, and chronic fatigue from anemia and malabsorption of nutrients. The stool may be greasy (steatorrhea) and foul-smelling. Older children can develop osteoporosis, delayed puberty, and dental enamel defects (Williams et al., 2022).

Treatment for chronic celiac disease includes a lifelong adherence to a gluten-free diet (Williams et al., 2022). Foods that contain gluten, together with other foods contaminated by these grains, should be completely removed from the diet. The Celiac Disease Foundation (2022) provides a variety of supports including a list of gluten-free foods and a guide to reading food labels. In general, foods made from corn, rice, soy, and potato (without contamination of gluten) as well as fresh fruits and vegetables are usually well tolerated (Williams et al., 2022). Nutritional deficiencies are treated with supplements. For the student with celiac disease, the school nurse may assist in maintaining a gluten-free diet while at school by developing a Section 504 plan. The school nurse should work with the cafeteria personnel to make gluten-free food options available.

Teachers and parents need to know what foods, medications, and commercially available clays for children (e.g., Play-Doh) contain gluten and should be avoided. Gluten cannot be absorbed through the skin; however, attention must be paid to the ingredients in toothpaste and lipstick that may contain gluten. Youth should be counseled that grain alcohols are made with the offending gluten products.

ALTERATIONS IN CELLULAR HEALTH: CANCER

Over 10,000 children under 15 years of age are diagnosed with cancer each year in the United States. Childhood cancers are the second leading cause of death, following accidents, in children ages 5 to 14 years (American Cancer Society, 2022). Although the number of childhood cancer diagnoses has risen, survival rates have dramatically improved (Schmidt et al., 2021). Over the last several decades, pediatric cancer 5-year survival rates have increased to approximately 85% (Siegel et al., 2020).

Cancer occurs when the body is unable to regulate cell division resulting in abnormal cells that proliferate without control (Marsh, 2022). Therefore, cancerous cells do not function normally, cannot fulfill their designated role, and in some cases may fail to mature (referred to as blast cells).

BOX 24-2

Individualized Healthcare Plan for a Student With Inflammatory Bowel Disease (IBD)

Name:
Teacher/Grade:
D.O.B.:
Address:
Parents:
Biographical Data:

Medical Diagnoses: Crohn's disease and ulcerative colitis >6 months
Physician:
Telephone:
Telephone:
Nursing Services:

Allergies:
As-needed (prn) Medication:

NURSING DIAGNOSIS	GOALS	NURSING INTERVENTIONS	EVALUATION
Risk for diarrhea related to gastrointestinal inflammation, infection	The student will participate in the classroom with accommodations.	1. Set guidelines for seeking assistance. • Indications of flare-up of bowel problems such as diarrhea, pain, fever, poor appetite, or weight loss. • Develop a way for the student to inform the teacher she is leaving to go to the bathroom without needing to attract attention of classmates. • Notify healthcare providers as needed.	■ Student will maintain academic progression in classes.
Risk for impaired comfort related to illness-related symptoms	The student will report an increased level of comfort after interventions	1. Work with student to develop consistent system to measure pain. 2. Identify measures that work to decrease discomfort. 3. Provide calm and private environment for student when in pain. 4. Obtain medication and any management measures that need to be done at school. 5. Provide easy access to a bathroom where privacy is ensured. 6. Educate appropriate school staff. • What is IBD and how does it affect the body? • Student's health status • Management measures that need to be done at school • Need for flexible educational programming such as use of the bathroom, past and advance assignments, temporary classroom and physical education adjustments, and rest periods • Encourage staff to ask questions or raise concerns if they have them.	■ Student will list indicators of a flare-up. ■ Student will be free of pain. ■ Student will take prn medication as prescribed.
Nutrition: less than body requirements (intake of nutrients insufficient to meet metabolic needs)	The student will make dietary selections that are nutritionally dense while avoiding trigger foods.	Educate student on appropriate dietary selections. Provide menus to student and parents/guardians. Have nutritionist work with food services to provide appropriate foods.	■ Student will maintain appropriate BMI.

Prepared by: _______ *(School Nurse)* Date: ___________

As these cells continue to rapidly proliferate, they have the ability to invade the surrounding tissue and to metastasize to other areas of the body.

Cancer in children differs from adult cancers. Childhood tumors grow faster than adult tumors because body tissues are normally in a state of rapid growth during childhood and adolescence. Therefore, cancers in children are often seen in body parts that normally experience the most growth: blood, lymph, brain and central nervous system (CNS), and bones. The incidence of cancer increases with age.

The specific cause of childhood cancer is unknown, although particular genetic factors and environmental exposures place children at risk. Cancer predisposition syndromes (CPSs), genetic syndromes that have increased risk of cancer, account for about 10% of childhood cancers, including neurofibromatosis type 1, trisomy 21, retinoblastoma, Noonan syndrome, Beckwith-Wiedemann syndrome, familial adenomatous polyposis, and children with a significant family history of cancer (Kagami et al., 2022). Environmental risk factors include infections that can promote oncogenic changes in the immune system, ionizing radiation exposure during the younger years, air and chemical pollution, smoking, and extremely low frequency magnetic fields (Schmidt et al., 2021).

In children ages 0 to 14 years, the most common types of cancer include leukemias, brain and CNS tumors, lymphomas, neuroblastoma, cancer in the kidney, and bone cancer (Siegel et al., 2021). In adolescents ages 15 to 19 years, the most common cancers are cancer of the brain and CNS, lymphomas, leukemias, thyroid cancer, gonadal (testicular and ovarian) cancer, and bone cancer (Siegel et al., 2021). Clinical manifestations are primarily related to the location of the cancer or tumor.

Leukemia

Leukemia is an unrestricted proliferation of white blood cells (WBCs) in the bone marrow and accounts for about 20% of all cancers in children (Siegel et al., 2017). The two main forms of leukemia in children are *acute lymphocytic leukemia* (ALL) and *acute myelogenous leukemia* (AML). In ALL, there is an increased number of lymphocytes. ALL is the most commonly diagnosed leukemia in children and adolescents. Most cases of ALL are diagnosed between the ages of 2 and 4 years, and in this age group the prognosis is excellent (Inaba & Pui, 2021). In AML, there is an increased number of myeloblasts. AML is more often diagnosed during the teenage years and tends to be challenging to treat (Reinhardt et al., 2022).

Leukemia has had dramatic improvements in survival rates. The 5-year survival rates for children approximate 90% for ALL and 65% to 70% for AML (American Cancer Society, 2019b). In leukemia, the WBCs do not mature and proliferate uncontrollably resulting in the abnormal presence of immature WBCs, or blast cells, in the bloodstream. Blast cells are not effective in fighting infection, and they compete for and deprive the healthy cells of essential nutrients needed for metabolism. Blast cells also "crowd out", or leave little room, for normal red blood cells (RBCs) and platelets. Bone marrow is normally composed of 5% blast cells. In leukemia the bone marrow may be up to 95% blast cells. Children and adolescents often speak of their decreasing blast cell count as a measure of how they are progressing in their treatment.

Leukemia in children often presents with frequent or recurrent infections, fever, upper respiratory infections, pharyngitis, and loss of appetite and weight loss. Other common manifestations include swollen lymph nodes, splenomegaly, and hepatomegaly. Students with associated anemia may present to the health office with pallor, fatigue, and weakness, as well as bleeding tendencies, including bruising and petechiae (American Cancer Society, 2019a). Bone pain is common as the bone marrow hypertrophies and students may present with limping, refusal to bear weight on their legs, or even pathological fractures. Weight loss and swollen lymph nodes may also be present.

Chemotherapy is the primary treatment for children with ALL. Bone marrow transplant may be required in cases of AML and recurrence of ALL (Inaba & Pui, 2021). There are numerous nursing implications for students with leukemia at school with immunocompromised state as the major concern. See Online Materials OM24-2 for an IHP for a student receiving chemotherapeutic treatment.

Lymphomas

Lymphomas are neoplasms in the lymphatic and hematopoietic systems. Lymphomas are categorized as *Hodgkin lymphoma* and *non-Hodgkin lymphoma.* The tumors of Hodgkin lymphoma contain large Reed-Sternberg cells, whereas non-Hodgkin lymphomas do not (Nemours KidsHealth, 2022). There is a strong association between the Epstein-Barr virus and the development of both Hodgkin lymphoma and non-Hodgkin lymphoma (Donzel et al., 2022).

Hodgkin lymphoma is the most common form of lymphoma diagnosed in children and young adults (Simonin et al., 2023). Hodgkin lymphoma is more common in white children than in children of other racial/ethnic groups (National Cancer Institute, 2022). Due to increased knowledge and treatment advances, the 5-year survival rate is 90% to 95% (Simonin et al., 2023).

Manifestations of Hodgkin lymphoma include painless enlargement of lymph nodes (especially cervical or supraclavicular), night sweats, fever of 100.4°F (38°C) or higher for 3 consecutive days, malaise, and unintentional weight loss (10% or more) over the preceding 6 months. Hodgkin lymphoma may metastasize to the spleen, liver, bone marrow, and lungs. The disease is staged according to the number of lymph node sites involved, the presence of extranodal disease, and history of other symptoms (Cheson et al., 2014).

Non-Hodgkin lymphoma is more diffuse, disseminates earlier, spreads more rapidly, and involves a different type of lymphocyte than Hodgkin lymphoma. As non-Hodgkin lymphoma more often presents in advanced stages, which may include metastasis, the 5-year survival rate is lower than for Hodgkin lymphoma (Sehn & Salles, 2021). Children with non-Hodgkin lymphoma have better outcomes than adults diagnosed with non-Hodgkin lymphoma (Sheikh et al., 2022). Nearly all non-Hodgkin lymphoma in children belongs to one of three types: lymphoblastic, Burkitt, or large cell. In non-Hodgkin lymphoma, masses can develop in the mediastinal area. Manifestations include symptoms related to the mass pressing on structures such as the spinal cord, trachea, esophagus, or intestines; dyspnea; pain; altered movement/mobility; abdominal pain; and nausea or vomiting. This cancer may also develop in the tonsils, cervical lymph nodes, or other lymph nodes. Non-Hodgkin lymphoma can spread quickly to the bone marrow, the surface of the brain, and/or the membranes that surround the lungs and heart (Sheikh et al., 2022). Treatment may include surgery to remove masses related to the lymphoma, in addition to chemotherapy and radiation.

Brain and Nervous System Cancer

CNS tumors, including brain tumors, are the most common solid tumor in children and lead to significant morbidity and mortality in children (Udaka & Packer, 2018). Radiation exposure is the only consistent known environmental risk factor for development of brain and CNS tumors (Partap & Monje, 2020). CNS tumors include glial tumors (ependymal, low- and high-grade gliomas, and glioneuronal) and nonglial tumors (embryonal, germ cell, choroid plexus, and craniopharyngioma) (Partap & Monje, 2020). CNS tumors cause symptoms by putting pressure on the neighboring tissue, invading and damaging normal structures, or blocking cerebrospinal fluid pathways. Morning headaches, vomiting, lethargy, visual changes, ataxia, or seizures may develop as the increased intracranial pressure (ICP) progresses. Headaches may be worse in the recumbent position or awaken the child at night. Visual changes may include blurry or double vision, dilated pupils that do not constrict, and cranial nerve IV palsy causing eye deviation. CNS tumors can affect the child's ability to concentrate, and thus academic performance frequently declines.

Neuroblastomas arise in the sympathetic nervous system (extracranial) from immature nerve cells; they are the most common tumors of the nervous system in children 5 years of age and younger (Mahapatra & Challagundla, 2023).

Treatment for central and peripheral nervous system cancers includes surgical removal of the tumor, when possible, as well as chemotherapy and radiation. Advances have been made in treatment for some types of CNS tumors, but most remain difficult to treat. Students may experience long-term effects from the treatment (Partap & Monje, 2020).

Bone Tumors

Osteosarcoma and Ewing sarcoma are the most common primary bone tumors in children and adolescents (Belayneh et al., 2021). Osteosarcoma primarily affects the femur, tibia, and humerus whereas Ewing sarcoma forms in a variety of bone tissues. Manifestations of bone tumors include bone pain, reduced range of motion, swelling or palpable mass, and pathological fracture from a minor injury. Overall prognosis is good; however, metastasis significantly reduces the 5-year survival rate for bone cancer (Belayneh et al., 2021). Treatment includes surgery to remove the tumor along with chemotherapy either before and/or after surgical intervention (Belayneh et al., 2021). Although complete amputation may be necessary, limb-sparing surgery may also be possible with the insertion of a bone prosthesis to preserve the limb.

Bone can be a primary source of cancer and can also be a site of metastasis from other types of cancer. Students with metastasis to the bone from another cancer may also experience bone pain and pathological fractures.

General Considerations for Students Being Treated for Cancer

Treatment for childhood cancer includes aggressive and ongoing treatments, including chemotherapy and radiation. Students may also be recovering from surgical intervention, hematopoietic stem cell transplantation, and immunotherapy. Children in active treatment may be in school; some treatment regimens may take several years to fully complete and involvement in school improves quality of life (Kwak et al., 2021). Frequently, students who are in active treatment phase have either central lines or may have implanted ports that may or may not be accessed during the school day. Central lines and accessed ports should have an intact, occlusive dressing to protect them from being pulled or exposed to trauma. Assessment of the accessed ports or central lines is important to ensure the integrity of the dressing. Extra occlusive dressings and hemostats (clamps) should be available at school. Additionally, the nurse should have orders from the healthcare provider for care of the central line that includes an order to change the dressing if needed. If the catheter is dislodged, there is bleeding from the site, or blood is backing up in the tubing, pressure should be applied, and the parent/guardian and healthcare provider immediately contacted.

Students who are actively in treatment or who have received stem cell transplant are at risk for infection due to immunosuppression (Patel & Green, 2020). Parent/guardians and the healthcare provider should be informed if the student develops fever, signs of infection, or has been potentially exposed to an infectious outbreak (Ruggiero, 2021). Students who are neutropenic or immunosuppressed may need to remain home for a period of time until the risk of infection is reduced or their immune status is stable. Good hand washing is essential and masking may be necessary to protect the student from infection. Students who are currently being treated for cancer may have an altered immunization schedule with some vaccines needing to be repeated and other vaccines deferred until treatment is complete (Close et al., 2020).

Fatigue is a common side effect of chemotherapy, so rest periods may be included in the IHP (Ruggiero, 2021). Nausea, anorexia, and constipation often occur with treatment and may be alleviated with medications and altering feeding to include smaller, frequent meals (Gerceker et al., 2022). Weight loss can be managed with feeding supplementation. Mouth sores also occur as a side effect of treatment and oral care is important (Gerceker et al., 2022). Be aware that even minor trauma may require frequent observation or medical attention if the student has a low platelet count as evidenced by petechiae. Psychosocial aspects related to treatment and diagnosis should be considered (Darcy et al., 2019). It may be necessary to provide education to the student's class or peers, especially if the student has experienced changes in body image such as alopecia, cushingoid appearance because of steroids, or if they have central lines.

Late Effects

Advances in chemotherapy and radiation have significantly improved survival rates for pediatric cancer. However, "late effects" of cancer treatment can develop, manifested by long-term adverse effects on normal, developing tissues that may not be evident for months or years after therapy or treatment has been completed (Landier et al., 2018). Approximately three out of five children who survive childhood cancer will develop late effects (Children's Oncology Group, 2022). Whenever a student has a history of past treatment for cancer, even if they have been free of the primary cancer for years, the school nurse must be observant for the development of additional conditions.

Late effects can affect the function of an organ, growth of structures, cognitive development, mental health, and even have socioeconomic consequences (Erdmann et al., 2021). Cognitively, comprehension and learning can be affected by radiation and chemotherapy. Radiation can physically damage organs causing them to become fibrotic and stiff, as well as affecting future growth of the organ or body system, including the musculoskeletal system (De et al., 2022). Cardiotoxicity can cause cardiomyopathy, fatigue, and damage to the valves and coronary arteries, and can lead to heart arrhythmias and even heart failure (Kendall et al., 2022). Pulmonary complications can develop from pulmonary fibrosis leading to shortness of breath and increased risk of lung infections (Nguyen et al., 2022). Other late effects may include abnormal tooth enamel, early loss of permanent teeth, and increased caries. Sensorimotor hearing loss and tinnitus (ringing in the ears), cataracts, and osteopenia can occur. Late effects also include the risk of developing a second malignancy or rejection of a bone marrow transplant. Bone marrow transplant rejection, called graft vs. host disease, can lead to significant health complications affecting all organs of the body.

Other late effects may be related to surgical intervention. These include the removal of lymph nodes and body parts, which can leave scar tissue, cause physical changes to the musculoskeletal system, increase the development of edema, and lead to body image concerns. Radiation treatments frequently cause the development of scar tissue resulting in pain and adhesions. Late effects from treatments can also alter and delay sexual development and increase risk of infertility.

Of primary concern in the school setting is the onset of neurocognitive late effects, which include learning disabilities and a decline in cognitive scores on comprehension and achievement tests (Daetwyler et al., 2022). Poor hand-eye coordination, attention and memory processing, and mental health concerns may develop. Often, neurocognitive late effects can be the result of chemotherapies administered intrathecally and radiation treatments to the head. The development of neurological effects, including seizures, headaches, and altered pituitary function, may also occur (Daetwyler et al., 2022).

There may come a time when treatment options have been exhausted. At this time, care of the child moves from focusing on a cure to providing comfort and quality of life. Physical fatigue, increased pain and discomfort, decreased mobility, change in body appearance, and decreased appetite are commonly seen in the terminal stages of cancer. Children may still want to continue to attend school during this time, and the school can provide support and assistance that helps keep them involved in the school community. See Chapter 21 for a discussion of *Do Not Attempt Resuscitation* orders in the school setting.

ALTERATIONS IN HEMATOLOGICAL/ IMMUNOLOGICAL HEALTH

Students may also be affected by chronic conditions of the hematological and immunological systems. These include conditions affecting the platelets, such as immune (idiopathic) thrombocytopenic purpura (ITP); conditions affecting clotting, such as hemophilia and von Willebrand disease; conditions affecting the RBCs, such as sickle cell disease and anemia; and conditions affecting immune function such as human immunodeficiency virus (HIV). The school nurse should have plans in place to manage these conditions since improved treatments mean more students are in school with these chronic conditions.

Students taking anti-inflammatory medications for hematological or immunological diseases are at risk for immunosuppression. Medications that can cause immunosuppression include long-term cortisone preparations for autoimmune conditions, ongoing chemotherapy treatments for cancer, and antirejection medications for the post–organ transplant period. Rarely, students may have primary immune deficiency conditions that put them at increased risk for infection, including agammaglobulinemia, DiGeorge syndrome, and deficiencies of specific cell lines.

Surveillance related to infection risk is an essential role for the school nurse. These students may not always demonstrate the typical symptoms of infection and illness. Cuts or signs of illness need prompt attention, immunizations may be deferred, and families need to be informed immediately if outbreaks of infectious diseases occur at school.

Hemophilia

Hemophilia is a genetic condition that causes a deficiency of clotting factors. The type of hemophilia is determined by the clotting factor affected. The most common types of hemophilia involve factor VIII (known as hemophilia A) and factor IX (known as hemophilia B or Christmas disease). Deficiencies can occur in any factor, but A and B are sex-linked. The defective gene is passed from mother to son, who will exhibit the bleeding disorder. There are about 30,000 males in the United States living with hemophilia; hemophilia A is four times more common than hemophilia B (CDC, 2022a). Females can become disease carriers when a father passes his affected X chromosome to his daughter, who may be healthy or may be mildly affected. Hemophilia may also result from new mutations with no known family history (Alblaihed et al., 2022). Deficiencies in other clotting factors can occur in either sex.

Regardless of the type of hemophilia, the result is an interference with the ability of the blood to appropriately clot, resulting in bleeding episodes. Depending on the amount of clotting factor in the blood, hemophilia ranges from mild to severe. Children with severe hemophilia present with significant bleeding episodes in the first 2 years of life, whereas those with mild hemophilia may go undiagnosed for years. Signs associated with hemophilia include excessive or prolonged bleeding and bruising after an injury, trauma, blood draw, or invasive medical procedure (Alblaihed et al., 2022). Hemarthrosis, or bleeding into the joints, can also result from injury and presents as warm, painful joints with decreased range of motion. Repeated joint bleeding can lead to irreversible damage causing arthritis, chronic pain, and reduced quality of life over time (Regling et al., 2022).

Intracranial bleeding, which can occur from even a minor head injury, is the most severe bleeding complication and leading cause of death in hemophilia (Alblaihed et al., 2022). Typical signs of intracranial bleeding include signs of increased intracranial pressure such as headache, vomiting, change in behavior, double vision, or seizures. Students with a history of intracranial bleeding may have ongoing disabilities including cognitive impairments and motor dysfunction.

New pharmacological therapies have greatly reduced bleeding episodes and improved the quality of life for individuals with hemophilia. Students with severe hemophilia or multiple joint bleeding episodes typically receive regular and routine prophylaxis with factor concentrates (recombinant or plasma derived) or nonfactor treatments (monoclonal antibody) (Regling et al., 2022). Studies show regular prophylaxis, compared with on demand factor treatment at the time of injury, has reduced bleeds and significantly reduced joint damage, improved quality of life, and increased life span. About one-third of those with hemophilia A develop neutralizing antibodies to factor VIII concentrates, leading to a decreased effectiveness (Regling et al., 2022). Other treatments include desmopressin acetate/vasopressin (DDAVP), antifibrinolytic medications, or newer gene therapy treatments. DDAVP, administered via nasal spray or injection, may be sufficient for treating mild hemophilia by increasing the level of factor VIII. Parents may be taught to administer factor concentrates via venous access or to administer nonfactor treatments by subcutaneous injection (Regling et al., 2022).

Nonpharmacological management includes rest, ice, compression, and elevation. Cold compresses applied to joints or areas of injury help to decrease bleeding and swelling. Elevating an affected extremity above the level of the heart and applying an elastic bandage and firm pressure for 10 to 15 minutes will help reduce bleeding. Bleeding that does not stop after 10 minutes should be referred for immediate care. Nosebleeds may require continuous pressure for 10 minutes or longer. Any head trauma requires a medical evaluation. All injuries and interventions require notification of the parent/guardian .

It is important that students maintain a BMI within normal range and exercise regularly to decrease extra weight on affected joints. A medical alert bracelet is recommended. An IHP should be developed, and an EAP outlining how to handle a bleeding situation in the absence of a nurse should be given to the student's teachers and need-to-know staff.

Von Willebrand Disease

Von Willebrand disease is the most common inherited bleeding disorder characterized by low levels of von Willebrand factor. Although von Willebrand disease occurs in both males and females, it disproportionately affects females due to hemostatic events such as menstruation and pregnancy (VanderMeulen et al., 2022). About 30% of von Willebrand disease is inherited, with the remaining cases as new mutations. Von Willebrand disease is considered a disorder of multiple genetic risk factors, with the type O blood group having a higher incidence (Sadler et al., 2022). It is suspected that the true number of cases of von Willebrand disease is underreported because symptoms may be mild in nature (Berntorp et al., 2022). Although clotting factors are produced in the liver, von Willebrand factor is a protein that is produced in the body tissue. It is released after trauma to the tissue and helps platelets stick together to form a blood clot; when it is deficient, the clot cannot develop, and bleeding ensues. Signs and symptoms of von Willebrand disease are similar to those of hemophilia (CDC, 2022c).

There are three types of von Willebrand disease. Most individuals have the mild form that responds well to medications such as DDAVP (Sadler et al., 2022). DDAVP is used to increase the release of von Willebrand factor from the endothelial lining of blood vessels. Individuals who are unable to take DDAVP or need more comprehensive treatment can receive von Willebrand factor replacement, which is given by IV infusion. Women who have heavy menstrual bleeding can use a combination of oral contraceptives, which helps increase von Willebrand factor, increase factor VIII in the blood, and prevent heavy menstrual flow (Eladly & Miesbach, 2022). School nurses should refer students with bleeding issues for medical evaluation, such as females with routinely heavy menstrual periods, or students who have frequent nose bleeds or who experience excessive or prolonged bleeding/bruising after injury.

Students with hemophilia or von Willebrand disease can lead active lives; however, precautions should be taken. The student's accommodations should be outlined in a Section 504 plan. The school nurse should develop an EAP that outlines how school staff should respond in the absence of a nurse if the student is injured or there is evidence of bleeding. Medical orders often indicate that contact sports should be avoided. Safe sports include swimming (but not diving), biking, golf, and walking. Medications that interfere with blood clotting, such as aspirin or ibuprofen, should be avoided. In the event of injury, the school nurse should complete a physical assessment even if the student is initially asymptomatic and monitor the student closely. Attention should be paid to minor cuts and trauma, especially head trauma due to the increased risk of intracranial bleeding.

Immune Thrombocytopenic Purpura

Immune thrombocytopenic purpura (ITP) is an acquired disorder resulting in platelet destruction. Manifestations include development of petechiae (tiny red/purple nonblanching lesions), purpura, ecchymosis, and mucosal (nose, mouth, and gingival) bleeding (Grace & Lambert, 2022). ITP is an autoimmune disease where the immune system attacks and destroys one's own platelets, often occurring 1 to 4 weeks after a viral infection. Treatment is supportive as ITP is self-limited and frequently resolves without treatment. However, in more severe cases, immunosuppression with corticosteroids, IV immunoglobulin, or platelet transfusions may be warranted (Grace & Lambert, 2022). As with other bleeding disorders, the school nurse should monitor for risk of bleeding after injury and refer to the healthcare provider as necessary.

Sickle Cell Disease

Sickle cell disease (SCD) is an autosomal recessive inherited disorder that causes the hemoglobin structure of the red blood cell to be altered. Individuals who inherit one gene are carriers, and those who inherit one gene from each parent have SCD. There are approximately 100,000 individuals living in the United States with SCD and most are identified by newborn screening programs (Kavanagh et al., 2022).

Hemoglobin (Hg) is a protein that allows RBCs to carry oxygen from the lungs throughout the body (Kavanagh et al., 2022). The sickle cell gene (S) makes an abnormal form of hemoglobin, referred to as hemoglobin S (HgbS), compared with hemoglobin (HgbA) that is normally present. People who have inherited two sickle cell genes (HgbSS) have the most severe manifestations of the disease, sickle cell anemia. Some individuals have a milder form of the disease (HgSC) in which they inherit a sickle cell gene (S) from one parent and an abnormal hemoglobin (C), from the other parent. An individual with only one copy of the HgSC gene is referred to as having sickle cell trait (SCT) and has limited symptoms except under extreme conditions (Kavanagh et al., 2022).

HgbS differs from HgbA in several ways. When deoxygenated in the capillary beds, HgbS changes shape from round biconcave to "sickle" or C shape, which causes the RBCs to clump together and obstruct small blood vessels, leading to ischemia. Sickling in the vessels is referred to as sickle cell crisis or *vaso-occlusive crisis*. HgbS also has increased adhesion molecules that bind to the endothelial wall allowing the RBCs to stick and collect more easily (Kavanagh et al., 2022). Additionally, RBCs with HgbS hemolyze more rapidly than RBCs with HgbA resulting in anemia (Kavanagh et al., 2022). There are several complications of SCD the school nurse should be familiar with, including vaso-occlusive crisis, acute chest syndrome, fever, sepsis, priapism, anemia, gallbladder disease, and stroke.

Symptoms of ***vaso-occlusive crisis*** can range from mild to severe and may require hospitalization. Pain is the hallmark symptom of a vaso-occlusive crisis. Pain episodes are unpredictable and may be rare, sporadic, or frequent depending on the severity of the student's disease and exposure to precipitating factors. Pain in SCD is complex and may begin with fatigue and body aches, progressing to localized pain, which can last for days (Kavanagh et al., 2022). Pain usually localizes in the hands, feet, abdomen, or long bones and is difficult to tolerate and manage, ranging from moderate to excruciating (Kavanagh et al., 2022). Pain management may include acetaminophen, ibuprofen, controlled substances, or referral to healthcare provider in cases of severe pain that cannot be controlled. Fatigue, chest pain, dizziness, sudden pain at any site without signs of redness or inflammation, shortness of breath, coldness in the hands and feet, and pallor are all signs and symptoms related to vaso-occlusive crisis (Kavanagh et al., 2022). School policies must be followed if controlled substances are prescribed. School attendance may be difficult for students due to pain and plans should be made for these instances.

Acute chest syndrome is a life-threatening emergency involving a sickle crisis in the heart and lungs causing dyspnea, coughing, and fever. Trouble breathing and chest pain may indicate acute chest syndrome, which requires immediate treatment in an acute care setting (Kavanagh et al., 2022).

Individuals with SCD are predisposed to infection and high risk for ***sepsis,*** contributing to increased mortality

(Kavanagh et al., 2022). Fever and infections should be treated promptly, and adherence to vaccination schedules and antibiotic prophylaxis is important. Many school-age children and adolescents have increased risk of infection due to having had a splenectomy or functional asplenia from obstruction and destruction of the spleen after years of SCD. Children with SCD should receive the pneumococcal, meningococcal, and annual influenza vaccines. Encouraging good hand hygiene is especially important for these students to decrease their risk for infection. Fever may be a sign of bacteremia and requires immediate medical evaluation because of the increased risk for overwhelming sepsis (Kavanaugh et al., 2022).

Priapism, a prolonged painful erection, affects about 40% of males with SCD and may require emergent care (Kavanagh et al., 2022). Due to the hypercoagulability of SCD, estrogen-containing contraceptives are contraindicated and progestin-only contraceptives or barrier methods are recommended (Kavanagh et al., 2022).

Acute anemia can develop due to destruction of the RBCs by the spleen as well as sequestration of sickled RBCs in the spleen leading to hypovolemia and shock (Kavanagh et al., 2022). *Chronic anemia* may be evident by persistently low hemoglobin levels. The school nurse may identify this in the student who appears to have fatigue and reduced energy for activity or for schoolwork. The anemia and its sequelae can severely limit an individual's ability to function and carry out normal tasks of daily living. Physical activity should be encouraged when the child has been cleared by the healthcare provider; however, physical education in school may need to be modified to because of anemia. Physical education also increases oxygen consumption and can precipitate hypoxia, leading to sickling.

Individuals with SCD are at risk for ***ischemic stroke*** if sickling occurs in a cerebral vessel. Symptoms of stroke include headache, seizures, weakness on one side of the body, limping, and sudden speech, vision, or hearing changes. Those at increased risk of stroke may require regular blood transfusions (Kavanagh et al., 2022). Development of gallbladder disease increases with age in those with SCD, often requiring cholecystectomy (Kavanagh et al., 2022).

The school nurse should ensure that health and education plans for students with SCD entail accommodations that support wellness and academic success by preventing and ameliorating conditions that cause sickling of the RBCs such as dehydration, acidosis, hypothermia, infection, and deoxygenation under physiological stress.

A Section 504 plan is indicated for students with SCD who are able to learn in the general curriculum. Students who experience chronic or acute pain, fatigue, and disablity require targeted accommodations to optimize participation at school. An IEP is needed for students who have mini-strokes or strokes that impair learning. At the beginning of each school year, the school nurse should meet with the family and student with SCD to ensure health information, treatment plans, medication schedule, and other considerations are up to date. From this information, the school nurse develops an IHP. The school nurse needs to be a part of the student support team for students with SCD and incorporate components of the current IHP and EAP into the child's IEP or Section 504 plan (Shannon & Holman, 2017). Plans for intermittent home instruction may need to be considered for students who are frequently hospitalized or miss significant school days due to sickle cell crisis. See Chapter 8 for a sample EAP (Box 8-3) and a sample Section 504 plan (Box 8-4) for a student with SCD.

Dehydration can occur during illness or overheating. Interventions in an acute care setting include the administration of oxygen and fluids, as well as pain management. Staying hydrated at school by drinking plenty of fluids is extremely important; students with SCD should have access to water and bathroom privileges as needed. Additional fluids will be necessary if the temperature outside is hot, if the child has a fever or pain, or if the child has an increase in activity level.

Cold weather causes vasoconstriction and contributes to sickling; therefore students may have more difficulty during winter months. The temperature in school transportation vehicles and decisions about going outside for recess will need to be considered. Swimming in cold water or playing in snow may trigger a pain episode. Weather and environmental considerations should be determined ahead of time as reflected in the medical orders and the school nurse's IHP and communicated to the educational team.

Parents/guardians should be called immediately for pain that does not resolve with medication and rest and for fever; abdominal pain or swelling, especially in the area of the spleen; increased fatigue; and a cough or mild chest pain. An EAP also should be in place for situations that arise during the school day with clear and concise directions with specific actions attached. Signs requiring emergency medical services include neurological changes, seizures, vision changes, numbness or inability to move a body part, difficulty breathing, prolonged priapism, and severe pain (Kavanagh et al., 2022).

Although SCD can be life-limiting, many individuals are living into middle age and beyond with good healthcare management. Preventing complications, maintaining good health, incorporating a healthy lifestyle into daily living, and finding ways to cope with pain are essential (Kavanagh et al., 2022). Medications for SCD include hydroxyurea, L-glutamine, crizanlizumab, and voxelotor. Hydroxyurea induces the development of fetal hemoglobin, which inhibits HgbS, and L-glutamine decreases the sickling of the RBC. Crizanlizumab reduces vaso-occlusion and voxelotor helps increase hemoglobin levels. Other treatments include blood transfusions, especially in the case of high risk for stroke or before surgery, bone marrow transplant, and gene therapies (Kavanagh et al., 2022). Many new treatments for SCD are under development, including gene therapy.

Human Immunodeficiency Virus Disease

Infection with the ***human immunodeficiency virus*** (HIV) causes primary immune system dysfunction, but also affects multiple organ and body systems beyond the immune system. Although new infections have decreased over the past decade, it is estimated there are over 1.1 million people in the United States living with HIV (Peterson, 2022). The prevalence in children 12 years and younger is low but increases markedly in adolescence and young adulthood (CDC, 2023b). There are two types of HIV: HIV-1 (most common in the United States and more aggressive) and HIV-2 (more common in West Africa).

HIV is a retrovirus that attacks the body's T helper (CD4) lymphocytes, which are part of the adaptive immune system. The adaptive immune system has memory and responds to pathogens through cell-mediated immune responses (T lymphocytes/cells) and the production of antibodies (B lymphocytes). T lymphocytes use chemical messengers (CD4 T helper cells) to activate the adaptive response to detect and kill viruses and tumor cells (CD8 killer cells). The CD4 helper cells are also responsible for activating B cells to make antibodies that match and attack the pathogen (Banasik et al., 2022). HIV attaches to the CD4 T helper cells, hijacking them and causing the CD4 cell to make more of the HIV virus. In this process, the CD4 cell is destroyed (Peterson, 2022). This loss of CD4 cells reduces messages to the CD8 and B cells resulting in a progressive immunodeficiency (Peterson, 2022). Monitoring the progression of HIV infection includes monitoring CD4 counts and viral load. Viral load is an indicator of how fast the virus is replicating in the host.

Students with a low CD4 count are at greater risk for infection because the immune system may not be able to mount an effective attack against an invading organism (Peterson, 2022); thus the virus significantly increases the risk of opportunistic infections. In individuals who are immunocompromised, the organisms become pathogens and cause disease. Families of students with HIV disease must be notified immediately if their child is exposed to infectious diseases in the school environment; the student may require passive antibody treatment to prevent infection or antibiotics to rapidly treat and control infections.

The classification system for pediatric HIV is primarily dependent on the CD4 count and the clinical manifestations present:

- Stage 0: early infection without symptoms
- Stage 1: CD4 count greater than 500 cells/mm^3
- Stage 2: CD4 count of 200 to 499 cells/mm^3
- Stage 3: CD4 count less than 200 cells/mm^3 with the development of opportunistic infections

Stage 3 is considered *acquired immune deficiency syndrome* (AIDS) (Elsevier Point of Care, 2022).

The World Health Organization's (2016) classification system for adolescents and adults uses signs and symptoms to categorize the stages from clinical stage 1 (asymptomatic) to clinical stage 4 (advanced disease). Even if HIV disease does not appear to be symptomatic, viral replication continues (increasing viral load) and CD4 cells continue to be destroyed. This latent period can be years in length. With preventive or proper treatment, viral replication should be decreased. The therapeutic goal is that this condition does not progress to AIDS.

Perinatal transmission of HIV has declined by more than 90% since the early 1990s. Routine HIV testing of all pregnant women is now a component of prenatal care and has been instrumental in identifying HIV-positive mothers. Early identification of HIV allows antiretroviral prophylaxis to be started. Upon delivery, the newborn is also started on antiretroviral prophylaxis, leading to a significant decrease in perinatal transmission.

Although the virus is relatively weak outside of the body and easily destroyed, it can be transmitted through contact with infected blood and body fluids, sexually through semen or vaginal secretions, or perinatally (Peterson, 2022). Although most children who are HIV+ were infected perinatally, children who are sexually abused are at risk for HIV and other sexually transmitted infections and should be screened often. Adolescents who have unprotected sex or inject drugs are at increased risk for HIV. Adolescents should have developmentally appropriate education and accurate information on how to reduce or eliminate the risk factors for HIV, including where free testing is available. Youth should be made aware of the privacy rules regarding HIV testing and notification in the state in which they reside.

The school nurse and school staff are not always aware of HIV status of students. The Occupational Safety and Health Administration (n.d.) requires schools to provide bloodborne pathogen training for all school staff. The school nurse is integral to educating the entire school community about practicing universal precautions to reduce the risk for transmission when encountering blood or body fluids.

HIV affects all body systems; however, GI manifestations are common in students infected with HIV (Peterson, 2022). GI symptoms include altered nutrition from chronic diarrhea, fungal infections of the oral mucosa, esophagitis, and abdominal pain. These conditions can result in malnutrition, malabsorption, and poor weight gain. In addition, the adverse effects of the HIV medication regimen can cause nausea, vomiting, and diarrhea. Some individuals respond well to lactose-free diets. Small, frequent meals are often more tolerable to those with GI concerns, and this intervention should be considered for the IHP and 504 plan.

Pulmonary complications remain a common cause of morbidity. *Pneumocystis carinii* pneumonia is the most common opportunistic infection among those with HIV. Students exhibiting fever, shortness of breath, dry cough, cyanosis, and hypoxemia should be evaluated for pneumonia. Early treatment of respiratory infections is essential.

Neurological effects can include encephalopathy, developmental and motor delays, cognitive deficits, and behavior deficits, which all put the child at academic risk. Neurological complications can range from subtle to severe psychiatric disturbances (Elsevier Point of Care, 2022). Metabolic abnormalities such as dyslipidemia, growth failure, nephropathy, cardiac disease, and development of lymphomas are known complications (Peterson, 2022).

Treatment goals include reducing viral replication/load, restoring and preserving immune function, maintaining growth and development, and reducing morbidity and mortality from HIV. Highly active antiretroviral therapy (HAART) is a treatment regimen that interferes with the replication process of HIV and decreases the viral load and prevents destruction of the immune system. HAART has resulted in delayed progression of HIV and a decline in mortality rates for individuals with AIDS. Students with HIV/AIDS are entering adulthood (Elsevier Point of Care, 2022).

Students with HIV disease benefit from school nurse–led case management. School nurses play an important role in the early identification of symptoms of infection, leading to prompt treatment. The school nurse can help the family maintain continuity of care at school by establishing a medication regimen that is consistent with the home routine. In addition, the school nurse is an important advocate for the family and child, especially ensuring that the child receives needed services. Confidentiality is an essential aspect of care for the individual with HIV. Social support and assisting with access to needed resources is another opportunity for the school nurse, as a parent may be ill with HIV or AIDS or may have already died. Significant stigma still surrounds having HIV. The school nurse plays an important role in making school a positive experience for these students.

ALTERATIONS IN NEURO/MUSCULOSKELETAL HEALTH

Cerebral Palsy

Cerebral palsy (CP) is the most common motor disability in childhood. It results from injury to the brain of the developing fetus or neonate (CDC, 2023d; Paul et al., 2022). CP results in a nonprogressive permanent motor disorder affecting movement, motor function, sensory function, and neurological function, causing disability (Paul et al., 2022). CP affects the brain's ability to communicate motor tasks to the body. Some individuals with CP also exhibit other learning and behavior problems. Despite medical advances, the prevalence of CP has not changed significantly in the last 30 years, affecting approximately 2 to 3 in every 1,000 live births (Paul et al., 2022).

In developed countries, CP is most commonly associated with prematurity and low birth weight of less than 2.5 kg (Paul et al., 2022). Other possible causes include hypoxic-ischemic encephalopathy, intrauterine infections, multiple gestations, genetic causes, malformation of the brain during the developmental period, and the health of the mother before conception. Healthy children can develop CP during childhood as a result of a head injury, illness, accident, or poisoning, typically before age 5 while the brain is still developing (Paul et al., 2022).

Many children with CP demonstrate delayed developmental milestones. Therefore assessment of motor development is essential, including muscle tone, reflexes, and posture throughout the infant period. Children with severe forms of CP may be diagnosed as early as 6 to 12 months, while children with less severe forms may be diagnosed later (Paul et al., 2022). The use of predictive tools, MRI, and clinical evaluation helps diagnose high-risk infants (premature and low birth weight). The goal is early intervention services to optimize the brain's plasticity and capacity for recovery. Early clinical signs include the following:

- Poor head control
- Hypotonic or hypertonic muscle tone
- Hand fisting beyond 3 months of age
- Lack of peripheral reflexes after 5 months
- Moro and atonic neck reflexes past 6 months
- Absent parachute reflex
- Leg scissoring in older infants and toddlers

The inability to walk and gait issues in young children are indicators that further evaluation is warranted (Paul et al., 2022).

CP is categorized according to the type of motor abnormality (spastic, dyskinetic, ataxic, mixed spastic/dystonic) and the area of presentation (quadriplegic, hemiplegic, diplegic, and monoplegic) (Paul et al., 2022).

Spastic CP occurs in approximately 80% of cases and is due to damage to the motor cortex that controls movement. It results in the presence of exaggerated stretch reflexes with resistance to movement and increased tone, in addition to persistent and primitive reflexes, including Moro, Babinski, and asymmetrical tonic neck reflexes (Paul et al., 2022). The increased tone continues to be present during sleep and results in the development of contractures. Some students receive botulinum toxin injections (Botox) to treat the spasticity and muscle tightness (Kaya Keles & Ates, 2022). Intrathecal baclofen, delivered directly into the spinal cord via an implanted pump, or oral antispasmodic medications may also be administered (Sheu et al., 2022).

Dyskinetic CP occurs in 6% to 15% of students with CP and is the result of injuries to the subcortical structures. Dyskinetic CP involves altered tone and uncontrolled involuntary movement, including dystonia and athetosis. Dystonia refers to either hypertonic or hypotonic muscle tone. Athetoid CP is associated with slow, writhing movements that appear to flow into each other. Athetoid movements combined with chorea movements (rapid, random, jerky movements) is choreoathetosis (Paul et al., 2022). Rigidity involving inflexibility and resistance to active or passive motion is rare in dyskinetic CP.

Ataxic CP is associated with damage to the cerebellum that inhibits or impairs movement and balance coordination, resulting in gait abnormalities. It accounts for about 5% to 10% of CP cases (Paul et al., 2022). In ataxic CP, muscle tone can range from hypotonic to atonic.

Mixed spastic/dystonic CP results from insults to various areas of the brain and involves more than one motor pattern (Sheu et al., 2022).

The school nurse should assess whether the student with CP experiences or is at risk for various associated health and wellness issues, including the following:

- Mobility impairments
- Learning disabilities
- Intellectual disability
- Visual, hearing, and speech/language deficits
- Feeding and eating difficulties
- Seizures
- Pain
- Bowel and bladder involvement
- Respiratory and cardiovascular involvement
- Skin integrity
- Safety issues
- Social issues

Decreased mobility and physical activity due to motor impairment pose risks associated with venous stasis, precipitating the development of deep vein thrombosis, and osteoporosis (Paul et al., 2022). Encouragement of physical activity and weight-bearing status is an important aspect of reducing risk of venous stasis and improving bone mineral density (Paul et al., 2022). The school nurse can be instrumental in facilitating physical activity and weight-bearing status.

In approximately 60% of children with CP, intelligence is not affected. However, learning problems and intellectual deficits affect many children with CP. Learning disabilities may be due to perceptual impairments (Blasco et al., 2022). See Chapter 26 for more information on nursing interventions for students with learning disorders and intellectual disabilities.

Vision problems are a concern in children with CP. The degree of vision impairment varies according to the location and severity of brain injury. Hearing impairments are also common in children with CP. Treatment for hearing loss includes the use of hearing aids that facilitate the transmission of sound to the brain. Speech and language impairments often occur because of muscle tone, motor problems, and decreased lung capacity. Computers and augmentive communication devices can assist children with speech impairments (Paul et al., 2022). Vision, hearing, and speech/language impairments are discussed later in this chapter.

Seizures are a common comorbidity in children with CP. Epilepsy in children with CP is often early onset and difficult to treat. The incidence of status epilepticus is significantly higher in individuals with CP (K et al., 2022). The primary mode of treatment includes oral anticonvulsant medications. See Chapter 27 for more information on seizures.

Pain is experienced by up to 75% of children with CP. Communication challenges and multiple pain etiologies complicate the management of pain in children with CP (Paul et al., 2022). Pain decreases quality of life, affects mood, and interferes with normal daily activities (Vinkel et al., 2022). Most complaints involve pain in the lower extremities and back, although communication or cognitive impairments make it difficult to verbalize the discomfort. Pain may be caused by muscle spasms, contractures, scoliosis, gastroesophageal reflux, constipation, corneal abrasions, and treatments for associated conditions. When a child enters school, it is important to ask parents/guardians how the child demonstrates pain.

Feeding and eating problems are common in children with CP. Students may benefit from therapeutic services of a school speech/language pathologist. Motor movements, such as chewing and swallowing, may be altered (Paul et al., 2022). Softer foods may be needed if the swallowing muscles are affected. Students with CP who have oral motor difficulties and/or gastroesophageal reflux are at risk for aspiration. Some children with CP need assistance with eating, ranging from placing food in the child's mouth to feeding through a percutaneous endoscopic gastrostomy/button gastrostomy or jejunostomy tube (see Chapter 25). Students should remain in an upright position after eating to promote digestion and reduce the risk for aspiration. Spasticity or movement disorders create increased caloric demands. Adequate nutrition must be maintained at school. The school nurse should monitor the weight and growth of students with CP.

Anencephaly and Microcephaly

Anencephaly is a severe birth anomaly in which the skull, forebrain, and cerebellum are absent; the remaining parts of the brain may be exposed. In the United States, anencephaly occurs in approximately 1 in every 4,600 births (CDC, 2023a). Most cases of anencephaly result in miscarriage, stillbirth, or death soon after delivery (Iskandar & Finnell, 2022).

Microcephaly is a congenital anomaly in which the skull and brain are significantly smaller than normal ranges. See Figure 24-1. In the United States, microcephaly occurs in about 1 in every 800 to 5,000 births (CDC, 2023c). The size of the head is related to the extent of neurodevelopmental disorder; the smaller the head size, the more severe the issues tend to be. Although severe microcephaly can be life-threatening, many children survive. Severe microcephaly is associated with the following:

- Seizures
- Developmental delay, such as problems with speech or other developmental milestones (e.g., sitting, standing, and walking)
- Intellectual disability (decreased ability to learn and function in daily life)
- Problems with movement and balance
- Feeding problems, such as difficulty swallowing
- Hearing loss
- Vision problems (CDC, 2023b, para. 3)

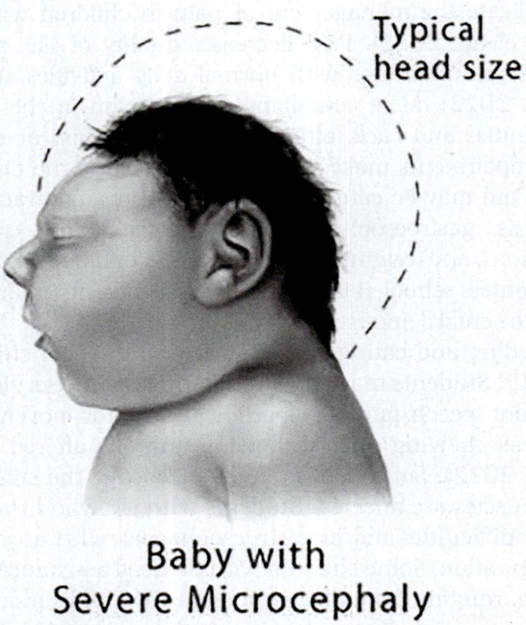

FIGURE 24-1. Microcephaly. *(CDC, 2023c).*

The causes of microcephaly are not well understood. Causes may be genetic; associated with intrauterine exposure to infection, malnutrition, or toxic substances; or due to impaired cerebral blood flow (CDC, 2023b). Students with microcephaly require therapeutic and educational programming.

Neural Tube Defects

Failure of the neural tube to fuse or close during the third week of gestation can lead to anencephaly or neural tube defects of the spine (Iskandar & Finnell, 2022).

Neural tube defects can be closed (spina bifida) or open (meningocele and myelomenigocele) (Vandertop et al., 2022). Supplementation with folic acid before conception reduces the incidence of neural tube defects. Some neural tube defects are able to be corrected with prenatal fetal surgery (Iskandar & Finnell, 2022). Neural tube defect severity varies based on the size and location of the defect, as well as the extent of spinal cord and nerve involvement. A complex relationship between genetic and environmental factors contributes to neural tube defects (Iskandar & Finnell, 2022).

Spina bifida refers to splitting of the vertebral arches. *Spina bifida occulta* indicates no protrusion of the meninges or meningeal sac. Spina bifida occulta is the mildest of the three forms of spina bifida resulting in a small gap in the vertebrae, small hairy patch, pigmented area, or dimpling with no spinal cord damage.

Meningocele is associated with protrusion of the meningeal sac resulting in an external pouch of spinal fluid with little or no damage. The meningeal sac does not contain the spinal cord and is usually repaired shortly after birth. ***Myelomeningocele,*** also referred to as open spina bifida, is the most severe form of neural tube defect (Norkett et al., 2016). In myelomeningocele, the spinal cord is found in the meningeal sac and protrudes through the vertebrae, exposing the tissue, spinal cord, and nerves. Surgical repair is required. Symptoms and clinical presentation vary based on the location and size of the spinal lesion, as well as the number of spinal nerves within the meninges or sac (Iskandar & Finnell, 2022). High lumbar or thoracic lesions present with sensorimotor deficits, paraplegia or lower extremity weakness, respiratory weakness, and absence of bowel and bladder control. Lower sacral lesions may have normal neurological examinations or mild lower extremity weakness (Iskandar & Finnell, 2022). See Figure 24-2.

Commonly, children with myelomeningocele also have a ***Chiari II malformation*** (Kuhn & Emmady, 2022). Chiari II is "characterized by downward displacement of the medulla, fourth ventricle and cerebellum into the cervical spinal canal, as well as elongation of the pons and fourth ventricle" (American Association of Neurologic Surgeons [AANS], 2023a, para. 7). Chiari II malformation impairs the flow of cerebrospinal fluid (CSF) between the ventricles of the brain and the spinal cord, commonly resulting in symptomatic hydrocephalus (Norkett et al., 2016).

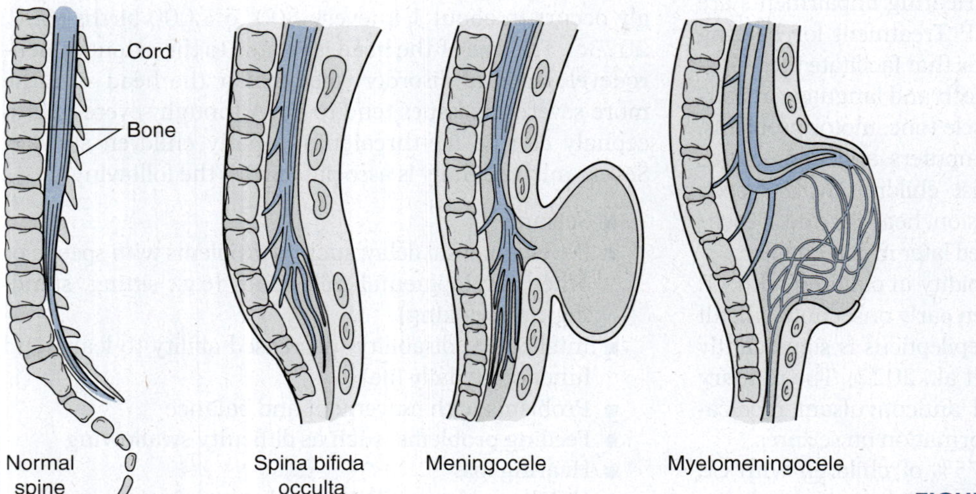

FIGURE 24-2. Neural tube defects.

Hydrocephalus

Hydrocephalus is a condition in which excess CSF accumulates in the ventricles, causing increased intracranial pressure (AANS, 2023b). Symptoms associated with hydrocephalus in school-age children include the following:

- Nausea and vomiting
- Swelling of the optic disc or papilledema
- Blurred or double vision
- Balance and gait abnormalities
- Slowing or loss of developmental progress
- Changes in personality
- Inability to concentrate
- Seizures
- Poor appetite
- Urinary incontinence (AANS, 2023b)

Congenital hydrocephalus is commonly managed by surgically implanting a ***ventriculoperitoneal shunt*** (VP shunt) during early life (AANS, 2023b). Some children with mild hydrocephalus can be treated conservatively. A small number undergo an endoscopic third ventriculostomy in which a neurosurgeon creates a new CSF pathway through an opening in the floor of the third ventricle (Norkett et al., 2016).

A VP shunt is a flexible tube with a one-way valve that diverts CSF from the brain to the peritoneal cavity to maintain stable intracranial pressure. Inserted in a lateral ventricle, the VP shunt leaves the skull behind the ear and tunnels under the skin to terminate in the peritoneum where the excess CSF is absorbed (AANS, 2023b). See Figure 24-3. VP shunts for students with myelomeningocele are typically required for their life spans. VP shunts need to be surgically revised as a child grows or when the shunt malfunctions resulting in symptomatic hydrocephalus. Note: VP shunts may also be required for other causes of increased intracranial pressure such as tumors, injury, or disease (AANS, 2023b).

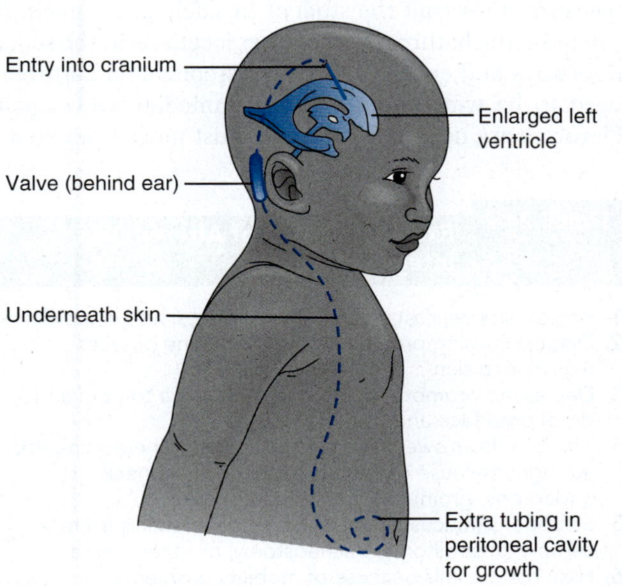

FIGURE 24-3. Child with ventriculoperitoneal (VP) shunt.

> ### Focus on the Framework
> **Care Coordination**
>
> School nurse–led case management entails serving as a liaison between the family, the school student support team, and healthcare providers to ensure that coordinated services are provided for students with special healthcare needs (National Association of School Nurses [NASN], 2021; NASN 2024). Hydrocephalus with increased intracranial pressure is potentially life-threatening. VP shunts can malfunction. The school nurse needs to be familiar with the baseline neurological status of students with ventricular shunts. Increased intracranial pressure can injure brain cells and impair cognitive and functional capacities. Accommodations at school include precautions to avoid head injury. Parents/guardians should be notified immediately, because alterations from baseline status or fever need prompt medical evaluation and treatment by specialists. The school nurse should develop an EAP for students with VP shunts so that school staff can quickly identify signs and symptoms of hydrocephalus and appropriately respond. Emergency medical services should be activated for any student displaying acute signs of increased intracranial pressure such as abnormal vital signs, decreased level of consciousness, or prolonged seizures.

Mobility services, occupational therapy, and physical therapy may need to provide adaptive equipment. When students with neural tube defects have paralysis or decreased sensation in the extremities or torso, special attention must be paid to safety concerns regarding heat, cold, and compression.

Children with neural tube defects have a high risk of **latex allergies** due to frequent exposure to latex medical products during procedures at an early age (Posanka, 2022). Symptoms of an allergic response range from a pruritic rash to urticaria, rhinitis, and even anaphylaxis (see Chapter 21). School nurses need to educate school staff that minimizing the risk of latex contact at school involves decreasing exposure to products that contain latex, such as toys, art supplies, rubber bands, swim goggles, paints and glues, pencil erasers, elastic in clothing, gym mats, and medical equipment (including gloves and adhesive bandage strips). A list of latex products and their alternatives is available from the Spina Bifida Association of America (2015).

Other health-related concerns for students with neural tube defects include spinal curvatures (scoliosis or kyphosis) caused by the initial lesion or the surgical correction and short stature, which may result in other medical issues. Children with lesions in the low lumbar region can walk but may need below-the-knee orthotics and forearm crutches, and those with high sacral lesions may walk with ankle or foot braces (Iskandar & Finnell, 2022). Students with spina bifida are at higher risk for obesity because of decreased physical activity. Adaptive physical education can include modifications that focus on strength training and energy expenditure. Vision problems may be related to hydrocephalus, refractive errors, or amblyopia. A comprehensive annual vision examination is essential.

Children with neural tube defects often require a number of surgeries and treatments throughout life, resulting in considerable absences from school and reduced opportunities for socialization. It is imperative the IHP meets the child's specific needs and promotes the highest level of independence and autonomy possible. See Online Materials OM 24-3 for an IHP for a student with spina bifida.

Additional Concerns

Children with CP and neural tube defects often experience issues with bladder and bowel control. *Neurogenic bladder* and *neurogenic bowel* are caused by impaired motor neuron innervation of genitourinary and gastrointestinal structures (Cerebral Palsy Guide, 2021; Stanton & Lavenbarg, 2017). It is not uncommon for children with neurogenic bladder and/or bowel to master toileting at a later age than their typical peers.

The goal of neurogenic bladder management is to prevent kidney and ureter damage, including urinary tract infections and incontinence (Iskandar & Finnell, 2022). Neurogenic bladder can present as follows:

- *Overactive bladder:* The bladder is unable to empty fully or begins to empty before the person can make it to the bathroom.
- *Overflow incontinence:* Urinary leakage occurs due to the bladder not emptying.
- *Stress incontinence:* The muscles that control urination do not function properly.
- *Urge incontinence:* Spasms of the bladder cause it to shrink before the person reaches the bathroom (Cerebral Palsy Guide, 2021, para. 9).

Students with neurogenic bowel are prone to constipation, impaction, or fecal leakage. Hydration, dietary fiber, and bowel training are mandatory in the prevention of fecal impaction and bowel obstruction. Children who have difficulty with voluntary bladder and bowel control may also be prone to bladder infections.

Diapering and toileting should be done in private in the least restrictive environment with minimal loss of instructional time. Often the least restrictive environment is in or close to the classroom and not in the school health office. Toileting routines should allow for privacy to avoid any embarrassment for the student and optimize self-esteem and success. For students who are continent but are not independently mobile or can manage self-care, a program of timed voids or bowel evacuation may be needed. Extra precautions should be taken for students in diapers and girls who are menstruating, especially if they are immobile.

Although the school nurse will monitor the student's health status, the tasks of diapering and assisting with toileting or menstrual care do not require nursing judgment and therefore can be done by unlicensed assistive personnel.

Some students require urinary catheterization at school. A nurse may be responsible for catheterizing the student. If appropriate and allowed by state nurse practice acts, routine catheterization may be delegated to unlicensed assistive school personnel under the nurse's supervision. See Chapter 30 for more discussion on delegation. See Chapter 25 for more information on urinary catheterization. In addition, students with altered mobility may be prone to bone demineralization, which can predispose the child to urinary calculi or stones.

The school nurse should monitor skin integrity. Many factors can cause altered skin integrity in students with neuromuscular disorders (Table 24-2). The goal of skin care is to keep areas clean and dry, as well as decrease pressure in areas that are prone to the development of skin breakdown. Chaffed areas and skin breakdown increase risk for infections and discomfort.

Decreased muscle tone may result in altered breathing pattern and increased energy expenditure from breathing, leading to fatigue and inability to clear secretions. Students with severe motor impairment may need mechanical ventilation to support their respiratory efforts. Direct care for a child with a tracheostomy and/or ventilator assistance includes suctioning and treatments to mobilize secretions with ongoing assessment to ensure the safety and well-being of the student (see Chapter 25). Many children who are ventilator-assisted attend school with the support of a licensed nurse caregiver in attendance. Federal legislation requires this level of support to be provided by the school system.

Safety is a concern for children and adolescents with altered mobility who are at greater risk for falls and injury than the general student population. Accessibility includes not only ramps and automatic door openers but also measures to permit the student to safely get to class, the cafeteria, the bathroom, and other locations in the school. Doorways and entrances into classrooms and bathrooms need to be wide enough to accommodate wheelchairs. Elevators are needed if the child must move from floor to

TABLE 24-2 External Causes of Altered Skin Integrity

1. Braces, splints, casts, positioning devices, and wheelchairs
2. Diapers causing pressure to skin and urine or feces exposed to skin
3. Decreased oromotor control causing saliva to pool and drool onto face and neck
4. Moisture from sweat production in areas where skin folds are tight because of joint contractures (i.e., neck, underarms, groin)
5. Secretions (mucus, stomach contents) draining from an ostomy, gastrostomy, tracheostomy, or other stoma
6. High risk for falls because of mobility problems

floor. Issues must be addressed related to congestion in the halls during change of class, obstacles such as book bags or debris on floors, and negotiating uneven or disrupted surfaces both indoors and outdoors. Changes in weather can pose additional risks for injury to the student with motor difficulties, requiring careful snow and ice removal and vigilant attention to wet floor surfaces indoors.

Additional safety interventions may include the use of protective helmets and safety-proofing the home and learning environments. The school nurse should identify potential areas in which specific strategies are necessary to ensure a safe environment for students. Accommodations should be included in the Section 504 plan or IEP. The school nurse must apprise teachers of the student's safety needs. A student with CP who has sensory, mobility, or cognitive impairment may need a staff member assigned to them during emergency situations (e.g., fire, violent intruder, evacuation scenarios).

Students with neuromuscular developmental disorders may also face challenges in developing peer relationships. They may not have the physical abilities or endurance to join in school activities and extracurricular events with other students. They may be dependent on others for many aspects of their life and develop less independence than their peers. Participating in a full day of classes can precipitate fatigue requiring rest periods in the school health office. Separation from the group for special education and/or therapeutic support services can limit opportunities to develop friendships. Students strive to be like their peers in every way, with their primary desire wanting to "fit in"; but they may be painfully aware when this is not the case. These students are at risk of bullying and victimization (physically, mentally, or financially) by individuals who might take advantage of their dependent status.

Students with neuromuscular disorders should be given opportunities to participate in social and extracurricular activities to the greatest extent possible. Outside of school, many activities are available to children and adolescents with motor and cognitive impairments, including adapted sports leagues and Special Olympics. These organizations offer opportunities for students to learn new skills, participate in activities at their own level, develop a sense of "team," gain a sense of accomplishment, and make new friends.

The school nurse serves as the case manager to coordinate services within the school and as a liaison with the healthcare provider. However, the IEP team is crucial in facilitating a coordinated plan for the health-related service delivery and educational enrichment. Working with families is essential when determining which strategies and interventions are helpful.

Muscular Dystrophy

Duchenne muscular dystrophy (DMD), an X-linked recessive disorder, is the most common and most severe form of muscular dystrophy in children (Venugopal & Pavlakis, 2023). The prevalence of DMD is 1 in 10,000 males ages 5 to 24 years (Romitti et al., 2015). DMD is caused by a mutation of the gene that encodes for dystrophin, a protein in skeletal muscle that when absent results in progressive skeletal muscle weakness (Venugopal & Pavlakis, 2023).

Most children reach expected developmental milestones until muscle weakness appears around age 2 to 3 years (Venugopal & Pavlakis, 2023). Families and caregivers may notice difficulty with motor activities such as running, riding a bike, and climbing stairs. Other clinical manifestations include a waddling Trendelenburg gait, lordosis, and frequent falls. Gower sign is the classic sign of DMD "wherein they 'climb up' their thighs with the aid of their hands to overcome the weakness of their pelvic and proximal lower limb muscles" (Sangam & Munakomi, 2023). Loss of ambulation begins between ages 7 and 13 years. Achilles tendons contract, causing children to toe walk. Calf muscle hypertrophy is noted in most children. By early adolescence, students with DMD typically require a wheelchair.

Progressive scoliosis in DMD develops once students lose their ability to walk and affects respiratory function (Venugopal & Pavlakis, 2023). By mid to late adolescence, DMD causes muscle weakness so severe it interferes with self-care activities. Progressive muscle deterioration leads to a compromise in cardiopulmonary function with cardiomyopathy, arrhythmias, and CHF during the second decade of life (Venugopal & Pavlakis, 2023). Weakness also affects respiratory muscles and coughing becomes ineffective, leading to increased respiratory infections. The school nurse should assess for hypoxia when the student complains of excessive fatigue, headache, and shortness of breath. Students with DMD are at risk for obesity from decreased activity levels (Venugopal & Pavlakis, 2023). Over time, difficulty eating and swallowing increases the risk of malnutrition. Students may need assistance with meals and eventually enteral nutrition through a feeding tube. The GI muscles may be affected resulting in constipation.

No effective treatment exists for DMD. The goal is to maintain optimum functioning in all muscles for as long as possible and prevent contractures. Treatments to meet these goals include physical, occupational, and aqua therapy; breathing exercises; bracing; and surgery to release contractures (Venugopal & Pavlakis, 2023). As DMD progresses, adaptive equipment should be used to meet the needs of these children. Occupational and physical therapy and any educational assists are important adjuncts to care. Treatment with glucocorticoids has been found to slow the rate of muscle fiber death, and angiotensin-converting enzyme inhibitors and/or beta blockers are helpful in slowing the progression of cardiomyopathy (Venugopal & Pavlakis, 2023). Gene therapies may provide promising alternatives (Markati et al., 2022).

As the disease progresses, death is due to respiratory or cardiac failure (Venugopal & Pavlakis, 2023). Older students with DMD and their families may be faced with difficult end-of-life decisions. It is imperative that the school nurse take a leadership role in preparing the school team to respect Do Not Attempt Resuscitation (DNAR) orders or Physician Orders or Medical Orders for Life Sustaining Treatment (POSLT or MOLST) (see Chapter 20). See Online Materials OM24-4 for a sample IHP for a child with muscular dystrophy.

Juvenile Idiopathic Arthritis

Juvenile idiopathic arthritis (JIA) is the most common rheumatic disease of children in the Western world, affecting females more often (Thatayatikom et al., 2023). JIA is considered idiopathic because it is not completely understood (National Institute of Arthritis and Musculoskeletal and Skin Diseases [NIAMS], 2021). The International League of Associations of Rheumatology divides JIA into seven categories (Table 24-3). JIA is a chronic autoimmune inflammatory disease that causes inflammation of the joints and other connective tissues. The symptoms begin before the age of 16, must last at least 6 weeks, and have an unknown cause.

The classic signs of joint inflammation in JIA include swelling, redness, warmth, pain, and decreased range of motion, especially in the morning (NIAMS, 2021). Chronic inflammation in the joint spaces (synovium) results in effusion, hypertrophy, or thickening of the synovial membrane, resulting in damage to the joint capsule, the cartilage, and ultimately the bone. In addition to joint pain and inflammation, uveitis (eye inflammation), skin changes/rashes, fever, and slowed growth may also occur.

The classic diagnostic picture for systemic JIA is a high fever daily for at least 2 weeks, fleeting macular salmon-colored rash, and generalized lymphadenopathy (NIAMS, 2021). Arthritis can appear during this attack or may not appear for months or years. Laboratory blood tests in JIA include erythrocyte sedimentation rate (ESR), C-reactive protein (CRP), autoantibodies, antinuclear antibody (ANA), and/or rheumatoid factor. However, these laboratory tests are not always positive in children.

The arthritis seen in polyarticular arthritis has an insidious onset; it is usually symmetrical and affects the large joints, usually the knees, elbows, wrists, and ankles. However, the spine and small bones of the hands and feet can be involved as well as temporomandibular joints and bones in the middle ear. The most common sequelae are joint damage and contractures. Clinical manifestations can include a limp, refusal to walk, or hip pain; an unexplained rash or fever (prolonged or cyclical); muscle weakness associated with rash; and multisystem disease (Thatayatikom et al., 2023). Manifestations at the time of onset through the first 6 months of the disease determine the classification of JIA.

TABLE 24-3 Classification System for Juvenile Idiopathic Arthritis

Category	Description
Systemic arthritis	Involves one or more joints and 2 weeks of fever, rash, lymphadenopathy, serositis, and hepatosplenomegaly
Oligoarticular	Involves one to four joints for the first 6 months of disease (persistent or extended)
Polyarticular: negative rheumatoid factor	Involves five or more joints in the first 6 months of the disease
Polyarticular: positive rheumatoid factor	Involves five or more joints in the first 6 months
Psoriatic arthritis	Arthritis with psoriasis or psoriasis in a first-degree relative and/or nail abnormalities
Enthesitis-related arthritis	Arthritis and/or enthesitis (inflammation at the tendon insertion site)
Other/ undifferentiated arthritis	Associated with at least two of the following: • + Sacroiliac or lumbosacral pain • + HLA-B27 antigen • + Arthritis in male older than 8 years • + Acute anterior uveitis • + Inflammatory bowel disease • + Reiter syndrome • + Acute anterior uveitis in a first-degree relative

National Institute of Arthritis and Musculoskeletal and Skin Diseases (2021).

Treatment goals include symptom control, prevention of joint damage, and maintenance of function. Early diagnosis and treatment provide the best outcome. Children with polyarticular JIA who have persistent joint swelling and a positive rheumatoid factor are more likely to experience joint damage and therefore require more aggressive treatment. The first line of treatment involves NSAIDs, such as ibuprofen or naproxen, to reduce pain and inflammation (NIAMS, 2021). NSAIDs should be taken with food because they can cause GI distress.

Disease-modifying drugs (DMARDs) to prevent joint destruction are added as a second-line treatment when arthritis does not respond to NSAID therapy. DMARDs include hydroxychloroquine (Plaquenil), sulfasalazine (Azulfidine), methotrexate (Rheumatrex), and medications known as *biologicals.* The biologicals include "anti-TNF agents" such as etanercept (Enbrel), infliximab (Remicade), and adalimumab (Humira), as well as abatacept (Orencia) and anakinra (Kineret). These drugs may be used in combination with oral DMARDs. Where only a single joint is involved, a steroid preparation can be injected into the joint before any additional medications are given (NIAMS, 2021).

A serious complication of JIA is uveitis, which is an inflammation of the iris and ciliary body leading to glaucoma, cataracts, and other damage to the eyes (NIAMS, 2021). The possibility of uveitis necessitates comprehensive eye examinations by an ophthalmologist at least twice a year. Contractures, altered joint physiology and the use of corticosteroids may lead to decreased or altered growth, discrepancies in the length of extremities and spinal curvature (Thatayatikom et al., 2023).

Students with JIA may have difficulty with school tasks such as writing, climbing stairs, carrying a tray in the cafeteria, tying shoes, or even raising their hands. Necessary accommodations in the Section 504 plan may include use of a wheelchair, modifications to locks on lockers, use of padding around pencils, and adaptive physical education. Children should be allowed to participate in all school activities to their fullest extent. Students on immunosuppressant medications may need to delay some immunizations and be excused if infectious outbreaks occur within the school. Students may require assistance in self-care behaviors. Arthritis flairs are especially painful. Youth with JIA can have delayed puberty; however, their need for sexuality education is the same as for their peers. It is important for girls to understand the potential impact of their medications on an unintended pregnancy, as some medications are teratogenic.

Early diagnosis and treatment is paramount to preserving joint function and reducing morbidity. Exacerbations and joint inflammation can damage the joint over time (NIAMS, 2021). The prognosis is dependent on the type of disease, symmetrical joint involvement, early hip involvement, and whether the child has a positive rheumatoid factor. With treatment, many children achieve periods of remission, and JIA may completely resolve (NIAMS, 2021). See Box 24-3 for an example of an IHP for a child with JIA.

Scoliosis

Scoliosis is defined as an abnormal lateral curvature of the spine, prevalent in 2% to 3% of the population and most often diagnosed between the ages of 10 and 15 years (AANS, 2023c). Scoliosis will affect pulmonary function with progression (Cheng et al., 2022). Most cases of scoliosis are considered idiopathic, while other cases may be related to congenital or neuromuscular conditions, such as cerebral palsy or Duchenne muscular dystrophy (discussed earlier in this chapter) (Menger & Sin, 2023). See Chapter 12 for posture screening guidelines. X-rays are needed to determine the angle of the curve (Cobb angle) and whether treatment is needed (Menger & Sin, 2023).

Scoliosis can cause lumbar back pain as well as cardiopulmonary compromise. Treatment aims to stop the curvature from progressing and improve lung function. For mild to moderate curves between 20% and 40%, bracing may prevent further curvature. The degree to which progression is slowed is directly proportional to the amount of time the student wears the brace (Sato et al., 2022). It is essential for the school nurse to monitor skin integrity, especially on pressure points. The student may feel self-conscious wearing the brace and may need emotional support. Clothing choices can be made to minimize the appearance of the brace.

Serious curvatures of more than 40% to 45% and those who have not responded to bracing may require a spinal fusion where bone is grafted from the iliac crest. This surgery consists of instrumentation of the spine with rods and screws to attain alignment and may be delayed until skeletal maturity is complete.

> **Did You Know?**
>
> ***Kyphosis*** is protrusion/convex angulation of the thoracic spine (commonly called "humpback") as if the person is bending forward. Kyphosis is commonly seen in the elderly with osteoporosis.
>
> ***Lordosis*** is accentuation of the lumbar curvature of the spine (commonly referred to as "swayback") with the back being arched. It is normal in toddlers and pregnant women.

Scoliosis can also be nonstructural. This nonprogressive form is considered to be functional; it is a function of factors such as one leg shorter than the other or always carrying one's books on one side (Claytor & Bazner-Chandler, 2017). Treatment for nonstructural scoliosis depends on the cause. Shoe lifts, postural exercises or even corrective lenses may be ordered if the problem is caused by poor vision that results in a head tilt. The curve will disappear with functional scoliosis when doing the Adams Forward Bend Test.

ALTERATIONS IN COMMUNICATION AND SENSORY HEALTH

The ability to communicate is paramount to a child's social, academic, and intellectual future (Pace et al., 2019). Communication is both receptive and expressive. Communication includes the ability to receive sensations, the ability to process sensations (decode, integrate, understand, and incorporate into memory), and the ability to express speech or language in some form. Communication disorders include disorders of speech (articulation, voice, resonance, fluency), dysfunction of the oral and facial motor muscles, disorders of cognition, and hearing loss.

Sensory deficits that can impair communication include difficulty with hearing, vision, speech and language, and sensation. These deficits can be categorized as congenital or acquired and as unilateral or bilateral. The causative factors of many speech and language deficits are unknown. Early intervention for speech and language deficits decreases the likelihood a problem will persist or worsen as the individual matures. Students with communication deficits can use assistive technology in the school setting to help them learn and accommodate for challenges with communication.

Speech/Language Disorders

Speech disorders include the inability to produce sounds and words fluently without stuttering, the inability to articulate and properly annunciate, and the inability to make sounds that can be heard (American Speech-Language-Hearing Association [ASHA], 2022c). Hearing

BOX 24-3

Individualized Healthcare Plan for a Student With Juvenile Idiopathic Arthritis

Name:	Medical diagnosis: Juvenile idiopathic arthritis	Allergies:
Teacher & Grade:	Physicians:	As-Needed (prn) Medications and Therapy:
D.O.B.:	Telephone:	Other:
Parents:	Nursing Services:	
Address:		Telephone:
Biographical Data:		

NURSING DIAGNOSIS	GOALS	NURSING INTERVENTIONS	EVALUATION
Chronic pain related to chronic musculoskeletal condition	The student will access comfort measures with limited interruption in instruction time.	1. Administer medications as ordered by physician during school day. 2. Heating pad, warm water hand soaks, hot packs as needed to minimize pain. 3. Modifications as needed to minimize pain during school/classroom activities.	■ Pain is managed during school day. ■ Student participates in classroom activities with modification as needed to minimize pain.
Risk for disuse syndrome related to pain	Student will receive needed assistance on regular or intermittent basis as condition warrants.	1. Assess for need for mobility assistance during flare-ups—elevator key, wheelchair, extended time to change classes, bus drop-off sites. 2. Modify emergency evacuation plan based on student's mobility issues and where situated in building.	■ Student will be able to manage mobility to and around school.
Risk for self-care deficit related to musculoskeletal impairment	Student to communicate when needs assistance.	1. Assist teachers and student to identify areas of modification for classroom. 2. Collaborate with physical therapy and occupational therapy. 3. Praise student for communicating need for assistance.	■ Student communicates need for assistance on a daily basis or as needed.
Risk for fatigue related to increase in physical symptoms	Student will be able to participate based on activity and energy level.	1. Provide clinic rest periods as needed. 2. Stretch breaks during class time (time to get up and walk or stretch to flex joints).	■ Student will successfully participate in the academic program.
Risk for ineffective coping related to uncertainty, inadequate opportunity to prepare for stressor, inability to conserve adaptive energies	Student will develop positive body image. Increased awareness of abilities and disabilities, knowledge, and skills	1. Encourage and provide process for communicating needs to nurse, teachers, peers, or others. 2. Explore and discuss ways alike/different to assist student toward realistic body image. 3. Facilitate communication between student/teacher, student/nurse, and other appropriate staff.	■ Student is able to identify strengths and weaknesses and describe body changes related to disease process and normal development. ■ Effective communication of feelings and needs. ■ Teachers are knowledgeable about impact of JIA on student's school performance and variability of disease process.

Prepared by: ______________________________ ***(School Nurse)*** **Date:** __________

disorders can cause speech delay because the child is unable to properly hear pronunciations and therefore cannot mimic sounds.

Speech disorders can also result from apraxia, hearing disorder, dysarthria, or stuttering, as defined in the following list:

- ***Apraxia*** is a neurological disorder affecting motor function, planning, and task performance, in the absence of apparent neurological insult to motor, sensory, or comprehension. It can result from various types of brain lesions, including stroke, dementia, tumors, neurocognitive disorders, and brain injuries (Gowda & Schneider, 2023, para. 1).
- ***Dysarthria*** is a neuromotor disorder that results from abnormalities in speed, strength, accuracy, range, tone, or duration required for speech control. Decreased speech intelligibility characterizes the disorder. The content of the spoken language remains intact, so the patient can write and comprehend spoken and written language (Jayaraman & Das, 2023, para. 1).
- ***Stuttering*** is a speech disorder characterized by repetition of sounds, syllables, or words; prolongation of sounds; and interruptions in speech known as blocks. Individuals who stutter know exactly what they would like to say but have trouble producing a normal flow of speech. These speech disruptions may be accompanied by struggle behaviors, such as rapid eye blinks or tremors of the lips. Stuttering can make it difficult to communicate with other people, which often affects a person's quality of life and interpersonal relationships (National Institute on Deafness and Other Communication Disorders, 2017, para. 1).

Language is the use of words to share ideas and is made up of subtle social nuances that determine the meaning of words, inflection of words, and sentence structure (ASHA, 2022c). Causes of language disorders include developmental delays, brain injuries, hearing loss, and prematurity. Children with language disorders may have trouble learning new words, have trouble putting sentences together, have trouble reading or writing, or may have selective mutism, refusal to talk in selective situations or places (ASHA, 2022c).

Early intervention by a speech-language therapist is essential for children with a speech and/or language delay. The student needs strategies to communicate to decrease frustration, allow socialization with peers, and help school staff meet the student's needs. There are many communication devices that can be used for a range of cognitive abilities including sign language, simple picture cards or boards, and augmentive communication devices that produce sounds.

Did You Know?

Language disorders are differentiated as expressive or receptive.

- *Expressive language disorders* involve difficulty sharing thoughts or ideas completely, typically through spoken language. Students struggle to say what they want to say (express) or to be understood by others.
- *Receptive language disorders* are characterized by difficulty understanding the meaning of words or language concepts, including nonverbal communication. Some students with receptive language disorders can speak clearly but not fully understand what their words mean.
- *Mixed receptive-expressive language disorders* are characterized by a combination of the above, wherein a child has difficulty both understanding and saying or conveying what they want to communicate (Understood Team, 2019).

Hearing Loss/Deafness

Unilateral or bilateral hearing loss affects about 20% of children to some degree before 18 years of age (Sommerfeldt & Kolb, 2023). Congenital hearing loss can be attributed to genetic disorders or maternal infection (e.g., cytomegalovirus or rubella). Other causes of early-onset hearing loss include prematurity, postnatal infection (e.g., meningitis, otitis media), ototoxic drugs, ear or head trauma, or structural abnormalities of the ears, head, and face. In addition, high noise levels can contribute to hearing loss.

Newborns are screened for hearing loss before hospital discharge (Sommerfeldt & Kolb, 2023). Hearing is fully developed at birth. Early identification of newborn hearing loss leads to early intervention to minimize language and communication delays. Early intervention within 6 months is paramount, because hearing affects speech development, communication, safety, academic success, and social relationships (Gustafson & Corbin, 2021). Hearing loss alone does not affect intellectual capacity or ability to learn. However, children with hearing impairment may qualify for special education services beginning at age 3 or a Section 504 plan to provide for their unique learning needs. Approximately 73,000 (1%) of students in U.S. public schools receive special education services based solely on having a hearing impairment (National Center for Education Statistics, 2023).

The *deaf community* is a cultural group that shares common experiences, concerns, and language. Deaf culture includes a reliance on eyesight and visual strategies including the use of visual language such as American Sign Language (National Deaf Center [NDC], 2022). The preferred terminology of this community is "deaf" and "hard of hearing." However, IDEA defines deafness in two categories, both of which are offered services, but are treated differently under the law. "Hearing impairment" is considered an impairment that affects education whereas "deafness" is a hearing impairment that is so severe the child cannot process language through hearing even with the help of amplification (NDC, 2022).

The three types of hearing loss are classified by their location within the auditory system: conductive, sensorineural, and mixed.

- ***Conductive hearing loss*** is common in younger children and involves a mechanical problem of the outer ear (wax, foreign body) or middle ear (chronic otitis media, chronic effusions, ossicle discontinuity, or tympanic membrane disorder) (Sooriyamoorthy & De Jesus, 2023). Conductive hearing loss often resolves if the underlying problem can be managed or treated. This type of hearing loss is most responsive to amplification measures, such as hearing aids, because it affects the loudness (amplitude and intensity) of sound, measured in decibels (dB).
- ***Sensorineural hearing loss,*** the most common type of hearing loss, occurs because of damage to the inner ear (cochlea) or the eighth cranial nerve leading to the brain from the inner ear (Tanna et al., 2023). This type of hearing loss is often caused by congenital or genetic disorders, noise trauma that damages the cochlear nerve, or ototoxic medications. Sensorineural hearing losses are permanent and irreversible, causing difficulty hearing and understanding speech. This involves the pitch or frequency of sound measured by sound cycles per second or hertz (Hz).
- ***Mixed hearing loss*** affects the outer, middle, and inner ear and is a combination of conductive and sensorineural hearing loss (Anastasiadou & Al Khalili, 2023).
- ***Auditory neuropathy spectrum disorder*** occurs when the brain is not able to interpret sound due to damage of the inner ear or the cochlear nerve (National Center on Birth Defects and Developmental Disabilities, 2022).

See Table 24-4 for causes of sensorineural and conductive hearing loss.

There are more than 400 inherited syndromes associated with hearing loss, some of which manifest during adolescence and early adulthood (Shave et al., 2022). Early identification of hearing loss is paramount to initiate effective treatment and services at school as indicated. The school nurse has an integral role in identifying these youth during school screenings. An audiogram measures both the pitch or frequency (Hz) and the loudness or intensity (dB). The softest level of the various frequencies that a student should hear as recorded on the audiogram is called the threshold. Hearing loss can range from mild to profound and is evaluated as a reduction in loudness, pitch, or both. The degree of hearing loss is identified by the decibel level (Table 24-5). For a child, 0 to 15 dB is within normal limits. A student with a hearing loss greater than 90 dB has a profound degree of hearing loss (ASHA, 2022c). Even a minimal hearing loss of 16 to 25 dB can have a significant effect on academic achievement (Leigh et al., 2016).

TABLE 24-4 Causes of Hearing Loss

Causes of Conductive Hearing Loss	Causes of Sensorineural Hearing Loss
Impacted cerumen	Diseases, especially brain infections
Otitis media or externa	Birth injury or head trauma
Foreign body in eardrum	Drugs toxic to auditory system
Fluid in middle ear caused by cold or allergies	Genetic syndromes
	Aging
Perforated eardrum	Noise exposure
	Tumors

American Speech-Language-Hearing Association (2022d).

Hearing Devices

The goal of sound amplification is to provide the student with the greatest amount of hearing possible while maintaining maximum comfort. There are different modes of amplification depending on the degree and cause of the hearing loss. Hearing aids are the most commonly used hearing devices (ASHA, 2022b). They are powered by either disposable or rechargeable batteries and pick up sound via a microphone and amplifier. The sound is then changed to electrical energy, which is converted by the receiver to acoustic energy so it can be heard. Hearing aids work best in quiet environments without additional background noise because hearing aids amplify all sound (ASHA, 2022b).

School audiologists and speech-language pathologists often provide services to students with hearing aids (ASHA, 2022b). However, a teacher or the school nurse may be responsible for checking the hearing aid settings and batteries daily at school to make certain the student gets the most out of the academic day. It is important to always keep extra batteries on hand (ASHA, 2022b).

The type of hearing aid may change as the child develops. The most common is the behind-the-ear hearing aid, which is a hard plastic case worn behind the ear that connects to a plastic earmold that fits inside the outer ear. Other common types are the receiver-in-canal or receiver-in-the-ear hearing aid, custom in-the-ear hearing aid, bone conduction and sound processor, and contralateral or bilateral routing of signal hearing aid (ASHA, 2022b).

Hearing aids can be analog or digital. Analog aids are the most affordable and convert the sound waves into electrical signals that are amplified (ASHA, 2022b). Digital aids convert sound waves into numerical codes like the binary code of a computer before amplifying them and are more effective in noisy environments. Digital hearing aids allow the audiologist to adjust the aid to multiple listening environments. Newer hearing aids also have connectivity options for smartphones and data logging ability to track wear time, which may help determine the usefulness of the device for the student (ASHA, 2022b).

TABLE 24-5 Sounds and Description of Hearing Loss at Specified Decibels

Decibel Level	Common Sounds at Specified Decibel Levels	Decibel Level Tested	Amount of Hearing Loss
0	Quietest sound	0–15	Normal
30	Whisper, quiet library	16–25	Slight hearing loss
60	Normal conversation, sewing machine	26–40	Mild hearing loss
90	Lawnmower, shop tools, truck traffic	41–65	Moderate hearing loss
100+	Chainsaw, pneumatic drill, snowmobile, firecracker	66–95	Severe hearing loss
		>95	Profound hearing loss

American Speech-Language-Hearing Association (2022a).

Hearing aids are expensive, small, and easily thrown out or lost; therefore students should not, in most cases, remove hearing aids themselves. Hearing aids should be maintained properly. They should be turned off when not in use, kept dry, and properly stored, and batteries need to be changed as needed. Earwax, ear drainage, moisture, hair products, and heat can damage the aid. Special care and cleaning of the earmold should be performed per the manufacturer's recommendation to preserve the longevity. Whistling sounds, feedback, and irritation caused by the hearing aid could indicate earwax buildup or an insufficient fit, which may require follow-up with a healthcare provider or audiologist. Hearing aids should be rechecked annually for proper fit and amplification (ASHA, 2022b).

Some students with hearing aids can also benefit from ***frequency-modulated transmission (FM) devices* or *digital modulation (DM) devices.*** These devices can be used within the classroom setting to improve hearing and separate out background noise from the teacher or speaker (ASHA, 2022b). The transmitter unit is clipped to the shirt of the speaker, and the student wears the receiver unit. The teacher can freely move around the room and the student does not have to stay focused on reading the teacher's lips. When changing classes, a student can give the teachers the transmitter to wear upon entrance into the classroom. A charging system for the FM system can be kept at school and checked daily to ensure proper functioning. The school nurse needs to be competent on the assistive communication devices so that problems can be identified early and handled properly.

Bone conduction hearing aids can be used for students with conductive hearing loss who do not respond to the standard hearing aid. A bone conduction hearing aid includes a 1-inch bone vibrating device held firmly against the mastoid bone with a headband or attached to the skull with a titanium screw. The vibration of sound bypasses the outer and middle ear and stimulates the inner ear via bone conduction (ASHA, 2022b).

Cochlear implants may benefit children with profound sensorineural hearing loss. Different from hearing aids that amplify sound, cochlear implants bypass damaged hair cells or sensory receptors of the ear; the existing auditory nerve fibers are stimulated, sending neuroimpulses to the brain to be interpreted as sound. Early implantation (less than 2 years of age) is a major variable leading to successful outcomes (McGregor & Goldman, 2022). With intensive speech therapy, children who receive cochlear implants at an early age can develop speech, language, and social skills according to typical developmental expectations. The school nurse should be aware that students with cochlear implants are at risk for development of acute otitis media and bacterial meningitis.

The receiver of the cochlear implant is surgically placed under the skin above the ear and inserted into the cochlea; the transmitter component easily attaches to the skull by a magnet to the receiver component (National Institute on Deafness and Other Communication Disorders, 2021). See Figure 24-4. School staff need to be educated by the school nurse that other strong magnets should not be near the child because they can deprogram the cochlear implant. Gaps in the effectiveness of the cochlear implant impair learning and result in loss of instructional time to visit the hearing specialist. Additionally, head injury should be reported to the healthcare provider to ensure the device has not been damaged. The school nurse should be aware that students with cochlear implants are at risk for development of acute otitis media and bacterial meningitis.

Communication Methods

Within the United States, *American Sign Language* (ASL) incorporates hand signals and facial and body gestures that correlate with words or concepts found in the English language. ASL is not universal and may differ across countries and even within regions; therefore it may not be universally understood by the deaf community (NDC, 2022). Family members, school nurses, teachers, and other school staff members should know important signs to communicate with the child. For example, the school nurse should learn signs for "pain," "toileting," "no"/"yes," "help," "where," "how long." Picture charts consistent with what is used in

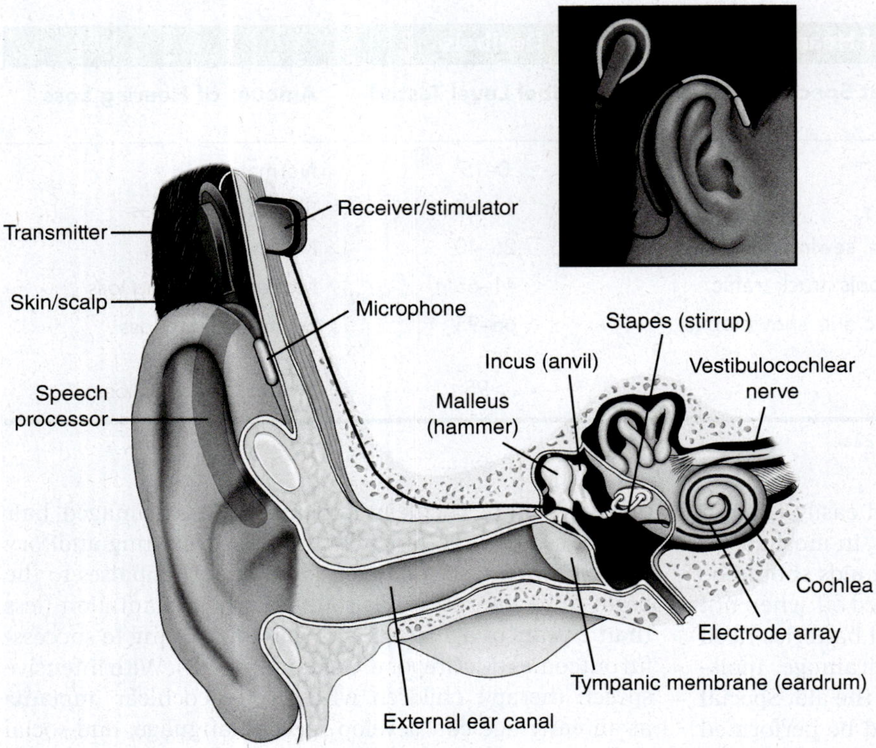

FIGURE 24-4. Student with a cochlear implant.

the classroom can facilitate communication between the student and the school nurse.

Some families believe that it is best for their child who is deaf to learn to communicate through a *total communication approach* that uses multiple modalities. This philosophy does not use sign language and depends on lip reading combined with cued speech, body language, and facial expression to communicate. Through lip reading, only about 40% of the words are understood, so it is helpful to add cued speech for greater communication. Cued speech uses hand signals to help differentiate between words that look similar when formed by lips.

Special Considerations

Hearing impairment and deafness are eligibility categories for special education services. The student's educational needs should be addressed by the IEP team. Students with hearing impairments will need educational assistance and related services to be successful in the classroom; these include speech, language, and/or auditory training. The school staff should take a comprehensive and consistent approach to communicating with these students. The approach should also be endorsed by the family and be respectful of cultural and language preferences. Staff education on the preferred communication method is imperative to help lower barriers to learning.

Students considered hearing impaired, hard of hearing, or deaf are at potential risk in the event of a school emergency, such as a fire or tornado. These students should have an emergency evacuation plan wherein a staff member is assigned to assist the student in the event of an emergency.

If a parent/guardian also is hearing impaired, the school should have a telecommunication device for the deaf (TDD). When a school does not have a TDD, a deaf relay service can provide telephone communication between a hearing person and a person with a TDD. Fax machines and e-mail may also be a useful source of communication. ASL or other appropriate interpreters should be available for parent/guardian meetings.

Students who are hard of hearing may benefit from the following accommodations from the educational staff:

- Provide preferential seating.
- Provide written instructions for assignments.

Practice Connection

It is estimated that noise-induced hearing loss accounts for 15.2% of children and adolescents with some degree of permanent damage to their hearing (Su & Chan, 2017). Additionally, adolescents living in rural locations report more noise exposures due to machinery, gunfire, power tools, and all-terrain vehicles with little use of hearing protection (Reel et al., 2022). *It's a Noisy Planet: Protect Their Hearing* is a national program sponsored by the National Institute on Deafness and Other Communication Disorders (2019) that promotes noise reduction to prevent hearing loss, especially in children ages 8 to 12 years. This program has activities and talking points about hearing loss prevention for parents, educators, and health professionals and other adults who care for children.

- Decrease ambient noise in the classroom.
- Face the student when talking to facilitate lip reading.
- Reduce glare from sunlight and avoid backlighting, which may make it difficult to see speakers or presented materials.

Vision Impairments

Most vision impairments can be corrected or greatly improved with glasses or contacts. Approximately 25% of children ages 2 to 17 years wear glasses or contacts (U.S. Department of Health and Human Services, 2021). Recent trends identify significant increases in myopia (nearsightedness) as well as a decline in vision screening since 2020 (Chauhan et al., 2023). Vision is an important aspect in social and intellectual development as well as quality of life during childhood (Lam & Suh, 2022). Untreated eye problems can worsen and affect learning, mental health, and adjustment in school.

Unlike hearing, vision reaches adult maturity by school age; therefore it is key to initiate early screening and referral so vision issues can be detected and treated as soon as possible. Schools provide an important link in visual care by providing vision screening services. Regular school-based vision screenings are key to identifying students who need a comprehensive eye examination to identify and treat the issue, as indicated. See Chapter 12 for more information on vision screening.

IDEA (2004) states that "***Visual impairment*** including blindness means an impairment in vision that, even with correction, adversely affects a child's educational performance. The term includes both partial sight and blindness" [§§300.8 (c)(13)]. ***Low vision*** is defined by the National Eye Institute (2023a) as "a vision problem that makes it difficult to do everyday activities. It can't be fixed with glasses, contact lenses, or other standard treatments like medicine or surgery" (para. 1). Common visual problems in childhood include refractive errors (i.e., myopia, hyperopia, astigmatism), amblyopia, strabismus, and retinoblastoma.

Common Vision Conditions

Refractive errors cause blurry vision and are commonly corrected by glasses or contacts. Refractive errors include myopia (nearsightedness), hyperopia (farsightedness), and astigmatism (irregular curvature of the lens). Students, especially younger students, may not recognize that they cannot see well. Signs and symptoms of refractive errors can include the following:

- Blurry vision
- Double vision
- Hazy vision
- Seeing glare or halo around lights
- Squinting
- Headaches
- Eye fatigue (eye rubbing)
- Closing one eye
- Difficulty focusing when reading or using a computer (National Eye Institute, 2023b)

Screening for refractive errors is generally accomplished through visual acuity screening.

Myopia, or nearsightedness, is when vision is clear close up but blurry in the distance. In myopia, the eyeball is too long or there is a high focusing power of the lens or cornea causing the light entering the eye to focus in front of the retina. Glasses or contact lenses with concave or divergent minus (−) lenses can be prescribed to improve vision (American Association for Pediatric Ophthalmology and Strabismus [AAPOS], 2023). Myopia typically worsens over time and plateaus until late adolescence or early adulthood.

Hyperopia, or farsightedness, is clear distance vision, but blurry near vision. In hyperopia, the eye is too short or has too little focusing power causing light entering the eye to fall behind the retina (AAPOS, 2023). Many young children have small degrees of hyperopia that do not require corrective lenses because children can naturally accommodate their focus. Hyperopia generally improves as children enter adolescence. More significant hyperopia is treated with converging or plus (+) powered lenses.

Astigmatism is a common refractive error in children that may run in families. In astigmatism, the eye is egg or oval shaped either horizontally (the eye is wider than tall) or vertically (the eye is taller than wide). This makes the cornea or lens asymmetrically curved causing the light entering the eye to focus at different points in front or behind the eye (AAPOS, 2023). Near and far distance vision are blurry. Astigmatism is associated with other eye examination abnormalities. Additionally, astigmatism can lead to amblyopia and vision loss if not treated (American Academy of Ophthalmology, 2023). See Figure 24-5 for images of refractive errors.

Amblyopia is a condition of abnormal vision development in infancy and early childhood causing decreased vision in one or both eyes (AAPOS, 2023). Though often called "lazy eye," amblyopia may not be an obvious eye problem. In amblyopia, the brain does not receive a proper image from the eye, and the neuropathways between the eye and the brain are not properly stimulated; therefore the brain does not "learn to see" in the affected eye(s). *Bilateral amblyopia* is treated with early prescription and consistent wear of corrective lenses. *Asymmetrical amblyopia* occurs when the vision in one eye is better than the vision in the other. Over time, the brain will rely on the stronger eye exclusively, allowing vision in the weaker eye to worsen. Amblyopia is associated with refractive errors and strabismus. Treatment for amblyopia involves forcing the weaker eye to work by patching the stronger eye or administering

Did You Know?

Amblyopia is a leading cause of permanent vision loss in childhood. It must be identified and treated early (AAPOS, 2023). Students younger than 7 years old are significantly more responsive to treatment than students between 7 and 13 years old (Holmes et al., 2011).

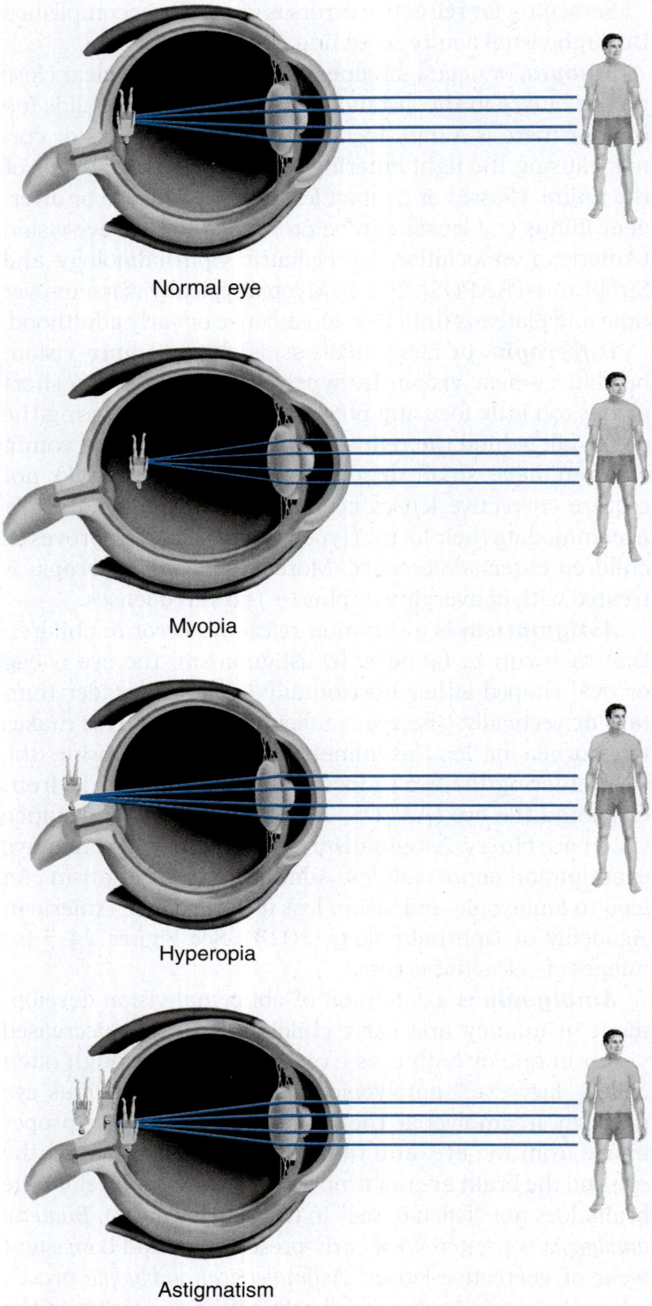

FIGURE 24-5. Refractive vision errors.

prescription eye drops in the stronger eye to blur vision (AAPOS, 2023; CDC, 2022b).

Strabismus is the misalignment of the eyes caused by a muscle imbalance where the eye(s) turns inward (esotropia) or outward (exotropia) (CDC, 2022b). Failure to correct strabismus can lead to reduced depth perception. Strabismus can be screened for by using the corneal light reflex test and cover/uncover test.

Less commonly, vision loss may be caused by congenital defects such as cataracts, retinoblastoma, brain tumors, medications, maternal infections, and trauma. Caused by a gene mutation, ***retinoblastoma*** is the most common intraocular cancer in childhood occurring in approximately 1 in 17,000 live births (Cruz-Galvez et al., 2022). Common symptoms of retinoblastoma include leukocoria (white pupil with absence of a red reflex), strabismus, or misaligned eyes. Retinoblastoma is highly treatable with a survival rate of 90% to 95%; however, vision loss and enucleation of the affected eye often occur.

Blindness

Students who are ***blind*** (no vision) or who are significantly visually impaired need an IEP with individualized and intensive services to facilitate development and learning. Remember that under IDEA (2004), all school-age children are entitled to a free and appropriate education in the least restrictive environment. For most students who are blind/severely visually impaired, this means learning in a regular classroom or a special education class with school-based services provided by itinerant vision teachers and other related service providers as indicated (Industries for the Blind and Visually Impaired, 2023). However, other students require an intensive level of services that can only be provided by a specialized school for the blind, especially in their early years of disability. Some parents prefer to home school their child. Comprehensive services for students who are blind or severely visually impaired may include the following:

- Instruction in Braille, the primary reading medium
- Use of a wide variety of assistive technology (e.g., optical scanners with speech output or Braille display)
- Orientation and mobility services so the student can be safe and navigate their environment
- Extended school year; vocational training and career education; and any other related services, as indicated

Deaf-Blindness

An individual considered deaf-blind typically has a varied range of loss in each of the affected senses. IDEA defines ***deaf-blindness*** as "concomitant hearing and vision impairments, the combination of which causes such severe communication and other developmental and educational needs that they cannot be accommodated in special education programs solely for children with deafness or children with blindness" (2004).

Certain genetic and congenital disorders are associated with deaf-blindness, including Usher syndrome, CHARGE syndrome, microcephaly, and prenatal infections such as rubella and herpes (National Center on Deaf-Blindness [NCDB], 2022). In deaf-blindness, there is usually a range of hearing and visual loss such that there may be some hearing or some vision (NCDB, 2022). In many cases, vision and/or hearing loss may or may not be present at birth but progressively develops as the child ages. There are over 10,000 children and youth younger than 21 years of age who have deaf-blindness (NCDB, 2022).

Individuals who are deaf-blind are a very diverse group; every case is individualized and needs to be treated and managed accordingly. The impact of deaf-blindness cannot be fully understood by adding the impact of the visual impairment to the impact of the hearing impairment, because each sense interacts in a fundamental way to support learning and development (Intini et al., 2022). Early identification and intervention will reduce the developmental disadvantages posed by deaf-blindness. A highly specialized collaborative team is needed to optimize outcomes.

Children who are deaf-blind learn to communicate in ways that use their dominant senses in combination with the highest level possible of their nondominant senses. The dominant senses are at a heightened level and are a resource for communication in deaf-blind individuals. Children who are deaf-blind can communicate using tactile signing, watching an interpreter at close range, following the signer by holding the signer's wrist and using their eyes to follow the signs, and placing their hand over the finger-spelling hand or signer's palm.

Color Vision Deficiency

"***Color vision deficiency*** is the inability to distinguish certain shades of color" (American Optometric Association, 2019, para. 1). Color vision deficiency occurs when the cones in the macula of the retina do not have one or more photosensitive pigments that transmit the perception of colors through the optic nerve in the brain. The majority of people with this condition can see colors, though many have difficulty discriminating between shades of reds and greens (more common) or blues and yellows (less common). Usually, color vision deficiency is an X-linked recessive inherited condition passed from mother to son; more boys (8%) are affected than girls (0.5%). However, damage to the retina or optic nerve caused by injury or certain diseases (e.g., diabetes, leukemia, or sickle cell) can also cause vision color deficiency. The term *color blindness,* or *achromatopsia,* refers to the rarer condition in which people are only able to see things in black and white or shades of gray (American Optometric Association, 2019). Though there is no cure, school nurses and teachers should be aware of which students have color vision deficiencies so educational accommodations and vocational counseling are offered.

ALTERATIONS IN ENDOCRINE HEALTH

The endocrine system is a network of glands that regulate the production and secretion of hormones into the bloodstream. These hormones, regulated by feedback systems and releasing hormones, affect various target organs throughout the body and regulate the body's growth, metabolism, and sexual development and function. The most common endocrine problem is diabetes mellitus, which is covered in Chapter 23. Other common endocrine conditions in children are discussed here.

Thyroid Conditions

The thyroid gland can be underactive (hypoactive) or overactive (hyperactive). Hypothyroidism results in a deficiency in secretion of thyroid hormone. *Hypothyroidism* can be congenital, presenting at birth, or it can develop later in childhood. ***Congenital hypothyroidism*** affects approximately 1 in 2,000 births in the United States and is primarily due to a defect in thyroid gland development (Bowden & Goldis, 2023). Newborn screening programs are essential as manifestations of congenital hypothyroidism are difficult to identify and lead to severe intellectual disability if left untreated. Children with congenital hypothyroidism need lifelong thyroid replacement to optimize neurodevelopment. Blood levels should be monitored regularly throughout childhood because doses need to be adjusted as the child grows (Bowden & Goldis, 2023).

Acquired hypothyroidism in childhood and adolescence is primarily due to Hashimoto thyroiditis and has a prevalence of about 3% in this population (Rodriguez et al., 2022). Hashimoto thyroiditis is an autoimmune disease that leads to the destruction of the thyroid gland resulting in low thyroid levels and a subsequent increase in thyroid-stimulating hormone (TSH). The preferred diagnostic laboratory test to diagnose and monitor treatment of hypothyroidism is serum TSH level (Rodriguez et al., 2022). Clinical manifestations of hypothyroidism include myxedematous skin changes (puffiness around the face, hands, and feet), dry skin, cold intolerance (feeling cold when other people feel warm), weight gain, constipation, and decreased energy. Children and adolescents may demonstrate problems with memory, attention, and a decline in academic performance. School nurses should be aware that children with Down syndrome have increased risk of hypothyroidism (Rodriguez et al., 2022). Treatment includes replacement of thyroid with monitoring of serum levels to optimize dosing as the child or adolescent grows. School nurses who notice symptoms of hypothyroidism or new academic difficulties should contact the student's parent/guardian or healthcare provider, especially if recent serum levels of TSH have not been obtained.

Hyperthyroidism results in excessive circulating thyroid hormone and is usually the result of Graves' disease, an autoimmune condition. In Graves' disease, the body produces antibodies that overstimulate the thyroid gland causing it to overproduce and release too much thyroid hormone (Vaidyanathan, 2022). The incidence is higher in females and can occur at any age during childhood but peaks during adolescence (Vaidyanathan, 2022). Manifestations of the disease may include tachycardia, nervousness/tremors, heat intolerance with increased sweating, weight loss, insomnia, and exophthalmos (protruding eyeballs). In contrast to hypothyroidism, TSH levels are low in Graves' disease with high levels of thyroid hormone. Treatment for hyperthyroidism includes medications to antagonize the thyroid gland or a thyroidectomy (Vaidyanathan, 2022). In cases where a thyroidectomy has been performed, the child will then need lifelong thyroid replacement. Medications such as atenolol or propranolol may be prescribed to help with symptomatic relief of palpitations or tremors (Vaidyanathan, 2022).

Thyroid storm (thyrotoxic crisis) is a life-threatening but rare emergency and results from a sudden increase or release of thyroid hormone. Signs and symptoms include an acute onset of high fever, tachycardia with cardiovascular decompensation, and mental status changes (Vaidyanathan, 2022). A thyroid storm may be precipitated by acute infection, trauma, or discontinuation of antithyroid therapy and requires emergent care.

Other Endocrine Conditions

Growth hormone deficiency, short stature, and constitutional growth delay are all reasons a student may be receiving treatment with recombinant human growth hormone (Danowitz & Grimberg, 2022). ***Growth hormone deficiency*** can be congenital or acquired. Congenital growth hormone deficiency is due to genetic abnormalities or anomalies of the pituitary gland; acquired growth hormone deficiency is likely from a tumor or head injury (Danowitz & Grimberg, 2022). ***Constitutional growth delay*** with familial short stature occurs in approximately 15% of children and is the leading cause of short stature and pubertal delay, affecting boys more often than girls (Aguilar & Castano, 2023). ***Short stature*** is defined as a height more than 2 standard deviations below the mean for age (less than the 3rd percentile) on growth charts. Constitutional growth delay is benign and is a diagnosis of exclusion; no treatment is needed; students typically catch up to their normal growth curve. *Familial short stature* is genetic and occurs when one or both parents are also of short stature. Growth hormone is selectively prescribed by endocrinologists for specific diseases associated with short stature: growth hormone deficiency, renal insufficiency, Turner syndrome, Prader-Willi syndrome, small for gestational age, and idiopathic short stature, among others (Aguilar & Castano, 2023). Treatment with growth hormone not only increases linear growth, but also positively affects lipid profile, cardiac performance, muscle mass, and bone density (Danowitz & Grimberg, 2022).

Diabetes insipidus is a disorder where there are decreased amounts of antidiuretic hormone (ADH) or vasopressin in the body (Hui et al., 2023). Vasopressin, made by the hypothalamus and stored in the pituitary gland, is a hormone that normally acts on the kidney to reduce urine output by increasing the concentration of the urine. In diabetes insipidus, the decrease in vasopressin causes the hallmark manifestations of passing large amounts of dilute urine and increased thirst. If untreated, hypovolemia, dehydration, and electrolyte disturbances can develop quickly. The cause of diabetes insipidus is often idiopathic or it may be the result of neurosurgery or a traumatic brain injury (Hui et al., 2023). Treatment includes the administration of DDAVP and ADH analogue. In the school environment, students with diabetes insipidus should have DDAVP available in the school nurse office and access to water. Students who exhibit thirst and polyuria should be evaluated immediately by the school nurse.

Precocious puberty is an endocrine condition where children show physical developmental signs of puberty early, before 8 years of age in girls and before 9 years of age in boys. The mechanism of precocious puberty is not fully understood; however, the number of children with the condition has globally increased over the last few decades and females are more frequently affected (Han et al., 2022). Factors associated with the development of precocious puberty include geographical region, family environment, endocrine disrupting chemicals such as pesticides, and personal nutritional factors. These factors appear to stimulate increased levels of gonadotropin-releasing hormone and gonadotropins, which leads to the early development of secondary sex characteristics. Precocious puberty leads to early epiphyseal plate closure, overall lifetime decreased linear height, and may increase risk of hypertension, diabetes, and even infertility in adulthood (Han et al., 2022). Early sexual development can lead to stigmas and psychosocial stresses due to body image changes (Turan Miral & Hotun Sahin, 2022). Treatment for precious puberty is aimed at reducing or blocking the secretion of gonadotropins either through medications or removal of tumors (Bakhtiani & Geffner, 2022).

ALTERATIONS IN GENITOURINARY HEALTH

Chronic Kidney Disease

Chronic kidney disease, also called chronic renal disease, can result in end-stage renal failure in childhood (Panzarino et al., 2022). Early identification and treatment are essential to limit devastating complications associated with renal failure.

Chronic kidney disease can be either genetic or acquired. Possible causes include the following:

- Polycystic kidney disease (genetic)
- Congenital renal and urinary tract malformations
- Glomerulonephritis (autoimmune)
- Nephrotic syndrome (autoimmune)
- Recurrent urinary tract infections associated with vesicoureteral reflux
- Chronic pyelonephritis
- Diabetes
- Hypertension
- Malignancies

Chronic kidney disease causes nephrotic destruction and occurs in a slow, progressive manner without symptoms until the disease is advanced (Panzarino et al., 2022). The kidneys have the ability to compensate and remain asymptomatic until approximately half of the nephrons are nonfunctional. As the disease progresses, the nephrons are no longer able to adjust and maintain fluid and electrolyte balance, at which point symptoms appear. Uremia occurs when the kidneys can no longer filter waste so it accumulates in the bloodstream. Chronic kidney disease is categorized in stages based on glomerular filtration rates with stages 4 to 5 the most severe (Panzarino et al., 2022).

The kidney has many functions including production of erythropoietin, fluid and electrolyte balance, filtering waste, vitamin D synthesis, and acid-base balance. Erythropoietin stimulates RBC development; therefore anemia is a common complication of chronic kidney disease. Early signs of anemia include decreased energy, secondary amenorrhea, and pallor. The decreased energy results in listlessness and a preference for sedentary play in children. The child with chronic kidney disease is more likely to experience infection, such as pneumonia, urinary tract infections, and septicemia.

As the kidneys' ability to filter waste declines and the glomerular filtration rate decreases, ***uremic syndrome*** develops (Panzarino et al., 2022). Symptoms of uremic syndrome include decreased appetite, headaches, muscle cramps, nausea, weight loss, malaise, dry and itchy skin, and decline in growth. Urine output will continue to decrease, leading to altered fluid balance, and blood pressure will continue to increase. Electrolyte imbalances develop resulting in hyperkalemia, hyperphosphatemia, hypocalcemia, and rickets. Metabolic acidosis may also develop as the kidneys are unable to balance the blood's pH by making bicarbonate (Panzarino et al., 2022).

During end-stage kidney failure, the student will need dialysis (hemodialysis or peritoneal dialysis) and eventually a kidney transplant. These treatments are life-altering decisions for the family and child that involve emotional, psychosocial, and financial stressors. The school environment may provide stability and some normalization for the child.

Dietary measures play an important role in the management of chronic kidney disease. The goal of dietary measures is to consume the requisite calories and protein for growth, while at the same time minimizing the actual demands for processing by the kidneys. Protein and phosphorous may need to be limited (Panzarino et al., 2022). It is not uncommon to see malnutrition in individuals with chronic renal failure. Milk and protein intake are monitored to maintain a calcium-phosphorus balance; vitamin D or calcium carbonate may be given to regulate this balance. A major concern is failure to grow, especially in the child who has not reached adolescence. Recombinant human growth hormone has been successful in accelerating growth in these children. Dental care is very important in the child with chronic kidney disease because of hypomineralization, hypoplasia, tooth discoloration, and altered size and shape of the teeth in students with chronic kidney disease.

Hypertension is common among those with kidney disease and may be managed with antihypertensive medications, reduced sodium intake, and fluid restrictions. The school nurse plays an important role in monitoring the child's blood pressure and providing medications as prescribed.

The student may also be prescribed erythropoietin to help with anemia. Antibiotics may be given at the first sign of infection as the child is at increased risk of infections. Vitamin D, calcium, and medications to reduce itching may also be part of the medication profile. Children who have had renal transplants may also be taking antirejection medications. Drugs that are excreted by the kidneys need to be closely monitored and may have adjusted dosing; nephrotoxic medications should be limited (Panzarino et al., 2022). Over-the-counter medications, particularly NSAIDs, should be used cautiously as some may be nephrotoxic and contraindicated in individuals with chronic kidney disease.

The student's Section 504 plan should provide for rest periods as needed so that the child can participate in learning activities to the fullest extent possible. If the student has shunts for dialysis, care must be taken to avoid trauma to the arm; blood pressure readings should not be taken in that arm. A medical alert bracelet is recommended so that medical professionals will be able to address the child's individual needs more quickly and precisely in case of an emergency. It is helpful to allow children as much responsibility in their treatment as possible.

CONCLUSION

Students with chronic conditions are children first. Although they have specific healthcare needs, students with chronic conditions have the right to participate fully in the school environment. The school nurse is the constant in the student's school experience over the years to provide holistic continuity of care in conjunction with the family, educational team, and healthcare providers.

The school nurse is in a unique position to provide school nurse–led case management, serving as a liaison and care coordinator between the family, the healthcare providers, and the school. Involving the family in developing the IHP, Section 504 accommodation plan, or IEP ensures a safe and productive educational experience. The school nurse plays an important role in providing information to the family related to available resources that can enhance the family unit. Ongoing communication with the student's teachers also supports the coordination of health and education goals for these students.

Students with chronic conditions are uniquely affected by their condition; some consider it a disability, others do not. Some students may need special accommodations, but all students with special healthcare needs require a school nurse to monitor their condition. Students with chronic conditions should be fully included in the learning environment and be accepted as important members of the school community.

References

Abdelghani, E., Cua, C. L., Giver, J., & Rodriguez, V. (2021). Thrombosis prevention and anticoagulation management in the pediatric patient with congenital heart disease. *Cardiology and Therapy, 10*(2), 325–348. https://doi.org/10.1007/s40119-021-00228-4

Aguilar, D., & Castano, G. (2023, June 26). *Constitutional growth delay*. StatPearls [Internet]. https://www.ncbi.nlm.nih.gov/books/NBK539780/

Alblaihed, L., Dubbs, S. B., Koyfman, A., & Long, B. (2022). High risk and low prevalence diseases: Hemophilia emergencies. *The American Journal of Emergency Medicine, 56*, 21–27. https://doi.org/10.1016/j.ajem.2022.02.045

American Academy of Ophthalmology. (2023). *What is astigmatism? Symptoms, causes, and treatment.* https://www.aao.org/eye-health/diseases/what-is-astigmatism

American Academy of Pediatrics. (2023, February 8). *Multisystem inflammatory syndrome in children (MIS-C): Interim guidance.* https://www.aap.org/en/pages/2019-novel-coronavirus-covid-19-infections/clinical-guidance/multisystem-inflammatory-syndrome-in-children-mis-c-interim-guidance/

American Association for Pediatric Ophthalmology and Strabismus. (2023). *Refractive errors in children.* https://aapos.org/glossary/refractive-errors-in-children

American Association of Neurologic Surgeons. (2023a). *Chiari malformation.* https://www.aans.org/en/Patients/Neurosurgical-Conditions-and-Treatments/Chiari-Malformation

American Association of Neurologic Surgeons. (2023b). *Hydrocephalus.* https://www.aans.org/en/Patients/Neurosurgical-Conditions-and-Treatments/Hydrocephalus

American Association of Neurologic Surgeons. (2023c). *Scoliosis.* https://www.aans.org/Patients/Neurosurgical-Conditions-and-Treatments/Scoliosis

American Cancer Society. (2019a). *Signs and symptoms of childhood leukemia.* https://www.cancer.org/cancer/leukemia-in-children/detection-diagnosis-staging/signs-and-symptoms.html

American Cancer Society. (2019b). *Survival rates for childhood leukemias.* https://www.cancer.org/cancer/leukemia-in-children/detection-diagnosis-staging/survival-rates.html

American Cancer Society. (2022). *Key statistics for childhood cancers.* https://www.cancer.org/cancer/cancer-in-children/key-statistics.html

American Optometric Association. (2019). *Color vision deficiency.* https://www.aoa.org/patients-and-public/eye-and-vision-problems/glossary-of-eye-and-vision-conditions/color-deficiency

American Speech-Language-Hearing Association. (2022a). *Degree of hearing loss.* https://www.asha.org/public/hearing/Degree-of-Hearing-Loss/

American Speech-Language-Hearing Association. (2022b). *Hearing aids for children.* https://www.asha.org/practice-portal/professional-issues/hearing-aids-for-children/

American Speech-Language-Hearing Association. (2022c). *Speech and language disorders.* https://www.asha.org/public/speech/disorders/childsandl/

American Speech-Language-Hearing Association. (2022d). *Types of hearing loss.* https://www.asha.org/public/hearing/types-of-hearing-loss/

Ananthakrishnan, A. (2015). Epidemiology and risk factors for IBD. *Nature Reviews Gastroenterology & Hepatology, 12*, 205–217. https://doi.org/10.1038/nrgastro.2015.34

Anastasiadou, S., & Al Khalili, Y. *Hearing loss.* (2023). StatPearls [Internet]. https://www.ncbi.nlm.nih.gov/books/NBK542323/#:~:text=Hearing%20loss%20that%20involves%20problematic,is%20called%20mixed%20hearing%20loss

Arvind, B., & Ramakrishnan, S. (2020). Rheumatic fever and rheumatic heart disease in children. *The Indian Journal of Pediatrics, 87*(4), 305–311. https://doi.org/10.1007/s12098-019-03128-7

Bakhtiani, P., & Geffner, M. (2022). Early puberty. *Pediatrics in Review, 43*(9), 483–492. https://doi.org/10.1542/pir.2021-005059

Banasik, J., Banasik, B. N., & Miller, B. J. (Eds.). (2022) *Pathophysiology* (7th ed., pp. 240–268). Elsevier.

Belayneh, R., Fourman, M. S., Bhogal, S., & Weiss, K. R. (2021). Update on osteosarcoma. *Current Oncology Reports, 23*(6), 71. https://doi.org/10.1007/s11912-021-01053-7

Bell, C. S., Samuel, J. P., & Samuels, J. A. (2019). Prevalence of hypertension in children: Applying the new American Academy of Pediatrics clinical practice guideline. *Hypertension, 73*(1), 148–152. https://doi.org/10.1161/HYPERTENSIONAHA.118.11673

Berntorp, E., Trakymienė, S. S., Federici, A. B., Holstein, K., Corrales-Medina, F. F., Pierce, G. F., Srivastava, A., Prondzinski, M. V. D., Johnsen, J. M., Zupan, I. P., Halimeh, S., Nummi, V., & Roberts, J. C. (2022). Sixth Åland Island Conference on von Willebrand disease. *Haemophilia: The Official Journal of the World Federation of Hemophilia, 28*(Suppl 5), 3–15. https://doi.org/10.1111/hae.14495

Blasco, M., García-Galant, M., Berenguer-González, A., Caldú, X., Arqué, M., Laporta-Hoyos, O., Ballester-Plané, J., Miralbell, J., Jurado, M. Á., & Roser Pueyo. (2022). Interventions with an impact on cognitive functions in cerebral palsy: A systematic review. *Neuropsychology Review*, 10.1007/s11065-022-09550-7. Advance online publication. https://doi.org/10.1007/s11065-022-09550-7

Bowden, S. A., & Goldis, M. (2023, June 5). *Congenital hypothyroidism.* StatPearls [Internet]. https://www.ncbi.nlm.nih.gov/books/NBK558913/

Bultas M. W., & Fuller, K. (2021). Multisystem inflammatory syndrome in children and COVID-19 infections. *NASN School Nurse, 36*(6), 341–345. https://doi.org/10.1177/1942602X211021136

Celiac Disease Foundation. (2022). *About celiac disease.* https://celiac.org/about-celiac-disease/what-is-celiac-disease/

Centers for Disease Control and Prevention. (2020, May 29). *Kawasaki disease.* https://www.cdc.gov/kawasaki/index.html

Centers for Disease Control and Prevention. (2022a, August 1). *What is hemophilia?* https://www.cdc.gov/ncbddd/hemophilia/facts.html

Centers for Disease Control and Prevention. (2022b). *Vision Health Initiative: Common eye disorders and diseases.* https://www.cdc.gov/visionhealth/basics/ced/index.html

Centers for Disease Control and Prevention. (2022c). *Von Willebrand disease.* https://www.cdc.gov/ncbddd/vwd/facts.html

Centers for Disease Control and Prevention. (2023a, June 28). *Anencephaly.* https://www.cdc.gov/ncbddd/birthdefects/anencephaly.html

Centers for Disease Control and Prevention. (2023b, October 2). *HIV in the United States by age: HIV diagnoses.* https://www.cdc.gov/hiv/group/age/diagnoses.html

Centers for Disease Control and Prevention. (2023c). *Microcephaly.* https://www.cdc.gov/ncbddd/birthdefects/data.html

Centers for Disease Control and Prevention. (2023d). *What is cerebral palsy?* https://www.cdc.gov/ncbddd/cp/facts.html

Cerebral Palsy Guide. (2021, January 29). *Cerebral palsy incontinence.* https://www.cerebralpalsyguide.com/blog/cerebral-palsy-incontinence/

Chauhan, M. Z., Elhusseiny, A. M., Samarah, E. S., Rook, B. S., Sallam, A. B., & Phillips, P. H. (2023). Five-year trends in pediatric vision screening and access in the United States. *Ophthalmology, 130*(1), 120–122. https://doi.org/10.1016/j.ophtha.2022.09.018

Cheng, T., Einarsdottir, E., Kere, J., & Gerdhem, P. (2022). Idiopathic scoliosis: A systematic review and meta-analysis of heritability. *EFORT Open Reviews, 7*(6), 414–421. https://doi.org/10.1530/EOR-22-0026

Cheson, B. D., Fisher, R. I., Barrington, S. F., Cavalli, F., Schwartz, L. H., Zucca, E., & Lister, T. A. (2014). Recommendations for initial evaluation, staging, and response assessment of Hodgkin and non-Hodgkin lymphoma: The Lugano classification. *Journal of Clinical Oncology, 32*(27), 3059. https://doi.org/10.1200/JCO.2013.54.8800

Cheung, T., de Zoeten, E. F., Hoffenberg, E. J., Liu, E., Pan, Z., Walker, T., & Stahl, M. (2022). Characteristics of children with inflammatory bowel disease and coexisting celiac disease seropositivity. *Journal of Pediatric Gastroenterology and Nutrition, 75*(6), 737–742. https://doi.org/10.1097/MPG.0000000000003613

Children's Oncology Group. (2022). *Late effects of treatment for children's cancer.* https://www.childrensoncologygroup.org/lateeffectsoftreatment

Choudhry, S., Puri, K., & Denfield, S. W. (2019). An update on pediatric cardiomyopathy. *Current Treatment Options in Cardiovascular Medicine, 21*(8), 36. https://doi.org/10.1007/s11936-019-0739-y

Chowdhury, S., Koziatek, C, & Rajni, M. (2023). *Acute rheumatic fever*. StatPearls [Internet]. https://www.ncbi.nlm.nih.gov/books/NBK594238/

Chu, P. Y., Li, J. S., Kosinski, A. S., Hornik, C. P., & Hill, K. D. (2017). Congenital heart disease in premature infants 25–32 weeks' gestational age. *The Journal of Pediatrics, 181*, 37–41. https://doi.org/10.1016/j.jpeds.2016.10.033

Claytor, C., & Bazner-Chandler, J. (2017). Musculoskeletal disorders. In C. Burns, A. Dunn, M. Brady, N. Starr, C. Blosser, & D. Garzon (Eds.), *Pediatric primary care* (pp. 1042–1081). Elsevier.

Close, E., McConnell, G., Cross, S., & Bradford, J. L. (2020). Immunogenicity of childhood vaccines after pediatric cancer. *American Family Physician, 102*(11). https://www.aafp.org/pubs/afp/issues/2020/1201/od1.html

Crohn's and Colitis Foundation. (2022). *Signs and symptoms of Crohn's disease*. https://www.crohnscolitisfoundation.org/what-is-crohns-disease/diagnosis-testing

Cruz-Gálvez, C. C., Ordaz-Favila, J. C., Villar-Calvo, V. M., Cancino-Marentes, M. E., & Bosch-Canto, V. (2022). Retinoblastoma: Review and new insights. *Frontiers in Oncology, 12*, 963780. https://doi.org/10.3389/fonc.2022.963780

Daetwyler, E., Bargetzi, M., Otth, M., & Scheinemann, K. (2022). Late effects of high-dose methotrexate treatment in childhood cancer survivors—A systematic review. *BMC Cancer, 22*(1), 1–12. https://doi.org/10.1186/s12885-021-09145-0

Danowitz, M., & Grimberg, A. (2022). Clinical indications for growth hormone therapy. *Advances in Pediatrics, 69*(1), 203–217. https://doi.org/10.1016/j.yapd.2022.03.005

Darcy, L., Enskär, K., & Björk, M. (2019). Young children's experiences of living an everyday life with cancer—A three-year interview study. *European Journal of Oncology Nursing, 39*, 1–9. https://doi.org/10.1016/j.ejon.2018.12.007

De, B., Florez, M. A., Ludmir, E. B., Maor, M. H., McGovern, S. L., McAleer, M. F., Grosshans, D. R., Chang, E. L., Mahajan, A., & Paulino, A. C. (2022). Late effects of craniospinal irradiation using electron spinal fields for pediatric patients with cancer. *International Journal of Radiation Oncology · Biology · Physics*. https://doi.org/10.1016/j.ijrobp.2022.06.055

Delaney, A., Baker, A. L., Bastardi, H., & O'Brien, P. (2017). The child with cardiovascular dysfunction. In M. J. Hockenberry, D. Wilson, & C. C. Rogers (Eds.), *Essentials of pediatric nursing* (10th ed., pp. 738–785). Elsevier.

de Loizaga, S. R., & Beaton, A. Z. (2021). Rheumatic fever and rheumatic heart disease in the United States. *Pediatric Annals, 50*(3), e98–e104. https://doi.org/10.3928/19382359-20210221-01

Diorio, C., Henrickson, S. E., Vella, L. A., McNerney, K. O., Chase, J., Burudpakdee,C., Lee, J. H., Jasen, C., Balamuth, F., Barrett, D. M., Banwell, B. L., Bernt, K. M., Blatz, A. M., Chiotos, K., Fisher, B. T., Fitzgerald, J. C., Gerber, J. S., Gollomp, K., Gray, C., . . . Bassiri, H. (2020). Multisystem inflammatory syndrome in children and COVID-19 are distinct presentations of SARS–CoV-2. *Journal of Clinical Investigation, 130*(11), 5967–5975. https://doi.org/10.1172/JCI140970

Donzel, M., Bonjour, M., Combes, J. D., Broussais, F., Sesques, P., Traverse-Glehen, A., & de Martel, C. (2022). Lymphomas associated with Epstein-Barr virus infection in 2020: Results from a large, unselected case series in France. *Eclinicalmedicine, 54*, 101674. https://doi.org/10.1016/j.eclinm.2022.101674

Eladly, F., & Miesbach, W. (2022). Von Willebrand disease—Specific aspects in women. *Hamostaseologie, 42*(5), 330–336. https://doi.org/10.1055/a-1891-9976

Elsevier Point of Care. (2022, November 2). *Clinical overview: HIV infection in children. Clinical Key*. https://www.clinicalkey.com

Erdmann, F., Frederiksen, L. E., Bonaventure, A., Mader, L., Hasle, H., Robison, L. L., & Winther, J. F. (2021). Childhood cancer: Survival, treatment modalities, late effects and improvements over time. *Cancer Epidemiology, 71*, 101733. https://doi.org/10.1016/j.canep.2020.101733

Farr, S. L., Downing, K. F., Riehle-Colarusso, T., & Abarbanell, G. (2018). Functional limitations and educational needs among children and adolescents with heart disease. *Congenital Heart Disease, 13*(4), 633–639. https://doi.org/10.1111/chd.12621

Flynn, J. T., Kaelber, D. C., Baker-Smith, C. M., Blowey, D., Carroll, A. E., Daniels, S. R., ... & Urbina, E. M. (2017). Clinical practice guideline for screening and management of high blood pressure in children and adolescents. *Pediatrics, 140*(3). https://doi.org/10.1542/peds.2017-1904

Fox, C. (2021). Pediatric hypertension. *Primary Care, 48*(3), 367–378. https://doi.org/10.1016/j.pop.2021.04.001

Garcia, R. U., & Peddy, S. B. (2018). Heart disease in children. *Primary Care: Clinics in Office Practice, 45*(1), 143–154. https://doi.org/10.1016/j.pop.2017.10.005

GBD 2017 Inflammatory Bowel Disease Collaborators. (2020). The global, regional, and national burden of inflammatory bowel disease in 195 countries and territories, 1990–2017: A systematic analysis for the Global Burden of Disease Study 2017. *The Lancet. Gastroenterology & Hepatology, 5*(1), 17–30. https://doi.org/10.1016/S2468-1253(19)30333-4

Gerceker, G. Ö., Yildirim, B. G., Sülün, A. A., Bektaş, M., Özdemir, H. H., & Malbora, B. (2022). The effect of chemotherapy on symptoms and nutritional status in children with cancer. *European Journal of Oncology Nursing, 61*, 102206. https://doi.org/10.1016/j.ejon.2022.102206

Gowda, S., & Schneider, L. K. (2023, August 14). *Apraxia*. StatPearls [Internet]. https://www.ncbi.nlm.nih.gov/books/NBK585110/#:~:text=Apraxia%20is%20a%20neurological%20disorder,neurocognitive%20disorders%2C%20and%20brain%20injuries

Grace, R. F., & Lambert, M. P. (2022). An update on pediatric ITP: Differentiating primary ITP, IPD, and PID. *Blood, 140*(6), 542–555. https://doi.org/10.1182/blood.2020006480

Gustafson, S. J., & Corbin, N. E. (2021). Pediatric hearing loss guidelines and consensus statements—Where do we stand? *Otolaryngologic Clinics of North America, 54*(6), 1129–1142. https://doi.org/10.1016/j.otc.2021.07.003

Han, X. X., Zhao, F. Y., Gu, K. R., Wang, G. P., Zhang, J., Tao, R., Yuan, J., Gu, J., & Yu, J. Q. (2022). Development of precocious puberty in children: Surmised medicinal plant treatment. *Biomedicine & Pharmacotherapie, 156*, 113907. https://doi.org/10.1016/j.biopha.2022.113907

Holmes, J. M., Lazar, E. L., Melia, B. M., Astle, W. F., Dagi, L. R., Donahue, S. P., Frazier, M. G., Hertle, R. W., Repka, M. X., Quinn, G. E., Weise, K. K.; Pediatric Eye Disease Investigator Group. (2011). Effect of age on response to amblyopia treatment in children. *Archives of Ophthalmology, 129*(11), 1451–1457. https://www.ncbi.nlm.nih.gov/pmc/articles/PMC3217111/

Hui, C., Khan, M., Khan Suheb, M. Z., & Radbel, J. M. (2023, June 1). *Diabetes insipidus*. StatPearls [Internet]. https://www.ncbi.nlm.nih.gov/books/NBK470458/

Inaba, H., & Pui, C. H. (2021). Advances in the diagnosis and treatment of pediatric acute lymphoblastic leukemia. *Journal of Clinical Medicine, 10*(9), 1926. https://doi.org/10.3390/jcm10091926

Individuals With Disabilities Education Improvement Act of 2004, 20 U.S. C. § 1400. (2004). http://idea.ed.gov/download/statute.html

Industries for the Blind and Visually Impaired. (2023). *Educational options for blind and visually impaired kids*. https://ibvi.org/blog/educational-options-for-blind-and-visually-impaired-kids/

Intini, M., Garrino, L., Conti, A., Dimonte, V., & Borraccino, A. (2022). Deaf-blindness through the voices and experiences of parents and educators. *Journal of Deaf Studies and Deaf Education, 27*(4), 373–384. https://doi.org/10.1093/deafed/enac014

Iskandar, B. J., & Finnell, R. H. (2022). Spina bifida. *The New England Journal of Medicine, 387*(5), 444–450. https://doi.org/10.1056/NEJMra2116032

Jayaraman, D. K., & Das, J. M. (2023, June 4). *Dysarthria*. StatPearls [Internet]. https://www.ncbi.nlm.nih.gov/books/NBK592453/

K, A., Saini, L., Gunasekaran, P. K., Singh, P., Sahu, J. K., Sankhyan, N., Sharma, R., Bhati, A., Yadav, J., & Sharawat, I. K. (2022). The profile of epilepsy and its characteristics in children with cerebral palsy. *Seizure, 101*, 190–196. https://doi.org/10.1016/j.seizure.2022.08.009

Kagami, L., Baldino, S., & MacFarland, S. P. (2022). Childhood cancer predisposition: An overview for the general pediatrician. *Pediatric Annals, 51*(1), e15–e21. https://doi.org/10.3928/19382359-20211207-01

Kavanagh, P. L., Fasipe, T. A., & Wun, T. (2022). Sickle cell disease: A review. *JAMA, 328*(1), 57–68. https://doi.org/10.1001/jama.2022.10233

Kaya Keles, C. S., & Ates, F. (2022). Botulinum toxin intervention in cerebral palsy-induced spasticity management: Projected and contradictory effects on skeletal muscles. *Toxins, 14*(11), 772. https://doi.org/10.3390/toxins14110772

Kendall, S. J., Langley, J. E., Crooks, B. N., Giacomantonio, N., Heinze-Milne, S., Johnston, W. J., ... & Grandy, S. A. (2022). The impact of exercise on cardiotoxicity in pediatric cancer survivors: A scoping review protocol. *Healthy Populations Journal, 2*(2). https://doi.org/10.3390/curroncol29090500

Kim, E. H., Lee, J. H., Song, I. K., Kim, H. S., Jang, Y. E., Yoo, S., & Kim, J. T. (2019). Accuracy of pulse oximeters at low oxygen saturations in children with congenital cyanotic heart disease: An observational study. *Pediatric Anesthesia, 29*(6), 597–603. https://doi.org/10.1111/pan.13642

Kleinhenz, J., & Wagner, E. (2022). Biologics in pediatric inflammatory bowel disease. *Pediatric Annals, 51*(2), e77–e81. https://doi.org/10.3928/19382359-20220113-01

Konrad, J., Eber, E., & Stadlbauer, V. (2022). Changing paradigms in the treatment of gastrointestinal complications of cystic fibrosis in the era of cystic fibrosis transmembrane conductance regulator modulators. *Paediatric Respiratory Reviews, 42*, 9–16. https://doi.org/10.1016/j.prrv.2020.12.001

Kuhn, J., & Emmady, P. D. (2022, May 8). *Chiari II malformation.* StatPearls. https://www.ncbi.nlm.nih.gov/books/NBK557498/

Kwak, Y., Kim, Y., Choi, E. S., & Im, H. J. (2021). Self-efficacy, post-traumatic growth, and quality of life of pediatric cancer survivors: A cross-sectional study. *European Journal of Oncology Nursing, 54*, 102019. https://doi.org/10.1016/j.ejon.2021.102019

Lam, M., & Suh, D. (2022). Screening, diagnosis, and treatment of pediatric ocular diseases. *Children, 9*(12), 1939. https://doi.org/10.3390/children9121939

Landier, W., Skinner, R., Wallace, W. H., Hjorth, L., Mulder, R. L., Wong, F. L., ... & Hudson, M. M. (2018). Surveillance for late effects in childhood cancer survivors. *Journal of Clinical Oncology, 36*(21), 2216. https://doi.org/10.1200/JCO.2017.77.0180

Leigh, I. W., Andrews, J. F., & Harris, R. (2016). *Deaf culture: Exploring deaf communities in the United States.* San Diego, CA: Plural Publishing.

Liamlahi, R., & Latal, B. (2019). Neurodevelopmental outcome of children with congenital heart disease. *Handbook of Clinical Neurology, 162*, 329–345. https://doi.org/10.1016/B978-0-444-64029-1.00016-3

Lipshultz, S.E., Law, Y.M. Asante-Korang, A., Austin, E.D., Dipchand, A.I., Everitt, M.D., Hsu, D.T., Lin, K.Y., Price, J.F., Wilkinson, J.D., & Colan, S.D. (2019). Cardiomyopathy in children: Classification and diagnosis: A scientific statement from the American Heart Association. *Circulation, 140*(1), e9-e68. On behalf of the American Heart Association Council on Cardiovascular Disease in the Young; Council on Clinical Cardiology; and Council on Genomic and Precision Medicine. https://doi.org/10.1161/CIR.0000000000000682

Mahapatra, S., & Challagundla, K. B. (2023, July 10). *Neuroblastoma.* StatPearls [Internet]. https://www.ncbi.nlm.nih.gov/books/NBK448111/

Markati, T., Oskoui, M., Farrar, M. A., Duong, T., Goemans, N., & Servais, L. (2022). Emerging therapies for Duchenne muscular dystrophy. *The Lancet. Neurology, 21*(9), 814–829. https://doi.org/10.1016/S1474-4422(22)00125-9

Marsh, J. D. (2022). Neoplasia. In J. Banasik, B. N. Banasik, & B. J. Miller (Eds.), *Pathophysiology* (7th ed., pp. 120–145). Elsevier.

Maternal and Child Health Bureau. (2022, June). *Children and youth with special healthcare needs: NCHS data brief.* Health Resources and Services Administration. https://mchb.hrsa.gov/sites/default/files/mchb/programs-impact/nsch-data-brief-children-youth-special-health-care-needs.pdf

McCrindle, B. W., Rowley, A. H., Newburger, J. W., Burns, J. C., Bolger, A. F., Gewitz, M., ... & Pahl, E. (2017). Diagnosis, treatment, and long-term management of Kawasaki disease: A scientific statement for health professionals from the American Heart Association. *Circulation, 135*(17), e927–e999. https://doi.org/10.1161/CIR.0000000000000484

McGregor, S., & Goldman, R. D. (2022). Language outcomes after cochlear implant. *Canadian Family Physician, 68*(10) 737–738. https://doi.org/10.46747/cfp.6810737

Menger, R. P., & Sin, A. H. (2023, April 3). *Adolescent and idiopathic scoliosis.* StatPearls [Internet]. https://www.ncbi.nlm.nih.gov/books/NBK499908/

National Association of School Nurses. (2021). *A model for school nurse–led case management.* https://www.nasn.org/blogs/nasn-profile/2021/08/24/manual-a-model-for-school-nurse-led-case-mgmt

National Association of School Nurses. (2024). *Framework for 21st century school nursing practice.* https://www.nasn.org/nasn-resources/framework

National Cancer Institute. (2022). *Cancer stat facts: Hodgkin lymphoma.* National Institutes for Health. https://seer.cancer.gov/statfacts/html/hodg.html

National Center for Chronic Disease Prevention and Health Promotion. (2017). *Research brief: Chronic health conditions and academic achievement.* Centers for Disease Control and Disease Prevention, Division of Population Health. https://www.cdc.gov/healthyschools/chronic_conditions/pdfs/2017_02_15-CHC-and-Academic-Achievement_Final_508.pdf

National Center for Education Statistics. (2023, May). *Students with disabilities.* https://nces.ed.gov/programs/coe/indicator/cgg/students-with-disabilities

National Center on Birth Defects and Developmental Disabilities. (2022, July 18). *Types of hearing loss.* Centers for Disease Control and Prevention. https://www.cdc.gov/ncbddd/hearingloss/types.html

National Center on Deaf-Blindness. (2022). *Deaf-blindness overview.* https://www.nationaldb.org/info-center/deaf-blindness-overview/

National Deaf Center. (2022). *The deaf community: An introduction.* https://nationaldeafcenter.org/resource-items/deaf-community-introduction/

National Eye Institute. (2023a). *Low vision.* https://www.nei.nih.gov/learn-about-eye-health/eye-conditions-and-diseases/low-vision

National Eye Institute. (2023b). *Refractive errors.* https://www.nei.nih.gov/learn-about-eye-health/eye-conditions-and-diseases/refractive-errors

National Institute of Arthritis and Musculoskeletal and Skin Diseases. (2021). *Juvenile idiopathic arthritis (JIA).* https://www.niams.nih.gov/health-topics/juvenile-arthritis

National Institute on Deafness and Other Communication Disorders. (2017, March 6). *Stuttering.* https://www.nidcd.nih.gov/health/stuttering

National Institute on Deafness and Other Communication Disorders. (2019). *It's a noisy planet: Tips for teaching kids about noise-induced hearing loss.* https://www.noisyplanet.nidcd.nih.gov/educators/tips-to-teach-kids

National Institute on Deafness and Other Communication Disorders. (2021). *Cochlear implants.* https://www.nidcd.nih.gov/health/cochlear-implants

National Organization for Rare Disorders. (2023, August 24). *Pediatric cardiomyopathy.* https://rarediseases.org/rare-diseases/pediatric-cardiomyopathy/

Nemours KidsHealth. (2022, February). *Lymphoma.* https://kidshealth.org/en/parents/cancer-lymphoma.html

Nguyen, H. N., McBee, M. P., Morin, C. E., Sharma, A., Patel, K. R., Silva-Carmona, M., & Guillerman, R. P. (2022). Late pulmonary complications related to cancer treatment in children. *Pediatric Radiology, 52*(10), 2029–2037. https://doi.org/10.1007/s00247-022-05391-x

Norkett, W., McLone, D. G., & Bowman, R. (2016). Current management strategies of hydrocephalus in the child with open spina bifida. *Spinal Cord Injury Rehabilitation, 22*(4), 241–246. https://doi.org/10.1310/sci2204-241

Occupational Safety and Health Administration. (n.d.). *Bloodborne pathogen and needlestick prevention.* U.S. Department of Labor. https://www.osha.gov/bloodborne-pathogens/resources

Pace, A., Alper, R., Burchinal, M. R., Golinkoff, R. M., & Hirsh-Pasek, K. (2019). Measuring success: Within and cross-domain predictors of academic and social trajectories in elementary school. *Early Childhood Research Quarterly, 46,* 112–125. https://doi.org/10.1016/j.ecresq.2018.04.001

Panzarino, V., Lesser, J., & Cassani, F. A. (2022). Pediatric chronic kidney disease. *Advances in Pediatrics, 69*(1), 123–132. https://doi.org/10.1016/j.yapd.2022.03.008

Partap, S., & Monje, M. (2020). Pediatric brain tumors. *CONTINUUM: Lifelong Learning in Neurology, 26*(6), 1553–1583. https://doi.org/10.1212/CON.0000000000000955

Patel, N., & Green, A. (2020). Cancer and antineoplastic therapies and the risk of infection in the pediatric cancer patient. In *Pediatric transplant and oncology infectious diseases* (pp. 22–33.e3). Elsevier.

Paul, S., Nahar, A., Bhagawati, M., & Kunwar, A. J. (2022). A review on recent advances of cerebral palsy. *Oxidative Medicine and Cellular Longevity, 2022,* 2622310. https://doi.org/10.1155/2022/2622310

Peterson, F. (2022). HIV disease and AIDS. In Banasik, B. N. Banasik, & B. J. Miller (Eds.), Pathophysiology (7th ed., pp. 240–268). Elsevier, Inc

Posanka, B. (2022). Adverse event leads to quality improvement plan: Learning from a classroom latex exposure. *NASN School Nurse, 37*(3), 132–135. https://doi.org/10.1177/1942602X221077234

Price, J. F. (2019). Congestive heart failure in children. *Pediatrics in Review, 40*(2), 60–70. https://doi.org/10.1542/pir.2016-0168

Reel, L. A., Hicks, C. B., & Arnold, C. (2022). Noise exposure and use of hearing protection among adolescents in rural areas. *American Journal of Audiology, 31*(1), 32–44. https://doi.org/10.1044/2021_AJA-20-00196

Regling, K., Callaghan, M. U., & Sidonio, R., Jr. (2022). Managing severe hemophilia A in children: Pharmacotherapeutic options. *Pediatric Health, Medicine and Therapeutics, 13,* 27–35. https://doi.org/10.2147/PHMT.S293246

Rehman, R., Pinkos, B., Shapiro, J. M., & Cerezo, C. (2022). Nutritional management of inflammatory bowel disease. *Rhode Island Medical Journal, 105*(10), 31–37.

Reinhardt, D., Antoniou, E., & Waack, K. (2022). Pediatric acute myeloid leukemia—past, present, and future. *Journal of Clinical Medicine, 11*(3), 504. https://doi.org/10.3390/jcm11030504

Rodriguez, L., Dinauer, C., & Francis, G. (2022). Treatment of hypothyroidism in infants, children and adolescents. *Trends in Endocrinology and Metabolism, 33*(7), 522–532. https://doi.org/10.1016/j.tem.2022.04.007

Rohit, M., & Budakoty, S. (2020). Approach to a child with congestive heart failure. *The Indian Journal of Pediatrics, 87*(4), 312–320. https://doi-org.ezp.slu.edu/10.1007/s12098-020-03255-6

Romitti, P. A., Zhu, Y., Puzhankara, S., James, K. A., Nabukera, S. K., Zamba, G. K. D., . . . Bolen, J. (2015). Prevalence of Duchenne and Becker muscular dystrophies in the United States. *Pediatrics, 135*(3), 513–521. https://doi.org/10.1542/peds.2014-2044

Rosen, R. (2022). Novel advances in the evaluation and treatment of children with symptoms of gastroesophageal reflux disease. *Frontiers in Pediatrics, 10,* 1–7. https://doi.org/10.3389/fped.2022.849105

Rowley, A. H. (2020). Understanding SARS-CoV-2-related multisystem inflammatory syndrome in children. *Nature Reviews Immunology, 20*(8), 453–454. https://doi.org/10.1038/s41577-020-0367-5

Ruggiero, K. (2021). Disorders in hematology and oncology commonly seen in pediatric primary care. In K. Ruggiero & M. Ruggiero (Eds.), *Fast facts handbook for pediatric primary care* (pp. 235–241). Springer Publishing.

Sadler, B., Castaman, G., & O'Donnell, J. S. (2022). Von Willebrand disease and von Willebrand factor. *Haemophilia: The Official Journal of the World Federation of Hemophilia, 28*(Suppl 4), 11–17. https://doi.org/10.1111/hae.14547

Sangam, S., & Munakomi, S. (2023, February 23). *Gower sign.* StatPearls [Internet]. https://www.ncbi.nlm.nih.gov/books/NBK540973/#:~:text=In%201879%2C%20neurologist%20Sir%20William,and%20proximal%20lower%20limb%20muscles

Sato, M., Ohashi, M., Tashi, H., Makino, T., Shibuya, Y., Hirano, T., & Watanabe, K. (2022). Association of success of brace treatment and various aspects of in-brace correction in patients with adolescent idiopathic scoliosis. *Journal of Orthopaedic Science,* S0949-2658(22)00285-8. Advance online publication. https://doi.org/10.1016/j.jos.2022.10.001

Schmidt, J. A., Hornhardt, S., Erdmann, F., Sánchez-García, I., Fischer, U., Schüz, J., & Ziegelberger, G. (2021). Risk factors for childhood leukemia: Radiation and beyond. *Frontiers in Public Health, 9,* 805757. https://doi.org/10.3389/fpubh.2021.805757

Scott, M., & Neal, A. E. (2021). Congenital heart disease. *Primary Care, 48*(3), 351–366. https://doi.org/10.1016/j.pop.2021.04.005

Sehn, L. H., & Salles, G. (2021). Diffuse large B-cell lymphoma. *The New England Journal of Medicine, 384*(9), 842–858. https://doi.org/10.1056/NEJMra2027612

Shannon, R.A., & Holman, C.F. (2017). Sickle cell disease. In S. Will, M.J. Arnold, & Zaiger, D.S. (Eds). *Individualized healthcare plans for the school nurse,* pp. 899-914. Sunrise River Press.

Shave, S., Botti, C., & Kwong, K. (2022). Congenital sensorineural hearing loss. *Pediatric Clinics, 69*(2), 221–234. https://doi.org/10.1016/j.pcl.2021.12.006

Sheikh, I. N., Elgehiny, A., Ragoonanan, D., Mahadeo, K. M., Nieto, Y., & Khazal, S. (2022). Management of aggressive non-Hodgkin lymphomas in the pediatric, adolescent, and young adult population: An adult vs. pediatric perspective. *Cancers, 14*(12), 2912. https://doi.org/10.3390/cancers14122912

Sheu, J., Cohen, D., Sousa, T., & Pham, K.L. (2022). Cerebral palsy: Current concepts and practices in musculoskeletal care. *Pediatrics in Review, 43*(10), 572–581. https://doi-org.ezp.slu.edu/10.1542/pir.2022-005657

Siegel, D. A., Henley, S. J., Li, J., Pollack, L. A., Van Dyne, E. A., & White, A. (2017). Rates and trends of pediatric acute lymphoblastic leukemia—United States, 2001–2014. *MMWR. Morbidity and Mortality Weekly Report, 66*(36), 950–954. https://doi.org/10.15585/mmwr.mm6636a3

Siegel, D. A., Richardson, L. C., Henley, S. J., Wilson, R. J., Dowling, N. F., Weir, H. K., Tai, E. W., & Buchanan Lunsford, N. (2020). Pediatric cancer mortality and survival in the United States, 2001–2016. *Cancer, 126*(19), 4379–4389. https://doi.org/10.1002/cncr.33080

Siegel, R. L., Miller, K. D., Fuchs, H. E., & Jemal, A. (2021). Cancer statistics, 2021. *CA: A Cancer Journal for Clinicians, 71*(1), 7–33. https://doi.org/10.3322/caac.21654

Sika-Paotonu, D., Beaton, A., Raghu, A., Steer, A., & Carapetis, J. (2017). Acute rheumatic fever and rheumatic heart disease. In J. J. Ferretti et al. (Eds.), *Streptococcus pyogenes: Basic biology to clinical manifestations* [Internet]. University of Oklahoma Health Sciences Center. https://www.ncbi.nlm.nih.gov/books/NBK425394/

Simonin, M., Jardin, F., Leblanc, T., Latour, S., & Parker, J. L. (2023). An update on molecular features and therapeutic perspectives of pediatric classical Hodgkin lymphoma. What the clinician needs to know? *European Journal of Medical Genetics,* 104672. https://doi.org/10.1016/j.ejmg.2022.104672

Soma, V. L., Shust, G. F., & Ratner, A. J. (2021). Multisystem inflammatory syndrome in children. *Current Opinion in Pediatrics, 33*(1), 152–158. https://doi.org/10.1097/MOP.0000000000000974

Sommerfeldt, J., & Kolb, C. M. (2023, February 27). *Hearing loss assessment in children.* StatPearls [Internet]. https://www.ncbi.nlm.nih.gov/books/NBK580492/

Sooriyamoorthy, T., & De Jesus, O. (2023, February 12). *Conductive hearing loss.* StatPearls [Internet]. https://www.ncbi.nlm.nih.gov/books/NBK563267/

Spina Bifida Association of America. (2015). *Latex in the home and community.* https://www.spinabifidaassociation.org/wp-content/uploads/latex-in-the-home-and-community-eng.pdf

Stanton, A., & Lavenbarg, T. (2017). The child with neuromuscular or muscular dysfunction. In M. J. Hockenberry, D. Wilson, & C. C. Rogers (Eds.), *Essentials of pediatric nursing* (10th ed., pp. 978–1006). Elsevier.

Su, B., & Chan, D. (2017). Prevalence of hearing loss in US children and adolescents. *JAMA Otolaryngology–Head & Neck Surgery, 143*(9), 920–927. https://doi:10.1001/jamaoto.2017.0953

Subedi, S., Behrle Yardley, A. L., & Shapiro, J. M. (2022). Inflammatory bowel disease in children and adolescents. *Rhode Island Medical Journal (2013), 105*(10), 8–13.

Tanna, R. J., Lin, J. W., & De Jesus, O. (2023, February 12). *Sensorineural hearing loss.* StatPearls [Internet]. https://www.ncbi.nlm.nih.gov/books/NBK565860/

Thatayatikom, A., Modica, R., & De Leucio, A. (2023). *Juvenile idiopathic arthritis.* StatPearls [Internet]. https://www.ncbi.nlm.nih.gov/books/NBK554605/

Turan Miral, M., & Hotun Sahin, N. (2022). Psychosocial adaptation to precocious puberty: A nursing support program. *Journal of Child and Adolescent Psychiatric Nursing: Official Publication of the Association of Child and Adolescent Psychiatric Nurses, Inc, 35*(3), 285–294. https://doi.org/10.1111/jcap.12376

Udaka, Y. T., & Packer, R. J. (2018). Pediatric brain tumors. *Neurologic Clinics, 36*(3), 533–556. https://doi.org/10.1016/j.ncl.2018.04.009

Understood Team. (2019). Understanding language disorders. In *Understood for learning and attention issues.* https://www.understood.org/en/learning-attention-issues/child-learning-disabilities/communication-disorders/understanding-language-disorders

U.S. Department of Health and Human Services. (2021). QuickStats: Percentage of children aged 2–17 years who wear glasses or contact lenses, by sex and age group—National Health Interview Survey, United States, 2019. *MMWR Morbidity and Mortality Weekly Report, 70*(23), 865. http://dx.doi.org/10.15585/mmwr.mm7023a4

U.S. Food and Drug Administration. (2021). *Grapefruit juice and some drugs don't mix.* https://www.fda.gov/consumers/consumer-updates/grapefruit-juice-and-some-drugs-dont-mix

Vaidyanathan, P. (2022). Update on pediatric hyperthyroidism. *Advances in Pediatrics, 69*(1), 219–229. https://doi.org/10.1016/j.yapd.2022.04.004

VanderMeulen, H., Arya, S., Nersesian, S., Philbert, N., & Sholzberg, M. (2022). What have we learned about the patient's experience of von Willebrand disease? A focus on women. *Hematology. American Society of Hematology. Education Program, 2022*(1), 631–636. https://doi.org/10.1182/hematology.2022000391

Vandertop, W. P., Buis, D. R., & Feller, R. (2022). Spina bifida. *The New England Journal of Medicine, 387*(17), 1628. https://doi.org/10.1056/NEJMc2211513

Venugopal, V., & Pavlakis, S. (2023). *Duchenne muscular dystrophy.* StatPearls [Internet]. https://www.ncbi.nlm.nih.gov/books/NBK482346/.

Vinkel, M. N., Rackauskaite, G., & Finnerup, N. B. (2022). Classification of pain in children with cerebral palsy. *Developmental Medicine and Child Neurology, 64*(4), 447–452. https://doi.org/10.1111/dmcn.15102

Watanabe, K., & Shih, R. (2020). Update of pediatric heart failure. *Pediatric Clinics of North America, 67*(5), 889–901. https://doi.org/10.1016/j.pcl.2020.06.004

Watkins, D. A., Beaton, A. Z., Carapetis, J. R., Karthikeyan, G., Mayosi, B. M., Wyber, R., ... & Zühlke, L. J. (2018). Rheumatic heart disease worldwide: JACC scientific expert panel. *Journal of the American College of Cardiology, 72*(12), 1397–1416. https://www.jacc.org/doi/abs/10.1016/j.jacc.2018.06.063

Williams, P. M., Harris, L. M., & Odom, M.R. (2022). Celiac disease: Common questions and answers. *American Family Physician, 106*(1), 36–43. https://www.aafp.org/pubs/afp/issues/2022/0700/celiac-disease.html

World Health Organization. (2016). *WHO clinical staging of HIV disease in adults, adolescents, and children.* https://www.ncbi.nlm.nih.gov/books/NBK374293/

Zhang, Y. Z., & Li, Y. Y. (2014). Inflammatory bowel disease: Pathogenesis. *World Journal of Gastroenterology, 20*(1), 91–99. https://doi.org/10.3748/wjg.v20.i1.91

Zimmerman, M. S., Smith, A. G. C., Sable, C. A., Echko, M. M., Wilner, L. B., Olsen, H. E., ... & Kassebaum, N. J. (2020). Global, regional, and national burden of congenital heart disease, 1990–2017: A systematic analysis for the Global Burden of Disease Study 2017. *The Lancet Child & Adolescent Health, 4*(3), 185–200.

Chapter 25

Students With Medical Complexity

Karen J. Madura ▪ Molly Hofmann

CHAPTER OUTLINE

The school health office was traditionally a low-tech environment, but now technology is everywhere in school nursing practice. Smartphones, tablets, and computers have become integral parts of the modern education system. For most people, technology makes life easier; but for some—it makes life possible. Today's school nurses must have a broad range of knowledge and skills, especially when caring for students with special healthcare needs supported by medical technology.

Children with special healthcare needs are broadly defined as "those who have or are at increased risk for a chronic physical, developmental, behavioral, or emotional condition and who also require health and related services of a type or amount beyond that required by children generally" (Health Resources and Services Administration [HRSA], 2022, p. 1). Approximately one in five children (19%) in the United States are reported to have a special healthcare need (Child and Adolescent Health Measurement Initiative, 2020–2021; Ghandour et al., 2022). Data from the *National Survey on Children's Health* conducted by the U.S. Census Bureau (2016–2019) indicated that of those children, prescription medication use was the most reported type of special healthcare need at 29.3%; 25.9% reported functional limitations, 26.8% reported both prescription medications and functional limitations, and 18% reported above routine use of specialized services (Ghandour et al., 2022).

Compared with children without special healthcare needs, these children are more likely to be male than female (21.8% vs. 17.1%), non-Hispanic black (23.4%), and live in poverty (20.6%). Only 15.4% of families report their child with special healthcare needs receives services (Child and Adolescent Health Measurement Initiative, 2020–2021). Additionally, 2019 to 2020 data demonstrated that children with special healthcare needs were nearly four times as likely to have unmet healthcare needs in the past year compared with children without special healthcare needs (8.8% vs. 2.3%) across categories of medical, dental, vision, hearing, and mental health care (HRSA, 2022).

Children with medical complexity are one subset of children with special healthcare needs. *Medical complexity* refers to children with the most intensive healthcare needs who are often medically fragile with complex chronic conditions and who have functional limitations, high healthcare use, and significant service needs. Children with medical complexity are estimated to comprise 3% of the U.S. population of children with special healthcare needs (Barnert et al., 2017).

Although students with chronic health conditions may require specific health-related procedures and medications, it does not necessarily mean they are "ill". Students can live healthy lives even though they are supported by medical technology. They are often well children because of their technology, treatments, and medications. Yet, students should not be defined by their condition, needs, or diagnoses. By placing the person first, the disability is no longer the defining characteristic of an individual, but just one of several aspects of the whole person. People-first language is an objective way of acknowledging, communicating, and reporting about disabilities (Centers for Disease Control and Prevention [CDC], 2022). School nurses should educate others and model *student-first language* to build dignity, respect, and trust. It is not appropriate to say a ventilator-dependent student or a traumatic brain injury student; it *is* appropriate to say a student with a ventilator or a student with a traumatic brain injury. Student-first language helps to destigmatize or "demedicalize" students with medical complexity in the educational setting. For instance, instead of saying it is time to catheterize a student or administer a gastrostomy tube feeding, the school nurse can simply say it is time to "toilet" or time for "lunch."

Medical technology is constantly changing and improving, with devices becoming smaller and more portable. School nurses need evidence-based skills to care for students with a range of medical technologies, including insulin pumps, vascular access devices, implanted cardiac pacemakers and defibrillators, gastrostomy tubes, tracheostomies, ventilators, and more.

The purpose of this chapter is to provide general considerations for some of the more common skills required to care for the needs of students with medical complexity at school. The school nurse will need to become familiar with the specific equipment used for an individual student and options for troubleshooting equipment problems. While this chapter provides generally accepted best practices, the content cannot replace nursing judgment, physician or other healthcare provider orders, state board of nursing regulations, or school district policies and protocols. Nursing care of students with chronic conditions such as allergies, asthma, diabetes, and seizures is discussed in other chapters of this textbook.

CARE COORDINATION

The *National Care Coordination Standards for Children and Youth With Special Health Care Needs* defines *care coordination* as follows:

> *Patient and family-centered, assessment-driven, team-based activities designed to meet the needs of the children and youth. Care coordination addresses interrelated medical, social, developmental, behavioral, educational, and financial needs to achieve optimal health and wellness outcomes and efficient delivery of health-related services and resources within and across systems. (National Academy for State Health Policy, 2020, p. 5)*

Care coordination is a relational and dynamic process that involves partnerships with families and interprofessional collaboration between many different individuals and disciplines to develop a shared plan of care that outlines care needs and goals. Well-coordinated care can lead to improvements in integrated care delivery across systems, reductions in duplicative or avoidable care and improvements in family quality of life.

According to the National Association of School Nurses' (NASN's) *School Nursing Practice Framework* (2024a) and the *Scope and Standards of School Nursing Practice* (NASN, 2022), the school nurse is responsible for care coordination for children with special healthcare needs in the school setting. Care coordination at school focuses on the health care needed at school for the student to remain present and ready to learn at school (Bobo et al., 2019) *Care coordination* within the school system is defined by NASN (2020a) as "the principle that brings student-centered-like activities together that are purposeful and deliberate in the delivery of health services over time" (p. 226).

Care coordination extends outside of the school setting to include the student's medical home or medical team, health insurance provider, or other community-based entity. Some students have care coordinators from a healthcare system who can partner with the school nurse. A partnership between care coordinators can enable the school nurse to maintain focus on care related to the educational setting, whereas the external care coordinator can focus on elements of care needed outside of school. Studies show students with chronic health conditions who received care coordination in school experienced better health and had greater academic success (Bobo et al., 2019).

Focus on the Framework

The following components are included under the **Care Coordination** principle of NASN's *School Nursing Practice Framework* (2024b):

- Provide direct care for emergent, episodic, and chronic mental and physical health needs.
- Connect student and family to available resources.
- Collaborate with families, school community, mental health team (including school counselors, social workers, and psychologists), and medical home.
- Develop and implement plans of care.
- Foster developmentally appropriate independence and self-advocacy.
- Provide evidence-based health counseling.
- Facilitate continuity of care with family during transitions.

Foundational to care coordination is *school nurse–led case management* that involves the child's personal health teams, including the family. According to NASN (2021):

> *Case management strategies help deal with, prevent, and/or reduce the occurrence of health problems to find solutions inside and outside of school and traditional healthcare systems, such as addressing transportation, housing, and food security concerns. The strategies are proactive, comprehensive, promote self-care and independence, and address both health and academic goals; and they are outlined in a student's individualized healthcare plan (IHP). (p. 2)*

See Chapter 20 for more detailed discussion of care coordination and case management.

Developing Student-Centered Plans

School nurses should establish consistent protocols for developing and implementing new plans of care for students with medical complexity according to the nursing process, as well as monitoring, evaluating, and updating these plans in communication with parents/guardians and healthcare providers. The health assessment completed by the school nurse with the family should begin as soon as the student is referred to or identified within the school system. Families and school staff need to actively contribute to the planning process with the school nurse. Students' needs may fluctuate, thereby necessitating ongoing assessments and care plan adjustments. Both health and education plans for students with special healthcare needs should consider the following questions (Ward & Ward, 2014, p. 19):

- Is the condition very complex but relatively stable with the appropriate interventions?
- Is the student's condition progressive and degenerative?
- Is the student's condition susceptible to going through periods of "wellness" (remission) with occasional bouts of serious symptoms, possibly requiring hospitalizations?

School nurses must use the most relevant evidence-based information to ensure their practices are current and supported by science. Textbooks, journals, and trusted online sources can provide current evidence. Healthcare providers from specialty clinics, primary care, home healthcare agencies, and healthcare equipment vendors are valuable resources that school nurses can utilize to learn about a student's care and the medical technology involved.

Many students supported by medical technology qualify for special education services under the *Individuals With Disabilities Education Improvement Act of 2004* (IDEA) and have an individualized education program (IEP). This process first requires that the school nurse develop an individualized healthcare plan (IHP). Other students supported by medical technology can achieve academically in the general curriculum and do not need an IEP. These students are protected against discrimination at school secondary to dependence on medical technology under the *Rehabilitation Act of 1973* and qualify for a Section 504 plan (U.S. Department of Education, Office for Civil Rights, 2016). It is the position of NASN that the school nurse is an essential member of IEP and Section 504 teams (NASN, 2023). See Chapter 7 for more information about laws protecting students with disabilities.

The school nurse develops an IHP to guide the daily nursing care for each student with special healthcare needs (NASN, 2020b). IHPs are nursing care plans for nurses. The IHP identifies the student's unique healthcare needs and details of nursing care. HP interventions reflect the current medical orders and evidence-based nursing practices while considering the cultural contexts, preferences, and needs of the family. IHPs should ensure that necessary supplies are available. If the student is at risk for an emergency or life-threatening event at school, the school nurse also develops an emergency action plan (EAP) for the educational staff and trains them to respond accordingly. The IHP and EAP may be referenced in the student's IEP or Section 504 plan as it relates to accessing the curriculum and meeting the student's needs at school in a nondiscriminatory way. See Chapter 8 for more information about developing health and educational plans for students with special healthcare needs.

Communication

The school nurse actively serves as liaison between the school, student and family, and healthcare providers, partnering with the involved parties to keep the lines of communication open. The principles of privacy and confidentiality must be respected in accordance with the *Health Insurance Portability and Accountability Act* (HIPAA) and the *Family Education Rights and Privacy Act* (FERPA) (Bergren, 2017). This includes sharing information with stakeholders and team members that need to know about the care students receive at home, daily routines, self-care skills, who the primary healthcare provider and specialists are, and how the student responds when unwell.

The family can be asked to demonstrate the usual healthcare procedures performed at home to help the school nurse learn how to provide care in a comfortable, familiar, and culturally sensitive manner. Parents/guardians need to inform the school nurse of changes in the student's status in a timely manner. Likewise, the school nurse must promptly communicate to families any concerns about the student's health status and educate them about standards of care as indicated.

Open communication between the school nurse and the family should be established to build trust, and contact information should be kept up to date. All families deserve to feel that school is a safe and caring place for their child. The school nurse emphasizes to school staff the importance of communication with the family about the child's various health, treatment, and educational activities throughout the day.

Clear communication with the primary care provider and/or specialists is also imperative, especially regarding the medical orders for care provided for a student during the school day. Written procedure orders need to stipulate the details of care, including routes, dosages, and time and frequency of the care or procedures, as well as unique instructions and management of adverse events. Home and school schedules need to be coordinated to meet the student's needs while minimizing disruptions to instructional time in the classroom. Providers and parents/guardians must work together to provide the medications, durable medical equipment, and other supplies needed for school.

Delegation

School nurses need to know the stipulations of their state's nurse practice act regarding whether delegation of medications or procedures to nonnurses, or unlicensed assistive personnel (UAP), is allowed and under what circumstances. In states that allow delegation, the school nurse is responsible for training and monitoring the UAP's delivery of the healthcare task. Delegation of healthcare tasks in the school setting should only be considered for routine medication and procedure administration if the student's status is stable and predictable. The nursing process and nursing judgment can never be delegated (National Council of State Boards of Nursing & American Nurses Association, 2019; Shannon & Kubelka, 2013a, 2013b). The school nurse remains responsible for the student's health care when care tasks are delegated. See Chapters 30 and 31 for further discussion of the principles of delegation in the school setting.

Students Requiring Personal Nursing Services

Some students with medical complexity have healthcare needs that require them to have continuous personal nursing care from a personal (one-on-one) nurse or a classroom nurse who may care for more than one student. Under the principle of a free and appropriate public education (FAPE), public school districts are responsible for the costs of providing the health care at school the student needs to access their education (see Chapter 7). Districts can hire personal nurses for students directly or contract with private nursing or home health agencies. Depending on the needs of the student, a registered nurse or a licensed vocational/practical nurse may be hired. School districts should have written and signed contracts or memorandum of understanding with the healthcare agency that clearly outlines the responsibilities of the personal nurse (Shannon & Minchella, 2015). School nurses may be unsure of their responsibilities for the student and their roles with the personal nurse. Although the student's direct care needs are administered by another nurse, the school nurse is still responsible for monitoring and supporting the health status of that student, as with all students on campus. It is important to foster communication with the personal nurse and explain the boundaries and expectations of care in the school. See Chapter 20 for further discussion of students requiring personal nursing services at school.

Transportation

Students with special healthcare needs may require individualized transportation plans included in their IEPs. Transportation is identified in IDEA (2004) as a related service including travel to and from school, travel in and around the school building, and special equipment such as adapted

Did You Know?

Financing for Caregiving Assistance in the Home

The school nurse can be an advocate, leader, and resource for both the student and family. School nurses can work with case managers and social workers to help reduce the financial burden for families of children with medical complexity. The school nurse can support and advocate for their students beyond the classroom by having a basic understanding of financing for caregiving assistance in the home.

State Medicaid programs are the most common form of payment for caregiving assistance for children with medical complexity in the home setting. Individuals enrolled in Medicaid who are under 21 years of age are entitled to Early and Periodic Screening, Diagnosis, and Treatment (EPSDT) benefits, which include home health services such as private duty nursing or personal care services (Simpser & Hudak, 2017).

In addition to EPSDT services, students may also be eligible for services through a *Home and Community Based Service (HCBS) Waiver* through their state's Medicaid Program. HCBS waivers are intended to provide services to individuals with long-term needs to help keep them in the home and out of institutions. The types of HCBS waivers, services available through the waiver, and eligibility vary by state. Income threshold requirements are waived in some states, meaning the eligible individual may live in a household that would not otherwise qualify for Medicaid. Waivers may also have caregiving assistance or funding to help support modifications needed to accommodate care in the home (Centers for Medicare and Medicaid Services, n.d.).

Although not commonly offered, many states are beginning to expand self-direction services available through waiver programs that allow family members or other types of caregivers to be paid for caregiving (Teshale et al., 2021). This caregiver expansion increased support to families who experience economic hardship as a result of caring for their child with special health care needs and provides additional support when nursing is not available.

Some private insurance plans offer coverage for private duty nursing or personal care services. These are plan specific and often depend on the ability to show reduction in cost of care from the more acute setting. See Chapter 32 for detailed information on Medicaid reimbursement for school health services.

buses, lifts, or ramps that are needed. School nurses should collaborate with parents/guardians and transportation services to develop safe and appropriate plans for students with medical complexity to be transported to and from school. The transportation plan should comply with state and federal laws, local guidelines, and policies related to transporting students with disabilities (O'Neil & Hoffman, 2018). Consultations can be requested from experts in transporting students with medical equipment to ensure implementation of the safest plan that meets the unique needs of the student.

Special considerations when developing a transportation plan include the following:

- Travel time on the bus: Does the student require the time on the bus to be limited due to medical needs, such as the last pick-up on the way to school and first drop-off on the way home?
- Child safety restraint system: What is the appropriate safety restraint system for the student's age, developmental level, and medical needs? Wheelchairs need to be secured with a four-point tie-down device facing forward (National Highway Traffic Safety Administration, n.d.). Wheelchair trays and other devices that pose a safety risk should be removed and secured on the bus for transport.
- Is supervision from an adult other than the bus driver needed for safety reasons? Does a nurse need to ride the bus with the student to provide medical procedures or emergency interventions, such as suctioning or oxygen administration?
- Transport of equipment: What arrangements are needed for the safe transportation of oxygen and other medical equipment on school buses? In the event of a crash, medical equipment can become a projectile to cause injury if it is not secured appropriately.
- Is the student sensitive to heat and cold, requiring air conditioning or heating during transportation?
- Emergency evacuations off the bus should be practiced at a minimum of once annually or as changes in the student's status or equipment warrant.

Transition to Adulthood

Transitioning from adolescence to adulthood for the student with special health care needs can be a time of great change. Adulthood brings transition from a school to a vocational or higher education setting. It can potentially mean transitioning to a new living environment with various levels of independence based on the youth's needs and abilities. It also is a time for transition from pediatric to adult healthcare providers and settings.

Health care transition is defined as "the process of moving from a child/family-centered model of health care to an adult/patient-centered model of health care, with or without transferring to a new clinician. It involves the planning, transfer, and integration into adult health care" (Got Transition, 2023, para. 1). Data from the National Survey on Children's Health shows that only 20% of children and youth with special healthcare needs receive the services necessary to transition to adult health, meaning 80% of these individuals and their families have unmet needs related to transition planning (Child and Adolescent Health Measurement Initiative, 2020–2021). Goals related to healthcare transition include improving the ability of youth and young adults with special healthcare needs to manage their own care to the fullest extent possible and outlining an organized process for integrating into adult-centered health care (Got Transition, 2023).

The school nurse has an important role in working with students and families in preparation for the transition to adult health care. Transition planning is best when it starts early, around age 12 to 14. IDEA requires that transition planning is in place by age 16. State laws vary, but many mandate that transition planning begins as early as age 14. School nurses can help establish goals that involve students in additional elements of their care to promote greater independence and self-care when possible and educate families on ways to prepare for transition readiness.

CLINICAL CONSIDERATIONS

Maintaining Privacy

The school nurse must take steps to ensure the privacy of all students during treatments, procedures, and conversations. Special education and related services, including nursing services, should be provided in the least restrictive environment (IDEA, 2004). The nurse needs to consider the proximity of the student and their classroom and the time away from instruction when identifying locations for providing private care or special procedures. For example, one student may want to have their gastrostomy tube (G-tube) feeding in the cafeteria with peers, while another may want lunch in the privacy of the health office.

Promoting Self-Care and Independence

Depending on their functional and developmental level, students supported by medical technology can learn self-care skills. The school nurse should write student-centered health goals and objectives in the IEP that focus on developing self-efficacy skills. For example, students who have G-tube feedings may start the road to independence by first holding the bolus syringe. A student can begin the self-care skills of catheterization by handing the nurse the supplies in the correct order. A student with a tracheostomy may take the self-care step of wiping secretions from a tracheostomy while looking in a mirror.

Sterile Versus Clean Procedures

Procedures that are conducted with sterile technique in a hospital setting can often be performed with a clean technique in the community setting of home and school. For example, in the hospital, urinary catheterization technique uses a sterile catheter and sterile gloves, whereas clean technique uses a clean catheter and clean gloves. In the home or school environment, clean technique is often the mainstay for managing neurogenic bladder in pediatric patients (Liu et al., 2022). However, infections may be indications for the use of sterile technique. The school nurse should clarify the level of care ordered for each student and monitor each student for ongoing response to that care.

Medical Equipment and Supplies

The family is responsible for providing the school nurse with the equipment and supplies needed during the school day and on the school bus. The list of supplies needed for healthcare procedures should include the type, size, and manufacturer of the equipment, and required backup equipment. It is the school nurse's responsibility to know how to clean and operate durable medical equipment at school. Systematic checks must be completed for battery power, cleanliness, service, and maintenance. The nurse needs to document the inventory and safety checks of all equipment.

All vital equipment, such as ventilator, tracheostomy, and emergency supplies, *must* be with the student at all times. Although the nurse should make sure that all equipment is in proper working order each day, maintenance of durable medical equipment (e.g., gastrostomy feeding pumps, suction machines) is the responsibility of the parent/guardian. Equipment and supplies may come with various warranties and maintenance requirements. If the school purchases equipment, the school nurse must be aware of maintenance, calibration, and warranty requirements. An identified systematic way should be in place to check equipment for battery power, function, and cleanliness. Oxygen tanks must be checked daily to certify that the supply is adequate. Cleaning of supplies, such as gastrostomy feeding extension tubing, should be done after each use according to the manufacturer's instructions.

Special attention should also be paid to the student's allergies so that supplies and equipment do not contain materials that can cause allergic or anaphylactic reactions. Many students with complex medical needs have had multiple medical procedures and surgeries that put them at increased risk for latex allergy via contact, inhalation, or ingestion. Children with spina bifida are at increased risk for latex allergies (American Academy of Allergy, Asthma, and Immunology, 2024). For these students, the school nurse should create a latex-safe environment that is absent of products and materials known to contain latex (Beierwaltes & Schoessler, 2017). See Chapter 21 for more information on students with allergies.

Positioning and Mobility Devices

Students who require musculoskeletal support need proper positioning and mobility devices to foster optimum functioning in the learning environment. Proper positioning can help to reduce muscle tension and pain and improve the ability to participate in learning. The school nurse should consult and collaborate with the school physical and occupational therapists to plan and implement optimal therapeutic positioning and function. Mobility specialists can assess the learning environment and make recommendations to improve the student's accessibility, safety, and independence.

Positioning support for students can include specially designed cushions, chairs, desks, standers, and other therapeutic equipment to provide musculoskeletal support. Many students wear orthotic devices to maintain proper hand, foot, or trunk alignment. Fitted harnesses, vests, head supports, belts, and straps may be needed to provide musculoskeletal support and ensure the safety of the student while using adaptive or mobility devices.

Many devices can be used to assist with mobility, lifting, and transferring in the school environment. Manual and motorized wheelchairs allow mobility at school on a temporary or long-term basis. The school nurse should evaluate the fit and effectiveness of adaptive equipment and frequently assess the student's skin integrity.

Transfer belts, transfer boards, and transfer sheets are examples of simple tools to support the process of lifting and transferring a student. Larger students may need to be transferred with the assistance of a hydraulic lift. It is critical that sufficient staff are available to help with moving a student to prevent injury to either the student or to staff members. All staff assisting in transferring students in and out of equipment must be appropriately trained in proper body mechanics and safe lifting and transferring techniques.

FEEDING TUBES

It is essential that school nurses are prepared to care for students with feeding tubes, also called *enteral tubes.* Children who require feeding tubes do so to maintain adequate nutritional intake needed for growth, development, and health. Without feeding tubes, these children may not be able to meet nutritional requirements due to the following causes:

- Congenital problems of the mouth, esophagus, stomach, or intestines
- Sucking or swallowing disorders
- Failure to thrive
- Severe gastrointestinal reflux
- Extreme problems with taking medications (Perkins & Paul, 2014)

Types

There are several different types of feeding tubes depending on where in the gastrointestinal system the tubes are placed. For temporary supplemental nutrition needs, a tube may be inserted in the nose via a nasogastric (NG) tube, nasoduodenal (ND) tube, or nasojejunal (NJ) tube (Cleveland Clinic, 2022a; Perkins & Paul, 2014). More commonly for long-term feeding needs, tubes are inserted in the stomach via a gastric (G) tube or button or into the duodenal or jejunal space via a jejunal (J) tube or a gastric jejunal (GJ) tube (Gillette Children's, 2023). See Figure 25-1.

To keep these tubes in place, a retention balloon located underneath the insertion site is filled with saline. In addition to the different locations of feeding tubes, there are many different types of tubes that are manufactured. Percutaneous endoscopic gastrostomy (PEG) tubes are long G-tubes that extend out from the site of insertion. Common types of skin-level feeding devices or *buttons* that lie flat against the body include MIC-KEY, AMT mini ONE, Bard G-tubes, and Nutri-ports (Perkins & Paul, 2014).

Some children have a feeding tube with both a G-port and a J-port (GJ-tubes). GJ-tubes are placed in the stomach just like G-tubes but have a thin, long tube that is threaded into the jejunal portion of the small intestine. The J-port is often used for feeding in children who have a higher risk of aspiration and cannot tolerate feedings in their stomach. With J-tubes, there is less chance of regurgitation because feeds are introduced lower in the GI tract. Jejunostomy tubes require a pump and cannot be administered as a bolus feeding (Anderson & Herring, 2022). The G-port is often used for venting and in many cases for medication administration. Both G- and J-tubes are sized by the diameter of the tube and the length of the tube's stem (Abdelhadi et al., 2016).

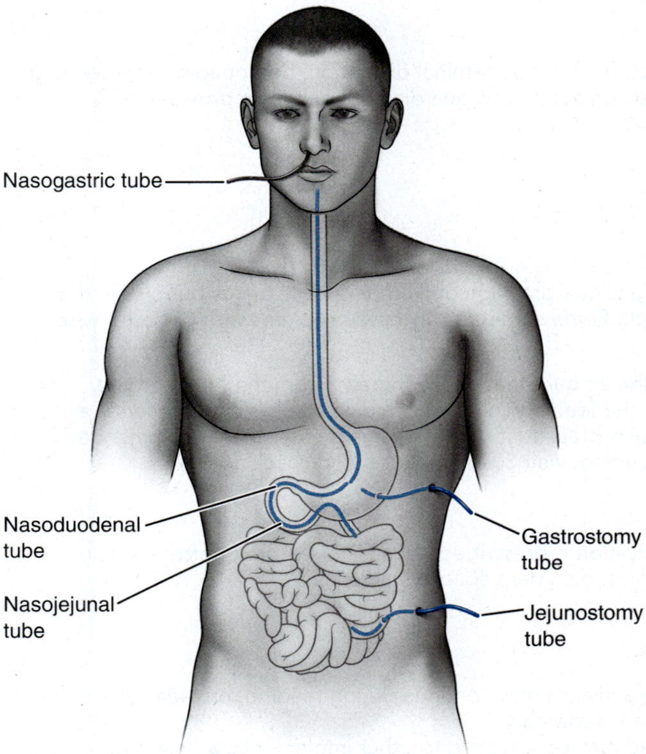

FIGURE 25-1. Gastrostomy and jejunostomy tubes.

Enteral Feeding Administration

Enteral feedings may be administered via intermittent boluses or continuous or episodic slow delivery per gravity drip or infusion pump. Some children only require medication administration through the feeding tube and take all their nutrition by mouth. The school nurse should assess the insertion site and condition of the device daily. According to medical orders, it may be necessary to perform site care and dressing changes, replace the device, or take appropriate action should the feeding tube become dislodged during the school day. The frequency of assessments will vary depending on whether and how often the student is fed during school hours.

The school nurse needs to know the procedures for administering both intermittent and continuous tube feedings and ensure that medical orders for feedings, medications, or other treatments are current. Feeding tube orders typically include the following:

- Type and size of feeding tube
- Type of feeding formula: rate (duration), frequency, and delivery method of feeding (pump, gravity drip, or bolus)
- Need for and frequency of checking for gastric residuals (not always indicated)
- Water flushes before or after administration or throughout the day
- Need for and frequency of venting (burping) of the G-tube to release gas or air
- Positioning and activity level during and after feeding
- Site care, such as topical creams or powders to be administered around the stoma site
- Orders for medications administered via feeding tube
- Whether the student can take food or drink by mouth
- Procedures to implement should the tube fall out (Corrigan et al., 2017)

Checking for residuals before feeds is *not* routinely done unless ordered by the provider. Medications administered via a feeding tube need to be in liquid form. Tablets should be crushed and diluted in water. Capsule contents must be fully dissolved in water before being administered in a feeding tube (Boullata, 2021). Feedings may be given as intermittent bolus feeds over a specified period or run continuously at a slow rate using a feeding pump over the course of hours. Feeding bags and extension tubing need to be primed before and after administering the feeding and at least every 8 hours for continuous feeds (Donoghue & Kraft, 2019). Both G- and J-tubes are clamped or capped between feedings to prevent leakage.

A variety of electronic pumps can deliver feedings and fluids over a specified time or continuously either by being plugged into an electric socket or powered by battery. Batteries should be checked for adequate charge. Pumps may be mounted on a pole or wheelchair or carried in a backpack while running on battery power. The pump settings control the rate and amount of flow, as well as the alarms for flow problems, feeding completion, and blockage or air in the line (Perkins & Paul, 2014).

Enteral formulas are usually administered at room temperature to avoid discomfort to the student. It is the school nurse's responsibility to know how long the feeding solution can be stored or refrigerated after being opened. Open formula must be refrigerated in a clean plastic sealed and labeled container and typically used within 24 to 48 hours according to the product label. Reusing feeding bags and tubes is not recommended as this can be a source of contamination and subsequent infection (Osland et al., 2021). Refer to the medical orders and equipment recommendations regarding cleaning, reuse, and disposal of extension tubing. See Table 25-1 for more information about G-tube feeding.

TABLE 25-1 Sample* Procedure for Gastrostomy Tube Feeding Bolus or Continuous Feeding Method by Pump

Procedure	Points to Remember
Review the healthcare provider's order before beginning the feeding process.	This will allow the nurse or UAP to familiarize themselves with nuances related to the procedure and student.
1. Wash hands. 2. Assemble equipment: • Formula at room temperature • 60-mL catheter-tipped syringe • Feeding pump and IV stand (optional) • Clamp or cap for end of tube (optional) • Water (if prescribed) • Feeding bag set • Tape • Gloves	Anticipating the tasks to be done, the risk involved, and the personal protective equipment needed. Identify size and type of G-tube. Some students get cramps if the feeding solution is too cold. Shake the can well to mix. Check expiration date. Some students may have powdered formula: follow the mixing instructions on the can, specifically pay attention to the type of water. Feeding pumps have alarms. Become familiar with meanings of alarms and how to respond to them. Water is used to flush tubing after feeding. Tape, pin, or velcro may be used to secure G-tube to clothing.
3. Explain the procedure to the student at their level of understanding. Encourage the student to participate as much as possible.	By encouraging the student to assist in the procedure, the caregiver helps the student achieve self-help skills.
4. Position student.	Student may be sitting or lying on right side with head elevated at a 30-degree angle. When positioning student, make sure clamp is not pressing on skin. The most significant risk with tube feedings is aspiration of liquid nutrition into the lungs.
5. Wash hands. Put on gloves.	
6. Assess the abdomen for signs of malposition or obstruction of gastronomy tube such as difference in external tube length compared with baseline measurements or abdominal distention. Compare external tube length to tube length measurements obtained after initial placement of tube, contact parent/guardian or healthcare provider if there is a discrepancy.	If the student has abdominal distention, do not administer feeding, instead contact parent/guardian or healthcare provider.
7. Vent G-tube if ordered. (Open G-tube to air.) Connect 30- to 60-mL catheter-tipped syringe with barrel removed.	Venting allows drainage of fluid or release of gas bubbles in the stomach. Some students may have problems with gas otherwise.
8. Unclamp the tubing and check residuals (if ordered) by inserting a catheter-tipped syringe and gently drawing back on the plunger to remove any liquid or medication that may be left in the stomach. Look at amount in tube and push fluid slowly back into stomach.	Note the amount that was withdrawn from the feeding tube. Adjust the feeding volume according to physician's orders if a residual is present. If the residual is greater than recommended, hold feeding, wait 30–45 minutes, and check again.
9. Pour feeding/fluids into the feeding bag and run feeding through bag and tubing to the tip. Let the formula run completely through the tubing to get rid of the air (prime the pump). Then clamp the tubing shut.	If medication is prescribed, administer before or after feeding, according to student-specific guidelines.
10. Hang bag on pole and place tubing into the pump mechanism and set for proper flow rate.	School activities may continue during feeding, provided the student is sedentary. The bag may be attached to other implements; a pole is not required.

TABLE 25-1 Sample* Procedure for Gastrostomy Tube Feeding Bolus or Continuous Feeding Method by Pump—cont'd

Procedure	Points to Remember
11. Insert tip of feeding bag tube into G-tube and unclamp G-tube.	
12. Open clamp of feeding bag tubing.	
13. For *continuous feeding* with pump, add more fluid to bag when empty.	Be alert to any unusual changes in the student's tolerance of the feeding. Nausea/vomiting, cramping, or diarrhea may indicate that the feeding is being given too quickly or the formula is too cold.
14. When *single feeding* is completed (bag empty), clamp feeding bag tubing and clamp G-tube.	
15. Disconnect feeding bag from G-tube.	
16. Unclamp G-tube and flush with water.	This clears the tube of any feeding fluid.
17. Clamp and cap G-tube.	
18. Remove gloves and wash hands.	
19. Make sure tubing is secure and tucked inside clothing, not inside diaper or underpants.	
20. Refer to student-specific guidelines regarding position and activity after feeding.	The feeding tube may be disconnected while the student is being transported to and from the school program.
21. Wash syringe and other reusable equipment in soapy water. Rinse thoroughly, dry, and store in a clean area.	Most open formula is good for 48 hours when refrigerated. The exceptions are some elemental formulas that are only good for 24 hours. Open formulas should be stored in clean, plastic, labeled containers (not the original can) in the refrigerator. Formula should be discarded after 48 hours.
22. Document feeding and/or medication, residual volumes, and feeding tolerance.	Report to family any change in the student's usual pattern.

*Procedures may vary according to medical orders, equipment/devices, and the student's unique needs.
Adapted from Bowden & Greenberg (2016); Children's Hospitals and Clinics of Minnesota (2014); Perkins & Paul (2014).

School nurses need to be aware of potential safety concerns and problems when a student attends school with a feeding tube. Feedings should be stopped immediately if a student begins to cough, choke, or show signs of aspiration or respiratory distress, including facial color changes or breathing difficulty. If symptoms do not resolve once the feeding is stopped, activate emergency medical services (EMS) and notify the student's parents/guardians (Corrigan et al., 2017).

Nonemergent problems with feeding tubes at school may include the following:

- Nausea, cramping, or agitation: Stop the feeding and contact the provider regarding the potential for complications, such as leaking of formula into the peritoneal space or the presence of ileus.
- Abdominal discomfort or distention: Attempt to relieve excess air or gas by venting the G-port.
- Vomiting: Stop the feeding and position the student on their side to prevent aspiration.
- Clogged or blocked tubes: Blockage may occur due to thick feeding fluid or inadequate flushing. Techniques to dislodge a blockage include rolling or squeeze the tubing toward the stomach to dislodge the blockage and/or drawing back with a catheter-tipped syringe to remove the clog then flushing the tubing with warm water.
- Infection at insertion site: Discomfort may indicate an infection around the tube site. Redness, swelling, or tenderness needs to be reported to the student's parents/guardians and healthcare provider.
- Confirming correct placement: If there is doubt about the correct placement of a feeding tube, contact both the student's parents/guardians and provider and do not proceed with the feeding. An x-ray is the evidence-based recommendation to confirm correct placement.
- Infusion pump malfunction: The school nurse can contact the parent/guardian or product manufacturer when feeding tube pumps are not working properly. Manufacturer representatives are a good resource for troubleshooting problems. Some pump companies have online video tutorials on how to operate and care for their products.
- Feeding tube falls out: A dislodged G-tube or button may be able to be reinserted *if* the school nurse has medical orders and has been trained on the procedure.

Backup tubes should always be kept in the nurse's office. If the tube cannot be reinserted, a urinary catheter can be used to keep the stoma patent until the student is transported to a tertiary care setting to have a new tube placed. If a catheter is not available, cover the site with a dry gauze dressing (Corrigan et al., 2017). GJ-tubes and J-tubes need to be replaced by a physician or interventional radiologist. Dislodged feeding tubes should be replaced within 2 hours to prevent closure at the stoma (Corrigan et al., 2017; Perkins & Paul, 2014).

OSTOMIES AND STOMAS

An *ostomy* is a surgical opening through the abdominal wall into the large intestine (colostomy), the small intestine (ileostomy), the bladder (urostomy), or ureters (ureterostomy). Children have ostomies to bypass nonfunctioning segments of the intestinal or urinary tract systems so that stool or urine can be eliminated from the body. The stoma forms the external portion of the opening. An ostomy is connected to a pouch that collects the stool or urine.

Ostomies in the Enteral Tract

Conditions that may require colostomies or ileostomies include obstruction, inflammatory bowel disease, cancer, abnormal motility, congenital anomalies, infections, and traumatic injury. The types of colostomies in the large intestine include descending or sigmoid colostomy, double-barrel transverse colostomy, or loop transverse colostomy. See Figure 25-2. Some children with colostomies have a second stoma called a mucus fistula that passes mucus ordinarily created within the colon (Cleveland Clinic, 2022b).

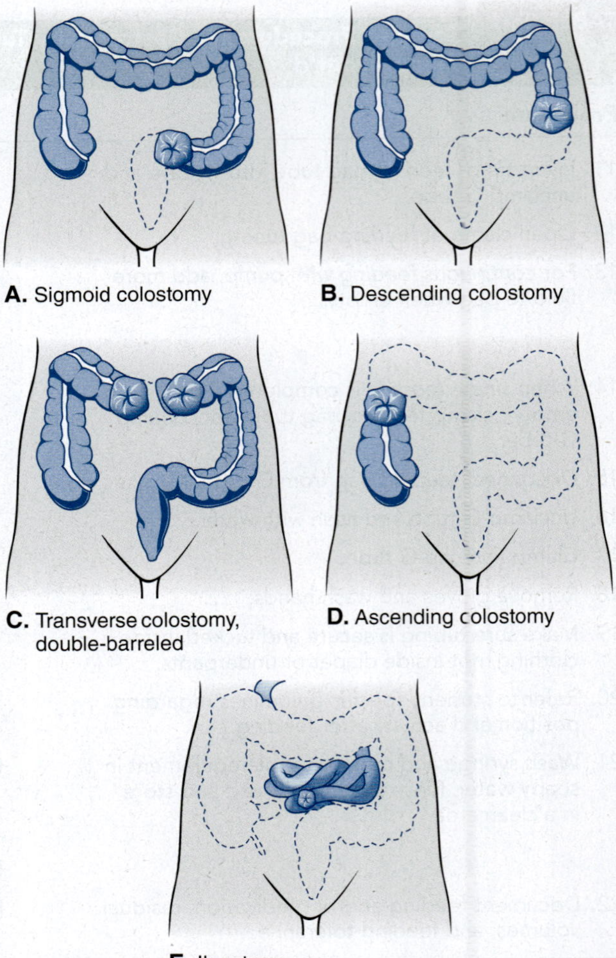

FIGURE 25-2. Ostomies in the enteral tract.

Ileostomies are created in the small intestine to drain feces when the large intestine has been damaged or removed due to injury, illness, or blockage or when there is a lack of innervations of nerves in the intestines. Students with ileostomies typically have more continuous drainage of stool of loose consistency than colostomies because the ostomy is in the small intestine where digestion is completed and most of the water entering through the GI tract is absorbed. The school nurse needs to be aware that the enzymes in liquid stool may be particularly caustic to the skin (Collado-Boira et al., 2021). Students may also need to be careful with their diets to prevent blockage of the ileostomy from partially digested foods. Foods that are commonly associated with blockages include popcorn, mushrooms, and nuts (Kirkland-Kyhn et al., 2018). Medical evaluation may be indicated for students with ileostomies who have vomiting, diarrhea, high fevers, or dehydration.

Ostomy pouches need to be emptied throughout the day depending on the type of ostomy, the student's diet, and how many hours the student attends school. The pouch should be emptied when it is one-third to one-half full to prevent too much weight within the pouch, which can cause leakage around the skin. Gas accumulation is also measured as content in a colostomy and ileostomy bag. Excessive gas accumulation can cause the bag to balloon and blow out, detaching from the stoma. Preventing leakage of ostomies is essential not only to prevent skin irritation and infection but to also protect the emotional well-being of the student. The school nurse should consider emptying the ostomy pouch after the student arrives at school and before the student leaves at the end of the day to prevent leakage (Grant & Quigley, 2014). The school nurse can assist students to learn self-care skills to empty ostomy pouches directly into the toilet, depending on their level of independence.

If an ostomy pouch needs to be changed at school, steps need to be taken to prevent irritation to the student's skin and leakage of pouch contents and to manage odors. Many different skin barriers are used to protect the skin where the ostomy pouch is attached. The stoma should be measured so the skin barrier can be cut to the appropriate size and configuration for providing skin protection and a stable surface to mount the ostomy appliance. Standard precautions should always be followed. See Table 25-2 for a sample of ostomy care procedures.

TABLE 25-2 Sample* Procedure for Changing a Colostomy Pouch

Procedure	Points to Remember
1. Assemble equipment: • Soft cloth or gauze • Clean pouch and belt, if needed • Skin barrier/wafer (if two-piece system) • Measuring guide, if needed • Disposable gloves, if pouch is to be changed by someone other than student • Tape, if needed • Scissors, if specified • Protective powder • Pectin ring or paste, if used	Each student should have a complete setup at school with a spare pouch and clip/pouch closure, although many pouches today have integrated pouch closures and no longer require separate clips. Some may have built-in air release filters. One-piece system: Pouch and wafer are made in one piece. *Two-piece system:* Pouch and wafer are separate. Each one has a plastic ring that clicks together, similar to closing a Tupperware container.
2. Wash hands and put on gloves.	Anticipating the tasks to be done, the risk involved, and the personal protective equipment needed will enhance protection of both the caregiver and student.
3. Explain procedure at the student's level of understanding. The student may already be an active participant.	By encouraging the student to assist in the procedure, the caregiver helps the student achieve maximum self-care skills.
4. Discuss with student what their ostomy care needs are and determine which steps they may do independently or with minimal assistance.	
5. Empty contents of pouch.	To prevent the spread of germs, hand hygiene should be performed before and after ostomy care.
6. Carefully remove the used pouch and skin barrier by gently pushing the skin away from the bag instead of pulling the bag off the skin.	This helps the skin not tent up and avoids skin irritation.
7. Inspect skin for redness, rash, bleeding, or blistering.	If there is skin irritation, check student-specific guidelines. Do not put medication, ointment, or adhesive on the damaged skin. Report skin irritation to school nurse and/or family or healthcare provider.
8. Wash the stoma area using clean cloth or gauze. Do not scrub. Cover the stoma with gauze, and then clean the skin around the stoma.	A small amount of pinpoint bleeding from stoma may occur; this is not uncommon. Avoid soap with moisturizers, emollients, and fragrance as this can be irritating and affect adherence to the skin.
9. If there is open, denuded skin, apply protective powder around stoma and then lightly pat the barrier protective wipes over the powder to form a protective film and seal it.	Powder helps absorb moisture from denuded skin; if there is no skin compromise, there is no need for layer of powder.
10. If a skin barrier wafer is used that requires fitting, measure stoma per student-specific guidelines. Place skin barrier on skin around stoma.	Some wafers are cut to fit and some are custom precut (usually students who have had a stoma for more than 6 months). The opening of the skin barrier wafer should fit close to the stoma without constricting blood supply and should not be too large to avoid exposure of excess skin, as well as to minimize the potential for skin irritation.
11. Peel off backing from adhesive on pouch and apply paste or pectin to skin or wafer portion of pouch, per student-specific guidelines.	May be used to fill in uneven skin creases or gaps to help prevent leakage and skin irritation. Also, can be used around flat, skin-level stomas.
12. Securely apply pouch closure to bottom of pouch.	Many pouches now manufactured with built-in velcro-type closures.
13. If a two-piece pouch system is used, attach the pouch to the plastic ring on the wafer before placing it on the abdomen.	Putting pouch and wafer together before placing over stoma may be more comfortable for the student.
14. Remove used gauze and discard in appropriate receptacle.	
15. Center the new pouch directly over the stoma.	
16. Firmly press the pouch to the skin barrier so there are no wrinkles and no leaks.	If indicated, open the pouch to allow in a small amount of air. If a belt is used to fasten pouch, attach to pouch.
17. Dispose of used pouch in appropriate receptacle.	

Continued

TABLE 25-2 Sample* Procedure for Changing a Colostomy Pouch—cont'd

Procedure	Points to Remember
18. Remove gloves and wash hands.	Refer to standard precautions.
19. Document completion of the procedure.	Report to the family any change in stool pattern, skin irritation, or tolerance of the procedure.
20. Recognizing complications	Dehydration signs and symptoms: • Losing more than 1,000 mL of liquid stool per 24-hour period • Excessive thirst, dark concentrated urine, weakness, or lethargy Blockage signs and symptoms of patients with a colostomy or ileostomy: • Thin and malodorous clear liquid stool • Abdominal cramping and pain • Reduced and concentrated urine output • Abdominal distention • Engorged stoma

*Procedures may vary according to medical orders, equipment/devices, and the student's unique needs.
Adapted from Grant & Quigley (2014); Kirkland-Kyhn (2018).

Ostomies in the Urinary Tract

A *urostomy* is created when the bladder has been removed or bypassed to drain the urine through a stoma in the abdominal wall. A urostomy joins the ureters to a piece of intestine to make the stoma. A *ureterostomy* connects one or both ureters directly to the surface of the abdomen. A *vesicostomy* is usually a temporary procedure creating a conduit to the bladder in the suprapubic space. In some cases, the surgeon can create an internal pouch out of the bladder, called a continent urostomy or vesicostomy, where the urine collects until drained via catheterization (Grant & Quigley, 2014). See Figure 25-3A–C.

Complications and Issues Related to Ostomies

It is important that the school nurse monitor an ostomy site closely, including the consistency, color, and amount of a student's stool or urine collected in the ostomy pouch. The following assessments need to be reported to both the student's parents/guardians and healthcare provider:

- Stool that appears to contain blood or is frequently watery
- Urine that appears to be cloudy, dark amber, or contains blood
- Red, blistered, or bleeding stoma and/or surrounding skin excoriation: Avoid applying medication, ointment, or adhesive to damaged skin.
- An enlarged stoma accompanied by cramping or vomiting. This may be a sign that the stoma has prolapsed and is a medical emergency (Kirkland-Kyhn et al., 2018).

Students with ostomies may have issues with body image. It is essential they are assured privacy and dignity in the school setting. All students with ostomies should keep a backup set of clothing available at school in the event of a leakage of stool or urine. The school nurse should educate staff about the needs of students with ostomies and advocate those students be supported to participate in all school activities, including physical education and extracurricular activities as they are able.

URINARY CATHETERIZATION

Urinary catheterization is the placement of a tube into the bladder. A continent ureterostomy or vesicostomy drains urine when a child does not have the capacity

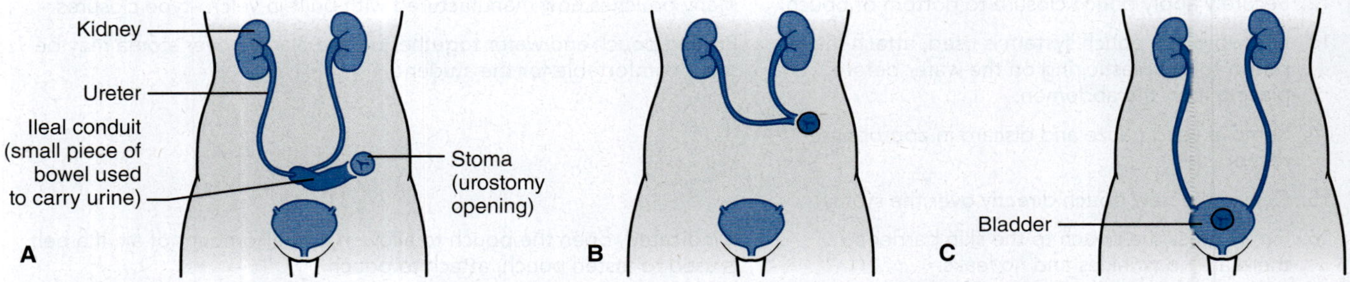

FIGURE 25-3. Ostomies in the urinary tract. A, Ileal conduit. B, Ureterostomy. C, Vesicostomy.

for spontaneous, controlled emptying of the bladder (Beauchemin et al., 2018). Catheterization can

- Prevent bladder overfilling
- Prevent urine leaking or incontinence
- Prevent reflux of urine back into the kidneys that can result in kidney damage
- Remove residual urine after spontaneous bladder emptying
- Be used to instill medication into the bladder

Neurogenic bladder is an example of a health condition in children that may require urinary catheterization secondary to an anomaly of the spine (myelodysplasia) that occurs commonly in spina bifida, spinal cord injury above the level of the sacral nerves, or urological surgery. Urinary catheterization is usually performed as clean intermittent catheterization (CIC) at home or at school (Tobias, 2017).

School nurses commonly need to catheterize students. CIC can be done in the school nurse's office or in a private bathroom with the student in a supine position on a cot or sitting on a toilet. When developmentally appropriate, students should learn to self-catheterize into a container or toilet. Catheterization supplies include a calibrated container to collect urine, water-soluble lubricant if the catheter is not self-lubricated, liquid soap and water, paper towels or wet wipes, gloves, catheters, absorbent towels, or pads (for supine CIC), and a storage receptacle for clean catheters (Tobias, 2017).

Using standard precautions, CIC for females and males begins with cleaning the urinary meatus with clean technique using soapy cotton balls or a student-specific cleaning solution. The catheter tip is lubricated and gently inserted through the meatus into the bladder until urine flows freely into the receptacle. Do not force the catheter (Newman, 2021). Figures 25-4 and 25-5 illustrate CIC for biological males and females.

Children with a continent ureterostomy or vesicostomy may also be catheterized by the school nurse or self-catheterized. The procedure is similar to CIC, but the catheter is inserted through the stoma to drain the urine (Cleveland Clinic, 2022c).

Did You Know?

Reusing catheters is an off-label use and is not recommended. There are no evidence-based guidelines on cleaning or disposing of reused catheters. This practice has changed and up to 200 catheters per month are now provided by many insurers to decrease urinary tract infections (UTIs). Some insurance plans and state Medicaid plans require prior authorization for more than 30 per month (Beauchemin et al., 2018). The school nurse can be an advocate for the student and their family regarding this practice and educate caregivers on how to reduce the likelihood of recurrent UTIs.

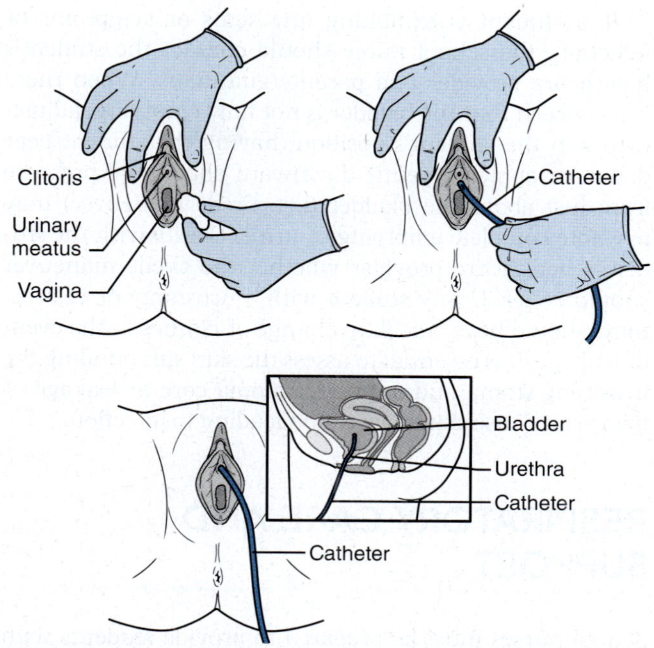

FIGURE 25-4. Clean intermittent catheterization—female.

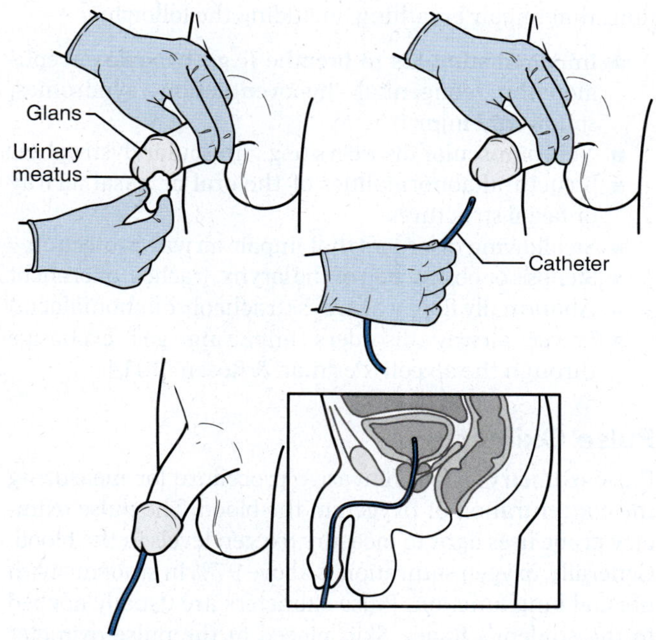

FIGURE 25-5. Clean intermittent catheterization—male.

The school nurse should be aware of the student's baseline urine characteristics to identify any concerning changes that may need intervention. Some problems that may occur with a student requiring CIC during school hours include the following:

- Difficulty emptying the student's bladder
- Difficulty passing the catheter into the bladder
- Urine leakage
- UTI symptoms

If a student is exhibiting any signs or symptoms of infection, the school nurse should contact the student's healthcare provider and parents/guardians. When there is a concern that the bladder is not fully emptying, adjustments in the student's position, having the student bear down, or applying gentle downward abdominal pressure from just above the bladder (i.e., Credé maneuver) may promote complete emptying of urine. Clarify with the student's healthcare provider whether the Credé maneuver should be used. Any student with a urostomy or vesicostomy should have a backup change of clothes in the event of leakage. It is essential to assess the skin surrounding the urostomy stoma and to provide stoma care as leakage of urine can cause skin maceration leading to infection.

RESPIRATORY CARE AND SUPPORT

School nurses must be prepared to provide students with respiratory care and support ranging from the need for oxygen to full mechanical ventilation. Children require respiratory care at school for a variety of chronic conditions that impair breathing, including the following:

- Impaired stimulus to breathe (e.g., hypoxic encephalopathy, congenital hypoventilation syndromes, spinal cord injury)
- Neuromuscular disorders (e.g., muscular dystrophy)
- Structural abnormalities of the oral or nasal airway or facial structures
- Swallowing disorders that impair airway protection
- Stenosis or obstruction of the larynx, trachea, or bronchi
- Abnormally floppy airways (tracheobronchomalacia)
- Lower airway disorders impairing gas exchange through the alveoli (Perlman & Rosen, 2014)

Pulse Oximetry

Pulse oximetry is a noninvasive procedure for measuring the concentration of oxygen in the blood. The pulse oximetry probe uses light to measure oxygen levels in the blood. Generally, oxygen saturation is above 97% in students with normal lung function. Pulse oximeters are usually applied to the student's finger. Skin placed in the pulse oximeter must be clean and dry for an accurate reading. The pulse oximetry readings are affected by motion, poor peripheral circulation, carbon monoxide poisoning, anemia, nail polish, cold fingers, and bright lights (Brown, 2017).

It is imperative for the school nurse to know a student's baseline acceptable oxygen saturation and typical vital sign parameters. A child who has respiratory or cardiac illness may have a low baseline level of oxygen saturation. These parameters should be listed in the student's medical orders and IHP along with frequency of monitoring, nursing interventions, and the emergency action plan for the student (Perlman & Rosen, 2014).

> **Practice Connection**
>
> Pulse oximetry is *not* a stand-alone assessment; it is an adjunct tool combined with other assessment data to establish the student's current respiratory status. Respiratory care of students includes frequent and thorough assessment by the school nurse, including subjective information, observation, auscultation of lung fields, and vital signs.

Oxygen

Oxygen is required by all cells in the body. Some students require continuous intermittent as-needed (prn) supplemental oxygen while at school for respiratory conditions; it relieves shortness of breath and reduces the workload of the heart. *Oxygen is considered a medication that requires medical orders.* Orders should include the diagnosis for which oxygen is required, how much oxygen to administer, parameters for administration (pulse oximetry readings, exercise), delivery device, and what constitutes an emergency for the child. Delivery methods in the school setting include continuous flow by nasal cannula, face mask, and tracheostomy mask. The school nurse should closely monitor the respiratory status of students requiring oxygen, including pulse oximetry (Perlman & Rosen, 2014).

Oxygen can be delivered from a cylinder in the form of gas or liquid or from an oxygen concentrator. Oxygen in gas cylinders, or tanks, come in a variety of sizes. Oxygen tanks have a gauge (regulator) attached, generally to the top of the tank. Some tanks are pulled around on wheels. Liquid oxygen comes in a tank that feels cool to touch and is filled by the caregiver at home. Always be sure to check the level of oxygen in the tank when the student arrives at school because improper filling of the tank at home can affect the oxygen supply. Keeping a backup tank and regulator at school is advisable. Often, humidification systems are needed to prevent drying of the student's mucosa (Perlman & Rosen, 2014).

An oxygen concentrator creates its own oxygen from the atmosphere. Though used less frequently in small children, it may be seen at school. Oxygen concentrators run on a battery and electrical power; they must be plugged in to maintain the battery charge in the event of a power outage (Perlman & Rosen, 2014).

School staff and families need to be aware of hazards associated with the delivery of oxygen and take precautions to prevent problems. Designated UAP, custodians, and principals should be included in training. Oxygen supports combustion, so sources of flame or high heat must be kept away from the student with oxygen such as cigarettes, candles, and Bunsen burners in the science laboratories. Combustible products should also be avoided around oxygen tanks, such as oils and oil-based petroleum products (e.g., petroleum jelly). Signs indicating that oxygen is in use should be posted in the classrooms. Oxygen should be stored away from direct sunlight and in an appropriate stabilizing stand that prevents accidental tipping and falling. The gauge on an oxygen cylinder should be protected from damage because the oxygen is under pressure; if the gauge fractures, the cylinder can become a projectile and injure others. Do not cover an oxygen tank. State and local regulations and statutes determine oxygen storage requirements. The local fire department should be notified that oxygen is used at school. It is also important to determine the seating of the student in the classroom relative to the oxygen supply and the length of tubing needed for the student to move safely within the learning environment (Perlman & Rosen, 2014).

The school nurse or the nurse in charge of the student's daily care should assess the length of time each oxygen container will last based on the oxygen flow rate being used and make plans for delivery of needed oxygen at appropriate intervals. Checks of oxygen levels in the tanks or liquid cylinders need to be documented daily to ensure adequate supply. If using a concentrator, the length of time an oxygen concentrator can run on battery power should be estimated. Plans for backup power in case of power outages or building evacuations should be in place. Enough oxygen must be available for the entire length of an outside school activity or field trip. Care must be taken to prevent oxygen tubing from being kinked, blocked, punctured, or disconnected (Perlman & Rosen, 2014).

Tracheostomies

A tracheostomy is an opening made in the trachea through which a tube is inserted to allow for air exchange and suctioning of secretions. See Figure 25-6. A tracheostomy is performed for many reasons in children, including muscular disease, recurrent aspiration, inability to protect one's airway, trauma, malformation of the facial or airway structures, and need for long-term mechanical ventilation.

Several types of tracheostomy tubes are used in children. Single-lumen uncuffed tracheostomy tubes made of silastic are the most common. Tracheostomy tubes are securely held in place by holders (ties or straps) fastened around the child's neck (Perlman & Rosen, 2014). An obturator fits inside the tracheostomy tube and guides its insertion into the trachea. An obturator is *never* left in place because it occludes the airway, but it must always stay with the student in case it is needed to reinsert the tube. Cuffed tracheostomy tubes are designed to prevent air leaks during mechanical ventilation. The cuff is inflated when the pilot balloon near the stoma is inflated. Always refer to the product information to determine whether the cuff is filled with air, saline, or sterile water and volume in the cuff. Cuffed tubes need to be deflated on a regular schedule determined by the physician. See Figure 25-7.

Some students have tracheostomies due to anatomical abnormalities of the upper airway but have normal pulmonary function and are able to cough and clear secretions from the tracheostomy independently; they may not need oxygen or respiratory assistance and may be typically active. However, most students with tracheostomies require personal nursing support in school. The standard of care for a child with a tracheostomy is to be monitored by an awake, trained caregiver 24 hours a day, 7 days per week (Sterni et al., 2016). If the student requires personal nursing care, a nurse travels with the student on the bus to and from school. If a parent/guardian chooses to drive the student to school, the nurse will meet the student at school. The student must travel with a backup tracheostomy tube the correct size as well as a tube one size smaller. The size of the tracheostomy tube is labeled on the box and the tube.

All students with tracheostomies need a speech evaluation and a communication plan from a speech therapist. The child may need to learn sign language, use a speaking valve on their tracheostomy tube, or use a technology-based communication device. The school nurse needs to be aware of how the student communicates and be familiar with medical orders involving the use of speaking valves. A student with a tracheostomy may have oral sensory issues affecting their enjoyment of food. Additionally, because the nose is bypassed by the tracheostomy, a student's sense of smell and taste may also be affected.

Since the tracheostomy tube bypasses the mouth and nose that normally humidify and protect the airway, a supplemental heat and moisturized exchanger device that protects the airway from dry and cold air and filters out

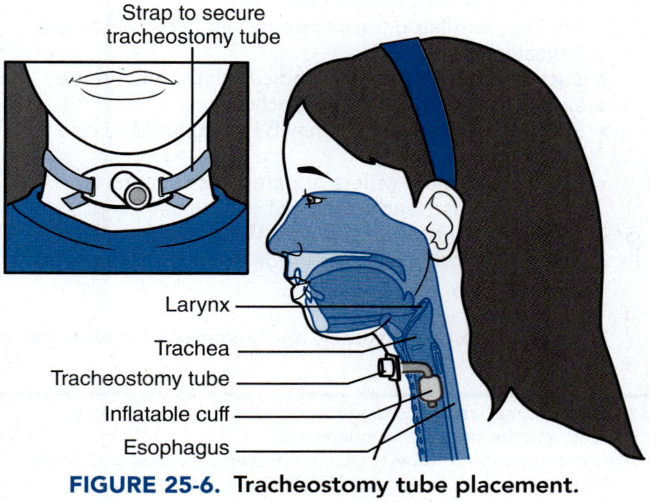

FIGURE 25-6. Tracheostomy tube placement.

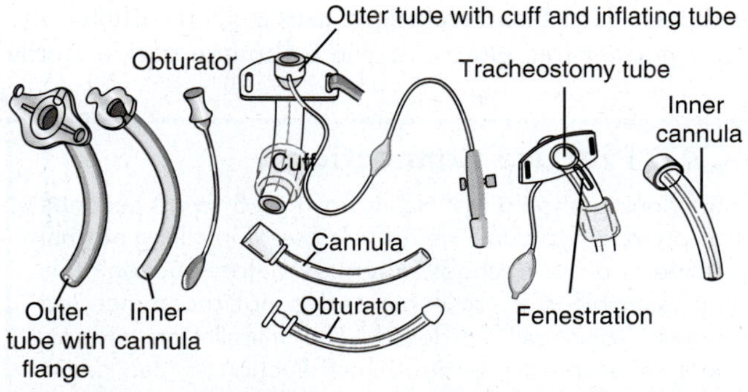

FIGURE 25-7. Tracheostomy tube and obturator. *(Wilkinson, JL & Van Leuven, K: Fundamentals of Nursing: Theory, Concepts & Applications. Vol. 1. 2007. Philadelphia: FA Davis.)*

particulate matter (dust) in the air is often used (Perlman & Rosen, 2014). The use of humidity allows secretions to remain thin and easier to suction and helps to prevent mucous plugs. The humidity device attaches over the tracheostomy tube and needs to be removed for suctioning or coughing so that mucus can be cleared. The school nurse should ensure that essential tracheostomy equipment always accompanies the student, including the following:

- Spare tracheostomy tube, one-size-smaller tracheostomy tube, obturator, ties
- Tracheostomy holders, blunt scissors, water-soluble lubricant or normal saline
- Portable suction device with appropriate suction catheters
- Manual resuscitator bag
- Syringe to inflate or deflate the tracheostomy cuff
- Heat and moisture exchanger
- Clean gloves (Perlman & Rosen, 2014)

Care of a Tracheostomy Tube

School nurses need to know about the care of tracheostomies, be competent in performing tracheal suctioning, and identify indications changing a trach tube. Suctioning the tracheostomy is one of the most common and important aspects of trach care. Suctioning is needed to remove mucus, maintain a patent airway, and prevent blockages. The frequency of suctioning varies by student individual needs. Indications for suctioning include the following:

- Audible or visual signs of secretions
- Signs of respiratory distress, such as increased work of breathing or color change
- Suspicion of blockage or partial obstruction of the tracheal tube
- Desaturation on pulse oximetry
- Ventilation pressure changes (if ventilated)
- Per request of the student (Jones, 2022)

The school nurse needs to be familiar with the student's individual suctioning instructions, including length of suction catheter insertion, pressure on the suction machine, and whether clean verses sterile technique should be used. In the home or school setting, clean technique is usually acceptable, but the level of technique is determined by medical orders. Clean technique uses a clean catheter and clean powder-free gloves. Sterile technique uses a sterile catheter and sterile gloves. A modified sterile technique uses a sterile catheter and clean gloves. See Table 25-3 for suctioning procedure instructions; Figure 25-8 highlights proper placement of the suction catheter. The size of the suction catheter is dependent on the size of the tracheostomy tube. Older students can learn to suction themselves if they are developmentally able. Oral secretions or

Practice Connection

Suctioning should last no more than 5 to 10 seconds to prevent hypoxia. The routine use of instilling normal saline into the tracheostomy tube before suctioning is *not* supported by research and is *not* recommended unless specifically ordered. The installation of normal saline before endotracheal suctioning can cause oxygen saturation to be reduced for up to 2 minutes (Anderson & Herring, 2022).

TABLE 25-3 Sample* Procedure for Tracheal Suctioning

1. **Reassure and position student as recommended.**
2. **Assemble equipment and supplies.**
   - Assemble suction supplies or suction catheter kit (if used) on clean surface.
   - Pour small amount of normal saline or water into disposable container.
   - Confirm premeasured length of catheter to be inserted.
   - Put on clean gloves.
   - Choose one hand (usually dominant hand) to keep clean for handling suction catheter and the other hand to manipulate nonclean equipment.
3. **Turn on suction machine.**
   - Confirm suction setting of 60 to 100 mm HG according to medical orders. Confirm proper connections between machine and collection canister
   - Open suction catheter and attach to suction machine (or prepare to insert closed system catheter).
4. **Suction the student.**
   - Remove ventilator, tracheostomy cap, filter, or valve as indicated and place on clean surface.
   - Place finger of clean hand at premeasured length of catheter.
   - Keeping the thumb off the suction control valve, gently insert catheter into tracheostomy to premeasured length. Place the thumb over the suction control valve to suction while gently twirling the catheter between the fingers to rotate catheter inside the trachea tube. (Note: Generally, suction catheters are inserted to only 0.5 cm beyond the end of the tracheostomy tube.)
   - Complete suctioning within 5 seconds (count "1-one thousand, 2-one thousand, . . .").
   - Rinse the catheter if needed with water or normal saline.
   - If moist, gurgling, or whistling noises are heard or if mucus is seen, repeat suctioning. Allow student to rest 30 to 60 seconds before repeating.
   - Replace ventilator, tracheostomy cap, filter, or valve as indicated.
   - Suction mouth and nose if indicated: Do NOT reuse suction catheter to suction trachea.
   - Specific suction catheter may be designated for the mouth/nose.
   - Follow procedure orders or parent instructions on cleaning, reuse, and storage of suction catheters.
5. **Dispose of catheter and gloves.** Wrap catheter around gloved hand and pull gloves inside out and dispose of gloves properly.
6. **Wash hands.**
7. **Note the color, consistency, and quantity of secretions.**
8. **Document.**

*Procedures may vary according to medical orders, equipment/devices, and the student's unique needs.
Adapted from Ann & Robert H. Lurie Children's Hospital of Chicago (2024b); Boroughs & Dougherty (2015); Perlman & Rosen (2014).

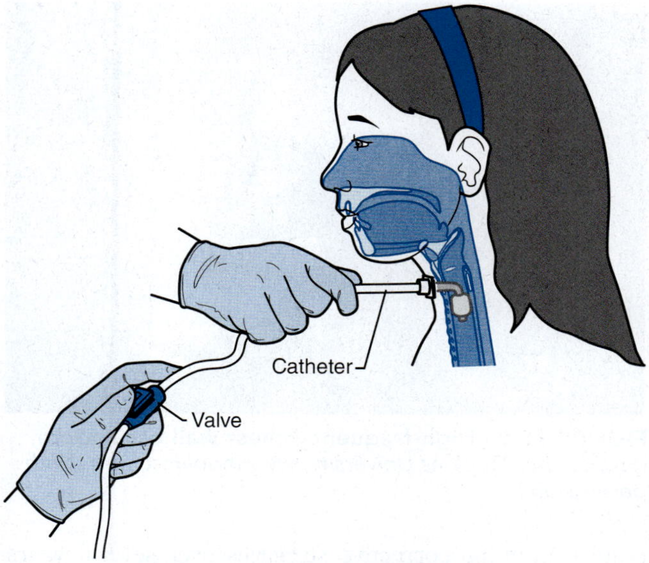

FIGURE 25-8. Tracheal suctioning.

secretions coughed up to the opening of the tracheostomy tube can be suctioned using a rigid plastic suction tip (e.g., Yankauer tube).

Tracheostomy tubes are changed regularly to help keep mucus and bacteria from building up over time (American Thoracic Society, 2016a). Routine tracheostomy tube changes are usually performed at home by a parent/guardian, home nurse, or trained caregiver. However, there may be times at school when an emergent tracheostomy tube change needs to be performed or when a dislodged tracheostomy tube needs to be replaced. Two people are involved in performing a tracheostomy tube change. If the same size tracheostomy tube cannot be reinserted (recannulated), attempt to insert a tube one size smaller. Failure to recannulate is a medical emergency requiring rescue breathing and activation of EMS for immediate assistance and to transport the student to the nearest emergency department.

Ventilators

Some students need either intermittent or continuous mechanical ventilation through a tracheostomy tube due to conditions that affect the lungs (i.e., underdeveloped lungs resulting from prematurity or other lung diseases), musculoskeletal or neurological conditions that lead to weak breathing, or conditions affecting the patency of the airway (American Thoracic Society, 2016b). Ventilators assist in respiration by

- Delivering oxygen and removing carbon dioxide
- Providing positive airway pressure that helps to keep airways open, prevents lung tissue from collapsing or compressing (atelectasis), and improves secretion clearance
- Reducing the work of breathing to help the student participate in activities (American Thoracic Society, 2016b)

Ventilators that are used at school are typically small, lightweight, and quiet. They should be relatively easy to use and troubleshoot. Internal and external battery power allows for portability (Noah & Budek, 2016). Sources of backup electrical and battery power are essential in case of primary battery failure. Having a backup oxygen supply is also crucial. Ventilators are frequently mounted to a mobility device, such as a wheelchair, or mounted on a moveable unit for students who are ambulatory (Perlman & Rosen, 2014).

The primary care provider or a specialist overseeing the student's care determines the ventilator settings and alarm parameters depending on the student's unique condition, lung function, and whether the student breathes spontaneously. Examples of ventilator settings include the following:

- Volume-controlled ventilation (VCV): Machine-delivered volume is the primary control. The inflation pressure generated depends on the respiratory system compliance and resistance.
- Pressure-controlled ventilation (PCV): The pressure change above the baseline is the primary control. The tidal volume delivered to the lungs depends on the respiratory system's compliance and resistance.
- PCV and VCV synchronize with the student's spontaeous breaths to support adequate respiration.
- Other advanced modes of mechanical ventilation are occasionally indicated (Sarnaik et al., 2016).

Students who need mechanical ventilation must be continuously monitored by a professional nurse with skills in managing the specific ventilator (Noah & Budek, 2016). However, the school nurse should be capable of caring for the student on a ventilator in case of an emergency or when the personal nurse is not available. The specifics of each ventilator can be taught by the personal nurse or learned by inviting the representative from the durable medical equipment company to provide in-service instruction. Family members can share information about the nuances and preferences of their child's ventilator care.

When an alarm occurs, it is important to critically assess the student first, rather than the machine. It is essential to determine whether the student needs suctioning or whether other causes of respiratory distress are contributing to acute changes, such as a blocked or dislodged tracheostomy tube, bronchospasm, or disconnection from the ventilator. Avoid assuming mechanical malfunction and discontinuing an alarm without performing a thorough physical assessment of the student. In the event of ventilator malfunction or if the student exhibits signs of acute distress, initiate assisted ventilation with a mechanical resuscitator bag or bag-valve mask device. Activate EMS for transport to the emergency department and contact the family (Bowden & Greenberg, 2016).

Percussion and Postural Drainage

Percussion and postural drainage may be needed at school for students who have chronic conditions that cause chest muscle weakness (e.g., cerebral palsy, muscular dystrophy, spinal muscle atrophy, amyotrophic lateral sclerosis) or thick, sticky mucus secondary to chronic pulmonary disease (e.g., cystic fibrosis, bronchiectasis, chronic pneumonia, primary ciliary dyskinesia). Percussion and postural drainage, also referred to as chest physical therapy (chest PT), assists the student to cough up secretions for expectoration or suctioning by loosening mucus in the airways and using gravity to facilitate removal of secretions (Bryant, 2022). Chest PT can be performed manually or with a high-frequency chest wall oscillation vest.

Medical orders should outline the frequency and duration of the chest PT, including the parameters for continuing or stopping the procedure. The school nurse (or delegated staff if allowed) must be trained in the prescribed procedure. Before performing the percussion and postural drainage, the nurse should auscultate the lungs and take a pulse oximetry reading and vital signs. The student must be continually observed during the procedure. If signs of respiratory compromise develop, stop the procedure, institute emergency interventions, and contact the parent/guardian and/or physician. Following the procedure, the nurse must repeat vital signs and pulse oximetry, and document the amount of mucus produced and the student's reaction to the procedure. Chest PT should not be done before meals or less than an hour after ingesting food. Both manual therapy and vest therapy should not be performed on bare skin; a light T-shirt is recommended (Cystic Fibrosis Foundation, n.d.a).

Traditional chest PT incorporates the cupping of hands to repeatedly clap the student's chest (percussion) for the prescribed length of time, followed by repeatedly vibrating the student's chest wall with flat firm hands. The cupped clapping and vibration are repeated in various specific positions meant to facilitate the drainage of the mucus out of the airways via gravity from each lung field (Cystic Fibrosis Foundation, n.d.b). The student should be positioned so that the mucus from that lung field will flow to the bifurcation of the bronchi by gravity.

A high-frequency chest wall oscillator is an inflatable device resembling a vest that is strapped around the child and attached via air tubes to an air pulse generator (Bryant, 2022). The air generator creates air pressure against the chest wall by rapidly inflating and deflating the vest, up to 20 times per minute, with an effect like percussion. The air pulse generator is operated at specific settings that cannot be changed. Treatments typically last about 20 to 30 minutes with stops every 5 minutes for the student to huff or cough out the loosened secretions (Cystic Fibrosis Foundation, n.d.b; see Figure 25-9).

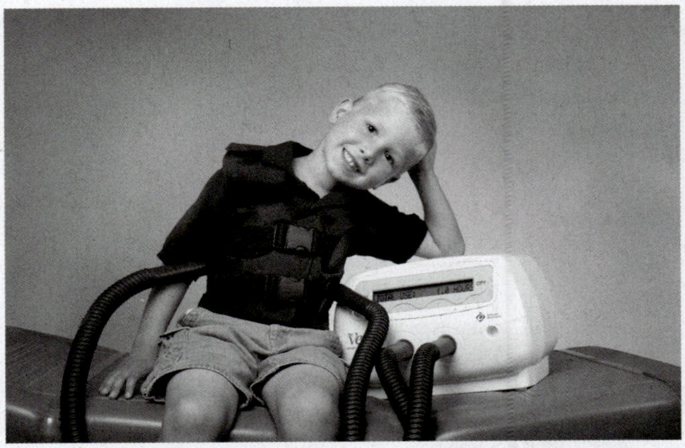

FIGURE 25-9. High-frequency chest wall oscillation. *(From Johns Hopkins University, www.hopkinscf.org. With permission.)*

CARDIOVASCULAR DEVICES

Students with congenital or acquired cardiac conditions may need complex monitoring and care by the school nurse. Students with significant congenital heart defects, such as tetralogy of Fallot or hypoplastic left heart syndrome, require multiple corrective surgeries over several years. Acquired conditions include congestive heart failure, cardiomyopathy, and abnormal heart rhythms (Schroeder et al., 2022). Cardiovascular devices include monitors, vascular access devices, pacemakers, pacer/defibrillators, and implantable defibrillators.

The school nurse needs to assess the student, obtain medical orders, and determine the level of care required throughout the school day. The school nurse should collaborate with the student (if developmentally appropriate), the family, and healthcare provider(s) to develop a detailed IHP and EAP. The EAP should include when to initiate cardiopulmonary resuscitation (CPR) by trained staff, location of an automated external defibrillator, and when to activate EMS. The school nurse is responsible for ensuring that educational staff are trained accordingly. Cardiology care team members, medical supply company staff, or private consultants can be enlisted to help train the school nurse and educational staff on the child's condition and healthcare needs at school.

Portable Cardiac Monitoring

Students may wear portable cardiac monitors for a period of time to determine whether symptoms such as dizziness, fatigue, palpitations, syncope, or chest pain are caused by cardiac issues (Seattle Children's Hospital Heart Center, 2017). Although there are no risks to wearing an event monitor, the school nurse needs to know the student's typical ranges for heart rate, blood pressure, and level of activity tolerance, and regularly assess the student for cardiac signs and symptoms. Parents/guardians should notify the school nurse that an event monitor is being used in school.

A *Holter monitor* records the heart rhythm for an extended period of time, from 24 hours up to weeks (Boston Children's Hospital, 2024a). Holter monitors are smaller than a deck of cards and are connected to the student via electrodes placed on the student's chest. The monitor is attached to the child via a strap or clipped to clothing.

A *cardiac event monitor* records the hearts electrical activity as the student goes about their everyday activities (American Heart Association [AHA], 2022a). Event monitors record the heart rhythm when the event button is pushed by the student (or responsible adult) when symptoms are felt, such as chest pain, dizziness, or palpitations. There are different types of event monitors. Some record the heart rhythm only when the device is activated (non-looping) or for a short period of time before the event button is pushed (memory loop recording). Autotrigger event monitors may be used to capture rare events or arrhythmias during sleep. Event monitors may be smaller than a mobile phone attached to the student's chest with electrocardiogram (ECG) stickers; the recording device is worn on the body via a pouch or fanny pack. Other monitors are smaller and worn as a patch on the wrist (Ann & Robert H. Lurie Children's Hospital of Chicago, 2024a). Events are recorded or sent electronically in real time and communicated to the physician. Some event monitors may be used up to a month with a medical order (Boston Children's Hospital, 2024a).

Students typically do not have any activity restrictions when on portable cardiac monitors. However, monitors must always be kept dry; students should avoid excessive sweating. Students should also avoid magnets, metal detectors, electric blankets, and handheld electrical appliances (e.g., hair dryers, electric razors, or electric toothbrushes) that may interfere with the recording (Boston Children's Hospital, 2024a).

Pacemakers and Implantable Cardioverter-Defibrillators

Pacemakers are small devices implanted under the skin in the abdomen or near the collarbone for cardiac conditions causing slowed heart rate such as bradycardia, sick sinus syndrome, and heart block. The device has wires or leads that are placed in or on the heart, continuously monitoring the heart to detect an abnormal ECG rhythm. When the pacemaker detects an abnormal heart rate, it sends an electrical signal that the student does not typically feel to stimulate the heart to resume a normal rhythm (Children's Wisconsin, 2023).

Implantable cardioverter-defibrillators (ICDs) are small devices implanted under the skin with wires that connect to the heart. ICDs differ from pacemakers because they detect rapid or erratic heartbeats, such as ventricular tachycardia or ventricular fibrillation. When the ICD detects an arrhythmia, it releases a stronger electrical shock to slow the heart rate, which the student may describe as feeling like a kick in the chest. Some ICDs also function as pacemakers (Children's National Health System, 2024).

Both pacemakers and ICDs have pulse generators with sealed lithium batteries lasting 5 to 7 years, depending on the device used (Bass & Gandelman, 2024). Symptoms such as exercise intolerance, fatigue, palpitations, dizziness, and syncope may indicate pacemaker or ICD malfunction/failure and require immediate medical evaluation. Students with implanted cardiac devices usually are encouraged to be active and engage in normal activities, though physicians may advise against contact sports to avoid impact to the chest and device area (Children's Wisconsin, 2023). If the student does receive a blow to the chest, follow-up with a healthcare provider is necessary. Students with a pacemaker or an ICD should wear a medical alert bracelet or necklace in case of emergency.

The school nurse needs to be familiar with warnings from the implanted cardiac device manufacturer about interference from other devices that may pose a risk when brought into proximity with a student's internally implanted cardiac device. While interference is rare, precautions should be taken; the most common sources of interference include cellphones and security systems (AHA, 2022b).

Vascular Access Devices

School nurses may care for students with vascular access devices to deliver fluids, medications, or blood products. They are indicated when peripheral vein access cannot be obtained, when peripheral vein administration is contraindicated, and/or when the duration of intravenous therapy is for an extended time. Indications include chemotherapy, long-term antibiotics, or total parenteral nutrition (TPN). Vascular access devices may also be used to obtain blood specimens (Brown, 2017).

Peripherally inserted central catheter (PICC) lines are used for short-term or moderate-term therapy. They are most often inserted above the antecubital space. PICC lines can be inserted by specially trained nurses (Anderson & Herring, 2022). Central venous access devices (CVADs) are typically used for more long-term therapy or for agents, such as TPN or chemotherapy, that are irritating when administered through a PICC line. CVADs are placed by interventional radiologists into the right subclavian vein and threaded into or near the heart, then secured to the

Did You Know?

Magnets and equipment containing magnets, such as cellphone headphones (ear-bud and clip-on versions), should be kept at least 6 inches away from the ICDs (AHA, 2022b). High-frequency cellphones, walkie-talkies, and CB radios that are less than 3 watts should be kept at least 6 inches from the pacemaker or ICD. Students who participate in vocational/machine shop classes should stay at least 2 feet away from power-generating equipment (e.g., welding equipment and jumper cables) and heavy machinery that may contain magnets. Microwave ovens, metal detectors, and other household appliances pose little to no risk of interfering with pacemakers and ICDs. However, students should be instructed to pass quickly through metal detectors or given accommodations to bypass the metal detector in case it is triggered by the implanted cardiac device (AHA, 2022b).

chest. They may have single, double, or triple lumens. Double- and triple-lumen CVADs allow for repeated blood sampling and infusion of more than one therapy to be instilled at the same time. PICC lines and CVADs may have an infusion port implanted under the skin that can be accessed with a needle when intermittent infusions are needed (e.g., chemotherapy), thereby eliminating the need for external tubing on the chest (Anderson & Herring, 2022).

The student with a vascular access device should have a school nurse available all day, every day. However, the school nurse is not responsible for accessing a PICC or CVAD port or administering medications through the venous access device during the school day. Schools should evaluate whether a student with a central line who is receiving long-term continuous therapy needs a personal nurse to care for them at school.

Protecting a student's venous access device from trauma in the school setting is essential. A smooth-edged clamp or hemostat should always be with the child in case the integrity of the line is compromised. If the line is broken or torn, take the following actions immediately to prevent an air embolism or blood loss:

- Immediately clamp the line with a smooth edge clamp or hemostat between the break/cut and the access site as close to the body as possible.
- Tape the catheter so that the uncapped/damaged site is resting above the level of the heart.
- Place the student on the left side in Trendelenburg position to help trap the air in the apex of the right atrium and prevent it from entering the right ventricle and moving into the lungs (McCarthy et al., 2016).
- Notify parents/guardians and providers. The student should be transported to a healthcare facility so that the line can be repaired or replaced as soon as possible.
- If the CVAD is pulled out, cover the catheter site with sterile gauze; apply direct, firm pressure; and activate EMS.
- Activate EMS for shortness of breath, hypotension, dyspnea, chest pain, tachycardia, anxiety, nausea, dizziness, or confusion, all of which are concerning symptoms that may indicate an air embolism or blood loss.

The school nurse should obtain medical orders regarding activity restrictions for students with vascular access devices. Measures to prevent a blow to the student's chest should be instituted, including avoiding contact sports. Any student with a central line who receives a forceful blow to the chest should immediately be evaluated by the school nurse. All visible intravascular devices should be secured to the student's body to prevent the device from being pulled out (Bowden & Greenberg, 2016).

Preventing infection is a priority for students with vascular access devices (Farou et al., 2021). The school nurse must be alert for signs of infection, including tenderness, swelling, redness, and warmth, and report symptoms to both the student's parents/guardians and provider. Avoid immersion of the catheter site in water to prevent infection. If the student has a dressing, the school nurse should know the proper dressing change techniques and have proper supplies should the dressing become loose or fall off during the school day. It is essential to use proper hand washing, gloves, and aseptic technique during manipulation of the access site.

Students who are receiving dialysis may have shunts in the forearm for hemodialysis or in the abdomen for peritoneal dialysis. These devices do not cause the student discomfort or require special care, but the school nurse should be aware of their presence. The school nurse may need to assess the function and patency of the dialysis shunt for an adequate bruit and thrill and notify the parent/guardian and provider of any problems. *Do not take a blood pressure in the arm with a hemodialysis shunt.* Impact to the dialysis shunt must be avoided.

Ventricular Assist Devices

The quality of life for children with end-stage heart disease may be significantly improved by a ventricular assist device (VAD). VADs may stabilize students with acute heart failure to stabilize awaiting heart transplant, to allow the heart to heal, or to support life for children who are not candidates for transplantation. Many children with VADs can return home from the hospital and participate in many normal daily activities, including school (Boston Children's Hospital, 2024b).

A VAD is a surgically implanted pump that supports the left ventricle, right ventricle, or both to pump blood to the body (Nemours KidsHealth, 2021). The VAD has an external driveline that exits the body through the abdomen and attaches to a battery pack. The battery pack can be carried like a purse with a strap that goes across the body (like a shoulder bag). The battery is charged by plugging into a wall outlet or car battery charger. Backup batteries and power sources are mandatory. Most patients with VADs do not have palpable pulses or blood pressures that can be measured (Nemours KidsHealth, 2021).

A personal nurse for a student with a VAD is indicated. Still, when a student with VAD plans to return to school, the school nurse needs to coordinate detailed plans of care and emergency preparation with the VAD healthcare team, school staff, EMS, the family, and the student. Comprehensive training for the school nurse and school staff should be done by the student's VAD team so that the student's healthcare needs can be met at school. Parents/guardians may request that end-of-life directives be respected at school (see Chapter 20).

CONCLUSION

Every child has the right to a free and appropriate public education (IDEA, 2004). The school nurse is integral to ensuring this right for students with medical complexity. Students with significant and rare conditions are now able to attend school thanks to advances in medical technology.

Medical technology changes rapidly, and it is challenging for the school nurse to remain current. Each school nurse is responsible for identifying their own learning needs and taking the appropriate steps to develop competencies required to deliver and coordinate care for these students.

Careful assessment, planning, caring, and communication are needed for the student with medical complexity. The school nurse serves as liaison between the student, educational staff, family, and healthcare providers to ensure a safe and supportive learning environment that meets the student's special healthcare needs in the least restrictive environment.

The Editors gratefully acknowledge the work of the previous chapter authors, Stephanie Porter, Dorothy Page, Heather Engholm, and Carrie Sompii.

References

Abdelhadi, R. A., Rahe, K., & Lyman, B. (2016). Pediatric enteral access device management. *Nutrition in Clinical Practice: Official Publication of the American Society for Parenteral and Enteral Nutrition, 31*(6), 748–761. https://doi.org/10.1177/0884533616670640

American Academy of Allergy, Asthma, and Immunology. (2024). *Latex allergy overview*. https://www.aaaai.org/conditions-and-treatments/allergies/latex-allergy

American Heart Association. (2022a). *Cardiac event recorder.* https://www.heart.org/en/health-topics/arrhythmia/prevention—treatment-of-arrhythmia/cardiac-event-recorder

American Heart Association. (2022b). *Devices that may interfere with ICDs and pacemakers.* https://www.heart.org/en/health-topics/arrhythmia/prevention—treatment-of-arrhythmia/devices-that-may-interfere-with-icds-and-pacemakers

American Thoracic Society. (2016a). *Use of a tracheostomy with a child.* https://www.thoracic.org/patients/patient-resources/resources/tracheostomy-in-child.pdf

American Thoracic Society. (2016b). *Using a home ventilator with a child.* https://www.thoracic.org/patients/patient-resources/resources/using-a-home-ventilator-with-a-child.pdf

Anderson, C., & Herring, R. (2022). Pediatric nursing interventions and skills. In D. L. Hockenberry, D. Wilson, & M. L. Winkelstein (Eds.), *Wong's essentials of pediatric nursing* (7th ed., pp. 551–618). Elsevier Mosby.

Ann & Robert H. Lurie Children's Hospital of Chicago. (2024a). *Pediatric Holter and event monitoring.* https://www.luriechildrens.org/en/specialties-conditions/holter-event-monitoring/

Ann & Robert H. Lurie Children's Hospital of Chicago. (2024b). *Tracheostomy care at home.* https://www.luriechildrens.org/en/specialties-conditions/pediatric-ent-otolaryngology/resources/tracheostomy-care-at-home/

Barnert, E. S., Coller, R. J., Nelson, B. B., Thompson, L. R., Chan, V., Padilla, C., Klitzner, T. S., Szilagyi, M., & Chung, P. J. (2017). Experts' perspectives toward a population health approach for children with medical complexity. *Academic Pediatrics, 17*(6), 672–677. https://doi.org/10.1016/j.acap.2017.02.010

Bass, P. F., & Gandelman, G. (2024). *A child living with a pacemaker or implantable cardioverter defibrillator (ICD).* University of Rochester Medical Center, Health Encyclopedia. http://www.urmc.rochester.edu/encyclopedia/content.aspx?ContentTypeID=90&ContentID=P01803

Beauchemin, L., Newman, D. K., Le Danseur, M., Jackson, A., & Ritmiller, M. (2018). Best practices for clean intermittent catheterization. *Nursing, 48*(9), 49–54. https://doi.org/10.1097/01.NURSE.0000544216.23783.bc

Beierwaltes, P., & Schoessler, S. (2017). Latex safe at school: A student-centered approach. *NASN School Nurse, 32*(6), 343–345. https://doi.org/10.1177/1942602X17715495

Bergren, M. D. (2017). HIPAA, FERPA and the privacy of student health information in individualized healthcare plans. In S. I. S. Will, M. Waldin, & D. S. Zaiger (Eds.), *Individualized healthcare plans for the school nurse: A comprehensive resource for school nursing management of health conditions* (2nd ed., pp. 59–65). Sunrise River Press.

Bobo, N., Maughan, E. D., Carr, D., & Tillman, A. (2019). School nurse-led care coordination. Proceedings from the national strategy to action roundtable. *NASN School Nurse, 34*(4), 229–234. https://doi.org/10.1177/194260X19825617

Boroughs, D., & Dougherty, J. (2015). Pediatric tracheostomy care: What home care nurses need to know. *American Nurse Today, 10*(3), 8–10.

Boston Children's Hospital. (2024a). *Holter and event monitors.* http://www.childrenshospital.org/conditions-and-treatments/treatments/holter-and-event-monitors

Boston Children's Hospital. (2024b). *Ventricular assist device program.* https://www.childrenshospital.org/programs/ventricular-assist-device-program

Boullata, J. I. (2021). Enteral medication for the tube-fed patient: Making this route safe and effective. *Nutrition in Clinical Practice, 36*(1), 111–132. https://doi.org/10.1002/ncp.10615

Bowden, V., & Greenberg, C. (2016). *Pediatric nursing procedures.* Wolters Kluwer Health.

Brown, T. L. (2017). The child who is hospitalized. In M. J. Hockenberry, D. Wilson, & C. C. Rodgers (Eds.), *Wong's essentials of pediatric nursing* (10th ed., pp. 575–635). Mosby Elsevier.

Bryant, R. (2022). The child with respiratory dysfunction. In D. L. Hockenberry, D. Wilson, & M. L. Winkelstein (Eds), *Wong's essentials of pediatric nursing* (11th ed., pp. 619–679). Elsevier Evolve.

Centers for Disease Control and Prevention. (2022, February 1). *Communicating with and about people with disabilities.* https://www.cdc.gov/ncbddd/disabilityandhealth/materials/factsheets/fs-communicating-with-people.html

Centers for Medicare and Medicaid Services. (n.d.). *Home and community-based services.* https://www.medicaid.gov/medicaid/home-community-based-services/home-community-based-services-authorities/home-community-based-services-1915c/index.html

Child and Adolescent Health Measurement Initiative. (2020–2021). *2020–2021 National Survey of Children's Health (NSCH) data query.* Data Resource Center for Child and Adolescent Health, U.S. Department of Health and Human Services, Health Resources and Services Administration, Maternal and Child Health Bureau. https://www.childhealthdata.org/

Children's Hospitals and Clinics of Minnesota. (2014). *A guide for parents: G-tube care at home.* https://www.childrensmn.org/references/PFS/homecare/gastrostomy-care-g-j-tube.pdf

Children's National Health System. (2024). *Pediatric pacemaker and defibrillator management.* https://childrensnational.org/choose-childrens/conditions-and-treatments/heart/pacemaker-implantation-treatment

Children's Wisconsin. (2023). *Living with a pacemaker.* https://childrenswi.org/medical-care/herma-heart/conditions/living-with-a-pacemaker

Cleveland Clinic. (2022a). *Nasogastric tubes.* https://my.clevelandclinic.org/health/treatments/24313-nasogastric-tube

Cleveland Clinic. (2022b). *Mucous fistula.* https://my.clevelandclinic.org/health/treatments/22844-mucous-fistula

Cleveland Clinic. (2022c). *Mitrofanoff procedure, purpose, process, and recovery.* https://my.clevelandclinic.org/health/treatments/23535-mitrofanoff-procedure

Collado-Boira, E., Boldo-Roda, P., Bernat-Adell, M., Morar, K., Ayora, A., & Medina, P. (2021). Effectiveness of semi occlusive sodium carboxymethyl cellulose fibers and hydrocolloid dressings for irritant peristomal dermatitis: A case series. *Advances in Skin & Wound Care, 34*(9), 493–497. https://doi.org/10.1097/01.ASW.0000767336.91651.67

Corrigan, M. L., Huang, S., Weaver, A., Keeler, D., Rahe, K., Balint, J., Marti, M., Goodman, B., Nagy, T., DeLano, V., & Bond, B. (2017). Resources for the provision of nutrition support to children in educational environments. *Nutrition in Clinical Practice, 32*(6), 834–843. https://doi.org/10.1177/0884533617718471

Cystic Fibrosis Foundation. (n.d.a). *Basics of postural drainage and percussion*. https://www.cff.org/Life-With-CF/Treatments-and-Therapies/Airway-Clearance/Basics-of-Postural-Drainage-and-Percussion

Cystic Fibrosis Foundation. (n.d.b). *Living with CF: Airway clearance, chest physical therapy*. https://www.cff.org/managing-cf/chest-physical-therapy

Donoghue, E. A., & Kraft, C. A. (2019). *Managing chronic health needs in childcare and schools: A quick reference guide*. American Academy of Pediatrics.

Farou, N., Lucas, C., & Olympia, R. P. (2021). School nurses on the front lines of healthcare: Children with medical devices—central venous access device malfunctions and infections. *NASN School Nurse, 36*(6), 328–332. https://doi.org/10.1177/1942602X20940393

Ghandour, R. M., Hirai, A. H., & Kenney, M. K. (2022). Children and youth with special health care needs: A profile. *Pediatrics, 149*, s1–s17. https://doi.org/10.1542/peds.2021-056150D

Gillette Children's. (2023). *Feeding tubes*. https://www.gillettechildrens.org/conditions-care/feedingtubes#:~:text=A%20feeding%20tube%20is%20a,and%20into%20the%20small%20intestine

Got Transition. (2023). *Six core elements of health care transition*. https://www.gottransition.org/six-core-elements/

Grant, R. H., & Quigley, S. (2014). Ostomy care. In S. M. Porter, P. A. Branowicki, & J. S. Palfrey (Eds.), *Supporting students with special health care needs: Guidelines and procedures for schools* (3rd ed., pp. 291–311). Paul H. Brookes Publishing Co.

Health Resources and Services Administration. (2022). *Children and youth with special health care needs*. National Survey on Children's Health Data Brief. Maternal and Child Health Bureau. https://mchb.hrsa.gov/sites/default/files/mchb/programs-impact/nsch-data-brief-children-youth-special-health-care-needs.pdf

Individuals With Disabilities Education Improvement Act of 2004 (Pub. L. 108-446). https://www.gpo.gov/fdsys/pkg/PLAW-108publ446/content-detail.html

Jones, S. (2022). *Clinical guidelines: Tracheostomy management*. The Royal Children's Hospital of Melbourne. https://www.rch.org.au/rchcpg/hospital_clinical_guideline_index/Tracheostomy_management/

Kirkland-Kyhn, H., Martin, S., Zaratkiewicz, S., Whitmore, M., & Young, H. (2018). Ostomy care at home. *American Journal of Nursing, 118*(4), 63–68. https://doi.org/10.1097/01.NAJ.0000532079.49501.ce

Liu, J., Bi, Y., Liu, Y., Tang, L., & Wang, A. (2022). Value of sufficient clean intermittent catheterization in urinary tract infection and upper urinary tract protection in children with neurogenic bladder. *Journal of Pediatric Urology, 18*(4), 499.e1–499.e6. https://doi.org/10.1016/j.jpurol.2022.04.011

McCarthy, C. J., Behravesh, S., Naidu, S. G., & Oklu, R. (2016). Air embolism: Practical tips for prevention and treatment. *Journal of Clinical Medicine, 5*(11), 93. http://doi.org/10.3390/jcm5110093

National Academy for State Health Policy. (2020). *National care coordination standards for children and youth with special health care needs*. https://eadn-wc03-8290287.nxedge.io/wp-content/uploads/2022/12/care-coordination-report-v5.pdf

National Association of School Nurses. (2020a). Framework for 21st Century School Nursing Practice—Clarifications and updated definitions. *NASN School Nurse, 35*(4), 225–233. https://doi.org/10.1177/1942602X20928372

National Association of School Nurses. (2020b). *Use of individualized healthcare plans to support school health services* [Position Statement]. Author. https://www.nasn.org/nasn-resources/professional-practice-documents/position-statements/ps-ihps

National Association of School Nurses. (2021). *A model for school nurse-led case management*. Author. https://learn.nasn.org/courses/33713/documents/48822

National Association of School Nurses. (2022). *School Nursing: Scope and Standards of Practice* (4th ed.). Author.

National Association of School Nurses. (2023). *IDEIA and Section 504 teams—The school nurse as an essential team member* [Position Statement]. Author. https://www.nasn.org/nasn-resources/professional-practice-documents/position-statements/ps-ideia

National Association of School Nurses. (2024a). A contemporary framework update for today's school nursing landscape: Introducing the School Nursing Practice Framework. *NASN School Nurse, 39*(3), 140–147. https://www.doi.org/10.1177/1942602X241241092

National Association of School Nurses. (2024b). School Nursing Practice Framework [Infographic]. https://higherlogicdownload.s3.amazonaws.com/NASN/8575d1b7-94ad-45ab-808e-d45019cc5c08/UploadedImages/PDFs/frameworkhorizontal_FINAL_4_3_24_V2.pdf

National Council of State Boards of Nursing & American Nurses Association. (2019). *National guidelines for nursing delegation*. https://www.ncsbn.org/NGND-PosPaper_06.pdf

National Highway Traffic Safety Administration. (n.d.). *School bus driver in-service safety series*. https://one.nhtsa.gov/people/injury/buses/UpdatedWeb/index.html

Nemours KidsHealth. (2021). *Ventricular assist device*. https://kidshealth.org/en/parents/vad.html

Newman, D. K. (2021). Intermittent self-catheterization patient education checklist. *Urologic Nursing, 41*(2), 97–109. https://doi.org/10.7257/1053-816X.2021.41.2.97

Noah, Z. L., & Budek, C. E. (2016). Chronic respiratory insufficiency. In R. M. Kliegman, B. F. Stanton, J. W. St. Geme, N. F. Schor, & R. E. Berhman (Eds.), *Nelson textbook of pediatrics* (20th ed., pp. 2146–2155e). Elsevier.

O'Neil, J., & Hoffman, B. D. (2018). School bus transportation of children with special health care needs. *Pediatrics, 141*(5), 1–7. https://doi.org/10.1542/peds.2018-0513

Osland, E. J., Andersen, S., Coleman, E., & Marshall, B. (2021). Revisiting the evidence for the reuse of enteral feeding equipment in ambulatory patients: A systematic review. *Nutrition in Clinical Practice: Official Publication of the American Society for Parenteral and Enteral Nutrition, 36*(1), 169–186. https://doi.org/10.1002/ncp.10574

Perkins, J. M., & Paul, F. (2014). Tube feeding. In S. M. Porter, P. A. Branowicki, & J. S. Palfrey (Eds.), *Supporting students with special health care needs: Guidelines and procedures for schools* (3rd ed., pp. 211–247). Paul H. Brookes Publishing Co.

Perlman, L., & Rosen, D. (2014). Respiratory care. In S. M. Porter, P. A. Branowicki, & J. S. Palfrey (Eds.), *Supporting students with special health care needs: Guidelines and procedures for schools* (3rd ed. pp. 2313–2385). Paul H. Brookes Publishing Co.

Rehabilitation Act of 1973 (Pub. L. 93-112). https://www.gpo.gov/fdsys/pkg/STATUTE-107/pdf/STATUTE-107-Pg718.pdf

Sarnaik, A. P., Clark, J. A., & Sanaik, A. A. (2016). Respiratory distress and failure. In R. M. Kliegman, B. F. Stanton, J. W. St Geme, N. F. Schor, & R. E. Berhman (Eds.), *Nelson textbook of pediatrics* (20th ed., pp. 528–545.e1). Elsevier.

Schroeder, M., Baker, A. L., Bastardi, H., & O'Brien, P. (2022). The child with cardiovascular dysfunction. In M. J. Hockenberry, D. Wilson, & C. C. Rodgers (Eds.), *Wong's essentials of pediatric nursing* (11th ed., pp. 733–782). Mosby Elsevier.

Seattle Children's Hospital Heart Center. (2017). *Event monitor*. www.seattlechildrens.org/clinics-programs/heart/what-to-expect/event-monitor

Shannon, R. A., & Kubelka, S. (2013a). Reducing the risks of delegation: Use of procedure skills checklists for unlicensed assistive personnel in schools, part 2. *NASN School Nurse, 28*(5), 222–226. https://doi.org/10.1177/1942602X13490030

Shannon, R. A., & Kubelka, S. (2013b). Reducing the risks of delegation: Use of procedure skills checklists for unlicensed assistive personnel in schools, part 1. *NASN School Nurse, 28*(4), 178–181. https://doi.org/10.1177/1942602X13489886

Shannon, R. A., & Minchella, L. (2015). Students requiring personal nursing care in school: Nursing care models and a checklist for school nurses. *NASN School Nurse, 30*(2), 76–80. https://doi.org/10.1177/1942602X15569781

Simpser, E., & Hudak, M. L. (2017). Financing of pediatric home health care. *Pediatrics, 139*(3), 1–6. https://doi.org/10.1542/peds.2016-4202

Sterni, L. M., Collaco, J. M., Baker, C., Carroll, J. L., Sharma, G. D., Brozek, J. L., Finder, J. D., Ackerman, V. L., Arens, R., Boroughs, D. S., Carter, J., Daigle, K. L., Dougherty, J., Gozal, D., Kevill, K., Kravitz, R. M., Kriseman, T., MacLusky, I., Rivera-Spoljaric, K., & Halbower, A. (2016). An official American Thoracic Society clinical practice guideline: Pediatric chronic home invasive ventilation. *American Journal of Respiratory and Critical Care Medicine, 193*(8), e16–e35.

Teshale, S., Fox-Grange, W., & Purington, K. (2021). *Paying family caregivers through Medicaid consumer-directed programs: State opportunities and innovations.* The National Academy for State Health Policy. https://www.nashp.org/wp-content/uploads/2021/04/paying-family-caregivers-April2021.pdf

Tobias, N. (2017). Practical considerations and current best practice for pediatric clean intermittent catheterization. *Continuing Nursing Education, 43*(6).

U.S. Department of Education, Office for Civil Rights. (2016). *Parent and educator resource guide to Section 504 in public elementary and secondary schools.* https://www2.ed.gov/about/offices/list/ocr/docs/504-resource-guide-201612.pdf

Ward, E., & Ward, M. (2014). Creating a positive school experience: Perspectives from the team. In S. M. Porter, P. A. Branowicki, & J. S. Palfrey (Eds.), *Supporting students with special health care needs: Guidelines and procedures for schools* (3rd ed., pp. 17–36). Paul H. Brookes Publishing Co.

part VI

Caring for Students With Neurological, Behavioral, and Mental Health Conditions

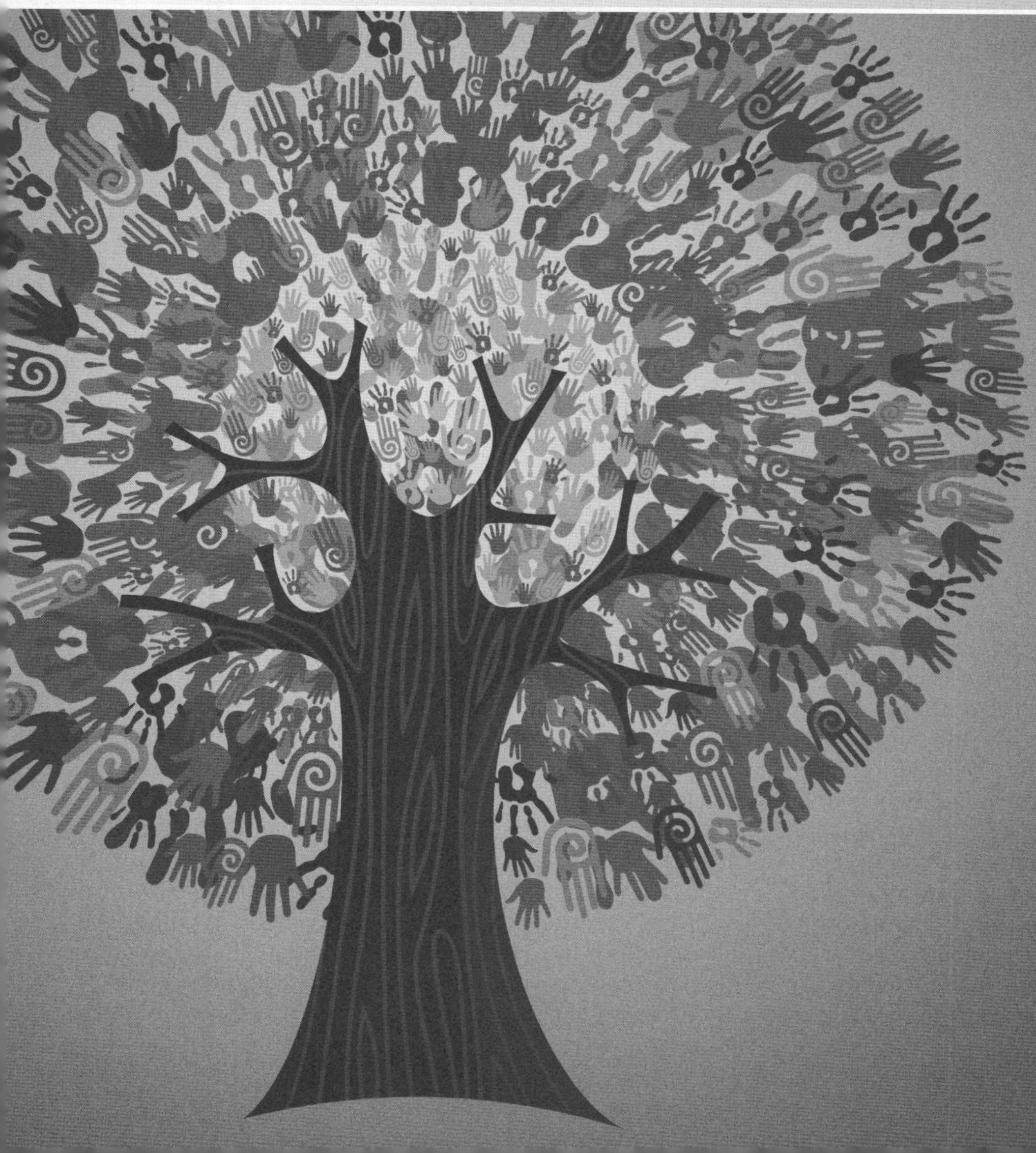

Chapter **26**

Students With Neurodevelopmental Disorders

Tracy J. Perron ▪ Diane Gillooly ▪ Kruti Acharya ▪ Robin Adair Shannon

CHAPTER OUTLINE

ATTENTION DEFICIT-HYPERACTIVITY DISORDER
- Diagnosis
- Causative Factors
- Comorbidities
- Treatment and Medications
- Alternative Therapies

LEARNING DISORDERS
- Specific Learning Disorders
- Diagnostic Process
- Interventions

AUTISM SPECTRUM DISORDER
- Causative Factors
- Clinical Presentation
- Screening and Diagnosis
- Associated Findings
- Interventions
- Considerations for School Nurses

INTELLECTUAL DEVELOPMENTAL DISORDERS
- Causative Factors
- Diagnostic Criteria
- Evaluation

FETAL ALCOHOL SPECTRUM DISORDER

GENETIC/CHROMOSOMAL ALTERATIONS
- Down Syndrome
- Fragile X Syndrome
- Klinefelter Syndrome
- Turner Syndrome
- Phenylketonuria

SPECIAL ISSUES
- Comorbidity/Dual Diagnosis
- Physical Activity
- Sexuality
- Victimization
- Ethical Issues
- School Nurse Care Coordination

CONCLUSION

REFERENCES

Federal laws enacted since the 1960s and 1970s, such as *Rehabilitation Act of 1973* and the *Individuals With Disabilities Education Improvement Act [IDEA]* (2004), led the way to the provision of more community and school-based services and support for persons with disabilities (Conrad, 2020). Society still struggles to provide full inclusion for persons with disabilities, including neurodevelopmental disabilities, into the community and school settings.

The *Diagnostic and Statistical Manual of Mental Disorders, Fifth Edition, Text Revision* (DSM-5-TR) characterizes conditions that result in neurodevelopmental disorders usually appearing before children enter elementary school (American Psychiatric Association [APA], 2022). Neurodevelopment disorders represent atypical brain processes that result in functional impairments in a student's social, academic, and occupational dimensions along a continuum from mild to severe. These conditions have long-term developmental implications and service needs. Among the conditions that the DSM-5-TR (APA, 2022) includes under neurodevelopmental disorders are intellectual developmental disorder (intellectual disability), specific learning disorders, autism spectrum disorder, attention deficit-hyperactivity disorder, communication disorders, and neurodevelopmental motor disorders. Also discussed in this chapter are common genetic or chromosomal disorders associated with atypical brain development. Many of these conditions may co-occur and are associated with a spectrum of comorbidities, such as musculoskeletal disorders, palsies, seizure syndromes, visual impairments, hearing impairments, and multiple congenital anomalies (McGuire et al., 2019).

Most students with neurodevelopmental disorders qualify for special education services under IDEA and have an individualized education program (IEP). The interdisciplinary support team provides comprehensive services based on the student's unique needs. The school nurse is an integral member on this team who monitors the student's health status, administers medications and special procedures as ordered, and serves as a liaison between the student's family, educational staff, and healthcare providers. The school nurse develops an individual healthcare plan for students with neurodevelopmental disorders who have special healthcare needs and ensures that school health services are reflected in the IEP. IDEA also stipulates that students with disabilities be offered transition planning at an appropriate secondary school age to prepare them for education and employment opportunities in adulthood. Depending on their individual needs, students with neurodevelopmental disabilities may qualify to receive a free and appropriate public education through the age of 21 (U.S. Office of Special Education and Rehabilitative Services, 2020).

Some students with neurodevelopmental disorders can achieve academically in the general curriculum and do not need an IEP. These students are protected against discrimination at school secondary to dependence on medical technology under the *Rehabilitation Act of 1973* and qualify for a Section 504 plan. See Chapter 7 for more information about laws protecting students with disabilities. See Chapter 8 for more information about developing health and educational plans for students with special healthcare needs. Chapter 20 discusses in depth supporting students with special healthcare needs.

Evidence-based school nursing services should always be delivered with sensitivity to the student's and family's cultural context, preferences, and priorities. The purpose of this chapter is to provide school nurses with an overview of prevalent neurodevelopmental disorders in students and the supports they need to learn and thrive at school.

ATTENTION DEFICIT-HYPERACTIVITY DISORDER

A significant number of school-age children have attention deficit-hyperactivity disorder (ADHD), which can influence their development and academic achievement (APA, 2022). School nurses interact with and care for students with ADHD both directly and indirectly. School nurses administer medications as ordered, assess for other health or emotional concerns, consult with and educate teaching staff, develop IEPs or Section 504 plans, and advocate for the needs of the student and family.

In children diagnosed with ADHD early, symptoms typically persist through the elementary and high school years and often into adulthood. Approximately 9.8% of individuals identified as having ADHD between the years 2016 and 2019 were between 3 and 17 years of age (Bitsko et al., 2022). Boys (13%) are more likely to be diagnosed than girls (6%); 62% of children diagnosed with ADHD take ADHD medications. Although ADHD is seen in all cultural groups, it is more commonly diagnosed in black non-Hispanic (12%) and white non-Hispanic children (10%), followed by Hispanic children (8%) and Asian non-Hispanic children (3%) (Bitsko et al., 2022).

Diagnosis

ADHD is defined as follows:

> *ADHD is a neurodevelopmental disorder defined by impairing levels of inattention, disorganization, and/or hyperactivity-impulsivity. Inattention and disorganization entail inability to stay on task, seeming not to listen, and losing materials necessary for tasks, at levels that are inconsistent with age or developmental level. Hyperactivity-impulsivity entails overactivity, fidgeting, inability to stay seated, intruding into other people's activities, and inability to wait—symptoms that are excessive for age or developmental level. (APA, 2022, Neurodevelopmental Disorders, para. 7)*

The ability to pay attention, have impulse control, and control activity levels is seen in most children and adolescents and matures with age as the student learns to self-regulate. Students with ADHD are distinguished from others because their behaviors impair functioning in academic, social, and/or familial arenas; their actions are often those of a younger age group. Symptoms must be present before 12 years of age and be seen in more than one setting (home, school, work) for a definitive diagnosis (APA, 2022). Students who may appear overactive on a playground but are able to settle down appropriately in the classroom would not fit these criteria. There are three diagnostic categories of ADHD: combined (ADHD-C), predominantly inattentive (ADHD-I), and predominantly hyperactive-impulsive (ADHD-HI). There are nine diagnostic criteria for the inattention category and nine diagnostic criteria for the hyperactivity-impulsivity category. See Box 26-1. The school setting is where most referrals for formal evaluation take place because symptoms frequently worsen in situations that require sustained attention.

The diagnosis for most students with ADHD is based on difficulties experienced in a structured school setting (Belanger et al., 2018). The educational evaluation of ADHD at school requires an interdisciplinary approach, including educational testing by a school psychologist. A thorough history of symptoms and behaviors is necessary to identify how the student's functioning is affected. The school nurse gathers a complete health history, including a prenatal history, and family medical and educational history (Belanger et al., 2018). Information about the home environment and living arrangements can be gathered in

BOX 26-1

Diagnostic Criteria for ADHD

A. A persistent pattern of inattention and/or hyperactivity-impulsivity that interferes with functioning or development, as characterized by (1) and/or (2):

1. Inattention: Six (or more) of the following symptoms have persisted for at least 6 months to a degree that is inconsistent with developmental level and that negatively impacts directly on social and academic/occupational activities.
   NOTE: The symptoms are not solely a manifestation of oppositional behavior, defiance, hostility, or failure to understand tasks or instructions. For older adolescents and adults (age 17 and older), at least five symptoms are required.
   a. Often fails to give close attention to details or makes careless mistakes in schoolwork, at work, or during other activities (e.g., overlooks or misses details, work is inaccurate).
   b. Often has difficulty sustaining attention in tasks or play activities (e.g., has difficulty remaining focused during lectures, conversations, or lengthy reading).
   c. Often does not seem to listen when spoken to directly (e.g., mind seems elsewhere, even in the absence of any obvious distraction).
   d. Often does not follow through on instructions and fails to finish schoolwork chores, or duties in the workplace (e.g., starts tasks but quickly loses focus and is easily sidetracked).
   e. Often has difficulty organizing tasks and activities (e.g., difficulty managing sequential tasks; difficulty keeping materials and belongings in order; messy, disorganized work; has poor time management; fails to meet deadlines).
   f. Often avoids, dislikes, or is reluctant to engage in tasks that require sustained mental effort (e.g., schoolwork or homework; for older adolescents and adults, preparing reports, completing forms, reviewing lengthy papers).
   g. Often loses things necessary for tasks or activities (e.g., school materials, pencils, books, tools, wallets, keys, paperwork, eyeglasses, mobile telephones).
   h. Is often easily distracted by extraneous stimuli (for older adolescents and adults, may include unrelated thoughts).
   i. Is often forgetful in daily activities (e.g., doing chores, running errands; for older adolescents and adults, returning calls, paying bills, keeping appointments).
2. Hyperactivity and impulsivity: Six (or more) of the following symptoms have persisted for at least 6 months to a degree that is inconsistent with developmental level and that negatively impacts directly on social and academic/occupational activities:
   NOTE: The symptoms are not solely a manifestation of oppositional behavior, defiance, hostility, or a failure to understand tasks or instructions. For older adolescents and adults (age 17 and older), at least five symptoms are required.
   a. Often fidgets with or taps hands or feet or squirms in seat.
   b. Often leaves seat in situations when remaining seated is expected (e.g., leaves his or her place in the classroom, in the office or other workplace, or in other situations that require remaining in place).
   c. Often runs about or climbs excessively in situations where it is inappropriate (NOTE: In adolescents or adults, may be limited to feeling restless).
   d. Often unable to play or engage in leisure activities quietly.
   e. Is often "on the go" acting as if "driven by a motor" (e.g., is unable to be or uncomfortable being still for extended time, as in restaurants, meetings; may be experienced by others as being restless or difficult to keep up with).
   f. Often talks excessively.
   g. Often blurts out an answer before a question has been completed (e.g., completes people's sentences; cannot wait for turn in conversation).
   h. Often has difficulty waiting his or her turn (e.g., while waiting in line).
   i. Often interrupts or intrudes on others (e.g., butts into conversations, games or activities; may start using other people's things without asking or receiving permission; for adolescents and adults, may intrude into or take over what others are doing).

B. Several inattentive or hyperactive-impulsive symptoms were present before age 12 years.

C. Several inattentive or hyperactive-impulsive symptoms are present in two or more settings (e.g., at home, school, or work; with friends or relatives; in other activities).

D. There is clear evidence that the symptoms interfere with, or reduce the quality of, social, academic, or occupational functioning.

E. The symptoms do not occur exclusively during the course of schizophrenia or another psychotic disorder and are not better explained by another mental disorder (e.g., mood disorder, anxiety disorder, dissociative disorder, personality disorder, substance intoxication or withdrawal).

Specify whether:

(F90.2) **Combined presentation:** If both Criterion A1 (inattention) and Criterion A2 (hyperactivity-impulsivity) are met for the past 6 months

(F90.0) **Predominantly inattentive presentation:** If Criterion A1 (inattention) is met but Criterion A2 (hyperactivity-impulsivity) is not met for the past 6 months

BOX 26-1

Diagnostic Criteria for ADHD—cont'd

(F90.1) **Predominantly hyperactive/impulsive presentation:** If Criterion A2 (hyperactivity-impulsivity) is met and Criterion A1 (inattention) is not met for the past 6 months

Specify if:

In partial remission: When full criteria were previously met, fewer than the full criteria have been met for the past 6 months, and the symptoms still result in impairment in social, academic, or occupational functioning.

Specify current severity:

Mild: Few, if any, symptoms in excess of those required to make the diagnosis are present, and symptoms result in no more than minor impairments in social or occupational functioning.

Moderate: Symptoms or functional impairment between "mild" and "severe" are present.

Severe: Many symptoms in excess of those required to make the diagnosis, or several symptoms that are particularly severe, are present, or the symptoms result in marked impairment in social or occupational functioning.

cooperation with the school social worker. A developmental history is essential, and a thorough health assessment can help identify other possible causes of behaviors that mimic ADHD symptoms such as sleep deprivation, adverse childhood experiences, anxiety, or other chronic conditions. With a scientific knowledge base related to normal growth and development, school nurses are an asset in the behavioral assessment of students through objective assessment of the student's behavior on more than one occasion in different social and learning environments at school.

Diagnostic assessments should be gathered using both structured and unstructured formats and in more than one setting. A number of parent/caregiver, teacher, and self-report rating scales are available to both measure and monitor signs and symptoms of ADHD (Table 26-1). Structured interviews can assist with diagnosis. Most assessments measure symptom frequency and the impact on the student's academic and social/emotional success compared with same-age neurodevelopmentally typical peers. Input from parents/guardians, teachers, the school nurse, and other support staff (e.g., the school counselor, social worker, and behavior specialists) is essential to the diagnostic process. The school nurse should screen for vision and hearing acuity and pay particular attention to those students with frequent health office visits, high accident rates, high impulsivity in unsafe situations, a history of insufficient sleep, and persistent discipline problems. Educational diagnosis of ADHD should be confirmed by a qualified doctor or healthcare provider (e.g., pediatrician, pediatric neurologist, psychiatrist, psychologist, nurse practitioner).

Causative Factors

Although there are no definitive causes of ADHD, there are multiple genetic, neuroanatomical, and neurobiological theories of etiology. There is a high prevalence of ADHD in parents/guardians and other relatives of students with ADHD, strongly implying a genetic basis for the disorder. Despite evidence linking several genes to ADHD, research establishing causality is inconsistent. Some studies have reported the important role of certain environmental

TABLE 26-1 Selected Behavior Rating Scales for Screening for ADHD and Monitoring the Efficacy of Treatment

Behavior Rating Scale Most Have Parent and Teacher Rating Scale Versions; Some Also Have Self-Assessments.	Validity Established in Ages (Years)
Achenbach Child Behavior Check List (Achenbach & Rescorla, 2001)	6–18
ADD–Hyperactivity Comprehensive Teacher Rating Scale, 2nd ed. (ACTeRs). (Ullmann et al., 2000)	5–14
ADHD Rating Scale–5 (DuPaul et al., 2016)	6–18
Behavior Assessment System for Children, 3rd ed. (BASC-3). (Reynolds & Kamphaus, 2015)	4–18
Conners 3 Parent and Teacher Rating Scales (Conners, 2008)	6–18
SNAP-IV Rating Scale–Revised (Bussing et al., 2008)	6–18
NIHQ Vanderbilt ADHD Diagnostic Scales (American Academy of Pediatrics & National Institute for Children's Healthcare Quality, 2002)	6–12

factors on the onset of developmental disorders including ADHD (Brikell et al., 2019). ADHD has also been associated with maternal factors that affect fetal development, such as smoking, maternal age at delivery, psychosocial stress, depression, and other mental health conditions (Chan & Mo, 2022; Zheng et al., 2020).

Comorbidities

Many students with ADHD may exhibit comorbid psychiatric disorders that can complicate both diagnosis and treatment (Radmanović & Burgić, 2021). Comorbidity of specific learning disorders (SLDs), conduct disorder (CD), oppositional defiant disorder (ODD), tic disorders, alcohol exposure in utero, and autism spectrum disorder have been frequently observed in students with ADHD (APA, 2022; Visser et al., 2020). Approximately 36.8% of students with ADHD have one coexisting condition, 26.8% have two, and 19.3% have three or more (Deavenport-Saman et al., 2022). Depression occurs in 20% to 30% of individuals with ADHD, and anxiety in more than 25% of individuals with ADHD (Mattingly et al., 2021).

Students with ADHD have a higher incidence of conduct disorders in adolescence and antisocial personality disorder in adulthood than the general pediatric population (Visser et al., 2020). Some children with ADHD are especially distracted by sensory sensitivities, such as being bothered by certain fabrics against their skin or the tags in the back of shirts. These can cause the student to focus only on these sensations rather than on what is going on in the classroom. If the nurse is astute to this possibility, a note home to the parents/guardians may resolve this bothersome stimulus. Parents/guardians report that turning shirts inside out is helpful, as is avoiding certain fabrics that have contact with the skin. It is important to keep in mind that students with autism spectrum disorder can also exhibit sensory sensitivities and hyperactive or inattentive behaviors that might potentially be misdiagnosed as ADHD (APA, 2022).

Treatment and Medications

Treatments for ADHD include medication, behavioral interventions, or a combination of the two (multimodal). According to the National Institute of Mental Health (NIMH; 2021), both pharmacological and behavioral/instructional interventions are effective to increase sustained attention, decrease disruptive behaviors, and increase academic outcomes among students diagnosed with ADHD. Generally, behavioral interventions (nonpharmacological) should be tried first, many of which are similar to those for individuals with specific learning disabilities. However, students with severe ADHD should be treated with medication in addition to other behavioral therapies (NIMH, 2021).

Pharmacological Interventions

Treatment should be determined based on the severity of the symptoms and the degree to which they interfere with the activities of daily living, including learning. ADHD medications help to reduce overactivity and improve self-regulation and attention, thereby improving academic outcomes.

A wide variety of medications with documented efficacy in treating students with ADHD currently exist. Stimulants, specifically extended release long acting, are the first-line drugs to treat students with ADHD without other comorbid diagnoses (Leahy, 2018). Stimulants have a paradoxical calming effect for individuals with ADHD by inhibiting the action of the dopamine transporter protein at the synapse, resulting in a decrease in hyperactivity and impulsivity and improved attention and focus (NIMH, 2022). Stimulants assist students to block out extraneous stimuli, thus making them more receptive to learning. Simply stated, this class of medications assist with *thinking and attention*, resulting in increased school-based productivity.

Over 30 medications are approved in the United States for the treatment of ADHD, most of which are stimulants that provide various means of delivery and duration of effects (Mattingly et al., 2021). See Table 26-2 for commonly prescribed ADHD psychostimulant medications. These medications are mainly recommended for students over 6 years of age; however, there is an increasing trend to begin stimulant therapy with preschool children (Leahy, 2018). Studies have shown that preschool children ages 3 to 5.5 years treated with methylphenidate had a significant improvement in ADHD symptoms compared with older students. However, preschool children had more significant side effects, such as irritability and fatigue, than did school-age children (Leahy, 2018). Therefore lower doses and close monitoring and follow-up of students are recommended (Mattingly et al., 2021). Students of all ages may respond differently to different stimulants. If a student does not respond to one stimulant medication, others should be prescribed. Often a second stimulant that includes both a methylphenidate and amphetamine may be prescribed. These trials should be explored before prescribing other classifications of medications (Leahy, 2018).

Stimulants begin having an effect within 20 to 30 minutes and can be administered in a variety of ways. Short-acting, intermediate-acting, and long-acting preparations are available and are equally efficacious (Cleveland Clinic, 2023). Short-acting medications usually require several daily doses; thus students usually need to come to the school nurse's office for a midday dose. Because of the short half-life of the short-acting stimulants, some students experience rebound effects or an increase in negative behaviors when the medication is wearing off (Leahy, 2018). If this is the case, it is recommended that the school nurse notify the parent/guardian and primary care provider so that the medication might be changed to a long-acting preparation, or the student may be ordered to take a second dose 1 hour before the rebound occurs.

The current standard of care is treatment with longer acting, sustained-release preparations that only require a morning dose; this provides more consistent coverage both

TABLE 26-2 **Psychostimulants Used for ADHD**

Drug	Formulation	Duration (hours)	Notes
Methylphenidate			
Ritalin or generic	Short-acting, immediate-release tablets	3–4	Abrupt onset and offset increase the number and severity of side effects.
Ritalin LA or generic	Extended-release capsule	3–4	Abrupt onset and offset increase the number and severity of side effects.
Methylin (liquid or generic)	Oral solution	3–4	Colorless, grape-flavored liquid; store at room temperature.
Methylphenidate HCl (Lupin)	Chewable tablet	3–4	Grape-flavored chewable tablet
Methylphenidate HCl	Extended-release tablets	6–8	Swallow whole; do *not* crush or chew.
Aptensio XR or generic	Extended release tablets	12	Capsule maybe opened and contents swallowed completely with applesauce.
Concerta or generic	Extended-release tablets	12	Must be swallowed whole; nonabsorbable shell may be passed in the stool.
Cotempla XRODT	Extended-release orally disintegrating tablet	12–13	Grape flavored; allow to dissolve in saliva.
Quillichew	Extended-release chewable tablet	8	Cherry flavored; may be taken with or without food.
Quillivant XR	Extended-release oral suspension	12	Fruit flavored; may be taken with or without food. Shake bottle for at least 10 seconds. May be stored at room temperature.
Jornay PM	Delayed-release extended-release capsule	12–14	Taken before sleep to provide early morning onset.
Daytrana—patch or generic	Transdermal patch	9	The time worn can be varied to control the duration of effects; monitor for skin rash or sensitivity. Discard patches appropriately.
Dexmethylphenidate			
Dexmethylphenidate HCl ER	Extended-release capsule	13	Capsule can be taken with or without food. Capsule may be opened and sprinkled into applesauce.
Focalin or generic	Short-acting immediate-release tablet	4–6	
Focalin XR or generic	Extended-release capsule	8–12	Capsule may be opened and beads swallowed completely in applesauce.
Serdexmethylphenidate and Dexmethylphenidate			
Azstarys	Once-daily capsule	13	Capsule can be taken with or without food. Capsule may be opened and sprinkled onto applesauce.
Dextroamphetamine			
Dexedrine or generic	Short-acting tablet	3–4	Take first dose upon awakening.
ProCentra or generic	Oral solution	3–6	Bubblegum flavored; may be taken with or without food. Shake bottle before preparing the dose. May be stored at room temperature.
Dexedrine ER or generic	Extended-release spansule	5–10	
Xelstrym	Transdermal patch	9	Patch may be applied to the upper arm, upper back, hip, chest, or flank area 2 hours before the effects of the medication are needed. Do not use more than one patch in a 24-hour period.
Zenzedi or generic	Immediate-release tablet	4–6	Take first dose upon awakening.

Continued

TABLE 26-2 **Psychostimulants Used for ADHD—cont'd**

Drug	Formulation	Duration (hours)	Notes
Mixed Amphetamine Salts and Dextroamphetamine			
Adderall or generic	Short-acting immediate-release tablets	4–6	May be taken with or without food.
Adderall XR or generic	Extended-release tablet	10–12	Capsule may be opened and beads swallowed with applesauce.
Dextroamphetamine/ amphetamine	Immediate-release tablet	5–8	
Dextroamphetamine/ amphetamine	Extended-release capsule	10–12	May open ER capsule but do not crush or chew.
Mydayis	Long-acting capsule	14–16	Capsules may be opened and beads swallowed whole with applesauce.
Amphetamine Sulfate			
Evekeo or generic	Immediate-release tablet	4–6	
Lisdexamfetamine			
Vyvanse	Long-acting capsule	10–13	Capsule may be opened and contents dissolved in water, yogurt, orange juice; use immediately after dissolving.
Vyvanse	Chewable tablet	10–13	Strawberry flavored; may be taken with or without food.
Amphetamine			
Desoxyn	2.5, 5	8–10	Not a first-line treatment
Lisdexamfetamine/Vyvanse (prodrug)	20, 30, 50, 60, 70	10–12	

*Capsules can be opened and sprinkled on food; do not chew the sprinkles.

Dupar & Dodson (2019).

during school hours and during after-school activities. Some students may need a short-acting dose in the early evening (Leahy, 2018). The capsules for some stimulants (e.g., Adderall) can be opened and sprinkled on food for students who are unable to swallow pills; granules should not be chewed because this destroys the long-acting function of the medication. If a student cannot swallow pills and has a difficult time with the granules, there are oral suspensions and disintegrating tablets available (e.g., ProCentra, QuilliChew, Cotempla).

A transdermal patch for methylphenidate (e.g., Daytrana) is also available. The patch is applied once daily in the morning, preferably 1 to 2 hours before school starts, and removed after 9 hours. The medication continues to work for another 3 hours after the patch is removed (Leahy, 2018). It is important to remove the patch in adequate time so that the child will be able to sleep at night. It is not uncommon for a mild erythema or pruritus, or both, to occur at the site because of a reaction to the adhesive. To minimize skin irritation, parents/guardians need to be reminded to alternate the hip on which the patch is applied daily and to apply the patch to different areas of the hip each day. Adhesive removers, oils, and lotions may be helpful to loosen the adhesive when removing the patch. Parents/guardians should not apply lotions or ointments before application of the patch because they may prevent the patch from adhering to the child's skin. If a child has an allergic reaction to the adhesive (significant redness or swelling that does not subside within a couple of hours after removal), the primary care provider should be notified (Leahy, 2018).

Another category of stimulants is *prodrug*. These medications are in their inactive form and become active once metabolized by the body. Lisdexamfetamine dimesylate (Vyvanse) is an example of a prodrug (Cleveland Clinic, 2023). It is suggested that Vyvanse may reduce the abuse of stimulants by students who do not have ADHD because it does not cause an immediate reaction.

Practice Connection

The school nurse should contact the parent/guardian when a student does not take their medication before school. Several doses can be kept at school with the accompanying healthcare provider's order to give as needed. The school nurse can write this accommodation into the student's individualized healthcare plan.

The dosage of stimulant medications is not usually related to body weight, as it is for most other medications; however, on initial induction, weight is used as a cursory starting point (Leahy, 2018). The recommended premise for dosage is to start with a low dose and to slowly titrate upward at intervals of approximately 1 week until the desired effects are achieved, the maximum dose is reached, or unacceptable side effects occur. The goal is to maximize the desired effect while at the same time minimizing the adverse effects of these medications.

Parents/guardians can be advised to make medication or dose changes on a Saturday, so they can observe the effects on their child over the weekend. Then school personnel can evaluate the student on Wednesday or Thursday so that the prescribing healthcare provider can be contacted on Friday to change the dosage by Saturday. The effectiveness of stimulants is measured by behavioral changes (e.g., decreased motor activity and increased attention span and concentration), as well as the onset of any new or increased side effects. Teacher input is essential in evaluating the effectiveness of this treatment. Teachers should be encouraged to notice the time of day when the medication effectiveness changes. The teacher's evaluation should be communicated to the parents/guardians by the school nurse along with the nurse's own observation. The parents/guardians can then notify the healthcare provider so that the appropriate dosage, time, and frequency of medication can be maintained or adjusted. The school nurse's role as a liaison between school and home is an integral part of successful pharmacological management of students with ADHD.

Adverse Effects

The most common negative side effects from stimulant medications include anorexia/appetite suppression, abdominal pain, headaches, and insomnia (American Academy of Child & Adolescent Psychiatry, 2020; American Academy of Pediatrics [AAP], 2019; Leahy, 2018). Others include gastrointestinal symptoms, growth delay, dizziness, irritability, and increased heart rate and blood pressure. All of these have implications for the school nurse when the student comes to the health office with one of these complaints. Insomnia can be especially troublesome because the behaviors associated with insomnia are similar to and exacerbate the behaviors associated with ADHD. If insomnia is a problem, dosing earlier in the day or using short-acting stimulants to avoid sleep problems may be helpful. If the insomnia continues, low doses of clonidine or melatonin may be helpful (Mehta et al., 2019). Students taking stimulant medication should be monitored for adverse effects at least monthly by their healthcare provider during the initiation of treatment; the school nurse will often see the student more frequently (Mehta et al., 2019).

If anorexia, nausea, or stomachache are problems, it may be helpful for students to take their medication with or just after meals, especially when combined with increased protein intake. it is essential to ensure that the student is getting enough quality calories to support growth if anorexia leads to weight loss and growth suppression. These students may need to be observed more closely during lunch because they may be easily distracted from meals and leave the table before they are finished eating, especially in the cafeteria. Supplements such as high-protein shakes or bars can boost caloric intake. The nurse should keep a careful record of the student's height and weight throughout the year. If a change in height or weight of 2 percentiles occurs within 6 months, the student should be referred to their primary care provider (Greenhill et al., 2020). Although stimulant medication may initially slow growth, especially if started at a young age, there are typically no significant differences in height by the time the child reaches adolescence (Leahy, 2018).

Many symptoms are mild and manageable and do not require medication for relief. A short break/rest in the health office or a calming location may help. However, a change in medication may be indicated if symptoms do not resolve within a reasonable amount of time or increase in intensity. Long-acting medications can help to avoid rebound, irritability, and dizziness (Leahy, 2018). If dizziness is a problem, the school nurse should monitor the student's blood pressure on a regular basis.

Contraindications to the use of stimulant medications include hypersensitivity to the drug or its components, structural cardiac defects, moderate-to-severe hypertension, and glaucoma. Students with the following diagnoses should not take stimulants:

- A diagnosed psychotic disorder: Stimulants may increase their symptoms.
- Active, moderate to severe substance abuse
- Hyperthyroidism, liver disease, and those prescribed monoamine oxidase inhibitors
- Tics: A rare side effect of stimulant medications is the development or worsening of tics; there is debate whether individuals with tic disorders should receive stimulants. New neuromuscular tics occur in 0.92% of those taking stimulant medication and usually indicate a need to decrease the dosage or change to a different stimulant (Preston et al., 2021).

A suggested link between stimulant use and cardiac adverse effects, specifically sudden cardiac death in students, has become a concern to healthcare providers prescribing stimulants and atomoxetine. Because these medications affect the sympathetic nervous system, they can cause an increase in heart rate (up to 10 beats per minute) and blood pressure (up to 5 mm Hg) without a change in electrocardiogram (ECG) parameters. A subset of youth with ADHD may have a marked increase in heart rate, especially during the first few months of treatment (Preston et al., 2021). Sudden cardiac death is a rare event in children with ADHD, occurring at rates no higher than those in the general pediatric population, and there is no evidence that having an ECG before starting stimulant therapy would prevent sudden death. Follow-up of many of the initial reports of sudden cardiac death found that most students who experienced a sudden cardiac death had an underlying cardiac anomaly or condition (Liu et al., 2019; Zhang et al., 2022). However, further evaluation before medications are prescribed is warranted for students with a family history of early cardiac arrhythmias or cardiac death or a personal history of cardiac structural abnormalities, including cardiomyopathy, chest pain, arrhythmias, or syncope of unclear origin (AAP, 2019).

Parents/guardians may choose to give their child a medication break. The provider may also suggest a medication break to allow the child's body to grow. Yet there are concerns with this approach. Families should understand that ADHD is still present, and the child may need to continue participating in academic and nonacademic activities that require attention. Standardized testing, and other demanding times at school when concentration is required, may also not be optimal times to pause medication. The education team should be informed if the medications are withheld so that appropriate accommodations are made. Parents/guardians may also worry that stimulant medications may lead to misuse or that children may become dependent. Research shows that this is unlikely if the medication is taken as prescribed (Mattingly et al., 2021).

While there may be many students in a school taking medications to treat ADHD, the school nurse is mindful that these medications are not innocuous and require continued, careful assessment, screening, and monitoring of vital signs and physical and mental health on a regular basis. It is important that the school nurse be included on the 504 or IEP team so that appropriate guidance is provided to the team and accommodations are included in the plan.

Nonstimulant Medications

For students who do not respond to stimulants or are unable to tolerate them even after trying different medications at different doses, it is important to reevaluate the diagnosis for other possible causes of the symptoms. If the provider is confident with the ADHD diagnosis, nonstimulant medications can be effective alternatives that are generally well tolerated and/or can enhance stimulants (Table 26-3).

Nonstimulant medications used to treat ADHD include atomoxetine (Strattera), guanfacine (Intuniv XR), viloxazine (Quelbree), and clonidine (Kapvay XR). The effects of nonstimulant medications may not be felt for several weeks of regular administration (Cleveland Clinic, 2023). These medications are not central nervous system stimulants and are often used in combination with stimulants. Adverse effects of the nonstimulants include gastrointestinal discomfort, especially pain and vomiting, leading to possible weight loss (AAP, 2019).

Clonidine and guanfacine do not improve attention, but they do help with behavioral difficulties, such as comorbid aggressive tendencies and tic disorders. Guanfacine (Tenex) is longer acting and less sedating than clonidine. Clonidine is available in a transdermal patch that lasts for 5 days; however, with the advent of the extended-release dose, transdermal use has been significantly reduced in students (Cutler et al., 2022). Clonidine is an antihypertensive; therefore baseline heart rate and blood pressure readings are recommended, together with periodic monitoring and evaluation of cardiac symptoms such as hypotension, dizziness, bradycardia, tachycardia, and palpitations. Students taking clonidine should not abruptly discontinue the medication. Instead, they should be weaned off the medication over a period of time to minimize negative side effects (Cutler et al., 2022).

Depression, anxiety, and tic disorders are comorbid psychiatric disorders often diagnosed in students with ADHD. Students who experience or display emotional lability, feeling disoriented, impaired awareness, a flat affect, exaggerated hyperactivity, or motor or vocal tics should have their medications or doses reevaluated. Severe mood disturbances have occurred in a very small number of patients. Both stimulant and nonstimulant drugs used to treat ADHD come with black box warnings of possible psychiatric events,

TABLE 26-3 Levels of Prevention in School Nursing

Drug	Formulation	Duration (hours)	Notes
Atomoxetine/Strattera	Long-acting capsule	24	Starts working in a few days to 1 week, but may take several weeks to achieve full effect. Swallow capsule whole.
Intuniv or generic guanfacine	Extended release	24	Swallow tablet whole. A high-fat diet may increase absorption to unhealthy levels.
Wellbutrin XL or generic	Extended release	24	Low efficacy; takes 8 weeks to fully develop benefits.
Qelbree	Extended release	24	Capsules may be swallowed whole or contents opened and the entire contents sprinkled into applesauce.
Clonidine ER Kapvay or generic	Extended release	12	Swallow tablet whole.

Dupar & Dodson (2019).

such as severe depression and suicidal ideation during the first few months of treatment (Preston et al., 2021). This is another reason why close monitoring by the school nurse and healthcare provider is important.

As with all medications, it is the school nurse's responsibility to understand the actions, doses, routes, duration, and effects and side effects of all medications administered to students.

School nurses often express concern when medications are prescribed off-label or are not Food and Drug Administration (FDA) approved for pediatric use. It is appropriate to request clarification from the prescribing provider and consult with the school psychologist, medical advisory committee, and administration and district legal counsel regarding the benefits/risks of off-label or non–FDA-approved medications or therapies, as well as the ethical and legal implications. As in the hospital setting, school nurses should question medication orders if something seems wrong and follow the stipulations of their state's nurse practice act.

Alternative Therapies

Many parents/guardians turn to alternative therapies due to fears and frustrations with the traditional ADHD treatment. Examples of alternate therapies include elimination diets; restrictions of preservatives, sugar, and food coloring; and dietary supplements such as omega-3 fatty acids, vitamins, and minerals. There have been some reports of small to medium effects from elimination diets such as eliminating dairy, gluten, citrus, corn and corn products, and processed foods (Wang et al., 2020). While elimination diets may be effective for a small number of students with ADHD, they require a large commitment by the parents/guardians and family to follow consistently. School nurses should recommend that any dietary restrictions include substitutions for nutrition lost in the diet. Before commencing this type of diet, parents/guardians should be encouraged to discuss their plans with their primary care provider and a registered dietitian.

Research related to fatty acid/omega-3 supplementation shows some benefit for students who have not responded to conventional treatment (Mazahery et al., 2019); however, there is not enough research related to side effects and adverse events. The school nurse should remind parents/guardians that these supplements should be discussed with the primary care provider because of risks for drug interactions, hepatotoxicity, and peripheral neuropathy.

Therapies such as yoga, massage, meditation and mindfulness, outdoor exercise, musical training, acupuncture, and chiropractic interventions have also been suggested to help students with ADHD (Kostova et al., 2019). Though there is little empirical evidence for the efficacy of these therapies, such interventions may be effective as adjunct therapy to help reduce stress (e.g., yoga and massage), assist with focus (e.g., meditation and mindfulness), increase cognitive function (e.g., acupuncture), and increase cognitive, social, and physical benefits (exercise).

School nurses should respect the student's and family's desire to explore alternative therapies to treat or complement treatment for ADHD. They can assist families to make informed decisions about the use of evidence-based interventions. School nurses should adhere to employer policies and their state nurse practice act when considering administration of alternative therapies to students.

LEARNING DISORDERS

There are many neurodevelopmental impairments that can interfere with a student's ability to learn at the same rate or in the same manner as their neurotypical peers. The school nurse needs to be knowledgeable about the manifestations of learning disorders and be an active member of the student support team in helping these students to grow and thrive. For students suspected of having learning disorders, it is essential to first rule out vision and hearing loss through routine screening.

Specific Learning Disorders

Specific learning disorders (SLDs) are persistent impairments (6 months or longer) in acquiring and applying the academic skills of reading (dyslexia), mathematics (dyscalculia), and/or written expression (dysgraphia). SLDs are present despite normal hearing and vision, intellectual abilities, or motor difficulties and adequate learning opportunities (APA, 2021, 2022). The prevalence of SLDs is between 5% and 15% in school-age children and is 2 to 3 times more common in males (APA, 2022), thereby constituting the largest category (34%) of students receiving special education services (National Center for Education Statistics [NCES], 2023). Dyslexia is the predominant form, affecting approximately 80% of students with SLDs.

The manifestations of SLDs vary widely and can be characterized as mild, moderate, or severe (APA, 2022). Unlike the early childhood developmental milestones that children master as the brain matures (CDC. 2022b), students must learn academic skills. SLDs are neurobiological disorders that do not result exclusively from poor teaching/learning environments. Students who have impairments in reading, spelling, written expression, and/or math consequently would be expected to have difficulties learning other subjects (science, history, social studies) that require these skills (APA, 2022).

Students may also commonly display avoidance behaviors, social/emotional stress, somatic complaints, and/or anxiety at school associated with the learning challenges. SLDs are thought to be present in early childhood but are typically diagnosed during the school-age years when the student falls significantly behind academic expectations for their grade level. SLDs typically persist throughout the life span; however, individuals can learn skills to compensate and manage the condition (APA, 2022). Students with learning disorders should receive special education services.

Did You Know?

According to the American Psychiatric Association (2021):

Specific learning disorder is a medical term used for diagnosis. It is often referred to as "learning disorder." "Learning disability" is a term used by both the educational and legal systems. Though learning disability is not exactly synonymous with specific learning disorder, someone with a diagnosis of specific learning disorder can expect to meet criteria for a learning disability and have the legal status of a federally recognized disability to qualify for accommodations and services in school. The term "learning difference" is a term that has gained popularity, especially when speaking with children about their difficulties, as it does not label them as "disordered" (para. 6).

There are no conclusive causes of SLD, but there are associated genetic and environmental risks. The relative risk for SLDs is significantly higher for students who have immediate family members with SLDs (e.g., 4 to 8 times higher for dyslexia; 5 to 10 times higher for dyscalculia) (APA, 2022). Studies have shown associations with neuroanatomical alterations or underactivity in the temporoparietal and occipital regions and overactivity in the frontal lobes, also suggesting dysfunction in cortical connectivity (Mascheretti et al., 2017). A myriad of environmental and perinatal factors are associated with SLDs, including childbirth-associated factors such as dystocia, hypoxia, anoxia, low birth weight, and preterm infants. Maternal tobacco, drug, and alcohol use during pregnancy are risk factors associated with SLDs. Environmental risk factors include low socioeconomic status and exposure to neurotoxins (e.g., air pollution, nicotine, flame retardants, and lead, among others) (APA, 2022).

Types of Specific Learning Disorders

Dyslexia refers to a student's difficulty with reading accuracy, rate or fluency, and comprehension. For these students, reading is slow, inaccurate, and requires great concentration. They may have difficulty recognizing, decoding, and spelling words resulting in challenges in understanding the meaning of what is read (APA, 2021).

Dyscalculia is an alternate term that refers to learning difficulties related to mathematics. It results in problems counting, performing, and understanding mathematical calculations such as measuring objects and space, telling time, counting money and giving change, and performing mental math and mathematical problem-solving (APA, 2021).

Dysgraphia is a commonly used term that refers to impairments in written expression, which may co-occur with dyslexia and/or dyscalculia. Students with dysgraphia may display a discrepancy between understanding and their written and verbal expression. They typically experience difficulties with grammar, spelling, and punctuation (APA, 2021). It is challenging for students with dysgraphia to organize and coherently express their thoughts in writing.

Other Types of Learning Disorders

School nurses may also encounter students diagnosed with ***auditory processing disorder,*** which describes difficulty understanding and processing information obtained through speech (Nemours KidsHealth, 2021). These issues can be especially pronounced in a poor listening environment with lots of ambient and competing sounds. Noisy situations are abundant in schools, such as in classrooms, auditoriums, lunchrooms, hallways, gyms, and playgrounds. Students with auditory processing disorder have normal hearing ability but have difficulty discriminating sounds (e.g., vowels or consonants) and have difficulties recalling information transmitted in an auditory manner. They may experience difficulties with spelling and phonics, understanding verbal directions, or following conversations (Nemours KidsHealth, 2021). They may have more difficulty learning from a lecture-style approach and benefit from seeing demonstrations, reading about the subject, and applying the information.

Diagnostic Process

There is no single test to diagnose SLDs, nor is there a list of specific characteristic behaviors or symptoms that are considered diagnostic for SLD. Generally, students with SLDs achieve below expectations for their grade level, and the learning issues cannot be attributed solely to external factors (e.g., chronic absenteeism, social or economic disadvantages, second-language learners). SLDs can also co-occur in children with other neurodevelopmental disorders that affect learning, such as ADHD and autism spectrum disorder, without other known neurological conditions, cognitive impairments, or intellectual disabilities.

The diagnosis of SLD is a clinical determination based on a synthesis of multiple factors (APA, 2021). A comprehensive assessment of the student must be conducted by the IEP team in all the indicated domains of the *full and individual evaluation* for special education services by qualified professionals as mandated by IDEA (2004). The school nurse is an integral member of the evaluation process with input regarding hearing and vision screening and the domains of normal child development, physical and mental health, and family functioning. See Chapter 8 for more information on the school nurse's role in special education processes.

In 2004, Congress made changes to IDEA (2004) and introduced a strong recommendation for the use of *response to intervention* (RTI) as one of the criteria for the diagnosis of SLD. The main premise of RTI is the use of evidence-based interventions together with measured outcomes to help determine optimal instruction techniques. According to IDEA, RTI *must* be in place *before* a diagnosis of SLD is made to ensure that the child's learning problems are not due to lack of adequate instruction in reading and math. See Chapter 7 for more information on RTI.

Interventions

RTI involves three tiers: Tier 1 is to identify students who are having difficulty or who are at risk for an SLD and provide supplemental interventions in the classroom. If these interventions are unsuccessful, Tier 2 involves a team that plans, implements, and evaluates targeted evidence-based interventions for the child over a 2- to 3-month period. Tier 3 calls for intensive interventions, often involving special education services (IDEA, 2004).

It should be remembered that a student with a high IQ might also have an SLD. Although not often identified because of poor academic performance, they still may demonstrate a significant difference between IQ scores and academic performance. These students deserve services the same as other students with SLDs.

SLDs are an education diagnosis, not a medical diagnosis. There is no medical treatment for SLDs, and medications are *not* usually part of the treatment plan. Each student with an SLD should have an individualized education program (IEP) that addresses their unique learning needs.

Educational interventions in the school setting may include using a multisensory approach, providing frequent cues and extended time for tasks, keeping instructions simple and short, assisting the students in deciding on tasks, providing close supervision, and developing rules for social behavior.

AUTISM SPECTRUM DISORDER

Autism spectrum disorder (ASD) is a neurodevelopmental condition characterized by social and communication challenges and restricted interests or repetitive behaviors (Centers for Disease Control and Prevention [CDC], 2022a). The term *spectrum* refers to the wide range of symptoms and severity that are seen in children with ASD. For example, some children with ASD have language impairment; others have age-appropriate or even advanced language skills. Similarly, some children have cognitive impairment or intellectual disability; others have age-appropriate cognition. Severity is determined by the intensity of supports a child requires to function in daily life (APA, 2022).

In 2000, the prevalence of ASD was estimated to be 1 in 150 children (CDC, 2022a). In 2020, ASD was estimated to affect approximately 1 in 35 children (CDC, 2023a). This increase could be due to a combination of factors such as changes in diagnostic criteria, increased awareness of ASD, and improved ascertainment. ASD prevalence was overall similar across racial and ethnic groups but is four times more common among boys compared with girls (CDC, 2023a).

Causative Factors

There is no single cause of ASD. Based on twin and family studies, there is strong evidence that ASD is highly heritable (i.e., runs in families). Hundreds of genes have been associated with ASD, which may help to explain the wide variety of presentations of the disorder (Lord et al., 2020). ASD causality is most likely multimodal with several causal pathways depending on the individual and the severity of the condition.

There are noncausal associations between environmental factors and ASD. For example, neonatal hypoxia, gestational diabetes, advanced parental age, and preterm birth are associated with an increased risk for ASD (Lord et al., 2020). Conversely, there are environmental factors that have clearly been shown *not* to be associated with an increased risk of ASD such as vaccination and assisted reproductive technology. Specifically, strong research evidence supports that there is no association between ASD and the measles, mumps, and rubella vaccine (DeStefano & Shimabukuro, 2019).

Clinical Presentation

According to DSM-5-TR (APA, 2022), children with ASD have functionally significant impairments in reciprocal social communication and interaction, as well as patterns of restricted and repetitive behaviors, interests, or activities. The symptoms must be present from early childhood and limit or impair everyday functioning. Symptoms may differ markedly in presentation, and severity ranges from mild to severe based on intensity of supports required.

Additionally, the diagnoses should be qualified by the level of support the child needs, whether or not the child has an accompanying intellectual and/or language impairment, and whether an associated genetic, medical, or other neurodevelopmental or mental/behavioral health problem is present (APA, 2022). See Box 26-2.

Intellectual disability affects approximately one-third of individuals with ASD (CDC, 2023a; Hyman et al., 2020). Students with ASD often have corresponding delays in developing self-care skills, such as toileting or dressing. Language development in students with ASD is also quite variable. Some toddlers with ASD meet language milestones on time but have rigid speech patterns; other children have uneven language development with robust vocabularies but limited receptive skills (National Institute on Deafness and Other Communication Disorders, 2020). Some students may be able to verbally express their needs and to make requests or talk about their preferred interest but cannot engage in back and forth conversations. Language delays in early childhood are frequently why families become concerned and seek medical evaluations and support.

BOX 26-2

Diagnostic Criteria for Autism Spectrum Disorder

A. Persistent deficits in social communication and social interaction across multiple contexts, as manifested by all of the following, currently or by history (examples are illustrative, not exhaustive; see text):

1. Deficits in social-emotional reciprocity, ranging, for example, from abnormal social approach and failure of normal back-and-forth conversation; to reduced sharing of interests, emotions, or affect; to failure to initiate or respond to social interactions.
2. Deficits in nonverbal communicative behaviors used for social interaction, ranging, for example, from poorly integrated verbal and nonverbal communication; to abnormalities in eye contact and body language or deficits in understanding and use of gestures; to a total lack of facial expressions and nonverbal communication.
3. Deficits in developing, maintaining, and understanding relationships, ranging, for example, from difficulties adjusting behavior to suit various social contexts; to difficulties in sharing imaginative play or in making friends; to absence of interest in peers.

B. Restricted, repetitive patterns of behavior, interests, or activities, as manifested by at least two of the following, currently or by history (examples are illustrative, not exhaustive; see text):

1. Stereotyped or repetitive motor movements, use of objects, or speech (e.g., simple motor stereotypies, lining up toys or flipping objects, echolalia, idiosyncratic phrases).
2. Insistence on sameness, inflexible adherence to routines, or ritualized patterns of verbal or nonverbal behavior (e.g., extreme distress at small changes, difficulties with transitions, rigid thinking patterns, greeting rituals, need to take same route or eat same food every day).
3. Highly restricted, fixated interests that are abnormal in intensity or focus (e.g., strong attachment to or preoccupation with unusual objects, excessively circumscribed or perseverative interests).
4. Hyper- or hyporeactivity to sensory input or unusual interest in sensory aspects of the environment (e.g., apparent indifference to pain/temperature, adverse response to specific sounds or textures, excessive smelling or touching of objects, visual fascination with lights or movement).

C. Symptoms must be present in the early developmental period (but may not become fully manifest until social demands exceed limited capacities, or may be masked by learned strategies in later life).

D. Symptoms cause clinically significant impairment in social, occupational, or other important areas of current functioning.

E. These disturbances are not better explained by intellectual developmental disorder (intellectual disability) or global developmental delay. Intellectual developmental disorder and autism spectrum disorder frequently co-occur; to make comorbid diagnoses of autism spectrum disorder and intellectual developmental disorder, social communication should be below that expected for general developmental level

Note: Individuals with a well-established DSM-IV diagnosis of autistic disorder, *Asperger's disorder,* or pervasive developmental disorder not otherwise specified should be given the diagnosis of autism spectrum disorder. Individuals who have marked deficits in social communication, but whose symptoms do not otherwise meet criteria for autism spectrum disorder, should be evaluated for social (pragmatic) communication disorder.

Specify current severity based on social communication impairments and restricted, repetitive patterns of behavior (see Table 2):

Requiring very substantial support
Requiring substantial support
Requiring support

Specify if:

With or without accompanying intellectual impairment
With or without accompanying language impairment

Specify if:

Associated with a known genetic or other medical condition or environmental factor (**Coding note:** Use additional code to identify the associated genetic or other medical condition.)
Associated with a neurodevelopmental, mental, or behavioral problem

Specify if:

With catatonia (refer to the criteria for catatonia associated with another mental disorder, p. 135, for definition) (**Coding note:** Use additional code F06.1 catatonia associated with autism spectrum disorder to indicate the presence of the comorbid catatonia.)
Severity levels for autism spectrum disorder (examples of level of support needs)

SEVERITY LEVEL	SOCIAL COMMUNICATION	RESTRICTED, REPETITIVE BEHAVIORS
Level 3 "Requiring very substantial support"	Severe deficits in verbal and nonverbal social communication skills cause severe impairments in functioning, very limited initiation of social interactions, and minimal response to social overtures from others. For example, a person with few words of intelligible speech who rarely initiates interaction and, when he or she does, makes unusual approaches to meet needs only and responds to only very direct social approaches.	Inflexibility of behavior, extreme difficulty coping with change, or other restricted/repetitive behaviors markedly interfere with functioning in all spheres. Great distress/difficulty changing focus or action.

BOX 26-2

Diagnostic Criteria for Autism Spectrum Disorder—cont'd

SEVERITY LEVEL	SOCIAL COMMUNICATION	RESTRICTED, REPETITIVE BEHAVIORS
Level 2 "Requiring substantial support"	Marked deficits in verbal and nonverbal social communication skills; social impairments apparent even with supports in place; limited initiation of social interactions; and reduced or abnormal responses to social overtures from others. For example, a person who speaks simple sentences, whose interaction is limited to narrow special interests, and who has markedly odd nonverbal communication.	Inflexibility of behavior, difficulty coping with change, or other restricted/repetitive behaviors appear frequently enough to be obvious to the casual observer and interfere with functioning in a variety of contexts. Distress and/or difficulty changing focus or action.
Level 1 "Requiring support"	Without supports in place, deficits in social communication cause noticeable impairments. Difficulty initiating social interactions, and clear examples of atypical or unsuccessful responses to social overtures of others. May appear to have decreased interest in social interactions. For example, a person who is able to speak in full sentences and engages in communication but whose to-and-fro conversation with others fails, and whose attempts to make friends are odd and typically unsuccessful.	Inflexibility of behavior causes significant interference with functioning in one or more contexts. Difficulty switching between activities. Problems of organization and planning hamper independence.

Approximately 20% of individuals with ASD have significantly decreased interaction with their surroundings, sometimes referred to as catatonic features in the literature (Vaquerizo-Serrano et al., 2021). ASD may involve impaired speech, lack of cooperation and negativism, agitation uninfluenced by external stimuli, aggression, posturing, echolalia, stereotypies (i.e., repetitive, abnormally frequent, non–goal-directed movements), odd social communication and difficulty identifying emotions or experiences, passivity in social interactions, and self-harming behaviors (APA, 2022; Vaquerizo-Serrano et al., 2021).

Impairments in social-emotional exchanges vary across development and have significant impact for students with ASD. Signs of impaired social communication and interaction, which are evident at a very early age, include the following:

- Avoids or does not keep eye contact
- Does not respond to name by 9 months of age
- Does not show facial expressions like happy, sad, angry, and surprised by 9 months of age
- Does not play simple interactive games like pat-a-cake by 12 months of age
- Uses few or no gestures by 12 months of age (e.g., does not wave goodbye)
- Does not share interests with others by 15 months of age (e.g., shows you an object that they like)
- Does not point to show you something interesting by 18 months of age
- Does not notice when others are hurt or upset by 24 months of age
- Does not notice other children and join them in play by 36 months of age
- Does not pretend to be something else, like a teacher or superhero, during play by 48 months of age
- Does not sing, dance, or act by 60 months of age (CDC, 2022c, para. 3)

Repetitive, routinized, and restricted behaviors can be seen in the play of children with ASD (CDC, 2022c). They may play with toys the same way each time and be attracted to parts of a toy rather than the whole object (e.g., playing with the wheels of a toy car rather than playing with the car functionally). They may line toys up rather than engaging in pretend play. Attempts to interrupt rigid nonfunctional behaviors or routines may trigger tantrums or aggressive behavior.

The interests of children with ASD can be intense and limited to specific topics (CDC, 2022c). They may focus on a typical childhood interest like dinosaurs or sports teams to the exclusion of other common childhood activities. They may readily engage in conversation about their preferred topic and steer conversations back to their topic of choice. For example, a child with ASD might fixate on dinosaurs, asking for dinosaurs for gifts, and wanting to collect different types of dinosaurs. Although such interests may be age-appropriate at first, children with ASD may maintain their interest (e.g., a specific cartoon) well past the time that peers have outgrown the same interest. Because children with ASD may not have insight into the fact that their peers no longer share their interest, this can also lead to social conflict. Changes in the classroom environment, such as rearranging furniture, or transitions from one activity to the next can also cause distress.

Children with ASD may also display impaired or inconsistent responsiveness to environmental sensations (CDC, 2022c). They may be hyposensitive or hypersensitive to sounds, textures, tastes, odors, sounds, or pain. For example, loud noises such as the ringing of school bell or school assemblies could be overwhelming. Children with ASD may not be able to tolerate wearing clothes with tags or constricting clothes like jeans because of tactile hypersensitivity. They may also have oral sensitivities and extremely restricted food preferences, sometimes even specifying the brand or color of food. Similarly, children with ASD may have unusual perceptions or expressions of illness or pain, or they may not be able to effectively communicate the cause for their distress. Whereas one student with ASD may display extreme reactions to minor discomfort or injury, another student with ASD may show little expression of pain in the face of significant discomfort or injury.

As students with ASD get older, they typically have difficulty making friends, initiating or sustaining conversations, and navigating social relationships (CDC, 2022c). These difficulties can lead to social isolation and peer victimization (i.e., bullying) (Forrest et al., 2020). When interpreting written and spoken language, students with ASD tend to be very literal. Understanding idioms, humor, sarcasm, or symbolism may be difficult, even for children with ASD who have average or above average IQs. Difficulty perceiving social cues may cause a student to miss or misinterpret nonverbal cues, directions, and rules of others, which may lead to unwarranted discipline problems and miscommunication. Safety issues are a significant concern when a student with ASD does not accurately perceive risks, dangers, and threats, such as wandering away from caregivers, jumping off playground equipment from an unsafe height, or acting aggressively when overstimulated in social situations.

Screening and Diagnosis

The American Academy of Pediatrics recommends screening all children for ASD with ASD-specific screening instruments at ages 18 and 24 months and through ongoing developmental surveillance (AAP, 2024). Early identification is key because it allows for early therapeutic intervention, which leads to improved long-term outcomes. There are several ASD screening instruments; however, the *Modified Checklist for Autism in Toddlers* (M-CHAT) is the most evidence informed and has been validated for use for children 16 to 30 months old (AAP, 2024; Center for Autism Research, 2022). Children who do not pass or score at risk for ASD on a screening instrument should be referred for a comprehensive diagnostic evaluation. It is essential that healthcare providers, including school nurses, communicate to parents/guardians that screening "positive" does not mean the child has ASD, but that further evaluation is needed. A positive screening result can be scary for families, and the fear they experience can be a barrier to seeking further diagnostic services. It should be noted that a definitive diagnosis of ASD is not required to qualify for early intervention or school-based services.

The other component of ASD screening is developmental surveillance, which is asking parents/guardians about concerns about their child's development and can take place during any interaction between providers and families (AAP, 2024). It is essential that healthcare providers, including school nurses, educate families on normal developmental milestones, including social and behavioral milestones in addition to the physical milestones (CDC, 2022b). It is important to note that intelligence testing has major limitations in accurately measuring the IQ of individuals with communication challenges; therefore results must be interpreted with caution.

ASD is diagnosed after extensive multimodal assessments that include clinical interviews of the child and parents/guardians; input from school professionals such as classroom teachers, school psychologist, and therapists; formal psychological testing; and formal observation of the child. Even though ASD can be reliably diagnosed as early as 14 months of age (Pierce et al., 2019), most children are not diagnosed until after 3 years of age. In a 2019 nationally representative sample, 23% of children were diagnosed with ASD before age 3, 44.5% were diagnosed between 3 and 5 years old, and 32% were after age 5 years of age (Child and Adolescent Health Measurement Initiative, 2019). Children with milder ASD symptoms and without language delays may not be identified until adolescence or adulthood when they are not able to meet the increased social demands and present with behavioral dysregulation (APA, 2022).

Did You Know?

The American Psychiatric Association's *Diagnostic and Statistical Manual of Mental Disorders, Fifth Edition, Text Revision* (DSM-5-TR) does not recognize "Asperger syndrome/disorder," "childhood disintegrative disorder," and "pervasive developmental disorder not otherwise specified" as separate childhood disorders. Children who may have previously been diagnosed with these disorders are now considered to have ASD (APA, 2022). Historically, Asperger syndrome/disorder was considered a less severe, higher-functioning form of autism in which individuals had intact and sometimes exceptional intellectual ability and verbal skills, although they often did not understand idiosyncratic language. Although there was a slight delay in the development of language, the primary challenge was a tendency to be awkward in social situations and have difficulty understanding and interpreting nonverbal cues, facial expressions, and voice tone of others (Evans, 2017).

Associated Findings

Several medical conditions co-occur with greater frequency in individuals with ASD. These include sleep problems, gastrointestinal problems, and seizure disorders (Hirota & King, 2023). Parent-reported sleep problems are significantly more common in preschoolers with ASD both with (47%) and without (57%) a comorbid developmental disability than typically developing peers or peers with a developmental disability without ASD features (Reynolds et al., 2019). Preschoolers with ASD were two and three times as likely to have parent-reported gastrointestinal symptoms (i.e., constipation, diarrhea) than children with other developmental disabilities and typically developing peers, respectively. Parent-reported gastrointestinal symptoms are also associated with greater sleep and behavior problems (Reynolds et al., 2019).

Psychiatric conditions also co-occur with greater frequency in individuals with ASD. The most frequent co-occurring psychiatric conditions associated with ASD over the life span are ADHD (28%) and anxiety disorders (20%) (Lai et al, 2019). Furthermore, the combined presentation of ADHD with both hyperactive/impulsive and inattentive features is commonly noted (78%) in children with ASD (Rau et al., 2020). Other frequently co-occurring psychiatric conditions include disruptive impulse-control disorders and conduct disorders (12%), depressive disorders (11%), obsessive-compulsive disorder (9%), bipolar disorders (5%), and schizophrenia (4%) (Lai et al., 2019). Children with ASD also have higher rates of anxiety, conduct, and depressive disorders compared with a nationally representative sample of children (Ghandour et al., 2019). Last, individuals with autism have increased odds of self-injurious behavior and suicidality.

Interventions

Early therapeutic intervention before 3 years old is key to positive outcomes for children with ASD. *Autism spectrum disorder* is an eligibility criteria for special education services under IDEA (2004), which ideally begins at ages 3 to 5 years through early childhood education as established in a student's IEP. Comprehensive school-based services include a small special education classroom learning environment as well as services the student needs such as occupational, physical, and speech therapy as indicated.

No single treatment or therapy is effective in all cases of ASD, but early intervention enhances the prognosis. A variety of therapeutic supports can benefit students with ASD. Some students benefit from structured behavioral plans (e.g., Applied Behavioral Analysis), whereas other students benefit from relationship-based therapeutic modalities (e.g., Floortime or Pivotal Response therapy) (Autism Research Institute, 2019). Occupational therapy can be particularly helpful in addressing sensory issues. For example, headphones can help reduce sensory overload from auditory stimuli. Speech therapy can address receptive and expressive language skills. Additionally, students with ASD who have limited verbal language can benefit from augmentive and alternative communication support such as picture exchange or a speech-producing device. Another popular technique used with students with ASD called "social stories" uses a narrative visual representation of an event or situation to teach the student what to expect and how to behave appropriately in social situations (Aldabas, 2019). Using social stories can help introduce new routines and help with transitions. For example, the school nurse could help prepare a student for a visit to the dentist by presenting a story about a child going to the dentist for the first time, describing what to expect, how to act, and how others might respond to them.

Over 80% of families of children with ASD have tried complementary and alternative medicine (CAM) and non–evidence-based treatments such as multivitamins (58.6%), gluten-free casein-free diet (54.8%), methyl B-12 injections (54.1%), and probiotics (52.2%) (Hopf et al., 2016). Other CAM treatments include amino acids and other nutritional supplements, prayer, massage therapy, detoxification therapy, hormone therapy, off-label use of antifungal or anti-inflammatory medications, and herbal therapy (Hopf et al., 2016). The school nurse should inquire about all treatments, special diets, and any CAM treatments the families may be seeking to help their child. In an effort to help their children, some families may be vulnerable to engaging in expensive alternative treatment regimens that have not been shown to be effective for ASD. While being respectful of the treatment options that families choose, the school nurse's role is to educate families on current evidence and to serve as a resource for teachers and families to understand treatment options.

Pharmacological intervention, when appropriate, should be tailored to an individual child's needs and monitored with a carefully constructed behavioral outcome plan. The school nurse should ensure that (1) a clear outcome plan that monitors improvements in behaviors is in place; (2) school staff are aware of possible side effects; and (3) there is a plan in place to report side effects. Medication is typically aimed at targeting troublesome symptoms that interfere with social and occupational functioning, such as self-injurious behaviors.

Irritability in students with ASD can present as tantrums, aggression, and self-injurious behavior. There are two FDA-approved antipsychotic medications to treat the irritability associated with ASD in children—risperidone and aripiprazole (Persico et al., 2019). Common side effects of risperidone and aripiprazole include an increase in appetite leading to weight gain and sedation. Children on these medications are at risk for metabolic syndrome and should have their body mass index (BMI) and laboratory tests (i.e., lipids) monitored regularly. There are several off-label medications such as guanfacine and clonidine that have been used to treat aggression and irritability in children with ASD. Co-occurring depressive, anxiety, or obsessive-compulsive disorders may also need pharmacological treatment. Children and adolescents with ASD may be more susceptible to side effects of selective serotonin reuptake inhibitors (SSRIs) than adults with ASD. When indicated, SSRIs should be trialed for a short duration at a low dosage (Persico, 2019). Along with medication, children and adolescents can participate in adapted cognitive-behavioral therapy to target anxiety symptoms (Lord et al., 2020). ADHD in children and adolescents with ASD can be treated with methylphenidate, atomoxetine, and guanfacine. The school nurse may need to monitor a complex set of medications and interventions to determine whether the desired student-centered goals are met and to ensure that unintended consequences do not occur.

Considerations for School Nurses

Careful observation and assessment are needed when the student with ASD presents to the health office. School nurses need to be aware of baseline behaviors and take a through history and physical assessment. It is imperative that the school nurse also have a good rapport with the parent/guardian to get accurate findings in a child with ASD. There can be a risk that typical health conditions, such as stomachaches and ear infections, may be missed or not treated. An injury, such as a broken bone that would hurt a typical peer, can seemingly go unnoticed in a student with ASD. The school nurse's care planning for a student with ASD involves working with families to identify and interpret how the student can or may express pain or discomfort. This should be part of the teaching for educators and support staff working with the student and included in the student's IHP.

INTELLECTUAL DEVELOPMENTAL DISORDERS

Historically, intelligence was thought to be a unitary trait on a continuum from very limited to extremely gifted. The APA (2018) defines *intelligence* as "the ability to derive information, learn from experience, adapt to the environment, understand, and correctly utilize thought and reason" (p. 1). Intellectual disability (ID) has been categorized under multiple classification systems to describe an affected individual's abilities and limitations. One of the most notable changes began in 2007 when the term *mental retardation,* as a disability category under IDEA, was changed to *intellectual disability* (also called *intellectual developmental disorder, IDD*). Concurrently, the American Association of Mental Retardation changed its name to the American Association of Intellectual and Developmental Disabilities (AAIDD). This change recognized that the term *mental retardation* was offensive and needed to be replaced with more positive terminology (Ziegler, 2020). In 2010, Congress passed *Rosa's Law* mandating that all references in federal laws to "mental retardation" be changed to *intellectual disability* and "mentally retarded individual" be replaced with an *individual with an intellectual disability* (Public Law 111-256; 111th Congress, 2010). Intellectual disability is one of the 13 disability categories for eligibility for special education services under IDEA (2004).

The terms *intellectual developmental disorder* (IDD) and *intellectual disability* (ID) are used interchangeably throughout the medical and research literature. The diagnosis of ID emphasizes both clinical judgment and standardized intelligence testing, with less emphasis on the intelligence quotient (IQ) score as was the case historically. The emphasis in classification is placed on either (1) the neurodevelopmental disorder or the resulting deficits in adaptive reasoning and functioning in academic, social, or practical settings or (2) the disability, functional deficits, and identification of needed supports, rather than the subtypes of mild, moderate, severe, or profound (APA, 2022).

ID is the fifth most prevalent type of disability served under the IDEA, Part B, in the public schools, preceded by specific learning disabilities, speech and language impairments, autism, and other health impairments (NCES, 2023). The number of students between the ages of 3 and 21 with ID served in the public schools with IEPs or during the 2020–2021 school year was 432,000 representing approximately 6% of the student population and between 5% and 7% of students receiving special education services (NCES, 2023). Approximately 1.2% of 8-year-olds qualified for an intellectual disability diagnosis (Patrick et al., 2021).

Although some children are diagnosed at birth, as in the case of children with Down syndrome, most children are not identified until preschool age when delays in speech and language skills and cognitive skills become apparent. The more profound the disability, the earlier the diagnosis usually occurs. Although IDD is usually a lifelong condition, the diagnosis can also be assigned when individuals lose previous cognitive and functional skills such as with severe traumatic brain injury, anoxia, meningitis or encephalitis, severe and chronic social deprivation, and lead or mercury poisoning, among others (APA, 2022).

Causative Factors

There are hundreds of causes of ID. Common associated conditions include prenatal causes, perinatal adverse outcomes of labor and delivery, postnatal injuries or illness affecting the brain, severe and prolonged social deprivation, and toxic exposure (APA, 2022). See Table 26-4.

Approximately 20% of causes are genetic or chromosomal in origin. These conditions include trisomies due to abnormal cell division (nondisjunction) at meiosis, translocation of genes, single gene transmission, gene deletions and breakages, or other anomalies.

Inborn errors of metabolism cause many cases of ID (Jansen et al., 2017; Ravindran et al., 2017; Stockler-Ipsiroglu et al., 2021). These metabolic disorders involve

TABLE 26-4 Selected Causes of Intellectual Disability

Chromosomal/Genetic Abnormalities	• **Angelman syndrome (AS):** Microdeletion on gene 15q11-q13, but passed by mother. Only the mother's chromosome 15 contains the activated UBE3A gene; if this gene is inactivated or absent, AS occurs. Characterized by microcephaly, hyperactivity, seizures, stiff and jerky gait, and speech impairment; generally happy disposition with frequent smiling and bouts of inappropriate laughter. May hand-flap and have sleep disturbances. Often misdiagnosed as cerebral palsy or autism. • **Cri du chat syndrome:** Microdeletion of short arm of chromosome 5 (typical region 5p15.3). Characteristics may include high-pitched catlike cry; low birth weight; failure to thrive; microcephaly; wide-set eyes; downward slanting eyelids; malformed ears; lag in speech/language; typically categorized as profound ID in the education setting with an IQ less than 20. • **Edwards syndrome (trisomy 18):** Typically does not survive past infancy. • **Fragile X syndrome:** Changes in *Fragile X Messenger Ribonucleoprotein 1 (FMR1)* gene in which the *FMR1* gene fails to make FMRP protein, which is necessary for brain development. Fragile X syndrome affects males and females but females display milder symptoms than males. Characteristics may include developmental delays such as not sitting, walking, or talking at expected age; learning disabilities; social and behavior problems such as failure to make eye contact, anxiety, trouble paying attention, hand-flapping, acting and speaking without thinking, and hyperactivity. • **Klinefelter syndrome (X chromosomal):** XXY-47 chromosomes (extra chromosome on the 23rd pair); only occurs in males. Characteristics may include gonadal dysgenesis, sterility, small testes, no secondary sex characteristics, gynecomastia caused by presence of estrogen, very tall and slim with long limbs, and moderate ID. • **Prader-Willi syndrome: Microdeletion** on chromosome 15 typically transmitted through the father. Characteristics may include mild to moderate ID, hypotonia, small hands and feet, narrow forehead, excessive eating leading to obesity, and a tendency for tantrums, stubbornness, and obsessive-compulsive disorder. • **Williams syndrome: Microdeletion** on chromosome 7. Characteristics may include mild to moderate ID, short forehead, dental problems, and extreme or overly affectionate interest in others, ADHD, anxiety, and phobias.
Genetic Metabolic Disorders/Inborn Errors of Metabolism (IEM)	• **Galactosemia:** IEM that causes impaired metabolism of carbohydrates causing undigested sugars to build up in the blood. Left undiagnosed or treated and depending on the type, may lead to ID, movement disorders, premature ovarian failure, cataracts, or pseudotumor of the brain. • **Homocystinuria:** A group of autosomal recessive IEM disorders in which the body is unable to process certain amino acids. This cystathionine beta-synthase deficiency, if left untreated with a specialized protein (methionine)-restricted diet from infancy, may cause ID, dislocation of the lens of the eye and nearsightedness, thromboembolic and cardiovascular disease, scoliosis, osteoporosis, and psychiatric comorbidities. • **Maple syrup urine disease:** An IEM in which the body is unable to process certain amino acids. A hallmark is dark, sweet-smelling urine noted in the neonatal period, poor feeding, vomiting, lethargy, and developmental delay. If untreated, it is fatal. • **Tay-Sachs disease:** IEM for lipids/fats resulting in the loss of both physical and mental abilities, blindness, and seizures; death by age 4. • **Phenylketonuria:** An IEM for amino acids that prevents the body from metabolizing phenylalanine. Newborn screening identifies most cases at birth. Treated with medication and strict dietary restrictions. Untreated cases can lead to ID, seizures, and behavior problems. • **Lesch-Nyhan disease:** An X-linked IEM (seen only in males) that causes a buildup of uric acid. Characteristics include neurological and behavioral problems, involuntary muscle movements, self-injury, arthritis, gout, kidney stones, and renal failure. Affected individuals usually cannot walk and typically do not survive past childhood.
Injuries/Abuse/Neglect	• **Head injuries:** Anoxia, hypoxia, bleeds • **Abusive head trauma (shaken baby syndrome):** Child abuse resulting in shearing of the vessels in the brain • **Malnutrition:** In early infancy, especially of the essential fatty acids
Environmental	• **Lead poisoning:** A neurotoxin that builds up in the body and brain. There is no safe level. Characterized by possible developmental delay, learning difficulties, sluggishness, hearing loss, and seizures • **Infection:** Meningitis, encephalitis; in utero infections (cytomegalovirus, toxoplasmosis, rubella)
Other Causes	• Extreme prematurity and intraventricular hemorrhage • Other neurological insults—untreated hydrocephalus; brain tumor; lack of brain development • Medications/drugs used in pregnancy—hydantoin (Dilantin), warfarin (Coumadin), oral isotretinoin (Accutane); drugs/alcohol • Microcephaly secondary to Zika virus infection in utero

Mayo Clinic (2019); National Center for Advancing Translational Sciences, Genetic and Rare Disease Information Center (n.d.).

flaws in enzymes or genes that assist in the degradation of products within the body (Jeanmonod et al., 2022). Brain injury may result if these enzymes are malfunctioning or deficient and by-products build up in the brain and cause damage, or if the genes are impaired. Some causes of inborn errors of metabolism can be detected with newborn screening, and with follow-up treatment the effect of the error can be reduced or eliminated (Arnold, 2018). For example, if a diagnosis of phenylketonuria (PKU) is made early, intellectual ability can be maintained with appropriate dietary measures (Dolan et al., 2017). With another condition of inborn errors of metabolism, Tay-Sachs disease, nothing can be done currently to prevent the neurological decay; therefore treatment focuses on comfort measures (National Organization for Rare Disorders [NORD], 2021).

A critical public health goal is early and continuous screening of infants and children. However, newborn screening requirements vary from state to state, with some mandating screening for as few as 32 conditions and others mandating as many as 77 conditions (Baby's First Test, 2022). Tests for PKU and congenital hypothyroidism can detect deficiencies, and treatment can prevent or lessen the resulting ID. The American College of Obstetricians and Gynecologists (2023) issued guidelines recommending prenatal diagnostic and screening testing to all pregnant women regardless of maternal age or other risk factors. School nurses should be aware of their state's condition-specific screening mandates (Steed et al., 2022).

Prenatal experiences and conditions may affect fetal outcomes. High-risk factors for the development of ID may include maternal behaviors during pregnancy (such as drug, alcohol, and/or tobacco use), maternal infections during pregnancy (such as rubella, cytomegalovirus, toxoplasmosis, or Zika virus), and maternal malnutrition. Cerebral dysgenesis in utero, such as in microcephaly, and untreated hydrocephalus are other physiological causes of ID during pregnancy (Zhu et al., 2021). Lack of prenatal care may result in delayed interventions for placental damage, hemorrhage, or hypertension and premature birth. Prenatal brain insults that may result in ID include intraventricular hemorrhage (common in premature and low-birth-weight infants), hypoxia, and anoxic injury (Zhu et al., 2021).

Postnatal causes of ID include untreated hyperbilirubinemia or hypothyroidism. Brain injury from head trauma and asphyxia can occur throughout childhood. ID can also be caused by degenerative neurological disorders, infections affecting the central nervous system (such as encephalitis and meningitis), lead poisoning, abusive head trauma (previously called shaken baby syndrome), and poor nutritional intake (especially deficiency of the essential fatty acids) during the first year of life.

A child raised in a low-stimulation or neglectful environment may also experience decreased development of neural pathways, resulting in a lack of neuronal response to stimuli. The neurobehavioral response to stimuli is a major component of cognition and memory that involves aspects of awareness, perception, reasoning, and learning. Early childhood programs and interventions may help to mitigate long-term risks for ID (Collins et al., 2017).

The most common syndromes associated with ID are autism spectrum disorder (ASD), trisomy 21 (Down syndrome), fragile X syndrome (FXS), and fetal alcohol spectrum disorder (The Arc, n.d.). While great strides have been made in understanding the causes of IDs, the causes of 35% to 40% of all cases with moderate to severe ID remain unknown (Jansen et al., 2017). Advances in genetic testing allow parents to make decisions regarding planning for future children.

Diagnostic Criteria

The current diagnostic criteria for *intellectual developmental disorder* (intellectual disability) in the DSM-5-TR are listed in Box 26-3.

IDD entails "deficits in general mental abilities (Criterion A) and impairment in everyday adaptive functioning, in comparison to an individual's age-, gender-, and socioculturally matched peers (Criterion B)" (APA, 2022, Intellectual Developmental Disorders, para. 3). Deficits can be categorized as being in the conceptual, social, and practical domains along a continuum from mild to moderate, severe, or profound.

Adaptive functioning includes those activities needed for developing personal independence and social responsibility, such as communication and social participation. The American Association on Intellectual and Developmental Disabilities (AAIDD) defines *adaptive behavior* as "the collection of conceptual, social and practical skills that all people learn in order to function in their daily lives" (2024a, para. 1). AAIDD uses a functional disability model focusing on the extent of the disability in various settings and considers the supports needed to allow for typical interactions within society (Schalock et al., 2021).

While the DSM-5-TR and AAIDD each provide different emphases, they both include deficits in intellectual and adaptive functioning in their definitions of ID. No one dimension alone is sufficient to describe a student with ID; a holistic approach must be taken, and all dimensions must be considered. A student with a disability is a person first (a valued member of society) who happens to have certain specific problems in functioning within society for a variety of reasons (classified as intellectual abilities, adaptive behavior, health, participation, and context) and who needs supports and services to function optimally as a member of society.

Evaluation

According to the APA (2022), "A comprehensive evaluation includes an assessment of intellectual capacity and adaptive functioning; identification of genetic and nongenetic etiologies; evaluation for associated medical conditions (e.g., cerebral palsy, seizure disorder); and evaluation

BOX 26-3

Diagnostic Criteria for Intellectual Developmental Disorder (Intellectual Disability)

Intellectual developmental disorder (intellectual disability) is a disorder with onset during the developmental period that includes both intellectual and adaptive functioning deficits in conceptual, social, and practical domains. The following three criteria must be met:

A. Deficits in intellectual functions, such as reasoning, problem solving, planning, abstract thinking, judgment, academic learning, and learning from experience, confirmed by both clinical assessment and individualized, standardized intelligence testing.

B. Deficits in adaptive functioning that result in failure to meet developmental and sociocultural standards for personal independence and social responsibility. Without ongoing support, the adaptive deficits limit functioning in one or more activities of daily life, such as communication, social participation, and independent living, across multiple environments, such as home, school, work, and community.

C. Onset of intellectual and adaptive deficits during the developmental period.

Note: The term intellectual developmental disorder is used to clarify its relationship with the WHO ICD-11 classification system, which uses the term Disorders of Intellectual Development. The equivalent term intellectual disability is placed in parentheses for continued use. The medical and research literature use both terms, while intellectual disability is the term in common use by educational and other professions, advocacy groups, and the lay public. In the United States, Public Law 111-256 (Rosa's Law) changed all references to "mental retardation" in federal laws to "intellectual disability."

Specify current severity (see Table 1):

(F70) Mild
(F71) Moderate
(F72) Severe
(F73) Profound

Severity levels for intellectual developmental disorder (intellectual disability)

SEVERITY LEVEL	CONCEPTUAL DOMAIN	SOCIAL DOMAIN	PRACTICAL DOMAIN
Mild	For preschool children, there may be no obvious conceptual differences. For school-age children and adults, there are difficulties in learning academic skills involving reading, writing, arithmetic, time, or money, with support needed in one or more areas to meet age-related expectations. In adults, abstract thinking, executive function (i.e., planning, strategizing, priority setting, and cognitive flexibility), and short-term memory, as well as functional use of academic skills (e.g., reading, money management), are impaired. There is a somewhat concrete approach to problems and solutions compared with age-mates.	Compared with typically developing age-mates, the individual is immature in social interactions. For example, there may be difficulty in accurately perceiving peers' social cues. Communication, conversation, and language are more concrete or immature than expected for age. There may be difficulties regulating emotion and behavior in age-appropriate fashion; these difficulties are noticed by peers in social situations. There is limited understanding of risk in social situations; social judgment is immature for age, and the person is at risk of being manipulated by others (gullibility).	The individual may function age-appropriately in personal care. Individuals need some support with complex daily living tasks in comparison to peers. In adulthood, supports typically involve grocery shopping, transportation, home and child-care organizing, nutritious food preparation, and banking and money management. Recreational skills resemble those of age-mates, although judgment related to well-being and organization around recreation requires support. In adulthood, competitive employment is often seen in jobs that do not emphasize conceptual skills. Individuals generally need support to make healthcare decisions and legal decisions, and to learn to perform a skilled vocation competently. Support is typically needed to raise a family.

Continued

BOX 26-3

Diagnostic Criteria for Intellectual Developmental Disorder (Intellectual Disability)—cont'd

SEVERITY LEVEL	CONCEPTUAL DOMAIN	SOCIAL DOMAIN	PRACTICAL DOMAIN
Moderate	All through development, the individual's conceptual skills lag markedly behind those of peers. For preschoolers, language and preacademic skills develop slowly. For school-age children, progress in reading, writing, mathematics, and understanding of time and money occurs slowly across the school years and is markedly limited compared with that of peers. For adults, academic skill development is typically at an elementary level, and support is required for all use of academic skills in work and personal life. Ongoing assistance on a daily basis is needed to complete conceptual tasks of day-to-day life, and others may take over these responsibilities fully for the individual.	The individual shows marked differences from peers in social and communicative behavior across development. Spoken language is typically a primary tool for social communication but is much less complex than that of peers. Capacity for relationships is evident in ties to family and friends, and the individual may have successful friendships across life and sometimes romantic relations in adulthood. However, individuals may not perceive or interpret social cues accurately. Social judgment and decision-making abilities are limited, and caretakers must assist the person with life decisions. Friendships with typically developing peers are often affected by communication or social limitations. Significant social and communicative support is needed in work settings for success.	The individual can care for personal needs involving eating, dressing, elimination, and hygiene as an adult, although an extended period of teaching and time is needed for the individual to become independent in these areas, and reminders may be needed. Similarly, participation in all household tasks can be achieved by adulthood, although an extended period of teaching is needed, and ongoing supports will typically occur for adult-level performance. Independent employment in jobs that require limited conceptual and communication skills can be achieved, but considerable support from coworkers, supervisors, and others is needed to manage social expectations, job complexities, and ancillary responsibilities such as scheduling transportation, health benefits, and money management. A variety of recreational skills can be developed. These typically require additional supports and learning opportunities over an extended period of time. Maladaptive behavior is present in a significant minority and causes social problems.
Severe	Attainment of conceptual skills is limited. The individual generally has little understanding of written language or of concepts involving numbers, quantity, time, and money. Caretakers provide extensive supports for problem solving throughout life.	Spoken language is quite limited in terms of vocabulary and grammar. Speech may be single words or phrases and may be supplemented through augmentative means. Speech and communication are focused on the here and now within everyday events. Language is used for social communication more than for explication. Individuals understand simple speech and gestural communication. Relationships with family members and familiar others are a source of pleasure and help.	The individual requires support for all activities of daily living, including meals, dressing, bathing, and elimination. The individual requires supervision at all times. The individual cannot make responsible decisions regarding well-being of self or others. In adulthood, participation in tasks at home, recreation, and work requires ongoing support and assistance. Skill acquisition in all domains involves long-term teaching and ongoing support. Maladaptive behavior, including self-injury, is present in a significant minority.

BOX 26-3

Diagnostic Criteria for Intellectual Developmental Disorder (Intellectual Disability)—cont'd

SEVERITY LEVEL	CONCEPTUAL DOMAIN	SOCIAL DOMAIN	PRACTICAL DOMAIN
Profound	Conceptual skills generally involve the physical world rather than symbolic processes. The individual may use objects in goal-directed fashion for self-care, work, and recreation. Certain visuospatial skills, such as matching and sorting based on physical characteristics, may be acquired. However, co-occurring motor and sensory impairments may prevent functional use of objects.	The individual has very limited understanding of symbolic communication in speech or gesture. He or she may understand some simple instructions or gestures. The individual expresses his or her own desires and emotions largely through nonverbal, nonsymbolic communication. The individual enjoys relationships with well-known family members, caretakers, and familiar others, and initiates and responds to social interactions through gestural and emotional cues. Co-occurring sensory and physical impairments may prevent many social activities.	The individual is dependent on others for all aspects of daily physical care, health, and safety, although he or she may be able to participate in some of these activities as well. Individuals without severe physical impairments may assist with some daily work tasks at home, like carrying dishes to the table. Simple actions with objects may be the basis of participation in some vocational activities with high levels of ongoing support. Recreational activities may involve, for example, enjoyment in listening to music, watching movies, going out for walks, or participating in water activities, all with the support of others. Co-occurring physical and sensory impairments are frequent barriers to participation (beyond watching) in home, recreational, and vocational activities. Maladaptive behavior is present in a significant minority.

for co-occurring mental, emotional, and behavioral disorders" (APA, Intellectual Developmental Disorders, para. 10). The APA (2022) recommends that cognitive and adaptive capacities be measured through a varied battery of neuropsychological testing and intellectual assessments that are appropriate for the student's age, sociocultural background, and primary language. Testing should be conducted and interpreted by trained professionals. Assessment of ID at school is typically the role of the school psychologist with supportive data from other qualified professionals on the multidisciplinary IEP team (teachers, occupational or physical therapists, etc.). The school nurse provides information regarding health history and current health status. With supportive therapies and special education services, intellectual and adaptive functioning can improve over time (APA, 2022).

There are multiple scales of intelligence and cognitive functioning, such as the *Wechsler Intelligence Scale for Children* (5th edition, ages 6 to17) and its companion instrument, the *Wechsler Preschool and Primary Scale of Intelligence* (4th edition, ages 2.6 to 7.7), which utilize developmentally appropriate activities to obtain a standard score for school-age children (Pearson, 2024). Other intelligence tests include the *Kaufman Brief Intelligence Scale* (KBIT-2), the *Reynolds Intellectual Screening Test* (RIST), and the *Wide Range Intelligence Test*. Originally, IQ was based on the ratio of tested mental age divided by the child's chronological age times 100 (Mensa International, 2022). The mean IQ was 100, with scores below 70 often associated with ID (Melby et al., 2020). Although the idea of a "quotient" was disbanded in favor of standard scores based on a normal curve with standard deviations, the results are still often referred to as IQ (Mensa International, 2022).

Adaptive or self-help and communication skills can be measured by a variety of adaptive behavior scales. Commonly used adaptive behavior scales include the *Scales of Independent Behavior* (SIB-R), the *Vineland Adaptive*

Behavior Scales (Vineland-3), the *Inventory for Client and Agency Planning*, and the *AAMD Adaptive Behavior Scale*. AAIDD (2024b) developed the *Diagnostic Adaptive Behavior Scale* (DABS) to provide a comprehensive standardized assessment of adaptive behavior. DABS provides a comprehensive standardized assessment of the adaptive behavior for individuals 4 to 21 years old and precise diagnostic information around the cutoff point where an individual is deemed to have "significant limitations" in adaptive behavior (one measure of ID) to determine the diagnosis of ID or related developmental disability (AAIDD, 2024b). Adaptive behavior is the collection of conceptual, social, and practical skills that all people learn in order to function in their daily lives. DABS measures three domains:

1. *Conceptual skills:* literacy; self-direction; and concepts of number, money, and time
2. *Social skills:* interpersonal skills, social responsibility, self-esteem, gullibility, naiveté (i.e., wariness), social problem-solving, following rules, obeying laws, and avoiding being victimized
3. *Practical skills:* activities of daily living (personal care), occupational skills, use of money, safety, health care, travel/transportation, schedules/routines, and the use of the telephone (AAIDD, 2024b, para. 4)

DABS is typically used by schools, forensic and clinical psychologists, psychometricians, social workers, occupational therapists, pediatricians, and disability-related government agencies to determine eligibility for special education services, home and community-based waiver services, Social Security Administration benefits, and appropriate treatment within the criminal justice system (AAIDD, 2024b).

Determining and describing the patterns of support needed by the student to accomplish typical daily tasks, such as communicating, caring for oneself, and interacting socially, gives a more accurate picture of a person with ID rather than an IQ score and a label of mild, moderate, or severe disability. Adaptive behavior scores are more useful for determining levels of assistance, education programs, and living situations needed by the individual (Zheng et al., 2021). The school nurse's health appraisal and recommendations are integral to the full and individual evaluation of a student diagnosed with or suspected of having ID.

The special education and related services a student with ID receives at school depend on the unique learning and functional needs of the student, not the disability label or level of disability. These services are outlined in the individualized education program (IEP) . For students who have ID and also have health needs at school, the school nurse develops an individualized healthcare plan (IHP) outlining how the student's school healthcare needs are to be met. The school nurse contributes to the IEP by developing student-centered health goals and objectives, stipulating nursing service minutes, and evaluating progress toward desired health and educational outcomes. Combining the care identified on the IHP and the services of the IEP will promote the highest level of independence and autonomy possible.

FETAL ALCOHOL SPECTRUM DISORDER

Fetal alcohol spectrum disorder (FASD) refers to a number of conditions related to prenatal alcohol ingested by the mother (National Center for Birth Defects and Developmental Disabilities [NCBDDD], 2023). Current research demonstrates that up to 5% of children in the United States have FASD (May et al., 2018). Most children with FASD appear normal at birth. Manifestation of FASD might include the following:

- Low body weight
- Poor coordination
- Hyperactive behavior
- Difficulty with attention
- Poor memory
- Difficulty in school (especially with math)
- Learning disabilities
- Speech and language delays
- Intellectual disability or low IQ
- Poor reasoning and judgment skills
- Sleep and sucking problems as a baby
- Vision or hearing problems
- Problems with the heart, kidneys, or bones
- Shorter-than-average height
- Small head size
- Abnormal facial features, such as a smooth ridge between the nose and upper lip (this ridge is called the philtrum) (NCBDDD, 2023, para. 8)

It is estimated that for every child born with FASD, three additional children are born without the physical characteristics of FASD but with neurobehavioral deficits of the condition that affect both learning and behavior.

Signs and symptoms of FASD range from mild to severe. Fetal alcohol syndrome represents the most severe form (NCBDDD, 2023). FASD is challenging for clinicians to definitively diagnose because mothers may not be forthcoming about their alcohol use during pregnancy and there are many other causes of the characteristics.

GENETIC/CHROMOSOMAL ALTERATIONS

Some causes of intellectual disability are genetic in etiology. Genetic conditions reflect changes in DNA and include mutations on one gene (single-gene defects), multifactorial conditions (more than one gene or more than one factor such as environment), or chromosomal abnormalities

(Queremel Milani & Tadi, 2023). Genes are sections of DNA that carry information for a particular trait, whereas chromosomes contain numerous genes. Therefore chromosome abnormalities tend to result in more severe and significant problems caused by an abnormal number of chromosomes or a structural problem of the chromosome (Queremel Milani & Tadi, 2023). Single-gene defects often have predictable patterns of inheritance and are considered dominant (requires only one gene to express the disorder), recessive (requires two genes to express the disorder), or X-linked (where the mutated gene occurs on the X chromosome). Mutated genes can be inherited or can be the result of a new mutation. The Human Genome Project has led to greater understanding of genetic conditions in the last couple of decades.

Down Syndrome

Down syndrome was first described in 1866 by an English physician, John Langdon Down. The chromosomal cause, trisomy 21, was identified more than 90 years later and the condition was named Down syndrome (Bull, 2020).

A *trisomy* indicates the individual received three chromosomes instead of two because one parent's pair failed to separate (nondisjunction) during meiosis (Queremel Milani & Tadi, 2022). Therefore the offspring has 47 chromosomes in every cell instead of 46; the extra chromosome appears on the number for the disorder's name. In addition to Down syndrome, other common autosomal trisomies include trisomy 13 (Patau syndrome) and trisomy 18 (Edwards syndrome) (Queremel Milani & Tadi, 2022). When a fetus is affected by either *trisomy 13 or 18*, the prognosis may result in a miscarriage, stillbirth, or a shortened life span. Children born with trisomy 13 or trisomy 18 are often severely disabled and require significant medical care. Clinical features include microcephaly, severe intellectual disability, congenital heart defects, and renal abnormalities (Queremel Milani & Tadi, 2022). Few of these children live past their first year of life due to life-threatening medical problems, and most will not survive to the school-age years.

Down syndrome is the most prevalent known cause of ID, but the incidence is decreasing, presumably because of advances in prenatal diagnosis and options available for termination of affected pregnancies. Prevalence in the United States is approximately one in 700 live births (CDC, 2020). These rates vary based on the age of the mother, with risk increasing with maternal age; the risk for Down syndrome increases from about one in 1,200 at age 25, to 1 in 900 at age 30, one in 350 at age 35, one in 100 at age 40, and one in 30 at age 45. Fifty-one percent of individuals with Down syndrome are born to mothers younger than 35 years (National Down Syndrome Society [NDSS], 2024).

Ninety-five percent of cases of Down syndrome are caused by nondisjunction in which the chromosome pairs fail to separate during meiosis, resulting in 47 chromosomes, or three chromosomes on the 21st pair, known as trisomy 21 (NDSS, 2024). Three percent of the cases are due to translocation, in which part of an extra 21st chromosome is attached to another chromosome. The remaining 2% are due to mosaicism, in which some cells have 46 and some have 47 chromosomes. The likelihood of having a second child with trisomy 21 is one in 100 up to the age of 40. The risk of recurrence of translocation is about 3% if the father is the carrier and 10% to 15% if the mother is the carrier (NDSS, 2024).

Associated Characteristics

Common physical features of Down syndrome include the following:

- Decreased or poor muscle tone
- Short neck, with excess skin at the back of the neck
- Flattened facial profile and nose
- Small head, ears, and mouth
- Upward slanting eyes, often with a skin fold that comes out from the upper eyelid and covers the inner corner of the eye
- White spots on the colored part of the eye (called Brushfield spots)
- Wide, short hands with short fingers
- A single, deep crease across the palm of the hand
- A deep groove between the first and second toes (Eunice Kennedy Shriver National Institute of Child Health and Human Development [EKSNICHHD], 2024, para. 2)

Students with Down syndrome experience a decreased linear growth velocity. Because the growth patterns are so unique, separate growth charts are available for children with Down syndrome (CDC, 2023b).

The hallmark characteristics of Down syndrome are mild to moderate cognitive and developmental impairments. Students with Down syndrome may exhibit issues with attention span, judgment, impulsivity, slow learning, and delays in language and speech development (EKSNICHHD, 2024). Studies indicate that the brain in individuals with Down syndrome is somewhat microcephalic and has a reduced volume of the frontal lobe and cerebellum. Students with Down syndrome typically have poor verbal and short-term memory skills. They have better performance on visual-spatial tasks than on verbal or auditory tasks and can usually learn to manage their self-care activities, although these skills are often delayed by 1 to 2 years (Da Cruz Netto et al., 2020; Fragoso et al., 2021; Rodrigues et al., 2019). Students with Down syndrome often enjoy participating in recreational activities and sports.

Language and speech development of students with Down syndrome is often significantly delayed, with short phrases not appearing until the preschool years (Milojevich & Lukowski, 2016). Some speak clearly, but many students have speech intelligibility difficulties. Most students with Down syndrome understand more than they can express verbally. Language skills are also often below cognitive abilities. The combination of articulation and expressive language difficulties often leads people to underestimate what students with Down syndrome can do. Exercises focused on the development of speech include feeding therapy, orofacial massage, and therapeutic exercises of the whole body. Children with Down syndrome who start speech therapy earlier in life (before age 5 years) achieve the best articulatory efficiency, whereas children who start later have more problems with swallowing, chewing, and biting (Nemours KidsHealth, 2022).

Although puberty may start somewhat later for boys, puberty and sexual development in students with Down syndrome progresses similarly at the same ages and sequences as their neurotypical peer. Most individuals with Down syndrome experience feelings of affection and desire for intimacy and sexual expression as they mature. However, the emotional and behavioral aspects of sexual maturity and judgment are typically underdeveloped (NDSS, 2022). Once mature, males with Down syndrome have a reduced sperm count and rarely father children. Females have regular menstrual periods and are capable of conceiving and carrying a baby to term. Sexual and reproductive health education should be part of educational programs and transition planning, with consideration for the learning style and cognitive level of the individual with Down syndrome. Therapeutic interventions can include activities of daily living with a focus on care during menstruation, sexual activity education, and reproductive health for teenagers with special needs (American Occupational Therapy Association, 2021). School nurses should keep in mind that these students are at increased risk for sexual abuse because of limitations in their problem-solving ability and their increased trust of others.

Comorbidities

Numerous health conditions are associated with Down syndrome, including heart defects in approximately 50% of cases, most commonly atrioventricular septal defects, as well as atrial septal defects, ventricular septal defects, and patent ductus arteriosus (Delany et al., 2021). The American Academy of Pediatrics published *Guidelines for Pediatricians for Health Supervision for Children With Down Syndrome* (Bull et al., 2022). The school nurse can refer to these guidelines to make sure that students are receiving recommended care. The guidelines may also offer useful information for school nurses when developing evidence-based IHPs for children with Down syndrome. According to this report, other medical conditions commonly seen in those with Down syndrome include the following:

- Hearing loss (75%)
- Obstructive sleep apnea (50% to 79%)
- Otitis media (50% to 70%)
- Eye problems (60% to 80%), including cataracts (less than 1% to 3%), nasolacrimal duct obstruction (3% to 36%), and strabismus and severe refractive errors (36% to 80%)
- Congenital heart defects (50%)
- Neurological dysfunction (1% to 13%)
- Gastrointestinal atresia (12%)
- Hip dislocation and hip abnormalities (2% to 8%)
- Symptomatic atlantoaxial instability (1% to 2%)
- Thyroid disease (24% to 50%), including Hashimoto thyroiditis (13% to 39%), with incidence dependent on age (Bull et al., 2022, Table 1)

Atlantoaxial instability is present in 6.8% to 27% of individuals with Down syndrome; however, less than 1% to 2% of individuals present with symptomatic atlantoaxial instability (Tomlinson et al., 2020). Atlantoaxial instability puts the student at risk for compression of cervical nerves. Symptoms can include neck pain, clumsiness, difficulty walking, having an abnormal gait, having sensory deficits, and being easily fatigued. Orthopedic problems may be caused by hypotonia and loose ligaments that may exacerbate the instability of the neck.

Cognitive function of individuals with Down syndrome deteriorates with age. During the adolescent years, behavior issues may arise, although typically people with Down syndrome experience fewer behavioral problems than people with ID of another cause, except for communication disturbance. Signs of aggression, depression, and psychiatric disorders have been found to occur at significantly higher rates in adolescents with Down syndrome (Dykens et al., 2015). Therefore physical causative factors need to be ruled out for older students with Down syndrome presenting with persistent behavior problems (Foley et al., 2016).

Interventions

School nursing services offered to students with Down syndrome should be included in the student's IEP. Interventions provided by the school nurse for these students may include the following:

- Complete routine hearing and vision screenings annually and follow-up on referrals to ensure that sensory deficits are not further affecting the student's ability to learn.
- Ensure at least semiannual dental checks and good dental hygiene in school to prevent periodontal disease.

> **Practice Connection**
>
> The American Academy of Pediatrics (2022) published guidelines for pediatricians for health supervision for children with Down syndrome. The school nurse can refer to these guidelines to make sure that students are receiving recommended care. The guidelines may also offer useful information for school nurses when developing evidence-based IHPs for children with Down syndrome.

- Ensure that radiographs are obtained for students involved in organized sports, such as the Special Olympics, before their participation to evaluate the status of the atlantoaxial subluxation/instability; discourage high-risk activities such as climbing trees or jungle gyms, contact sports, and somersaults.
- Be aware that because of deficiencies in the immune systems, students should be immunized against pneumococcus and hepatitis, in addition to maintaining full coverage for the other preventable communicable diseases.
- Coordinate physical therapy, occupational therapy, and speech therapy if appropriate; sign language may assist some students with communication problems to communicate important concepts (i.e., hungry, pain, juice, toilet).
- Promote a healthy diet and an exercise program because of students' predisposition to constipation and obesity; assess for signs of type 2 diabetes.
- Teach self-help skills related to hygiene, toileting, and menses.
- Teach sex education at the developmentally appropriate level; include content on dating, boundaries, and sex abuse prevention; obtain parental consent for nonmandated sex education topics.
- Be attentive to signs of physical illness because these students have an increased incidence of upper respiratory and ear infections.

A few families have opted for plastic surgery to reshape the eyes or to take a wedge out of the tongue so that it better fits into the small oral cavity. It is thought that this will decrease the stigma associated with Down syndrome and help with the problems associated with a protruding tongue, such as drooling and difficulties in eating, breathing, and speech. However, others believe that to alter their child's facial features would be to disrespect the child's individuality and identity (Tornali et al., 2021). The school nurse can assist by being nonjudgmental and using a shared plan of care model and working with families to promote their child's self-esteem. Education and role modeling by adults at school can foster acceptance of a student's physical differences and acceptance by peers.

Life expectancy for individuals with Down syndrome is longer than previously reported, yet still shorter than a typical life span. Persons with Down syndrome will usually live to age 60 (NDSS, 2022). Many enjoy life in supported living environments and find satisfaction in gainful employment, recreational activities, and meaningful social relationships.

Interestingly, individuals with Down syndrome have an 80% risk reduction of vascular anomalies and a reduced risk for development of solid tumors, except testicular cancer (Hasle et al., 2016). This protective effect is most likely because of increased gene product from the extra copy of chromosome 21. However, adults with Down syndrome are at increased risk for dementia and Alzheimer disease, with symptoms typically developing in the second decade of life; symptoms include decreased memory, social skills, and intelligence (NDSS, 2024). Families and individuals with Down syndrome require life span information about the health risks and other factors, so they can effectively develop and transition as they age.

Fragile X Syndrome

Fragile X syndrome (FXS) is the most common inheritable form of ID and the principal known single-gene disorder associated with autism (CDC, 2022d). FXS results from a fragile pinched-off or broken section of the lower arm of the sex-linked X chromosome.

According to the National Fragile X Foundation (NFXF; 2023), it is estimated that fragile X occurs in one in 4,000 males and one in 8,000 females. FXS is caused by a full mutation of the *FMR1* gene, with 200 to a few thousand repeats on this area of the chromosome; normally there are six to less than 50 repeats of the three nucleotides cytosine–guanine–guanine (CGG). This causes the gene to become methylated, resulting in deactivation and failure to send out the message to make proteins necessary for brain development.

There are three fragile X–associated disorders: FXS, fragile X–associated tremor/ataxia syndrome, and fragile X–associated primary ovarian insufficiency (NFXF, 2023). FXS involves the *FMR1* (the fragile X mental retardation 1) gene at Xq27.3, which is responsible for the production of a protein that is needed for brain and neurological development and function. The cognitive ability of those with FXS ranges from learning disabilities to ID. Delays in speech and language development are common, as are a variety of physical and behavioral characteristics discussed in the associated findings (NFXF, 2023). Fragile X–associated tremor/ataxia syndrome causes balance, tremor, and memory problems in some older males and a few female carriers of the *FMR1* gene (NFXF, 2023). Fragile X–associated primary ovarian insufficiency can lead to infertility and early menopause in some female carriers of the *FRM1* gene. It is possible to carry the gene for these variants and have no apparent signs.

Associated Characteristics

Although FXS occurs in both sexes, the symptoms are more severe in males (CDC, 2022d). Many individuals with FXS have a normal facial appearance; however, common atypical physical characteristics include the following:

- Long, narrow face with a high forehead and protruding large tongue
- Prominent jaw and high, arched palate, increasing the risk for recurrent sinus infections and otitis media, which can result in conductive hearing loss
- Connective tissue changes with hypotonia that may cause mitral valve prolapse, joint laxity with hyperextensibility of finger joints, low muscle tone, an

increased risk for hernias, joint dislocations, strabismus and refractive errors, and flat feet

- Large testicles after puberty
- Short stature for age (NFXF, 2023)

Students with FXS are usually healthy and have normal life spans. Additional comorbidities may include seizures (20%), ocular disorders, and sleep issues (CDC, 2022d).

Fragile X may be diagnosed after presentation of other concerns, such as delayed acquisition of developmental motor tasks; delayed speech or not speaking clearly; mild to severe learning disabilities; a dislike of bright lights, loud noises, and the texture of certain items; and dissatisfaction with being touched and making eye contact (NFXF, 2023).

The degree of cognitive impairment is correlated with the amount of *FMR* protein produced. Both genders present with a wide range of learning problems in the context of IQ and show a decline in IQ scores and adaptive functioning as they age. Sixty-eight percent of males have an IQ score lower than 50, while 18% have a score above 70. This decrease in IQ does not result in a loss of skills, but rather a slower acquisition of newer skills. In addition, nearly all people with FXS have behavioral symptoms, with males tending to present with ADHD and aggression, whereas females are more prone to shyness and withdrawal in social situations (Lozano et al., 2022). Functional impairments include delayed motor and speech development, short attention span, hyperactivity, dislike of change, anxiety, and poor auditory learning skills (Lozano et al., 2022).

The strengths of individuals with FXS include a developed sense of humor and good long-term memory, especially when a task is learned by seeing or doing. They can perform the activities of daily living and achieve more than would be expected based on their IQ. However, typically, they also have several limitations such as difficulty with short-term auditory or visual memory tasks, which impede sequential thinking. Although students with FXS generally have a good vocabulary, they have weaker communication and socialization skills and may engage in echolalia and perseverative and poorly articulated speech (NFXF, 2023). Temper tantrums are common during times of transition and during increased sensory stimulation (NFXF, 2023).

Of individuals with FXS, 16% of females and 46% of males also have a diagnosis of autism spectrum disorder, with symptoms including hand flapping, gaze aversion, and echolalia. However, less than 10% of those with autism have fragile X (NFXF, 2023). A checklist of phenotypic criteria has been established to identify individuals with developmental delay who would be appropriate candidates for molecular testing. Not all children with FXS have the apparent physical features of FXS, and some students who have learning disabilities may have undiagnosed FXS. Therefore evidence-based practice standards indicate that all students with developmental delay, ID, or autism receive a genetic evaluation for FXS (NFXF, 2023).

Interventions

There are several appropriate evidence-based approaches for individual and group educational teaching that are recommended for students with FXS and other IDs. These interventions include the following:

- Present all parts of a task at the same time because these students learn best in this manner (NFXF, 2023). (This is different from teaching strategies used for students with other causes of ID.)
- Stress activities with a concrete functional approach, for example, teaching numbers by counting out medication or counting the number of times one does an exercise.
- Provide a structured learning environment with smaller classrooms with decreased noise levels and minimal changes.
- Provide the use of headphones, either alone or attached to music, to assist in decreasing distraction and stimulation.
- Maintain a behavior chart; use positive reinforcement.
- Give clear, concrete directions, with visual cues if possible.
- Be aware that children with FXS have sleep difficulties with frequent wakefulness, which can affect cognitive outcomes in school. Communication with families will help the school be aware of days when the student needs a period of rest.
- For those with significant language problems, specific individualized communication plans are required. Interventions may include speech and language therapy or the use of sign language.
- Routinely screen for potential cardiac, orthopedic, dental, and neurological problems.
- When developmentally appropriate, students with FXS should receive reproductive and genetic counseling regarding their reproductive options.

Klinefelter Syndrome

Students with Klinefelter syndrome are males with an extra X chromosome (47,XXY). The XXY is due to nondisjunction or failure of the 23rd chromosome pair to separate in either the mother (XX) or father (XY) during meiosis, resulting in 47 chromosomes. Klinefelter syndrome is a common chromosomal abnormality and affects approximately one in 500 to 1,000 males (NORD, 2024). It is important to note that not all XXY males exhibit signs or symptoms associated with Klinefelter syndrome; up to 75% of XXY males go undetected during their lifetime.

Klinefelter syndrome typically results in decreased testosterone and elevated gonadotropin levels that can affect physical, developmental, behavioral, and cognitive functioning. Symptoms of Klinefelter syndrome that may prompt parents/guardians to have their child evaluated in infancy include hypospadias, small penis or testicles, or developmental delay (NORD, 2024). During the elementary school-age years, students with Klinefelter syndrome may have less muscle tone, difficulty with coordination, and a lower energy level than typical peers. The intelligence of most students with Klinefelter syndrome is not typically affected; however, without treatment they may have associated speech/language delays, ADHD characteristics, and learning disabilities (NORD, 2024). Behavioral concerns (e.g., anxiety, frustration, and an inability to clearly explain and communicate) may be evident (Butler et al., 2022).

Due to altered androgenic hormone production, preadolescent and adolescent males with Klinefelter syndrome exhibit alterations in pubertal development including lack of body and facial hair, lack of voice change, and lack of growth spurt (NORD, 2024). Other symptoms of concern are small testes, gynecomastia, little or no sperm upon ejaculation, disproportionately long growth of arms and legs, and extremely tall body stature.

Students with Klinefelter syndrome may need psychological support as social skills may take longer to develop resulting in isolation, preference to being alone, or difficulties with coping and verbalizing feelings (Butler et al., 2022). Esteem and body image issues may also complicate psychosocial development. Special education services through an IEP can help to address the constellation of learning and behavior challenges at school.

Hormone replacement therapy is a treatment option for adolescents with Klinefelter syndrome, consisting of monthly intramuscular injections of exogenous androgen or testosterone at the onset of puberty. Hormone replacement therapy helps bring on the development of secondary sex characteristics; however, risks include the development of aggressive behavior, increased risks for cancer in the genital regions, and early-onset male pattern baldness. Breast tissue enlargement may remain even with hormone replacement therapy and may require surgical resolution for body image concerns (Butler et al., 2022). As adults, individuals with Klinefelter syndrome have significantly decreased fertility rates and increased risk of metabolic syndrome, type 2 diabetes, obesity, dyslipidemia, and cardiovascular disease.

Turner Syndrome

Turner syndrome is the most common sex chromosome abnormality in females. *Turner syndrome* is the result of a deletion of a chromosome (monosomy) of an X chromosome (XO), leaving only 45 chromosomes due to nondisjunction. In some cases, the individual may only lack a part of one sex chromosome. The true occurrence of the syndrome is not known as many individuals with mild phenotypes may remain undiagnosed (Steiner & Saenger, 2022). The defining characteristics of Turner syndrome include short stature, ovarian dysgenesis resulting in infertility, and webbing of the neck. Associated problems include heart and kidney anomalies, autoimmune disorders, hearing loss, thyroid disorders, and hypertension. Diagnosis can be confirmed with chromosome confirmation. Upon diagnosis, the child should be evaluated for cardiovascular comorbidities, including hypertension, and renal abnormalities (Steiner & Saenger, 2022). The risk of osteoporosis and cardiovascular morbidity is increased due to the ovarian failure.

Most girls with Turner syndrome have normal intelligence. However, some may experience deficits in social cognition, difficulty with nonverbal problem-solving (mathematics), increased risk of attention deficit disorder, and psychomotor difficulties including visual-spatial organization (Steiner & Saenger, 2022). Verbal abilities are generally strong (Steiner & Saenger, 2022).

Students with Turner syndrome are followed by pediatric endocrinologists so growth hormone injections can be started to increase the child's height (Steiner & Saenger, 2022). A separate growth chart specific to Turner syndrome is available to plot stature for age percentiles. Estrogen replacement therapy starts after the age of 10 to help develop breast tissue and prevent osteoporosis (Steiner & Saenger, 2022).

Phenylketonuria

Phenylketonuria (PKU) is an inborn error of metabolism inherited as an autosomal recessive trait. PKU affects approximately 450,000 individuals worldwide (Elhawary et al., 2022). It is caused by a deficiency in the hepatic enzyme, phenylalanine hydroxylase, which is necessary to metabolize the essential amino acid found in proteins, phenylalanine. As a result of this deficiency, excessive amounts of phenylalanine accumulate in the bloodstream causing damage to the central nervous system, resulting in significant intellectual disability and epilepsy. An amino acid produced by the metabolism of phenylalanine, tyrosine, is absent in PKU. Tyrosine is needed to form melanin; therefore individuals with PKU typically have blond hair, blue eyes, and fair skin that is susceptible to eczema and sunburn (Elhawary et al., 2022).

With the early identification of PKU through universal newborn blood screening in the United States, profound cognitive impairments of PKU could now be averted (Elhawary et al., 2022). Treatment for PKU is lifelong and involves restricting phenylalanine in the diet to maintain a safe range (2 to 6 mg/dL up to 12 years and 2 to 10 mg/dL

Practice Connection

Rare Genetic, Chromosomal, and Congenital Conditions

School nurses are challenged when students have conditions that are rare and for which there is limited professional literature. The National Organization for Rare Disorders is an excellent resource for information for both the school nurse and the family (https://rarediseases.org/).

through adolescence). The diet must be supplemented with Phenex-2, a specially prepared phenylalanine-free formula for children and adults. It is essential for the school nurse to know what to look for on food labels and to have the dietary department involved in the care of children with PKU. In some cases, additional supplementation may be needed. Individuals with PKU should grow and develop typically as long as they maintain phenylalanine levels within the safe range.

SPECIAL ISSUES

Comorbidity/Dual Diagnosis

Students with neurodevelopmental disorders may also have coexisting conditions. Comorbid or associated conditions may include cerebral palsy, sensory impairments, seizure disorders, communication impairments, feeding difficulties, behavior/psychiatric disorders, ADHD, and thyroid disease. A significant portion of students with ID have sensory impairments, increasing as the severity of intellectual disability increases and with vision problems being the most common (Werkman et al., 2022). Speech-language and feeding problems are also associated with ID, as are some psychiatric and mood disorders.

It is important for school personnel, and especially school nurses, not to make assumptions based on the student's diagnoses; each student is unique. For example, some students with ASD may function at low intellectual levels; yet other students with ASD excel in reading and computation skills and grow up to be independent and highly successful. Approximately 32.9% of persons with ID report experiencing mental distress, though the association between ID and mental distress may be missed (Cree et al., 2020).

Physical Activity

Students who have neurodevelopmental disorders are often overweight, especially when associated with lower physical activity levels. They may also have predisposing factors for obesity related to comorbidity of certain genetic syndromes or medication adverse effects. Increased physical activity often results in an improved mental attitude and state of well-being (Herbert et al., 2020). Mobility issues may increase the challenges of a student with neurodevelopmental disabilities participating in physical education classes. The IEP should note whether the student requires specially designed (adaptive) physical education or accommodations (Assistance to States for the Education of Children With Disabilities and Preschool Grants for Children With Disabilities; Final Rule, 2006). Exercise is also a social activity; it allows individuals to participate with others in a nonacademic setting. The Special Olympics (n.d.) and the National Center on Health, Physical Activity, and Disability (2024) have been especially effective in providing a forum for individuals with disabilities to physically compete and be rewarded for their efforts. Competition promotes participation and exercise.

Sexuality

Students with neurodevelopmental disabilities need repeated information and practice related to everyday hygiene, self-care during menses, and sex education. There are numerous reports of individuals with neurodevelopmental disorders being more vulnerable to sexual abuse (Hughes et al., 2020). Their risk may be exacerbated by their need to be part of a social group and to be liked or difficulty with problem-solving or social skills. School nurses may be asked to teach students with neurodevelopmental disorders at any grade level about their bodies and address sexuality when students reach adolescence. School nurses, health educators, and healthcare professionals should strive to empower these students with the knowledge necessary to make responsible decisions about their own sexual behavior in a healthy and responsible manner. If students can understand the facts and associated concepts and make decisions, then they are equipped to give informed consent, avoid dangerous situations, or refuse unwanted sexual contact. To live healthy and safe lives, people with ID need the following:

- Regular social lives so they can make friends
- Education about their own bodies, sexuality, and reproductive health, including prevention of sexually transmitted diseases and unwanted pregnancy
- A means to communicate their sexual needs
- Opportunities for sexual expression and relationships
- Privacy
- The right to make mistakes

Supporting people with intellectual and developmental disabilities to live full lives means supporting them to live a full sexual life as well, if they desire.

Victimization

Most schools take active measures to establish a safe and inclusive culture for students. Yet students with developmental disabilities are at increased risk for bullying and abuse compared with students with typical development. It should be noted that individuals with neurodevelopmental disorders may also play the role of the bully toward more vulnerable students. Adolescents with neurodevelopmental disorders have significantly higher levels of coping with bullying if they participate in social activities, if they do not watch violent movies, and if their school counselor organized activities to prevent bullying (Aldrich et al., 2016).

Students with neurodevelopmental disabilities may also be physically or psychologically abused or neglected by their own families. Mental health concerns associated with abuse and neglect are a factor as students transition from adolescence to adulthood (Raya et al., 2013). School nurses may be the first to suspect abuse and may be the trusted adult to whom the student confides that they are being victimized. School personnel should take a team approach to ensure these students, as well as students with other differences, are considered part of the school population and are treated with the same respect, dignity, and expectations as other students. All school personnel have mandated reporter responsibilities. See Chapter 11 for more information on student exposure to trauma and bullying.

Ethical Issues

Children and youth are considered a vulnerable group regarding ethical human rights issues. This vulnerability increases when the minor has physical, intellectual, or emotional challenges or disabilities. Discrepancies between diagnostic criteria of some disorders and varying levels of acumen by healthcare providers and school professionals can create challenges to appropriately diagnosing neurodevelopmental disabilities. Diagnoses have serious implications for the student and family, the school district placement and services, and even court systems and social services eligibility. For example, in the criminal justice system, an adolescent with ID should be judged and sentenced in developmentally appropriate ways; a person with ID cannot be executed for murder (Death Penalty Information Center, 2024). The courts and psychiatric, psychological, and education associations agree that high-stakes decisions should never be made on the basis of a single test score. These same principles should apply to discipline in the school setting in accordance with IDEA.

School Nurse Care Coordination

Students with neurodevelopmental disabilities require care coordination and an advocate. Care coordination is a pillar of National Association of School Nurses' (NASN's) *School Nursing Practice Framework* (2024). School nurses are the ideal healthcare professionals to provide care coordination and school nurse–led case management for students with disabilities (NASN, 2021). School nurses serve as liaisons between the student, educational team, family, community social support services, and healthcare providers to ensure continuity of care and appropriate interventions at school. The professional school nurse possesses knowledge of the laws pertaining to education, health, and family that are essential for providing effective advocacy, as well as addressing the medical complexities of the specific condition. For many school districts, this paradigm shift must include fostering a team approach and empowering the school nurse to provide comprehensive care coordination services.

It is imperative that the student's IEP and IHP be integrated to ensure that comprehensive health services include preventive, educational, acute care, and long-term care. School nurses should be a part of the student's IEP team from the initial assessment through development of the IEP and implementation of services, including related nursing/health services as indicated (NASN, 2023). The student's IHP should reflect the health interventions at school and care coordination measures by the school nurse. Depending on the condition and comorbidities, students with neurodevelopmental disabilities may require more intensive monitoring and screenings than is mandated, such as biannual growth measurements and annual vision and hearing screening.

Dental care is often neglected for students with special needs. The school nurse can host mobile dental clinics to provide services at school and can develop a list of local dentists who care for students with special needs. The school nurse should educate students and families about the importance of daily oral hygiene and promote the necessity for routine primary oral care. Students with intellectual and developmental disorders should have as much information as possible about their health needs.

CONCLUSION

The school nurse is an integral member of the multidisciplinary team that supports the optimal health, education, and well-being of students with neurodevelopmental disabilities and their families. The school nurse uses tailored instructional strategies to teach students developmentally appropriate information about their health and provide their families and school staff with information about the student's unique needs. As care coordinator, the school nurse advocates for the rights of these students, while planning, implementing, and evaluating evidence-based care aligned with the unique needs and cultural contexts of each child with neurodevelopmental disabilities.

The Editors gratefully acknowledge the work of the previous chapter authors, Marie Foley, Linda Crawford, and Susan Whitehead. A special thank you to Romy Zemer for her assistance.

References

Achenbach, T. M., & Rescorla, L. A. (2001). *Manual for the ASEBA school-age forms & profiles.* University of Vermont, Research Center for Children, Youth, and Families.

Aldabas, R. (2019). Effectiveness of social stories for children with autism: A comprehensive review. *Technology and Disability, 3*(1, 2), 1–13. https://doi.org/10.3233/TAD-180218

Aldrich, H., Jankowski, C., Lyden, K., & Ganoe-Cleveland, B. (2016). Objective physical activity measurement for a child with special health care needs. *Journal of Pediatric Nursing, 31*(5), 548–553. http://dx.doi.org/10.1016/j.pedn.2016.05.007

American Academy of Child & Adolescent Psychiatry. (2020). *Attention-deficit hyperactivity disorder (ADHD): Parent's medication guide.* American Psychiatric Association. https://www.aacap.org/App_Themes/AACAP/docs/resource_centers/resources/med_guides/ADHD_Medication_Guide-web.pdf

American Academy of Pediatrics. (2019). *Clinical practice guideline for the diagnosis, evaluation, and treatment of attention-deficit/hyperactivity disorder in children and adolescents.* Ahttps://publications.aap.org/pediatrics/article/144/4/e20192528/81590/Clinical-Practice-Guideline-for-the-Diagnosis

American Academy of Pediatrics. (2022). Health supervision for children and adolescents with Down syndrome. *Pediatrics, 149*(5), e2022057010. https://doi.org/10.1542/peds.2022-057010

American Academy of Pediatrics. (2024, March 18). *How is autism diagnosed?* Healthy Children.org https://www.healthychildren.org/English/health-issues/conditions/Autism/Pages/Diagnosing-Autism.aspx?_gl=1*k1zaso*_ga*OTcwNDgyMzg5LjE2OTcxMjE0MzY.*_ga_FD9D3XZVQQ*MTcxMjIzMjA4OC4xOS4xLjE3MTIyMzIxNTguMC4wLjA

American Academy of Pediatrics & National Institute for Children's Healthcare Quality. (2002). *NICHQ Vanderbilt assessment scales: Used for diagnosing ADHD*. https://www.nichq.org/sites/default/files/resource-file/NICHQ_Vanderbilt_Assessment_Scales.pdf

American Association on Intellectual and Developmental Disabilities. (2024a). *Adaptive behavior.* https://www.aaidd.org/intellectual-disability/definition/adaptive-behavior

American Association on Intellectual and Developmental Disabilities. (2024b). *DABS: What is DABS?* http://aaidd.org/dabs

American College of Obstetricians and Gynecologists. (2023). *Current AGOC guidance.* https://www.acog.org/advocacy/policy-priorities/non-invasive-prenatal-testing/current-acog-guidance

American Occupational Therapy Association. (2021). *Occupational therapy and autistic females.* https://www.aota.org/-/media/Corporate/Files/Publications/CE-Articles/CEA_August_2021.pdf

American Psychiatric Association. (2018). *Intelligence, definition.* https://dictionary.apa.org/intelligence

American Psychiatric Association. (2021). *What is specific learning disorder?* https://www.psychiatry.org/patients-families/specific-learning-disorder/what-is-specific-learning-disorder

American Psychiatric Association. (2022). *Diagnostic and statistical manual of mental disorders, fifth edition, text revision* (DSM-5-TR). American Psychiatric Publishing.

Arnold, G. L. (2018). Inborn errors of metabolism in the 21st century: Past to present. *Annals of Translational Medicine, 6*(24), 467. https://doi.org/10.21037/atm.2018.11.36

Assistance to States for the Education of Children With Disabilities and Preschool Grants for Children With Disabilities; Final Rule. 34 CFR Federal Register 300 and 301. (2006).

Autism Research Institute. (2019). *Behavioral treatment.* https://www.autism.com/aba

Baby's First Test. (2022). *Conditions screened by state.* https://www.babysfirsttest.org/newborn-screening/states

Belanger, S., Andrews, D., Gray, C., & Korczak, D. (2018). ADHD in children and youth: Part 1—Etiology, diagnosis, and comorbidity. *Paediatrics & Child Health, 23*(7), 447–453. https://doi.org/10.1093/pch/pxy109

Bitsko, R. H., Claussen, A. H., Lichstein, J., Black, L. I., Jones, S. E., Danielson, M. L., Hoenig, J. M., Davis Jack, S. P., Brody, D. J., Gyawali, S., Maenner, M. J., Warner, M., Holland, K. M., Perou, R., Crosby, A. E., Blumberg, S. J., Avenevoli, S., Kaminski, J. W., & Ghandour, R. M. (2022). Mental health surveillance among children—United States, 2013–2019. *MMWR Supplement, 71*(2), 1–48.

Brikell, I., Kuja-Halkola, R., & Larsson, H. (2019). Heritability of attention-deficit hyperactivity disorder across the lifespan. *European Neuropsychopharmacology, 29*(3), 757–758. https://doi.org/10.1016/j.euroneuro.2017.06.106

Bull, M. J. (2020). Down syndrome. *The New England Journal of Medicine, 382*(24), 2344–2352. https://doi.org/10.1056/NEJMra1706537.

Bull, M. J., Trotter, T., Santoro, S. L., Christensen, C., & Grout, R. W. (2022). Health supervision for children and adolescents with Down syndrome. *Pediatrics, 149*(5), e2022057010. https://doi.org/10.1542/peds.2022-057010

Bussing, R., Fernandez, M., Harwood, M., Hou, W., Garvan, C. W., Eyberg, S. M., & Swanson, J. M. (2008). Parent and teacher SNAP-IV ratings of attention deficit hyperactivity disorder symptoms: Psychometric properties and normative ratings from a school district sample. *Assessment, 15*(3), 317–328.

Butler, G., Srirangalingam, U., Faithfull, J., Sangster, P., Senniappan, S., & Mitchell, R. (2022). Klinefelter syndrome: Going beyond the diagnosis. *Archives of Disease in Childhood,* archdischild-2020-320831. Advance online publication. https://doi.org/10.1136/archdischild-2020-320831

Center for Autism Research. (2022). *Modified checklist for autism in toddlers (M-CHAT).* https://www.research.chop.edu/car-autism-roadmap/modified-checklist-for-autism-in-toddlers-m-chat

Centers for Disease Control and Prevention. (2020). *Birth defects.* https://www.cdc.gov/ncbddd/birthdefects/downsyndrome/data.html

Centers for Disease Control and Prevention. (2022a). *What is autism spectrum disorder?* https://www.cdc.gov/ncbddd/autism/facts.html

Centers for Disease Control and Prevention. (2022b). *Developmental milestone resources for early head start and head start programs.* https://www.cdc.gov/ncbddd/actearly/headstart.html

Centers for Disease Control and Prevention. (2022c). *Signs and symptoms of autism spectrum disorder.* https://www.cdc.gov/ncbddd/autism/signs.html

Centers for Disease Control and Prevention. (2022d). *What is fragile X syndrome?* https://www.cdc.gov/ncbddd/fxs/facts.html

Centers for Disease Control and Prevention. (2023a). *Data and statistics on autism spectrum disorder.* https://www.cdc.gov/ncbddd/autism/data.html

Centers for Disease Control and Prevention. (2023b). *Growth charts for children with Down syndrome.* https://www.cdc.gov/ncbddd/birthdefects/downsyndrome/growth-charts.html

Chan, T. M., & Mo, Y. H. (2022). Parent–child interactive stress in Chinese families with children who have attention-deficit hyperactivity disorder. *Child and Adolescent Social Work Journal, 39*(4), 485–497. https://doi.org/10.1007/s10560-021-00744-1

Child and Adolescent Health Measurement Initiative. (2019). *National Survey of Children's Health.* Health Resources and Services Administration, Maternal and Child Health Bureau. https://nschdata.org/browse/survey/results?q=8180&r=1

Cleveland Clinic. (2023). *ADHD medications.* https://my.clevelandclinic.org/health/treatments/11766-adhd-medication

Collins, P. Y., Pringle, B., Alexander, C., Darmstadt, G. L., Heymann, J., Huebner, G., Kutlesic, V., Polk, C., Sherr, L., Shih, A., Sretenov, D., & Zindel, M. (2017). Global services and support for children with developmental delays and disabilities: Bridging research and policy gaps. *PLoS Medicine, 14*(9), e1002393. https://doi.org/10.1371/journal.pmed.1002393

Conners, C. K. (2008). *Conners third edition (Conners 3).* Los Angeles, CA: Western Psychological Services.

Conrad, J. A. (2020). On intellectual and developmental disabilities in the United States: A historical perspective. *Journal of Intellectual Disabilities, 24*(1), 85–101. https://doi.org/10.1177/1744629518767001

Cree, R. A., Okoro, C. A., Zack, M. M., & Carbone, E. (2020). Frequent mental distress among adults, by disability status, disability type, and selected characteristics—United States, 2018. *MMWR Morbidity and Mortality Weekly Report, 69*(36), 1238–1243. http://dx.doi.org/10.15585/mmwr.mm6936a2external icon

Cutler, A. J., Suzuki, K., Starling, B., Balakrishnan, K., Komaroff, M., Castelli, M., ... & Childress, A. C. (2022). Efficacy and safety of dextroamphetamine transdermal system for the treatment of attention-deficit/hyperactivity disorder in children and adolescents: Results from a pivotal phase 2 study. *Journal of Child and Adolescent Psychopharmacology, 32*(2), 89–97. https://doi.org/10.1089/cap.2021.0107

Da Cruz Netto, O. L., Rodrigues, S. C. M., de Castro, M. V., da Silva, D. P., da Silva, R. R., de Souza, R. R. B., de Souza, A. A. F., & Bissaco, M. A. S. (2020). Memorization of daily routines by children with Down syndrome assisted by a playful virtual environment. *Scientific Reports, 10*(1), 3144. https://doi.org/10.1038/s41598-020-60014-5

Death Penalty Information Center. (2024). *Intellectual disability.* https://deathpenaltyinfo.org/policy-issues/intellectual-disability

Deavenport-Saman, A., Vanderbilt, D. L., Harstad, E., Shults, J., Barbaresi, W., Bax, A., Cacia, J., Friedman, S., LaRosa, A., Loe, I., Mittal, S., & Blum, N. (2022). Association of coexisting conditions, attention-deficit/hyperactivity disorder medication choice, and likelihood of improvement in preschool-age children: A Developmental Behavioral Pediatrics Research Network study. *Journal of Child and Adolescent Psychopharmacology, 32*(6), 328–336. https://doi.org/10.1089/cap.2022.0009

Delany, D. R., Gaydos, S. S., Romeo, D. A. Henderson, H. T., Fogg, K. L., McKeta, A. S., Kavarana, M. N., & Costello, J. M. (2021). Down syndrome and congenital heart disease: Perioperative planning and management. *Journal of Congenital Heart Disease, 5*(7). https://doi.org/10.1186/s40949-021-00061-3

DeStefano, F., & Shimabukuro, T. T. (2019). The MMR vaccine and autism. *Annual Review of Virology, 6*(1), 585–600. https://doi.org/10.1146/annurev-virology-092818-015515

Dolan, B. E., Koch, R., Bekins, C., & Schuett, V. (2017). Purpose and approach of the guidelines. *National PKU News.* https://pkunews.org

Dupar, L., & Dodson, W. (2019). The ultimate guide to ADHD medication. *New Hope Media,* 12–15.

DuPaul, G. J., Power, T. J., Anastopoulos, A. D., & Reid, R. (2016). *ADHD rating scale? 5 for children and adolescents: Checklists, norms, and clinical interpretation.* Guilford Publications.

Dykens, E. M., Shah, B., Davis, B., Baker, C., Fife, T., & Fitzpatrick, J. (2015). Psychiatric disorders in adolescents and young adults with Down syndrome and other intellectual disabilities. *Journal of Neurodevelopmental Disorders, 7*(1), 9. https://doi.org/10.1186/s11689-015-9101-1

Elhawary, N. A., AlJahdali, I. A., Abumansour, I. S., Elhawary, E. N., Gaboon, N., Dandini, M., Madkhali, A., Alosaimi, W., Alzahrani, A., Aljohani, F., Melibary, E. M., & Kensara, O. A. (2022). Genetic etiology and clinical challenges of phenylketonuria. *Human Genomics, 16*(1), 22. https://doi.org/10.1186/s40246-022-00398-9

Eunice Kennedy Shriver National Institute of Child Health and Human Development. (2024, February 16). *What are the symptoms of Down syndrome?* https://www.nichd.nih.gov/health/topics/down/conditioninfo/symptoms

Evans, B. (2017). *The metamorphosis of autism: A history of child development in Britain.* Chapter 5: How do you measure a social impairment? Manchester University Press. https://www.ncbi.nlm.nih.gov/books/NBK436844/

Foley, K., Taffe, J., Bourke, J., Einfeld, S. L., Tonge, B. J., Trollor, J., & Leonard, H. (2016). Young people with intellectual disability transitioning to adulthood: Do behaviour trajectories differ in those with and without Down syndrome. *PLoS One, 11*(7). http://dx.doi.org/10.1371/journal.pone.0157667

Forrest, D. L., Kroeger, R. A. & Stroope, S. (2020). Autism spectrum disorder symptoms and bullying victimization among children with autism in the United States. *Journal of Autism and Developmental Disorders, 50*(2), 560–571. https://doi.org/10.1007/s10803-019-04282-9

Fragoso, D. C., Nunes, D. M., Maia, A. C. M., Garcia, L. A. L., Alves, H. C. B. R., da Silva, C. J., & Leite, C. C. (2021). What we should not forget about Down syndrome. *Neurographics, 11*(3), 149–165.

Ghandour, R. M., Sherman, L. J., Vladutiu, C. J., Ali, M. M., Lynch, S. E., Bitsko, R. H., & Blumberg, S. J. (2019). Prevalence and treatment of depression, anxiety, and conduct problems in US children. *The Journal of Pediatrics, 206,* 256–267. https://doi.org/10.1016/j.jpeds.2018.09.021

Greenhill, L. L., Swanson, J. M., Hechtman, L., Waxmonsky, J., Arnold, L. E., Molina, B. S., ... & MTA Cooperative Group. (2020). Trajectories of growth associated with long-term stimulant medication in the multimodal treatment study of attention-deficit/hyperactivity disorder. *Journal of the American Academy of Child & Adolescent Psychiatry, 59*(8), 978–989. https://doi.org/10.1016/j.jaac.2019.06.019

Hasle, H., Friedman, J., Olsen, J. H., & Rasmussen, S. A. (2016). Low risk of solid tumors in persons with Down syndrome. *Genetics in Medicine,* 1–7. https://www.nature.com/gim/journal/vaop/ncurrent/pdf/gim201623a.pdf

Herbert, C., Meixner, F., Wiebking, C., & Gilg, V. (2020). Regular physical activity, short-term exercise, mental health, and well-being among university students: The results of an online and a laboratory study. *Frontiers in Psychology, 11,* 509.

Hirota, T., & King, B.H. (2023). Autism spectrum disorder: A review. *JAMA, 329*(2), 157–168. doi:10.1001/jama.2022.23661

Hopf, K. P., Madren, E., & Santianni, K. A. (2016). Use and perceived effectiveness of complementary and alternative medicine to treat and manage the symptoms of autism in children: A survey of parents in a community population. *The Journal of Alternative and Complementary Medicine, 22*(1), 25–32. https://doi.org/10.1089/acm.2015.0163

Hughes, R. B., Robinson-Whelen, S., Goe, R., Schwartz, M., Cesal, L., Garner, K. B., Arnold, K., Hunt, T., & McDonald, K. E. (2020). "I really want people to use our work to be safe" ... Using participatory research to develop a safety intervention for adults with intellectual disability. *Journal of Intellectual Disabilities, 24*(3), 309–325. https://doi.org/10.1177/1744629518793466

Hyman, S. L., Levy, S. E., Myers, S. M., Kuo, D. Z., Apkon, S., Davidson, L. F., ... & Bridgemohan, C. (2020). Identification, evaluation, and management of children with autism spectrum disorder. *Pediatrics, 145*(1).

Individuals With Disabilities Education Improvement Act of 2004 (Pub. L. 108-446). https://www.gpo.gov/fdsys/pkg/PLAW-108publ446/content-detail.html

Jansen, S., Geuer, S., Pfundt, R., Brough, R., Ghongane, P., Herket, J. C., . . . de Vries, B. B. (2017). DeNovo truncating mutations in the last and penultimate exons of PPM1D cause an intellectual disability syndrome. *The American Journal of Human Genetics, 100,* 650–658. https://doi.org/101016/athg.2017.02.005

Jeanmonod, R., Asuka, E., & Jeanmonod, D. (2022). *Inborn errors of metabolism.* In: StatPearls [Internet]. https://www.ncbi.nlm.nih.gov/books/NBK459183/

Kostova, Z., Levin, L., Lorberg, B., & Ziedonis, D. (2019). Mindfulness-based interventions for adolescents with mental health conditions: A systematic review of the research literature. *Journal of Child and Family Studies, 28*(10), 2633–2649. https://doi.org/10.1007/s10826-019-01477-7

Lai, M. C., Kassee, C., Besney, R., Bonato, S., Hull, L., Mandy, W., ... & Ameis, S. H. (2019). Prevalence of co-occurring mental health diagnoses in the autism population: A systematic review and meta-analysis. *The Lancet Psychiatry, 6*(10), 819–829.

Leahy, L. G. (2018). Diagnosis and treatment of ADHD in children vs adults: What nurses should know. *Archives of Psychiatric Nursing, 32*(6), 890–895. https://doi.org/10.1016/j.apnu.2018.06.013

Liu, H., Feng, W., & Zhang, D. (2019). Association of ADHD medications with the risk of cardiovascular diseases: A meta-analysis. *European Child & Adolescent Psychiatry, 28*(10), 1283–1293. https://doi.org/10.1007/s00787-018-1217-x

Lord, C., Brugha, T. S., Charman, T., Cusack, J., Dumas, G., Frazier, T., Jones, E. J. H., Jones, R. M., Pickles, A., State, M. W., Taylor, J. L., & Veenstra-VanderWeele, J. (2020). Autism spectrum disorder. *Nature Review Disease Primers, 6*(1). https://doi.org/10.1038/s41572-019-0138-4

Lozano, R., Thompson, T., Dixon-Weber, J., Erickson, C. A., Berry-Kravis, E., Williams, S. ... & Hessl, D. (2022). Observable symptoms of anxiety in individuals with fragile X syndrome: Parent and caregiver perspectives. *Genes, 13*(9), 1660.

Mascheretti, S., De Luca, A., Trezzi, V., Peruzzo, D., Nordio, A., Marino, C., & Arrigoni, F. (2017). Neurogenetics of developmental dyslexia: From genes to behavior through brain neuroimaging and cognitive and sensorial mechanisms. *Translational Psychiatry, 7,* 1–15. e987. https://doi.org/10.1038/tp.2016.240

Mattingly, G. W., Wilson, J., Ugarte, L., & Glaser, P. (2021). Individualization of attention-deficit/hyperactivity disorder treatment: Pharmacotherapy considerations by age and co-occurring conditions. *CNS Spectrums, 26*(3), 202–221. https://doi.org/0.1017/S1092852919001822

May, P.A., Chambers, C.D, & Kalberg, W.O. et al. (2018). Prevalence of fetal alcohol spectrum disorders in 4 US communities. *JAMA, 319*(5), 474–482. doi:10.1001/jama.2017.21896

Mayo Clinic. (2019). *Lead poisoning.* https://www.mayoclinic.org/diseases-conditions/lead-poisoning/symptoms-causes/syc-20354717

Mazahery, H., Conlon, C. A., Beck, K. L., Mugridge, O., Kruger, M. C., Stonehouse, W., ... & von Hurst, P. R. (2019). A randomized controlled trial of vitamin D and omega-3 long chain polyunsaturated fatty acids in the treatment of irritability and hyperactivity among children with autism spectrum disorder. *The Journal of Steroid Biochemistry and Molecular Biology, 187*, 9–16.

McGuire, D. O., Tian, L. H., Yeargin-Allsopp, M., Dowling, N. F., & Christensen, D. L. (2019). Prevalence of cerebral palsy, intellectual disability, hearing loss, and blindness, National Health Interview Survey, 2009–2016. *Disability and Health Journal, 12*(3), 443–451. https://doi.org/10.1016/j.dhjo.2019.01.005

Mehta, T. R., Gurung, P., Nene, Y., Fayyaz, M., & Bollu, P. C. (2019). Sleep and ADHD: A review article. *Current Developmental Disorders Reports, 6*(4), 228–234. https://doi.org/10.1007/s40474-019-00178-6

Melby, L., Indredavik, M. S., Løhaugen, G., Brubakk, A. M., Skranes, J., & Vik, T. (2020). Is there an association between full IQ score and mental health problems in young adults? A study with a convenience sample. *BMC Psychology, 8*(1), 7. https://doi.org/10.1186/s40359-020-0372-2

Mensa International. (2022). What is IQ? *GWS Media.* https://www.mensa.org/iq/what-iq

Milojevich, H., & Lukowski, A. (2016). Recall memory in children with Down syndrome and typically developing peers matched on developmental age. *Journal of Intellectual Disability Research, 60*(Part 1), 89–100. http://dx.doi.org/10.1111/jir.12242

National Association of School Nurses. (2021). *A model for school nurse-led case management.* https://learn.nasn.org/courses/33713

National Association of School Nurses. (2023). *IDEIA and Section 504 teams—The school nurse as an essential team member* (Position Statement). Author. https://www.nasn.org/nasn-resources/professional-practice-documents/position-statements/ps-ideia

National Association of School Nurses. (2024). A contemporary framework update for today's school nursing landscape: Introducing the School Nursing Practice Framework. *NASN School Nurse, 39*(3), 140–147. https://www.doi.org/10.1177/1942602X241241092

National Center for Advancing Translational Sciences, Genetic and Rare Disease Information Center. (n.d.). *Diseases.* https://rarediseases.info.nih.gov/diseases

National Center for Birth Defects and Developmental Disabilities. (2023, October). *Fetal alcohol spectrum disorders.* Centers for Disease Control and Prevention. https://www.cdc.gov/ncbddd/fasd/facts.html

National Center for Education Statistics. (2023). *Students with disabilities.* https://nces.ed.gov/programs/coe/indicator/cgg

National Center on Health, Physical Activity, and Disability. (2024). *NCHPAD: Building healthy inclusive communities.* https://www.nchpad.org/

National Down Syndrome Society. (2022, June 17). *Relationships & sexuality: Sexuality and Down syndrome.* https://ndss.org/resources/relationships-sexuality#:~:text=AND%20EMOTIONAL%20DEVELOPMENT-,Children%20with%20Down%20syndrome%20experience%20the%20same%20sequence%20of%20physical,do%20not%20have%20Down%20syndrome

National Down Syndrome Society. (2024). *About Down syndrome?* https://ndss.org/about

National Fragile X Foundation. (2023). *What is fragile X syndrome?* https://fragilex.org/

National Institute of Mental Health. (2021). *Attention-deficit/hyperactivity disorder in children and teens: What you need to know.* [Brochure].

National Institute of Mental Health. (2022). *Attention-deficit/hyperactivity disorder (ADHD): Mental health medications.* https://www.nimh.nih.gov/health/topics/mental-health-medications

National Institute on Deafness and Other Communication Disorders. (2020). *Autism spectrum disorder: Communication problems in children.* National Institutes of Health. https://www.nidcd.nih.gov/health/autism-spectrum-disorder-communication-problems-children

National Organization for Rare Disorders. (2021, May 20). *Tay Sachs disease.* https://rarediseases.org/rare-diseases/tay-sachs-disease/

National Organization for Rare Disorders. (2024, March 29). *47, XXY (Klinefelter syndrome).* https://rarediseases.org/rare-diseases/47-xxy-klinefelter-syndrome/

Nemours KidsHealth. (2021, February). *Auditory processing disorder.* https://kidshealth.org/en/parents/central-auditory.html

Nemours KidsHealth. (2022, March). *Speech-language therapy.* https://kidshealth.org/en/parents/speech-therapy.html

Patrick, M. E., Shaw, K. A., Dietz, P. M., Baio, J., Yeargin-Allsopp, M., Bilder, D. A., Kirby, R. S., Hall-Lande, J. A., Harrington, R. A., Lee, L. C., Lopez, M. L. C., Daniels, J., & Maenner, M. J. (2021). Prevalence of intellectual disability among eight-year-old children from selected communities in the United States, 2014. *Disability and Health Journal, 14*(2), 101023. https://doi.org/10.1016/j.dhjo.2020.101023

Pearson. (2024). *Intelligence scales.* https://www.pearsonassessments.com/search.html?aq=Intelligence%20scales

Persico, A. M., Ricciardello, A., & Cucinotta, F. (2019). The psychopharmacology of autism spectrum disorder and Rett syndrome. *Handbook of Clinical Neurology, 165*, 391–414.

Pierce, K., Gazestani, V. H., Bacon, E., Barnes, C. C., Cha, D., Nalabolu, S., Lopez, L., Moore, A., Pence-Stophaeros, S., & Courchesne, E. (2019). Evaluation of the diagnostic stability of the early autism spectrum disorder phenotype in the general population starting at 12 months. *JAMA Pediatrics, 173*(6), 578–587. https://doi.org/10.1001/jamapediatrics.2019.0624

Preston, J. D., O'Neal, J. H., Talaga, M. C., & Moore, B. A. (2021). *Child and adolescent clinical psychopharmacology made simple.* New Harbinger Publications.

Public Law 111-256; 111th Congress, 124 STAT. 2643 U.S. Congress 111–256 (2010).

Queremel Milani, D. A., & Tadi, P. (2023, April 24). *Genetics, chromosome abnormalities.* StatPearls [Internet]. https://www.ncbi.nlm.nih.gov/books/NBK557691/

Radmanović, M. B., & Burgić, S. S. (2021). Comorbidity in children and adolescents with ADHD. *ADHD. From Etiology to Comorbidity.* IntechOpen.

Rau, S., Skapek, M. F., Tiplady, K., Seese, S., Burns, A., Armour, A. C., & Kenworthy, L. (2020). Identifying comorbid ADHD in autism: Attending to the inattentive presentation. *Research in Autism Spectrum Disorders, 69*, 101468. https://doi.org/10.1016/j.rasd.2019.101468

Ravindran, E., Hu, H., Yuzwa, S. A., Nernandez-Miranda, L. R., Kraemer, N., Ninnemann, O., . . . & Kaindl, A. M. (2017). Homozygous ARHGEF2 mutation causes intellectual disability and midbrain-hindbrain malformation. *PLOS Genetics, 13*(4), 1–24. https://doi.org/10.1371/journal.pgen.1006746

Raya, A. F., Ruiz-Olivares, R., Pino, J., & Herruzo, J. (2013). Parenting styles and parenting practices in disabled children and its relationship with academic competence and behavior problems. *Procedia–Social and Behavioral Sciences, 89*, 702–709. www.sciencedirect.com

Rehabilitation Act of 1973 (Pub. L. 93-112). https://www.gpo.gov/fdsys/pkg/STATUTE-107/pdf/STATUTE-107-Pg718.pdf

Reynolds, A. M., Soke, G. N., Sabourin, K. R., Hepburn, S., Katz, T., Wiggins, L. D., ... & Levy, S. E. (2019). Sleep problems in 2- to 5-year-olds with autism spectrum disorder and other developmental delays. *Pediatrics, 143*(3). https://doi.org/10.1542/peds.2018-0492

Reynolds, C., & Kamphaus, R. (2015). *Behavior assessment system for children* (3rd ed.). Bloomington, MN: Pearson.

Rodrigues, M., Nunes, J., Figueiredo, S., Martins de Campos, A., & Geraldo, A. F. (2019). Neuroimaging assessment in Down syndrome: A pictorial review. *Insights Into Imaging, 10*, 1–13.

Rosa's Law (Pub. L. 111-256). (2010). https://www.congress.gov/111/plaws/publ256/PLAW-111publ256.pdf

Schalock, R. L., Luckasson, R., & Tassé, M. J. (2021). An overview of intellectual disability: Definition, diagnosis, classification, and systems of supports. *American Journal on Intellectual and Developmental Disabilities, 126*(6), 439–442.

Special Olympics. (n.d.). *What we do.* https://www.specialolympics.org/what-we-do?locale=en

Steed, H., O'Toole, D., Lao, K., Nuñez, B., Surani, K., & Stuart-Cassel, V. (2022). *ChildTrends*. https://www.childtrends.org/publications/state-laws-on-school-nursing-outline-copious-responsibilities-for-nurses

Steiner, M., & Saenger, P. (2022). Turner syndrome: An update. *Advances in Pediatrics, 69*(1), 177–202. https://doi.org/10.1016/j.yapd.2022.03.004

Stockler-Ipsiroglu, S., Potter, B. K., Yuskiv, N., Tingley, K., Patterson, M., & van Karnebeek, C. (2021). Developments in evidence creation for treatments of inborn errors of metabolism. *Journal of Inherited Metabolic Disease, 44*(1), 88–98. https://doi.org/10.1002/jimd.12315

The Arc. (n.d.). *Intellectual disability*. www.thearc.org

Tomlinson, C., Campbell, A., Hurley, A., Fenton, E., & Heron, N. (2020). Sport preparticipation screening for asymptomatic atlantoaxial instability in patients with Down syndrome. *Clinical Journal of Sport Medicine, 30*(4), 293–295. https://doi.org/10.1097/JSM.0000000000000642

Tornali, C., Migliore, M., Polizzi, A., Bragazzi, N. L., Martini, M., Ruggieri, M., Praticò, A. D., & Vecchio, I. (2021). Reconstructive surgery in children with Down syndrome: Bioethical implications. *Journal of Pediatric Neurology, 19*(1), 1–6. https://doi-org.ezproxy.tcnj.edu/10.1055/s-0040-1709510

Ullmann, R. K., Sleator, E. K., & Sprague, R. L. (2000). *ACTeRS teacher and parent forms manual*. Champaign, IL: Metritech, Inc.

U.S. Office of Special Education and Rehabilitative Services. (2020). *A transition guide to post-secondary education and employment for students and youth with disabilities*. United States Department of Education. https://www2.ed.gov/about/offices/list/osers/transition/products/postsecondary-transition-guide-may-2017.pdf?utm_name=

Vaquerizo-Serrano, J., Salazar De Pablo, G., Singh, J., & Santosh, P. (2021). Catatonia in autism spectrum disorders: A systematic review and meta-analysis. *European Psychiatry, 65*(1), e4. doi:10.1192/j.eurpsy.2021.2259

Visser, L., Kalmar, J., Linkersdörfer, J., Görgen, R., Rothe, J., Hasselhorn, M., & Schulte-Körne, G. (2020). Comorbidities between specific learning disorders and psychopathology in elementary school children in Germany. *Frontiers in Psychiatry, 11*, 292. https://doi.org/10.3389/fpsyt.2020.00292

Wang, C., Li, K., Seo, D. C., & Gaylord, S. (2020). Use of complementary and alternative medicine in children with ADHD: Results from the 2012 and 2017 National Health Interview Survey. *Complementary Therapies in Medicine, 49*, 102352. https://doi.org/10.1016/j.ctim.2020.102352

Werkman, M. F., Landsman, J. A., Fokkens, A. S., et al. (2022). The impact of the presence of intellectual disabilities on sensory processing and behavioral outcomes among individuals with autism spectrum disorders: A systematic review. *Review Journal of Autism and Developmental Disorders*. https://doi.org/10.1007/s40489-022-00301-1

Zhang, L., Yao, H., Li, L., Du Rietz, E., Andell, P., Garcia-Argibay, M., ... & Chang, Z. (2022). Risk of cardiovascular diseases associated with medications used in attention-deficit/hyperactivity disorder: A systematic review and meta-analysis. *JAMA Network Open, 5*(11), e2243597–e2243597.

Zheng, S., LeWinn, K., Ceja, T., Hanna-Attisha, M., O'Connell, L., & Bishop, S. (2021). Adaptive behavior as an alternative outcome to intelligence quotient in studies of children at risk: A study of preschool-aged children in Flint, MI, USA. *Frontiers in Psychology, 12*, 692330. https://doi.org/10.3389/fpsyg.2021.692330

Zheng, Y., Pingault, J. B., Unger, J. B., & Rijsdijk, F. (2020). Genetic and environmental influences on attention-deficit/hyperactivity disorder symptoms in Chinese adolescents: A longitudinal twin study. *European Child & Adolescent Psychiatry, 29*(2), 205–216. https://doi.org/10.1007/s00787-019-01346-0

Zhu, C., Chen, C., & Thornton, C. (2021). Editorial: Experimental and clinical approaches in the pursuit of novel therapeutic strategies for perinatal brain injury and its neurological sequelae. *Frontiers in Cellular Neuroscience, 15*, 762111. https://doi.org/10.3389/fncel.2021.762111

Ziegler, M. E. (2020). Disabling language: Why legal terminology should comport with a social model of disability. *Boston College Law Review, 61*, 1183.

Chapter 27

Students With Seizures and Epilepsy

Nancy Santilli ▪ Patricia Gellasch ▪ Robin Adair Shannon

CHAPTER OUTLINE

Seizure disorders are the most common and serious neurological conditions among children (Hauser, 2016). The standing definition of a *seizure* is "a transient occurrence of signs and/or symptoms due to abnormal excessive or synchronous neuronal activity in the brain" (Fisher et al., 2005, p. 741). Seizures are unexpected, stereotypical, and repetitive time-limited events that can cause alterations in autonomic, sensory, motor, or psychic function. They can alter consciousness, emotional state, memory, cognition, and behavior (Kiriakopoulos, 2019).

Seizures and epilepsy are not the same. A seizure is an event; epilepsy is a neurological condition that predisposes an individual to seizures. *Epilepsy* is defined as "a disorder of the brain characterized by an enduring predisposition to generate epileptic seizures and by the neurobiologic, cognitive, psychological, and social consequences of this condition. The definition of epilepsy requires the occurrence of at least one epileptic seizure" (Fisher et al., 2005, p. 471). The abnormal electrical activity in the brain that causes seizures can be due to general dysfunction of the biochemical mechanisms within bilaterally distributed networks of the brain (generalized) or from specific areas of one hemisphere of the brain (focal) (Fisher et al., 2017).

The Centers for Disease Control and Prevention (CDC; 2024) estimates there were approximately 2.9 million adults and 456,000 children, or 1% of the U.S. population, with seizure disorders or epilepsy in 2021. It is estimated that at least 10% of the population will experience one seizure (Rizvi et al., 2017). There is a 70% increased risk of having subsequent seizures in the first 2 years following the first seizure when high-risk clinical features are present, such as electroencephalograms (EEGs), prior brain insult, and nocturnal seizures. Most adults with epilepsy had their first seizure in childhood. Students with seizures have a higher prevalence of comorbidities, including various mental health, developmental, physical, and functional disorders, than students without seizures (Jennum et al., 2021). These comorbidities can have a significant impact on educational access, school functioning, social development, mental health, and safety for students living with seizure disorders.

The purpose of this chapter is to give school nurses an overview of the various types, presentations, and management of seizures and epilepsy. Best practices in meeting of the healthcare needs of children and youth with seizures at school will be discussed.

CLASSIFICATION OF SEIZURES AND EPILEPSY

The etiology of seizures may or may not be known, or there may be more than one cause. A thorough evaluation of seizures will help accurately diagnose epilepsy. In 2017, the International League Against Epilepsy (ILAE) determined a new framework for the classification of seizures and epilepsies (Fisher et al., 2017). The ILAE reclassified seizure types into three groups based on onset: *focal, generalized,* and *unknown.* See Figure 27-1. These categories have been

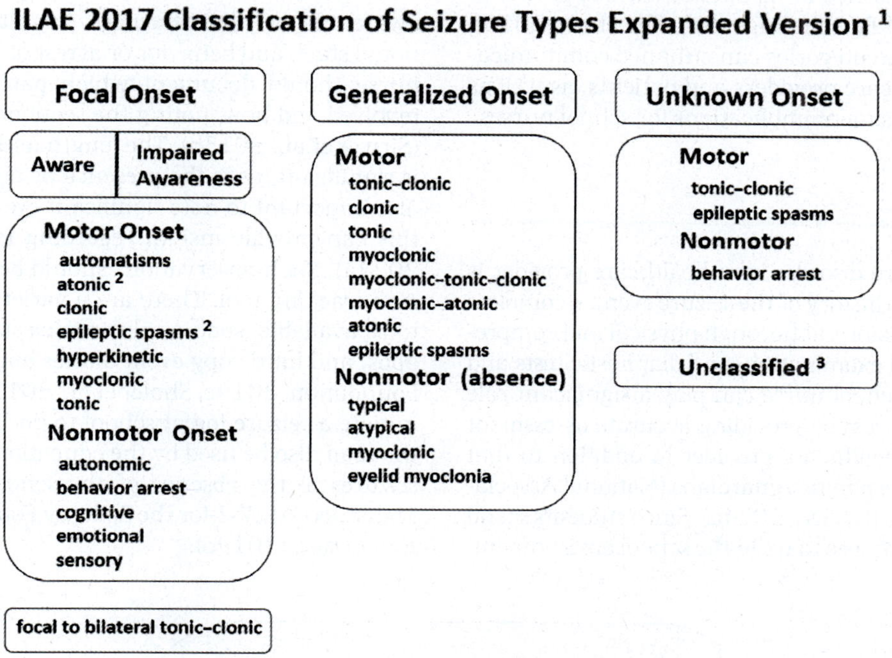

Figure 2.

The expanded ILAE 2017 operational classification of seizure types. The following clarifications should guide the choice of seizure type. For focal seizures, specification of level of awareness is optional. Retained awareness means the person is aware of self and environment during the seizure, even if immobile. A focal aware seizure corresponds to the prior term simple partial seizure. A focal impaired awareness seizure corresponds to the prior term complex partial seizure, and impaired awareness during any part of the seizure renders it a focal impaired awareness seizure. Focal aware or impaired awareness seizure optionally may further be characterized by one of the motor-onset or nonmotor-onset symptoms below, reflecting the first prominent sign or symptom in the seizure. Seizures should be classified by the earliest prominent feature, except that a focal behavior arrest seizure is one for which cessation of activity is the dominant feature throughout the seizure. A focal seizure name also can omit mention of awareness when awareness is not applicable or unknown and thereby classify the seizure directly by motor onset or nonmotor-onset characteristics. Atonic seizures and epileptic spasms would usually not have specified awareness. Cognitive seizures imply impaired language or other cognitive domains or positive features such as déjà vu, hallucinations, illusions, or perceptual distortions. Emotional seizures involve anxiety, fear, joy, other emotions, or appearance of affect without subjective emotions. An absence is atypical because of slow onset or termination or significant changes in tone supported by atypical, slow, generalized spike and wave on the EEG. A seizure may be unclassified due to inadequate information or inability to place the type in other categories. [1]Definitions, other seizure types and descriptors are listed in the accompanying paper and glossary of terms. [2]Degree of awareness usually is not specified. [3]Due to inadequate information or inability to place in other categories.

Epilepsia © ILAE

FIGURE 27-1. ILAE 2017 classification of seizure types—expanded version. *(Fisher et al., 2017) Used with permission.*

recognized by the Epilepsy Foundation. Note that the terms "simple partial," "complex partial," and "convulsion" are no longer used (Fisher et al., 2017).

Identification of the acute seizure type can then be used to further classify the type of epilepsy based on whether the etiology can be determined by clinical evaluation. The etiology of epilepsy can be differentiated into six groups: genetic, structural, metabolic, immune, infectious, and unknown (Scheffer et al., 2016). See Figure 27-2. *Genetic epilepsies* are inherited, in which seizures are the core symptom of the disorder; however, the causative gene mutation may not be known (Scheffer et al., 2016). Epilepsies of *unknown cause* are epilepsies for which the underlying cause has not been determined; the term "idiopathic" is no longer used (Scheffer et al., 2017). An *epilepsy syndrome* is diagnosed in the presence of distinctive clinical presentations and associated EEG findings (Scheffer et al., 2016). Understanding these categories can enhance communication between healthcare providers and patients, as well as awareness of management implications for school nurses.

DIAGNOSIS

Diagnosis of a seizure disorder by a healthcare provider is based on an accurate history of the seizure event, a complete medical and social history, a thorough physical and comprehensive neurological examination, and diagnostic tests and consultations. The school nurse can play a significant role in the diagnostic process by providing accurate assessment information to the healthcare provider in addition to that communicated by the parents/guardians (National Association of School Nurses [NASN], 2024a). Since students spend the better part of their weekdays in the school environment, school nurses and school personnel are likely to witness students (or adults) having seizures in school.

If a suspected seizure event is witnessed at school, the school nurse should provide a detailed history of the event including descriptions of what occurred before, during, and after the episode. Parents/guardians and healthcare providers can use these reports to aid the diagnostic process. It is important to know when the episode occurred or if there was a preceding event, such as sleep deprivation, illness, trauma, or a specific stimulus (i.e., visual stimuli, flickering lights, or reading). A report should include the signs and symptoms that occurred during the seizure activity and whether the episode was stereotypical (same as previous events). The report should note if there was a localized or generalized alteration in motor or nonmotor functions.

The school nurse should detail the student's level of awareness or consciousness, cognition, memory, emotional state, and behavior or arrest of behavior. The school nurse should document which parts of the body were involved and how, noting the sequence of the progression (Sirven et al., 2013b). The length and frequency of events is significant, as is the presence of a postictal period. It is also important to note significant eye or head deviation as this can provide insight regarding localization (Wilfong, 2022a). Such observations should be compiled into a seizure tracking tool. There are a variety of seizure tracking tools available, such as electronic seizure diary or tracker apps, and hard copy event diaries and calendars (Epilepsy Foundation, 2019c; Shafer et al., 2013). School nurses can initiate a seizure log at school to document seizure events that can also be used by the educational staff who witness seizures in the absence of the school nurse. See Online Materials OM27-1 for the Epilepsy Foundation's *My Seizure Event Diary* (2019c).

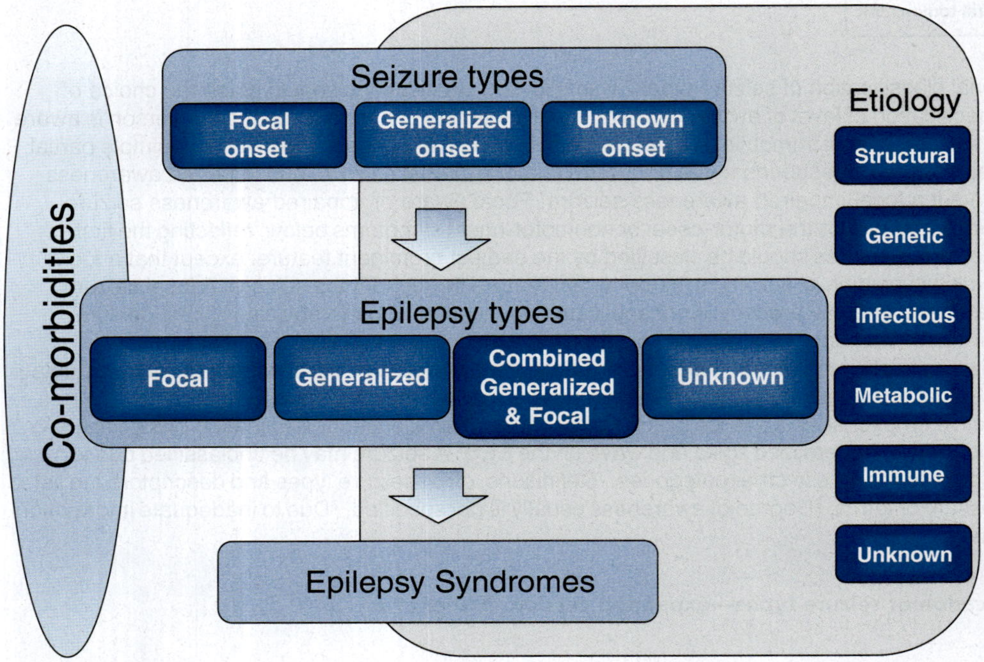

FIGURE 27-2. Framework for epilepsy classification. *(Scheefer et al., 2016) Used with permission.*

Data collection includes whether there is a history of seizures (including febrile seizures), labor and delivery complications, delayed developmental milestone, serious infections or illnesses, head trauma (especially resulting in loss of consciousness), drug or alcohol abuse, and family history related to epilepsy (Wilfong, 2022a). If the parent/guardian indicates that the student has had seizure activity at home, the school nurse can encourage the parent/guardian and relatives to video record any abnormal neurological activity that is suspected to be a seizure. This will enable the healthcare provider to visualize the activity and assist in determining a potential seizure diagnosis (Ricci et al., 2021).

A pediatric neurologist is the ideal healthcare provider to evaluate and diagnose a child who has experienced a seizure and to determine whether the child has epilepsy. The school nurse can facilitate this process of referral by connecting the parent/guardian with a local pediatric neurologist. This should be done in conjunction with the primary healthcare provider, who guides care in the medical home model. In rural areas where access to pediatric neurologists may not be available, the school nurse should collaborate with the student's primary healthcare provider to develop a realistic and feasible plan to have the student assessed by the most qualified healthcare provider who has clinical expertise in pediatric neurology.

The clinical expert in pediatric neurology will perform a complete physical and neurological examination to determine whether there are any abnormalities. An electrocardiogram should also be obtained as part of the complete physician assessment if any concern exists about a cardiogenic cause for the abnormal activity (Wilfong, 2022a). An EEG should be performed while both awake and asleep, as epileptiform activity is typically present only in one state (usually sleep). The findings on the EEG often enable the healthcare provider to determine the type of seizure activity. Knowing the type of seizure activity helps in the selection of antiseizure medications (ASMs) and treatment options.

Further testing may be indicated if the EEG is inconclusive in determining the presence of epileptiform activity. Brain magnetic resonance imaging (MRI) may be ordered to rule out the presence of brain lesions or damage that may precipitate seizure activity (Mountz et al., 2017). Genetic and metabolic screening may be indicated depending on the presenting symptoms, development, and history. If clinically indicated, routine blood work and a lumbar puncture may be a part of the diagnostic evaluation. The school nurse may help explain procedures in easily understandable language to help prepare students and families for diagnostic experiences.

TYPES OF SEIZURES

There are many different types of seizures. The sensations and presentations of seizure activity are unique to each individual and the type of epilepsy they have. Generally, seizures evolve over three phases (Epilepsy Foundation, 2019a).

The first is the ***beginning phase*** during which some people experience a prodromal stage and/or an aura (Epilepsy Foundation, 2019a). During a *prodromal stage*, a person senses hours or days before that a seizure is pending. They may experience signs such as mood changes, anxiety, light-headedness, insomnia, difficulty focusing, or other behavior changes. Some students may also experience *auras* during the beginning phase, which are thought to be the early part of a seizure. Auras are unusual feelings or sensations that come on abruptly and indicate that a seizure is about to occur. Students may get a feeling of *déjà vu* (i.e., "already seen" in French), or the illusion that something has happened before. Some students experience *jamais vu* (i.e., "never seen" in French) which is the feeling that a familiar situation is unfamiliar or is being experienced for the first time. Other aura sensations may include odd smells, sounds, or tastes; dizziness; visual disturbances; numbness or tingling; nausea; headache; and intense panic or fear (Epilepsy Foundation, 2019a). Students are typically very aware of their prodromal symptoms and auras. Reports by students with epilepsy of unusual sensations should be taken very seriously so that steps to prevent or limit a seizure can be taken immediately at school.

The middle or ***ictal phase*** denotes the time of the active electrical seizure activity in the brain (Epilepsy Foundation, 2019a). Depending on the type of seizure and epilepsy, signs and symptoms of the ictal phase may include altered or loss of consciousness; confusion; difficulty hearing; odd sensory phenomena (e.g., unusual smells, sounds, tastes); difficulty talking or saying strange words or utterances; tachycardia; respiratory distress; or other stereotypical seizure movements or manifestations. Different types and presentations of seizures are detailed below. During an active seizure, the school nurse or trained school personnel must activate the student's seizure action plan, initiate seizure first aid, and administer rescue seizure medications if ordered by a licensed prescriber (NASN, 2023, 2024b).

The ending or ***postictal phase*** is the period when the brain recovers from the ictal phase and the person experiences the physical and mental aftermath of the seizure activity (Epilepsy Foundation, 2019a). Again, depending on the type, intensity, and duration of the seizure, the postictal period may be brief, or it may take some time for the brain to return to baseline functioning. Students may display the following signs or symptoms after a seizure: altered levels of consciousness; confusion; thirst; weakness; sore muscles; complete or partial immediate memory loss; exhaustion or fatigue; and fear, anxiety, frustration, shame, or embarrassment. During the postictal phase the school nurse carefully assesses the student for injuries and determines the student's disposition according to their status and seizure action plan: whether the student can rest in the health office and return to class, whether the student should go home, whether immediate medical follow-up is needed, or whether emergency medical services (EMS)

> **Practice Connection**
>
> NASN's *School Nursing Evidence-Based Clinical Practice Guideline: Students With Seizures and Epilepsy* (2023) provides school nurses with current practice recommendations for providing high-quality care to students with seizure disorders. The guideline is a decision-making tool to help improve the health and safety of students with seizure disorders based on the most current, relevant, and highest quality of information available. Accompanying this clinical practice guideline, NASN has developed the *School Nursing Evidence-Based Clinical Practice Guideline: Students With Seizures and Epilepsy Implementation Toolkit* (2024b). This toolkit offers a robust compendium of resources to support quality nursing care and support services for these children at school, such as assessment and intake checklists and forms, sample individualized healthcare plans (IHPs), tips for developing individualized education programs (IEPs) and Section 504 plans, emergency action plans, training guides, and more. Visit the NASN webpages linked under *Resources* at the end of this chapter.

should be activated for transport to the nearest emergency department.

Focal Onset Seizures

Focal onset seizures originate in a distinct area of the cerebral cortex that can vary in location and presentation (Scheffer et al., 2017). The school nurse should note whether the student appears to be aware of their surroundings when experiencing a focal seizure. *Focal onset aware* seizures (previously called "simple partial seizures") occur when a student is awake and able to recall events during the seizure. Students displaying changes in their level of consciousness are experiencing *focal onset impaired awareness seizures* (previously called "complex partial seizures") (Fisher et al., 2017).

Motor symptoms of focal onset seizures include the following:

- *Clonic*—jerking
- *Atonic*—muscle limpness or weakness
- *Tonic*—muscle rigidity or tenseness
- *Myoclonic*—brief muscle twitching
- *Epileptic spasms*—brief flexion and extension of a leg, arm, or the head
- *Automatisms*—lip smacking, chewing, clapping, hand rubbing, running, verbal outbursts (Kiriakopoulos & Schafer, 2022b)

Nonmotor symptoms of focal onset seizures do not involve involuntary movements, but the person may be aware of sudden and unusual sensations such as the following:

- Changes in thinking or emotions
- Autonomic sensations (e.g., gastrointestinal sensations, hot or cold waves, goose bumps, tachycardia)
- Behavior arrest (e.g., all movement stops, staring) (Kiriakopoulos & Shafer, 2022b)

Generalized Onset Seizures

Generalized onset seizures occur when the eruption of abnormal brain activity involves both cerebral hemispheres, classified as motor or nonmotor (absence) (Scheffer et al., 2017). Students may experience complete loss of consciousness with no memory of the seizure (Fisher et al., 2017). There are three various types of generalized seizures: *atonic, tonic-clonic,* and *absence.*

- ***Atonic seizures*** cause students to lose muscle tone in all or part of their body. The loss of tone can be as minor as a drooping eyelid or as dangerous as falling to the floor (Kiriakopoulos & Shafer, 2022a). Atonic seizures are sometimes called "drop seizures."
- ***Tonic-clonic seizures*** include a stiffening and rhythmic jerking of a student's body. The onset of this type of seizure follows a process (Kiriakopoulos & Shafer, 2017). First, the *tonic* phase begins, causing the student's body to stiffen and lose consciousness. Then follows the *clonic* phase when the student's body jerks rhythmically and rapidly. Students may display apnea, cyanosis, incontinence, upper eye deviation, or increased salivation during the seizure (Sarkis et al., 2015). Following the conclusion of a generalized onset seizure, students display varied and individualized responses ranging from confusion and an inability to be aroused, to profound agitation; this is referred to as the *postictal period* (Chelse et al., 2013).
- ***Absence seizures*** are a type of generalized onset seizure that can be either *typical* or *atypical.* Students experiencing *typical absence seizures* are completely unresponsive and display a brief, 10- to 20-second blank stare with or without small movements such as fluttering of the eyelids or smacking of the lips (Pearl & Holmes, 2016). Absence seizures have an abrupt onset and ending, with total unresponsiveness but no loss of consciousness. Although consciousness is maintained, there is no memory of the event, and the individual usually resumes activity once the seizure ends (Kiriakopoulos & Shafer, 2019). *Atypical absence seizures* present similarly to *typical absence* seizures; however, the student may be able to interact with others during the seizure (Pearl & Holmes, 2016).

Unknown Onset Seizures

Unknown seizures are a diagnosis of exclusion, meaning healthcare providers can confirm a student has epilepsy, but test results are inconclusive or there is insufficient clinical information to determine whether the seizures are focal or generalized (Fisher et al., 2017; Scheffer et al., 2017). The seizure onset may not have been observed because the person was alone or asleep, or witnesses were not able to accurately observe or describe the seizure due to the stress or chaos surrounding the event. A diagnosis of unknown seizures may be temporary because further medical evaluation can often clarify the nature of the seizure disorder.

Several episodic phenomena involving motor, autonomic, sensory, and behavioral functions can mimic the presentation of epileptic seizures. These disorders include syncopes (convulsive, cardiac, orthostatic, and reflex), hyperventilation attacks, and psychogenic nonepileptic seizures (Romantseva & Lin, 2020; Stainman & Kossoff, 2020). Migraine headache presentation can mimic a seizure. In fact, migraine headaches and seizures commonly coexist (Gupta et al., 2015). Due to the unique nature of the antecedents to and etiologies of psychogenic seizures, as well as other related disorders, school nurses should collaborate with the student's healthcare providers to discuss approaches to assessment and management of these nonepilepsy disorders.

Seizure Presentations

Most seizure events present as a *single seizure* with stereotypical movement, meaning that they present similarly each time. There are instances when a seizure begins focally and progresses into a generalized seizure. An individual may have more than one seizure type. Seizures may be triggered by certain events, sounds, visual experiences, or general health status. Stress in general can be a precipitant of seizures (McKee & Privitera, 2017). When possible, it is important to identify triggers and to take steps to avoid or minimize them. The school nurse should ask about triggers to minimize exposure. The school nurse should also inform the healthcare team and a parent/guardian should any triggers be identified in the school environment. Potential triggers and risk factors can be found in Box 27-1.

BOX 27-1

Common Seizure Triggers

COMMONLY REPORTED SEIZURE TRIGGERS INCLUDE THE FOLLOWING:

- Specific time of day or night
- Sleep deprivation—overtired, not sleeping well, not getting enough sleep, disrupted sleep
- Illness (both with and without fever)
- Flashing bright lights or patterns
- Alcohol—including heavy alcohol use or alcohol withdrawal
- Drug use—use of cocaine and other recreational drugs such as Ecstasy/MDMA
- Stress
- Menstrual cycle or other hormonal changes
- Not eating well, long times without eating, dehydration, not enough fluids, low blood sugar, vitamin and mineral deficiencies
- Specific foods, excess caffeine or other products that may aggravate seizures
- Use of certain medications
- Missed medications

Epilepsy Foundation (2024a, para. 3).

Cluster seizures are a group of seizures that occur over a defined period of time of 6 to 24 hours that are different from the stereotypical single seizure event. They vary in number, length, and/or pattern. During cluster seizures the individual returns to baseline between seizures. Cluster seizures can occur with any seizure type. Forty-six percent of individuals with active seizures have a history of clusters (Detyniecki et al., 2018). Cluster seizures can evolve into status epilepticus or other seizure emergencies.

Status epilepticus is defined as a "a seizure that lasts more than 5 minutes or when seizures occur very close together and the person doesn't recover consciousness between them" (Singh, 2023, para. 1). Status epilepticus is a medical emergency requiring prompt treatment. There are two types of status epilepticus: convulsive status and nonconvulsive status. Even though the term "convulsion" is no longer used in the classification of seizures, it is still applied to status epilepticus.

Convulsive status epilepticus is when a person has a tonic, clonic, or tonic-clonic seizure lasting longer than 5 minutes. It can also present as a series of tonic-clonic seizures over a period of 5 minutes or longer where the person does not return to baseline between events. The dangers of status epilepticus are decreased oxygenation (resulting in acidosis), decreased cerebral perfusion, increased intracranial pressure, and hypoglycemia that can lead to morbidity and mortality (Rosenblum & Blosser, 2017). Status epilepticus is a medical emergency requiring prompt treatment with rescue medication(s) and activation of EMS for possible transfer to an emergency department. Sustained seizures lasting more than 30 minutes increase the risk of sudden unexpected death in epilepsy (SUDEP) (Singh, 2023).

Nonconvulsive status epilepticus describes "a single or repeated absence or focal impaired awareness seizures during which the person is not able to respond but is not displaying any movement or shaking of the body for longer than 10 minutes" (Singh, 2023, para. 7). These seizures may persist unless emergency treatment is initiated. Symptoms can be subtle in the absence of major motor activity. There may be associated confusion and lack of ability to communicate or respond appropriately. Treatment intervention is individualized based on the individual's presentation, underlying neurological condition, and interference in activities of daily living.

EPILEPSY SYNDROMES

Epilepsy syndromes are identified by characteristic seizure types, symptoms, and EEG findings (Specchio et al., 2022). Several features define each epileptic syndrome, including age of onset, family history, seizure type, genetic findings, and associated neurological signs and symptoms. Identification of an epileptic syndrome can guide healthcare providers in addressing seizures with medication or nonpharmacological treatments. Communication from the school nurse about seizure durations and characteristics can aid healthcare providers in identifying specific epileptic syndromes. Within the three categories of epilepsies (focal, generalized, and unknown), there are many epileptic syndromes with onset in childhood.

The ILAE reclassification of seizure types (Scheffer et al., 2017) led to the renaming of epilepsy syndromes (Specchio et al., 2022). Epilepsy syndromes are categorized into three groups: *self-limiting focal epilepsies, generalized epilepsies,* and *developmental and/or epileptic encephalopathies.* However, some epileptic syndromes not categorized by these three labels are considered *special syndromes.* Many epilepsy syndromes of childhood carry good prognoses. Some syndromes that emerge during the neonatal period resolve well before a child starts school (Scheffer et al., 2017).

Self-Limiting Focal Epilepsies

Self-limiting focal epilepsies include syndromes characterized by age-dependent occurrence in otherwise neurotypical children (Specchio et al., 2022). It is thought that genetic factors have an important role. Cognition and neurological functions are usually not affected. Almost all children with self-limiting focal epilepsies will experience remission by puberty. Examples of self-limiting focal epilepsy syndromes include the following:

- *Self-limited epilepsy with centrotemporal spikes* (SeLECTS)—formerly known as childhood epilepsy with centrotemporal spikes, (benign) Rolandic epilepsy, or (benign) epilepsy with centrotemporal spikes
- *Self-limited epilepsy with autonomic seizures* (SeLEAS)—formerly known as Panayiotopoulos syndrome, or early onset (benign) occipital epilepsy
- *Childhood occipital visual epilepsy* (COVE)—formerly known as late onset (benign) occipital epilepsy or idiopathic childhood occipital epilepsy–Gastaut type
- *Photosensitive occipital lobe epilepsy* (POLE)—formerly known as idiopathic photosensitive occipital lobe epilepsy (Specchio et al., 2022)

Generalized Epilepsy Syndromes

Generalized epilepsy syndromes are rare and associated with complex genetic origins. They may or may not be associated with environmental factors. Examples of generalized epilepsy syndromes include the following:

- *Childhood absence seizure* (CAE)—formerly known as pyknolepsy, or petit mal
- *Epilepsy with eyelid myoclonia* (EEM)—formerly known as Jeavons syndrome
- *Epilepsy with myoclonic absences* (EMA)—formerly known as Bureau and Tassinari syndrome (Specchio et al., 2022)

Did You Know?

The *Epilepsy Foundation* Web site (https://www.epilepsy.com) has a wealth of information, resources, forms, and links to help school nurses provide safe and quality care to students with seizures and epilepsy.

Developmental and/or Epileptic Encephalopathies

Developmental and/or epileptic encephalopathies (DEEs) represent epilepsies with developmental stagnation or progressive neurological deterioration that typically present in infancy. Developmental and/or epileptic encephalopathies are commonly associated with genetic causes (Specchio et al., 2022). Affected students have a range of cognitive, behavioral, and physical difficulties. Angelman syndrome and 15q inversion-deletion are examples of genetic causes associated with DEEs. Students with DEEs may have frequent seizures and multiple seizure types (multifocal) including epileptic spasms, tonic or atonic seizures, and myoclonic seizures. Examples of developmental and/or epileptic encephalopathies include the following:

- *Epilepsy with myoclonic atonic seizures* (EMAtS)—formerly known as Doose syndrome
- *Lennox–Gastaut syndrome* (LGS)
- *Developmental epileptic encephalopathy with spike-and-wave activation in sleep* (DEE-SWAS); epileptic encephalopathy with spike-and-wave activation in sleep (EE-SWAS)
- *Landau-Kleffner syndrome*
- *Febrile infection-related epilepsy syndrome* (FIRES)
- *Hemiconvulsion–hemiplegia–epilepsy syndrome* (HEE) (Specchio et al., 2022)

Due to advances in symptomatic and supportive management, many individuals with epilepsy associated with progressive neurological deterioration are living into adulthood (Gorodetsky & Fasano, 2022).

PHARMACOLOGICAL TREATMENT

Epilepsy treatment does not cure seizures or epilepsy. The goal of treatment is to allow the individual to lead an age-appropriate, typical lifestyle with optimal seizure control without or with minimal side effects. A variety of treatment options for seizures and epilepsy are available, including pharmacological, nonpharmacological, surgical, and alternative treatments. Pharmacological treatments have grown to include many types of antiseizure medications (ASMs). These medications are specifically targeted to treat various types of seizures and epilepsies (Vossler & Gidal, 2020). Approximately 30% of persons have epilepsy that is nonresponsive to at least two first-line antiseizure medications (Kumar, 2021). Nonpharmacological treatments, including dietary regimens, neurostimulation, and epilepsy surgery, are often indicated for these students.

In some cases, families may choose to use non–Food and Drug Administration (FDA)–approved herbal preparations, nutritional supplements, and medical marijuana in lieu of, or in combination with, approved medical therapies. The school nurse should initiate collaborative communication with the healthcare provider to be well informed of any epilepsy treatments, regardless of type, that a student may be receiving. The school nurse should always use nursing judgment to deliver school health services within the scope of practice standards, in accordance with the state's nurse practice act, and in compliance with federal and state legal rules and regulations (NASN, 2023).

Pharmacological treatment is typically the first line of treatment for children who experience two unprovoked seizures with medications tailored to each student's individual need (Kanner et al., 2018a). The healthcare provider must consider seizure type(s), adverse effects, dosing, compliance, and the parents'/guardians' fears and misconceptions about drug treatment (Swisher & Radtke, 2016). Healthcare providers aim to select an ASM with a minimal/manageable side-effect profile and that does not worsen comorbid conditions and/or behavioral concerns.

Antiseizure Medications

Monotherapy (single drug) is the ideal goal with pharmacological treatment, but it is not always possible for seizures that are difficult to control. Individuals receiving monotherapy are found to have better compliance, fewer adverse effects, and a decreased risk for potential drug interactions with other prescribed medications (Kanner et al., 2018a). When using polytherapy (two or more drugs), there is the possibility of increased negative side effects, drug interactions, and more complicated pharmacokinetics. Polytherapy is indicated after two failed monotherapies are trialed in succession, or if the first ASM is well tolerated, but fails to completely control seizure activity (Swisher & Radtke, 2016).

A variety of well-established medications are available to treat seizure disorders (Kanner et al., 2018b). New generation ASMs have been found to have equal or better efficacy and tolerability than the previous generation ASMs and in some instances are more beneficial for specific seizure syndromes. The new generation ASMs have simpler pharmacokinetics and less effects on liver metabolism (Abou-Khalil, 2022). Not all ASMs are FDA approved for use in children or for first-line treatment. However, many pediatric epilepsy centers prescribe these medications based on evidence that supports their efficacy and safety (Wilfong, 2021). See Table 27-1 for a list of frequently prescribed ASMs and side effects.

The school nurse must be aware of any and all medications the student is taking to assess for complications and monitor for adverse effects, regardless of whether or not the medications are administered during the school day (NASN, 2023). Some medications such as psychoactive, cardioactive, and analgesic drugs may decrease the efficacy of ASMs (Abou-Khalil, 2022), resulting in increased seizure activity or additional or more serious side effects.

Negative ASM side effects vary and may include sedation, fatigue, somnolence, lethargy, headaches, dizziness,

TABLE 27-1 Antiseizure Medications

Drug, Formulation, DEA Scheduling, FDA Indication, Dosing	Possible Adverse Reactions	Contraindications, Warnings, and Precautions
Brivaracetam (BRV) *Tablet; oral solution* *Focal onset; ≥4 yr* *By weight; bid*	Sedation, N/V, dizziness, anger, depression, anxiety, psychosis and disturbance in gait/coordination	Bronchospasm, angioedema, hepatic impairment
Cannabidiol (CBD) *Oral solution* *LGS, TSC, or DS; ≥1 yr* *By weight; bid*	Somnolence, decreased appetite, weight loss, diarrhea, rash, pruritus, angioedema	Monitor: ALT, AST, total bilirubin
Carbamazepine (CBZ) *IR/ER tablet, ER capsule, chewable, oral solution* *Focal onset, GTCS, mixed seizure types* *By weight; bid-qid*	Sedation, diplopia, ataxia, dizziness, blurred vision, hyponatremia, N/V, low WBC counts, decreased T3, T4, increased liver enzymes, worsens GTCS in PWE with absence seizures	SJS and TENS, aplastic anemia, agranulocytosis, DRESS Contraindicated: bone marrow suppression
Cenobamate (CNB) *Tablet* *LGS; adjunctive TX; ≥2 yr* *By weight; bid*	Sedation, fever, URI, drooling, constipation, UTI, insomnia, irritability, depression, dependence, withdrawal effects, vomiting, ataxia, bronchitis, pneumonia	Rash; use with opioid can cause profound sedation, respiratory depression, coma, and death

Continued

TABLE 27-1 **Antiseizure Medications—cont'd**

Drug, Formulation, DEA Scheduling, FDA Indication, Dosing	Possible Adverse Reactions	Contraindications, Warnings, and Precautions
Clonazepam (CZP) Schedule IV *Tablet, ODT tablet* *LGS, myoclonic and absence seizures* *By weight: divided 2 to 3 doses/day*	Sedation, dizziness, ataxia, hypersalivation, respiratory depression, porphyrogenic; impaired judgment, cognition, or motor skills Paradoxical agitation, irritability, anger, anxiety, nightmares, hallucination, psychosis, depression, dependence, tolerance	Use with opioid can cause profound sedation, respiratory depression, coma, and death Contraindications: acute narrow angle glaucoma, significant liver disease, sensitivity to BDZs
Ethosuximide (ESM) *Capsule (gel), oral solution* *Absence* *By weight; bid*	N/V, abdominal pain, anorexia, weight loss, diarrhea, sedation, dizziness, ataxia, leukopenia, HA, behavior changes, sleep disturbance, depression, hyperactivity, irritability, psychosis, hallucination, gingival hypertrophy, tongue swelling	SJS, rash, DRESS, leukopenia, agranulocytosis, pancytopenia, eosinophilia, systemic lupus erythematosus; abnormal liver and renal function tests
Everolimus (EVL) *Tablets for suspension* *TSC-associated focal; adjunctive TX; ≥2 yr; qd*	Stomatitis, noninfectious pneumonitis Bacterial, fungal, viral, and protozoal infection, including opportunistic infection Myelosuppression, embryofetal toxicity, pneumonia, irregular menses, fever, diarrhea, rash	Impaired wound healing, hypersensitivity, renal failure, thrombocytopenia, embryofetal toxicity
Felbamate (FBM) *Tablet, suspension* *LGS; adjunctive TX; ≥2 yr* *By weight; tid or qid*	HA, insomnia, N/V, abdominal pain, anorexia, weight loss, facial edema, anxiety, acne, rash, constipation, diarrhea, hypophosphatemia, rhinitis, infection, somnolence, ataxia, dizziness, tremor	Aplastic anemia, hepatic failure Contraindicated: history of blood dyscrasia or hepatic dysfunction
Fenfluramine (FEN) *Oral solution* *Schedule IV* *DS; ≥2 yr* *By weight; bid*	Decreased appetite, weight loss, diarrhea, somnolence, sedation, lethargy, increased blood pressure, angle closure glaucoma	Valvular heart disease, pulmonary arterial hypertension (REMS program is mandatory)
Gabapentin (GBP) *Capsule, tablet, refrigerated oral solution* *Focal onset; adjunctive TX; ≥3 yr* *By weight and age; tid*	Drowsiness, sedation, fatigue, ataxia, dizziness, nystagmus, diplopia, peripheral edema, fever, viral infection, nausea, vomiting, tremor	DRESS, anaphylaxis, angioedema; respiratory depression when used with CNS depressants, including opioids, or in the setting of underlying respiratory impairment; cognitive impairment; neuropsychiatric changes in children ages 3–12 yr
Lacosamide (LCM) *Tablet, oral solution (10 mg/mL)* *Schedule V* *Focal onset; ≥4 yr* *By weight; bid*	Dizziness, ataxia, diplopia, HA, nausea, atrial fibrillation, atrial flutter, and ventricular arrhythmias	Bradycardia, AV block and ventricular tachyarrhythmia, rarely resulting in asystole, cardiac arrest, and death; syncope (especially with diabetes), DRESS
Lamotrigine (LTG) *Tablet (standard, chewable, dispersible, orally disintegrating, ER)* *Focal onset: withdrawal to monotherapy; ≥16 yr* *Focal onset, LGS, primary TCS: adjunctive TX; ≥2 yr* *By weight; bid*	Dizziness, HA, diplopia, ataxia, nausea, vomiting, somnolence, insomnia in high doses, aseptic meningitis	Rash, SJS, TEN, DRESS

TABLE 27-1 Antiseizure Medications—cont'd

Drug, Formulation, DEA Scheduling, FDA Indication, Dosing	Possible Adverse Reactions	Contraindications, Warnings, and Precautions
Levetiracetam *(LEV)* *IR/ER tablet, oral solution* *Focal onset: ≥1 month* *Myoclonic in JME: adjunctive TX; ≥12 yr* *Primary TCS: adjunctive TX; ≥6 yr* *By weight and age; bid*	Somnolence, fatigue, asthenia, dizziness, infection, ataxia, incoordination, anemia, pancytopenia, leukopenia, neutropenia, agranulocytosis, thrombocytopenia	SJS and TEN, rhabdomyolysis, angioedema, anaphylaxis Irritability, aggression, depression, suicidal ideation, psychotic symptoms (especially in children)
Oxcarbazepine *(OXC)* *IR/ER tablet, oral suspension* *Focal onset* *Monotherapy: ≥4 yr* *Adjunctive TX: ≥2 yr* *By weight and age: bid*	Dizziness, cognitive problems, somnolence, fatigue nausea, HA, diarrhea, vomiting, URI, constipation, dyspepsia, ataxia, coordination problems, nervousness, pancytopenia, agranulocytosis, leukopenia; hyponatremia	SJS and TEN, DRESS; anaphylaxis, angioedema, cross hypersensitivity with CBZ
Perampanel *(PER)* *Schedule III* *Tablet, oral solution (0.5 mg/mL)* *Focal onset: ≥4 yr* *Primary GTCS: adjunctive TX; ≥12 yr* *Fix dosing: qd*	Dizziness, vertigo, somnolence, fatigue, irritability, hostility, aggression, anger, mental status changes, HA, ataxia, anxiety, paranoia, euphoric mood, agitation, falls, nausea, vomiting, weight gain, abdominal pain	Homicidal ideation, suicidal thoughts, DRESS
Phenobarbital *(PB)* *Schedule IV* *Tablets, elixir* *Focal onset and generalized onset* *By weight and age: qd*	Sedation, cognitive slowing, HA, depression, N/V, tolerance, dependence, confusion, decreased REM sleep, hepatic dysfunction, osteoporosis, megaloblastic anemia with chronic use, hypoventilation, bradycardia, and hypotension With pain: agitation or delirium Children: irritability, hyperactivity, reduced IQ	SJS, TEN, DRESS, rash, angioedema, respiratory depression, synergistic effects with ETOH or sedatives, psychological and physical dependence; barbiturate withdrawal can cause convulsions and delirium and may be fatal
Phenytoin *(PHT)* and fosphenytoin *(FOS)*: *PHT delayed-release capsule, suspension* *Focal onset, GTCS* *By weight; bid or tid*	Nystagmus, ataxia, coordination impairment, dysarthria, cognitive slowing, gingival hyperplasia, rash, hypertrichosis, lymphadenopathy, pseudolymphoma, lymphoma, Hodgkin disease, thrombocytopenia, leukopenia, pancytopenia, osteoporosis, decreased vitamin D level activates porphyrogenia	SJS and TEN, DRESS, angioedema, hepatotoxicity
Pregabalin *(PGB)* *Schedule V* *Capsule, oral solution* *Focal onset; adjunctive TX; ≥1 month* *By weight; bid or tid*	Dizziness, somnolence, dry mouth, peripheral edema, blurred vision, weight gain, ataxia, attention and concentration problems	Angioedema (face, mouth, throat, larynx), hives, dyspnea, wheezing; respiratory depression with concomitant CNS depressants or with underlying respiratory impairment
Primidone *(PRM)* *Schedule IV* *Tablet* *Focal onset and TCS; monotherapy* *By weight and age; tid or qid*	Diplopia, nystagmus, drowsiness, ataxia, vertigo, N/V, fatigue, irritability, emotional disturbance, impotence	Rash, RBC hypoplasia and aplasia, agranulocytosis, megaloblastic anemia Contraindicated: porphyria, PB allergy

Continued

TABLE 27-1 Antiseizure Medications—cont'd

Drug, Formulation, DEA Scheduling, FDA Indication, Dosing	Possible Adverse Reactions	Contraindications, Warnings, and Precautions
Rufinamide *(RUF)* ***Tablet*** ***LGS; adjunctive TX; ≥1 yr*** ***By weight; bid***	Leukopenia HA, N/V, dizziness, fatigue, ataxia, gait disturbances, somnolence, coordination problems	DRESS, Rash, SE
Stiripentol *(STP)* ***Capsule, powder for suspension*** ***DS; adjunctive TX with clobazam; ≥2 yr*** ***By weight; bid***	Somnolence, decreased weight and appetite, neutropenia, thrombocytopenia, agitation, ataxia, hypotonia, nausea, tremor, dysarthria, insomnia	Alcohol and other CNS depressants may increase sedation and somnolence
Tiagabine *(TGB)* ***Tablet*** ***Focal onset; adjunctive TX; ≥12 yr*** ***bid***	Dizziness, N/V, somnolence, fatigue, tremor, cognitive slowing, anxiety, diarrhea, abdomen pain	Serious rash, moderately severe generalized weakness
Topiramate *(TPM)* ***Tablet, capsule (IR and ER), sprinkle*** ***Focal onset and GTCS; ≥2 yr*** ***LGS: adjunctive TX; ≥2 yr*** ***qpm or bid***	Language and cognitive (confusion, memory, word-finding, attention, concentration) disturbances Kidney stones Paresthesia, anorexia, weight loss, fatigue, somnolence, dizziness, anxiety, depression or mood problems, abnormal vision, fever, taste perversion, diarrhea, hypoesthesia, nausea, abdominal pain, URI	SJS and TEN; acute myopia with secondary angle closure glaucoma and vision loss, visual field defects; oligohydrosis and hyperthermia (especially in children); chronic untreated MA may lead to decreased growth in children, increased alkaline phosphatase level, hypophosphatemia, and osteomalacia
Valproic acid *(VPA)* and divalproex sodium ***Tablet (IR and ER), capsule, sprinkle*** ***Focal onset and absence; monotherapy*** ***Multiple seizure types that include absence; adjunctive TX*** ***By weight; qd for ER; bid or tid***	Hyperammonemia, thrombocytopenia, coagulopathy, hypothermia Abdomen pain, alopecia, blurred vision, anorexia, ataxia, amnesia, asthenia, back pain, constipation, depression, diarrhea, diplopia, dizziness, dyspepsia, dyspnea, emotional lability, fever, infection, HA, increased appetite, insomnia, N/V, nervousness, nystagmus, peripheral edema, pharyngitis, rash, rhinitis, abnormal thinking, tinnitus, tremor, weight gain or loss	DRESS, pancreatitis Substantial risk of major congenital malformations with gestational exposure Contraindications: women of childbearing potential and pregnancy
Zonisamide *(ZNS)*Capsule ***Focal onset; adjunctive TX; ≥16 yr*** ***qd***	Somnolence, fatigue, anorexia, weight loss, dizziness, ataxia, agitation, irritability, depression, psychosis, speech or language disturbance, psychomotor slowing, kidney stones, rash, hyperammonemia, and encephalopathy Acute myopia and secondary angle closure glaucoma	SJS, TEN, DRESS, hepatic necrosis, agranulocytosis, decreased WBC counts, aplastic anemia, oligohydrosis and hyperthermia in children, hyperchloremic MA Chronic untreated MA may lead to decreased growth rate in children, increased risk of kidney stones, increased alkaline phosphatase level, hypophosphatemia, osteomalacia

ALT, Alanine aminotransferase; *AST,* aspartate aminotransferase; *bid,* twice a day; *BP,* blood pressure; *CNS,* central nervous system; *DEA,* Drug Enforcement Administration; *DRESS,* drug reaction with eosinophilia and systemic symptoms (multiorgan hypersensitivity); *DS,* Dravet syndrome; *ECG,* electrocardiogram; *ER,* extended release; *GTCS,* generalized tonic-clonic seizure; *HA,* headache; *IR,* immediate release; *JME,* juvenile myoclonic epilepsy; *LGS,* Lennox-Gautaut syndrome; *MA,* metabolic acidosis; *N/V,* nausea and vomiting; *ODT,* oral disintegrating tablet; *PWE,* person with epilepsy; *qd,* once daily; *qpm,* every afternoon or evening; *REM,* rapid eye movement; *REMS,* risk evaluation and mitigation strategies; *SJS,* Stevens-Johnson syndrome; *TEN,* toxic epidermal necrolysis; *tid,* three times a day; *TCS,* tonic-clonic seizure; *TSC,* tuberous sclerosis complex; *TX,* treatment; *URI,* upper respiratory infection; *UTI,* urinary tract infection; *WBC,* white blood cell.
See drug manufacturer product information for details.
Adapted from Vossler & Gidal (2020).

insomnia, anorexia, and gastrointestinal upset (Verotti et al., 2020). The school nurse should work with families and teachers to ensure appropriate accommodations are in place to meet the needs of students experiencing adverse side effects from ASM treatment so that impairment in school function is minimized.

Students experiencing somnolence and fatigue should be allowed to briefly rest in the health office, which may be all they need to continue with their day. Headaches and dizziness can also be negative side effects of ASMs. These symptoms may require medical orders for ibuprofen or acetaminophen for resolution. The presence and severity of ASM side effects and prescribed medication at school to address side effects should be recorded and reported to parents/guardians and healthcare providers at scheduled intervals so that appropriate changes to the medication regimen may be made. A change in medication may be needed if the side effects significantly affect learning, increase in intensity, change behavior, or do not resolve within a reasonable amount of time.

If insomnia is a problem, dosing earlier in the day to avoid sleep problems may be helpful. If anorexia, nausea, or gastrointestinal problems occur, it may be helpful for students to take their medication with or just after meals (if not contraindicated). If anorexia leads to weight loss and growth suppression, it is essential to ensure that the student is getting quality calories to support growth. Dietary supplements such as nutritional shakes or high-protein bars may be indicated. The school nurse should monitor the student's weight and height every few months and notify the prescribing healthcare provider if any significant deviations from expected growth parameters are observed. Dosage and type of medication prescribed may also need to be adjusted as the student grows and enters puberty. The school nurse can assist in tracking the need for medication adjustment by monitoring the presence of breakthrough seizures and any other changes in symptoms.

School nurses should provide education and reminders to students and parents/guardians about important considerations related to the student's prescribed medication regimen. For example, good dental hygiene is imperative for students taking phenytoin, which may cause gingival hyperplasia. Divalproex sodium may result in hair loss or breakage and platelet dysfunction resulting in excessive bruising/bleeding; a multivitamin with zinc and selenium may be recommended for brittle hair (Vossler & Gidal, 2020). To establish the most effective dose, the healthcare provider will periodically order blood work to monitor serum concentrations of certain ASM medications, as well as detect alterations in liver or kidney function and determine the extent of medication compliance. It is important for therapeutic levels of ASMs to be maintained; thus it may be helpful to have an extra dose of medication available at school (accompanied by appropriate clinician order) for days a home dose is missed.

Both epilepsy and long-term ASM therapy are associated with decreased bone density and subsequent osteoporosis, which increases the risk for fractures. Students taking ASMs are also at risk for impaired bone growth and vitamin D deficiency (Vossler & Gidal, 2020). The school nurse should encourage bone protective interventions for students, including adequate exposure to sunlight, a balanced diet, and maintaining optimal levels of physical activity (Ziemba, 2022).

Warnings and Precautions Associated With Antiseizure medications

All ASMs carry a specific warning for suicide. The school nurse should immediately report signs of the emergence or worsening of depression, suicidal ideation, self-harm, or other unusual changes in mood or behavior to the parent/guardian and healthcare provider. Specific use of opioids with other central nervous system depressants, such as benzodiazepines, increases the risk of life-threatening overdose (Laing et al., 2021; Liu et al., 2021). Concomitant use of benzodiazepines and opioids may result in profound sedation, respiratory depression, coma, and death.

Some ASMs can decrease the effectiveness of hormonal birth control medications (Bangar, 2016). Additionally, there is an increase in the incidence of birth defects in pregnant individuals who take ASMs, especially when treated with polytherapy. Therefore the school nurse should counsel students with epilepsy who are engaging in sexual activity to speak with their healthcare provider about effective contraception methods and family planning.

Seizure Rescue Medications

Rescue medications are typically ordered for seizure clusters and when a seizure lasts more than 5 minutes (status epilepticus). Parameters for seizure emergencies vary by individual student and will typically be outlined by the healthcare provider in the student's seizure action plan (SAP) discussed in more detail later in this chapter. The rescue medications of choice are benzodiazepines because of their fast action. Until 2019, rectal diazepam (Valium) was the only FDA-approved rescue medication prescribed for students with refractory seizures at school (Dean et al., 2021). Rectal diazepam (Diastat®) is FDA approved for use in children ages 2 years and older. It may be the preferred rescue medication for some children, especially those under 6 years old.

However, for obvious reasons, the administration of rectal valium presents issues related to the student's privacy and dignity. Additionally, when a nurse is not immediately available, the delegation of rectal valium administration can be complicated. State nurse practice acts and state legislation vary widely across states regarding the delegation of healthcare tasks and whether the administration of rescue seizure medications in the school setting is allowed. Delegation requires careful assessment, planning, and training of unlicensed assistive personnel (UAP) by the school nurse. However, many school personnel are not comfortable with administering a controlled substance or a medication rectally. See Chapters 6, 30, and 31 for more detailed discussions of the principles of delegation.

Fortunately, in recent years intranasal forms of benzodiazepines have been approved by the FDA for children. Intranasal diazepam (Valtoco®) is FDA approved for children 6 years of age and older (Neurelis Inc., 2021). Midazolam nasal spray (Nayzilam®) is FDA approved for children ages 6 and older (UCB Inc., 2021). Although the school nurse must still carefully plan and train UAP (when permitted), these intranasal rescue medications are easier to administer, do not require partially undressing the student, and have established safety profiles.

Oral, buccal, or sublingual benzodiazepines (e.g., lorazepam, clonazepam) are not FDA approved as seizure rescue medications for children; however, the school nurse may see these medications prescribed off-label. Oral routes for these medications have limitations including the risk of harm to the person administering the drug and risks for the student, namely increased oral secretions and aspiration (Gidal et al., 2020).

The school nurse should communicate closely with the family and licensed prescriber and advocate that the least invasive and most effective seizure rescue medication is ordered for school (NASN, 2023). A list of seizure rescue medications, potential adverse events, and clinical implications can be found in Table 27-2.

NONPHARMACOLOGICAL TREATMENT

Roughly one-third of individuals with epilepsy have a refractory form, which means that adequate trials of two well-tolerated, appropriately chosen ASM regimens have not been effective in maintaining adequate seizure control (Sultana et al., 2021). Nonpharmacological therapies such as neurostimulation, seizure alert devices, dietary regimens, and epilepsy surgery may be considered for therapeutic management of refractory seizures and epilepsy.

Vagus Nerve Stimulators

The *vagus nerve stimulator* (VNS) is an implantable device, often used in conjunction with ASMs, for individuals age 4 years or older with refractory focal seizures who are not candidates for surgical resection (FDA, 2017). The aim of the VNS is to reduce the frequency and/or severity of seizures. This system consists of two internal components (an implantable battery powered pulse generator [a pacemaker-like device] and stimulating leads) and three external components (programming wand, programming device, and magnet). The pulse generator is placed under the left chest wall with the lead tunneled from the device to the left vagus nerve in the neck where it is attached by a coiled electrode. See Figure 27-3.

The device is turned on in the operating room or at the child's first appointment after surgery with the neurologist. The neurologist or seizure specialist will postoperatively (within 2 weeks) program the device to deliver the desired strength and timing of impulses and will readjust the settings on an outpatient basis. New generation VNS therapy can be programmed to control seizures in different modes via a wireless device (LivaNova, 2024). *Normal mode* helps to prevent seizures by delivering stimulation at regular programmed intervals during the day. *AutoStim mode* delivers stimulation in response to rapid increases in heart rate, which may indicate a seizure.

Magnet mode manually delivers stimulation when a handheld magnet (i.e., wand) is swiped or briefly held over the

TABLE 27-2 Seizure Rescue Medications

Drug, Indication, Schedule	Route and Form	Potential Side Effects and Important Considerations
Diazepam (Diastat®) *Schedule IV* *Dosed by weight and age* *FDA approved for children ≥2 yr*	Rectal gel	Sedation, dizziness, depression, fatigue, motor and cognitive impairment; use with opioids can cause respiratory depression, coma, and death; contraindicated in narrow-angle glaucoma; maintain privacy and dignity by shielding procedure from view
Diazepam (Valtoco®) *Schedule IV (individual spray units = 5 mg, 10 mg, 15 mg, 20 mg)* *Dosed by weight and age* *FDA approved for children ≥6 yr*	Intranasal spray	Central nervous system (CNS) depression, somnolence, headache, nasal discomfort; use with opioids can cause respiratory depression, coma, and death; contraindicated in narrow-angle glaucoma
Midazolam (Nayzilam) *5 mg* *Schedule IV* *FDA approved for children ≥12 yr*	Intranasal spray	CNS depression, somnolence, impaired cognition, headache, nasal discomfort, runny nose, throat irritation; use with opioids can cause respiratory depression, coma, and death; contraindicated in narrow-angle glaucoma

See drug manufacturer product information for details.
Adapted from Vossler & Gidal (2020).

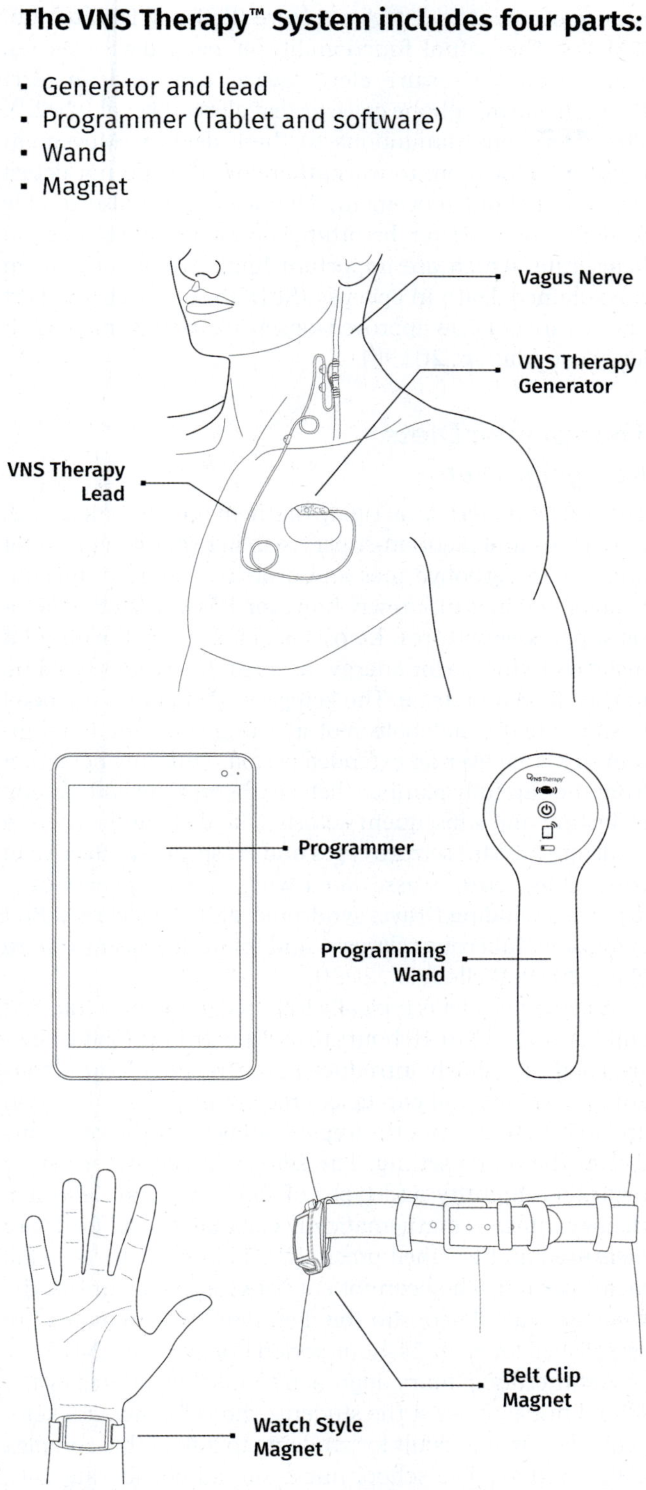

FIGURE 27-3. The vagus nerve stimulator therapy system. *(Liva Nova, 2022. With permission.).*

generator either by the patient or a witness to stop or decrease the duration of the seizure. Typically, the VNS magnet is worn on the student's wrist or attached to the student's belt or book bag. Swiping the magnet across the device gives an extra "dose" of stimulation. The magnet is swiped from the middle of the chest across the device at the onset of a seizure or on presentation of an aura (an unexpected sensory or perceptual experience before the start of a seizure) or a focal aware seizure. This can result in preventing the seizure from occurring, shortening the duration of the seizure, or shortening the length of the postictal period. Each swipe should be the amount of time it takes to say "one-one thousand." The swiping procedure can be done every 1 to 2 minutes as directed by provider orders. Swiping the device with the magnet can be done numerous times throughout the day without injury to the student (LivaNova, 2022). However, if the seizure does not stop as expected, a rescue seizure medication can be administered if indicated (see Table 27-1). A student's seizure action plan (SAP) should identify the appropriate actions to take if the seizure or seizure cluster does not stop, including any emergency protocols that should be put into place (NASN, 2023).

The mechanism of action of VNS therapy is not well understood. However, it is known that the VNS does alter activity in several regions of the brain (medulla, cerebellum, and thalamus), causes brain wave synchronization as visualized on EEG, and alters the concentrations of various neurotransmitters within the central nervous system (Wang et al., 2021). Approximately 60% of pediatric patients with VNS stimulators report a reduction or improvement in seizure activity at 24 months after implant (LivaNova, 2024).

The negative side effects of a VNS are typically mild and commonly include hoarseness, coughing, throat pain, shortness of breath, tingling, and muscle pain. Coughing improves if the parameters of the stimulation device are adjusted. Tolerability of side effects typically improves over time. Surgical site infection occurs in about 5% of cases and is typically treated with systemic antibiotics (FDA, 2017). Vocal cord paralysis may also occur after surgery. VNS therapy can potentially exacerbate obstructive sleep apnea, which may result in poor seizure control (Joshi et al., 2013). Certain medical or imaging procedures, such as MRI or radiation treatment, can potentially damage the generator or leads. Electric devices with a strong magnetic field or electric current, such as some tablet computers, should be kept at least 6 inches from the chest where the generator is implanted (LivaNova, 2022).

The VNS can also be turned off by taping the magnet over the device on the left chest wall. This is done if the stimulation is uncomfortable, negative side effects occur that do not resolve, or the student wants to speak without being interrupted by hoarseness. Once the magnet is removed from the device, the stimulation process resumes at the predetermined parameters. The healthcare provider will provide instructions regarding use of the VNS and the circumstances in which the device may be turned off; a parent/guardian should be notified if the device is turned off.

The ideal candidate for VNS therapy is an individual who is capable of manipulating the magnet independently at the onset of a seizure (Joshi et al., 2013). However, motor or cognitive disabilities do not exclude individuals from being treated with VNS therapy. In this case, the caregiver would activate the device upon the onset of a seizure. If state nurse practice act delegation rules allow, the nurse may teach UAP to use the device if a school nurse is not readily available.

Other Neurostimulation Modalities

Less commonly, school nurses may care for students with other neurostimulation modalities, such as responsive neurostimulation or deep brain stimulation (Starnes et al., 2019). A *responsive neurostimulation* (RNS) device continuously monitors brain waves and responds to unusual electrical activity. When unusual electrical activity is detected, the device responds within milliseconds by giving a small amount of stimulation to an area of the brain. The objective is to deliver the small burst of stimulation and assist brainwaves to return to normal before clinical symptoms occur (Iyengar & Shafer, 2017). The RNS® System is FDA approved for individuals 18 years of age and older with focal or partial seizures. The device is adjustable and reversible. The stimulator is positioned in the skull. Very small wires going from the stimulator are placed in one or two places on top of the brain where seizure activity may begin. The exact placement and programming of an RNS is individualized. Programming may need to be adjusted based on seizure activity (Iyengar & Shafer, 2017). Although the RNS device is not currently approved for individuals less than 18 years of age, there have been published case reports of off-label implantation in pediatric patients with evidence showing significant reduction in seizure activity (Kokoszka et al., 2018; Nagahama et al., 2021; Singhal et al., 2018).

Deep brain stimulation (DBS) includes the placement of a device in the brain with thin wires that carry electrical impulses from the neurostimulator device directly to the brain. The purpose of DBS is to stop brain signals that cause seizures. The device is programmed to deliver the stimulation in a preset cycle. Therefore DBS does not directly respond to a seizure. The DBS device can record and report information from the brain that may be useful when making future treatment decisions. DBS is currently FDA approved for individuals 18 years of age and older (Kiriakopoulos, 2018). Randomized controlled trials are lacking in pediatric patients. Systematic reviews and some case reports have presented findings from the off-label use of DBS in patients younger than 18 years of age showing a reduction in seizures (Benabid et al., 2002; Khan et al., 2021; Tykocki et al., 2021; Valentín et al., 2017; Velasco et al., 2006; Yan et al., 2021).

Seizure Alert Devices

Seizure alert devices do not stop or prevent a seizure from happening, but they can alert others that the student is about to have a seizure by detecting repeated shaking movements. Mattress, watch, camera, or motion devices are available. They work best in individuals with tonic-clonic or focal motor seizures because seizure alert devices need movement to detect a seizure (Epilepsy Foundation, 2019b). The actual functionality of each device varies. Many available seizure alert devices can send an alert through alarms, phone calls, or text alerts (Li et al., 2022). There are some limitations to these devices. Movement is required for them to work; therefore they do not detect seizures without movement. The devices are also unable to detect or alert for breathing problems or changes in heart rate, which are important implications for sudden unexplained death in epilepsy (SUDEP). Last, seizure alert devices are not FDA approved for seizure management (Epilepsy Foundation, 2019b).

Therapeutic Diets

Ketogenic Diet

The *ketogenic diet* is a rigid, mathematically calculated, physician- and dietitian-supervised diet that is high in fat and low in carbohydrates and protein. The exact mechanism of action is unknown; however, it is known that ketosis suppresses seizures. Ketosis is achieved by burning fat instead of glucose for energy; as a result, ketones build up in the blood and urine. The ketogenic diet allows the body to simulate the metabolism of a fasting state and to maintain this state over an extended period. Thus any deviation from the carefully planned diet can disrupt the body's state of fasting and subsequent ketosis. The diet can be used in all drug-resistant seizure types and is especially effective in controlling seizures associated with several epilepsy syndromes, including Dravet syndrome, glut-1 deficiency, Rett syndrome, tuberous sclerosis, and infantile spasms (Meira et al., 2019; Wells et al., 2020).

A ketogenic diet is typically initiated in the hospital. The child fasts for 24 to 48 hours to assist with developing ketosis. Foods are slowly introduced over the next 3 days. Parents/guardians and caretakers receive in-depth education and instruction about the implementation of the ketogenic diet in the home setting. The ketogenic diet is very strict regarding quantity and types of food and drink allowed. Dietary intake is mathematically calculated, and foods are measured and weighed precisely. Children eat three small meals per day. They cannot eat between meals unless the foods are calculated into the diet. Fluid requirements are established for each 24-hour period (Meira et al., 2019).

An interdisciplinary approach should be initiated by the school nurse to assist the student who is following a ketogenic diet. It is difficult for students to follow this complex diet at school. The school nurse should collaborate with the healthcare provider, dietitian, teachers, staff, parent/guardian, and child, if appropriate, in developing appropriate accommodations at school (NASN, 2023). Classroom teachers, paraprofessionals, specialists, dietary staff, and other school community members involved in the student's care and activities must be educated about the diet so that they are aware of the restrictions. The school nurse must emphasize that even a small deviation from the carefully calculated meal plan, such as a single piece of candy or cookie, can reset the body's ketotic state, thus eliminating the antiseizure effects of the diet for about 2 weeks (Meira et al., 2019; Ruan et al., 2022; Wells et al., 2020).

The teacher and school nurse should have ketogenic diet–compliant snacks that the student can eat in the event that parties or special occasions are celebrated in school; however, this should be discussed in advance with a parent/guardian to ensure that any supplemental intake is calculated into the student's meal plan for the day. The complexities involved with implementation of a ketogenic diet call for the school nurse, healthcare provider, parent, and school to work collaboratively to develop a mutually agreed upon plan to ensure that the regimen is adhered to. For young students, this may involve assigning a paraprofessional to assist with and monitor meal intake as prepared by the parent/guardian. Any potential or actual deviations should be communicated to the school nurse and parent/guardian immediately.

Side effects of the ketogenic diet include gastrointestinal upset (nausea, vomiting, diarrhea, and constipation), hypercholesterolemia, and kidney stones (Newmaster et al., 2022). The school nurse should monitor the student for the presence of gastrointestinal side effects and kidney stones and communicate observations to the parent/guardian and healthcare provider. Students should have their urine checked for ketones several times per week (Newmaster et al., 2022). If the parents/guardians are unable to consistently check ketones at home, medical orders for ketone checks at school may need to be obtained and incorporated into the student's IHP. Any deviation from expected urine ketone parameters should immediately be reported to the parents/guardians and healthcare provider. Students on ketogenic diets are at risk of falling into lower height and weight percentiles. The school nurse should monitor height and weight and report any abrupt or significant changes. These students also need to be monitored for severe dehydration, especially in warmer weather; indoor recess may be recommended during hot weather.

The ketogenic diet should be tried for 3 months to determine its efficacy in seizure control. Approximately 50% of children with drug-resistant epilepsy experience a decrease in seizures by the first year on the diet (Newmaster et al., 2022). Students on a ketogenic diet can usually decrease the frequency and dose of ASMs. Despite efficacy, up to 50% of individuals discontinue the diet within the first 6 months and less than 10% continue to follow the diet after 1 year (Martin-McGill et al., 2020). This is likely due to the challenges related to maintaining an extremely structured, restrictive diet for school-age children and families.

Modified Diets

The *modified Atkins diet* (MAD) and the *low glycemic index treatment* (LGIT) are two other diets used for epilepsy. The MAD diet was developed in an attempt to have a more palatable and less restrictive diet than the ketogenic approach. Carbohydrates are initially restricted to 10 g/day for the first month and then slowly increased to 15 to 30 g/day as tolerated based on seizure control. Fats are encouraged. There are no protein, calorie, or fluid restrictions (Wells et al., 2020). The LGIT diet considers the glycemic index of foods to address epilepsy. The glycemic index is the measure of a food's tendency to increase the glucose level in the blood. Numerous factors affect the glycemic index, such as particle size, type of starch, starch gelatinization, presence of fat, acidity, and fiber content of foods. In the LGIT diet, the individual is allowed 40 to 60 g/day of low-glycemic carbohydrates with a glycemic index of less than 50. Fats are encouraged, but there are no protein, calorie, or fluid restrictions. A dietitian gives general guidelines for this diet, but the student and family must read food labels. Adherence to this diet is typically much easier (Wells et al., 2020). Both the MAD and LGIT diets have the potential for similar side effects as the ketogenic diet, and students on these diets must receive regular consultation from clinicians and dietitians, as well as monitoring by the school nurse.

Epilepsy Surgery

Epilepsy surgery is a treatment option for individuals whose seizures are refractory to other treatment options. An individual with a single, well-localized focus of epileptiform activity is the ideal candidate for epilepsy surgery (Joshi et al., 2013). Uncontrolled seizures in children are associated with increased mortality as well as poor cognitive and psychosocial outcomes (Fine & Wirrell, 2020). Therefore surgery should be considered early for students with drug-resistant epilepsy because of the potential for improved health and quality of life outcomes. Prospective surgical candidates undergo a detailed history and physical, noninvasive EEG and video EEG, structural and functional neuroimaging, cognitive testing, and a family social work evaluation (Joshi et al., 2013). Healthcare providers must also consider family and student perceptions of seizure control before a decision is made to proceed with epilepsy surgery.

Depending on the location of the epilepsy, surgical options include anterior temporal lobectomy, focal resection, corpus callosotomy, hemispherectomy, and subpial transections. Outcomes vary depending on the surgery performed and the type of epilepsy and seizures being treated. Approximately 70% of infants, children, and youth obtain a seizure-free postoperative outcome (Jayalakshmi et al., 2017). Overall, younger age at surgery or onset of epilepsy is predictive of favorable postoperative seizure outcomes (Ryvlin et al., 2014).

While positive developmental, cognitive, and quality of life outcomes can be expected in many cases, epilepsy surgery may be accompanied by significant adverse outcomes, including perioperative death and the development of postoperative neurological deficits (Jayalakshmi et al., 2017). Although a surgeon will provide education related to the procedure, the school nurse may be called on as a resource to educate the staff regarding risks and benefits of treatment, as well as to plan for any sequelae that affect the child when returning to the school setting. Continuation of ASM therapy is typically recommended for at least 6 months postoperatively with subsequent reassessment for the need for pharmacotherapy. If seizures persist but are better controlled than before surgery, the goal is to wean the ASM regimen to a lower dose and ultimately achieve seizure control with monotherapy (Wilfong, 2022b).

Alternative Treatments

Since the early 2000s, the treatment of seizures using alternative treatments, such as herbal preparations, supplements, and homeopathic remedies, has significantly increased. Little is known about the efficacy and adverse effects of these preparations. Furthermore, because herbals and homeopathic medications are not regulated by the FDA, preparation and labeling are not consistent and independently evaluated by a regulatory body. Lack of information on these substances makes it difficult for healthcare providers to give proper advice regarding use.

Examples of herbals used in the treatment of epilepsy include valerian root, kava, and black cohosh. Homeopathic remedies used to treat seizures include mistletoe, American hellebore *(Veratrum viride)*, and skullcap *(Scutellaria lateriflora)* (Bell, 2015). School nurses should provide culturally competent care and respect parents'/guardians' choices regarding complementary or alternative therapy that aligns with their culture. However, it is important for the school nurse to stress to parents/guardians the need to discuss the use of herbal preparations and supplements with the healthcare team because of risks for significant negative side effects, drug interactions, nephrotoxicity, hepatotoxicity, and worsening of the existing condition.

Medical marijuana is increasingly considered as an alternative treatment, with several open-label research studies in progress to explore the potentially beneficial effects of cannabidiol (the nonpsychoactive compound of cannabis) in controlling seizures (Patel, 2018). Students with long-term drug-resistant epilepsy may be involved in such studies. Although many states have legalized medical and/or recreational marijuana, the FDA has yet to approve smoked or ingested marijuana (containing THC) for any medicinal purposes (DeWitt-Parker, 2016; FDA, 2020).

Cannabidiol (CBD) oral solution (Epidiolex) is the first FDA-approved drug that contains a purified drug substance derived from marijuana. This medication is FDA approved as a Schedule V medication to treat seizures associated with Lennox-Gastaut syndrome and Dravet syndrome in patients 2 years of age and older (FDA, 2018). CBD is considered a Schedule V controlled substance, which means that it can be administered by nurses if ordered (U.S. Drug Enforcement Administration, 2018).

If a parent/guardian requests that the school nurse administer a homeopathic treatment, herbal remedy, or another non–FDA-approved medical marijuana product at school, the school nurse should encourage the parent/guardian to consult with the healthcare provider to schedule adjunctive therapies to be taken at home. State laws, nurse practice acts, and school policies in most states prohibit the presence of marijuana on school grounds. Administration of medical marijuana at school (other than Epidiolex) would violate these regulations. Additionally, the school nurse must understand the active ingredients, actions, dosing, and side effects of any administered therapeutic agent. Because most alternative medications are not ordered by a healthcare provider and are not FDA approved, most states prohibit school nurses from administering them. According to NASN (2022),

> *When deciding whether or not to incorporate the use of non-FDA approved therapies or dietary supplements into school nurse practice, it is important that the school nurse first determine what is known about the product, such as ingredients, precautions, recommended dose, and any potential adverse effects. Secondly, determine whether administration is allowable under federal and state law, including applicable state nurse practice acts, and district policy. (para. 4)*

Well-meaning school nurses who administer alternative therapeutic agents at school can inadvertently put their students at risk of harm and themselves at risk for liability.

PROGNOSIS

Different outcomes and responses to treatment may be expected across epileptic syndromes. Most epilepsies can be well controlled with pharmacological management, and many children may eventually discontinue their antiseizure medications (Beghi et al., 2015). Approximately 65% of children with epilepsy achieve complete remission, defined as freedom from medications and seizures for at least 5 years (Berg et al., 2014). Among children diagnosed with seizure onset before the age of 2 years, 53% are seizure free (i.e., defined as no seizure activity for 2 years or longer) by the age of 7 (Stödberg et al., 2022).

Numerous factors can indicate a poor prognosis for seizure cessation, including epilepsy onset after 10 years old, developmental delays, history of generalized tonic-clonic seizures, and generalized abnormalities on the EEG (Berg et al., 2014). Although teachers and other students may misunderstand the capabilities of students with epilepsy (Kolar Sridara Murthy et al., 2016), most students with epilepsy are able to participate in all school activities.

Sudden Unexplained Death in Epilepsy

Sudden unexplained death in epilepsy (SUDEP) is when death following a seizure is not caused by drowning, trauma, status epilepticus, or other potential causes (Harden et al., 2017). SUDEP is rare. The annual incidence rate of SUDEP is 1.16 cases per 1,000 individuals with epilepsy (Thurman et al., 2014). Seizure freedom is strongly associated with reduced risk of SUDEP (Harden et al., 2017). Students with uncontrolled generalized tonic clonic seizures and seizures that occur at night are at greatest risk for SUDEP. Missing medication doses and drinking alcohol may also result in suboptimal seizure control and increase the student's risk for SUDEP (Scorza et al., 2020; Sveinsson et al., 2020). Empowering students and families with knowledge about strategies to reduce the risk of SUDEP is an important preventive measure (Mesraoua et al., 2022). School nurses can educate students and families about the importance of taking their seizure medication as prescribed (right dose and right time) and avoiding seizure triggers to reduce the number of seizures. School nurses are also well-positioned to discuss the importance of not using alcohol with their students who have epilepsy.

SCHOOL NURSING CONSIDERATIONS

Whether a student has their first seizure at school, has frequent seizures at school, or their seizures are well managed and they rarely or never have a seizure at school—school nursing care of students with seizures is complicated and requires expertise and extensive planning.

School Nurse Case Management

School nurses provide case management of students with seizures and epilepsy. School nurse–led case management is a collaborative and interdisciplinary approach involving the student, their family, healthcare team, and the school team (NASN, 2021). Case management is a comprehensive, holistic, and evidence-based strategy to providing high-quality school health services for these students. See Chapter 20 for general principles of case management and caring for students with special healthcare needs.

Fortunately, NASN and the Epilepsy Foundation provide robust resources to support school nurses to fulfill this professional responsibility. School nurses should employ the practice recommendations outlined in NASN's *School Nursing Evidence-Based Clinical Practice Guideline: Students With Seizures and Epilepsy* (2024a) to foster the health, safety, and education of students with seizure disorders. In addition, a compendium of resources and strategies can be found in the *School Nursing Evidence-Based Clinical Practice Guideline: Students With Seizures and Epilepsy Implementation Toolkit* (2024b). This toolkit has practical documents such as assessment checklists, intake forms, sample IHPs, tips for developing IEPs and Section 504 plans, emergency action plans, training guides, and more.

Further, funded by the CDC and the U.S. Department of Health and Human Services, NASN is engaged in the *Coordinated Support System for Students With Epilepsy* (2024a). "The project's goal is to build school nurse capacity and confidence to assess and address the physical, emotional, and social needs of students with epilepsy—and to connect students and families with a network of community-based supports, resources, and self-management programs" (para. 3).

Focus on the Framework

The *Coordinated Support System for Students With Epilepsy* puts each of NASN's School Nursing Practice Framework (2024c) principles into action.

Care Coordination

- Provide case management for students with epilepsy.
- Develop individualized healthcare plans (IHPs), emergency action plans/emergency care plans (EAPs/ECPs), and emergency evacuation plans (EEPs).
- Participate in the development of 504 plans.
- Educate students on self-management, including medications, safety plans, and stigma.
- Coordinate with students, families, healthcare professionals, and school personnel to assess for and address any gaps in accessing health care.
- Share resources such as community support groups for student and families.
- Provide transition planning.
- Identify and educate school staff on potentially stigmatizing/bullying school experiences.

Community/Public Health

- Facilitate access to specialty care.
- Educate school staff and student peers in the classroom on disease management.
- Address stigma associated with seizures and find advocates to support students with epilepsy as they progress through their education.
- Provide culturally effective health care to students and address social needs that affect health equity, including access to medical insurance, medications, shelter, food, and other social needs.

Leadership

- Lead policy development addressing chronic disease management, transition planning, and stigma/bullying for students with epilepsy.
- Implement healthcare transition planning and speak about stigma in IEP and 504 meetings.

Quality Improvement

- Track health outcome trends and evaluate interventions designed to improve the health and quality of life of students with epilepsy.
- Document and track health office visits.
- Assess for signs and symptoms of mental health challenges, including comments from students that may point to stigma and bullying, such as anxiety, fear, or avoidance of certain classes or school activities.

Continued

Focus on the Framework—cont'd

- Track patterns in seizure activity at school and report to families and healthcare providers.

Standards of Practice

- Maintain competence, including being knowledgeable of and implementing NASN's *School Nursing Evidence-Based Clinical Practice Guideline: Students With Seizures and Epilepsy* (https://learn.nasn.org/courses/63321#).
- Follow the state nurse practice act.
- Use critical thinking in the care of students with epilepsy (NASN, 2024c, p. 4).

Visit the webpages linked under *Resources* at the end of this chapter to access these resources.

Health and Education Plans

The appropriate accommodations to meet the health, safety, and educational needs of a student with epilepsy should be outlined in the student's Section 504 plan or individualized education program (IEP). The type of plan depends on whether the individual student needs accommodations to participate in the regular curriculum (Section 504) or special education services (IEP); yet the nursing services in either plan may look similar. Student goals in the IEP or Section 504 plan are individualized according to the student's unique needs. Examples of student goals related to nursing services might include the following:

- Decreased unnecessary emergency room visits
- Increased return to class when safe and appropriate (e.g., student returns to baseline)
- Decreased number of inpatient hospital admissions among students with seizures and epilepsy who receive rescue medication in the school setting, when indicated
- Decreased number of school absences
- Increased safe inclusion in as many school activities as possible
- Facilitated identification and allocation of resources for students with epilepsy who may have developmental or learning needs
- Decreased time spent out of the classroom
- Improved student academic success
- Increased opportunities for full participation in all school activities
- Improved quality of life
- Improved mental well-being
- Decreased social isolation
- Improved transition from pediatric to adult care (NASN, 2023, pp. 6–7)

It is the school nurse's responsibility to have an IHP and a seizure action plan (SAP) on file for every student with epilepsy. The IHP should be based on the student's current health status and medical orders. Remember that IHPs are nursing care plans written by nurses for nurses. IHPs are written in nursing language and contain protected health information and therefore are not suitable for distribution to lay staff.

Seizure Action Plans

A *seizure action plan* is "seizure-specific treatment plan signed by the healthcare provider which includes parameters for emergency care in the event of a prolonged seizure, prescribed rescue medications and instructions for use, as well as emergency contact information" (NASN, 2023 p. 9). A SAP from the Epilepsy Foundation (or other professional organization) can be used as part of the IHP (Sirven et al., 2013a).

The student's SAP is based on the principles of seizure first aid and serves as an easy-to-understand guide for unlicensed school staff to follow in the absence of a school nurse. The SAP organizes all the information about the student's epilepsy treatment in one place. It provides individualized guidance from the student's healthcare provider about parameters for returning to the classroom, when to be sent home, when to administer a rescue medication if prescribed, when to seek emergency services, and/or when the student should go to the emergency department. The SAP is developed in collaboration with the input of the healthcare provider, the family, the student if developmentally appropriate, and the school nurse (Dean et al., 2021; Sirven et al., 2013a). The SAP helps school personnel know what to do to prevent an emergency and/or how to respond in emergency situations. The key components of an SAP include the following:

- Student and emergency contact information
- Seizure information: type and typical presentation
- Types of protocols indicated at school
- Seizure first aid
- When rescue therapy is needed and what to do
- Care after the seizure
- Special instructions for first responders and the emergency department
- Daily seizure medications
- Other health information, such as seizure triggers, allergies, surgeries, neurostimulator device, diets, and so on

- Healthcare contacts
- Signatures of parents/guardians and healthcare provider (Epilepsy Foundation, 2020a)

The school nurse can initiate an SAP on behalf of a student and work in collaboration with the healthcare team, parents/guardians, and student (as appropriate) to finalize it. School nurses are responsible for making sure all of the key elements are included in the SAP and updated by the healthcare provider when management strategies change. School nurses are also responsible for making sure school personnel responsible for responding to a student's seizure have access to the SAP and that they understand the specific directions. SAP templates are available from organizations such as the Epilepsy Foundation (see Resources), Epilepsy Alliance, and Seizure Action Plan Coalition. Templates help to present the information in a uniform manner so that school nurses and school personnel know where to look for the information that they need when the student has a seizure or an emergency arises. Individual school districts may also have a preferred SAP template (Dean et al., 2021). Annual review and update of the student's SAP is necessary if a change in health status or seizure control occurs.

The school nurse should carefully consider with whom and how the SAP is shared at school, keeping in mind that it contains confidential protected health information and more details than most school personnel need to know. Additionally, medication changes during the academic year may make it challenging to keep the SAP current. The school nurse should consult with parents/guardians before a student's seizure diagnosis is shared at school. The school nurse must consider whether administration of prescribed rescue medication by UAP adheres to the parameters of the state regulations, the state's nurse practice act, and the principles of delegation.

When delegation is not appropriate, or for school or transportation personnel who are only expected to give basic seizure first aid (see following section), the school nurse can develop a very simple and brief emergency action plan (EAP). The EAP outlines for school personnel: IF YOU SEE THIS (symptoms/seizure activity)—then DO THIS (specific seizure first-aid step). The school nurse also should take advantage of teaching opportunities to educate school personnel about epilepsy, handling seizure emergencies, and methods to empower and support students with epilepsy. Students with epilepsy have the right to positive social and educational experiences despite their disability. The school nurse should keep a record of who is in receipt of an SAP or EAP, what training has been done, and who has participated.

Barriers to managing seizures in the school setting include the absence of a school nurse and insufficient education of school personnel (Terry et al., 2016). School nurses can overcome these barriers by collaborating with clinicians, families, and school personnel to ensure that appropriate medical orders and action plans are developed and implemented appropriately in the school setting (Butler et al., 2020; Dean et al., 2021). See Chapter 8 for detailed discussion of developing IHPs, Section 504 plans, IEPs, and EAPs for students with special healthcare needs.

Seizure First Aid

No one can predict if, when, and where a student will have a seizure. Therefore all school personnel should be prepared. The primary goal of seizure first aid is to keep the student safe during a seizure (Epilepsy Alliance America, 2024). It is the school nurse's responsibility to make sure that school staff members are trained to respond to a student appropriately. General first aid principles apply to all seizures, regardless of type. A student should never be left alone during a seizure and should always be supported by an individual appropriately trained in seizure first aid. A plan should be in place to maintain the student's privacy and keep other students or unnecessary observers away, especially if the seizure occurs in the classroom. A seizure record, observation record, or electronic tracking application can be used to record thorough observations of the seizure. The school nurse should educate teachers, school staff, and bus drivers and transportation aides about first aid for seizures. The Epilepsy Foundation (2024) has flyers that can be posted or distributed (Fig. 27-4) containing first aid considerations to guide teaching of school staff. Refer to the school district policy regarding how to handle medical emergencies that occur on the school bus.

It is not necessary to contact EMS for every seizure that occurs in the school setting. The healthcare provider will indicate what constitutes a seizure emergency for an individual student on the student's SAP. For students with known epilepsy and seizure disorders, most seizures do not require a visit to an emergency department if it is within the parameters of the student's typical seizure activity. When exhibiting typical seizure activity, sending a student to the emergency department is unnecessary and inconvenient, and it places undue financial burden on the family and healthcare system for a costly ambulance transport and emergency evaluation. A seizure is generally considered an emergency in the following circumstances:

- Seizure lasts longer than 5 minutes
- Repeated seizures
- Difficulty breathing
- Seizure occurs in water
- Person is injured, pregnant, or sick
- Person does not return to their usual state
- First-time seizure
- The person asks for medical help (Shafer, 2022, When to call for emergency help)

Injury Prevention

Students with epilepsy are at risk of being injured during a seizure. Seizures can lead to abrupt falls with loss of protective reflexes and loss of consciousness, potentially

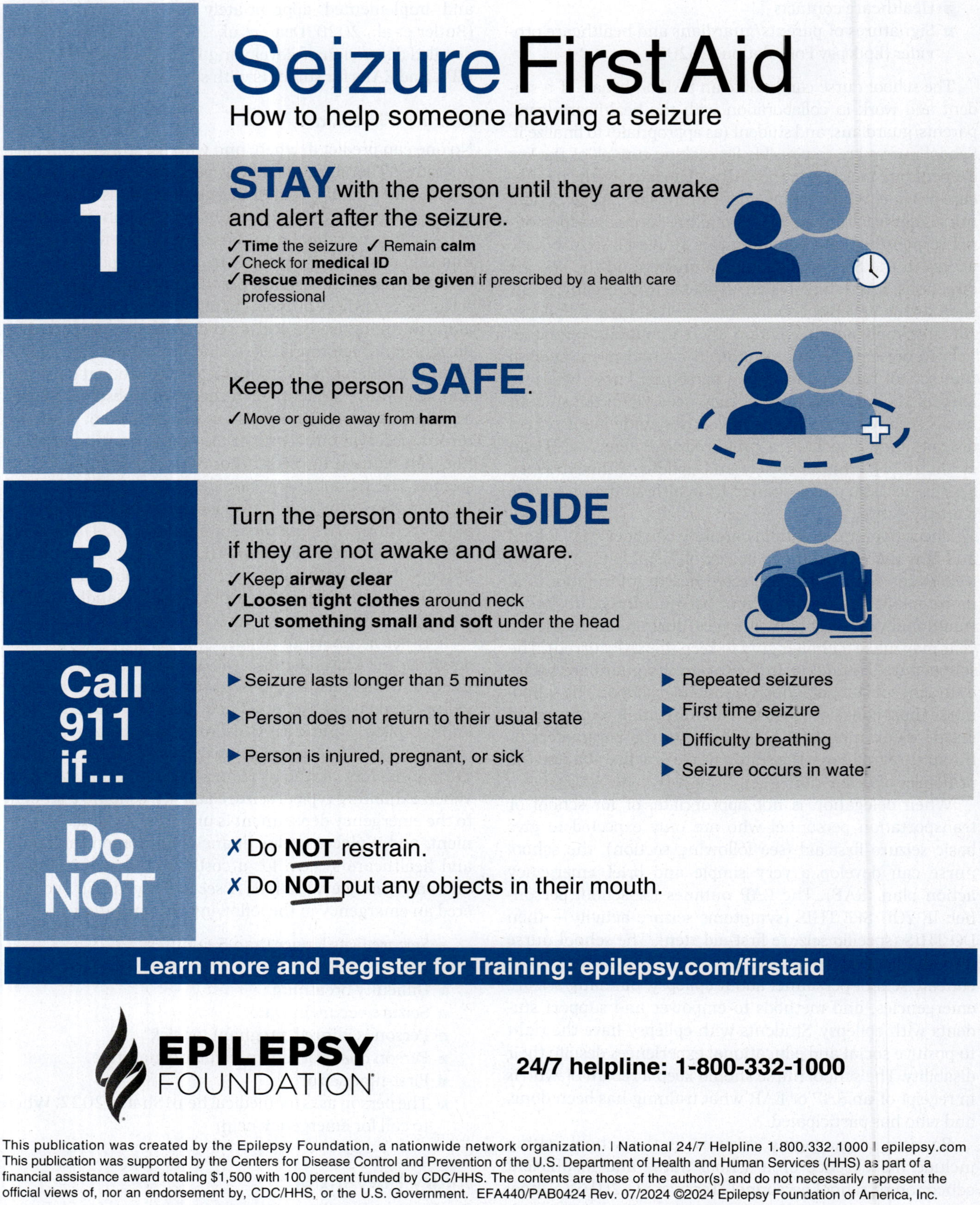

Seizure First Aid

How to help someone having a seizure

1 — **STAY** with the person until they are awake and alert after the seizure.

- ✓ **Time** the seizure ✓ Remain **calm**
- ✓ Check for **medical ID**
- ✓ **Rescue medicines can be given** if prescribed by a health care professional

2 — Keep the person **SAFE**.

- ✓ Move or guide away from **harm**

3 — Turn the person onto their **SIDE** if they are not awake and aware.

- ✓ Keep **airway clear**
- ✓ **Loosen tight clothes** around neck
- ✓ Put **something small and soft** under the head

Call 911 if...

- ▶ Seizure lasts longer than 5 minutes
- ▶ Person does not return to their usual state
- ▶ Person is injured, pregnant, or sick
- ▶ Repeated seizures
- ▶ First time seizure
- ▶ Difficulty breathing
- ▶ Seizure occurs in water

Do NOT

- ✗ Do **NOT** restrain.
- ✗ Do **NOT** put any objects in their mouth.

Learn more and Register for Training: epilepsy.com/firstaid

EPILEPSY FOUNDATION®

24/7 helpline: 1-800-332-1000

This publication was created by the Epilepsy Foundation, a nationwide network organization. | National 24/7 Helpline 1.800.332.1000 | epilepsy.com
This publication was supported by the Centers for Disease Control and Prevention of the U.S. Department of Health and Human Services (HHS) as part of a financial assistance award totaling $1,500 with 100 percent funded by CDC/HHS. The contents are those of the author(s) and do not necessarily represent the official views of, nor an endorsement by, CDC/HHS, or the U.S. Government. EFA440/PAB0424 Rev. 07/2024 ©2024 Epilepsy Foundation of America, Inc.

FIGURE 27-4. Seizure first aid. *(Epilepsy Foundation, 2024b). Used with permission.*

resulting in burn, orthopedic, dental, soft tissue, head, and submersion injuries (Lagunju et al., 2016). Generally, exercise does not trigger seizures. Being active and participating in sports benefits the physical and mental health of students with seizures as it does for all students. Students with epilepsy are not at greater risk than other students of being injured during sports. Efforts should be made to allow students with epilepsy full participation in school activities. However, students with active seizures may need to limit participation in certain sports and school activities to ensure their safety (Sirven et al., 2013c). A school nurse should work with the student's healthcare team to identify accommodations to maximize engagement at school.

School nurses should educate students, families, and school staff members about seizure precautions in special circumstances, including heights, high heat, water, using mechanical equipment and heavy machinery, and driving. Safety precautions for each student should be evaluated and applied on an individual basis. However, general safety precautions to avoid injury are generally the same for all students with seizures. Table 27-3 suggests precautions for physical activities for students with severe seizure disorders; adult supervision is required for all special activities listed.

If an adult's presence is not expected, a responsible "buddy" should accompany the student during the activity when developmentally appropriate. There must be a balance between safety and providing the student with the best possible life experiences, including enjoying social and physical activities with peers. School nurses can work with other school staff and administrators to ensure these safety measures are a standard part of the student's accommodations at school.

Mental and Behavioral Health Considerations

Approximately one in three individuals with epilepsy has a mental health comorbidity (Lu et al., 2021). Mood and anxiety disorders are most common in adult patients, while attention deficit-hyperactivity disorder is the most common coexisting diagnosis for school-age children (Auvin et al., 2018). The school nurse is positioned to identify mental health issues in students with epilepsy. As a trusted professional in the school setting, the nurse may be the first person to whom a student confides their feelings. Appropriate referrals and collaboration with the primary healthcare provider, mental health provider, parent/guardian, teachers, school social worker, counselor, and school psychologist can assist the student by tailoring medical regimens and school accommodations to improve mental health outcomes for students with epilepsy.

TABLE 27-3 Safety Considerations for Students With Active Seizures

Concern	Activity	Precautions
Height	Rope climbing, rock climbing, parallel bars	Wear a fitted helmet
		Ensure soft ground (e.g., mulch) is beneath equipment
	Playground	
	Bunk bed use	Select bottom bunk
Heat	Oven and stove use	Turn pot and pan handles inward, toward the center of the stove
	Bunsen burner use and campfires	Ensure student is far enough away from flame that the student would not fall into flame if a seizure occurs
Water	Swimming	Never swim alone; 1:1 adult assigned in pool
		Keep student's head above water in event of a seizure, remove from water as soon as possible.
		Initiate cardiopulmonary resuscitation (CPR) if student stops breathing.
		Call emergency services for any seizure activity in water
Mechanical equipment/ heavy machinery	Mechanical or electrical power tool use	1:1 supervision required
	Driving	Laws related to licensure, physician report to state, or need for a seizure-free period before driving vary; see http://www.epilepsy.com/driving-laws for state-specific information
Sports/physical activity	Climbing, biking, roller blading/ skating, ice skating, horseback riding, ice hockey	Wear a fitted helmet
	Boxing	Participation not recommended; suggest wrestling

Source: Adapted from Epilepsy Foundation (2013b).

Depression is also a common comorbid mental health condition occurring with epilepsy. The prevalence rate of depression among individuals with controlled epilepsy is 10% to 20%, and 20% to 60% in those with intractable epilepsy (Leeman-Markowski & Schachter, 2015). Depression is not well recognized in individuals with epilepsy and is often undertreated. Furthermore, as noted earlier, antiseizure medications carry *black box warnings* regarding potential increased risk for suicide. Given these facts, suicide is 10 times more common in people with epilepsy compared with the general population (Leeman-Markowski & Schachter, 2015). See Chapter 28 for a discussion on depression in children and youth and the emergency interventions that must be taken to protect students with suicidal ideation.

Individuals with seizure disorders also have an increased risk of psychosis compared with those without epilepsy. Interictal (between seizures) psychosis is the most common form of psychosis found in individuals with epilepsy, whereas postictal (after a seizure) psychosis is less common (Akanuma et al., 2020). Individuals with interictal psychosis typically respond better to treatment with medication. Postictal psychosis is characterized by hallucinations, paranoia, and delusional thoughts. The symptoms usually begin within several days of a cluster of seizures (Leeman-Markowski & Schachter, 2015).

Anxiety disorders affect approximately 20% to 40% of individuals with epilepsy (Rocamora et al., 2021). Anxiety disorders are most seen between seizures, usually manifested as a generalized anxiety disorder. Interictal anxiety disorders can occur during seizure freedom and are not necessarily related to seizure frequency. Both pharmacological and behavioral approaches to treatment may be helpful to students with seizures and anxiety (Holmes, 2021; Leeman-Markowski & Schachter, 2015).

Impulsive and aggressive behaviors also may manifest interictally. Preictal irritability or actual aggression can occur minutes, hours, or days before a seizure event (Leeman-Markowski & Schachter, 2015). Ictal aggression is rare, but may be manifested as purposeful, aggressive, or violent behaviors during a seizure event. Postictal aggression can be manifested as "resistive violence," which results from being physically restrained during a seizure. Violent behaviors can also be seen with a postictal psychosis. Assessing, monitoring, and communicating the manifestations of coexisting mental health disorders are integral to quality school nursing interventions and psychological well-being of students with epilepsy.

Quality of Life

Epilepsy can have a significant impact on academic achievement, family and social relationships, and social and emotional wellness. The school nurse and educational team must consider the psychosocial, cultural, educational, and occupational effects of an epilepsy diagnosis. Optimal seizure control supports student and family well-being in all aspects of quality of life, not just physical health (Austin, 2016; Fayed et al., 2021; Rozensztrauch & Kołtuniuk, 2022).

Decreases in quality of life for students with epilepsy and their families are associated with healthcare utilization, hospital admissions, and increased healthcare costs (Ryan et al., 2016). Therefore identifying any negative effects on a student's quality of life following a diagnosis of epilepsy is essential to supporting optimal wellness and minimizing lost instructional time.

Students with epilepsy are at risk for developing learning problems, cognitive impairment, and social or familial isolation secondary to epilepsy and its treatment (Austin, 2016; Beghi et al., 2015). School nurses take a leading role in identifying the health barriers to learning associated with epilepsy and ensuring that the appropriate health and education plans are implemented for eligible students.

A thorough assessment of quality of life can aid the school nurse in identifying problems that affect the student and family. Many questionnaires have been developed and validated to assess quality of life in students with epilepsy. These tools examine social experiences, academic functioning, psychological or behavior changes, and issues encountered as a family and in the community (Austin, 2016). They can also measure levels of stigma, engagement in social activities, and unexpected fatigue (Goodwin et al., 2015).

Data obtained from a comprehensive quality of life evaluation can assist the school nurse and school support professionals (e.g., social workers, counselors) to collaborate with the student's healthcare team to make appropriate adjustments in treatment, identify educational needs, make necessary referrals for mental health and other services, and assist with social skills and opportunities to achieve optimal medical, developmental, social, and educational outcomes.

Transition Planning

School nurses guide families and support students during periods of transition. Transition planning is appropriate and necessary when students reenter the school environment after a prolonged absence or hospitalization, move between schools, or prepare for life after their school years such as postsecondary education or employment. A clearly defined and coordinated transition plan helps to ensure the student does not experience gaps in their medical care or academics. Periods of transition can be challenging for the student and the family. Students may experience increased stress, behavior changes, and reduced quality of life (NASN, 2019). For students with epilepsy, becoming more independent with self-management and increasing knowledge of their disease may be overwhelming (Wilson et al., 2022). At the same time, families may struggle to give the student more independence for fear of negative consequences (Goselink et al., 2022).

Each student has their known individual medical and academic needs, but unplanned situations can also arise during a time of transition (Pieters et al., 2021). The challenges associated with transition planning appear to increase for students moving from pediatric to adult settings or secondary- to post–secondary-school environments (Epilepsy Foundation, 2018; Pieters et al., 2021). The school nurse and the student support team can help facilitate a seamless transition by speaking with the student and family about their medical and academic goals and coordinating and communicating a systematic plan of transition with all stakeholders, such as the student, family, healthcare providers, academic partners, and employers (NASN, 2019).

Employment

Many factors can contribute to lack of employment among youth with epilepsy, especially for those with uncontrolled seizures. Many individuals with epilepsy face employment discrimination. The Americans With Disabilities Amendment Act (ADA) was enacted in 2008 to fight job discrimination against those with chronic conditions. The original purpose of the ADA was to assist individuals with epilepsy and other disabilities to obtain and retain employment. Many jobs are safe for students with epilepsy, but others may pose risks. Before accepting a job position, an adolescent with epilepsy should have a realistic discussion with their family and healthcare provider about the safety of jobs that involve dangerous machinery, power tools, height requirements, or other potential injuries (Epilepsy Foundation, 2013a). See Chapters 7, 8, and 20 for more discussion on transition planning.

Seizure Safe Schools Legislation

The Epilepsy Foundation (2022) is leading an initiative to ensure that all schools in the United States are prepared and equipped to provide a safe learning environment for students with epilepsy. Being prepared and equipped means that schools have trained personnel (e.g., nurses, teachers, staff, coaches, volunteers) to recognize and respond to a student experiencing a seizure and the tools necessary for successful management (Epilepsy Foundation, 2022). The initiative includes a foundation for state-level legislative bills based on the following five key elements:

- School staff (anyone working with the student) are required to complete training on seizure recognition and first-aid response training.
- The student's file must include the SAP, and the plan must be made available to any school staff or volunteers responsible for the student.
- FDA-approved medications prescribed by the student's provider can be administered even when the school nurse is not available.
- Educating and raising awareness among the school community about epilepsy and first-aid response.
- A Good Samaritan clause for those acting in good faith in response to a student having a seizure.

These elements may vary between states. School nurses need to stay informed about school seizure legislation in the state where they practice (Epilepsy Foundation, 2022). If these essential elements of seizure safe schools are not state mandated, school nurses can contact their state lawmakers and work with their NASN state affiliate to lobby for enactment of this important legislation. If seizure safe school legislation is in place, school nurses should take the lead to ensure that the school district is compliant with the required policies, protocols, and procedures.

CONCLUSION

Seizures and epilepsy are common neurological disorders of childhood; students have seizures at school. School nurses must be competent regarding seizures and epilepsy diagnosis, treatment, prognosis, and quality of life issues. Effective management of seizures in the school setting requires school nurses to actively engage in every step of the nursing process. The school's readiness to respond to seizures and support the student's safety in the learning environment decreases anxiety for the students, parents/guardians, staff, and classmates. School nurses act as healthcare providers, health educators, case managers, liaisons, and advocates. They improve coordinated care for students with epilepsy by fostering open lines of communication among the student, the family, the school staff, and the healthcare team. The role of the school nurse in seizure management is integral to improving both health and educational outcomes for students with seizure disorders.

The Editors gratefully acknowledge the work of the previous chapter authors, Brenna Quinn and Angela Lepkowski.

Resources

Centers for Disease Control and Prevention. *Epilepsy guidance for schools.* https://www.cdc.gov/epilepsy/php/guidance-for-schools/?CDC_AAref_Val=https://www.cdc.gov/epilepsy/groups/schools.htm

Epilepsy Alliance America. (2024). *On-demand seizure first aid training for school personnel.* https://www.epilepsyallianceamerica.org/seizure-safety/seizure-first-aid-training-for-school-personnel-your-way/on-demand-seizure-first-aid-training-for-school-personnel/

Epilepsy Foundation. https://www.epilepsy.com/

Epilepsy Foundation. (2020a). *Seizure action plan.* https://www.epilepsy.com/sites/default/files/atoms/files/SCHOOL%20Seizure%20Action%20Plan%202020-April7_FILLABLE.pdf

Epilepsy Foundation. (2024). *Seizure first aid.* SeizureFirstAidPoster%20Rev07-2024.pdf

National Association of School Nurses. (2023). *School nursing evidence-based clinical practice guideline: Students with seizures and epilepsy.* Author. https://learn.nasn.org/courses/63321/documents/94882

National Association of School Nurses. (2024a, January). *Coordinated support system for students with epilepsy.* https://learn.nasn.org/courses/54876

National Association of School Nurses. (2024b, February 5). *School nursing evidence-based clinical practice guideline: Students with seizures and epilepsy implementation toolkit.* Author. https://learn.nasn.org/courses/63450

References

Abou-Khalil, B. W. (2022). Update on antiseizure medications 2022. *Continuum (Minneapolis, Minn.), 28*(2), 500–535. https://doi.org/10.1212/CON.0000000000001104

Akanuma, N., Adachi, N., Fenwick, P., Ito, M., Okazaki, M., Hara, K., Ishii, R., Sekimoto, M., Kato, M., & Onuma, T. (2020). Individual vulnerabilities to psychosis after antiepileptic drug administration. *BMJ Neurology Open, 2*(2), e000036. https://doi.org/10.1136/bmjno-2019-000036

Americans With Disabilities Amendment Act (ADAA) of 2008. (2009). 42 U.S.C. § 12101–12102. https://www.ada.gov/regs2016/adaaa.html

Austin, P. (2016). Quality of life in children with epilepsy. In J. M. Pellock, D. R. Nordli, R. Sankar, & J. Wheless (Eds.), *Pellock's pediatric epilepsy: Diagnosis and therapy* (4th ed., pp. 1135–1146). New York, NY: Demos Medical Publishing.

Auvin, S., Wirrell, E., Donald, K. A., Berl, M., Hartmann, H., Valente, K. D., Van Bogaert, P., Cross, J. H., Osawa, M., Kanemura, H., Aihara, M., Guerreiro, M. M., Samia, P., Vinayan, K. P., Smith, M. L., Carmant, L., Kerr, M., Hermann, B., Dunn, D., & Wilmshurst, J. M. (2018). Systematic review of the screening, diagnosis, and management of ADHD in children with epilepsy. Consensus paper of the Task Force on Comorbidities of the ILAE Pediatric Commission. *Epilepsia, 59*(10), 1867–1880. https://doi.org/10.1111/epi.14549

Bangar, S. (2016). Women with epilepsy: Clinically relevant issues. *Functional Neurology, 31*(3), 127. https://doi.org/10.11138/fneur/2016.31.3.127

Beghi, E., Giussani, G., & Sander, J. W. (2015). The natural history and prognosis of epilepsy. *Epileptic Disorders, 3*, 243–253. https://doi.org/10.1684/epd.2015.0751

Bell, W. (2015). Alternative therapies. In A. M. Husain (Ed.), *Practical epilepsy* (pp. 358–364). New York, NY: Demos Medical.

Benabid, A. L., Minotti, L., Koudsié, A., de Saint Martin, A., & Hirsch, E. (2002). Antiepileptic effect of high-frequency stimulation of the subthalamic nucleus (corpus luysi) in a case of medically intractable epilepsy caused by focal dysplasia: A 30-month follow-up: Technical case report. *Neurosurgery, 50*(6), 1385–1392. https://doi.org/10.1097/00006123-200206000-00037

Berg, A. T., Rychlik, K., Levy, S. R., & Testa, F. M. (2014). Complete remission of childhood-onset epilepsy: Stability and prediction over two decades. *Brain, 137*(12), 3213–3222. https://doi.org/10.1093/brain/awu294

Butler, S. M., Boucher, E. A., Tobison, J., & Phan, H. (2020). Medication use in schools: Current trends, challenges, and best practices. *Journal of Pediatric Pharmacology and Therapeutics, 25*(1), 7–24. https://doi.org/10.5863/1551-6776-25.1.7

Centers for Disease Control and Prevention. (2024, May 15). *Epilepsy facts and stats.* https://www.cdc.gov/epilepsy/data-research/facts-stats/index.html

Chelse, A. B., Kelley, K., Hageman, J. R., & Koh, S. (2013). Initial evaluation and management of a first seizure in children. *Pediatric Annals, 42*(12), 244–248. https://doi.org/10.3928/00904481-20131122-08v

Dean, P., O'Hara, K., Brooks, L., Shinnar, R., Bougher, G., & Santilli, N. (2021). Managing acute seizures: New rescue delivery option and resources to assist school nurses. *NASN School Nurse, 36*(6), 346–354. https://doi.org/10.1177/1942602X211026333

Detyniecki, K., O'Bryan, J., Choezom, T., Rak, G., Ma, C., Zhang, S., Bonito, J., & Hirsch, L. J. (2018). Prevalence and predictors of seizure clusters: A prospective observational study of adult patients with epilepsy. *Epilepsy & Behavior, 88*, 349–356. https://doi.org/10.1016/j.yebeh.2018.09.035

DeWitt-Parker, C. (2016). Medicinal use of marijuana: What school nurses need to know. *NASN School Nurse, 3*(3), 170–176. https://doi.org/10.1177/1942602X16638815

Epilepsy Alliance America. (2024). *On-demand seizure first aid training for school personnel.* https://www.epilepsyallianceamerica.org/seizure-safety/seizure-first-aid-training-for-school-personnel-your-way/on-demand-seizure-first-aid-training-for-school-personnel/

Epilepsy Foundation. (2013a). *Safety at work.* https://www.epilepsy.com/preparedness-safety/staying-safe/safety-work#:~:text=General%20Safety%20Tips&text=If%20seizures%20are%20not%20controlled,to%20call%20for%20emergency%20care

Epilepsy Foundation. (2013b). *Staying safe with exercise and sports.* https://www.epilepsy.com/preparedness-safety/staying-safe/safety-exercise-and-sports

Epilepsy Foundation. (2018). *Epilepsy strategies: Transitioning to college.* https://www.epilepsy.com/stories/epilepsy-strategies-transitioning-college

Epilepsy Foundation. (2019a). *Seizure phases.* https://epilepsyfoundation.org.au/understanding-epilepsy/seizures/seizure-phases/?pdf=727#:~:text=Seizures%20take%20on%20many%20different,(post%2Dictal)%20stage

Epilepsy Foundation. (2019b). *The role of seizure alerts.* https://www.epilepsy.com/complications-risks/early-death-sudep/role-seizure-alerts

Epilepsy Foundation. (2019c). *Using seizure diaries.* https://www.epilepsy.com/manage/tracking/seizure-diaries

Epilepsy Foundation. (2020a). *Seizure action plan.* https://www.epilepsy.com/sites/default/files/atoms/files/SCHOOL%20Seizure%20Action%20Plan%202020-April7_FILLABLE.pdf

Epilepsy Foundation. (2022). *Advocacy: Seizure safe schools.* https://www.epilepsy.com/advocacy/priorities/seizure-safe-schools

Epilepsy Foundation (2024a). *Common seizure triggers.* https://www.epilepsy.com/what-is-epilepsy/seizure-triggers#What-are-some-commonly-reported-triggers

Epilepsy Foundation. (2024b). *Seizure first aid.* https://www.epilepsy.com/sites/default/files/atoms/files/SFA%20Flier_HQ_8.5x11_PDF.pdf

Fayed, N., Garrone, J. N., Russell, D. J., & Ronen, G. M. (2021). Quality of life (QOL) narratives of growing up with epilepsy from youth and family perspectives. *Epilepsy & Behavior, 114*(Pt A), 107613. https://doi.org/10.1016/j.yebeh.2020.107613

Fine, A., & Wirrell, E. C. (2020). Seizures in children. *Pediatrics in Review, 41*(7), 321–347. https://doi.org/10.1542/pir.2019-0134

Fisher, R. S., Boas, W. v. E., Blume, W., Elger, C., Genton, P., Lee, P., & Engel, J. (2005). Epileptic seizures and epilepsy: Definitions proposed by the International League Against Epilepsy (ILAE) and the International Bureau for Epilepsy (IBE). *Epilepsia, 46*(4), 470–472. https://doi.org/10.1111/j.0013-9580.2005.66104.x

Fisher, R. S., Cross, J. H., French, J. A., Higurashi, N., Hirsch, E., Jansen, F. E., Lagae, L., Moshé, S. L., Peltola, J., Roulet Perez, E., Scheffer, I. E., & Zuberi, S. M. (2017). Operational classification of seizure types by the International League Against Epilepsy: Position Paper of the ILAE Commission for Classification and Terminology. *Epilepsia, 58*(4), 522–530. https://doi.org/10.1111/epi.13670

Food and Drug Administration. (2017). *Summary of safety and effectiveness data. Stimulator, automatic nerve, implanted for epilepsy.* https://www.accessdata.fda.gov/cdrh_docs/pdf/p970003s207b.pdf

Food and Drug Administration. (2018, June 25). *FDA approves first drug comprised of an active ingredient derived from marijuana to treat rare, severe forms of epilepsy.* https://www.fda.gov/NewsEvents/Newsroom/PressAnnouncements/ucm611046.htm

Food and Drug Administration. (2020). *FDA and cannabis.* https://www.fda.gov/news-events/public-health-focus/fda-and-cannabis-research-and-drug-approval-process

Gidal B., Klein P., & Hirsch L. J. (2020). Seizure clusters, rescue treatments, seizure action plans: Unmet needs and emerging formulations. *Epilepsy & Behavior, 112*, Article 107391.

Goodwin, S. W., Lambrinos, A. I., Ferro, M. A., Sabaz, M., & Speechley, K. N. (2015). Development and assessment of a shortened Quality of Life in Childhood Epilepsy Questionnaire (QOLCE-55). *Epilepsia, 56*(6), 864–872. https://doi.org/10.1111/epi.13000

Gorodetsky, C., & Fasano, A. (2022). Developmental and epileptic encephalopathies in adults: An evolving field. *Neurology, 99*(3), 89–91. https://doi.org/10.1212/WNL.0000000000200190

Goselink, R. J. M., Olsson, I., Malmgren, K., & Reilly, C. (2022). Transition to adult care in epilepsy: A systematic review. *Seizure, 101*, 52–59. https://doi.org/10.1016/j.seizure.2022.07.006

Gupta, S. N., Gupta, V., & Fields, D. (2015). Spectrum of complicated migraine in children: A common profile in aid to clinical diagnosis. *World Journal of Clinical Pediatrics, 4*(1). https://doi.org/10.5409/wjcp.v4.i1.1

Harden, C., Tomson, T., Gloss, D., Buchhalter, J., Cross, J. H., Donner, E., French, J. A., Gil-Nagel, A., Hesdorffer, D. C., Smithson, W. H., Spitz, M. C., Walczak, T. S., Sander, J. W., & Ryvlin, P. (2017). Practice guideline summary: Sudden unexpected death in epilepsy incidence rates and risk factors. Report of the guideline development, dissemination, and implementation subcommittee of the American Academy of Neurology and the American Epilepsy Society. *Neurology, 88*(17), 1674–1680. https://doi.org/10.1212/WNL.0000000000003685

Hauser, W. A. (2016). Epidemiology of epilepsy in children. In D. R. Nordli, J. M. Pellock, R. Sankar, & J. W. Wheless (Eds.), *Pellock's pediatric epilepsy: Diagnosis & therapy* (pp. 177–206). Springer Publishing Company.

Holmes, G. L. (2021). Drug treatment of epilepsy neuropsychiatric comorbidities in children. *Paediatric Drugs, 23*(1), 55–73. https://doi.org/10.1007/s40272-020-00428-w

Iyengar, S., & Shafer, P. O. (2017, November 28). *Responsive neurostimulation (RNS)*. https://www.epilepsy.com/treatment/devices/responsive-neurostimulation

Jayalakshmi, S., Vooturi, S., Gupta, S., & Panigrahi, M. (2017). Epilepsy surgery in children. *Neurology India, 65*(3), 485–492. https://doi.org/10.4103/neuroindia.NI_1033_16

Jennum, P., Debes, N. M. M., Ibsen, R., & Kjellberg, J. (2021). Long-term employment, education, and healthcare costs of childhood and adolescent onset of epilepsy. *Epilepsy & Behavior, 114*(Pt A), 107256. https://doi.org/10.1016/j.yebeh.2020.107256

Joshi, S. M., Singh, R. K., & Shellhaas, R. A. (2013). Advanced treatments for childhood epilepsy: Beyond antiseizure medications. *JAMA Pediatrics, 167*(1), 76–83. https://doi.org/10.1001/jamapediatrics.2013.424

Kanner, A. M., Ashman, E., Gloss, D., Harden, C., Bourgeois, B., Bautista, J. F., Abou-Khalil, B., Burakgazi-Dalkilic, E., Llanas Park, E., Stern, J., Hirtz, D., Nespeca, M., Gidal, B., Faught, E., & French, J. (2018a). Practice guideline update summary: Efficacy and tolerability of the new antiepileptic drugs I: Treatment of new-onset epilepsy: Report of the guideline development, dissemination, and implementation subcommittee of the American Academy of Neurology and the American Epilepsy Society. *Neurology, 91*(2), 74–81. https://doi.org/10.1212/WNL.0000000000005755

Kanner, A. M., Ashman, E., Gloss, D., Harden, C., Bourgeois, B., Bautista, J. F., Abou-Khalil, B., Burakgazi-Dalkilic, E., Llanas Park, E., Stern, J., Hirtz, D., Nespeca, M., Gidal, B., Faught, E., & French, J. (2018b). Practice guideline update summary: Efficacy and tolerability of the new antiepileptic drugs II: Treatment-resistant epilepsy: Report of the guideline development, dissemination, and implementation subcommittee of the American Academy of Neurology and the American Epilepsy Society. *Neurology, 91*(2), 82–90. https://doi.org/10.1212/WNL.0000000000005756

Khan, M., Paktiawal, J., Piper, R. J., Chari, A., & Tisdall, M. M. (2021). Intracranial neuromodulation with deep brain stimulation and responsive neurostimulation in children with drug-resistant epilepsy: A systematic review. *Journal of Neurosurgery: Pediatrics*, 1–10. https://doi.org/10.3171/2021.8.PEDS21201

Kiriakopoulos, E. (2018). *Deep brain stimulation*. Epilepsy Foundation. https://www.epilepsy.com/treatment/devices/deep-brain-stimulation

Kiriakopoulos, E. (2019, October 1). *Understanding seizures*. Epilepsy Foundation. https://www.epilepsy.com/what-is-epilepsy/understanding-seizures

Kiriakopoulos, E., & Shafer, P. O. (2017). *Tonic-clonic seizures*. Epilepsy Foundation. https://www.epilepsy.com/what-is-epilepsy/seizure-types/tonic-clonic-seizures

Kiriakopoulos, E., & Shafer, P. O. (2019). *Absence seizures*. Epilepsy Foundation. https://www.epilepsy.com/what-is-epilepsy/seizure-types/absence-seizures

Kiriakopoulos, E., & Shafer, P. O. (2022a). *Atonic seizures*. Epilepsy Foundation. http://www.epilepsy.com/learn/types-seizures/atonic-seizures

Kiriakopoulos, E., & Shafer, P. O. (2022b). *Focal onset impaired awareness seizures (complex partial seizures)*. Epilepsy Foundation. http://www.epilepsy.com/learn/types-seizures/focal-onset-impairedawareness-seizures-aka-complex-partial-seizures

Kokoszka, M. A., Panov, F., La Vega-Talbott, M., McGoldrick, P. E., Wolf, S. M., & Ghatan, S. (2018). Treatment of medically refractory seizures with responsive neurostimulation: 2 pediatric cases. *J Neurosurgery Pediatrics, 21*(4), 421–427. https://doi.org/10.3171/2017.10.PEDS17353

Kolar Sridara Murthy, M., Govindappa, L., & Sinha, S. (2016). Outcome of a school-based health education program for epilepsy awareness among schoolchildren. *Epilepsy & Behavior, 57*, 77–81. https://doi.org/10.1016/j.yebeh.2016.01.016

Kumar, G. (2021) Evaluation and management of drug resistant epilepsy in children. *Pediatric and Adolescent Health Care, 51*(7), 1-10. https://doi.org/10.1016/j.cppeds.2021.101035

Lagunju, I. A., Oyinlade, A. O., & Babatunde, O. D. (2016). Seizure-related injuries in children and adolescents with epilepsy. *Epilepsy & Behavior, 54*, 131–134. https://doi.org/10.1016/j.yebeh.2015.11.019

Laing, M. K., Ti, L., Marmel, A., Tobias, S., Shapiro, A. M., Laing, R., Lysyshyn, M., & Socías, M. E. (2021). An outbreak of novel psychoactive substance benzodiazepines in the unregulated drug supply: Preliminary results from a community drug checking program using point-of-care and confirmatory methods. *The International Journal on Drug Policy, 93*, 103169. https://doi.org/10.1016/j.drugpo.2021.103169

Leeman-Markowski, B. A., & Schachter, S. C. (2015). Psychiatric comorbidity of epilepsy. In E. Wyllie (Ed.), *Treatment of epilepsy: Principles and practice* (6th ed., pp. 88–193). Lippincott Williams & Wilkins.

Li, W., Wang, G., Lei, X., Sheng, D., Yu, T., & Wang, G. (2022). Seizure detection based on wearable devices: A review of device, mechanism, and algorithm. *Acta Neurologica Scandinavica, 146*(6), 723–731. https://doi.org/10.1111/ane.13716

Liu, S., O'Donnell, J., Gladden, R. M., McGlone, L., & Chowdhury, F. (2021). Trends in nonfatal and fatal overdoses involving benzodiazepines—38 states and the District of Columbia, 2019–2020. *MMWR, 70*(34), 1136–1141. https://doi.org/10.15585/mmwr.mm7034a2

LivaNova. (2022). *VNS therapy: Sentiva technical guide*. https://www.livanova.com/epilepsy-vnstherapy/getmedia/a0f9e731-f117-4948-896e-abcfb377eb3f/im-7601065-epi_sentecgd19u1-rev-b_sentival-technical-guide.pdf

LivaNova. (2024). *What is VNS therapy and how does it work?* https://www.livanova.com/epilepsy-vnstherapy/en-us

Lu, E., Pyatka, N., Burant, C. J., & Sajatovic, M. (2021). Systematic literature review of psychiatric comorbidities in adults with epilepsy. *Journal of Clinical Neurology, 17*(2), 176–186. https://doi.org/10.3988/jcn.2021.17.2.176

Martin-McGill, K. J., Bresnahan, R., Levy, R. G., & Cooper, P. N. (2020). Ketogenic diets for drug-resistant epilepsy. *The Cochrane Database of Systematic Reviews, 6*(6), CD001903. https://doi.org/10.1002/14651858.CD001903.pub5

McKee, H. R., & Privitera, M. D. (2017). Stress as a seizure precipitant: Identification, associated factors, and treatment options. *Seizure, 44*, 21–26. https://doi.org/10.1016/j.seizure.2016.12.009

Meira D, I., Romão, T. T., Pires do Prado, H. J., Krüger, L. T., Pires, M. E. P., & da Conceição, P.O. (2019). Ketogenic diet and epilepsy: What we know so far. *Frontiers in Neuroscience, 13*, 5. https://doi.org/10.3389/fnins.2019.00005

Mesraoua, B., Tomson, T., Brodie, M., & Asadi-Pooya, A. A. (2022). Sudden unexpected death in epilepsy (SUDEP): Definition, epidemiology, and significance of education. *Epilepsy Behavior, 132*, 108742. https://doi.org/10.1016/j.yebeh.2022.108742

Mountz, J. M., Patterson, C. M., & Tamber, M. S. (2017). Pediatric epilepsy: Neurology, functional imaging, and neurosurgery. *Seminars in Nuclear Medicine, 47*(2), 170–187. https://doi.org/10.1053/j.semnuclmed.2016.10.003

Nagahama, Y., Zervos, T. M., Murata, K. K., Holman, L., Karsonovich, T., Parker, J. J., Chen, J. S., Phillips, H. W., Fajardo, M., Nariai, H., Hussain, S. A., Porter, B. E., Grant, G. A., Ragheb, J., Wang, S., O'Neill, B. R., Alexander, A. L., Bollo, R. J., & Fallah, A. (2021). Real-world preliminary experience with responsive neurostimulation in pediatric epilepsy: A multicenter retrospective observational study. *Neurosurgery, 89*(6), 997–1004. https://doi.org/10.1093/neuros/nyab343

National Association of School Nurses. (2019). *Transition planning for students with healthcare needs* [Position Statement]. MD: Author. https://www.nasn.org/nasn-resources/professional-practice-documents/position-statements/ps-transition

National Association of School Nurses. (2021). *A model for school nurse-led case management*. https://learn.nasn.org/courses/33713

National Association of School Nurses. (2022). *Complementary and integrative therapies* [Position Statement]. Author. https://www.nasn.org/nasn-resources/professional-practice-documents/position-statements/ps-therapies

National Association of School Nurses. (2023). *School nursing evidence-based clinical practice guideline: Students with seizures and epilepsy*. Author. https://learn.nasn.org/courses/63321/documents/94882

National Association of School Nurses. (2024a, January). *Coordinated support system for students with epilepsy*. https://learn.nasn.org/courses/54876

National Association of School Nurses. (2024b, February 5). *School nursing evidence-based clinical practice guideline: Students with seizures and epilepsy implementation toolkit*. Author. https://learn.nasn.org/courses/63450

National Association of School Nurses. (2024c, May). A contemporary framework update for today's school nursing landscape: Introducing the School Nursing Practice Framework. *NASN School Nurse, 39*(3), 140–147. https://www.doi.org/10.1177/1942602X241241092

Neurelis Inc. (2021). *Valtoco (diazepam nasal spray)*. https://www.valtoco.com/sites/default/files/pdf/Prescribing_Information.pdf

Newmaster, K., Zhu, Z., Bolt, E., Chang, R. J., Day, C., Mhanna, A., Paudel, S., Farooq, O., Swaminathan, A., Acharya, P., Cheungpasitporn, W., Gupta, S., Samanta, D., Mahfooz, N., Mainali, G., Carney, P. R., & Naik, S. (2022). A review of the multi-systemic complications of a ketogenic diet in children and infants with epilepsy. *Children (Basel, Switzerland), 9*(9), 1372. https://doi.org/10.3390/children9091372

Patel, A. (2018, July 3). *Medical marijuana and epilepsy*. http://www.epilepsy.com/learn/treating-seizures-and-epilepsy/other-treatment-approaches/medical-marijuana-and-epilepsy

Pearl, P., & Holmes, G. (2016). Childhood absence epilepsies. In J. M. Pellock, D. R. Nordli, R. Sankar, & J. Wheless (Eds.), *Pellock's pediatric epilepsy: Diagnosis and therapy* (4th ed., pp. 309–322). Demos Medical Publishing.

Pieters, H., Watson, M., & Baca, C. M. (2021). Pediatric and adult epileptologist perspectives and experiences of pediatric to adult epilepsy care transition: "Saying goodbye and opening a door." *Epilepsy Behavior, 120*, 107981. https://doi.org/10.1016/j.yebeh.2021.107981

Ricci, L., Boscarino, M., Assenza, G., Tombini, M., Lanzone, J., Di Lazzaro, V., Casciato, S., D'Aniello, A., Morano, A., Di Gennaro, G., & Epilepsy Study Group of the Italian Neurological Society. (2021). Clinical utility of home videos for diagnosing epileptic seizures: A systematic review and practical recommendations for optimal and safe recording. *Journal of Neurological Sciences, 42*(4), 1301–1309. https://doi.org/10.1007/s10072-021-05040-5

Rizvi, S., Ladino, L. D., Hernandez-Ronquillo, L., & Téllez-Zenteno, J. F. (2017). Epidemiology of early stages of epilepsy: Risk of seizure recurrence after a first seizure. *Seizure*. https://doi.org/10.1016/j.seizure.2017.02.006

Rocamora, R., Chavarría, B., Pérez, E., Pérez-Enríquez, C., Barguilla, A., Panadés-de Oliveira, L., Principe, A., & Zucca, R. (2021). Mood disturbances, anxiety, and impact on quality of life in patients admitted to epilepsy monitoring units. *Frontiers in Neurology, 12*, 761239. https://doi.org/10.3389/fneur.2021.761239

Romantseva, L., & Lin, N. (2020). Acute seizures—work-up and management in children. *Seminars in Neurology, 40*(6), 606–616. https://doi.org/10.1055/s-0040-1718718

Rosenblum, R., & Blosser, C. (2017). Neurologic disorders. In C. Burns, A. Dunn, M. Brady, N. Starr, C. Blosser, & D. Garzon (Eds.), *Pediatric primary care* (6th ed., pp. 660–702). Elsevier.

Rozensztrauch, A., & Kołtuniuk, A. (2022). The quality of life of children with epilepsy and the impact of the disease on the family functioning. *International Journal of Environmental Research and Public Health, 19*(4), 2277. https://doi.org/10.3390/ijerph19042277

Ruan, Y., Chen, L., She, D., Chung, Y., Ge, L., & Han, L. (2022). Ketogenic diet for epilepsy: An overview of systematic review and meta-analysis. *European Journal of Clinical Nutrition, 76*(9), 1234–1244. https://doi.org/10.1038/s41430-021-01060-8

Ryan, J. L., McGrady, M. E., Guilfoyle, S. M., Follansbee-Junger, K., Peugh, J. L., Loiselle, K. A., Arnett, A. D., & Modi, A. C. (2016). Quality of life changes and health care charges among youth with epilepsy. *Journal of Pediatric Psychology, 41*(8), 888–897. https://doi.org/10.1093/jpepsy/jsv098

Ryvlin, P., Cross, J. H., & Rheims, S. (2014). Epilepsy surgery in children and adults. *The Lancet. Neurology, 13*(11), 1114–1126. https://doi.org/10.1016/S1474-4422(14)70156-5

Sarkis, R. A., Thome-Souza, S., Poh, M. Z., Llewellyn, N., Klehm, J., Madsen, J. R., Picard, R., Pennell, P. B., Dworetzky, B. A., Loddenkemper, T., & Reinsberger, C. (2015). Autonomic changes following generalized tonic clonic seizures: An analysis of adult and pediatric patients with epilepsy. *Epilepsy Research, 115*, 113–118. https://doi.org/10.1016/j.eplepsyres.2015.06.005

Scheffer, I. E., Berkovic, S., Capovilla, G., Connolly, M. B., French, J., Guilhoto, L., Hirsch, E., Jain, S., Mathern, G. W., Moshé, S. L., Nordli, D. R., Perucca, E., Tomson, T., Wiebe, S., Zhang, Y. H., & Zuberi, S. M. (2017). ILAE classification of the epilepsies: Position paper of the ILAE Commission for Classification and Terminology. *Epilepsia, 58*(4), 512–521. https://doi.org/10.1111/epi.13709

Scheffer, I. E., French, J., Hirsch, E., Jain, S., Mathern, G. W., Moshé, S. L., Perucca, E., Tomson, T., Wiebe, S., Zhang, Y. H., & Zuberi, S. M. (2016). Classification of the epilepsies: New concepts for discussion and debate—Special report of the ILAE Classification Task Force of the Commission for Classification and Terminology. *Epilepsia Open, 1*(1–2), 37–44. https://doi.org/10.1002/epi4.5

Scorza, C. A., Guimarães-Marques, M., Girão, E. R. C., Nejm, M., Finsterer, J., Girão, M. J. B. C., Younes, R. N., Laranjeira, R. R., & Scorza, F. A. (2020). Alcohol and sudden unexpected death in epilepsy: Do not pop the cork. *Clinics, 75*, e1770. https://doi.org/10.6061/clinics/2020/e1770

Shafer, P. O. (2022). *General first aid for seizures*. Epilepsy Foundation https://www.epilepsy.com/recognition/seizure-first-aid

Shafer, P. O., Fisher, R., & Schachter, S. C. (2013). *Using seizure diaries*. Epilepsy Foundation. https://www.epilepsy.com/manage/tracking/seizure-diaries

Singh, R. (2023, May 12). *Status epilepticus*. Epilepsy Foundation. https://www.epilepsy.com/complications-risks/emergencies/status-epilepticus

Singhal, N. S., Numis, A. L., Lee, M. B., Chang, E. F., Sullivan, J. E., Auguste, K. I., & Rao, V. R. (2018). Responsive neurostimulation for treatment of pediatric drug-resistant epilepsy. *Epilepsy & Behavior Case Reports, 10*, 21–24. https://doi.org/10.1016/j.ebcr.2018.02.002

Sirven, J. I., Shafer, P. O., & Schachter, S. (2013a). *Seizure action plans*. https://www.epilepsy.com/preparedness-safety/action-plans

Sirven, J. I., Shafer, P. O., & Schachter, S. (2013b). *Seizure observation*. https://www.epilepsy.com/manage/tracking/observation

Sirven, J. I., Shafer, P. O., Schachter, S. (2013c). *Staying safe with exercise and sports*. https://www.epilepsy.com/preparedness-safety/staying-safe/safety-exercise-and-sports

Specchio, N., Wirrell, E. C., Scheffer, I. E., Nabbout, R., Riney, K., Samia, P., Guerreiro, M., Gwer, S., Zuberi, S. M., Wilmshurst, J. M., Yozawitz, E., Pressler, R., Hirsch, E., Wiebe, S., Cross, H. J., Perucca, E., Moshé, S. L., Tinuper, P., & Auvin, S. (2022). International League Against Epilepsy classification and definition of epilepsy syndromes with onset in childhood: Position paper by the ILAE Task Force on nosology and definitions. *Epilepsia, 63*(6), 1398–1442. https://doi.org/10.1111/epi.17241

Stainman, R. S., & Kossoff, E. H. (2020). Seizure mimics in children: An age-based approach. *Current Problems in Pediatric and Adolescent Health Care, 50*(12), 100894. https://doi.org/10.1016/j.cppeds.2020.100894

Starnes, K., Miller, K., Wong-Kisiel, L., & Lundstrom, B. N. (2019). A review of neurostimulation for epilepsy in pediatrics. *Brain Sciences, 9*(10), 283. https://doi.org/10.3390/brainsci9100283

Stödberg, T., Tomson, T., Anderlid, B. M., Andersson, T., Henry, O., Åmark, P., & Wedell, A. (2022). Outcome at age 7 of epilepsy presenting in the first 2 years of life. A population-based study. *Epilepsia, 63*(8), 2096–2107. https://doi.org/10.1111/epi.17314

Sultana, B., Panzini, M. A., Veilleux Carpentier, A., Comtois, J., Rioux, B., Gore, G., Bauer, P. R., Kwon, C. S., Jetté, N., Josephson, C. B., & Keezer, M. R. (2021). Incidence and prevalence of drug-resistant epilepsy: A systematic review and meta-analysis. *Neurology, 96*(17), 805–817. https://doi.org/10.1212/WNL.0000000000011839

Sveinsson, O., Andersson, T., Mattsson, P., Carlsson, S., & Tomson, T. (2020). Pharmacologic treatment and SUDEP risk: A nationwide, population-based, case-control study. *Neurology, 95*(18), e2509–e2518. https://doi.org/10.1212/WNL.0000000000010874

Swisher, C., & Radtke, R. (2016). Principles of treatment. In A. Husain (Ed.), *Practical epilepsy* (pp. 253–262). Demos Medical.

Terry, D., Patel, A. D., Cohen, D. M., Scherzer, D., & Kline, J. (2016). Barriers to seizure management in schools: Perceptions of school nurses. *Journal of Child Neurology, 31*(14), 1602–1606. https://doi.org/10.1177/0883073816666738

Thurman, D. J., Hesdorffer, D. C., & French, J. A. (2014). Sudden unexpected death in epilepsy: Assessing the public health burden. *Epilepsia, 55*(10), 1479–1485. https://doi.org/10.1111/epi.12666

Tykocki, T., Mandat, T., Kornakiewicz, A., Koziara, H., & Nauman, P. (2021). Deep brain stimulation for refractory epilepsy. *AMS, 8*(5), 805–816. https://doi.org/10.5114/aoms.2012.31135

UCB Inc. (2021). *NAYZILAM® (midazolam nasal spray)*. https://www.ucb-usa.com/_up/ucb_usa_com_kopie/documents/Nayzilam_PI.pdf

U.S. Drug Enforcement Administration. (2018, September 27). *FDA-approved drug Epidiolex placed in schedule V of Controlled Substance Act.* https://www.dea.gov/press-releases/2018/09/27/fda-approved-drug-epidiolex-placed-schedule-v-controlled-substance-act

Valentín, A., Selway, R. P., Amarouche, M., Mundil, N., Ughratdar, I., Ayoubian, L., Martín-López, D., Kazi, F., Dar, T., Jiménez-Jiménez, D., Hughes, E., & Alarcón, G. (2017). Intracranial stimulation for children with epilepsy. *European Journal of Paediatric Neurology, 21*(1), 223–231. https://doi.org/10.1016/j.ejpn.2016.10.011

Velasco, A. L., Velasco, F., Jiménez, F., Velasco, M., Castro, G., Carrillo-Ruiz, J. D., Fanghänel, G., & Boleaga, B. (2006). Neuromodulation of the centromedian thalamic nuclei in the treatment of generalized seizures and the improvement of the quality of life in patients with Lennox-Gastaut syndrome. *Epilepsia, 47*(7), 1203–1212. https://doi.org/10.1111/j.1528-1167.2006.00593.x

Verrotti, A., Lattanzi, S., Brigo, F., & Zaccara, G. (2020). Pharmacodynamic interactions of antiepileptic drugs: From bench to clinical practice. *Epilepsy & Behavior, 104*(Pt A), 106939. https://doi.org/10.1016/j.yebeh.2020.106939

Vossler, D. G., Gidal, B. E., & The AES Treatments Committee. (2020). *A summary of antiseizure medications available in the United States: 2020 update.* https://www.aesnet.org/docs/default-source/pdfs-clinical/2020-september-aes_summary_of_asms.pdf?sfvrsn=c1a0ed0b_2

Wang, Y., Zhan, G., Cai, Z., Jiao, B., Zhao, Y., Li, S., & Luo, A. (2021). Vagus nerve stimulation in brain diseases: Therapeutic applications and biological mechanisms. *Neuroscience and Biobehavioral Reviews, 127*, 37–53. https://doi.org/10.1016/j.neubiorev.2021.04.018

Wells, J., Swaminathan, A., Paseka, J., & Hanson, C. (2020). Efficacy and safety of a ketogenic diet in children and adolescents with refractory epilepsy—a review. *Nutrients, 12*(6), 1809. https://doi.org/10.3390/nu12061809

Wilfong, A. (2021). Management of convulsive status epilepticus in children. *UpToDate.* https://www.uptodate.com/contents/management-of-convulsive-status-epilepticus-in-children

Wilfong, A. (2022a). Seizures and epilepsy in children: Initial treatment and monitoring. *UpToDate.* https://www.uptodate.com/contents/seizures-and-epilepsy-in-children-initial-treatment-and-monitoring

Wilfong, A. (2022b). Seizures and epilepsy in children: Refractory seizures and prognosis. *UpToDate.* http://www.uptodate.com/contents/seizures-and-epilepsy-in-children-refractory-seizures-and-prognosis

Wilson, N., Whittaker, K., Arnott, J., Burke, L., Beresford, M. W., & Peak, M. (2022). Stuck in transit: A qualitative study of the transitional care needs of young people with epilepsy and juvenile idiopathic arthritis. *J Child Health Care,* 13674935221074777. Advance online publication. https://doi.org/10.1177/13674935221074777

Yan, H., Siegel, L., Breitbart, S., Gorodetsky, C., Gonorazky, H. D., Yau, I., Go, C., Donner, E., Kalia, S. K., Fasano, A., Weil, A. G., Fallah, A., & Ibrahim, G. M. (2021). The child & youth comprehensive longitudinal database for deep brain stimulation (CHILD-DBS). *Child's Nervous System, 37*(2), 607–615. https://doi.org/10.1007/s00381-020-04880-4

Ziemba, K. (2022). *Bone health.* Epilepsy Foundation. https://www.epilepsy.com/complications-risks/bone-health

Chapter **28**

Students With Behavioral/Mental Health Concerns and Conditions

Connie R. Kartoz ▪ Liza Woods ▪ Jennifer S. Graber

CHAPTER OUTLINE

Childhood and adolescence are critical periods when brain development and cognitive and emotional skill acquisition occur, potentially affecting lifelong mental health (World Health Organization [WHO], 2022a). All children and adolescents experience anger, joy, and many other emotions; as they grow, they learn to identify their emotions and their respective causes. They also develop adaptive coping mechanisms to learn to regulate their emotions effectively. However, recent surveys reveal that 16.5% of those 6 to 17 years old have a mental health disorder, with only about half receiving treatment (National Alliance on Mental Illness [NAMI], 2023). Most mental health disorders present before adulthood, with one-half of all chronic mental health disorders beginning by age 14 and 75% by age 24 (NAMI, 2022a). While advances have been made, mental health disorders are still seen as a stigmatizing condition for many, and not all healthcare providers are adequately prepared to evaluate and treat them. Both the American Academy of Pediatrics (AAP) and the National Alliance on Mental Illness (NAMI) have declared that child and adolescent mental health is at a crisis level in the United States (AAP, 2021a; NAMI, 2021).

Good mental health is crucial to a student's well-being and affects many domains, including physical health, school performance, sense of connectedness and overall engagement in learning (National Association of School Psychologists, 2021; WHO, 2021). Concern around student mental health is amplified as today's students face increasing demands to function autonomously and navigate increasingly complex social demands; these concerns were further exacerbated by the COVID-19 pandemic (AAP, 2021b). Interdisciplinary teams within the school and community can promote student mental health and well-being and address student mental health concerns.

As critical members of these teams, school nurses can help support student mental health (National Association of School Nurses [NASN], 2022a). School nurses are positioned to design and deliver preventive programs, identify and triage students at risk for mental health concerns, provide evidence-based interventions, coordinate referrals to mental health providers in the school and community, and support ongoing care coordination (Bohnenkamp et al., 2019; Hoskote et al., 2023; NASN, 2022a). Outcomes are more successful for those treated by a proactive, multidisciplinary, patient-centered care team, which includes the school nurse (Anttila et al., 2020; Hoover & Bostic, 2022; NASN, 2024).

CLARIFICATION OF TERMS

Just as the definition of health is more than the absence of disease, so is mental health more than just the absence of a mental health disorder; mental health exists on a continuum (Centers for Disease Control and Prevention [CDC], 2023b; WHO, 2022b). The WHO defines *mental health* as "a state of well-being that enables people to cope with the stresses of life, realize their abilities, learn well and work well, and contribute to their community" (2022b, para. 1). Mental health is essential to a person's well-being and relationships and is important in every stage of life, including childhood and adolescence.

Although mental health and behavioral health are often used interchangeably, *behavioral health* is a broader term that includes mental health. The CDC states that behavioral health "describes the connection between a person's behaviors and the health and well-being of the body and mind" (2023b, para. 10). The Substance Abuse and Mental Health Services Administration [SAMHSA] defines *behavioral health* as the "promotion of mental health, resilience and wellbeing; treatment of disorder; and support of individuals and families who experience these disorders" (2019, p. 2). Thus behavioral health includes not only ways to treat alterations in mental health but also includes ways to prevent them. The term *behavioral health* more accurately encompasses the role of school nurses in providing population and individual nursing interventions. Behavioral well-being is fostered through systems that address the promotion of social and emotional health, as well as the prevention of mental health and substance use disorders through identification and supportive services. Schools are major systems that support healthy behavior in students in the United States. The *Behavioral Health and Wellness of Students* position statement of the National Association of School Nurses (NASN) states the following:

> *Student behavioral health and wellness must be prioritized for students to successfully access and engage in educational opportunities. It is imperative that school systems respond to, and address, student behavioral health and wellness to ameliorate disparities to the social determinants of health. School nurses are often the initial access point to identify concerns, determine interventions, and link families to school and/or community resources. (NASN, 2022a, p. 1)*

Good behavioral and mental health are imperative to learning in the school setting, and school nurses can use assessment skills to identify those at risk (NASN, 2022a; Rosvall, 2020).

The terms *mental illness* and *mental disease* have now been replaced by *mental health* and *mental disorder.* The *Diagnostic and Statistical Manual of Mental Disorders, 5th Edition, Text Revision* [DSM-5-TR] defines a *mental disorder* as "a syndrome characterized by clinically significant disturbance in an individual's cognition, emotion regulation, or behavior that reflects a dysfunction in the psychological, biological, or developmental processes underlying mental functioning" (American Psychiatric Association [APA], 2022, p. 14). These disorders are usually associated with significant distress. The DSM-5-TR designates the criteria required to be diagnosed with any given mental disorder. When only some symptoms are present, the term *mental health concern* is used.

Persistent symptoms that impair one's functioning across multiple spheres (e.g., not getting along with family, difficulty sustaining peer relationships, failure to make effective educational progress despite intellectual abilities) are usually acknowledged as *behavioral health concerns.* When children experience distress that interferes with the functions of daily living (e.g., trauma, adverse childhood experiences, grief), rapid intervention and support by the adults familiar with the child, including the school nurse, can help to diminish the impact of the adverse events and the development of mental health concerns.

It should be noted that the *Individuals With Disabilities Education Improvement Act of 2004* (IDEA) uses the category *emotional disturbance* as a qualifying category for special education services. *Emotional disturbance* is defined as

> *a condition exhibiting one or more of the following characteristics over a long period of time and to a marked degree that adversely affects a child's educational performance:*
>
> *(A) An inability to learn that cannot be explained by intellectual, sensory, or health factors*
> *(B) An inability to build or maintain satisfactory interpersonal relationships with peers and teachers*
> *(C) Inappropriate types of behavior or feelings under normal circumstances*
> *(D) A general pervasive mood of unhappiness or depression*
> *(E) A tendency to develop physical symptoms or fears associated with personal or school problems*
> *(ii) Emotional disturbance includes schizophrenia. The term does not apply to children who are socially maladjusted. [IDEA, 2017, §300.89(c)(4)]*

PREVALENCE OF MENTAL HEALTH DISORDERS

The mental health crisis has never been more prominent in today's youth. Almost 18% of U.S. children ages 2 to 17 years have a diagnosed mental, behavioral, or developmental disorder. The urgency is highlighted by the fact that suicide is the second leading cause of death among youth ages 10 to 14 and the third leading cause of death among those ages 15 to 24. One in five youth felt that the COVID-19 pandemic had a significant impact on their mental health (CDC, 2023b; NAMI, 2022a). The most recent Youth Risk Behavior Survey (CDC, 2023c) found that over 40% of high school students were debilitated by feelings of sadness and hopelessness and almost 30% experienced poor mental health.

Behavioral disorders occur across the developmental spectrum. The most common mental disorders diagnosed include attention deficit-hyperactivity disorder (ADHD; 9.8%), anxiety (9.4%), behavior problems (8.9%), and depression (4.4%; CDC, 2023b). These statistics increase in youth ages 12 to 17 years with over 15% being diagnosed with major depression. Comorbidity, the co-occurrence of more than one mental disorder or a mental health disorder in association with another health or neurodevelopmental condition, is common in children and adolescents. The DSM-5-TR

> *recognizes that mental disorders do not always fit completely within the boundaries of a single disorder. Some symptom domains, such as depression and anxiety, involve multiple diagnostic categories and may reflect common underlying vulnerabilities for a larger group of disorders. (APA, 2022, p. 10)*

For example, 70% of children with autism spectrum disorder have another mental disorder and 41% will have two or more additional diagnoses, including anxiety, ADHD, and oppositional defiant disorder (Young et al., 2020).

Mental health concerns in youth often go unrecognized or untreated, even though effective therapies are available (WHO, 2022a). For all youth, there are a variety of barriers to accessing services. It is estimated that almost 80% of children and adolescents diagnosed with a mental disorder do not get the treatment they need, increasing the burden on schools to address and support the needs of these students (U.S. Department of Education [USDOE], 2021). This is especially true for minority populations where delays in accessing treatment are multifactorial, including decreased access to mental health care, not seeking care, not receiving appropriate care needed, and ending treatment early (Perzichilli, 2020). Students' unknown and untreated mental health problems can lead to behavior issues at school. However, students of color experience reactive and exclusionary discipline rather than interventions or additional support, resulting in children and youth of color having poorer outcomes than white peers (USDOE, 2021). The evidence and research, while troubling, create an opportunity to reconceptualize and prioritize how to provide school- and program-based mental health supports. Left unaddressed, students with mental health challenges, especially students of color and marginalized groups, can experience multiple negative outcomes in their young life, including trouble making friends, learning, concentrating, and completing work, as well as poor grades, absences, suspension, expulsion, contact with the juvenile justice system, and even suicide (Cohen, 2019; Houri & Kincade, 2021).

CAUSATIVE FACTORS

The reason for the high prevalence of mental health concerns is unknown, although many hypotheses have been proposed. Genetics may predispose young people to developing mental health problems. Other potential contributing variables include experiencing trauma, physical or sexual abuse, neglect, long-term illness or disability problems with family members, problems with peers, sexual identity and orientation concerns, sleep problems, obesity, concerns about body image, and, more recently, effects of COVID-19 (NAMI, 2022b; USDOE, 2021; WHO, 2022b). Many of these traumatic events, particularly those related to abuse, household challenges, and neglect, are termed *adverse childhood experiences* (ACEs; CDC, 2023a). School nurses and all school staff need general knowledge of ACEs, their impact, and opportunities for early intervention, as research has highlighted the influence of traumatic events experienced by children on physical and mental health and well-being that extends into adulthood. See Chapter 11 for more information on ACEs. Additional proposed causes for the development of mental health concerns include environmental toxins (such as high lead levels), fetal alcohol exposure, and the stress caused by chronic poverty (American College of Obstetricians and Gynecologists Committee on Obstetric Practice, 2021). There are also pressures from within the school setting, including the pressure to excel and to do well on standardized testing. Social pressures related to social relationships are high in later elementary, middle school, and high school, with social media having a significant impact (NAMI, 2022b). Ineffective parenting and household chaos may exacerbate or cause emotional responses (Marsh et al., 2020). Ultimately, successful school performance rests on a foundation of good mental health.

SELECTED MENTAL HEALTH DISORDERS

The *Diagnostic and Statistical Manual of Mental Disorders, 5th edition text revision* outlines the diagnostic criteria for significant mental health disorders affecting school-age children (APA, 2022). Several mental health disorders experienced by students are discussed in this section, with anxiety and depression being the most common. ADHD and neurodevelopmental disorders are discussed in Chapter 26.

Anxiety Disorders

Anxiety is a normal emotion and is usually used to describe stress. However, these feelings are not the same. Stress describes external pressure, whereas anxiety describes the internal emotional response to stress. Anxiety disorders can include excessive fear (response to an imminent threat) and anxiety (anticipation of a future threat). Fear is more closely related to the body's fight-or-flight response, while anxiety is more associated with "muscle tension and vigilance in preparation for future danger and cautious or avoidant behaviors" (APA, 2022, p. 216). Fear also includes the fear response we call panic. Panic attacks are common in those with anxiety disorders but are not limited to them. Avoidance behaviors are also common and often used as a control measure for these disorders.

To be classified as an anxiety disorder, the fears and worries are more frequent than typically experienced, last longer, and interfere with life activities (APA, 2022). Anxiety disorders are among the most common forms of psychiatric disorders in children and adolescents, affecting about 9.4% of all youth, with girls diagnosed twice as frequently as boys (CDC, 2023b). The most prevalent anxiety disorders in children and adolescents include separation anxiety disorder, social anxiety disorder, selective mutism, specific phobias, panic disorder, and generalized anxiety disorder (APA, 2022).

There are a variety of etiological considerations for anxiety, and without proper treatment, the disorder will progress into adulthood. Demographic factors such as being female, low educational attainment, and low or unsatisfactory household income are associated with higher rates of anxiety. Effects of pathophysiological factors are relevant as youth with two parents impaired by at least one anxiety disorder are at substantially higher risk for the development of anxiety problems compared with peers with unaffected parents (APA, 2022). Psychobiological factors, particularly negative temperament, are associated with sensitivity to anxiety-provoking responses and decreased ability to tolerate distress (APA, 2022). High levels of parental rejection and authoritarianism are also associated with increased susceptibility to anxiety disorders. Childhood adversities such as death, loss, parental separation, exposure to violence, and other traumatic events confer additional risks, which are discussed later in this chapter.

Generalized Anxiety Disorder

Generalized anxiety disorder is found in about 0.9% of U.S. adolescents and 2.9% of adults and is twice as prevalent in females as males. It is more common in those of European descent and those who live in high-income countries. General anxiety disorder is nonspecific, chronic worry in more than one area of life accompanied by at least one somatic symptom (APA, 2022). Worries associated with generalized anxiety disorder are pervasive and excessive and typically concern social situations, natural phenomena, and school performance. Suicidal thoughts and behaviors are also associated with this disorder. Genetics account for one-third of the risk for this disorder and overlap with other factors such as behavioral inhibition and negative affectivity. Childhood trauma and overprotective/controlling parenting have also been associated with generalized anxiety disorder. In school or sporting events, generalized anxiety disorder may manifest as concern over competence or quality of performance despite the fact that the student is not being evaluated. The overwhelming worry experienced by those with general anxiety disorder saps the individual of energy and impairs their ability to work efficiently at home, school, and work. These individuals often miss school due to the symptoms of their condition, resulting in poor school performance. This disorder also is associated with increased use of medical resources and increased risk of coronary morbidity.

Treatment for anxiety disorders generally consists of cognitive behavioral therapy with or without medication. Some research supports the combination of therapy and medication as the most effective for children from ages 7 to 17 years. Most children and adults are treated with selective serotonin reuptake inhibitors (SSRIs), with benzodiazepines used less frequently. Children and adolescents should be monitored for side effects such as headache, stomachache, and difficulty sleeping. While rare, some youth will experience suicidal thoughts, which needs to be addressed immediately.

Separation Anxiety Disorder

Separation anxiety disorder is common in young school-age children and is perhaps the first type of anxiety identified by parents, especially at the start of the school year. Separation anxiety disorder is estimated to affect approximately 4% of children under age 12 (Feriante et al., 2023). Children and youth may worry about caregivers when apart from them; their fears may be specific (e.g., accidents, mugging, death) or general concerning dangers that could compromise the safety of either party (APA, 2022). The concerns are developmentally inappropriate, excessive, and interfere with social and academic functioning. There is some evidence to support the heritability of this disorder, and it may be seen across families. Cultural variation should always be considered as anxiety may be related to the high value that is placed on family interdependence by the family or culture rather than an anxiety disorder. Youth with a separation anxiety disorder may exhibit persistent refusal behaviors or demonstrate a reluctance to attend school. Anxiety may present as *school refusal*, which affects 2% to 5% of children and peaks in ages 5 to 6 and again from 10 to 11 (Kawsar et al., 2022). School refusal is not a diagnosis but a symptom.

Students with separation anxiety may visit the nurse's office frequently and present with somatic complaints, such as stomachache, nausea, abdominal discomfort, headache, shortness of breath, sweating, crying, chills, and a general feeling of "I don't feel good" with a request to go home and school refusal. Untreated anxiety symptoms are associated with increased academic failure, interpersonal difficulties, emotional problems, and behavioral impairments.

Social Anxiety Disorder

Social anxiety disorder affects approximately 7% of individuals with about 75% having an onset between ages 8 and 15 (APA, 2022). The main feature of social anxiety disorder is the intense fear or anxiety experienced in social situations in which the individual feels they are being negatively evaluated or scrutinized by others. Their behaviors may be misinterpreted as being "shy" or socially inhibited and may be exacerbated by bullying and public embarrassment (APA, 2022). The condition is heritable and more common in those who exhibit high negative affectivity (neuroticism) and low extroversion. The effects of various types of trauma, such as bullying, maltreatment, and the impact of ethnic discrimination and racism, are associated with social anxiety disorder, although the causal path is unknown. Consequences associated with social anxiety include serious academic and psychological impairments similar to other anxiety disorders. Social anxiety may result in friendship challenges, school refusal, loneliness, depression, and substance use in older adolescents (Spence et al., 2017).

Selective Mutism

Selective mutism is a rare disorder and therefore is not easily tracked. Selective mutism is the failure to speak in *specific* social situations where there is an expectation of speaking, such as in school (APA, 2022). Families may report that students who display selective mutism at school talk "normally" at home. It is diagnosed when the condition lasts more than a month and is not attributed to a communication disorder or comfort with the language. The onset is usually seen before age 5 but may not be diagnosed until the child enters the school system. Children seem to "outgrow" their mutism; however, it may reveal underlying social anxiety disorder. Some data suggest that it is more common in girls than boys and that those who are required to speak in a nonnative language are at risk for developing selective mutism. Parents who are socially inhibited or overprotective are more likely to have children with selective mutism. It has not been shown to be heritable but, due to the overlap with social anxiety disorder, may have a genetic component. Children with selective mutism often have continued difficulty in social situations and can become isolated and unable to share their needs with peers and school staff. This can result in poor peer relationships and low academic performance.

Specific Phobias

Specific phobias are developmentally inappropriate and disproportionate fears and/or anxiety about a specific situation or object that persist for a minimum of 6 months (APA, 2022). Perceived fears are commonly unrealistic compared with the actual danger of the triggering stimulus (e.g., the beetle will attack me and chase me for miles). Overall, 5% of children and 16% of adolescents have a specific phobia (APA, 2022). Phobias fall into one of five subtypes: animal, natural environment (such as storms or heights), blood-injection-injury, situational (e.g., enclosed spaces), and other types (e.g., costumed characters). Affected youth avoid the feared stimulus and exhibit significant distress (e.g., crying, tantrums, freezing, clinging behaviors) when made to endure it (APA, 2022). As with other anxiety disorders, impairments from phobias can have deleterious effects on academic, emotional, and social functioning and result in comorbid anxiety and mood disorders.

Panic Disorder

Panic disorder occurs in about 2% to 3% of adolescents and in less than 0.4% of children under 14, with the median age of onset between 20 and 24 years (APA, 2022). Women are affected by panic disorder at a rate of 2:1 compared with men. Non-Latinx whites have the highest prevalence of panic disorder compared with Latinx, African American, and Asian Americans. However, American Indian people have the highest prevalence of panic disorder ranging from 2.6% to 4.1%. The diagnosis is characterized by recurrent panic attacks with concern about having another attack and worry about the consequences of an attack. Panic attacks are marked by surges of fear and worry that peak within minutes of onset during which at least 4 of 13 identified somatic or cognitive symptoms are present, such as chest pain, sweating, or fear of dying (APA, 2022). Intense experiences of physical symptoms can manifest as persistent somatic complaints, high absenteeism, and frequent medical visits. Consequently, high levels of physical and social impairments are associated with panic disorder, as is academic difficulty, in addition to higher economic costs related to hospital visits compared with other anxiety conditions.

Post-Traumatic Stress Disorder

Post-traumatic stress disorder (PTSD) is categorized as a mental health problem in the form of a stress response that develops after experiencing or witnessing a traumatic event such as actual or threatened serious injury/death or sexual violence (APA, 2022). Symptoms may develop over time, resulting in an initial diagnosis of acute stress disorder followed later by a PTSD diagnosis as the symptoms persist or increase to meet the diagnostic criteria. Prevalence of PTSD has been estimated to be between 6.1% and 8.3% in the United States. Children as young as 1 year old have been diagnosed with PTSD, although the diagnostic criteria differ for those less than 6 years of age. Black, Indigenous, and Latinx individuals are more likely to experience PTSD symptoms compared with whites. PTSD is also more common in those whose vocation increases the likelihood that they will experience trauma (e.g., emergency personnel).

Symptoms of PTSD fall into four categories. Those suffering from PTSD may experience some or all of the symptoms depending on various personal factors such as temperament, past experiences, and support systems. Each case is personal and as unique as the person experiencing the symptoms. Symptoms include the following:

- Intrusive or recurrent memories of the trauma. This symptom is a result of the way the mind and body manage post-traumatic stress. The brain is unable to process memories as it usually does, which can lead to nightmares and flashbacks or vivid memories of the event that feel like they are real. This can be triggered by environmental cues, smells, or something that reminds the individual of where the traumatic event occurred (APA, 2022).

- Avoidance of trauma reminders. Those who are experiencing PTSD are constantly screening their environment to avoid potential triggers. This can interfere with the ability to attend school or interact with others. Conversely, they may over engage in work or other activities to avoid thinking about triggering events (APA, 2022).
- Feeling sad, angry, or numb. Negative emotions are more prevalent in people with PTSD and can include feeling sadness, anger, and a loss of pleasure in things that used to make them happy. To limit intense negative emotions and suppress memories, individuals may become emotionally numb, shuttering away feelings, or use alcohol or other drugs (APA, 2022).
- Feeling "on edge," or other changes in reactivity or arousal. This is directly related to the physiological arousal changes that occur in response to trauma where one may be more jittery than normal, feel or act impatient, or be irritable. This can cause difficulty with sleeping and concentrating (APA, 2022).

Many of these symptoms can be interrelated and can be cyclical in their ability to be treated. For example, if nightmares are keeping a student up all night or causing them to avoid sleep because they are afraid of experiencing nightmares, then they are irritable and fatigued during the day, making it difficult to function or achieve a positive outlook (APA, 2023).

Symptoms of PTSD can be found in children but they may also experience a different presentation than what is seen in adults. Preschool children may show signs of traumatic stress in the form of separation fear and anxiety, crying or screaming excessively, poor appetite or weight loss, and nightmares. School-age children (ages 5 to 12) may not have flashbacks or problems remembering parts of the trauma the way adults with PTSD often do, but they might put events of the trauma in the wrong order. Children might make associations that there were signs the trauma was going to happen, leaving them on high alert so that they can avoid future traumas. Children also demonstrate signs of PTSD in their play by repeating part of the trauma or reenacting it. However, this play does not make their worry or distress go away (National Center for PTSD, 2022). Elementary school children often display stress by becoming anxious or fearful, feeling guilt or shame, having difficulty concentrating, and having difficulty sleeping (National Institute of Mental Health [NIMH], 2022). Many signs of PTSD or complex trauma often mimic symptoms of ADHD or oppositional defiant disorder, such as the following (Miller et al., 2023):

- Hyperarousal and being unable to sit calmly and pay attention
- Being distracted by intrusive thoughts of the traumatic event that cannot be mentally processed
- A negative view of others and perceiving most people as hostile, causing them to act impulsive or oppositional
- Difficulty with executive functions such as planning how to complete a task or homework, managing emotions, or thinking things through before acting on impulse

Teens (ages 12 to 18) begin to experience symptoms that are more like PTSD in adults but often show more impulsive and aggressive behaviors than younger children or adults do in response to trauma. Middle and high school students often can feel depressed or alone, develop eating disorders or self-harming behaviors, begin abusing alcohol or drugs, or engage in risky sexual behavior (NIMH, 2022). Sexually abused children often have problems with fear, worry, sadness, anger, feeling alone and apart from others, low self-worth, and difficulty trusting others. Behaviors such as aggression, inappropriate sexual behavior, self-harm, and abuse of drugs or alcohol are also signs of trauma (National Center for PTSD, 2022). See Chapter 11 for further discussion of trauma.

Trauma affects children, teens, and adults with lasting and serious impact. Research has shown that child trauma survivors may experience learning problems, including lower grades and more suspensions and expulsions, increased use of health and mental health services, increased involvement with child welfare and the juvenile justice system, and long-term health problems (NIMH, 2022). Trauma is a risk factor for nearly all behavioral health and substance use disorders. Early intervention is key to assisting school-age children to develop resilience and coping skills, which are essential for post-traumatic growth. Having a supportive caregiving system and adults in their lives who are consistent and work to get them connected to support are protective factors that could mean a life-changing difference in their outcome trajectory. Advocacy and providing a consistent supportive environment can make the difference.

Trauma-Informed Care

Trauma-informed care is an approach that provides the tools and guidance needed to understand how students (or anyone) who has experienced trauma and adversity can heal and thrive. Trauma-informed care shifts the reaction from "what is wrong with this student" to "what happened to this student" (The Institute on Trauma and Trauma-Informed Care [ITTIC], 2022). Using a trauma-informed approach ensures that you are part of the solution to help someone instead of making a situation worse, even when you are not sure that trauma has occurred. Increased awareness of the prevalence of trauma has aligned with neuroscientific advancement to better understand the neurobiology of trauma (Bargeman et al., 2022). From this research, it is clear that childhood trauma can disrupt normal neurocognitive development and often can lead to long-term negative health outcomes. However, experiencing the toxic stress of adverse experiences does not necessarily mean that these children must experience lifelong problems. Empirical literature shows promising evidence regarding the effectiveness of using trauma-informed services in comparison to traditional services to help mitigate the impact of trauma and toxic stress and promote resilience and post-traumatic growth (Bargeman et al., 2022). Trauma-informed care has six guiding principles and is an approach to interacting with others to promote environments and interactions of healing and recovery rather than practices that may inadvertently retraumatize (ITTIC, 2022). See Figure 28-1.

Adopting a trauma-informed approach is not accomplished through any one single avenue. It is a method that requires attention, caring awareness, sensitivity, and often a cultural change. Being trauma-informed means that you integrate SAMHSA's (2022) "Four R's" of a trauma-informed approach: realize, recognize, respond, and resist. *Realize* the widespread impact of trauma and understand potential paths for recovery; *recognize* the signs and symptoms of trauma in students and others; *respond* by fully integrating knowledge about trauma into policies, procedures, and practices; and above all *resist* retraumatization. A trauma-informed approach is more than a list of tasks to accomplish. It is a paradigm shift that is deliberate and intentional. Being trauma-informed is an ongoing process rather than a destination and should be instilled into policies, procedures, and practices as often as possible for better student and staff outcomes.

> **Focus on the Framework**
>
> **Care Coordination**
>
> The Framework principle of **Care Coordination** includes the school nurse's role in providing direct care for emergent episodic and chronic mental and physical health needs. **E.V.E.N.T.** is an easy-to-remember acronym that school nurses can use to respond to someone in a trauma-informed way.
>
> **E. Empathy**—for the feelings and respect for the worth of the person, with no effort to change them.
>
> **V. Validation**—recognition and acceptance of the person's thoughts, feelings, and behaviors as understandable.
>
> **E. Equal**—treating the person as an equal; entering communication with mutual respect without hierarchy.
>
> **N. Normal**—acknowledging that the person's feelings or behaviors are a normal response to trauma and they are not alone.
>
> **T. Trust**—maintaining respectful and professional boundaries.
>
> Sebton (2020).

Obsessive-Compulsive Disorders

Youth with *obsessive-compulsive disorder* (OCD) are preoccupied with obsessions and/or compulsions that occupy a large percentage of their time. Approximately 2% of individuals in the United States are affected by OCD, with males more likely to develop OCD in adolescence or earlier, 30% more likely to develop a lifetime tic disorder, and 25% of all cases starting by age 14 (APA, 2022; Nazeer et al., 2020). *Obsessions* are intrusive and include repetitive

6 GUIDING PRINCIPLES TO A TRAUMA-INFORMED APPROACH

The CDC's Office of Public Health Preparedness and Response (OPHPR), in collaboration with SAMHSA's National Center for Trauma-Informed Care (NCTIC), developed and led a new training for OPHPR employees about the role of trauma-informed care during public health emergencies. The training aimed to increase responder awareness of the impact that trauma can have in the communities where they work. Participants learned SAMHSA'S six principles that guide a trauma-informed approach, including:

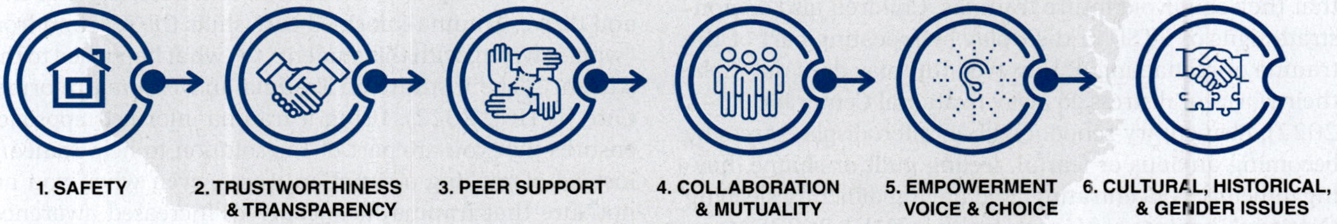

Adopting a trauma-informed approach is not accomplished through any single particular technique or checklist. It requires constant attention, caring awareness, sensitivity, and possibly a cultural change at an organizational level. On-going internal organizational assessment and quality improvement, as well as engagement with community stakeholders, will help to imbed this approach which can be augmented with organizational development and practice improvement. The training provided by OPHPR and NCTIC was the first step for CDC to view emergency preparedness and response through a trauma-informed lens.

FIGURE 28-1. Six guiding principles to a trauma-informed approach. *(CDC, 2022)*

thoughts, urges, and images that often result in attempted compensatory behaviors. *Compulsions* are repetitive acts completed to reduce feelings of distress or attempt to prevent threatening events from occurring and are often observable and easier to diagnose in youth. Indeed, families may first notice compulsive behaviors rather than hear or discern obsessions in the student. Compensatory activities can include cognitive behaviors (e.g., hand washing, checking doors, doing something exactly the same way or a certain number of times) and mental activities (e.g., praying, counting to certain numbers, saying certain words) and are excessive and/or ineffective at neutralizing the trigger in a meaningful way (APA, 2022).

Research regarding the cause of OCD is limited, but genetic, temperamental, and environmental characteristics have been identified as likely risk factors. Childhood onset of OCD is associated with development of OCD in other first-degree relatives (APA, 2022). Temperamental risk factors include negative affect, behavioral inhibition, and high internalizing symptoms, while environmental influences include exposure to trauma and physical or sexual abuse. In cases of sudden onset in children, postinfectious autoimmune syndrome and other infectious agents have been implicated (APA, 2022).

Clinically significant OCD symptoms can contribute to substantial academic and interpersonal impairments. Avoidance of situations perceived as threatening or spending excessive amounts of time occupied with symptoms can lead to decreased time in instructional settings, diminished academic productivity, and limited opportunities for socialization (Nazeer et al., 2020). Long-term prognosis varies across life domains with respect to problem severity but increased financial difficulties, few significant relationships, and reduced quality of life have long been associated with untreated symptoms of OCD (APA, 2022).

Did You Know?

Since the 1980s, cases of children with sudden onset of neurological and psychiatric behaviors following *Streptococcus* infections have been noted (APA, 2022). These children, between 3 years old and puberty, develop symptoms such as vocal and motor tics, obsessions, and compulsions seemingly overnight (Genetic and Rare Diseases Information Center, 2024). The condition, pediatric autoimmune neuropsychiatric disorders associated with *Streptococcus* (PANDAS), is not well known and sometimes treated skeptically as it can present with over 24 different neurological and/or psychological symptoms. In addition, while PANDAS is associated with *Streptococcus* infection, children do not always present with sore throat, making the connection more difficult. School nurses can educate and collaborate with the school team to identify and refer students with new psychiatric symptoms for further evaluation (Boyd et al., 2024).

Treatment of OCD includes exposure and response prevention therapy, a type of cognitive behavioral therapy, along with medication if needed (International OCD Foundation, n.d.). Selective serotonin reuptake inhibitors (SSRIs) are most commonly used with the precaution of monitoring the child for the development of suicidal thoughts. Depending on the need, treatment can be delivered in residential centers, day programs, and outpatient and inpatient settings. Support groups are also available for children, youth, and families. Treatment for children and youth with OCD is generally successful.

Trichotillomania

Trichotillomania is a related impulse control disorder usually involving compulsive hair pulling but may include other repetitive "impulses" that cannot be resisted (APA, 2022). Only 1% to 2% of the adults and youth will exhibit this type of behavior with an equal female:male distribution in children with a 2:1 gender ratio in adults. Affected youth may pull hair from the scalp, eyelids, and eyebrows, as well as from the less common pubic and axillary areas. Trichotillomania is usually associated with other repetitive behaviors such as biting nails or skin picking (APA, 2022). Students may do well controlling the impulse to pull hair for weeks but subsequently have a difficult interval for just a few minutes where they pull out significant amounts of hair and leave a bald spot clearly visible to others. There is evidence of genetic and physiological influence in the development of trichotillomania, as onset typically occurs in conjunction with puberty. Anxiety and depression are highly comorbid with trichotillomania in youth, partly attributable to chronic symptoms coupled with significant distress.

The psychotherapeutic treatment of choice for trichotillomania is habit reversal training, which also integrates relaxation strategies to support management of stress. Psychoeducation emphasizes the core elements of self-monitoring, stimulus control, and habit reversal used to disrupt hair-pulling patterns. The skills are taught in a strategic sequence to support the youth's development of competing responses (e.g., fist clinching, use of manipulatives) that activate muscle groups used for hair-pulling behaviors. Thus youth are trained to engage in fist clenching, pencil flipping, and other competing activities rather than problematic behavior when pulling urges first appear.

Depressive Disorders

There are a number of different types of depressive disorders, including major depressive disorder, persistent depressive disorder (dysthymia), and disruptive mood dysregulation disorder. Common to all of these is the presence of a sad, empty, or irritable mood, accompanied by "related changes that significantly affect the individual's capacity to function" (APA, 2022, p. 178). The types of depression differ by duration and timing. The diagnosis of major depression has increased for youth, with about 9% of children and 15% of teenagers meeting the criteria for depression at any given time and almost 19% of adolescents having seriously considered attempting suicide (CDC, 2023b). Additional symptoms that might indicate depression include decreased appetite that may be associated with significant weight loss or failure to make expected weight gain, changed sleeping habits (insomnia or hypersomnia), increased or decreased activity, significant fatigue, concentration difficulties, diminished feelings of self-worth, excessive or inappropriate guilt, and recurrent thoughts of death or suicidal ideation (APA, 2022).

The causes of depressive disorders include genetic influences; biochemical factors, especially related to neurotransmitters such as serotonin, norepinephrine, and dopamine; and environmental factors such as stress and loss (Boland et al., 2022). The presence of stressors, such as abuse, neglect, exposure to violence, parental separation, and ongoing conflicts, adds to the risk (APA, 2022; NIMH, 2022).

Major Depressive Disorder

Major depressive disorder in youth presents as at least 2 weeks of a persistent change from normal mood, characterized as exhibiting a depressed or irritable mood much of the time, most days, and/or loss of interest or pleasure in previously pleasurable activities, plus several additional symptoms such as weight loss, altered sleep patterns, decreased ability to concentrate, feeling worthless or guilty, and having recurrent thoughts of death (APA, 2022). It can occur as a single episode or as a chronic recurrent condition and results in identifiable impairment in functioning across life settings, such as decreased academic performance or interpersonal challenges.

Persistent Depressive Disorder

Persistent depressive disorder, formerly known as dysthymia, is recognized as a persistent, long-term change in mood that is less intense but more chronic than major depressive disorder. Students with persistent depressive disorder will present with depressed mood or irritability for most of the day over the course of most days over the course of a year (2 years in adults). The individual must also demonstrate at least two other symptoms, such as change in eating or sleeping, problems with concentration or decision making, low self-esteem, low energy, or decreased hope (APA, 2022). Without appropriate treatment, persistent depressive disorder is associated with relationship difficulties, occupational challenges such as academic failure, substance use and abuse, and general medical problems. Additionally, students with persistent symptoms are susceptible to the development of anxiety, mood disorders, and major depressive disorder.

Disruptive Mood Dysregulation Disorder

The diagnosis of *disruptive mood dysregulation disorder* was developed to differentiate depression from bipolar disorder in children. The key distinction is that bipolar disorder requires distinct, unusual episodes of manic symptoms, whereas disruptive mood dysregulation disorder represents unremitting symptoms of severe irritability, with frequent verbal or physical angry outbursts an average of three or more times per week and chronically negative mood states between episodes (APA, 2022). The prevalence of disruptive mood dysregulation disorder is unclear; however, based on its core feature, between 2% and 5% of children and adolescents are estimated to have this disorder. The onset is before age 10 and not before age 6. The developmentally inappropriate manifestations of irritability in disruptive mood dysregulation disorder are present across two or more life settings, such as home and school, apparent throughout the day and observable by others (APA, 2022). Disruptive mood dysregulation disorder is now used to describe those children who persistently display profound irritability. Children who have an episode lasting weeks followed by long intervals of months without such profound mood irritability are characterized as having bipolar disorder. Disruptive mood dysregulation disorder cannot be diagnosed if symptoms occur during manic or hypomanic episodes; in these cases, investigation of bipolar disorder is warranted (APA, 2022).

Academic and interpersonal challenges are common among those affected, often resulting in low academic performance and difficulty sustaining friendships. Disruptive mood dysregulation disorder is not a comorbidity of oppositional defiant disorder, but is highly correlated with other disruptive behavior, mood, and anxiety disorders. Extremely low frustration tolerance and severe angry outbursts also contribute to the increased likelihood of aggressive behavior, suicidal ideation, self-harm attempts, and psychiatric hospitalizations compared with nonaffected peers (APA, 2022).

Depressive disorders in children and adolescents are treated with cognitive behavioral therapy. A mood diary can be used to help the child or teen to identify situations and thoughts that trigger their feelings. Adolescents can also benefit from interpersonal psychotherapy, which is more directed and meant to address problematic relationships or specific issues that are causing the most recent episode of depression. SSRIs are generally not used in children with depression but can be used in adolescents. Monitoring for side effects and suicidal ideation is required any time youth are prescribed SSRIs. Students with disruptive mood dysregulation disorder may be treated with cognitive behavioral therapy and "off-label" treatment with stimulants or atypical antipsychotic medications to provide some symptom relief. Parents and caregivers may also benefit from training on how to respond to their child's behavior including rewards for positive behavior (NIMH, 2023b).

Bipolar Disorder

Bipolar I disorder is a condition in which the episodes of depression are interspersed with periods of mania and characterized by "a distinct period of abnormally and persistently elevated expansive, or irritable mood lasting at least 1 week" (APA, 2022, p. 141). Additionally, hypomanic and depressive episodes can precede and/or follow manic episodes. Although pediatric *bipolar disorder* is difficult to disentangle, about 3% of adolescents exhibit symptoms of the disorder (APA, 2022). Characteristics of mania include inflated self-esteem, significantly decreased need for sleep, talkativeness with a pressured speech that is difficult to interrupt, being easily distracted, and feeling as if one's thoughts are racing (APA, 2022). Individuals experiencing a manic episode may also demonstrate increased goal-directed activity or increased agitation and engage in pleasurable but risky behaviors that have a high probability of negative outcomes. A hallmark symptom of childhood mania is episodes of seemingly unprovoked intense rage that can last up to 2 to 3 hours with symptoms that may resemble those of a child with severe ADHD, oppositional defiant disorder, or conduct disorder. Notably, there is a high degree of comorbidity between these conditions and bipolar disorder (APA, 2022).

The presence of hypomanic episodes and the absence of mania distinguishes *bipolar II disorder* from bipolar I. Hypomanic periods are distinct and characterized by elevated or irritable mood and energy or activity levels that are markedly different from the individual's typical presentation. Symptoms persist for most of the day over at least 4 consecutive days and are apparent to others. A minimum of three of the following symptoms will also be present: grandiosity, decreased sleep, pressured speech, flight of ideas, distractibility, goal-directed activity, or excessive involvement in potentially dangerous activities (APA, 2022). Unlike mania in bipolar I, hypomanic episodes do not require hospitalization or result in significant functional impairment. Hypomania coupled with interspersed major depressive disorder results in a diagnosis of bipolar II.

Genetic and physiological factors, as well as environmental influences, contribute to the development of bipolar I and bipolar II. Family history is consistently the most significant risk factor, as individuals with affected family members are on average 10 times more likely to develop bipolar disorder than the general population (APA, 2022). Research suggests that subclinical but high-risk symptoms associated with bipolar disorder are evident 10 years before onset in youth predisposed by genetics. This being the case, early screening and intervention efforts are crucial and may effectively change the development of bipolar I and II in youth.

Treatment plans for bipolar disorder are carefully developed by the provider alongside the child or adolescent and family (NIMH, 2023a). Consistency and adherence to the plan are important aspects of care for those with bipolar conditions. Antipsychotic medications are most often prescribed for the treatment of manic episodes. Mood stabilizer medications and atypical antipsychotic medications can also be used, but long-term use of these medications is not well tested and comes with the potential for significant side effects such as metabolic syndrome (Leibenluft, 2024). The treatment plan can also include cognitive behavioral and family-focused therapy to assist with symptom management.

Schizophrenia Spectrum Disorders

Schizophrenia falls on a spectrum of severity of illness and is characterized by problems in one or more of five domains: delusions (fixed false beliefs), hallucinations (sensory perception disturbances), disorganized thinking (impairments in speech), disorganized or abnormal motor movements (agitation to catatonia), and negative symptoms (diminished emotional expression and avolition; APA, 2022). Only about 1% of the population has this diagnosis, but it is a progressive chronic illness that can cause severe impairment in functioning. Schizophrenia develops in four phases and symptoms usually first appear in adolescence. Phase I is the premorbid phase and is characterized by shyness, withdrawal, lack of friends, and poor school performance. The prodromal phase, or phase II, can last from 2 to 5 years and is a worsening of premorbid symptoms with social withdrawal, cognitive impairment, depressive symptoms, and deterioration in overall functioning (APA, 2022). In phase III, active psychotic phase, the person is experiencing an acute schizophrenic episode and will meet the criteria for schizophrenia according to the DSM-5-TR. Phase IV is the residual phase where the person is in remission and the acute psychosis is either gone or diminished with some residual negative symptoms remaining (APA, 2022). Genetics plays a key role in the development of schizophrenia; those who have relatives with the same condition are more likely to develop schizophrenia.

Early intervention is the key to improved outcomes for students with a diagnosis of schizophrenia. School nurse awareness of the earlier phases of the disorder can help to identify the possibility of schizophrenia early on. In his seminal work, Dr. William McFarlane (2011) describes the Portland Identification and Early Referral (PIER) model to detect, intervene, and prevent psychosis. This model was implemented at schools and colleges in multiple states and is still the best option today for decreasing the cognitive decline seen in schizophrenia (McFarlane, 2011; Parham et al., 2019). Treatment for schizophrenia almost always includes atypical antipsychotic medications to address acute episodes but also as a maintenance therapy to improve socialization and self-care (Patel et al., 2014). The relapse rate for those who stop taking their medication is 60% to 80% versus those who continue to take their medication (18% to 32%). Long-acting injectable antipsychotic agents are now available and have been shown to prevent hospitalizations more effectively than oral agents. Concomitant psychotherapy, including individual and group therapy along with cognitive behavioral therapy, is also found to assist patients in preventing relapses and help with medication monitoring.

Eating Disorders

Eating disorders include several diagnoses related to behaviors around food and overall energy balance that lead to unhealthy outcomes for sufferers that range from altered growth and development to life-threatening electrolyte deficiencies and increased risk of suicide (Hornberger et al., 2021). Identification, treatment, and support of students affected by an eating disorder are made more complicated by the necessity of eating for human life, cultural focus on physical appearance and body size, and stigma related to behavioral health disorders. Despite the intersectional nature of these forces, school nurses must be knowledgeable about eating disorders and assist in early identification and referral, as early treatment may have better outcomes (Hornberger et al., 2021).

The prevalence of eating disorders diagnosed per the DSM-5-TR reveals anorexia to affect about 1% of females by age 20 and 0.1% to 0.3% of males. When including bulimia and binge eating, the rate for females approaches 5% (National Eating Disorder Association [NEDA], 2023). Related symptoms and unhealthy eating behaviors that do not meet diagnostic criteria are far more common in children and adolescents. Exact epidemiological information on eating disorders is difficult to ascertain due to a range of diagnostic criteria and a lack of wide survey data. For example, the CDC does not track eating behaviors in the Youth Risk Behavior Survey. One of the most recent and large ($N = 14,322$) national surveys of 18- to 24-year-olds found unhealthy eating behaviors in 15.4% of women and 7.5% of men with BMIs in the normal range. For those with a BMI greater than 25, the rate nearly doubled to 29.3% and 15.8%, respectively (Nagata et al., 2018). Body image concerns and unhealthy weight control behaviors are not isolated to adolescents and young adults. A variety of studies suggest that up to 50% of 6- to 12-year-olds experience poor body image and begin to alter their eating habits at this age (Pursey et al., 2021).

The most familiar diagnoses in the eating disorder spectrum are anorexia and bulimia nervosa. *Anorexia nervosa* symptoms include restricted calories leading to low body weight, a fear of gaining weight despite being underweight, and altered body image (APA, 2022). Students affected by *bulimia nervosa* may experience binge eating, which is uncontrollable eating of large amounts in a set period of time. Concomitantly, students engage in behaviors to limit weight gain such as self-induced vomiting, misuse of laxatives, diuretics, or other medications. Other calorie balance behaviors include fasting or excessive exercise. Individuals with this condition often feel that their self-worth is related to body size/shape (APA, 2022).

The DSM-5-TR includes disorders closely related to these longstanding diagnoses. *Binge-eating disorder* involves binge eating without compensatory behaviors and includes guilt and anguish regarding binge-eating episodes. Diagnoses related to restrictive eating include *avoidant/restrictive food intake disorder* (AFRID) and *atypical anorexia*. In the latter, the criteria for anorexia may be met, but weight is in the normal range. In AFRID, school nurses may notice students who are not gaining the expected weight or have psychosocial difficulty related to food restriction. The selective eating by these students is related to a lack of interest in eating or a significant sensory sensitivity to food (Eddy, n.d.). Students may not attend social gatherings or may isolate themselves during lunch periods. Risk factors for eating disorders are difficult to identify; however, there are some data to support a heritable link (APA, 2022). Student athletes may be at increased risk, especially in weight-sensitive sports such as dancing and wrestling (NEDA, 2023). Individuals with eating disorder often have comorbidities such as anxiety and depression. Other mental health disorders such as depression, anxiety, and substance use are also associated with individuals with eating disorders (NIMH, 2024). The role of the school nurse in caring for students affected by eating disorders ranges from identification and referral to supportive care to education of teachers and staff and community-level prevention programming.

School nurses may identify a student at risk for eating disorders during routine height and weight checks. This may also include student statements that may indicate body dysphoria or measurements that indicate unexpected changes in weight. As with suicide, asking a student about unhealthy eating behaviors will not worsen the disorder (NEDA, 2022). While the U.S. Preventive Services Task Force (USPSTF; 2022) does not recommend screening asymptomatic students for an eating disorder, those with weight changes, inadequate growth, menstrual irregularities, or pubertal delay may be screened or referred for screening. See Box 28-1 for an assessment mnemonic

BOX 28-1

Recognizing Students With Eating Disorders at School Using BONES

Bundled-up: Wearing layers or bulky clothes to hide weight loss and/or stay warm.

Observable physical changes: Fluctuations in weight (up or down), dry skin, thinning hair, blue hands/feet, brittle nails, swelling around salivary glands, fine hair on the body (lanugo), muscle weakness, poor wound healing, dental changes (if vomiting).

Not feeling well: Nonspecific gastrointestinal complaints, dizziness on standing, syncope, difficulties concentrating, headache, fatigue, weakness, menstrual irregularities.

Extremes: Mood swings (e.g., guilt, disgust, depression, irritability), compulsive behaviors, isolating or withdrawing from social situations, reluctant to ask for help, preoccupation with body size and shape, "fat" talk, drinks excessive amounts of water, frequent bathroom trips, rigid exercise regimen.

Skipping, skimming, or structuring meals: Dieting, restricting whole categories of food, appearing uncomfortable eating around others, skipping meals (e.g., going to the library or doing homework during lunch), or taking small portions.

Source: Lucas et al. (2022, p. 86).

created specifically for school nurses to recognize students who may have an eating disorder.

Treatment of eating disorders and unhealthy eating and weight control behaviors is complex and often requires an interprofessional team. Treatment may range from inpatient hospitalization for students who are suicidal, at critically low body weights, or who have life-threatening electrolyte abnormalities to intensive partial hospital therapy to counseling and pediatrician-managed care. Most patients will receive family or individual psychotherapy, often cognitive behavioral therapy. Therapy, as well as medications such as antidepressants, antipsychotics, and mood stabilizers, are also used to treat comorbid conditions that may be contributing to the eating disorder.

The school nurse may be asked to weigh students with an eating disorder periodically. As with all height and weight checks, this should be done in private, and the school nurse should not comment on the findings (NEDA, 2022). The frequency and process for weight checks should be clearly discussed with the treatment team as the reasons and frequency differ depending on the type of clinical protocol being used to support the student (Waller & Mountford, 2015). For example, whether the student faces the scale or not, and what amount of clothing is permitted are all relevant questions for the treatment team. See Table 28-1 for additional eating disorder resources.

Oppositional Defiant Disorder

It can be normal for children and adolescents to have trouble controlling their emotions and behaviors. However, when there is evidence of a child with a persistent pattern of angry or irritable mood, argumentative or defiant behaviors, or vindictiveness toward others, these behaviors move beyond the scope of normal child development and into a diagnosis of oppositional defiant disorder (Aggarwal & Marwaha, 2022). The overall prevalence of this disorder is estimated at about 3.3% and is found only slightly more in boys than in girls, with the difference waning by adolescence. *Oppositional defiant disorder* (ODD) is a type of childhood disruptive behavior disorder that primarily involves problems with self-control of emotions and behaviors. ODD may be assessed in a child as young as 5 years of age. However, they are usually identified before 8 years of age but no later than 12 years of age, with these behaviors occurring much more consistently and intensely than other age-related peers without a diagnosis (CDC, 2024a).

The exact causes of ODD are unknown, but it is clear there is intersectionality between biological, psychological, environmental, and social factors at play with children diagnosed with ODD (American Academy of Child and Adolescent Psychiatry [AACAP], 2009). Additionally, childhood maltreatment and harsh, inconsistent parenting are commonly found in families of children with ODD (Aggarwal & Marwaha, 2022). Social factors such as peer rejection, deviant peer groups, poverty, neighborhood violence, and other unstable social or economic factors are known to have negative effects on children's behaviors and may contribute to the development of ODD. In terms of genetic factors, it is estimated that heritability of ODD is around 40% and there is a substantial genetic overlap with conduct disorder (Aggarwal & Marwaha, 2022).

ODD refers to a recurrent pattern of developmentally inappropriate levels of negativistic, defiant, and hostile behavior that causes serious problems at home, in school, or with peers (CDC, 2024a). For a diagnosis of ODD to be made, the behavior must persist for at least 6 months and be characterized by the frequent occurrence of at least four of the following behaviors in an interaction with someone who is not a sibling:

- Loses temper often
- Easily annoyed or touchy
- Often angry or resentful
- Regularly argues with authority figures; for children this can mean an adult
- Refuses or actively defies rules or requests from authority figures
- Deliberately annoys others
- Blames others for their mistakes
- Is spiteful and vindictive at least two times in last 6 months

TABLE 28-1 Eating Disorder Resources

Organization	Resource	Web site/URL
Anorexics and Bulimics Anonymous (ABA)	12-step support group	https://aba12steps.org/
Eating Disorder Hope	Private, large Web site with resources for patients	https://www.eatingdisorderhope.com/
National Alliance for Eating Disorders	Treatment, support groups, help for family	https://www.allianceforeatingdisorders.com/
National Eating Disorder Association (NEDA)	Educator Toolkit: signs and symptoms, tips for nurses, holistic assessment form	https://www.nationaleatingdisorders.org/sites/default/files/Toolkits/EducatorToolkit.pdf
National Institute of Mental Health	Information and access to current clinical trials/research	https://www.nimh.nih.gov/health/topics/eating-disorders

For an ODD diagnosis there must be evidence of impairment at either the individual level, social level with peers, or with educational, family, or other important areas of functioning but tends to be more noticeable at home or school. ODD has three severity classifications: *mild*, where symptoms occur in only one setting, such as home, school, work, or with peers; *moderate*, where symptoms occur in at least two settings; and *severe*, where symptoms occur in three or more settings (APA, 2022). The most common behaviors that children and adolescents with ODD exhibit are defiance, spitefulness, negativity, hostility and verbal aggression (Aggarwal & Marwaha, 2022). Students diagnosed with ODD have difficulty remaining in the classroom due to their disruptive behaviors and often become quickly acquainted with disciplinary staff in school. These students can disrupt the classroom by yelling, starting fights, and not listening to instructions, and may even go so far as to throw desks or rip up their assignments.

Several psychological evaluation surveys are available to assist in the diagnosis of ODD. The surveys generally assess the student in various settings and collect parental input. Treatment requires a combination of approaches (AACAP, 2009). Treatment can include parent management training, family therapy, cognitive problem-solving skills training, social skill, and school-based programs, as well as pharmacotherapy.

Conduct Disorder

Unlike ODD, *conduct disorder* is a pervasive disorder with clinically significant antisocial behaviors that show an ongoing pattern of aggression toward others and serious violations of rules and social norms (CDC, 2024a). Conduct disorder is a DSM-5-TR diagnosis assigned to individuals who habitually violate the rights of others and will not conform their behavior to the law or social norms appropriate for their age (APA, 2022). Specifications for the disorder include limited prosocial emotions; lack of remorse, guilt, or empathy; shallow or deficient affect; or a lack of concern about performance that is often blamed on others. Conduct disorder often brings a young person into contact with the juvenile justice system or other disciplinary action from parents or school administration (APA, 2022). Similar to ODD, the severity of conduct disorder is specified as mild, moderate, and severe. This disorder is also divided into subtypes based on the age at onset. Risk factors for conduct disorder are undercontrolled infant temperament, low verbal IQ, parental rejection, harsh discipline, neglect, and other forms of child maltreatment, including sexual abuse.

The prevalence of conduct disorder increases from childhood to adolescence with higher rates seen among males (APA, 2022). Behaviors can start as early as preschool years with ODD, a common premorbid condition, which, if unaddressed, may progress to a diagnosis of conduct disorder. Middle childhood to middle adolescence is where conduct disorder symptoms are most apparent and is when it most often comes to parental, educational, or clinical attention (APA, 2022). The estimated lifetime prevalence of conduct disorder in the United States is 9.5%, with 12% in males and 7.1% in females, with a median age of onset of 11.6 years (Patel et al., 2018). Males may be more frequently diagnosed due to the tendency to act out violently, while girls tend to act out in interpersonal relationships. There is some evidence of a genetic component with apparent predispositions for youth with parents (biological or adopted) who have substance use disorder, mood disorder, schizophrenia, ADHD, and conduct disorder. The potential role of an imbalance of neurotransmitters has also been asserted, as have frontal lobe and executive functioning issues (Boland et al., 2022). This interferes with a child's ability to play, manage impulses, stay away from harm, and learn from negative experiences (Johns Hopkins, 2022).

Conduct disorder is divided into four main groupings: aggression toward people and animals, destruction of property, deceitfulness or theft, and serious violation of rules (APA, 2022). To diagnose conduct disorder, at least three of the following behaviors must be present in the past 12 months with at least one in the past 6 months. In addition to these items, the individual must also experience significant impairment in functioning to warrant a diagnosis.

- Often bullies, threatens, or intimidates others
- Often initiates physical fights
- Has used a weapon that can cause serious physical harm to others (e.g., bat, brick, broken bottle, knife, gun)
- Has been physically cruel to people
- Has stolen while confronting a victim (e.g., mugging, purse snatching, extortion, armed robbery)
- Has forced someone into sexual activity
- Has deliberately engaged in fire setting with the intention of causing serious damage
- Has deliberately destroyed others' property (other than by fire setting)
- Has broken into someone else's house, building, or car
- Often lies to obtain goods or favors or to avoid obligations (i.e., "cons" others)
- Has stolen items of nontrivial value without confronting a victim (e.g., shoplifting, but without breaking and entering; forgery)
- Often stays out at night despite parental prohibitions, beginning before age 13 years
- Has run away from home overnight at least twice while living in the parental or parental surrogate home or once without returning for a lengthy period
- Is often truant from school, beginning before age 13 years

There is a high degree of comorbidity between conduct disorder and ODD and other mental health conditions such as mood disorders, intermittent explosive disorder, and especially ADHD and substance use (Patel et al., 2018). Therefore medications, which are not usually prescribed to treat conduct disorder, may be indicated to treat comorbid concerns. Treatment approaches need to intervene at many levels, and an ideal treatment plan should integrate the individual, family, school, and community (CDC, 2024a). Parent management training and classroom behavior management have demonstrated efficacy in the treatment of conduct disorder and ODD. Parent behavior training supports the development of positive parenting strategies (e.g., positive attending, increased monitoring), problem-solving, communication, reinforcement (e.g., praise for prosocial behavior), and consistent discipline practices. Youth with conduct disorder and ODD also benefit from a complementary set of cognitive behavioral skills training, including problem-solving, calming/relaxation, and communication skills to address negative attribution styles and promote effective responses to stressful situations.

In school, teachers or counselors may apply group management techniques with emphasis on reinforcement and use of consistent discipline practices. A behavior intervention plan should be in place that describes the steps that should be taken when acting out occurs. It is essential for the school nurse to follow the steps on the behavior plan. The *Good Behavior Game* is an exemplary program and targeted intervention used to teach social-emotional awareness, encourage self-regulation, and promote prosocial skills (PAXIS Institute, 2021). Conduct disorder is a strong prognostic indicator for both antisocial personality disorder and psychoactive substance use disorders in adulthood if therapeutic interventions are not successful.

SUICIDAL IDEATION AND BEHAVIOR

Suicide among youths continues to be a serious and ongoing problem. The rates of suicidal ideation, attempt, and completion are on the rise, according to the 2021 *Youth Risk Behavior Survey* (CDC, 2023c) of high school students across the United States. Suicide is the third leading cause of death among youth ages 15 to 19 (CDC, 2024b). The number of youth and young adults who die of suicide exceeds the number who die of cancer, heart disease, AIDS, birth defects, stroke, pneumonia, influenza, and chronic lung disease combined (Jason Foundation, 2022). In 2022, 493 children ages 10 to 14 and 6,528 youth and young adults ages 15 to 24 reportedly died from suicide (Curtin et al., 2022). This is likely an under accounting of the total number of suicide deaths in children and youth.

In 2021, approximately 22% of high school–age students (30% females, 14% males) seriously considered attempting suicide, and 10% of high school students attempted suicide (13% females, 7% males). Although girls may be more likely to consider attempting suicide, boys are more likely to die of suicide (Miranda-Mendizabal et al., 2019). Rates of suicide attempts and suicide deaths are rising in students of color, especially among Latinx and black girls (CDC, 2023c).

Risk Factors

A history of previous mental health disorder, substance use disorder, and exposure to interpersonal violence are common risks for suicidal behavior in adolescents and young adults of any gender identity (Miranda-Mendizabal et al., 2019). However, in slightly more than half of suicides in children and youth, there was no identified mental health condition (Stone et al., 2018). Depression, exposure to violence, impulsivity, bullying, feelings of hopelessness or helplessness, and acute loss and rejection increase the risk of suicidal thoughts or actions (AACAP, 2024). Teens who engaged in intentional nonsuicidal self-injury had almost 27 times higher risk of suicide within the next year (Poudel et al., 2022). However, students can inflict self-harm without the intention of suicidal behavior. Students with a family history of psychiatric illness are also at high risk. The children of parents who attempted suicide are six times more at risk of suicide than those whose parents did not attempt suicide.

Youth are also at risk by the nature of their developmental and social stages. The judgment and decision-making abilities of youth and young adults are a function of the prefrontal cortex, the brain's executive control center, which does not fully develop until one's mid-20s. This leads youth to be more impulsive and less able to weigh risks, consequences, and values in the same way as mature adults (Cohen, 2022). Certain risk factors for suicidal behaviors are more likely to be seen in males than females (Table 28-2).

Suicide is especially high among youth who identify as sexual minorities. There was a significant decrease in

TABLE 28-2 Suicide Risk Factors More Likely to Be Associated With Female and Male Youth

	Risks for Suicide *Attempt*	Risks for Suicide *Death*
Females	• Eating disorders • Post-traumatic stress disorder • Bipolar disorder • Victim of dating violence • Depressive symptoms • Interpersonal problems • Previous abortion	Insufficient research literature to determine
Males	• Disruptive behavior/conduct problems • Hopelessness • Parental separation/divorce • Friend's suicidal behavior • Access to means	• Substance abuse • Externalizing disorders • Access to means

Miranda-Mendizabal et al. (2019).

suicide attempts in the lesbian, gay, bisexual, transgender, queer, plus (LGBTQ+) population in the immediate years following the passage of same-sex marriage policies in the United States in 2015 (Raifman et al., 2017); however, this trend has not been sustained. In 2021, youth who identified as LGBTQ+ youth were approximately three times more likely to seriously consider attempting suicide than youth who identified as heterosexual and almost four times more likely to attempt suicide (CDC, 2023c). Comprehensive intervention strategies within schools and communities are needed with the express goal of reducing violence and victimization and preventing suicide risk among LBGTQ+ and other marginalized youths.

School nurses need to understand the risks and signs of suicidal thoughts and interventions that help youth avoid the decisive or impulsive action of suicide with devastating consequences (AACAP, 2024). Reducing deaths by suicide in youth is an urgent public health goal, especially in light of emerging data that suggest that the COVID-19 pandemic further increased youth rates of death by suicide and increased emergency department visits for suicide attempts (Berk, 2022). Issues of intersectionality, inclusion, and systemic inequities need to be at the forefront of discussions on how to address the problem of youth suicide.

Signs and Symptoms

Suicidal ideation, that is, suicidal thoughts or ideas, is a broad term to describe a range of contemplation related to suicidal thinking, preoccupations, and behavior (Harmer et al., 2022). Many people who are considering suicide do not appear outwardly upset or depressed (Cohen, 2022). The stigma of mental illness can be a barrier to seeking help. Regularly and proactively checking in with students to let them know you are available to listen can help be a proactive way to intervene around independent and self-reliant students.

Warning signs associated with suicide can be similar to other mental health conditions, including the following:

- Changes in eating or sleeping habits
- Frequent or pervasive sadness
- Withdrawal from friends, family, and regular activities
- Frequent complaints about physical symptoms often related to emotions, such as stomach aches, headaches, fatigue, feeling "sick," and so on
- Decline in the quality of schoolwork
- Preoccupation with death and dying
- Stops planning and talking about the future
- Giving away important possessions (AACAP, 2024)

Students who make comments such as "I can't take this anymore," "They'll be better off without me around," "I wish I was dead," or "I won't be a problem for you much longer" are in crisis and may be demonstrating active suicidal intention that requires immediate intervention to prevent them from carrying out a suicide plan. Thoughts of killing oneself without a specific plan or intent to follow through with a plan are early warning signs that the student needs further evaluation and intervention. Although many people feel uncomfortable talking about suicide, school nurses should directly ask a student whether they are thinking about suicide and if they have a suicide plan (AACAP, 2024). The National Institute of Mental Health (2020) offers a simple tool, the *Ask Suicide-Screening Questions (ASQ) Toolkit,* to help determine the level of a person's suicide risk and next steps to take. See Figure 28-2.

There is no evidence that talking about suicide increases the risk or gives students the idea to engage in suicidal behavior. Opportunities to intervene may be missed if students are not asked directly what they are experiencing. Asking students about their thoughts and feelings lets them know that someone cares and gives them an opportunity to talk to someone about the problems they are facing (AACAP, 2024). Any person thinking about suicide during the past month needs significant attention and follow-up. When suicidal thoughts and statements arise, it is always best practice to err on the side of caution and safety and have the student evaluated immediately by a trained and qualified mental health professional (AACAP, 2024).

Intervention

The school nurse collaborates with the other professionals on the student support team who have mental health expertise such as licensed school social workers, counselors, and psychologists to get students the appropriate level of intervention (NASN, 2022a). Protocols and procedures for intervening need to be in place before there are issues. All team members need to understand their delineated roles. When and how to contact parents/guardians, minor confidentiality laws, and referral resources for both inpatient and outpatient psychiatric services should be clearly outlined. Students with a history of suicidal ideation need a safety plan developed by a therapist or social worker that the student agrees to follow and that is supported by the school. A safety plan outlines the student's warning signs, coping mechanisms, professionals to contact when indicated, and how to make the student's environment as safe as possible (Jones, 2020). Students who receive special education services under the qualifying characteristic of emotional disturbance should have a *behavioral intervention plan* (see Chapter 8).

School nurses can demonstrate that they are comfortable talking about suicide and other mental health topics by having mental health literature and posters in the health office. Mental health assessment and screening should be a normal part of student assessment. This helps to reduce the stigma of mental health and communicate to students that they can get help in the school health office.

Prevention

The AAP and American Foundation for Suicide Prevention (AFSP), in collaboration with experts from NIMH, created a *Blueprint for Youth Suicide Prevention* as an educational resource to support pediatric health clinicians and other

NIMH TOOLKIT

asQ Suicide Risk Screening Tool

Ask Suicide-Screening Questions

Ask the patient:

1. In the past few weeks, have you wished you were dead? ❍ Yes ❍ No
2. In the past few weeks, have you felt that you or your family would be better off if you were dead? ❍ Yes ❍ No
3. In the past week, have you been having thoughts about killing yourself? ❍ Yes ❍ No
4. Have you ever tried to kill yourself? ❍ Yes ❍ No

   If yes, how? ____________________________

   When? ____________________________

If the patient answers **Yes** *to any of the above, ask the following acuity question:*

5. **Are you having thoughts of killing yourself right now?** ❍ Yes ❍ No

   If yes, please describe: ____________________________

Next steps:

- If patient answers "No" to all questions 1 through 4, screening is complete (not necessary to ask question #5). No intervention is necessary *(*Note: Clinical judgment can always override a negative screen).*
- **If patient answers "Yes" to any of questions 1 through 4, or refuses to answer, they are considered a positive screen. Ask question #5 to assess acuity:**
  - ☐ **"Yes"** to question #5 = **acute positive screen** (imminent risk identified)
    - **Patient requires a STAT safety/full mental health evaluation. Patient cannot leave until evaluated for safety.**
    - Keep patient in sight. Remove all dangerous objects from room. Alert physician or clinician responsible for patient's care.
  - ☐ **"No"** to question #5 = **non-acute positive screen** (potential risk identified)
    - **Patient requires a brief suicide safety assessment to determine if a full mental health evaluation is needed. If a patient (or parent/guardian) refuses the brief assessment, this should be treated as an "against medical advice" (AMA) discharge.**
    - Alert physician or clinician responsible for patient's care.

Provide resources to all patients

- 24/7 National Suicide Prevention Lifeline, 988
- 24/7 Crisis Text Line: Text "HOME" to 741741

asQ Suicide Risk Screening Toolkit NATIONAL INSTITUTE OF MENTAL HEALTH (NIMH) NIH 2/6/2024

FIGURE 28-2. Ask Suicide-Screening Questions (ASQ) Toolkit. *(National Institute of Mental Health, 2020)*

health professionals in identifying strategies and key partnerships to support youth at risk for suicide (AAP, 2023). The *Blueprint* provides information, strategies, and concrete examples to help schools and community partners work together toward youth suicide prevention efforts. Specific behavioral targets such as reducing bullying, violence, and substance abuse through education and strategic community efforts can help create safe school environments and can help reduce incidents of suicide.

No single strategy works best to prevent suicide. Prevention programs can target at-risk students either individually or collectively as groups of students. Prevention program strategies include developing protocols for students at risk for suicide, training of staff, and parent/guardian education. The student population should be empowered to assist their peers by sharing their concerns with adults in the school. Families and communities can be educated that restricting access to lethal means, such as firearms, is associated with a decrease in suicide (Zalsman et al., 2016). Treating depression and other mental health conditions is key to prevention.

Training can help school staff feel better prepared to identify students at risk for suicide by outlining actionable steps to take once students have been identified as a risk. The National Suicide Prevention Lifeline (n.d.) has a campaign funded by SAMHSA that promotes the acronym *ACT—Acknowledge, Care, and Tell,* which is a resource for school faculty and staff when talking with students who are suspected of having suicidal ideation (Box 28-2).

Mental Health First Aid is a skills-based training that teaches participants how to help someone who is developing a mental health problem or experiencing a mental health crisis. The training covers warning signs; provides information on common mental health issues such as depression, anxiety, trauma, and addiction; and provides a five-step action plan to help someone obtain professional help along with self-help (National Council for Mental Wellbeing, 2023). See Resources for additional trainings that can help professionals build skills to help prevent suicide.

BOX 28-2

ACT: Acknowledge, Care, Tell

A resource for faculty and staff to facilitate conversations with struggling students.

ACT: Acknowledge, Care, Tell when concerned about a student, or approached by students asking for help:

Acknowledge: Whether a student asks for help directly, or you have concerns, acknowledge that the situation is serious and that you're worried about their well-being. Remember, there's no harm in asking a student if they're suicidal.

Example: "I really value your input in class and appreciate x, y, and z, but I've noticed a few changes in your behavior and wanted to check-in to see how you're doing." [As the conversation progresses] "Has it gotten so bad that you've thought about suicide?"

Care: Show you care by listening nonjudgmentally to what the student says; observe their demeanor and avoid making the student feel embarrassed or guilty. Offer words of encouragement, but do not promise to keep a secret. Acting to prevent suicide overrides any confidentiality between faculty/staff and students.

Example: "It sounds like you are really struggling. I would never want you to be hurting like this."

Tell: Advise the student that you must tell your school's mental health contact and that you will accompany them to their office.

Example: "There are people at this school who know how to help kids that are dealing with big issues like this. Let's walk down to the counseling suite together."

Whether or not you believe a student is suicidal, alert your school's mental health contact about your concerns and your conversation with the student.

Help is always available. The National Suicide Prevention Lifeline provides 24/7, free and confidential support at 1-800-273-TALK (8255).

National Suicide Prevention Lifeline (n.d.).

When There Is a Suicide in the School Community

The suicide of a student or staff has a significant impact on the entire school community. It is essential to have plans in place in anticipation of this traumatic event. An excellent resource is *After a Suicide: A Toolkit for Schools* from the Suicide Prevention Resource Center (AFSP& Suicide Prevention Resource Center [SPRC], 2018). It recommends that all student deaths be treated the same way, whether by suicide or by cancer. When suicide is glamorized, there is the risk of other students copying the behavior, leading to a cluster of suicides (i.e., three or more deaths).

Following a student suicide, the school's crisis response team should be mobilized. At the appropriate time, the death can be announced to the students, preferably in small groups rather than over the public address system. However, the cause of death should not be disclosed until the family has been consulted. Once suicide is identified as the cause, information and resources about suicide should

Did You Know?

- **National Suicide Prevention Lifeline**
- **Dial 988 for the National Suicide Prevention Hotline**
- **Text "HOME" to 741741 for the National Crisis Text Hotline**

School nurses can post flyers in the school health office with this information.

be provided to students and staff. It is essential to monitor social media and to pay attention to students who may be having difficulty with the death. These students should be encouraged to talk with counselors, the school nurse, or other staff (AFSP & SPRC, 2018). The services of the district crisis team or grief counselors can be employed.

CHILDHOOD BEREAVEMENT AND GRIEF

Many students experience loss, whether it be a family member, friend, or other significant person. The death of a staff member or classmate can also result in grieving, as can divorce, relocating, or a natural disaster. The school nurse is often in the position of comforting students experiencing grief and loss. According to the Society of Pediatric Psychology,

> *Bereavement refers to the objective experience of losing a loved one by death, whereas grief refers to one's subjective experience. In other words, grief represents the emotional, cognitive, behavioral, physical, and spiritual reactions that a bereaved child or adolescent experiences following the death of their loved one. Mourning is the cultural experience or observation of the loss. (Thompson et al., 2019, para. 1)*

The Childhood Bereavement Estimation Model approximates that in the United States, one in 12 students will grieve the death of a parent or sibling by age 18, accounting for over 6 million children and youth. Losing a parent/guardian or sibling is traumatic for school-age children and considered an adverse childhood event (ACE); it is undoubtedly one of the hardest experiences a child can experience (Judi's House, 2024). Rates of childhood bereavement vary widely between states with West Virginia having the highest rate (13.7%) and Nebraska having the lowest (6.7%). These rates escalated during the COVID-19 pandemic; it is estimated that approximately 216,600 U.S. children lost a member of their household between May 2020 and May 2022. Children and youth of color were twice as likely as white students to lose the only caregiver with whom they lived (Treglia et al., 2023). Isolation and interruptions in the normal systems of support, such as school, exacerbated the bereavement process during the pandemic for many students. With the increased prevalence of violent incidents and suicide, students may have to face the loss of a peer. The school nurse is often in the position of comforting students experiencing grief and loss.

Grieving is a normal life process after a loss. Elizabeth Kubler-Ross seminally described the *Five Stages of Grief* in 1996: denial, anger, bargaining, depression, acceptance, and hope (Elizabeth Kubler-Ross Foundation, 2010). Students grieve differently depending on many factors, including the circumstances of the death, family dynamics, developmental level, cultural contexts, and personality/temperament (Thompson et al., 2019). The school nurse may encounter elementary school students who regress; for example, incontinence may occur in students who previously had no issues with bowel or bladder control.

Signs and Symptoms

Subclinical, typical grief symptoms include emotional lability (sadness, crying, irritability), confusion, anger (outbursts), worry, and anxiety. Students often have difficulty concentrating on schoolwork; academic performance can decline (Thompson et al., 2019). Somatic complaints and difficulty sleeping can also impair focus in the classroom. Some students will avoid talking about their grief; others may use maladaptive coping behaviors, such as misusing alcohol or drugs. Over time, grief gradually resolves without therapeutic intervention as students come to accept the loss and find an equilibrium in routine living, though it is normal to experience moments of profound sadness triggered by memories, death anniversaries, and special events.

Atypical Grief Reactions

There are many different types of grief reactions (Table 28-3). Symptoms that worsen or persist for more than 6 months are indicative of childhood traumatic grief, complicated grief, or other atypical grief reactions. Approximately 5% to 10% of students will experience depression, PTSD, and/or prolonged grief disorder. In *prolonged grief disorder* the symptoms of grief are overwhelming and do not lessen over time (APA, 2022). Such intense and prolonged feelings of grief cause disabling impairments in daily living and require intensive treatment, including cognitive behavioral therapy. Symptoms of prolonged grief disorder include the following:

- Identity disruption (such as feeling as though part of oneself has died)
- Marked sense of disbelief about the death
- Avoidance of reminders that the person is dead
- Intense emotional pain (such as anger, bitterness, sorrow) related to the death
- Difficulty with reintegration (such as problems engaging with friends, pursuing interests, planning for the future)
- Emotional numbness (absence or marked reduction of emotional experience)
- Feeling that life is meaningless
- Intense loneliness (APA, 2022)

The risk for long-term depression, PTSD, and prolonged grief disorder varies depending on the type, scope, or intensity of the loss, coping skills, and social and family support. Losses that are sudden, unexpected, and traumatic increase the risks (APA, 2022). A study of students involved directly or indirectly in a fatal school bus accident found that 70% had prolonged grief reactions (Giannopoulou et al., 2021). Reexperiencing the event, increased arousal, negative cognitions such as self-blaming, and avoidance are correlated with stress-related anxiety and depressive disorders.

TABLE 28-3 Types of Grief Reactions

Type of Grief	Description
Anticipatory	Grief that occurs when death or loss is expected; occurs before the loss
Disenfranchised	Experience of a mourner's grief response being socially invalidated, unacknowledged, or discouraged
Complicated/chronic/prolonged	Significant grief that is impactful for more than 6 months
Traumatic	A condition in which trauma symptoms interfere with adaptive child grieving
Cumulative	Losses sustained over time affect response to loss
Masked	The person does not admit they are experiencing grief
Distorted	For example, prolonged and extreme anger may appear stuck in one phase of grief
Absent	The outward appearance of grief is not present; little to no sign of grief is present

Adapted from Dutil (2019); Glazer & Clark-Foster (2019); Wilson et al. (2022). From Edwards et al. (2023). Used with permission.

Support for Grieving Students

Cultures support different mourning customs and rituals that need to be respected and supported. Culture influences the "acceptable" length of the grieving process, as well as behaviors that are "expected" during grieving (which may actually be a cause of distress for the bereaved if they do not adhere to expectations). School nurses provide culturally sensitive care by assessing the student's family, social, religious, and community contexts and inquiring about the student's and family's expectations and priorities (see Chapter 10).

The school nurse can provide psychoeducation to students, families, and school staff related to normal grieving processes and potential treatment options for students experiencing atypical grief reactions. The National Child Traumatic Stress Network houses resources and tools in a wide range of languages that can be shared with youth, caregivers, school-based staff, and mental health providers.

The school nurse can provide support by actively listening, acknowledging normal grief responses, or simply sitting quietly with a student. Students should be encouraged to ask questions, express feelings (including crying), and share memories of their departed loved one. Students should be reassured that they did not cause the death, nor could they have prevented it. In cases of terminal illness where death is anticipated, the school nurse can support anticipatory grieving and suggest books and resources that are age-appropriate to help cope.

Because the school is perceived as a physically and psychosocially safe place, it can be a communal site where large numbers of students and staff may gather in vigil or remembrance and share the grieving process. Counselors are often brought into schools where tragedies have occurred to assist students in the grieving process. In some cases, the community is also invited to participate in this process. This demonstrates that the school community is caring and responsive to the larger community and continues to be a place of safety. The school nurse should be involved in any large-scale bereavement activities. Psychological first aid following large scale emergencies and disasters is discussed in Chapter 15.

School nurses should perform a self-assessment to ensure they are capable of supporting grieving students and staff. Depending on the personal impact of the loss, school nurses may need to defer their responsibilities to another professional until they are able to cope and function in their role at school. Frequently, district-based or local crisis response teams are available to help students through the initial grieving process.

SCHOOLS AND BEHAVIORAL/ MENTAL HEALTH

Schools play pivotal roles in addressing the substantial impact of student mental health concerns. The National Alliance on Mental Illness and the American Academy of Pediatrics, in partnership with the National Center for School Mental Health (NCSMH), call for organized, comprehensive, family-centered services that provide smooth connections with pediatric clinicians in the community in an effort to reduce the burden of mental health concerns (AAP, 2021b). Central components of such a system include addressing school climate, promotion of healthy socioemotional development, and prevention and treatment of mental health disorders. Addressing mental health is congruent with a school's mission to ensure a safe and healthy learning environment for students to promote academic success. Survey data indicate that approximately one-third of students who access mental health care did so solely through school (Ali et al., 2019). Policies that support positive student mental health and well-being are related to academic success (National Association of School Psychologists, 2021).

Schools should work to provide and fund individualized mental health care, positive school climates, and comprehensive school mental health systems (National Center for School Mental Health and MHTTC Network Coordinating Office, 2019; Zabek et al., 2023). Such comprehensive school mental health systems support the competencies of school mental health providers, including school nurses, school counselors, school psychologists, and school social workers, within a multitiered system of supports and services (see Chapter 7). Key features of comprehensive school mental health systems include

> *(a) well-trained specialized support personnel, (b) family–school–community collaboration, (c) needs assessment and resource mapping, (d) multitiered systems of support (MTSS) approach, (e) mental health screening, (f) evidence-based practice, (g) effective use of data, and (h) culturally responsive and equitable mental health practices. (Zabek et al., 2023, p. 2)*

Many of these activities intersect with competencies of NASN's *School Nursing: Scope and Standards of Practice* (2022b), including community collaboration, quality improvement activities that require data collection, use of evidence-based guidelines, and the development of student-centered plans of care (Zabek et al., 2023).

Student Behavior Assessment and Intervention

Mental health concerns in students are displayed over a continuum from developmentally appropriate behaviors in age groups to behaviors that signal a student is at risk for or is experiencing serious mental health issues. Educators, administrators, and school support team professionals need to establish what behaviors are expected at school of all students and how to identify and intervene when a student is displaying behaviors of concern.

Practice Connection

School nurses in an urban Midwestern city incorporated MTSS into the health office to address the socioemotional health of their students and decrease lost instructional time. Students were reporting to the health office with somatic complaints and the nursing staff realized the symptoms could be minimized using the MTSS approach. Tier 1 included a standardized assessment of the physical and emotional status of each student upon arrival in the health office. Students were taught self-regulating calming strategies as needed that could be implemented in the classroom, decreasing the need to come to the health office. Tier 2 was instituted for a smaller portion of students who needed additional support. It included Tier 1 strategies as well as more targeted interventions such as daily check-ins and involvement of other school team members. Tier 3 included more intensive interventions, and contact with parents and healthcare providers to clarify the source of the student's socioemotional concerns and a written plan to address them (Lytle et al., 2024).

School-Wide Positive Behavior Intervention and Supports

School-Wide Positive Behavior Intervention and Supports (PBIS) is an evidenced-based systematic approach to establishing norms for school behavior and outlining supports that children need to succeed academically and socially (Center on Positive Behavioral Interventions and Supports [CPBIS], 2024). It is a strategic framework endorsed by the U.S. Office of Special Education Programs that supports the development of positive school climates by preventing undesired behaviors and promoting behaviors in students associated with academic success and social well-being.

> *Positive Behavioral Interventions and Supports (PBIS) is an evidence-based, tiered framework for supporting students' behavioral, academic, social, emotional, and mental health. When implemented with fidelity, PBIS improves social emotional competence, academic success, and school climate. It also improves teacher health and wellbeing. It is a way to create positive, predictable, equitable and safe learning environments where everyone thrives. (CPBIS, 2024, p. 1)*

PBIS needs to be sensitive to the cultural contexts of diverse students. As of 2023, approximately 25,500 schools employ PBIS as the best practice approach to challenging behavior (CPBIS, 2024).

The interplay of five implementation elements is considered in all decisions: *equity, systems, data, practices,* and *outcomes.* PBIS follows the public health model of primary, secondary, and tertiary prevention. According to the CPBIS (2024):

- Tier 1 interventions include strategies for *all* students that are developed to provide academic, behavioral, and social/emotional support that meets students' needs. It engages families, educators, and school staff to implement equitable school-wide behavior strategies to prevent problem behaviors from developing in the student population. Tier 1 goals focus on promoting resiliency and safety and creating a supportive and respectful school environment. For example, Tier 1 strategies would outline student expectations and consequences in the learning environment, including classrooms and communal school spaces such as hallways, lunchrooms, playgrounds, assemblies, and after-school activities.
- Tier 2 targets the approximately 10% to 15% of students identified as being at risk for developing severe challenging behavior. Tier 2 strategies target identified problems at the school or classroom level in a subset of students, such as a small group of students who are having difficulty getting along and disrupting learning. The Tier 2 intervention includes focused practices that provide additional support to individual students, such as additional practice on behavioral, social/emotional, and academic competencies.
- Tier 3 of PBIS focuses on the approximately 1% to 5% of the student population who need intensive

individual assessment and behavioral support plans beyond Tier 1 and 2 strategies. Tier 3 interventions should be provided to any student with intensive mental health needs, whether or not they have additional services outlined in an IEP or Section 504 plan. Tier 3 involves functional behavior assessment, a comprehensive coordinated approach by the multidisciplinary educational and student support team, and individualized student-centered strategies. Problematic behaviors in students require careful assessment by the team to inform effective behavior plans (CPBIS, 2024).

Functional Behavior Assessment

Functional behavior assessment (FBA) is a systematic data collection process that student support teams can use to identify environmental events or stimuli that predict when and why persistent challenging behaviors (e.g., aggression, opposition, or self-injury) will occur and repeat (CPBIS, 2022). According to the CPBIS:

> *For students with more persistent and intensive challenges, function-based Tier 3 interventions are based on a formal Functional Behavioral Assessment (FBA) process used to (a) define and prioritize challenging behavior, (b) understand aspects of the environment that occasion and maintain the behavior, and (c) create an individualized multi-component behavior support plan (BSP) designed to address the function of student behavior. (2022, p. 4)*

An assumption of functional behavioral assessment and analysis is that all behaviors, including problem behaviors, serve a purpose or a function for the student who carries out the behavior. Challenging behaviors can happen for students with mental health or neurodevelopmental concerns because of environmental stimuli and events associated with the behavior. The student carries out the behavior to change something in the environment. FBA is widely accepted as a best practice approach for developing classroom behavioral interventions for any student displaying significant behavior problems. Under IDEA (2004), FBA is required under certain circumstances for students receiving special education services.

The school nurse contributes to the FBA by conducting interviews and reviewing records such as incident reports, academic reports, discipline and attendance records, the health record, history of health office visits, medical records and orders, and previous behavior plans. Interviews with teachers (past and present) and support staff (e.g., playground or cafeteria monitors and bus drivers) may shed light on the function of the behavior. Interviewing parents/guardians or family members will offer valuable insight into the dynamics of the behavior, including cultural and community contexts. The multidisciplinary educational team examines and interprets the FBA data before developing a *behavior support plan* (CPBIS, 2022).

A popular approach to data collection in behavior assessment is to examine what are commonly referred to as the *ABCs:* antecedent (A), behavior (B), and consequence (C). This approach considers the relationships between the factors that trigger behavior and the reactions of others. The antecedent (A) is the activating event. It consists of a trigger that occurs immediately before the behavior. A situation, person, request, or even a spoken word may be the stimulus that triggers a specific behavioral response in a student. For example, the teacher turns the classroom lights on and off to indicate clean-up time; then the student throws themself to the floor in a tantrum. In this case, the lights indicating the transition serve as the antecedent. Before the antecedent there may be additional components called *motivating operations.* Motivating operation events make a student more vulnerable to the antecedent (Kaiser & Rasminsky, 2017).

The physical and verbal behaviors (B) associated with the maladaptive behavior are examined. The behavior must be described in accurate objective detail so that it can be clearly identified, observed, and measured consistently (Kaiser & Rasminsky, 2017). The behavior should not be described as "The student responds poorly to directions" but rather "The student throws themself to the floor and tantrums for 5 minutes when the classroom lights are flashed to indicate it is time to clean up."

Consequences (C) are what happens in the environment as a result of the behavior. How did the students respond? How did the teacher react? Any response (adaptive or maladaptive) could reinforce and maintain challenging behaviors (Kaiser & Rasminsky, 2017).

The interdisciplinary team examines the factors thought to be sustaining the behavior and the function the behavior serves for the student. For instance, the student might misbehave to gain attention from their teachers or peers or to escape from unpleasant classroom activities by being sent to the office. Once the function of the behavior is identified, then the factors can be manipulated to reduce the unwanted behaviors and replace them with new positive behaviors (CPBIS, 2022). For example, a student is struggling in a class. During a math lesson, they become extremely frustrated, act out, and are sent to the dean's office. The misbehavior serves several functions for the student: they gain the attention of the teacher and peers and get out of the unpleasant class. Once in the dean's office, the student gains attention from the office staff, dean, and parents/guardians who are notified of the misconduct.

Mental Health Screening Tools and Referral

Physical or mental health assessment findings outside of the normal range should prompt school nurses to consider specific screening tools to gather more information. *Behavioral health screening tools* have been used in a variety of healthcare settings, including primary care and specialty psychiatric care, and some are applicable to the school setting for use by qualified professionals, such as social workers, counselors, school workers, and/or the school nurse. Screening tools are not used for diagnosis but are useful in identifying individuals who may need referral for further evaluation and treatment.

Clinical judgment must be used in deciding when to incorporate formal mental health screening tools at school. *Before screening is initiated, the student support team should determine how they will respond to students who screen positive and warrant referral and evaluation for treatment.* The school nurse must know whether state and district laws and policies allow formalized mental health screening and whether parent/guardian permission is required. Policies and resources should be in place to refer students who screen positive to a mental health practitioner or to an outpatient or inpatient mental health facility when immediate intervention is indicated. The school nurse serves as a liaison between the student, school, family, and providers to support identification, referral, and follow-up (NASN, 2022a).

A variety of valid and reliable questionnaires, checklists, and rating scales are available to mental and behavioral health specialists to screen and assess children for behavior problems. Many of these inventories are copyrighted, must be purchased, and are administered at school by a school psychologist, social worker, or counselor with specialized training. See Online Materials OM28-1 for selected youth mental health screening tools.

Endorsed by the American Academy of Pediatrics (2018), the *Pediatric Symptom Checklist* is a free, quick, 35-item screening tool that can easily be administered by school support team professionals, including the school nurse in the health office. The Pediatric Symptom Checklist is a "psychosocial screen designed to facilitate the recognition of cognitive, emotional, and behavioral problems so that appropriate interventions can be initiated as early as possible" (Bright Futures, n.d., p. 1). There are two versions: a parent-completed version for young children (PCS) and the youth self-report (Y-PSC). A significant score indicates that the student should be referred for further mental health evaluation.

A well-informed approach to screening by the school nurse should be done in consultation with the school support team and in communication with the student and family. Issues of consent and confidentiality must be considered carefully, especially regarding sensitive issues surrounding behavioral and mental health concerns.

The USPSTF and the AAP recommend screening for depression annually starting at age 12 (Zuckerbrot et al., 2018). Students who have a regular source of primary care may already be screened. Although there is no perfect depression screening tool, one method is to use a simplified two-item tool called the Patient Health Questionnaire (PHQ-2). The questions are as follows: Over the past 2 weeks, how often have you been bothered by any of the following problems?

1. Little interest or pleasure in doing things
2. Feeling down, depressed, or hopeless

The answers are measured on a 3-point scale from "not at all" (0) to "nearly every day" (3). Students who score more than 3 points should have additional screening and evaluation. Depending on school policy, the nurse can proceed, or refer the student. The PHQ-9 (Kroenke et al., 2001) has seven additional questions that can be asked:

1. Trouble falling or staying asleep, or sleeping too much
2. Feeling tired or having little energy
3. Poor appetite or overeating
4. Feeling bad about yourself—or that you are a failure or have let yourself or your family down
5. Trouble concentrating on things, such as reading the newspaper or watching television
6. Moving or speaking so slowly that other people could have noticed; or the opposite—being so fidgety or restless that you have been moving around a lot more than usual
7. Thoughts that you would be better off dead, or of hurting yourself in some way

School Nurse Care Coordination

School nurses are integral members of student support teams that promote positive school environments and programs essential for improving student mental and behavioral health (NASN, 2022a; Rosvall, 2020). School nurses provide holistic perspectives of behavior problems in students. When students display inappropriate behaviors, school nurses may be approached by parents or teachers to assist in behavior assessments to provide recommendations regarding the development of behavior support plans and/or the need for further mental health evaluation. School nurses often assist in the ongoing monitoring of behavior management interventions for students during the school day.

The management of mental/behavioral health issues is a large part of the school nurse's role regardless of the reason for a student's visit to the health office. The health office is often viewed as a safe zone, and the school nurse is often among the most trusted individuals in the school. "To be trusted in the school community, one must be available, visible, and consistent with the care provided" (Kaskoun & McCabe, 2022, p. 43). Given the prevalence of mental health disorders, school nurses must consider that a mental health concern is the underpinning reason for the visit to the office for somatic complaints or for an absence from school. Steps to explore explicit or implicit mental health concerns include assessment, specific screening, brief intervention, and referral and care coordination.

Referral and care coordination are a substantial component of the school nurses' responsibility regarding mental health care. In order to do so, the school nurse must know school and state policies regarding when to refer and be equipped with a list of responsive providers and service organizations. Identification of school team members who assist with mental health care and having regularly scheduled meetings can streamline care coordination. As with any team, coordination requires clear delineation of roles.

Assessment

Identifying mental health symptoms early enhances the school nurse's capacity for meeting the behavioral health needs of students and improves outcomes for students and families. Assessment and screening should be integrative, considering the physical and mental health status of the student (Perron et al., 2021). An assessment may unfold over several school nurse visits. Using an integrative approach allows the nurse to assess both the physical and mental health status of students simultaneously.

Additional components of a therapeutic relationship beyond trust include genuine interest, empathy, good listening skills, acceptance, positive regard, nonjudgmental attitude, and interventions appropriate to the student's developmental level and sociocultural background (Townsend & Morgan, 2021).

Motivational Interviewing

Motivational interviewing is "collaborative communication style that can be integrated into everyday practice to improve conversations and serve as a catalyst for behavior change" (Beckwith & Beckwith, 2020, p. 1). It is a therapeutic technique based on an empathetic, warm relationship with the student that draws out their feelings and unique story through conversation. Motivational interviewing goes beyond collecting data; it is a counseling style that school nurses can use to promote behavior change by allowing an individual to resolve uncertainty and gain self-efficacy. The school nurse listens intently and lets the student direct where the narrative will go. During a motivational interview, the school nurse expresses empathy for the student by being nonjudgmental and accepting while exploring the student's perspectives. Open-ended questions such as "What do you think about what is happening for you right now?" can give the student an opportunity to express themselves. A therapeutic relationship is established in which the student feels safe to self-identify their own motivations, reasons for their actions, and their willingness to change. As a core competency of specialty practice, school nurses can seek training in motivational interviewing (Beckwith & Beckwith, 2020; Moberg et al., 2022).

Observation in the Learning Environment

Gaining the full picture of a student's mental health status requires the school nurse to assess the student beyond the health office by observing the student in different instructional and social settings at school. Direct observation of the student can offer insight into classroom behavior as well as identify possible signs or symptoms of health conditions. A limitation of direct observation is that the student may alter their behavior in response to the observer's presence. The student who chronically misbehaves in a classroom setting may not demonstrate the same behaviors when aware that they are being watched by the school nurse or a school behavior specialist. During any time in the assessment process, the school nurse should immediately consult with the parents when an outside professional medical or mental health evaluation is warranted.

Common Factors Approach

Engaging students and families in partnering and planning to address mental health disorders can be challenging. Many barriers exist surrounding stigma, parental permission, and the inherent hopelessness of some of the conditions discussed here. The *common factors approach* provides school nurses with a framework to provide positive interactions and specific treatment skills. The common factors approach focuses on the process of care, including how to facilitate positive communication and interactions between students and providers as well as skills used by providers to influence behavior change (Barth & Lee, 2014; Skeen et al., 2019).

Specific common factors skills that are particularly applicable for school nursing practice are promoting calm and respectful communication, effectively eliciting mental health concerns, motivating students and families to listen and seek additional help, and addressing barriers to engaging in care (Barth & Lee, 2014). Data from a meta-analysis of mental health programs for adolescents reveal that addressing interpersonal skills enhances mental health wellness (Skeen et al., 2019). The AAP (2021b) offers the acronym HEL^2P^3 (hope; empathy; language and loyalty; and permission, partnering, and plan) to utilize this model. School nurses can offer expressions of hope that treatment or interventions are available, use the students' preferred language for their symptoms, and advocate for that student to receive individualized mental health support at school.

Psychoeducation

Students and families have varying understanding of the mental condition and available treatments. Students of any age may not understand why they feel or act in a certain way. School nurses are on the front line of providing brief therapeutic interventions for students with mental and behavioral health concerns (NASN, 2022a). *Psychoeducation* is an empirically supported strategy across a range of mental health concerns that includes education about the disorder and interventions. The school nurse can actively teach a student about their disorder to dispel myths, misinformation, and disinformation about their mental health diagnosis and treatment. Educating the student and family at their learning level about symptoms of a specific disorder can be helpful for enhancing self-care and reducing shame or guilt (Motlova et al., 2017). Typically, psychoeducation is applied at the onset of treatment and is foundational to effective intervention with youth. Psychoeducation should be presented in a developmentally appropriate and engaging manner. Evidence-based psychoeducation can also be developed

Did You Know?

There are many free resources available in the public domain that school nurses can use to educate teachers, families, and students about anxiety and other mental health issues. Explore the following examples:

- The Minnesota Association for Children's Mental Health (2024) includes reader-friendly fact sheets about anxiety symptoms and suggested classroom strategies (https://macmh.org/youth-and-family/).
- The Anxiety Canada Web site (2024) is a dynamic, interactive Web site for youth that houses a wealth of information that can support the implementation of the intervention strategies (www.anxietycanada.com).

school-wide (e.g., workshops and assemblies about mental health disorders).

Confidentiality and Privacy

The school nurse may find it difficult to have effective, confidential communication in the health office because of the presence of other students or staff (Bohnenkamp et al., 2019). Concern about confidentiality was one of three main themes revealed in an integrative review of school nurses' perceptions of their role related to mental health (Kaskoun & McCabe, 2022). Decisions about when to consult other members of the team (counselors, peer nursing staff, teachers, parents) can be difficult, especially with adolescents. School nurses may feel a level of burden knowing about a student's mental health status but not being able to share or process the information.

When a student needs more time or privacy to share concerns, the school nurse can schedule a time to meet when they will not be interrupted. If the student's concern or behavior needs immediate attention, then either the office door should be closed with a sign directing students to go to the main office or it may be necessary to hand off the student to another qualified staff member. Honoring the time and place of agreements of the meeting builds trust.

Care for the School Nurse as Caregiver

School nurses must take care of themselves while also caring for those in need. Janeway (2020) notes that caregiving is not only physically draining but also emotionally exhausting, and it is easy to feel burnt out, with almost half of all nurses feeling this way. This burnout, or compassion fatigue, can lead to irritability, tiredness, body aches and pains, weight gain, and getting sick more frequently (Wei, 2018). According to Wei (2018), there are five essential ways to make sure you are caring for yourself while also caring for others:

- Self-compassion—be kind to yourself, give yourself grace, and take some extra time for you.
- Practice breath awareness for 10 minutes every day.
- Try mind-body practice—this could be yoga, meditation, or deep relaxation exercises.
- Eat well and get quality sleep—this should be a priority.
- Remain connected and get support when needed—reach out to your friends and coworkers.

School nurse self-care can help ensure that the nurse is able to maintain a healthy environment for students, which in turn helps them learn better. Modeling proper self-care can demonstrate to students the importance of socioemotional balance for all. School nurses must take care of their physical and emotional needs to be well and serve the children, families, and school communities under their care.

CONCLUSION

Schools increasingly are the primary site for identification, referral, and intervention for students with behavioral health concerns. There is growing evidence that school mental health programs improve educational outcomes by decreasing absences, decreasing discipline referrals, and improving test scores (Houri & Kincade, 2021; Kawsar et al., 2022; Mitchell et al., 2021). As integral members of the multidisciplinary behavioral health team, school nurses should work to identify students with mental health needs, provide supportive counseling, help students to cope and problem-solve, and educate staff, students, and families on mental health concerns. School nurses serve as liaisons between the school, family, and healthcare providers to optimize communication and coordinate care for students with mental/behavioral health disorders. School nurses have an important role in promoting, coordinating, and supporting the social-emotional health of children toward improved education and quality of life outcomes.

School nurses should advocate for behavioral health resources that promote inclusive and supportive school environments. They should actively promote educational programming that prevents behavior problems and promotes social and emotional well-being in students and school communities. School nurses contribute valuable assessment data to the student support team and collaborate in the development of behavior improvement plans. By establishing trusting relationships with students, school nurses can affect positive behavior change on behalf of better health and educational outcomes for all students.

Resources

The free and confidential resources in the following table can help you connect with a skilled, trained mental health professional. These resources were obtained through the Centers for Disease Control and Prevention. Additional resources and links can be found in Online Materials OM28-2.

Type of Issue	Helplines
Crisis hotlines and text lines for urgent situations	• Call 911 • 988 Suicide and Crisis Lifeline (formerly known as the National Suicide Prevent on Lifeline): 988 for English or Spanish, or Lifeline Chat. TTY users can use their preferred relay service or dial 711 then 988. • Crisis Text Line: Text SIGNS to 741741 for 24/7, anonymous, free crisis counsel ng • Disaster Distress Helpline: CALL or TEXT 1-800-985-5990 (press 2 for Spanish)
Abuse/assault/violence	• National Domestic Violence Hotline: 1-800-799-7233 or text LOVEIS to 22522 • National Child Abuse Hotline: 1-800-4AChild (1-800-422-4453) or text 1-800-422-4453 • National Sexual Assault Hotline: 1-800-656-HOPE (4673) or Online Chat
LGBTQ+	• Trans Lifeline: 1-877-565-8860 (para español presiona el 2) • The Trevor Project's TrevorLifeline: 1-866-488-7386
Finding treatment	• FindTreatment.gov—Find a provider treating substance use disorders, addiction, and mental illness • American Psychiatric Association Foundation—Find a Psychiatrist • American Academy of Child and Adolescent Psychiatry—Child and Adolescent Psychiatrist Finder • American Psychological Association—Find a Psychologist
Opioid treatment	• Buprenorphine Treatment Practitioner Locator • Opioid Treatment Program Directory by State
Veterans/active-duty military	• Veterans Crisis Line: 988, then select 1, or Crisis Chat or text: 838255 • U.S. Department of Veterans Affairs Mental Health Resources • Help for Military Service Members and Their Families

The editors gratefully acknowledge the work of previous chapter authors: Brittany R. Patterson, Jill Bohenkamp, Sharon Hoover, Jeff Bostick, Janice Selekman.

References

Aggarwal, A., & Marwaha, R. (2022). *Oppositional defiant disorder.* [StatPearls]. National Center for Biotechnology. National Institute of Health. https://www.ncbi.nlm.nih.gov/books/NBK557443/

Ali, M. M., West, K., Teich, J. L., Lynch, S., Mutter, R. & Dubenitz, J. (2019). Utilization of mental health services in educational settings by adolescents in the United States. *Journal of School Health, 89,* 393–401. https://doi.org/10.1111/josh.12753

American Academy of Child and Adolescent Psychiatry. (2009). *ODD: A guide for families by the American Academy of Child and Adolescent Psychiatry.* https://www.aacap.org/App_Themes/AACAP/docs/resource_centers/odd/odd_resource_center_odd_guide.pdf

American Academy of Child and Adolescent Psychiatry. (2024). *Suicide in children and teens.* https://www.aacap.org/AACAP/Families_and_Youth/Facts_for_Families/FFF-Guide/Teen-Suicide-010.aspx

American Academy of Pediatrics. (2018). *Bright Futures tools and resource kit: Developmental, behavioral, psychosocial, screening, and assessment forms.* https://brightfutures.aap.org/materials-and-tools/tool-and-resource-kit/Pages/Developmental-Behavioral-Psychosocial-Screening-and-Assessment-Forms.aspx

American Academy of Pediatrics. (2021a). *AAP-AACAP-CHA declaration of a national emergency in child and adolescent mental health.* https://www.aap.org/en/advocacy/child-and-adolescent-healthy-mental-development/aap-aacap-cha-declaration-of-a-national-emergency-in-child-and-adolescent-mental-health/

American Academy of Pediatrics. (2021b). *Supporting mental health in schools.* https://downloads.aap.org/dochw/dshp/Supporting_Mental_Health_in_Schools_Final_Report-June_2021.pdf

American Academy of Pediatrics. (2023). *Blueprint for youth suicide prevention: Strategies for community and school settings for youth suicide prevention.* https://www.aap.org/en/patient-care/blueprint-for-youth-suicide-prevention/strategies-for-community-and-school-settings-for-youth-suicide-prevention/

American College of Obstetricians and Gynecologists Committee on Obstetric Practice. (2021). Reducing prenatal exposure to toxic environmental agents. *Obstetrics and Gynecology, 138*(1), e40–e54.

American Foundation for Suicide Prevention & Suicide Prevention Resource Center. (2018). *After a suicide: A toolkit for schools* (2nd ed.). https://sprc.org/online-library/after-suicide-toolkit-schools

American Psychiatric Association. (2022). *Diagnostic and statistical manual of mental disorders* (5th ed., text rev.). Author.

American Psychological Association. (2023). *PTSD treatment: Information for patients and families.* https://www.apa.org/ptsd-guideline/patients-and-families

Anttila, M., Tlitalo, M., Kukri, M. H., Hipp, K., & Valimaki, M. (2020). School nurses' perceptions, learning needs and developmental suggestions for mental health promotion: Focus group interviews. *International Journal of Environmental Research and Public Health, 17*(24), 9503. https://www.doi.org/10.3390/ijerph17249503

Anxiety Canada. (2024). *Resources, relief & results.* https://www.anxietycanada.com/

Bargeman, M., Belson, J., Mulvale, G., Niec, A., Theuer, A., & Moll, S. (2022). Understanding the conceptualization and operationalization of trauma-informed care within and across systems: A critical interpretive synthesis. *Milbank Quarterly, 100*(3), 785–853.

Barth, R. P., & Lee, B. R. (2014). Common elements and common factors approaches to evidence-informed children's services. In A. Shlonsky & R. Benbenishty (Eds.), *Evidence to outcomes in child welfare: An international reader* (pp. 59–82). Oxford University Press.

Beckwith, V. Z., & Beckwith, J. (2020). Motivational interviewing: A communication tool to promote positive behavior change and optimal health outcomes. *NASN School Nurse, 35*(6), 344–351. https://doi.org/10.1177/1942602X20915715

Berk, M. S. (2022). Editorial: Suicide prevention in youth. *The Association for Child and Adolescent Mental Health, 27*(4), 325–327. https://doi.org/10.1111/camh.12604

Bohnenkamp, J. H., Hoover, S., Connors, E. H., Wissow, L., Bobo, N., & Mazyck, D. (2019). The mental health training intervention for school nurses and other health providers in schools. *Journal of School Nursing, 35*(6), 422–433.

Boland, R., Verduin, M. L., & Ruiz, P. (2022). *Kaplan & Sadock's synopsis of psychiatry* (12th ed.). Wolters Kluwer.

Boyd, T. M., Moyer, S. M., & Lambert, D. (2024). Interdisciplinary collaboration to care for students diagnosed with PANDAS: An education and referral intervention. *The Journal of School Nursing, 40*(4), 452-459. https://doi.org/10.1177/1059840522112955

Bright Futures. (n.d.). *The Pediatric Symptom Checklist.* https://www.brightfutures.org/mentalhealth/pdf/professionals/ped_sympton_chklst.pdf

Center on Positive Behavioral Interventions and Supports. (2022). *Tier 3 brief functional behavior assessment (FBA) guide.* U.S. Department of Education, Office of Special Education Programs and Office of Elementary and Secondary Education. www.pbis.org

Center on Positive Behavioral Interventions and Supports. (2024). *Positive behavioral interventions & supports.* https://www.pbis.org/pbis/what-is-pbis

Centers for Disease Control and Prevention. (2022). *6 guiding principles to a trauma-informed care approach.* [Infographic.] https://stacks.cdc.gov/view/cdc/56843

Centers for Disease Control and Prevention. (2023a). *Fast facts: Preventing adverse childhood experiences (ACEs).* https://www.cdc.gov/violenceprevention/aces/fastfact.html

Centers for Disease Control and Prevention. (2023b). *Improving children's behavioral health.* https://www.cdc.gov/childrensmentalhealth/features/child-mental-health.html

Centers for Disease Control and Prevention. (2023c). *Youth risk behavior survey: Data summary & trends report 2011–2021.* https://www.cdc.gov/healthyyouth/mental-health/index.htm

Centers for Disease Control and Prevention. (2024a). *Behavior or conduct problems in children.* https://www.cdc.gov/children-mental-health/about/about-behavior-or-conduct-problems-in-children.html?CDC_AAref_Val=https://www.cdc.gov/childrensmentalhealth/behavior.html

Centers for Disease Control and Prevention. (2024b). *Underlying cause of death, 2018–2022, single race results, deaths occurring in 2022.* https://wonder.cdc.gov/controller/datarequest/D158;jsessionid=72AE6A5059278602FECEF4617C58

Cohen, C. (2019, April 1). *Data on disabilities: Good news, bad news on graduation rates.* National School Board Association. Data on Disabilities (nsba.org)

Cohen, S. (2022). *Suicide rate highest among teens and young adults.* UCLA Health. https://connect.uclahealth.org/2022/03/15/suicide-rate-highest-among-teens-and-young-adults/

Curtin, S. C., Garnett, M. F., & Ahmad, F. B. (2022). Provisional numbers and rates of suicide by month and demographic characteristics: United States, 2021. *NVSS Vital Statistics Rapid Release.* https://dx.doi.org/10.15620/cdc:120830

Dutil, S. (2019). Adolescent traumatic and disenfranchised grief: Adapting an evidence-based intervention for Black and Latinx youths in schools. *Children & Schools, 41*(3), 179–187.

Eddy, K. (n.d.). *Avoidant restrictive food intake disorder.* National Eating Disorder Association. https://www.nationaleatingdisorders.org/avoidant-restrictive-food-intake-disorder-arfid/?gad_source=1&gclid=Cj0KCQjw8pKxBhD_ARIsAPrG45mi5SMSyb3pFJnlotsfDoyvBwP7M_Lsw8f2uCPqlAVasgVl2hK8qOEaAombEALw_wcB#blog_posts

Edwards, J., Stone, M., Bartlett, H., Wallace, M., & Ventura, A. (2023). Grief in school-aged youth. *NASN School Nurse, 38*(4),171–175. https://doi.org/10.1177/1942602X231161332

Elizabeth Kubler-Ross Foundation. (2010). *5 stages of grief.* https://www.ekrfoundation.org/5-stages-of-grief/5-stages-grief/

Feriante J., Rorrico, T. J., & Bernstein, B. (2023). Separation anxiety disorder. *StatPearls.* https://www.ncbi.nlm.nih.gov/books/NBK560793/

Genetic and Rare Diseases Information Center. (2024). *PANDAS.* National Center for Advancing Translational Sciences. U.S. Department of Health & Human Services. https://rarediseases.info.nih.gov/diseases/7312/pediatric-autoimmune-neuropsychiatric-disorders-associated-with-streptococcus-infections

Giannopoulou, I., Richardson, C., & Papadatou, D. (2021). Peer loss: Posttraumatic stress, depression, and grief symptoms in a traumatized adolescent community. *Clinical Child Psychology and Psychiatry, 26*(2), 556–568. https://doi.org/10.1177/1359104520980028

Glazer, H. R., & Clark-Foster, M. (2019). *Understanding the journey: A lifespan approach to working with grieving people.* Charles C Thomas.

Harmer, B., Lee, S., Duong, T. H., & S, A. (2022). Suicidal ideation. *StatPearls Publishing,* https://pubmed.ncbi.nlm.nih.gov/33351435/

Hoover, S., & Bostic, J. (2022). Schools as a vital component of the child adolescent mental health system. *Psychiatric Services, 72*(1), 37–48. https://doi.org/10.1176/appi.ps.201900575

Hornberger, L. L., Lane, M. A., Lane, M., Breuner, C. C., Alderman, E. M., Grubb, L. K., ... & Baumberger, J. (2021). Identification and management of eating disorders in children and adolescents. *Pediatrics, 147*(1). https://doi.org/10.1542/peds.2020-040279

Hoskote, A. R., Croce, E., & Johnson, K. E. (2023). The evolution of the role of the U.S. school nurses in adolescent mental health at the individual, community, and systems level: An integrative review. *The Journal of School Nursing, 39*(1), 51–71. https://doi.org/10.1177/10598405211068120

Houri, A., & Kincade, L. (2021). *The connection between mental health and academic success.* Groves Learning Organization. https://www.groveslearning.org/connection-between-mental-health-academic-success/

Individuals With Disabilities Education Improvement Act. (2017). 20 U.S. Code § 1400. https://sites.ed.gov/idea/regs/b/a/300.8

Individuals with Disabilities Education Improvement Act of 2004 (Pub. L. 108-446). https://www.gpo.gov/fdsys/pkg/PLAW-108publ446/content-detail.html

The Institute on Trauma and Trauma-Informed Care. (2022). *What is trauma-informed care?* University at Buffalo, Buffalo Center for Social Research. https://socialwork.buffalo.edu/social-research/institutes-centers/institute-on-trauma-and-trauma-informed-care.html

International OCD Foundation. (n.d.). *How is OCD treated?* https://kids.iocdf.org/what-is-ocd-kids/how-is-ocd-treated/

Janeway, D. (2020). The role of psychiatry in treating burnout among nurses during the Covid-19 pandemic. *Journal of Radiology Nursing, 39*(3), 176–178. https://doi.org/10.1016/j.jradnu.2020.06.004

Jason Foundation. (2022). *Youth suicide statistics. The parent resource program.* https://prp.jasonfoundation.com/youth-suicide-statistics/

Johns Hopkins. (2022). *What is conduct disorder in children?* https://www.hopkinsmedicine.org/health/conditions-and-diseases/conduct-disorder

Jones, K. (2020). *What happens when your child's school reports suicidal ideation.* National Alliance on Mental Illness. https://www.nami.org/criminal-justice-and-legal/what-happens-when-your-childs-school-reports-suicidal-ideation/

Judi's House. (2024). *Childhood bereavement estimation model: National report 2024.* https://judishouse.org/download/2024-cbem-national-report/?wpdmdl=7509&_wpdmkey=66785e56c591a

Kaiser, B., & Rasminsky, J. (2017). *Challenging behavior in young children: Understanding, preventing, and responding effectively* (4th ed.). Boston, MA: Pearson.

Kaskoun J., McCabe E. (2022). Perceptions of school nurses in addressing student mental health concerns: An integrative review. *The Journal of School Nursing, 38*(1), 35–47. https://doi.org/10.1177/1059840521104622

Kawsar, M. D. S., Yilanli, M., & Marwaha, R. (2022, June 5). School refusal. *StatPearls.* https://www.ncbi.nlm.nih.gov/books/NBK534195/

Kroenke, K., Spitzer, R., & Williams, J. (2001). The PHQ-9: Validity of a brief depression severity measure. *Journal of General Internal Medicine, 16*(9), 606–613.

Liebenluft, E. (2024). *Effective medications for kids with bipolar disorder.* Child Mind Institute. https://childmind.org/article/what-medications-are-most-effective-in-children-with-bipolar-disorder/

Lucas, C., Brady, J., & Olympia, R. P. (2022). School nurses on the front lines of healthcare: Recognizing "BONES" and knowing when to pick up the phone: Eating disorders among students in the school setting. *NASN School Nurse, 37*(2), 83–88. https://doi.org/10.1177/19426 02X20942531

Lytle, M., Rau, W., & Stoner, S. (2024). The role of the school nurse in social-emotional assessment and intervention using the MTSS framework. *NASN School Nurse* [online first]. https://doi.org/ 10.1177/1942602X241240499

Marsh, S., Dobson, R., & Maddison, R. (2020). The relationship between household chaos and child, parent, and family outcomes: A systematic scoping review. *BMC Public Health, 20*(1), 513.

McFarlane, W. R. (2011). Prevention of the first episode of psychosis. *Psychiatric Clinics of North America, 34*(1), 95–107.

Miller, C., Mendel, C., & Howard. J. (2023). *Is it ADHD or trauma?* Child Mind Institute. https://childmind.org/article/is-it-adhd-or-trauma/

Minnesota Association for Children's Mental Health. (2024). *Fact sheets.* https://macmh.org/youth-and-family/

Miranda-Mendizabal, A., Castellví, P., Parés-Badell, O., Alayo, I., Almenara, J., Alonso, I., Blasco, M. J., Cebrià, A., Gabilondo, A., Gili, M., Lagares, C., Piqueras, J. A., Rodríguez-Jiménez, T., Rodríguez-Marín, J., Roca, M., Soto-Sanz, V., Vilagut, G., & Alonso, J. (2019). Gender differences in suicidal behavior in adolescents and young adults: Systematic review and meta-analysis of longitudinal studies. *International Journal of Public Health, 64*(2), 265–283. https://doi. org/10.1007/s00038-018-1196-1

Mitchell, R., McMaugh, A., Schniering, C., Cameron, C., Lystad, R., Badgery-Parker, T. & Nielssen, O. (2021). Mental disorders and their impact on school performance and high school completion by gender in Australia: A matched population-based cohort study. *Australian & New Zealand Journal of Psychiatry, 56*(12), 1602–1616. https://doi. org/10.1177/00048674211061684

Moberg, M., Lindqvist, H., Andermo, S., & Norman, Å. (2022). Sometimes it felt great, and sometimes it just went pear-shaped: Experiences and perceptions of school nurses' motivational interviewing competence: A convergent mixed-methods study. *Clinics and Practice, 12*, 333–349. https://doi.org/10.3390/clinpract12030039

Motlova, L. B., Balon, R., Beresin, E. V., Brenner, A. M., Coverdale, J. H., Guerrero, A. P. S., Louie, A. K., &Roberts, L. W. (2017). Psychoeducation as an opportunity for patients, psychiatrists, and psychiatric educators: Why do we ignore it? *Academic Psychiatry, 41*, 447–451. https://doi.org/10.1007/s40596-017-0728-y

Nagata, J. M., Garber, A. K., Tabler, J. L., Murray, S. B., & Bibbins-Domingo, K. (2018). Prevalence and correlates of disordered eating behaviors among young adults with overweight or obesity. *Journal of General Internal Medicine, 33*(8), 1337–1343. https://doi.org/ 10.1007/s11606-018-4465-z

National Alliance on Mental Illness. (2021). *Child mental health emergency: Rising numbers put pediatricians on alert.* https://nami.org/ Press-Media/In-The-News/2021/Child-mental-health-emergency-Rising-numbers-put-pediatricians-on-alert

National Alliance on Mental Illness. (2022a). *Mental health by the numbers.* https://nami.org/mhstats

National Alliance on Mental Illness. (2022b). *Mental health in schools: Where we stand.* https://www.nami.org/Advocacy/Policy-Priorities/ Improving-Health/Mental-Health-in-Schools

National Alliance on Mental Illness. (2023). *Mental health by the numbers.* https://www.nami.org/about-mental-illness/mental-health-by-the-numbers/#:~:text=22.8%25%20of%20U.S.%20adults%20 experienced,represents%201%20in%2020%20adults

National Association of School Nurses. (2022a). NASN position statement: The behavioral health and wellness of students. *NASN School Nurse, 37*(2), 103–105. https://doi.org/10.1177/ 1942602X211066656

National Association of School Nurses. (2022b). *School nursing: Scope and standards of practice* (4th ed.) Author.

National Association of School Nurses. (2024). A contemporary framework update for today's school nursing landscape: Introducing the School Nursing Practice Framework. *NASN School Nurse, 39*(3), 140–147. https://www.doi.org/10.1177/1942602X241241092

National Association of School Psychologists. (2021). *Comprehensive school-based mental and behavioral health services and psychologists* [handout]. Author.

National Center for PTSD. (2022). *PTSD basics.* U.S. Department of Veterans Affairs. https://www.ptsd.va.gov/understand/what/ptsd_ basics.asp

National Center for School Mental Health and MHTTC Network Coordinating Office. (2019). *Trainer manual, national school mental health curriculum.* MHTTC Network Coordinating Office.

National Council for Mental Wellbeing. (2023). *Mental health first aid for youth.* https://www.mentalhealthfirstaid.org/population-focused-modules/youth/

National Eating Disorder Association. (2022). *NEDA toolkit for educators.* https://www.nationaleatingdisorders.org/sites/default/files/Toolkits/ EducatorToolkit.pdf

National Eating Disorder Association. (2023). *Statistics and research on eating disorders.* https://www.nationaleatingdisorders.org/statistics-research-eating-disorders

National Institute of Mental Health. (2020). *Suicide risk screening tool.* screening_tool_asq_nimh_toolkit.pdf (nih.gov)

National Institute of Mental Health. (2022). *Post-traumatic stress disorder.* https://www.nimh.nih.gov/health/topics/post-traumatic-stress-disorder-ptsd

National Institute of Mental Health. (2023a). *Bipolar disorder in children and teens.* U.S. Department of Health and Human Services. https://www.nimh.nih.gov/sites/default/files/documents/health/ publications/bipolar-disorder-in-children-and-teens/bipolar-disorder-in-children-and-teens.pdf

National Institute of Mental Health. (2023b). *Disruptive mood dysregulation disorder: The basics.* U.S. Department of Health and Human Services. https://www.nimh.nih.gov/health/publications/disruptive-mood-dysregulation-disorder

National Institute of Mental Health. (2024). *Eating disorders.* U.S. Department of Health and Human Services. https://www.nimh.nih. gov/health/topics/eating-disorders

National Suicide Prevention Lifeline. (n.d.). *Act: Acknowledge, care, tell.* Substance Abuse and Mental Health Services Administration. U.S. Department of Health and Human Services. https://cdnsm5-ss18. sharpschool.com/UserFiles/Servers/Server_520831/File/Prevention% 20Programs/SOS_ACT_Handout.pdf

Nazeer, A., Latif, F., Mondal, A., Azeem, M. W., & Greydanus, D. (2020). Obsessive-compulsive disorder in children and adolescents: Epidemiology, diagnosis and management. *Translational Pediatrics*, S76-S93. https://doi.org/10.21037/tp.2019.10.02

Parham, L. D., Roush, S., Downing, D. T., Michael, P. G., & McFarlane, W. R. (2019). Sensory characteristics of youth at clinical high risk for psychosis. *Early Intervention in Psychiatry, 13*, 264–271. https://doi. org/10.1111/eip.12475

Patel, K. R., Cherian, J., Gohil, K., & Atkinson, D. (2014). Schizophrenia: Overview and treatment options. *Pharmacy and Therapeutics, 39*(9), 638–645.

Patel, R. S., Amaravadi, N., Bhullar H., Lekireddy, J., &Win, H. (2018). Understanding the demographic predictors and associated comorbidities in children hospitalized with conduct disorder. *Journal of Behavioral Sciences, 8*(9), 80. https://doi.org/10.3390/bs8090080

PAXIS Institute. (2021). *An international prevention science company.* https://www.paxis.org/school-based-programming/

Perron, T., Jakubowski, T., Razzi, C., & Kartoz, C. (2021). Mental health assessment of the frequent visitors in the school setting—Part 1: An overview. *NASN School Nurse, 36*(4), 197–204. https:// doi:10.1177/1942602X21996442

Perzichilli, T. (2020). The historical roots of racial disparities in the mental health system. *Counseling Today.* https://ct.counseling. org/2020/05/the-historical-roots-of-racial-disparities-in-the-mental-health-system/

Poudel, A., Lamichhane, A., Rana Magar, K., & Prasad Khanal, G. (2022). Non suicidal self injury and suicidal behavior among adolescents: Co-occurence and associated risk factors. *NIH BMC*

Psychiatry, 22, 96. https://www.ncbi.nlm.nih.gov/pmc/articles/PMC8827284/

Pursey, K. M., Burrows, T. L., Barker, D., Hart, M., & Paxton, S. J. (2021). Disordered eating, body image concerns, and weight control behaviors in primary school aged children: A systematic review and meta-analysis of universal-selective prevention interventions. *International Journal of Eating Disorders, 54*(10), 1730–1765. https://www.doi.org/10.1002/eat.23571

Raifman, J., Moscoe, E, Austin B., & McConnell, M. (2017). Difference-in-differences analysis of the association between state same-sex marriage policies and adolescent suicide attempts. *JAMA Pediatrics, 174*(4), 350–356.

Rosvall, P. (2020). Perspectives of students with mental health problems on improving the school environment and practice. *Education Inquiry, 11*(3), 159–174. https://doi.org/10.1080/20004508.2019.1687394

Sebton, S. (2020). *Trauma informed care advocate course.* University Health, San Antonio, Texas.

Skeen, S., Laurenzi, C. A., Gordon, S. L., du Toit, S., Tomlinson, M., Dua, T., Fleischmann, A., Kohl, K., Ross, D., Servili, C., Brand, A. S., Dowdall, N., Lund, C., van der Westhuizen, C., Carvajal-Aguirre, L., de Carvalho, C. E., & Melendez-Torres, G. J. (2019). Adolescent mental health program components and behavior risk reduction: A meta-analysis. *Pediatrics, 144*(2), 1–13. https://doi-org.ezproxy.tcnj.edu/10.1542/peds.2018-3488

Spence, S. H., Donovan, C. L., March, S., Kenardy, J. A., & Hearn, C. S. (2017). Generic versus disorder specific cognitive behavior therapy for social anxiety disorder in youth: A randomized controlled trial using internet delivery. *Behaviour Research and Therapy, 90,* 41–57. https://doi.org/10.1016/j.brat.2016.12.003

Stone, D. M., Simon, T. R., Fowler, K. A., Kegler, S. R., Yuan, K., Holland, K. M., Ivey-Stephenson, A. Z., & Crosby, A. E. (2018). Vital signs: Trends in state suicide rates—United States, 1999–2016 and circumstances contributing to suicide—27 states, 2015. *MMWR Morbidity and Mortality Weekly Report, 67*(22), 617–624.

Substance Abuse and Mental Health Services Administration. (2019). *Behavioral health integration.* https://www.samhsa.gov/sites/default/files/samhsa-behavioral-health-integration.pdf

Substance Abuse and Mental Health Services Administration. (2022). *Suicide prevention resource center.* https://www.samhsa.gov/suicide-prevention-resource-center-sprc

Thompson, A. L., Gardner, M. A., Russell, C. D., & Steinberg, D. M. (2019). *Fact sheet: Grief in children and adolescents.* https://pedpsych.org/fact_sheets/grief-children-and-adolescents/

Townsend, M. C., & Morgan, K. I. (2021). *Davis advantage for psychiatric mental health nursing* (10th ed.). F.A. Davis.

Treglia, D., Cutuli, J. J., Arasteh, K., & Bridgeland, J. (2023). Parental and other caregiver loss due to COVID-19 in the United States: Prevalence by race, state, relationship, and child age. *Journal of Community Health, 48*(3), 390–397. https://doi.org/10.1007/s10900-022-01160-x

U.S. Department of Education. (2021). *Supporting child and student social, emotional, behavioral, and mental health needs.* Office of Special Education and Rehabilitative Services. https://www2.ed.gov/documents/students/supporting-child-student-social-emotional-behavioral-mental-health.pdf

U.S. Preventive Services Task Force. (2022). Screening for eating disorders in adolescents and adults: US Preventive Services Task Force recommendation statement. *JAMA, 327*(11), 1061–1067. https://doi.org/10.1001/jama.2022.1806

Waller, G., & Mountford, V. A. (2015). Weighing patients within cognitive-behavioral therapy for eating disorders: How, when and why. *Behaviour Research and Therapy, 70,* 1–10. https://doi.org/10.1016/j.brat.2015.04.004

Wei, M. (2018, October 17). *Self-care for the caregiver.* Harvard Health Blog. https://www.health.harvard.edu/blog/self-care-for-the-caregiver-201810171716

Wilson, D. M., Darko, E. M., Kusi-Appiah, E., Roh, S. J., Ramic, A., & Errasti-Ibarrondo, B. (2022). What exactly is "complicated" grief? A scoping research literature review to understand its risk factors and prevalence. *OMEGA—Journal of Death and Dying, 86*(2), 471–487.

World Health Organization. (2021). *Adolescent mental health.* https://www.who.int/news-room/fact-sheets/detail/adolescent-mental-health

World Health Organization. (2022a). *Improving the mental and brain health of children and adolescents.* https://www.who.int/activities/improving-the-mental-and-brain-health-of-children-and-adolescents

World Health Organization. (2022b). *Mental health.* https://www.who.int/news-room/fact-sheets/detail/mental-health-strengthening-our-response

Young, S., Hollingdale, J., Absoud, M., Bolton, P., Branney, P., Colley, W., C raze, E., Dave, M., Deeley, Q., Farrag, E., Gudjonsson, G., Hill, P., Liang, H., Murphy, C., Mackintosh, P., Murin, M., O'Regan, F., Ougrin, D., Rios, P., ... Woodhouse, E. (2020). Guidance for identification and treatment of individuals with attention deficit/hyperactivity disorder and autism spectrum disorder based upon expert consensus. *BMC Medicine, 18*(146), 1–29. https://doi.org/10.1186/s12916-020-01585-y

Zabek, F., Lyons, M. D., Alwani, N., Taylor, J. V., Brown-Meredith, E., Cruz, M. A., & Southall, V. H. (2023). Roles and functions of school mental health professionals within comprehensive school mental health systems. *School Mental Health, 15*(1), 1–18. https://doi.org/10.1007/s12310-022-09535-0

Zalsman, G., Hawton, K., Wasserman, D., van Heeringen, K., Arensman, E., Sarchiapone, M., ... & Zohar, J. (2016). Suicide prevention strategies revisited: 10-year systematic review. *Lancet Psychiatry, 3*(7), 646–659. https://doi.org/10.1016/S2215-0366(16)30030-X

Zuckerbrot, R., Cheung, A., Jensen, P., Stein, R., Laraque, D., & GLAD-PC Steering Group. (2018). Guidelines for adolescent depression in primary care (GLAD-PC): Part 1. Practice, preparation, identification, assessment, and initial management. *Pediatrics, 141*(3). http://pediatrics.aappublications.org/content/141/3/e20174081

Chapter 29

Students Engaging in Risk-Taking Behaviors

Ellen M. McCabe ▪ Beth E. Jameson ▪ Robin Adair Shannon

CHAPTER OUTLINE

Risk-taking behaviors in children and youth can lead to significant morbidity and mortality during adolescence and can set young people on a trajectory for disease, dysfunction, and chronic illness in adulthood. Many types of risk behaviors place youth at risk for poor health outcomes, such as the use of alcohol, tobacco, and other drugs; sexual behaviors that contribute to sexually transmitted infections and unintended pregnancy; body modification; gambling and gaming; as well as Internet and social media misuse.

The challenge for school nurses is to assist young people to understand the risks they face and make healthy choices to avoid or reduce them. This chapter will review the risk and protective factors that influence youths' involvement in risky behaviors and the interventions school nurses and schools may consider for addressing risky behaviors in their students.

PERSPECTIVES OF RISK-TAKING BEHAVIORS

Neurobiological and Developmental Perspectives

There are multiple theories as to why adolescents engage in high-risk behaviors. Theories include the adolescent's need to test the limits of childhood, rebel against adult authority, develop their own identity, cope with psychosocial issues, or experience sensation and stimulation. *Sensation seeking* has been defined by Zuckerman (2007) as "seeking of varied, novel, complex, and intense sensations and experiences, and the willingness to take physical, social, legal, and financial risks for the sake of such experience" (p. 49).

Contrary to the common stereotype that youth see themselves as invincible to the negative consequences of risk, the decision to engage in risky behaviors is driven by a complex risk–reward assessment influenced by emotional and social cues. In other words, adolescents are cognitively adept at assessing their vulnerability to the consequences of engaging in risky behaviors under favorable circumstances. However, because the area of the brain responsible for impulse control, the prefrontal cortex, is slower to develop than regions responsible for pleasure and rewards (select areas of the midbrain and prefrontal cortex), adolescent decision making tends to be driven more by social factors and emotion than reason. The emotional rewards of participating in risky behavior may outweigh the young person's cognitive assessment of risk (McCloskey & Johnson, 2019). For example, although most adolescents can objectively describe the adverse effects of drinking alcohol, they are more likely to override this assessment if they are at a party surrounded by peers drinking. The social rewards of fitting in override the cognitive understanding of danger (McCloskey & Johnson, 2019).

Adolescence is classified by the World Health Organization (WHO; 2017) as the age range from 10 to 19 years. It is the second most rapid time of biological and psychological change after infancy (Sawyer et al., 2018). This developmental period is marked by physical (e.g., puberty), neurobiological (e.g., unevenly developing regions of the brain), cognitive (e.g., development of abstract thinking skills), and social/emotional (e.g., identity formation, increased influence of peers) changes.

Health-risk behaviors are not limited to adolescents and may also occur in elementary school students. Therefore consideration must be made for those who start puberty early. Nurses in these settings increasingly need to understand how to address high-risk behaviors in all students.

Population-Focused Perspectives

Much of what is known about trends in adolescent risk-taking and school-level prevention and intervention efforts comes from public health surveillance systems, notably the *Youth Risk Behavior Survey* (YRBS). The YRBS is conducted at the national level in middle and high schools every 2 years to monitor students' health behaviors, conditions, and experiences (Centers for Disease Control and Prevention [CDC], 2023b). Students answer questions about the leading causes of morbidity and mortality during adolescence, including alcohol and other drug use, tobacco use, sexual behaviors, unintentional injury, and violence (e.g., suicide attempts, weapon carrying, driving without a seatbelt), unhealthy diets, and physical inactivity. Results from this survey allow experts to identify and address emerging and continued adolescent behaviors and trends in health risks from a population-focused perspective. Interactive YRBS data per state and participating school districts can be used to plan and monitor program outcomes, support health policy, provide support for grant funding, and inform future surveys (National Academies of Sciences, Engineering, and Medicine, 2019).

Risk Factors and Protective Factors

Risky behaviors are defined as actions that "increase the risk of disease or injury, which can subsequently lead to disability, death, or social problems" (Tariq & Gupta, 2022, para. 1).

Resilience is both intrinsic (association with personality and genetic makeup of the individual) and extrinsic (external to the person and may exist at multiple levels of influence, including individual, family, school, community, and policy levels). Resilience is viewed as adaptive functioning after an adverse event (Malhi et al., 2019). Practitioners examining resiliency incorporate a strengths-based approach to help young people succeed despite adversity rather than focusing on deficits. Dual approaches that simultaneously seek to reduce risk while promoting protective factors are examples of incorporating a resilience-based perspective (Malhi et al., 2019).

Some youths are more resilient and can adjust to situations better than others (Malhi et al., 2019). One's resilience is determined by the presence of risk and *protective factors*, which make one more or less likely to engage in high-risk behaviors. Risk and protective factors can be either internal/intrinsic or external/extrinsic. Some risk and protective factors are more amenable to intervention than others. For example, intrinsic factors such as temperament or genetic predisposition toward certain behaviors and health outcomes are not easily modifiable (Malhi et al., 2019). Effective prevention focuses on reducing risk factors and strengthening protective factors that are most closely related to the problem being addressed (Substance Abuse and Mental Health Services Administration [SAMHSA], 2022c). Risk factors change with the developmental stage of the child and are often the absence of protective factors. Some risk factors are related to *social determinants of health*, including poor environmental conditions, housing and food insecurity,

> **Focus on the Framework**
>
> The National Association of School Nurses' (NASN's) *School Nursing Practice Framework* (2024) recognizes **community/public health** *nursing* as a key principle of school nursing. As public health nurses, school nurses have essential roles in implementing interventions at a systems level to address elements associated with the social determinants of health that affect student risk-taking behaviors and health outcomes.

poverty, neighborhood violence, lack of healthcare availability, discrimination, and racism (Healthy People 2030, n.d.; Morone, 2017). See Chapter 2 for more information on social determinants of health. Research suggests certain extrinsic protective factors or resources promote resilience and prevent various health risk behaviors across gender and racial/ethnic groups (SAMHSA, 2022c). Examples of external protective factors include the following:

- Connectedness to parents/guardians, family, prosocial peers, extrafamilial adults (e.g., teachers), school, and community organizations where the student feels accepted and respected
- Emotional support outside of the home
- Prevention education provided at home and school

School connectedness is one of the strongest extrinsic protective factors against risky behaviors and depression (CDC, 2022c; McCabe et al., 2022). Students feel connected to school when they feel accepted, respected, included, and supported by others in the school social environment. For decades, studies have consistently shown that students with higher levels of school connectedness are more likely to succeed academically and less likely to engage in a variety of health risk behaviors, including substance use, violence and gang involvement, and early initiation of sex (CDC, 2021b). The immediate goal for families, schools, and school nurses is to assist students in identifying strengths and building resiliency to make choices regarding high-risk behaviors. School nurses should remember that advocacy, policy development, enforcement, risk reduction strategies, and other public health nursing interventions can be implemented on a systems level.

SUBSTANCE USE IN YOUTH: OVERVIEW

Adolescent substance misuse and abuse, including alcohol, tobacco, marijuana, illegal drugs, and prescription drug misuse, is a significant public health concern (Mehta et al., 2022). Approximately 70% of high school students have used at least one substance (e.g., alcohol, tobacco, marijuana, cocaine) in their lifetime (CDC, 2021a). Substance use often co-occurs with other health risk behaviors and conditions, such as depression, bullying, and obesity, making it necessary for school nurses to address the behaviors holistically.

> **Did You Know?**
>
> School nurses should model the use of correct and consistent terms when referring to substance use in youth.
>
> - ***Substance use:*** The use—even one time—of any substance
> - ***Substance misuse:*** The use of any substance in a manner, situation, amount, or frequency that can cause harm to users or those around them. For some substances or individuals, any use would constitute misuse (e.g., underage drinking, injection drug use).
> - ***Substance use disorder*** (SUD): Substance use disorder occurs when the recurrent use of a substance (alcohol and/or other drugs) causes clinically significant impairment, including health problems, disability, and failure to meet major responsibilities at work, school, or home.
>
> SAMHSA (2021b, p. 2).

The risk factors for substance use often transcend the type of substance used. Adolescence itself is a risk factor for substance use, given that it is a time of rapid development and exploration. Social concerns have a substantial influence on adolescents' decision to use substances, including family, school, and community norms around substance use. Additional considerations should include access to alcohol, the use of media and advertising, and the portrayal of substance use as fun, relaxing, and glamorous. Although adolescence is a time of separating from parents/guardians and becoming more independent, parents/guardians remain critically influential in a young person's choices to use or not use substances.

The *Youth Risk Behavior Survey* (YRBS) (CDC, 2023b) and the *Monitoring the Future* study (Miech et al., 2023) routinely survey nationally representative samples of students in traditional schools regarding substance use. There is consistency between findings from the two groups to provide an accurate overview of youth substance use. Prevalence estimates may underestimate the scope of adolescent substance use in America.

ALCOHOL

Adolescents use alcohol more often than any other drug, including tobacco or marijuana (National Institute on Alcohol Abuse and Alcoholism [NIAAA] 2021b). In 2021, the YRBS indicated that 23% of teens reported they currently drink alcohol (CDC, 2023b). In 2019, 24.6% of 14- and 15-year-olds reported in their lifetime having at least one drink of alcohol (NIAAA, 2020). In 2019, 59% of 12th graders reported consuming alcohol once in their lifetime, indicating a decrease of 28% from 82% (SAMHSA, 2021a). In 2019, 7.0 million youth ranging from ages 12 to 20 had more than a few sips of alcohol in the prior month (NIAAA, 2020). In 2019, 15.0% of teens reported drinking alcohol before age 13 (SAMHSA, 2021a).

These findings are significant because the earlier a person starts using alcohol, the more likely they are to become involved in other risky behaviors and to become alcohol dependent later in life. For example, those who begin using alcohol before age 15 are 5.6 times more likely to have an alcohol use disorder (AUD) in the past year than those who wait until age 21 or later (NIAAA, 2020).

Alcohol and the Developing Brain

Alcohol consumption can interfere with the development of the adolescent brain, both in its structure and function (Lees et al., 2020; NIAAA, 2021a). Mounting evidence suggests that adolescent binge drinking negatively affects areas of the brain that contribute to language, memory, awareness, and attention. For example, alcohol consumption behaviors in youth of 12 to 14 years old predict that these youths later in life could have decreased educational achievements (Lees et al., 2020). Alcohol use by pregnant women of all ages can significantly affect the fetus's developing brain, with sequelae ranging from a slight lowering of intelligence to profound intellectual disability.

Binge Drinking

Adolescents tend to drink less often than adults; however, when they do drink, it is often in greater amounts than adults (NIAAA, 2021a). More than 90% of the alcohol drunk by youth between the ages of 12 and 20 is consumed by binge drinking. Importantly, in 2019, 825,000 youth disclosed binge drinking five or more days in the prior month (NIAAA, 2021c). Definitions of binge drinking differ by gender and are based on approximating how much it takes for a person's blood alcohol concentration (BAC) to reach 0.08%, or 80 mg/dL. For males, binge drinking generally occurs after five drinks in about a 2-hour time frame; females are involved in binge drinking if they have four or more drinks on the same occasion (NIAAA, 2021c). Youth surveys often measure binge drinking as five or more drinks on one occasion for males and four or more drinks for females (CDC, 2022b).

In the 2019 YRBS, 13.7% of high school students reported recently having five or more drinks of alcohol in a row, and 4.4% reported having 10 or more drinks in a row within a couple of hours (CDC, 2022b). More than 10 drinks in a row for males and more than eight drinks in a row is classified as *extreme binge drinking*, or high-intensity drinking, and poses exceptionally high risks for short- and long-term problems. This extreme binge drinking peaks among college-age students (NIAAA, 2021c).

Underage alcohol use differs by region of the country. In 2014, the highest reported levels were in the Northeast (28.3%), followed by the Midwest (24.5%), West (24.5%), and South (22.3%) (SAMHSA, 2021a). The highest levels of binge drinking in 2019 were among youth who identified as biracial or multiracial (7.7%), with the lowest levels found among black (2.8%) and Asian (2.8%) youth. Among White youth, binge drinking was 5.5%, and among Hispanic youth binge drinking was 4.8% (SAMHSA, 2021a). Research reports that 14-year-olds who are white, black, and Hispanic would be equally likely to drink alcohol, while 18-year-old whites and Hispanics are twice as likely to drink alcohol as black 18-year-olds (NIAAA, 2020). One reason for this shift is due to higher rates of school dropout among youth of color, as youth are more likely to use alcohol and other drugs (An et al., 2017). Therefore it is important for school nurses to recognize racial and ethnic differences. Although binge drinking among youth has declined, it remains a significant public health concern due to the number of youths who use alcohol in large quantities.

Alcohol Poisoning

Youth who binge drink place themselves at risk for alcohol poisoning or alcohol overdose, which is a life-threatening emergency. Alcohol poisoning occurs when the blood alcohol concentration is so high that brain regions responsible for fundamental life-support functions start to shut down, including heart rate, breathing, and temperature control (NIAAA, 2021a). Confusion, vomiting, clammy skin, trouble staying conscious, slow heart rate, seizures, difficulty breathing, and dulled responses (e.g., no gag reflex) are all symptoms of alcohol poisoning and require immediate medical intervention (NIAAA, 2021a).

The effects of too much alcohol *cannot* be reversed by walking, drinking hot coffee, or having a cold shower, but instead could make it worse (NIAAA, 2021a). School nurses should ensure that students know that these are not effective or safe ways to handle the effects of too much alcohol. Even after someone has lost consciousness, the blood alcohol concentration can continue to increase as alcohol in the stomach and intestine is absorbed into the bloodstream. One should never assume that an unconscious person can simply sleep off the effects of too much alcohol. In these situations, the absence of a gag reflex coupled with the increased risk of vomiting due to an irritated stomach increases the risk of aspiration and death (NIAAA, 2021a).

There are many well-established risks for underage drinking (i.e., consuming alcohol before age 21) (SAMHSA, 2021a). The CDC estimates that, on average, alcohol is a factor in 3,900 deaths each year among youth

Did You Know?

Alcohol equivalents for common alcoholic beverages:

12 ounces of beer = 5 ounces of wine = 1.5 ounces of 80-proof distilled spirit

under age 21, including nearly 1,600 from motor vehicle accidents, 1,300 from homicides, 500 from suicides, and 245 from accidents such as alcohol poisoning, burns, drowning, and falls (CDC, 2022b). Impaired judgment may make youth more likely to engage in other risky behaviors such as abusing other drugs and having unprotected sex (CDC, 2022b; SAMHSA, 2021a). For example, in 2019, 17.0% of high-school students had ridden in a car during the past month with someone who had been drinking alcohol, and 5.0% had driven under the influence of alcohol, thus increasing their risk of being in a motor vehicle accident (CDC, 2022b). Additionally, underage drinking negatively affects brain development during this crucial period of life and increases the risk for school, social, and legal problems, and assault (both sexual and physical).

Addressing Alcohol Use

Despite the risks of underage drinking, alcohol continues to be the drug of choice for adolescents and is more popular than tobacco or marijuana (CDC, 2022b). Although the law is clear that it is illegal to sell alcohol to minors or drink alcohol before age 21 (except for religious reasons), underage alcohol use remains a pervasive part of American culture that is influenced by norms around drinking in the United States overall and in youth culture specifically.

The National Institute on Alcohol Abuse and Alcoholism published *A Pocket Guide for Alcohol Screening and Brief Intervention for Youth* to address drinking problems (Johnston et al., 2011). In the first step, providers ask two screening questions: one about the student's drinking behavior and another about their friends' drinking behaviors. The wording and order of these questions are modified slightly depending on whether the student is in elementary (9 to 11 years), middle (11 to 14 years), or high school (14 to 18 years). Step two differs based on whether the adolescent does or does not drink alcohol. If the student does not report alcohol use, the provider should praise the choice, elicit reasons to continue abstaining from alcohol, and educate about alcohol risks. In the case where the student does not report alcohol use but that friends use, the provider should explore how the student plans to abstain from alcohol in the presence of friends who drink. The provider should also advise against riding in a car with a driver under the influence. In step three, the provider uses motivational interviewing techniques to advise and assist students who drink. The guidance provided depends on the level of risk determined during step two. Finally, step four provides follow-up and continued support to youth who drink. This support can happen during visits intended for following up on alcohol use or during other health visits (NIAAA, 2021b).

School nurses can be an ideal resource for families to provide materials and promote alcohol awareness programming. Interventions and health promotion activities should begin well before students enter high school. It is essential to identify students' areas of strength and resiliency to promote protective factors in decision making. The school nurse should accurately assess the student who presents to the health office with complaints of headache or gastrointestinal upset and suspicious of an alcohol problem. Other telltale signs might be the heavy use of mints or mouthwash, hand tremors, sweating, slurred speech, and unsteady gait.

SAMHSA provides the following suggestions for addressing substance use. The school nurse can assist in these school-level measures by advocating for students, addressing zero-tolerance policies, and increasing awareness.

- Provide an environment that allows students to explore and develop their talents.
- Inform parents/guardians and students about the consequences of underage drinking.
- Implement evidence-based programs aimed at preventing underage drinking.
- Provide and promote venues where adolescents can gather with friends where alcohol is unavailable (SAMHSA, 2021b).

Additional measures that schools can take to protect youth from underage drinking include the following:

- Encourage student involvement in school.
- Help students explore their talents and follow their passions, whether academic, musical, sports, or social or community causes.
- Provide opportunities for students to know that they matter and belong.
- Mentor students in behaviors and activities that result in positive outcomes, including how to handle peer pressure.
- Provide information to parents/guardians regarding school policies on alcohol use, consequences of alcohol use, and available community resources.
- Recognize that those who mature earlier or later than their peers may be at increased risk.

Practice Connection

SAMHSA (2020) has a free booklet called *Focus on Prevention* that helps communities plan and deliver substance use prevention strategies. It covers conducting needs assessments, identifying partners, and creating effective strategies for marketing and program evaluation. It includes a community assessment to identify the community's needs, issues, trends, and resources.

SAMHSA (2022b) provides resources for parents/guardians and caregivers to start and continue the conversation about the dangers of drinking alcohol and using other drugs at a young age. The myriad of materials for parents/guardians and caregivers offers recommendations to monitor children's substance use, including alcohol.

TOBACCO

Tobacco products, such as cigarettes, cigars, smokeless tobacco, cloves, and electronic cigarettes, are hazardous to health. Tobacco use during adolescence remains a major public health concern due to its evolving nature and associated morbidity and mortality. For example, the current use of other tobacco products, such as electronic cigarettes (e-cigarettes) and e-hookahs, has increased among middle and high school students (CDC, 2022a). Flavorings added to these products increase their appeal among youth. In 2014, over half (56%) of middle school students and nearly three-fourths (73%) of high school students who used tobacco in the prior 30 days used a flavored tobacco product (CDC, 2022a). While the percentage of students who use cigarettes has decreased, there has been a steep increase in nicotine use via electronic appliances (Hall et al., 2021). The decrease in smoking cigarettes among teens may also be in response to an increase in the perceived risk for sequelae, price increases, and age restrictions on the purchase of cigarettes. However, some underage youth circumvent laws by ordering cigarettes over the Internet. School nurses should ask students about their use of nicotine products rather than just their use of cigarettes.

Risk factors related to youth tobacco use include social and environmental factors, biological and genetic factors, mental health, personal perceptions, and family and personal factors. Youth may be more likely to smoke if exposed through advertising, perceive it as an everyday activity as portrayed in the media, have peers who use tobacco, or have parents who smoke (CDC, 2017a). Youth who expect positive outcomes from smoking, such as weight management or stress reduction, may be more likely to smoke. Depression, stress, and anxiety are also strongly related to more youth smoking (CDC, 2017b).

Other important factors related to youth tobacco use include low resistance skills, low self-esteem, low academic achievement, low parental involvement and support, and ease of access to tobacco (e.g., low prices and wide availability) (CDC, 2017b). Some evidence suggests that youth may be sensitive to nicotine and, compared with adults, may become dependent on it faster. Some youth may also find it harder to quit smoking due to genetic factors (CDC, 2017b). Although all states have age restrictions on buying tobacco products, youth find other methods to access tobacco.

Cigarettes

Nearly 90% of adults (87%) who reported being daily smokers tried their first cigarette by age 18 (American Lung Association, 2017a). The percentage of adolescents experimenting with cigarettes, even one puff, has decreased significantly, from 70% in 1991 to 58.4% in 2003 to 28.9% in 2017 (CDC, 2017b). Results from the 2022 *Monitoring the Future* study note that cigarette smoking among youth is at its lowest level in 41 years. Older students were more likely to report cigarette use, with 4.0% of 12th graders, 1.7% of 10th graders, and 0.8% of eighth graders reporting smoking in the past month (Miech et al., 2023). Of concern, 7.5% of children smoked before their 13th birthday (CDC, 2017b). The proportion of students reporting frequent cigarette use (i.e., smoking on 20 or more days in the month before the survey) also continued to decline, down to 3.4% of students (Kann et al., 2018). By comparison, 16.8% of students reported frequent cigarette use in 1999.

Cigarette smoke contains almost 7,000 chemicals, 69 of which cause cancer, including tar (American Lung Association, 2017a). Primary ingredients in cigarettes include tar and nicotine (Tabuchi, 2021). Tar is a sticky black liquid that sticks to cells in the lung tissue and allows other carcinogens in the cigarette to stick to it and accumulate in that site; its amount varies from 1 to 15 mg per cigarette, most of which is in the last third of the cigarette (Tabuchi, 2021). Nicotine, among the most addictive substances, increases the release of acetylcholine neurotransmitters that suppress the appetite, enhance pleasure, and assist in relaxation. Each cigarette contains 8 to 20 mg of nicotine, of which 1 mg is absorbed. The drug acts within seconds of being inhaled.

According to the U.S. Surgeon General, the developing adolescent brain is particularly vulnerable to the adverse effects of exposure to nicotine, affecting attention, learning, mood, and impulse control (Hwang & O'Neil, 2020). Youth are at higher risk for becoming dependent on nicotine if they use multiple tobacco products (CDC, 2017b). Carbon monoxide is another major component of cigarette smoke, which can interfere with hemoglobin function.

In addition, 58 million nonsmokers are exposed to second-hand smoke. In children, second-hand smoke increases the risk of sudden infant death syndrome (SIDS) and can cause ear and respiratory infections (e.g., pneumonia, bronchitis), respiratory symptoms (e.g., shortness of breath, sneezing, coughing), and more severe and frequent asthma attacks (CDC, 2017b). In adults, exposure to second-hand smoke can cause heart disease, lung cancer, and stroke (CDC, 2017b). Ample evidence shows that smoke-free policies have widespread public support without negatively affecting the economy (CDC, 2017b).

Almost every organ in the body is negatively affected by smoking. About 90% of lung cancer deaths and 80% of chronic obstructive pulmonary disease, including chronic bronchitis and emphysema, are directly caused by cigarette smoking (American Lung Association, 2017a). Scientists have identified causal links between smoking and a variety of other diseases, including coronary artery disease, stroke, diabetes mellitus, rheumatoid arthritis, and a variety of cancers such as colorectal cancer and cancers of the larynx, mouth, esophagus, stomach, pancreas, kidney, bladder, cervix, and blood (American Lung Association, 2017a).

Electronic Cigarettes

According to the National Institute on Drug Abuse (NIDA; 2020b), electronic cigarettes or *e-cigarettes* (also known as *electronic nicotine delivery systems* [ENDS], *e-cigs, e-hookahs, hookah pens, vapes, vape pens, Juuls,* or *mods*) are "battery-operated devices that people use to inhale an aerosol, that typically contains nicotine (though not always), flavorings, and other chemicals" (para. 1). E-cigarettes have surpassed conventional cigarettes as the most commonly used tobacco product among American youth (Cooper et al., 2022). In 2022, a study by the U.S. Department of Agriculture and the CDC found that 14.1% of high school and 3.3% of middle school students reported current e-cigarette use (Cooper et al., 2022).

The *Monitoring the Future* survey differentiated students who vaped to inhale nicotine and those who did not. Their findings showed that most students who vaped did not do so to inhale nicotine (Miech et al., 2023). Among those who reported using vape flavoring in the past 30 days were 4.9% of eighth graders, 7.4% of 10th graders, and 8.3% of 12th graders. In 2022, nicotine was vaped by 7.1% of eighth graders, 14.2% of 10th graders, and 20.7% of 12th graders, whereas marijuana was vaped by 4.2% of eighth graders, 10.3% of 10th graders, and 14.8% of 12th graders (Miech et al., 2023). Older youth are more likely than younger youth to use e-cigarettes, and Hispanic and white youth are more likely than black youth to use these products (CDC, 2022h). It appears that the e-cigarette trend may be leveling off.

With over 460 brands and 7,700 flavors currently on the market, e-cigarettes can look like traditional tobacco products (e.g., pipes, cigars, and cigarettes), other everyday items like USB memory sticks, mascara containers, or pens, or a variety of other designs (CDC, 2022a). Regardless of the design, most e-cigarettes have four different parts: a reservoir or cartridge that stores a liquid solution containing nicotine, flavorings, and other chemicals; a mouthpiece that is used to inhale the liquid solution; an atomizer (heating element); and a power source—typically a battery. When the user puffs on the mouthpiece, the heating element is activated and vaporizes the liquid into a vapor or aerosol that can be inhaled—otherwise known as *vaping*. E-cigarettes can also be used for *dripping*, where e-liquid drops are placed directly onto atomizer coils and heated to produce a vapor that can be inhaled (CDC, 2022a). One in four high school students reports practicing dripping and engaging in these activities for reasons such as creating a thicker vapor, improving flavors, and producing a stronger throat hit (i.e., contraction of the throat, which creates a pleasing sensation) (Cooper et al., 2022). E-cigarette products can also be used to deliver cannabinoids and potentially to deliver other illicit drugs (CDC, 2022a). The liquid in the cartridge is created by extracting nicotine from tobacco and mixing it with a base (e.g., propylene glycol); colorings, flavorings, and other chemicals may also be added. What chemicals are contained in various vaping products is not generally known. Laboratory tests demonstrate that harmful substances that can be breathed in and exhaled include nicotine; ultrafine particles that can be inhaled deep into the lungs; flavorings such as diacetyl, a chemical linked to serious lung disease; volatile organic compounds; cancer-causing chemicals; and heavy metals such as nickel, tin, and lead (CDC, 2022a).

Flavors are often used for marketing these products to young adults. One concern for school nurses is that unlike the telltale sign of smoking cigarettes in the school bathroom—a distinctive odor—the primary odor emanating from electronic cigarettes is the flavoring itself (Selekman, 2019). In 2020, the Food and Drug Administration (FDA) prioritized enforcement and marketing of electronic nicotine delivery systems that target youth or promote the use of ENDS by youth. The sale of prefilled cartridges in any flavor other than tobacco or menthol is prohibited, unless authorized by the FDA. While flavorings are not outright prohibited, the FDA will regulate and require by law an application to the FDA that the product meets standards in the law and provides for the protection of public health. The policy also includes a ban on marketing and/or advertising that targets youth using images of items that appeal to youth such as kid-friendly characters on food products, such as cereals (FDA, 2020a). Despite this recent legislation, in the most recent tobacco use survey, among middle and high school students who use e-cigarettes, 84.9% of students who reported using e-cigarettes used flavored varieties (Cooper et al., 2022).

E-cigarettes are often marketed as a harm-reduction strategy to help current adult smokers quit because the levels of toxic substances they contain have been found to be lower than what is present in conventional cigarettes (CDC, 2022a). Evidence supports a strong association between the use of e-cigarettes and other tobacco products among young people; longitudinal evidence suggests that nonsmoking adolescents and young adults in the United States who start using e-cigarettes are more likely to progress to smoking conventional cigarettes (Aleyan et al., 2018).

Evidence supporting the negative impact of e-cigarette use on youth, along with continued uncertainty about long-term use, has prompted policies to protect youth. In 2016, the FDA extended its regulatory authority to include e-cigarettes, allowing it to regulate the manufacturing, distribution, and marketing of these products under the auspices of the Family Smoking Prevention and Tobacco Control Act (FDA, 2017b). Before this, the federal government had no legal authority to prevent the sale of e-cigarettes to youth under the age of 18 and to penalize manufacturers who market flavored e-cigarettes that appeal to children (FDA, 2017b). Additionally, products must carry a warning about nicotine, and sales through vending machines in facilities that admit youth are prohibited (FDA, 2017b).

Smokeless Tobacco

In 2022, the CDC reported that 1.6% of high-school students used smokeless tobacco products such as chewing tobacco, snuff, or dip on at least 1 day in the past month.

The gender disparity in smokeless tobacco use is substantial, with 2.3% of males and 0.9% of females reporting using a smokeless tobacco product in the past month (CDC, 2022e). Additionally, white adolescents (2.2%) were more likely than Hispanic adolescents (1.3%) to use smokeless tobacco (CDC, 2022e).

Smokeless tobacco includes chewing tobacco, snuff, dip, and snus (rhymes with goose). *Snuff* is finely ground tobacco sold in tins or sachets, and *chew* is a leafier form of tobacco sold in pouches; both are held in the mouth between the cheek and gums, sometimes for hours. The nicotine is absorbed directly into the mucous membranes, resulting in the need to spit out the juices and saliva that accumulate in the mouth (American Cancer Society, 2020). *Snus* is a similar smoke-free and spit-free tobacco product in a teabag-like pouch; it is used for 30 minutes and then discarded.

Smokeless tobacco is not a safe alternative to smoking. Health consequences from smokeless tobacco include nicotine addiction; cancer of the mouth, esophagus, and pancreas; other diseases of the mouth (e.g., the recession of the gums, gum disease, tooth decay); and an increased risk of death from stroke and heart disease (American Cancer Society, 2020).

Strategies for Addressing Youth Tobacco Use

The FDA's *Youth Tobacco Prevention Plan* focuses on three aspects: preventing access (i.e., acting against retailers selling tobacco to underage individuals), curbing marketing (i.e., policy on enforcement against unauthorized flavored e-cigarette), and educating youth on the dangers while educating retailers of their position in protecting youth (FDA, 2020b).

CDC's guidelines for school health programs recommend that tobacco use be prohibited in all school facilities and at all school events (CDC, 2022e). Consistent with these guidelines, a *tobacco-free environment* is mandated in most schools. Still, tobacco use occurs at school. For example, students will smoke or vape in school bathrooms. If anyone enters the bathroom, the student can quickly flush the cigarette or e-cigarette down the toilet. This suggests that faculty and staff should routinely monitor the bathrooms between classes. Be advised that electronic cigarettes may only smell like the flavoring being used.

On an individual level, the "5 A's"—*Ask, Advise, Assess, Assist, Arrange*—can be used to assess tobacco dependence and intervention planning (Price et al., 2019). The steps include the following:

Ask about the person's smoking status with questions such as the following:

- Have you ever tried to quit but could not?
- Do you ever have strong cravings to smoke or felt like you really needed a cigarette?
- When you try to stop or stop for a while, do you find it hard to concentrate, or feel more irritable or nervous?

Advise the person to stop smoking.

Assess their willingness to quit.

Assist and *Arrange* for a brief intervention and follow-up.

Practice Connection

School nurses should be aware of the risk of the lithium-ion batteries of e-cigarettes exploding and causing severe burns, bleeding, and localized injury. It can occur with overheating, exposure to water, and contact with metallic objects, such as keys, and improper charging (Cummings et al., 2018). If this injury should occur, Cummings et al. (2018) recommend *using mineral oil for initial wound irrigation to remove any remaining alkaline material left on the tissues.* Immediate medical attention is warranted. The exploding e-cigarettes might also be a fire hazard for the school. There are also increased reports of young children swallowing the nicotine-laced liquid used in the e-cigarette, known as e-juice; these have resulted in calls to poison control centers and visits to emergency departments for nicotine poisoning (Cummings et al., 2018).

Prevention Approaches

Few teens stop smoking without external intervention. Although many psychosocial interventions have produced short-term success, for many students participating in cessation interventions is not sustained for the long-term (Duncan et al., 2018). This points to the importance of primary prevention in preventing dependence on tobacco and the development of tobacco-related illnesses. Nonsmokers should be praised for making smart choices, and alternatives should be provided for those who have just begun smoking. Some states have used tobacco settlement monies to sponsor youth groups committed to promoting the prevention and control of tobacco, such as the *Kick Butts Generation*, which involves more than 12,000 youth (Whitten et al., 2020).

The American Lung Association (2017b) supports a teen mentoring program called *Teens Against Tobacco Use.* It helps teens develop leadership skills and encourages younger children to avoid tobacco. *Tar Wars* is another tobacco-free education program designed by the American Academy of Family Physicians (2019) for fourth- and fifth-grade students. This free online program includes a preactivity exercise, a 1-hour classroom presentation, and a follow-up poster contest.

Smoking Cessation

Multiple programs are available to assist those who want to stop smoking. Programs grounded in social and cognitive-based approaches, such as cognitive behavioral therapy, are common. For example, the American Lung Association *Not on Tobacco* (N-O-T) program is one of the most successful and frequently used smoking cessation programs and is listed as a model program by SAMHSA

(American Lung Association, 2022b). N-O-T has been thoroughly evaluated and deemed effective for youth (Blank et al., 2017). It is user-friendly, youth-focused, gender-sensitive, and can easily be used in school. The program consists of 10 weekly sessions (50 minutes each) and follow-up sessions (at 2-week intervals) that are grounded in social cognitive theory. Most groups are limited to only one sex, including the leader (Blank et al., 2017).

The sessions include motivational issues, smoking history, and stress management; nicotine addiction; physical, psychological, and social consequences of smoking; preparing to quit; dealing with urges and cravings; relapse prevention; dealing with family and peer pressure; recognizing social, cultural, and media ploys; increasing healthy lifestyle behaviors; and accessing resources and support (Blank et al., 2017). In one study, pairing N-O-T with exercise (NoT+FIT) resulted in a lower likelihood of smoking at 3-month follow-up (Blank et al., 2017). Recruitment into smoking cessation programs is more successful if the programs are held during the day rather than after school. Where available, school-based health centers are an ideal location for smoking cessation programs. Tobacco use continues to be the leading cause of preventable death in America, and it usually begins during adolescence, making this a crucial time for primary and secondary prevention efforts (CDC, 2022e).

CAFFEINE AND ENERGY DRINKS

Children and adolescents are at-risk populations for caffeine use. Caffeine (1, 3, 7-trimethylxanthine) is a psychostimulant found in coffee, tea, cacao beans (source for cocoa and chocolate), and has been identified in over 60 other plant species. It is the most widely used psychoactive drug in the world (Samoggia & Rezzaghi, 2021; Soós et al., 2021). Trends in caffeine use data from the National Health and Nutrition Examination Survey (NHANES) show that over 75% of children (age greater than 5 years) and adolescents (ages 12 to 17 years) consume caffeine regularly (Meigs et al., 2022).

In adults, 400 mg/day of caffeine or less is generally considered safe (FDA, 2018). However, due to the lack of research to understand caffeine's effects on youth, the maximum safe amount of caffeine is unknown in children and adolescents (Soós et al., 2021). In 2018, the American Academy of Pediatrics (AAP) reaffirmed policy research that caffeine and stimulant substances have no place in the diet of children and adolescents (Temple, 2019). While other countries regulate, restrict, or even ban the sales of energy drinks to children (Meigs et al., 2022), the FDA (2018) has not provided federal guidelines for caffeine use in children and adolescents.

The primary source of caffeine in children and adolescents is soda (30 to 40 mg per 12-ounce can), followed by coffee (80 to 100 mg per 8-ounce cup), and tea (30 to 50 mg per 8-ounce cup) (Temple, 2019; FDA, 2018). The FDA limits caffeine in soda to 71 mg per 12 fluid ounces (FDA, 2018). Energy drinks are high in caffeine (40 to 250 mg per 8 ounces) and are used by 30% to 50% of all teens (Meigs et al., 2022; Samoggia & Rezzaghi, 2021; Soós et al., 2021). With brand names such as Red Bull, Monster Energy, and Full Throttle, energy drinks are listed as nutritional supplements; as such, they do not have to limit the caffeine to 71 mg per 12 fluid oz , as per the U.S. Food and Drug Administration for sodas (FDA, 2018). Additionally, caffeine is consumed in pill-form products that assist one in staying awake (e.g., No Doz, Vivarin), which may be added as an ingredient to food and beverages. Anhydrous (powdered) caffeine, often marketed as an energy supplement, can also be added to other products, thereby increasing the risk of overdose. One teaspoon of anhydrous caffeine equals the caffeine in about 25 cups of coffee (Wellershoff, 2018).

Caffeine has dose-dependent effects. Within 4 minutes of consumption, caffeine levels are noted in the blood (Samoggia & Rezzaghi, 2021). Levels peak approximately 40 to 120 minutes after ingestion, and the half-life is 3 to 7 hours (Samoggia & Rezzaghi, 2021). The most widely noted physiological effects of caffeine are decreased fatigue and sleepiness (Soós et al., 2021).

School nurses should be alert for signs and symptoms of excessive caffeine use. High caffeine doses (greater than 400 mg) are associated with impaired sleep and sleep quality; in turn, sleep impairment can negatively affect academic performance and is associated with growth hormone deficiencies. Other signs of excess caffeine include dehydration, tachycardia, increased blood pressure, and cardiac arrhythmias (Soós et al., 2021; Suppiah et al., 2021; FDA, 2018). Acute overdose symptoms include hyperactivity, irritability, dizziness, tremor, tachycardia, and headache (Soós et al., 2021; Suppiah et al., 2021).

Withdrawal symptoms begin 12 to 24 hours after sudden cessation of caffeine intake and peak in 1 to 2 days (Meigs et al., 2022; Samoggia & Rezzaghi, 2021; Yu et al., 2022). Withdrawal symptoms include headaches, impaired concentration, drowsiness, irritability, and muscle aches (Yu et al., 2022).

High caffeine consumption in youth is associated with other risk-taking behaviors: increased consumption of alcohol, increased tobacco use, and irrational choices (Grant & Chamberlain, 2018; Temple, 2019). Emerging research also suggests that caffeine is associated with increased body mass index in adolescents (Yu et al., 2022).

PRESCRIPTION AND OVER-THE-COUNTER DRUGS

Prescription drug misuse and abuse are defined as "taking a medication in a manner or dose other than prescribed; taking someone else's prescription, even if for a legitimate medical complaint such as pain; or taking a medication to feel euphoria (i.e., to get high)" (NIDA, 2020b, para. 1). Prescription and over-the-counter (OTC) medications are the most commonly abused and misused legal drugs. As the most quickly growing drug problem in America, prescription drug misuse has become a national public health problem, and young people are not immune to it (NIDA, 2020b). See Box 29-1 for commonly misused OTC drugs.

Youth may use legal drugs for their intended purpose but not at the dosage or by the person for whom they are prescribed. They may use drugs to relieve anxiety, enhance concentration, stay up late to complete assignments, improve athletic performance, lose weight, sleep, or get high (U.S. Drug Enforcement Administration [USDEA], 2018b). Though illegal, youth report sharing or trading prescription drugs. Youth report that it is easy to obtain drugs from home medicine cabinets and those of grandparents and friends: 53% of people ages 12 and older who misused pain relievers in the past year got the drug for no cost from a relative or friend, 21% obtained a prescription from a doctor, 11% bought the drug from a relative or friend, and 4% obtained the drug from a dealer or stranger (USDEA, 2018b).

Many teens do not perceive OTC and prescription drug abuse as illegal or risky and have less shame in using these drugs than nonprescribed illicit drugs (USDEA, 2018b). The USDEA (2018b) resource, *Prescription for Disaster: How Teens Abuse Medicine,* provides an extensive overview of the prescription and OTC drugs commonly abused by youth, including the signs of abuse and what adults can do to help youth who misuse medications.

Stimulants

Amphetamines are stimulants prescribed for medical conditions, such as attention deficit-hyperactivity disorder (ADHD) and narcolepsy. They are classified as Schedule II stimulants, meaning they have limited medical use and a high potential for abuse (USDEA, 2020a).

BOX 29-1

Commonly Abused and Misused Legal Drugs

Opioids: codeine, hydrocodone/Vicodin, oxycodone/OxyContin
Psychiatric medications: benzodiazepines (e.g., alprazolam [Xanax], clonazepam [Klonopin], diazepam [Valium], zolpidem [Ambien], quetiapine [Seroquel])
Stimulants used for ADHD: (e.g., amphetamine, dextroamphetamine mixed salts [Adderall], methylphenidate [Ritalin])
Cough and cold medications containing dextromethorphan or codeine

SAMHSA (2023).

Methamphetamine is also a Schedule II drug; there is one FDA-approved brand for children and youth (Desoxyn) (USDEA, 2022b). Otherwise, methamphetamine is an illegal street drug (discussed in the next section). With side effects such as insomnia, anorexia, and weight loss (Proebstl et al., 2018), amphetamines are abused by students to stay awake or diet. Other adverse effects include tachycardia, hypertension, nausea, vomiting, abdominal tics, agitation, increased body temperature, hallucinations, seizures, and death (Proebstl et al., 2018).

Cough and Cold Medications

Cough syrups and cold medications are examples of OTC drugs that young people commonly misuse because they are easy to access and can be drunk alone or with alcohol or soda (USDEA, 2018b). Brands that include *dextromethorphan* can cause mild distortions of color, visual hallucinations, dissociative out-of-body sensations, and loss of motor control. Of concern is the teen practice of *robo-tripping,* where teens take eight to 12 Robitussin cough medicine pills to get an intense buzz and euphoria that lasts for a few hours. The active ingredient is dextromethorphan with street names such as robo, DXM, triple C, tussin, or skittles. Dextromethorphan can also be purchased online and is an ingredient in more than 100 medicines. Another dangerous youth fad is called *sizzurp,* or *purple drank,* which involves mixing a cough syrup containing the antihistamine, promethazine, and codeine in a cup with fruit-flavored hard candy and any fruit-flavored soda (USDEA, 2018b). The amount of cough syrup may be more than 25 times the recommended dose (Miuli et al., 2020).

ILLEGAL DRUGS AND SUBSTANCE USE

Illegal substances, or *street drugs,* are non–FDA-approved drugs that can cause devastating health and social consequences for young people. Users often combine illegal street drugs with alcohol and tobacco. In addition, the legal consequences of selling and possessing these drugs place youth at significant risk of becoming justice-involved.

Marijuana

The terms *marijuana* and *cannabis* are commonly used interchangeably, but there are distinctions between the two. According to the National Center on Complementary and Integrative Health (2019, para. 1):

- The word "cannabis" refers to all products derived from the plant *Cannabis sativa.*
- The cannabis plant contains about 540 chemical substances.
- The word "marijuana" refers to parts of or products from the plant Cannabis sativa that contain

substantial amounts of tetrahydrocannabinol (THC). THC is the substance that's primarily responsible for the effects of marijuana on a person's mental state. Some cannabis plants contain very little THC. Under U.S. law, these plants are considered industrial hemp rather than marijuana.

Marijuana is classified as an illegal substance by the federal government (CDC, 2021a). Historically, criminalization of marijuana has disproportionately penalized and incarcerated individuals from black and brown populations versus white populations. Such inequities have contributed to negative stereotyping and racist perceptions of black and brown people and marijuana users. However, societal attitudes toward marijuana use are evolving rapidly. In recent years, many states have decriminalized the possession of small amounts of marijuana. Medical cannabis, in some form, is legal in almost all states (Ryan et al., 2021). The number of states that have legalized adult use of recreational marijuana and allow it to be sold in specially licensed dispensaries is increasing. Nevertheless, recreational marijuana is illegal for minors (CDC, 2021a). The use of medicinal marijuana at school for students with select medical conditions, such as seizures, may be allowed in some states, though it remains controversial. See Chapter 30 for more information on the administration of medicinal marijuana in schools.

In 2019, nearly 36.8% of high school students reported having tried marijuana; 21.7% reported using it within 30 days of taking the Youth Risk Behavior Study (YRBS). Marijuana is called by many slang names, such as *pot, herb, reefer, grass, weed, Mary Jane, Aunt Mary, skunk, boom, gangster, kif,* and *ganja,* among others. Dried marijuana leaf or flower can be rolled into a *joint, bone, nail cigarette,* or *blunt* (cigar) or smoked in a pipe (bowl) or water pipe (bong). Marijuana can be ingested as *edibles* by infusing it into beverages or mixed or baked into food or candy. It can also be put in some e-cigarette devices and vaped (CDC, 2021a; USDEA, 2020b).

Hashish, or hash, is a greenish-gray concentrated THC-rich product derived from the resin of marijuana flowers, which is typically smoked or eaten in an edible form to produce an intense high. Hash oil is a liquid extract of hash that can be added to or dabbed on other substances or products. It is estimated that a drop or two of hash oil on a cigarette has a similar effect to smoking an entire marijuana joint (USDEA, 2020b).

The concentrate of marijuana is an oil with potent THC levels of 40% to 80%. This cannabinoid oil (called 710, which is OIL spelled backward and upside down) can be smoked or vaped; and because it is odorless, it is harder to detect. It can also be mixed with other illicit drugs, alcohol, or food (Laestadius et al., 2019).

Synthetic cannabinoids, also known as *synthetic marijuana* or *fake weed,* have increased in popularity among young people. Common brand names include *Spice, K2, Black Mamba, Joker, Kush, Kronic, Mojo, Cloud 9,* and *herbal incense* (Griffith et al., 2019). Synthetic marijuana has become the second most used illicit drug after marijuana. Synthetic marijuana products can contain various manufactured chemicals that can be smoked, vaped, or ingested. They have no known medical benefits and a high potential for abuse; therefore it is illegal to buy, sell, or possess some of the chemicals found in synthetic marijuana. However, manufacturers are continually altering their chemical formulas to circumvent these laws. There are many different structures of synthetic cannabinoids, and more structures are being synthesized that have unknown contaminants and produce variable responses in users (Griffith et al., 2019).

THC must be differentiated from *cannabidiol,* commonly called CBD, which comes from the hemp varieties of the cannabis plant. CBD is a nonpsychoactive ingredient in products such as oils, ointments, pills, and medications; it does not produce a high similar to THC (CDC, 2021a). CBD is used for its purported benefits in relieving pain, anxiety, depression, nausea, post-traumatic stress disorder, and some types of seizure disorders (Healthline, 2019; Leafbuyer, 2018). More research is needed to determine the health effects of using CBD.

Effects and Health Effects

There are hundreds of chemical compounds in cannabis plants, 80 to 100 of which are cannabinoids. A *cannabinoid* is a "chemical substance, regardless of structure or origin, that joins the cannabinoid receptors of the body and brain and that have similar effects to those produced by the Cannabis sativa plant" (Drug and Alcohol Foundation, 2022, p. 1). The most common cannabinoids are delta-9 tetrahydrocannabinol (THC) and cannabidiol (CBD). The main psychoactive ingredient in marijuana is THC (USDEA, 2020b). Marijuana acts on specific cell receptors in the brain to induce pleasure sensations, relaxation, increased appetite, distorted perceptions of time, and enhanced sensations of taste and smell (NIDA, 2019c). Cannabinoids are absorbed and stored in fatty tissue, from which they are eliminated very slowly (CDC, 2021a). After one use, it can still be detected in urine samples several days later; in chronic users, it can be detected in the urine for weeks (NIDA, 2019c).

The effects of marijuana depend on the potency of the THC and vary widely between individuals (USDEA, 2020b). THC is rapidly absorbed into the bloodstream when smoked (CDC, 2021a). The "high" that occurs with smoking marijuana occurs within minutes and lasts 1 to 3 hours (NIDA, 2019c). Marijuana edibles may take up to 2 hours to take effect, peak in 4 hours, and last as long as 10 hours (Alaska Division of Public Health, 2023).

Marijuana use can interfere with short-term memory and may result in difficulty handling complex tasks (CDC, 2021a). It results in a slower reaction time, making driving dangerous. Marijuana negatively affects learning, memory, concentration, coordination, reaction time, emotions, and decision making. Some users may experience an anxiety reaction when using marijuana. About half of those who use it experience tachycardia, hypertension, and bloodshot eyes. The drug also exerts a mild antiemetic effect. Smoking marijuana can exacerbate respiratory problems such as asthma, and long-term use can cause adverse health outcomes similar to smoking cigarettes (CDC, 2021a).

Youth who use marijuana early and regularly are at increased risk for long-term effects including altered brain development, school dropout, other illicit drug use, lower IQ, cognitive impairment, chronic bronchitis, and psychosis disorders such as schizophrenia in predisposed individuals (Lovell et al., 2020). Students who use marijuana frequently from a young age are especially at risk for developing *marijuana use disorder,* which affects approximately 3 in 10 people (National Center for Injury Prevention and Control, 2020). Similar to addiction, the signs of marijuana use disorder include the following:

- Using more marijuana than intended
- Trying but failing to quit using marijuana
- Spending much time using marijuana
- Craving marijuana
- Using marijuana even though it causes problems at home, school, or work
- Continuing to use marijuana despite social or relationship problems
- Giving up important activities with friends and family in favor of using marijuana
- Using marijuana in high-risk situations, such as while driving a car
- Continuing to use marijuana despite physical or psychological problems
- Needing to use more marijuana to get the same high
- Experiencing withdrawal symptoms when stopping marijuana use (National Center for Injury Prevention and Control, 2020, para. 2)

Like natural cannabinoids found in marijuana, synthetic cannabinoids bind to both type 1 and type 2 cannabinoid receptors that are found primarily in the central nervous system (NIDA, 2019c). Users experience effects similar to marijuana, such as relaxation, altered mood and perception, and possibly symptoms of psychosis (e.g., confusion, extreme anxiety, paranoia, hallucinations). However, synthetic cannabinoids bind to cannabinoid receptors with a greater affinity than THC. Therefore they can have a more powerful and unpredictable effect on the brain and can also be addictive. Synthetic marijuana also acts on benzodiazepine and opioid receptors and binds nonspecifically to other cellular membranes. It also binds to peripheral tissues such as the kidneys, liver, and lungs (NIDA, 2019c).

Youth who are curious about marijuana but afraid of the social and legal consequences may also be enticed to try synthetic marijuana (NIDA, 2019c). In fact, youth should be warned that the effects of synthetic marijuana can be unpredictable and even life-threatening. Users can experience a variety of effects, such as kidney damage, elevated blood pressure, reduced blood supply to the heart, seizures, violent behavior, suicidal thoughts, and death (Griffith et al., 2019; NIDA, 2019c).

Cocaine

Also called *blow, coke, cola, snow, crack,* or *rock,* cocaine is a stimulant that comes in the form of a fine, white powder that can be snorted, injected, or rubbed on the gums to obtain a high likened to a sense of euphoria and exhilaration. The annual prevalence of cocaine use in 2022 was 0.5% for eighth graders, 0.35% for 10th graders, and 1.5% for 12th graders (NIDA, 2022b). Cocaine also comes in the form of a rock crystal, called crack, that can be smoked (NIDA, 2021). Sometimes cocaine is combined with heroin and injected, which is referred to as a *speedball.* Intranasal snorting requires the user to first chop the cocaine and line it up on a table, often with a razor blade, and then snort it through a straw or rolled-up bill. Cocaine is often used in binges to maintain a high. The high from snorting lasts 15 to 30 minutes, whereas smoking or injecting cocaine results in the quickest and strongest but shortest high of 5 to 10 minutes (NIDA, 2021).

Cocaine is a highly addictive drug, increasing dopamine to produce mental alertness, extreme energy, and happiness (NIDA, 2021). It can also result in hallucinations; paranoia; irritability; confusion; anxiety; hypersensitivity to sound, sight, and touch; and loss of touch with reality. Short-term physiological effects include elevated heart rate and blood pressure, dilated pupils, higher body temperature, restlessness, and muscle twitches or tremors (NIDA, 2021).

Long-term effects vary based on how cocaine is used. Individuals who snort cocaine may experience nosebleeds, difficulty swallowing, and reduced sense of smell (NIDA, 2021). Those who orally ingest cocaine may experience bowel decay. Those who inject cocaine place themselves at higher risk for infectious diseases such as human immunodeficiency virus (HIV) and hepatitis C from the use of dirty needles and engaging in risky sexual behaviors resulting from impaired judgment. All cocaine users are at risk for malnourishment due to a suppressed appetite (NIDA, 2021).

Methamphetamine

One subclass of amphetamines, methamphetamine, is a highly addictive and dangerous illicit drug that is also known as *meth, speed, ice, crystal, crank,* and *chalk.* Methamphetamine can be injected, snorted, swallowed, inhaled, or smoked (NIDA, 2019b). It is sometimes used to add to, or *cut,* other drugs. One form of meth is crystal methamphetamine, or *ice,* which can be smoked much like crack cocaine (NIDA, 2019b).

In 2022, 0.2% of eighth graders, 0.3% of 10th graders, and 0.5% of 12th graders reported using methamphetamines (Miech et al., 2023). Methamphetamine must be differentiated from the amphetamines used to treat ADHD. Amphetamines function by increasing the amount of dopamine released, a deficit of the condition (NIDA, 2019b); these medications are not addictive for the ADHD population.

Methamphetamine is cheap and easy to make using a variety of methods in clandestine labs that have evolved but continue to pose a great risk to the community due to the highly volatile nature of the chemicals used to cook it. Short-term effects of methamphetamines include increased alertness, energy, euphoria, self-confidence, activity, strength, talkativeness, sexual pleasure, and sense of well-being. Higher doses of this drug increase the potential for violence and can result in motor symptoms, such as tremors, spasms, tics, and athetoid movements. Because methamphetamine decreases the amount of saliva, side effects include teeth grinding and clenching of the jaws, which may lead to dental decay and what is called *meth mouth*. Other symptoms of meth abuse include slurred speech, agitation, paranoia, and hallucinations, including a feeling of insects creeping on the skin (NIDA, 2019b).

Another form of methamphetamine is called *Flakka* or *gravel*. This synthetic cathinone is highly addictive and unpredictable (Palamar et al., 2019). It produces delirium and euphoria as it floods the brain with dopamine; its side effects can be more deadly than cocaine and bath salts. This strain may cause increased vital signs, aggression, paranoia, and hallucinations, sometimes leading to heart attack, homicide, and death; symptoms may persist for days (Palamar et al., 2019).

Opioids and Fentanyl

Opioids are highly addictive and dangerous drugs. In the 2019 YRBS, 7.2% of adolescents reported misusing prescription opioids (Jones et al., 2020). Heavily marketed as safe by the pharmaceutical industry in the 2000s, prescriptions for opioid pain medications tripled, as did their nonmedical use. Increased public awareness and restrictions on providers have decreased this prescribing trend (Levy, 2019). However, because they are commonly found in the home, prescription opioids often find their way into the hands and bodies of children and youth.

FDA-approved ***fentanyl*** is a Schedule II narcotic; it is a synthetic opioid used as an anesthetic or analgesic for severe pain (USDEA, 2022a). Fentanyl is 100 times more potent than morphine and 50 times more potent than heroin. The effects on the body include relaxation, euphoria, pain relief, sedation, confusion, dizziness, nausea, vomiting, urinary retention, constricted pupils, and respiratory depression. FDA-approved forms of fentanyl include oral transmucosal lozenges, buccal or sublingual tablets, sublingual or nasal sprays, transdermal patches, and injectable formulations (USDEA, 2022a).

In recent years, illegally manufactured fentanyl has proliferated in counterfeit prescription medications and other illicit drugs, resulting in a dramatic rise in overdoses and overdose deaths among youth. These drugs can be bought through social media sources with relative ease, thereby contributing to their increasing availability (Tanz et al., 2022). They are sold by street names such as *Apache, China Girl, China Town, Dance Fever, Friend, Goodfellas, Great Bear, He-Man,* and *Jackpot,* to name a few (USDEA, 2022a).

Illicit fentanyl can be used in a variety of ways: injected, snorted, sniffed, smoked, or spiked onto blotter paper. Oral counterfeit pills or tablets that look like prescription pain medication (oxycodone) are readily available and often marketed in bright colors attractive to children and youth. The gel from fentanyl patches can be ingested or injected. A lethal dose of fentanyl powder can fit on the tip of a pencil lead (USDEA, 2022a).

Signs and symptoms of fentanyl overdose include stupor, pinpoint pupils, cold/clammy skin, respiratory depression, and coma (USDEA, 2022a). Immediate rescue response with the opioid antagonist, *naloxone*, is required to prevent death. Naloxone can be administered by intramuscular or subcutaneous injection and nasal spray. In March of 2023, the FDA approved 4-mg naloxone hydrochloride nasal spray for use without a prescription, making it available for anyone and requiring minimal training (FDA, 2023). Additional doses can be repeated in 2 to 3 minutes until emergency medical services arrive and assume responsibility for care (Cash et al., 2018). Many states have passed legislation allowing schools to stock naloxone for undesignated emergency use. Stock nasal naloxone can easily be included in the same wall-mounted cabinet with the school's automated external defibrillator (Davis et al., 2023). See Chapter 30 for more information on stock emergency medications.

From 2019 to 2021, overdose deaths among adolescents (10 to 19 years of age) increased by 109% (Tanz et al., 2022). Approximately 90% of these deaths were opioid overdoses. Of these deaths, 84% involved illegally manufactured fentanyl—with evidence of counterfeit pill ingestion in 25% of cases. In this group of adolescents, approximately 41% had evidence of mental health conditions, but only 35% had a known history of opioid use. A potential bystander was present in two-thirds of adolescent overdose deaths, but no overdose response was provided (Tanz et al., 2022).

Opioid deaths may be underreported. These shocking statistics represent the unacceptable loss of at least 1,800 adolescents from 2019 to 2021 in the United States (Tanz et al., 2022). Urgent efforts are needed to address this personal and public health crisis. The school nurse must advocate for school substance use prevention and harm reduction programs, including emergency response training for students and staff.

> *It is the position of the National Association of School Nurses (NASN) that the safe and effective management of opioid-related overdoses in schools must be incorporated into the school emergency preparedness and response plans. The registered professional school nurse (hereinafter referred to as school nurse) provides leadership in all phases of emergency preparedness and response. When emergencies happen, including drug-related emergencies, proper management of these incidents at school is vital to positive*

outcomes. The school nurse is essential to the school team and is responsible for developing and implementing emergency response procedures. School nurses in this role should facilitate access to naloxone for quick response in the management of opioid-related overdoses in the school setting. (NASN, 2020, para. 1)

Due to the complicated issues surrounding naloxone use in schools, NASN (2023) has developed the *Naloxone Education in Schools Toolkit* that provides resources to assist school nurses and school districts with developing a naloxone program and campus protocols for emergency naloxone administration.

Heroin

Heroin, also known as *smack* or *horse*, is a derivative of opium (NIDA, 2022c). It is processed from morphine extracted from the Asian poppy plant. It is usually injected but can be snorted and smoked. The effects of heroin include a "rush" of euphoria; dry mouth; warm, flushed skin; a state of drowsiness; and a depressed central nervous system. Its dangers include addiction, blood-borne infections contracted from contaminated needles, and vascular infections and their sequelae. Overdoses from heroin have increased dramatically in the United States over the last decade (NIDA, 2022c). This alarming trend is also linked to the increasing presence of fentanyl cut into illicit drugs.

Although heroin use among high school students has remained relatively low, with less than 1% of teens reporting using heroin in 2022 (NIDA, 2022c), many areas of the country have seen its use increase in epidemic proportions. Its addiction rate is high, with a significant risk of overdose and death.

Club/Party/Designer Drugs

A *club drug* is a general term that refers to illicit drugs, primarily synthetic, that are most commonly encountered at nightclubs and all-night dance parties with loud and repetitive electronic music, called *raves*. The drugs include MDMA (methylenedioxymethamphetamine; Ecstasy), ketamine, GHB (gamma-hydroxybutyrate), Rohypnol (flunitrazepam), LSD (lysergic acid diethylamide), PCP (phencyclidine), methamphetamine, and, to a lesser extent, cocaine and psilocybin mushrooms. Some of these drugs have gained popularity as a result of the false perception that they are not as harmful or as addictive as drugs such as heroin. GHB, Rohypnol, and ketamine are club drugs not yet popular among teens (Williams & Lundahl, 2019).

Designer drugs are drugs manufactured in underground laboratories as modified versions of substances controlled by the U.S. Food and Drug Administration (2016) to supply the illegal market with street drugs that technically are not illegal. Because of their manufacturing method, there are inconsistencies in dosages and purity. The USDEA (2018a) refers to these drugs as controlled substance analogs. Most cannot be detected in the urine after a few hours of use.

MDMA is also called *Ecstasy, Molly, X, XTC, Adam, Clarity,* and *Lover's Speed.* MDMA is classified as a Schedule I drug (a substance with high abuse potential, no accepted medical use, and illegal to possess) (USDEA, n.d.). Chemically similar to stimulants and hallucinogens, it produces dose-dependent stimulants and mild hallucinogenic effects (NIDA, 2022a).

MDMA's effects last 3 to 6 hours; many users take another dose when the effects from the first dose start to wear off (NIDA, 2022a). Irritability, depression, sleep and memory problems, impulsiveness, aggression, and decreased appetite can occur for a week after a moderate dose (NIDA, 2022a). Ecstasy increases the level of serotonin released by brain cells, producing euphoria and heightened feelings of empathy, emotional warmth, and self-acceptance, prompting its nicknames of *hug drug* or *love drug* (NIDA, 2022a). However, as the brain is depleted of serotonin, processes that are regulated by it, such as mood, sleep, appetite, and cognition, are affected (NIDA, 2022a). Adverse effects include diaphoresis, rapid and irregular heartbeats, hypertension, fatigue, muscle aches, involuntary muscle contraction such as jaw clenching, and insomnia (NIDA, 2022a). Many users suck pacifiers or lollipops to ease the tight jaw muscles (NIDA, 2022a).

MDMA can be deadly at high doses. It allows the user to dance for hours, which may result in elevated body temperature, dehydration, muscle breakdown, liver and cardiovascular failure, strokes, and seizures. Because MDMA is neurotoxic, chronic use damages the neurons that release serotonin and can result in long-term memory impairment (NIDA, 2022a).

In 2022, an estimated 0.6% of eighth graders, 0.7% of 10th graders, and 1.4% of 12th graders reported having used MDMA in the past 12 months (NIDA, 2022a). Rohypnol (flunitrazepam) is a central nervous system depressant related to benzodiazepines. It is tasteless and odorless and dissolves easily in carbonated beverages. Rohypnol is often used in sexual assaults (date rape) because a dose as small as 1 mg can impair a victim for 8 to 12 hours and cause profound anterograde amnesia (Thompson, 2021). Street names include *roofies, rophies, roche,* and the *forget-me pill.* Other adverse effects include hypotension, drowsiness, visual disturbances, dizziness, confusion, and urinary retention. In 2016, it was used by 0.5% to 1.1% of eighth through 12th graders (NIDA, 2022a).

Hallucinogens

The 2019 YRBS revealed that 38% of high school students indicated they had tried LSD, PCP or angel dust, mescaline, or mushroom at least once (NIDA, 2019a). *Lysergic acid diethylamide* (LSD), often called *acid,* is a hallucinogen that induces abnormalities in sensory perception (NIDA, 2019a). Sold in tablet, capsule, and liquid forms, LSD is also placed on blotter paper placed in the mouth. Within

30 minutes, the pupils dilate, diaphoresis occurs, and there are increases in body temperature, heart rate, and blood pressure. Loss of appetite may progress to nausea, numbness, weakness, or trembling. Long-term sequelae associated with LSD include psychosis and flashbacks, now called *hallucinogen-persisting perception disorder.* After a rise in use in the 1990s, the prevalence of LSD use has decreased to 0.8% of eighth graders, 2.1% of 10th graders, and 3.0% of 12th graders (NIDA, 2019a).

Other hallucinogens include phencyclidine, which goes by the names of *PCP, angel dust, crystal,* or *hog.* Phencyclidine is often sprayed on leaf material and smoked. *Psilocybin-containing mushrooms,* often called *shrooms,* are typically ingested or used to make tea to produce hallucinogenic effects (NIDA, 2019a). Adolescents also report using morning glory seeds and a type of sage called *salvia* (Salvia divinorum) for their hallucinogenic effects (NIDA, 2019a). Chewed or smoked, these drugs result in a short but intense hallucinogenic effect lasting 30 minutes (NIDA, 2019a). During this time, the individual has a decreased ability to interact with their surroundings. In 2016, less than 2% of high school students reported using salvia (NIDA, 2019a).

Inhalants

Inhalants are common household products that can be breathed in to get high, such as the contents of aerosol spray cans, paints, commercial chemicals, or propellants such as nitrous oxide from whipped cream dispensers (Mustonen et al., 2018). Inhalants such as glue, nail polish remover, gasoline, solvents, butane, or Freon found in older model air conditioners can also be sniffed or *huffed.* They may be sniffed directly from an open container or huffed from a rag soaked in the substance and held to the face. Students may place the rag in a bag and let the vapors concentrate before inhaling from the bag. Among teens, the most common inhalants are felt-tip pens/markers or magic markers, glue, spray paints, gasoline/lighter fluid, and computer cleaners (Mustonen et al., 2018).

Inhalants cause an immediate high and are cheap, legal, and available to younger children. The effects of inhalant intoxication resemble those of alcohol inebriation: loss of inhibition and euphoria/giddiness followed by depression, distorted perceptions of time and space, and decreased motor coordination such as slurred speech and unsteady gait (NIDA, 2020a). They also can cause headaches, dizziness, vomiting, and drowsiness. Chronic use of inhalants can cause permanent brain damage and localized damage to the bone marrow, lungs, and kidneys. When impairment from inhalants is suspected, school nurses should assess for the odor of the product on a student's breath or remnants of the inhaled substance near their mouth or nose (NIDA, 2020a).

New Psychoactive Substances

New psychoactive substances, also known as *designer drugs* or *legal highs,* are a heterogeneous group of synthetic mind-altering (psychoactive) substances that mimic the effects of illegal drugs such as stimulants, cannabis, sedatives/hypnotics, dissociative drugs, or hallucinogenic drugs. New psychoactive drugs are a major public health threat. Makers continually alter the chemical profiles of these drugs to avoid using officially banned substances. While these drugs may not be criminalized, they are also not regulated by the FDA and pose significant health risks, including poisoning and death (Sajwani, 2023).

Bath salts are synthetic psychoactive stimulants that are addictive. Brand names include *Bloom, Cloud Nine, Flakka, Lunar Wave, Scarface, White Lightning,* and *Vanilla Sky* (USDEA, 2018a). Bath salts are typically sold online or in drug paraphernalia stores in small foil or plastic packages in the form of a crystal-like brown or white powder. Bath salts are not considered illegal because they are labeled "not for human consumption," sometimes coming in packages labeled as *phone screen cleaner, jewelry cleaner,* or *plant food.* Bath salts can be snorted, injected, swallowed, smoked, or mixed with food or drink. Bath salts cause a high similar to methamphetamine or up to 10 times more potent than cocaine, which can result in extreme agitation, paranoia, hallucinations, increased sociability and sex drive, panic attacks, violence, and hypertension. Bath salts should not be confused with products used for bathing, such as Epsom salts, which do not contain psychoactive ingredients (USDEA, 2018a).

Performance-Enhancing Drugs

Social and environmental influences can drive youth to use performance-enhancing drugs, known as *ergogenic drugs,* such as anabolic steroids and creatine (Alonso & Fernández-García, 2020). Ergogenic drugs enhance the body's energy use, often at the expense of various body systems. Adolescent athletes are acutely aware of the impact of muscle, speed, and endurance in attaining athletic prowess (Siegmund, 2022). Some students are told they have college athletic potential but need to be bigger or stronger or "bulk up." Some students believe that being more muscular makes them more attractive.

Ergogenic products or aids are synthetically produced variants of testosterone, which are often considered nutritional supplements and therefore do not fall under the FDA's regulations. Thus there is no guaranteed consistency in the potency from one batch to another. Such products claim to increase lean body mass, decrease fat mass, and increase energy. Research on their effects has not been conducted in individuals younger than 18. Many build muscle mass effectively when combined with rigorous training (Alonso & Fernández-García, 2020). However, no evidence supports the idea that these products aid in recovery from sports injuries. Students need to be educated that the heart is also a muscle; therefore increasing muscle size may increase heart size, leading to cardiomyopathy (White et al., 2018). Other adverse effects and morbidity of anabolic steroids include infertility, hypertension, acne, and aggression (Siegmund, 2022).

ADDRESSING SUBSTANCE ABUSE IN SCHOOLS

According to the National Center for Education Statistics, "In 2019, about 22 percent of students in grades 9–12 reported that illegal drugs were offered, sold, or given to them on school property during the previous 12 months" (2022, para. 1). The school nurse is often the first to recognize or hear about a student who is abusing drugs. Some students brag about their drug use on social media. Warning signs might include decreased school performance, truancy, withdrawal from usual activities, increased disciplinary issues, or symptoms of depression or irritability. Schools should have policies and procedures in place to respond when a student is suspected of being under the influence of alcohol or drugs at school. Such policies need to consider the student's rights in congruence with federal, state, and local laws (Endsley, 2023).

Impaired Mental Status Assessment

The school nurse's focused assessment for altered mental status should prioritize the safety of the student and focus on subjective and objective data. Determinations of whether the student is intoxicated or impaired should be avoided and cannot be confirmed without medical evaluation. School nurses should communicate the assessment findings to the "need to know" school staff in terms of whether the student is safe to stay in school, needs to go home, or requires immediate medical care or emergency medical services. The student's right to confidentiality must be maintained. The school nurse must be alert for other causes of altered mental status such as sleep deprivation, prescribed or OTC medication side effects/adverse effects, epilepsy/seizures, hypoglycemia/hyperglycemia, uremia, concussion/head trauma, infections, psychiatric conditions, or shock (e.g., hypovolemic, septic, anaphylactic, cardiac) (Endsley, 2023; Patterson et al., 2017).

It is outside the scope of school nursing practice to participate in searches involving students or their possessions, nor should school nurses be involved in disciplinary actions regarding students' suspected drug/alcohol use.

Screening for Substance Use

The Substance Abuse and Mental Health Services Administration (2023) and the American Academy of Pediatrics (Levy & Williams, 2016) support screening for substance use in pediatric populations as a routine part of health care. However, these recommendations are not specifically for schools. AAP recommends widespread implementation of the *screening, brief intervention, and referral to treatment* (SBIRT) model using evidence-based tools (Levy & Williams, 2016; SAMHSA, 2022d). Schools should have protocols in place regarding screening students for substance use issues.

One short validated clinical assessment tool to screen for adolescent substance-related risks and problems is CRAFFT (CRAFFT, 2018, 2020; Fernald et al., 2023; Shenoi et al., 2019). CRAFFT stands for *Car, Relax, Alone, Forget, Friends, Trouble.* Adolescents may be more candid if they answer the tool themselves (self-administer), rather than having the questionnaire administered by an adult. See Figure 29-1. In addition to screening questions about alcohol and drugs, the CRAFFT+N (2.1) also screens for the use of tobacco products and vaping.

The school must be prepared to respond if a student is screened at risk on the CRAFFT or other substance use screening tool. Supporting students with substance use issues requires leadership from the school nurse, as well as collaboration with the interdisciplinary student-support team, including trained mental health professionals such as school social workers and counselors. The school team must be prepared to offer appropriate school services (e.g., education, counseling) and communicate with the family regarding referral resources for community mental health and substance use treatment as indicated. When a student needs treatment or the family requests help with substance abuse, the school nurse should have a list of local resources and the requirements for treatment (e.g., age parameters, therapeutic setting and duration, estimated costs, and types of health insurance accepted). The school nurse works as a liaison between school mental health professionals, primary care providers, local health systems, and public health departments to identify sites that provide services to low-income youth with substance use disorders and associated mental health conditions.

The school nurse can help the student's family understand that substance use disorders are complex and affect the brain of the developing child. No single treatment program is appropriate for everyone. Treatment may be lengthy (at least 3 months), and multiple attempts may be needed before the road to recovery begins. Keep in mind that students who abuse drugs or alcohol are at greater risk for engaging in other risky behaviors or may have mental health concerns that also must be assessed. The school nurse should also be attuned to students who are concerned that their parent/guardian is using or abusing drugs. Of primary concern is whether the student is safe in the home environment; involving child protective services or social services may be needed.

Remember that the privacy and confidentiality of protected and sensitive student health information must be maintained according to the Family Educational Rights and Privacy Act (FERPA) (U.S. Department of Health and Human Services & U.S. Department of Education, 2019). Therefore relevant findings should only be communicated with school personnel with a legitimate educational interest. The school nurse would communicate with parents the same as with any health concerns about their child.

Drug Testing in Schools

Multiple modalities can be used to screen for substance use, such as urine and hair analyses for multiple drugs and breath and saliva tests for alcohol. The detection

The CRAFFT+N Questionnaire

To be completed by patient

Please answer all questions **honestly**; your answers will be kept **confidential**.

During the PAST 12 MONTHS, on how many days did you:

1.	Drink more than a few sips of beer, wine, or any drink containing **alcohol**? Put "0" if none.	____ # of days
2.	Use any **marijuana** (cannabis, weed, oil, wax, or hash by smoking, vaping, dabbing, or in edibles) or "**synthetic marijuana**" (like "K2," "Spice")? Put "0" if none.	____ # of days
3.	Use **anything else to get high** (like other illegal drugs, pills, prescription or over-the-counter medications, and things that you sniff, huff, vape, or inject)? Put "0" if none.	____ # of days
4.	Use a **vaping device* containing nicotine and/or flavors**, or use any **tobacco products**†? Put "0" if none. **Such as e-cigs, mods, pod devices like JUUL, disposable vapes like Puff Bar, vape pens, or e-hookahs. †Cigarettes, cigars, cigarillos, hookahs, chewing tobacco, snuff, snus, dissolvables, or nicotine pouches.*	____ # of days

READ THESE INSTRUCTIONS BEFORE CONTINUING:

- **If you put "0" in ALL of the boxes above, ANSWER QUESTION 5 BELOW, THEN STOP.**
- **If you put "1" or more for Questions 1, 2, or 3 above, ANSWER QUESTIONS 5-10 BELOW.**
- **If you put "1" or more for Question 4 above, ANSWER ALL QUESTIONS ON BACK PAGE.**

		Circle one	
5.	Have you ever ridden in a CAR driven by someone (including yourself) who was "high" or had been using alcohol or drugs?	**No**	**Yes**
6.	Do you ever use alcohol or drugs to RELAX, feel better about yourself, or fit in?	**No**	**Yes**
7.	Do you ever use alcohol or drugs while you are by yourself, or ALONE?	**No**	**Yes**
8.	Do you ever FORGET things you did while using alcohol or drugs?	**No**	**Yes**
9.	Do your FAMILY or FRIENDS ever tell you that you should cut down on your drinking or drug use?	**No**	**Yes**
10.	Have you ever gotten into TROUBLE while you were using alcohol or drugs?	**No**	**Yes**

NOTICE TO CLINIC STAFF AND MEDICAL RECORDS:
The information on this page is protected by special federal confidentiality rules (42 CFR Part 2), which prohibit disclosure of this information unless authorized by specific written consent.

FIGURE 29-1. The CRAFFT+N Questionnaire.

The following questions ask about your use of any **vaping devices containing nicotine and/or flavors**, or use of any **tobacco products***. Circle your answer for each question.

	Circle one	
1. Have you ever tried to quit using, but couldn't?	**Yes**	**No**
2. Do you vape or use tobacco now because it is really hard to quit?	**Yes**	**No**
3. Have you ever felt like you were addicted to vaping or tobacco?	**Yes**	**No**
4. Do you ever have strong cravings to vape or use tobacco?	**Yes**	**No**
5. Have you ever felt like you really needed to vape or use tobacco?	**Yes**	**No**
6. Is it hard to keep from vaping or using tobacco in places where you are not supposed to, like school?	**Yes**	**No**
7. When you haven't vaped or used tobacco in a while (or when you tried to stop using)…		
a. did you find it hard to concentrate because you couldn't vape or use tobacco?	**Yes**	**No**
b. did you feel more irritable because you couldn't vape or use tobacco?	**Yes**	**No**
c. did you feel a strong need or urge to vape or use tobacco?	**Yes**	**No**
d. did you feel nervous, restless, or anxious because you couldn't vape or use tobacco?	**Yes**	**No**

**References:*

Wheeler, K. C., Fletcher, K. E., Wellman, R. J., & DiFranza, J. R. (2004). Screening adolescents for nicotine dependence: the Hooked On Nicotine Checklist. *J Adolesc Health*, *35*(3), 225–230;

McKelvey, K., Baiocchi, M., & Halpern-Felsher, B. (2018). Adolescents' and Young Adults' Use and Perceptions of Pod-Based Electronic Cigarettes. *JAMA Network Open*, *1*(6), e183535.

NOTICE TO CLINIC STAFF AND MEDICAL RECORDS:
The information on this page is protected by special federal confidentiality rules (42 CFR Part 2), which prohibit disclosure of this information unless authorized by specific written consent.

FIGURE 29-1.—cont'd

period varies with the drug and the method used to test for the presence of drugs (NIDA, 2019a). For example, drugs that are smoked or inhaled are almost instantly absorbed into the body's systems and then excreted, whereas oral ingestion of a drug results in slower absorption and excretion (NIDA, 2019a). Urine testing is the most common and economical means of testing (AAP, 2015). Urine samples have the highest concentration of a drug about 6 hours after ingestion, with most of it being excreted in 48 hours (SAMHSA, 2022a). Some prescription and OTC medications may affect the results of drug testing; therefore the use of these products must be considered (NIDA, 2019a).

The right of schools to require random drug testing was upheld by the U.S. Supreme Court in 1995 for middle and high school–age students involved in interscholastic sports and in 2002 for students involved in extracurricular activities (Waldman, 2023). Random drug and/or alcohol testing programs in schools are not widely implemented but are still required in some districts for participation in interscholastic sports or extracurricular activities, especially at the high school level. In some states, school districts collaborate with high school athletic associations, which oversee drug screening programs to promote fair participation in interscholastic activities and competitions. The rationale for randomized drug screening is the assumption that if students think they may be randomly tested and penalized for drug or alcohol use, they will be less likely to use these substances. However, research evidence to support the effectiveness of random drug testing in schools is inconclusive.

Random drug/alcohol testing is highly controversial. Many legal experts believe that it is an invasion of students' right to privacy; others fear that it can lead to racial profiling of historically marginalized groups of students. Parental consent for testing should be active (opt-in). Parents may object to the testing of their students about whom there is no suspicion of a drug/alcohol use problem. Students may be pulled out of class to provide specimens, resulting in lost instructional time. Random drug/alcohol screening is expensive, typically costing between 15 and 30 dollars per student.

The American Academy of Pediatrics (2015) does not support school-based drug testing for many reasons. Not all psychoactive substances may be detected by the drug screening tests used, and many have a short window for detection; therefore negative screens may provide false assurances. Positive test results are not diagnostic and do not necessarily indicate a substance use problem. Secondhand exposure, such as to marijuana smoke, can result in positive results. False positives may result in unfairly being banned from participating in activities or being subject to unfounded disciplinary action, including possible suspension or expulsion.

Students can find ways of evading drug detection (AAP, 2015). They may switch to using drugs reported to be undetectable. They may tamper with specimens (urine) or submit someone else's specimen. The temperature of urine samples should be immediately tested to see if it correlates with body temperature. The toilet bowl water in the collection area should be dyed blue to detect dilution. The only sure way to avoid tampering is to directly observe the student voiding to collect the specimen, which is inappropriate in school. Additionally, students may ingest dangerous chemicals believed to mask, or "clean", the urine of traceable substances, which can result in severe injury or illness. For some students, the threat of drug testing may result in a paradoxical increase in illicit drug use (AAP, 2015).

Accurate results of drug tests depend on interpretation by a specially trained clinician or provider. They are informed by knowing protected health information about the student, such as baseline medical status and prescribed medications (AAP, 2015). Initial positive results should be confirmed with more sensitive testing, which increases costs. The student should be interviewed to ascertain if they divulge or deny the use of illegal substances. Positive tests should be shared with the parents of students who are minors, but school drug testing policies should clearly outline how and with whom positive test results should be shared (AAP, 2015).

School nurses should carefully consider these factors when determining whether they have a professional role in random drug/alcohol screening programs. Importantly, schools with substance use screening programs should have intervention programs available for the students should they test positive. As health experts, school nurses are integral members of their school's student support team to provide wrap-around services and resources for students affected by drug/alcohol use. School nurses can be instrumental in ensuring that school policies, processes, protocols, and programs related to drugs and alcohol are evidence-based and protect the best interests of students.

Substance Use Prevention Efforts

The school nurse can play a significant role in substance use prevention education. Drug and alcohol education must begin in elementary school; the age range of 9 to 12 years is an ideal time to expand on and reinforce previous education provided. Programs that begin in elementary schools have been more effective in decreasing drug and alcohol use

Did You Know?

The National Education Association (2023, p. 44) "believes that mandatory drug or alcohol testing of students without probable cause is an unwarranted and unconstitutional invasion of privacy and opposes such testing. The Association also believes that schools must immediately notify parents/guardians of students suspected of abusing drugs, alcohol, and/or performance-enhancing dietary herbal supplements and must provide information about support services."

Practice Connection

Drug-Prevention Resources

Explore the following Web sites for more information and student resources for drug use prevention:

1. *Brain Power* is a science-based drug abuse information program for sixth through ninth graders. The Teacher's Guide and materials are free and are available online from the NIH (2022).
2. *The Mind Matters* series includes a teacher's guide developed by the National Institute on Drug Abuse (n.d.) "designed to help students in grades 5 -8 understand the biological effects of drug misuse on the brain and body, along with identifying how these drug-induced changes affect both behaviors and emotions. There is no more important time to address these issues with adolescents than in the middle school years, when they are forming opinions about the health risks of drugs" (p. 3).

during the middle school years. Prevention programs should enhance protective factors while reducing risk factors and address all forms of substance use, particularly those most prevalent in the local community (NIDA, 2019b).

Education of parents/guardians, students, and staff is critical to preventing the misuse of drugs. This includes how to safeguard medications at home, why medication should not be used by those for whom it was not prescribed, and the dangers of mixing medications. Parents/guardians and adults living in the household must monitor how many pills are in a prescription and keep track of refills. All medications in the home should be secured and preferably locked. Expired medications should be discarded safely; they should *not* be flushed down the toilet to prevent them from entering the water supply. It is recommended that the medication first be mixed with coffee grounds or kitty litter to make it undesirable so that teens do not extract them from the trash. Remove prescription labels before discarding medication containers. Many communities have drug disposal programs through police departments, pharmacies, or health systems.

The school nurse can provide drug prevention information on bulletin boards, the school Web site, pamphlets in the health office, or newsletters to parents/guardians. School nurses can assist in organizing educational offerings for families in the evening. Parents/guardians should be empowered to look for drugs in the home, including in their children's rooms, and should be made aware of school policies regarding drug possession and use in the school. Parents/guardians need to have clear rules about drug use.

SEXUAL ACTIVITY

Sexual development reaches its peak during the teenage years. While sexual curiosity is expected (see Chapter 9), sexual activity during adolescence is risky. According to the 2021 Youth Risk Behavior Survey (CDC, 2023b), between 2011 and 2021, the percentage of high school students who have ever had sex trended down from 47% to 30%. See Figure 29-2. Yet this good news is tempered by the data showing that fewer youth in 2021 (52%) reported using condoms during the last sexual intercourse compared with 2011 (60%). In 2021, approximately only one-third of youth (33%) reported using effective hormonal birth control and only 10% reported using both condoms and hormonal birth control. See Online Materials 29-1 for resources related to common methods of contraception and birth control methods.

The total number of teen pregnancies has also decreased in the United States since its peak in 1990, although there was a slight increase in 2006 and 2007 (CDC, 2023b). Despite decreases in teen pregnancy, disparities remain. In 2019, the birth rates for Hispanic teens (25.3 per 1,000) and non-Hispanic black teens (25.8 per 1,000) were more than 2 times higher than the rate for non-Hispanic white teens (11.4 per 1,000). The birth rate of American Indian/Alaska Native teens (29.2 per 1,000) was the highest among all races/ethnicities (CDC, 2023b). See Chapter 19 for more information on students who are pregnant and parenting.

The reasons adolescents give for having intercourse include the need to be loved, the need to be popular and accepted by peers, the need to feel grown up, peer pressure, curiosity, and because it is a pleasurable experience (Evans-Paulson et al., 2021). The media also influences the development of sexuality (Merrill & Liang, 2019). Children and adolescents are repeatedly exposed to sexual images in magazines, movies, TV, and on the Internet and social media. The news is often filled with stories of rape, sexual abuse, and adultery by influential adults, as well as advertisements for drugs to enhance sexual performance. With a click of a mouse, children can access free pornography Web sites displaying graphic and sometimes disturbing sexual acts. Parents/guardians are advised to apply content control limitations to Internet browsers on their children's computers, tablets, and smartphones that block adult-only materials.

Dating behaviors are often dictated by the family, the school, or community culture; this includes the age at which dating is allowed, whether dating implies an exclusive relationship with one person, and the activities that are included in dating behaviors (e.g., kissing, touching, or intercourse) (Wright et al., 2019). Positive parental relationships and parental monitoring are related to fewer sex partners, later sexual debut, and higher condom use among adolescents.

BODY DECORATION AND MODIFICATION

There are many forms of body decoration. There is body painting, including face painting of young children, body painting by football game fans, and temporary tattoos for children. There is also cutting and painting nails, applying makeup, and wearing jewelry. Ear piercing is the norm for

The Percentage of High School Students Who:*	2011 Total	2013 Total	2015 Total	2017 Total	2019 Total	2021 Total	Trend
Ever had sex	47	47	41	40	38	30	In right direction
Had four or more lifetime sexual partners	15	15	11	10	9	6	In right direction
Were currently sexually active	34	34	30	29	27	21	In right direction
Used a condom during last sexual intercourse†	60	59	57	54	54	52	In wrong direction
Used effective hormonal birth control†,‡	—	—	—	—	—	33	—
Used a condom and effective hormonal birth control (dual use)†,‡	—	—	—	—	—	10	—
Were ever tested for HIV	13	13	10	9	9	6	In wrong direction
Were tested for STDs during the past year§	—	—	—	—	9	5	In wrong direction

*For the complete wording of YRBS questions, refer to the appendix.

†Among sexually active students.

‡Survey question changed in the 2021 national YRBS; therefore, trends are not available.

§Variable introduced in 2019.

In wrong direction

No change

In right direction

FIGURE 29-2. **Youth Risk Behavior Survey 10-year trends for sexual activity.** *(CDC [2023b].)*

many adolescents and young adults, as are multiple piercings. Body piercing is perceived by some youth as another means to wear jewelry. Body adornment might also include temporary measures that last a few weeks, such as henna decorations.

Adolescents give multiple reasons why they engage in body adornment and modification. At its core, it can be seen as a way to reflect feelings as emotional expressions (Stanescu & Romascanu, 2020). Some youth indicate that body decoration is art and that the body is a canvas; others feel that it enhances their sexuality or enhances the pleasure of their partner (Desai & Breuner, 2022). For most, it is simply to enhance their appearance. Some say it is a social bonding act, something that friends do together. It may be a way to get attention, provide a sense of control and a sense of permanence, define oneself and feel unique, and transmit personal messages (Stanescu & Romascanu, 2020). Tattooing is used by some individuals to permanently commemorate the loss of a loved one.

Piercing and Tattooing

Piercing can be done to almost any part of the body. The entire area of the ear can be pierced, as can the tongue, nose, lips, eyebrows, cheeks, nipples, and navel, and even the genitals and flat areas of skin, such as along the forearm or on the back. Some youth place grommets (round metal eyelets), often called *gauges* or *stretching tapers*, into already pierced and healed tissues, especially the earlobes, to enlarge the hole to approximately 0.5 to 1 cm or more. Once these heal, the individual can either wear a curved barbell piece of jewelry in the grommet or attach chains through the grommet to piercings placed in other parts of the body. If the site becomes infected, it is essential to leave the piercing in while the infection is being treated and not remove the jewelry. Removal will put the student at risk for development of an abscess. If it appears that the student is allergic to the jewelry of the piercing, the jewelry must be removed.

Tattoos are increasingly popular among youth. There are no federal laws regulating tattoos. However, all 50 states have statutes that stipulate the minimum legal age to get a professional tattoo (Ink Different Tattoo School, 2023). The U.S. Food and Drug Administration (2017a) does not regulate practices in tattoo parlors and has not approved any inks for injection into the skin. Some teens use common household products to tattoo themselves, using sewing needles, straight pins, forks, paper clips, and pens to inject pigments, such as charcoal, soot, mascara, or carbon, into their skin, most of which are a series of uneven dots in black or brown (Atli et al., 2022).

The pigments used in professional tattooing are mostly from metallic salts (e.g., iron and titanium dioxide, India ink, and synthetic organic dyes). Tattoos are applied using an electrically powered instrument with a vertically vibrating solid needle that injects pigment up to 3,000 times/minute into the dermis at a depth of 1 to 2 mm (Kluger, 2019). A bandage is kept on only for a few hours. The tattoo should be patted dry rather than rubbed, and the student needs to avoid direct sunlight to avoid losing the sharpness of the image.

Tattoo removal is much more complicated, expensive, and painful than applying a tattoo. A laser breaks up the tattoo into particles that can be eliminated through the normal skin cleansing process (Boardman, 2019). Multiple treatments are usually required. Some colors are easier to remove than others.

Embedding, branding, and scarification are more risqué and permanent behaviors (Borgerson & Schroeder, 2018), in which youth cut or burn a design in the skin that will be unique to them. This is different than *cutting*, which is a self-harm behavior that should be addressed as mental health concern. Embedding is the insertion of shaped objects under the skin, resulting in projections or designs on the skin surface; these are usually made of a material, such as Teflon, which does not cause an immune response. Branding and scarification result in second- and third-degree burns. A design is burned into the skin with a hot implement, such as an Italian cookie iron or an electric wood-burning kit (Borgerson & Schroeder, 2018).

Complications of body modification may include scarring, disfigurement, keloid development, rejection and migration of piercings, interference with magnetic resonance imaging, and infection (localized and hepatitis B and C). Tattoos may result in a delay in the diagnosis of skin cancer later in life. Nipple piercing in females can obstruct ducts and interfere with later lactation (La Leche League International, 2023). Piercings in the mouth (i.e., cheeks, lips, and tongues) appear to cause the greatest number of complications, including receding gums, periodontitis, chipped teeth, increased spacing between teeth, and speech impediments (Passos et al., 2022). *Grills* are decorative covers of gold or silver that clip onto one or more teeth or are permanently applied. Grills can damage the teeth and gums and trap food and debris, resulting in bad breath and dental caries (Passos et al., 2022).

Tanning

Tanning is popular among youth. Tanning devices include sunbeds and sun tanning lamps that deliver ultraviolet (UV) rays to those who use them. These devices deliver both ultraviolet A (UVA) and ultraviolet B (UVB) rays, although UVA rays tend to be greater (Environmental Protection Agency [EPA], 2022). Whereas UVB rays penetrate the top layers of the skin and are most responsible for sunburns, UVA rays penetrate deeper layers of the skin (EPA, 2022). The International Agency for Research on Cancer (part of the World Health Organization) concluded that tanning beds are carcinogenic to humans (the highest cancer risk category) and more dangerous than had previously been thought (CDC, 2022d). Health risks include skin cancer (e.g., melanoma, basal cell carcinoma, squamous cell carcinoma), eye diseases that can cause blindness (e.g., cataracts, ocular melanoma), and premature skin aging such as age spots and wrinkles (CDC, 2022d).

Contrary to the messages marketed by the indoor tanning industry, indoor tanning is not safer than tanning outside in the sun; it is not a safe way to get vitamin D, and there is no safe base tan. Furthermore, results from a 2014 meta-analysis suggest that newer models of tanning beds are not safer to use than older ones (CDC, 2022d). The American Academy of Dermatology (2023) cites evidence that up to 400,000 cases of skin cancer each year can be attributed to indoor tanning, and women under age 30 who tan indoors are six times more likely to develop melanoma. Just one indoor tanning session increases the risk of basal cell carcinoma by 29% and squamous cell carcinoma by 67%, and individuals who use indoor tanning before age 24 are at increased risk of having basal cell carcinoma by age 50.

Frequent use of indoor tanning booths and sunlamps may result in a significant increase in the incidence of skin cancer (CDC, 2022d). In 2017, 5.6% of high school students reported using an indoor tanning device; females (7.5%) were more likely than males (3.5%) to report indoor tanning. Older female adolescents reported higher levels of indoor tanning than young females: 12.9% among 12th-grade females and 5.0% among ninth-grade females. Although the negative press has decreased the use of tanning salons, it should be noted that 57.2% of ninth through 12th graders reported sunburn in the past year; for white female teens, the percentage was 78.8% (CDC, 2022d).

Restrictions on indoor tanning for minors continue to become more widespread, given the consistent evidence of the link between indoor tanning and skin cancer. The CDC (2023b) identified 15 states and some counties and cities that have banned minors from using indoor tanning services. Parental consent for using tanning devices is also required in many states. School nurses can increase parental awareness of this issue to consider the consequences for their child's health before signing permission.

The school nurse can educate students both before and after they have engaged in body modification. This is an ideal time to ensure students have updated tetanus and hepatitis immunizations.

GAMBLING, GAMING, AND RISKY GAMES

Gambling, or *gaming*, is the practice of playing games of chance or betting to win money or something of value; it involves risk and uncertainty. It is estimated that 80% of adolescents have gambled, whether with cards, dice, board games, pool, or wagers on sports games. Most are social gamblers; however, 2.1% to 2.6% of adolescents in North America are estimated to be involved in problem gambling (Calado et al., 2017). Pathological gambling, or gambling disorder, is "gambling that results in adverse consequences for individuals, families, and communities," including "impaired mental health, physical health, relationship and family dysfunction, financial problems, employment difficulties, and legal issues" (Dowling et al., 2017, p. 110).

Gambling

Gambling behaviors usually precede other high-risk behaviors. Children are at risk for gambling at younger ages if their parents/guardians have gambling problems (Forrest & McHale, 2021). Pathological gambling will affect the student's academic performance and may result in stealing the money to place a bet. These young people are also at risk for the associated use of alcohol and other drugs. Counselors report examples of high school students who owe thousands of dollars in bad bets.

Schools need to be aware that gambling is inadvertently promoted by activities such as selling raffle tickets as fundraisers, where someone is picked as the winner. The school nurse can identify potentially inappropriate messages being given to students as activities are planned. However, many governments are dependent on gambling activities for revenue, such as lotteries and casinos. Parents/guardians must be made aware of the problems of gambling by youth; they need to be aware of the money earned by their teens, the money being spent, and the Internet sites visited. Counseling may be considered for youth involved in severe gambling.

Video/Online Gaming and Internet Addiction

Internet and gaming addiction is a growing concern because of the increased amount of time young people engage in these activities. For most youth, playing games online or spending time in social chat rooms with friends is a preferred leisure activity and a lifestyle choice (Stockdale & Coyne, 2018). In fact, children and adolescents spend more time using media in various forms (e.g., television, social media, computers/tablets, cellphones) than they do. Prosocial uses of media can increase connectedness and knowledge while improving health, but when misused, it can contribute to various risks and health problems (Odgers & Jensen, 2020).

Without parental controls, children and youth can easily access gambling, pornography, and sexual connections on the Internet. Long periods on the computer can lead to musculoskeletal problems, vision problems, sedentary lifestyles, and other potentially harmful problems (Park et al., 2020). It may result in a lack of sleep, translating into decreased academic performance. The problem is more common among teens with game systems in their bedrooms; parents/guardians need to limit how much time teens are online.

Sexting (the act of sending, receiving, or forwarding sexually explicit messages, pictures, or videos via a mobile device) is a high-risk behavior among youth. Sexting occurs via instant messaging and other social media applications, such as *Snapchat*. Sexting behaviors are correlated with dating and using alcohol and drugs before sexual activity (Strasburger et al., 2019). It has also led some youth to suicide. A discussion of sexting should occur when a child receives their first cellphone.

The American Academy of Pediatrics Council on Communications and Media (Guram & Heinz, 2018) recommends no more than 1 to 2 hours a day of screen time, which includes television and the Internet. They also recommend that two questions be asked at each well-child visit.

1. How much recreational screen time does your child or teenager consume daily?
2. Is there a TV set or Internet-connected device (computer, iPad, cellphone) in the child's or teenager's bedroom?

School nurses can also ask these questions when they are concerned about sleep deprivation/disturbances and other mental health issues surrounding excessive or inappropriate screen time on a variety of devices. Because adolescents are less likely to have well-child visits than younger children, the school nurse may be well positioned to screen adolescents for potential problems with media use.

Internet Challenges and Risky Games

The Internet and social media abound with viral online trends involving risky games or "challenges" aimed at children and youth and are a growing phenomenon on platforms such as TikTok.

The *choking game* made the news in 2007 when 82 cases of children and adolescents ages 6 to 19 were identified who had either strangled themselves or were strangled by another person to achieve a brief euphoric state, similar to taking drugs, which results from the cerebral hypoxia (Michel et al., 2019). This activity is also called the *blackout game, pass out game, scarf game,* and *space monkey*. There are reports of young people engaging in this risky activity during parties, but some children have tried it alone in their bedrooms. Possible sequelae include accidental disability and death (Michel et al., 2019). Deaths from the choking game are often classified as accidental deaths or suicide rather than taking into consideration that the youth was engaged in a deliberate attempt to temporarily asphyxiate themselves for pleasure (Michel et al., 2019). A similarly dangerous trend involves children challenging each other to hold their breath until they faint or lose consciousness.

Parents/guardians and educators must become aware of the existence of this activity and its warning signs. Physical signs include bloodshot eyes, flushed face, frequent headaches, hoarseness, petechiae on the face and near the eyes, unexplained cuts or bruises, covering the neck with clothing, and grogginess—particularly after spending time alone (Michel et al., 2019). Psychological signs may include a change in attitude or mood, irritability, aggression, or an unusual need for more privacy. Environmental signs might include missing or unusual placement of items, such as belts, scarves, neckties, bed sheets, bungee cords, ropes, T-shirts, or dog leashes tied around hooks, furniture, or doorknobs (Michel et al., 2019).

The list of dangerous trending Internet challenges is long and constantly expanding. Adults need to stay current with the risk-taking trends that youth may participate in and know that some may reappear once gone for a while. One recurrent trend involves challenges related to eating foods spiced with capsaicin, rated high on the Scoville heat unit scale, or eating an extremely hot pepper. For example, children challenge each other to see how many chips covered in a chili pepper mixture one can consume. The *One Chip Challenge* dares an individual to eat a large tortilla chip spiced with extremely hot Carolina Reaper and Scorpion peppers and see how long they can go without drinking or eating anything to relieve the extreme discomfort. The *Ghost Pepper Challenge* entails children daring each other to eat chips dipped in very hot salsa made with ghost peppers. Eating foods high in capsaicin can lead to mouth irritation and burning sensation, nausea, vomiting, diarrhea, and intestinal discomfort. Serious health effects may include chest pain, esophageal damage and heart problems (National Poison Control Center, 2024).

Other risky viral trends include dangerous stunts. One example is *the Bird Box Challenge*, where children wear blindfolds and engage in different activities while being videotaped. These may include outdoor activities that put them in danger of falls and motor vehicle accidents. New risky games are emerging constantly. When students present with unusual or unexplained injuries or complaints, the school nurse can inquire if the student has participated in any viral challenges. School nurses should collaborate with school counselors and educational staff to educate students, parents/guardians, and staff about the health and safety dangers of these risky activities to prevent untoward and even tragic outcomes.

DRIVING AS A HIGH-RISK BEHAVIOR

Unintentional injuries are the leading cause of death among adolescents. At only 7% of the U.S. population, adolescents ages 15 to 19 accounted for 11% of the costs associated with motor vehicle injuries in 2013 (CDC, 2022f). Data show that 227,000 adolescents ages 16 to 19 years were treated in emergency departments for injuries related to motor vehicle accidents, and 2,800 died in motor vehicle accidents during 2020 (CDC, 2022f). Newly licensed adolescents are at especially high risk of being in an accident. The crash rate for 16- to 17-year-olds is three times higher than the crash rate for 18- to 19-year-olds, and drivers between the ages of 16 and 19 are almost three times as likely to be in a fatal crash as drivers who are at least 20 years old (CDC, 2022g). Males and adolescents driving with other adolescent passengers are also at higher risk for motor vehicle accidents (CDC, 2022g). Adolescents are at greatest risk for motor vehicle accidents because they underestimate dangerous situations, do not recognize hazardous situations, make critical decision errors, exceed the speed limit, allow shorter headways, and do not always use seatbelts. Of drivers ages 15 to 30 years, 35% of males and 19% of females were speeding at the time of a crash involving fatalities.

Over one-half (56%) of adolescents ages 16 to 19 who died in motor vehicle accidents in 2020 were not wearing a seatbelt, despite evidence showing that seatbelts can reduce serious injuries and death by about half (CDC, 2022g). Although teens are taught about the consequences of driving under the influence of alcohol, they also need to be aware of *drugged driving*, which is the effect of recreational drug use, such as the use of marijuana, on driving.

Distracted driving is a growing public health crisis. According to the National Highway Traffic Safety Administration, "distracted driving is any activity that diverts attention from driving, including talking or texting on your phone, eating and drinking, talking to people in your vehicle, fiddling with the stereo, entertainment or navigation system—anything that takes your attention away from the task of safe driving" (n.d., para. 1). In 2021, 3,522 people were killed in crashes involving distracted drivers (Stewart, 2023). A higher percentage of drivers ages 15 to 20 were distracted than drivers age 21 and older (CDC, 2022g). Thirty-nine percent of surveyed teens responded that they had texted or e-mailed while driving a car during the last 30 days (CDC, 2022f).

Important vehicle accident prevention efforts include promoting use of seatbelts, discouraging drinking or texting while driving, and having graduated driver licensing

Did You Know?

Drinking or using substances while driving increases the risk for teen drivers and passengers. Here are some sobering statistics from the CDC (2022g):

- 5.4% of students reported drinking while driving in the last 30 days, and 17% reported that they rode with a driver who had been drinking.
- 29% of drivers ages 15 to 20 killed in motor vehicle crashes had been drinking.
- 17% of drivers ages 15 to 20 involved in fatal motor vehicle crashes had a BAC of 0.08% or higher—a level that is illegal for adults in all U.S. states. (Note: Utah has a BAC limit of 0.05%.)
- 62% of drivers ages 15 to 20 who were killed in motor vehicle crashes after drinking and driving were not wearing a seatbelt.
- 24% of male drivers ages 15 to 20 years and 17% of female drivers ages 15 to 20 years who were involved in fatal crashes had been drinking before the crash.

programs. Graduated licensing provides more extended practice periods behind the wheel, limitations for driving under high-risk conditions (e.g., nighttime, number of passengers), and greater participation by the parent in the teen's process of learning to drive. At the community level, the CDC (2022g) recommends enforcing zero-tolerance laws for drivers younger than 21 and laws regarding the minimum legal drinking age.

Although all states now have some type of graduated driver's license programs, the more comprehensive ones have reduced fatal crashes by 26% to 41% and overall crashes by 16% to 22% (CDC, 2022g). School nurses should be involved in school-wide campaigns to increase the risk awareness of teen drivers and advocate that health and driver education curricula include safe driving practices.

HIGH-RISK BEHAVIOR PREVENTION AND INTERVENTIONS

Programs addressing high-risk behaviors aim to prevent children and adolescents from engaging in high-risk activities. It is also clear that no single treatment or intervention program is appropriate or effective for all individuals. Intervention programs that address risky behaviors fall into the public health approach of primary, secondary, and tertiary prevention. Most programs developed for schools that address high-risk behaviors focus on primary prevention directed to all youth, regardless of risk.

School nurses can integrate academic, behavioral, and social-emotional efforts utilizing *multitiered systems of support* (MTSS) as a means to collaboratively work to implement evidence-based practices supporting the academic achievement and inclusion of all students in health promotion and prevention practices related to high-risk behaviors in students. MTSS is a proactive framework that also includes community and parent engagement. In the high-risk behavior context, MTSS Tier 1 would begin with universal screening of all students. Research has demonstrated that MTSS is critical for supporting student development across domains of functioning and supporting the prevention of high-risk behaviors (Briesch et al., 2022; Charlton et al., 2018; Rau & Lytle, 2020). See Table 29-1 for a description of types of prevention in schools.

TABLE 29-1 Three Levels of Youth Risk Behavior Prevention

Public Health Level of Prevention	Multitiered System of Support	Definition	Example
Primary prevention	Tier 1	Preventing the initial development of a disease or injury before it occurs. Typically, a population-based approach that is widely applied to the entire student body such as evidence-based education.	Texting and driving prevention campaigns; immunizations (e.g., human papillomavirus [HPV] or hepatitis B); substance use prevention programs; sex and reproductive health education.
Secondary prevention	Tier 2	Screening and early detection of at-risk students. Applied to subgroups of students known to be at risk or to have risk factors to engage in risky behaviors.	Programs that target students who have tried drugs, alcohol, or cigarettes. Programs that target students who have experienced sexual encounters but have not yet suffered consequences from these behaviors.
Tertiary prevention	Tier 3	Preventing consequences in those who have already developed signs and symptoms of risky behaviors or disease. In students with high-risk behaviors, the goal is to decrease their use/behavior and prevent further sequelae.	Programs led by qualified trained personnel at school and by health providers. Programs include teen support groups, therapeutic school settings, and substance use rehabilitation programs.

Practice Connection

As the expert in school health, the school nurse can provide leadership when schools decide which prevention and intervention programs are most relevant to the student population. Yet the options to choose from can be overwhelming. The CDC's Division of Adolescent and School Health (CDC, 2023a) has featured resources on school health strategies and programs that promote healthy behaviors in children and youth. Visit the CDC's *Adolescent and School Health Website* to learn more.

CONCLUSION

Adolescence is an incredible time of growth and experimentation when students experience many new feelings and temptations. Yet the developing brains of youth are not always mature enough to make informed and wise decisions. Many students engage in unsafe and sometimes dangerous behaviors that risk their immediate safety or long-term health. The school nurse is often the professional at school to suspect, identify, or respond to risky behaviors in youth. Although risky behaviors increase in prevalence as students advance through their school years, elementary school students can be influenced in many ways to engage in or be predisposed to take health and safety risks.

Students must have the education to make more mature decisions and a social environment that empowers them to act on that knowledge to make healthy choices. The need for information begins before elementary school and intensifies as children enter adolescence. The goal is for young people to have the information and skills to make informed and responsible decisions to be healthy and productive adults.

School nurses must stay informed of current trends in youth risk behavior and advocate for evidence-based prevention programs and intervention strategies in their schools. School nurses must coordinate with students, families, and educational teams, as well as community and primary care providers, to ensure that students engaging in risky behaviors have access to and receive the health care, social services, and education they deserve.

The Editors gratefully acknowledge the work of the previous chapter authors: Karen Johnson & Janice Selekman. Thank you to Samira Adams for assisting with the literature search.

References

Alaska Division of Public Health. (2023). *Get the facts about marijuana: Marijuana edible safety.* https://health.alaska.gov/dph/director/pages/marijuana/edibles.aspx

Aleyan, S., Cole, A., Qian, W., & Leatherdale, S. T. (2018). Risky business: A longitudinal study examining cigarette smoking initiation among susceptible and non-susceptible e-cigarette users in Canada. *BMJ Open, 8*(5), 1–7. https://doi.org/10.1136/bmjopen-2017-021080

Alonso, M. R., & Fernández-García, B. (2020). Evolution of the use of sports supplements. *PharmaNutrition, 14*(2020), 1–14. https://doi.org/10.1016/j.phanu.2020.100239

American Academy of Dermatology. (2023). *Indoor tanning.* https://www.aad.org/media/stats-indoor-tanning

American Academy of Family Physicians. (2019). *Tar wars.* https://www.aafp.org/patient-care/public-health/tobacco-nicotine/tar-wars.html

American Academy of Pediatrics. (2015). Technical report: Adolescent drug testing policies in schools. *Pediatrics, 135*(4), e1107–e1112. https://doi.org/10.1542/peds.2015-0055

American Cancer Society. (2020). *Health risks of smokeless tobacco.* https://www.cancer.org/content/dam/CRC/PDF/Public/7967.00.pdf

American Lung Association. (2017a). *Health effects of smoking.* http://www.lung.org/stop-smoking/smoking-facts/health-effects-of-smoking.html

American Lung Association. (2017b). *TATU teen teachers.* http://www.lung.org/local-content/nevada/our-initiatives/tatu-teen-teachers.html

American Lung Association. (2022b). *Not on tobacco (N-O-T).* http://www.lung.org/local-content/california/stop-smoking/not-on-tobacco.html

An, B. P., Loes, C. N., & Trolian, T. L. (2017). The relation between binge drinking and academic performance: Considering the mediating effects of academic involvement. *Journal of College Student Development, 58*(4), 492–508. https://doi.org/10.1353/csd.2017.0039

Atli, A., Akkaya, M., & Şad, S. N. (2022). Tattooing: A popular way of self-expression among university students. *Current Psychology, 41*(12), 8965–8974. https://doi.org/10.1007/s12144-021-01389-0

Blank, M., Ferris K., Metzger, A., Amy, G., Duncan, C., Jarrett T., & Dino, G. (2017). Physical activity and quit motivation moderators of adolescent smoking reduction. *American Journal of Health Behavior, 41*(4), 419–429. https://doi.org/10.5993/AJHB.41.4.6

Boardman, C. (2019). An insight into laser tattoo removal: Reasoning, methods and limitations. *Journal of Aesthetic Nursing, 8*(8), 377–381. https://doi.org/10.12968/joan.2019.8.8.377

Borgerson, J. L., & Schroeder, J. E. (2018). Making skin visible: How consumer culture imagery commodifies identity. *Body & Society, 24*(1–2), 103–136. https://doi.org/10.1177/1357034X187609

Briesch, A. M., Chafouleas, S. M., Iovino, E. A., Abdulkerim, N., Sherod, R. L., Oakes, W. P., Lane, K. L., Common, E. A., Royer, D. J., & Buckman, M. (2022). Exploring directions for professional learning to enhance behavior screening within a comprehensive, integrated, three-tiered model of prevention. *Journal of Positive Behavior Interventions, 24*(4), 278–288. https://doi.org/10.1177/10983007211050424

Calado, F., Alexandre, J., & Griffiths, M. D. (2017). Prevalence of adolescent gambling: A systematic review of recent research. *Journal of Gambling Studies, 33*, 397–424. https://doi.org/10.1007/s10899-016-9627-5

Cash, R. E., Kinsman, J., Crowe, R. P., Rivard, M. K., Faul, M., & Panchal, A. R. (2018). Naloxone administration frequency during emergency medical service events—United States, 2012–2016. *Morbidity and Mortality Weekly Report, 67*(31), 850–853. https://www.cdc.gov/mmwr/volumes/67/wr/pdfs/mm6731a2-H.pdf

Centers for Disease Control and Prevention. (2017a). *Secondhand smoke (SHS) facts.* https://www.cdc.gov/tobacco/data_statistics/fact_sheets/secondhand_smoke/general_facts/index.htm

Centers for Disease Control and Prevention. (2017b). *Youth and tobacco use.* https://www.cdc.gov/tobacco/data_statistics/fact_sheets/youth_data/tobacco_use/index.htm

Centers for Disease Control and Prevention. (2021a). *Marijuana: What we know.* https://www.cdc.gov/marijuana/factsheets/pdf/marijuanafactsheets-whatweknow-508compliant.pdf

Centers for Disease Control and Prevention. (2021b). *Sexually transmitted diseases: Adolescents and young adults.* https://www.cdc.gov/std/life-stages-populations/adolescents-youngadults.htm

Centers for Disease Control and Prevention. (2022a). *E-cigarette, or vaping, products visual dictionary.* https://www.cdc.gov/tobacco/

basic_information/e-cigarettes/pdfs/ecigarette-or-vaping-products-visual-dictionary-508.pdf

Centers for Disease Control and Prevention. (2022b). *Binge drinking.* https://www.cdc.gov/alcohol/fact-sheets/binge-drinking.htm

Centers for Disease Control and Prevention. (2022c). *School connectedness helps students thrive.* https://www.cdc.gov/healthyyouth/protective/school_connectedness.htm

Centers for Disease Control and Prevention. (2022d). *Skin cancer.* https://www.cdc.gov/cancer/skin/basic_info/what-is-skin-cancer.htm

Centers for Disease Control and Prevention. (2022e). *Smokeless tobacco product use in the United States.* https://www.cdc.gov/tobacco/data_statistics/fact_sheets/smokeless/use_us/index.htm#youth

Centers for Disease Control and Prevention. (2022f). *Teen drivers: Get the facts.* https://www.cdc.gov/transportationsafety/teen_drivers/teendrivers_factsheet.html

Centers for Disease Control and Prevention (2022g). *Top ten leading causes of death in the U.S. for ages 1–44 from 1981–2020.* https://www.cdc.gov/injury/wisqars/animated-leading-causes.html

Centers for Disease Control and Prevention. (2022h). *Quick facts on the risks of e-cigarettes for kids, teens, and young adults.* https://www.cdc.gov/tobacco/basic_information/e-cigarettes/Quick-Facts-on-the-Risks-of-E-cigarettes-for-Kids-Teens-and-Young-Adults.html?s_

Centers for Disease Control and Prevention. (2023a). *About e-cigarettes.* https://www.cdc.gov/tobacco/e-cigarettes/about.html

Centers for Disease Control and Prevention. (2023b). *Youth risk behavior survey: Data summary & trends report: 2011–2021.* https://www.cdc.gov/healthyyouth/data/yrbs/yrbs_data_summary_and_trends.htmhttps://www.cdc.gov/healthyyouth/data/yrbs/pdf/YRBS_Data-Summary-Trends_Report2023_508.pdf

Charlton, C. T., Sabey, C. V., Dawson, M. R., Pyle, D., Lund, E. M., & Ross, S. W. (2018). Critical incidents in the scale-up of state multi-tiered systems of supports. *Journal of Positive Behavior Interventions, 20*(4), 191–202. https://doi.org/10.1177/ 1098300718770804

Cooper, M., Park-Lee, E., Chunfeng, R., Cornelius, M., Jamal, A., Cullen, K. A., & Ren, C. (2022). Notes from the field: E-cigarette use among middle and high school students—United States, 2022. *Morbidity & Mortality Weekly Report, 71*(40), 1283–1285. https://doi.org/10.15585/mmwr.mm7140a3

CRAFFT (Car, Relax, Alone, Forget, Friends, Trouble). (2018). *About the CRAFFT.* Boston Children's Hospital. http://crafft.org/about-the-crafft/

CRAFFT 2.1+N. (2020). *The CRAFFT 2.1*+N Questionnaire. Boston Children's Hospital. https://crafft.org/wp-content/uploads/2021/07/CRAFFT_2.1N-HONC_Self-administered_2021-07-03.pdf

Cummings, K. M., Morris, P. B., & Benowitz, N. L. (2018). Another article about e-cigarettes: Why should I care? *Journal of the American Heart Association, 7*(14), e009944.

Davis, C. R., Plotkin, M., & Kelly, N. (2023). Action plan and model to reduce potential opioid overdose deaths on K-12 campuses. *NASN School Nurse, 39*(1). doi:10.1177/1942602X231185718

Desai, N., & Breuner, C. C. (2022). Tattoos and piercings in female adolescents and young adults. *Journal of Pediatric and Adolescent Gynecology, 36*(1), 14–17. https://doi.org/10.1016/j.jpag.2022.08.007

Dowling, N. A., Merkouris, S. S., Greenwood, C. J., Oldenhof, E., Toumbourou, J. W., & Youssef, G. J. (2017). Early risk and protective factors for problem gambling: A systematic review and meta-analysis of longitudinal studies. *Clinical Psychology Review, 51*, 109–124. https://doi.org/10.1016/j.cpr.2016.10.008

Drug and Alcohol Foundation. (2022). *Cannabinoids.* https://adf.org.au/drug-facts/cannabinoids/#:~:text=What%20are%20cannabinoids%3F,-The%20word%20cannabinoid%20refers%20to

Duncan, L. R., Pearson, E. S., & Maddison, R. (2018). Smoking prevention in children and adolescents: A systematic review of individualized interventions. *Patient Education and Counseling, 101*(3), 375–388. https://doi.org/10.1016/j.pec.2017.09.011

Endsley, P. (2023). Conducting substance use screenings. In C. A. Resha & V. L. Taliaferro, *Legal resource for school health services* (2nd ed., pp. 501–511). SchoolNurse.com

Environmental Protection Agency. (2022). *Ultraviolet (UV) radiation tanning equipment.* https://www.epa.gov/radtown/ultraviolet-uv-radiation-tanning-equipment

Evans-Paulson, R., Widman, L., Brasileiro, J., Maheux, A. J., & Choukas-Bradley, S. (2021). Examining the link between sexual self-concept and sexual communication among adolescents. *Communication Quarterly, 69*(5), 525–543. https://doi.org/10.1080/01463373.2021.1969585

Fernald, M., Cassidy, B., Ren, D., Mitchell, A., & Kameg, B. (2023). An evaluation of documentation and follow-up on the use of SBIRT in an outpatient behavioral health clinic through the use of the CRAFFT tool. *Journal of Child and Adolescent Psychiatric Nursing, 36*(1), 28–34. https://doi.org/10.1111/jcap.12395

Forrest, D., & McHale, I. G. (2021). Transmission of problem gambling between adjacent generations. *Journal of Gambling Studies, 37*(2), 711–722. https://doi.org/10.1007/s10899-020-09977-8

Grant, J. E., & Chamberlain, S. R. (2018). Caffeine's influence on gambling behavior and the types of impulsivity. *Addictive Behaviors, 76*, 156–160. https://doi.org/10.1016/j.addbeh.2017.08.007

Griffith, C., La France, B., & Griffith, H. (2019). How does synthetic marijuana (K2) mimic the effects of naturally occurring chemical compound found in THC? *International Journal of Collaborative Research on Internal Medicine & Public Health, 11*(1), 869–877.

Guram, S., & Heinz, P. (2018). Media use in children: American Academy of Pediatrics recommendations 2016. *Archives of Disease in Childhood–Education and Practice, 103*(2), 99–101. http://dx.doi.org/10.1136/archdischild-2017-312969

Hall, W., Gartner, C., & Bonevski, B. (2021). Lessons from the public health responses to the U.S. outbreak of vaping-related lung injury. *Addiction, 116*(5), 985–993. https://doi.org/10.1111/add.15108

Healthline. (2019). *Seven (7) benefits and uses of CBD oil.* https://www.healthline.com/nutrition/cbd-oil-benefits

Healthy People 2030. (n.d.). *Social determinants of health.* https://health.gov/healthypeople/priority-areas/social-determinants-health

Hwang, C., & O'Neil, J. (2020). E-cigarette use among adolescents. *The Journal for Nurse Practitioners, 16*(6), 453–456. https://doi.org/10.1016/j.nurpra.2020.02.021

Ink Different Tattoo School. (2023). *The 2022 state by state guide to tattoo laws in the United States.* https://tattooschool.com/2022-tattoo-laws-across-the-united-states/

Johnston, L. D., O'Malley, P. M., Bachman, J. G., & Schulenberg, J. E. (2011). *Monitoring the future national survey results on adolescent drug use: Overview of key findings, 2010.* Institute for Social Research, The University of Michigan. http://files.eric.ed.gov/fulltext/ED528077.pdf

Jones, C. M., Clayton, H. B., Deputy, N. P., Roehler, D. R., Ko, J. Y., Esser, M. B., Brookmeyer, K. A., & Hertz, M. F. (2020). Prescription opioid misuse and use of alcohol and other substances among high school students—Youth Risk Behavior Survey, United States, 2019. *MMWR Supplements, 69*(1), 38–46. https://doi.org/10.15585/mmwr.su6901a5

Kann, L., McManus, T., Harris, W. A., Shanklin, S. L., Lowry, R., Chyen, D., Whittle, L., Thornton, J., Lim, C., Bradford, D., Yamakawa, Y., Leon, M., Brener, N., Ethier, K. A., Flint, K. H., & Queen, B. (2018). Youth Risk Behavior Surveillance—United States, 2017. *MMWR Surveillance Summary, 65*(6), 1–114. https://www.cdc.gov/mmwr/volumes/67/ss/ss6708a1.htm

Kluger, N. (2019). An update on cutaneous complications of permanent tattooing. *Expert Review of Clinical Immunology, 15*(11), 1135–1143. https://doi.org/10.1080/1744666X.2020.1676732

Laestadius, L. I., Guidry, J. P., Greskoviak, R., & Adams, J. (2019). Making "weedish fish": An exploratory analysis of cannabis recipes on Pinterest. *Substance Use & Misuse, 54*(13), 2191–2197. https://doi.org/10.1080/10826084.2019.1638410

La Leche League International. (2023). *Nipple piercings.* https://www.llli.org/breastfeeding-info/nipple-piercings/

Leafbuyer. (2018). *Heal vs. high: Effects and benefits of CBD edibles.* https://www.leafbuyer.com/blog/heal-vs-high-effects-and-benefits-of-cbd-edibles/

Lees, B., Meredith, L. R., Kirkland, A. E., & Bryant, B. E. (2020). Effect of alcohol use on the adolescent brain and behavior. *Pharmacology, Biochemistry, and Behavior, 192*, 1–11. https://doi.org/10.1016/j.pbb.2020.172906

Levy, J. L., & Williams, J. F. (2016). American Academy of Pediatrics clinical report: Substance use screening, brief intervention, and referral to treatment. *Pediatrics, 138*(1). https://doi.org/10.1542/peds.2016-1211

Levy, S. (2019). Youth and the opioid epidemic. *Pediatrics, 143*(2), e20182752. https://doi.org/10.1542/peds.2018-2752

Lovell, M. E., Akhurst, J., Padgett, C., Garry, M. I., & Matthews, A. (2020). Cognitive outcomes associated with long-term, regular, recreational cannabis use in adults: A meta-analysis. *Experimental and Clinical Psychopharmacology, 28*(4), 471. https://doi.org/10.1037/pha0000326

Malhi, G. S., Das, P., Bell, E., Mattingly, G., & Mannie, Z. (2019). Modelling resilience in adolescence and adversity: A novel framework to inform research and practice. *Translational Psychiatry, 9*(1), 1–16. https://doi.org/10.1038/s41398-019-0651-y

McCabe, E. M., Davis, C., Mandy, L., & Wong, C. (2022). The role of school connectedness in supporting the health and well-being of youth: Recommendations for school nurses. *NASN School Nurse, 37*(1), 42–47. https://doi.org/10.1177/1942602X211048481

McCloskey, K., & Johnson, B. T. (2019). Habits, quick and easy: Perceived complexity moderates the associations of contextual stability and rewards with behavioral automaticity. *Frontiers in Psychology, 10*(1556). https://doi.org/10.3389/fpsyg.2019.01556

Mehta, C. M., Burke, P. E., & Shrier, L. A. (2022). Contexts of marijuana use and cessation among frequently-using youth in primary care. *Youth & Society, 54*(1), 43–67. https://doi.org/10.1177/0044118X20951060

Meigs, J. M., Bartolomeo, V. R., & Wolfson, A. R. (2022). Methodological review of caffeine assessment strategies with a focus on adolescents. *Sleep Medicine Reviews, 62*. https://doi.org/10.1016/j.smrv.2021.101587

Merrill, R. A., & Liang, X. (2019). Associations between adolescent media use, mental health, and risky sexual behaviors. *Children and Youth Services Review, 103*, 1–9. https://doi.org/10.1016/j.childyouth.2019.05.022

Michel, G., Garcia, M., Aubron, V., Bernadet, S., Salla, J., & Purper-Ouakil, D. (2019). Adolescent mental health and the choking game. *Pediatrics, 143*(2). https://doi.org/10.1542/peds.2017-3963

Miech, R. A., Johnston, L. D., O'Malley, P. M., Bachman, J. G., Schulenberg, J. E., & Patrick, M. E. (2023). *Monitoring the future national survey results on drug use, 1975–2022: Volume I, secondary school students*. Institute for Social Research, The University of Michigan. https://monitoringthefuture.org/wp-content/uploads/2022/12/mtf2022.pdf

Miuli, A., Stigliano, G., Lalli, A., Coladonato, M., D'Angelo, L., Esposito, F., Cappello, C., Pettorruso, M., Martinotti, G., Schifano, F., & Di Giannantonio, M. (2020). "Purple drank" (codeine and promethazine cough syrup): A systematic review of a social phenomenon with medical implications. *Journal of Psychoactive Drugs, 52*(5), 453–462. https://doi.org/10.1080/02791072.2020.1797250

Morone, J. (2017). An integrative review of social determinants of health assessment and screening tools used in pediatrics. *Journal of Pediatric Nursing, 37*, 22–28. https://doi.org/ 10.1016/j.pedn.2017.08.022

Mustonen, A., Niemelä, S., McGrath, J. J., Murray, G. K., Nordström, T., Mäki, P., Miettunen, J., & Scott, J. G. (2018). Adolescent inhalant use and psychosis risk—A prospective longitudinal study. *Schizophrenia Research, 201*, 360–366. https://doi.org/10.1016/j.schres.2018.05.013

National Academies of Sciences, Engineering, and Medicine. (2019). *Implementing strategies to enhance public health surveillance of physical activity in the United States*. The National Academies Press. https://doi.org/10.17226/25444

National Association of School Nurses. (2020). *Naloxone in the school setting* (Position Statement). Author. https://www.nasn.org/nasn-resources/professional-practice-documents/position-statements/ps-naloxone

National Association of School Nurses. (2023, September 9). *Naloxone education for school nurses toolkit*. https://learn.nasn.org/courses/58011

National Association of School Nurses. (2024). A contemporary framework update for today's school nursing landscape: Introducing the School Nursing Practice Framework. *NASN School Nurse, 39*(3), 140-147. https://www.doi.org/10.1177/1942602X241241092

National Center for Education Statistics. (2022). *Marijuana use and illegal drug availability*. https://nces.ed.gov/programs/coe/indicator/a15/marijuana-use-drug-availability

National Center for Injury Prevention and Control. (2020, October 19). *Marijuana and public health: Addiction (marijuana or cannabis use disorder)*. Centers for Disease Control and Prevention. https://www.cdc.gov/marijuana/health-

National Center on Complementary and Integrative Health. (2019). *Cannabis (marijuana) and cannabinoids: What you need to know*. https://www.nccih.nih.gov/health/cannabis-marijuana-and-cannabinoids-what-you-need-to-know

National Education Association. (2023). *2022–2023 NEA resolutions: C-19. Drug or alcohol testing of students*. https://www.nea.org/sites/default/files/2022-08/nea-resolutions_2022-2023.pdf

National Highway Traffic Safety Administration. (n.d.). *Distracted driving: Overview*. U.S. Department of Transportation. https://www.nhtsa.gov/risky-driving/distracted-driving

National Institute on Alcohol Abuse and Alcoholism. (2020). *Underage drinking*. U.S. Department of Health and Human Services, National Institutes of Health. https://www.niaaa.nih.gov/sites/default/files/publications/NIAAA_Underage_Drinking_1.pdf

National Institute on Alcohol Abuse and Alcoholism. (2021a). *Alcohol overdose: The dangers of drinking too much*. U.S. Department of Health and Human Services, National Institutes of Health. https://www.niaaa.nih.gov/sites/default/files/publications/Alcohol_overdose_0.pdf

National Institute on Alcohol Abuse and Alcoholism. (2021b). *Underaged drinking*. U.S. Department of Health and Human Services, National Institutes of Health. https://www.niaaa.nih.gov/publications/brochures-and-fact-sheets/underage-drinking

National Institute on Alcohol Abuse and Alcoholism. (2021c). *Understanding binge drinking*. U.S. Department of Health and Human Services, National Institutes of Health. https://www.niaaa.nih.gov/publications/brochures-and-fact-sheets/binge-drinking

National Institute on Drug Abuse. (n.d.). *Mind matters*. https://nida.nih.gov/sites/default/files/NIDA_MindMatters_TeachersGuide_2022.pdf

National Institute on Drug Abuse. (2019a). *Preventing drug use among children and adolescents*. https://www.drugabuse.gov/publications/preventing-drug-abuse-among-children-adolescents-in-brief/prevention-principles

National Institute on Drug Abuse. (2019b). *Methamphetamine facts*. https://nida.nih.gov/publications/drugfacts/methamphetamine

National Institute on Drug Abuse. (2019c). *Synthetic cannabinoids*. U.S. Department of Health and Human Services, National Institutes of Health. https://nida.nih.gov/publications/drugfacts/cannabis-marijuana

National Institute on Drug Abuse. (2020a). *Inhalants drug facts*. https://nida.nih.gov/publications/drugfacts/inhalants

National Institute on Drug Abuse. (2020b). *Misuse of prescription drug research report*. U.S. Department of Health and Human Services, National Institutes of Health. https://nida.nih.gov/publications/research-reports/misuse-prescription-drugs/overview

National Institute on Drug Abuse. (2021). *What is cocaine?* U.S. Department of Health and Human Services, National Institutes of Health. https://nida.nih.gov/publications/drugfacts/cocaine

National Institute on Drug Abuse. (2022a). *What is MDMA?* U.S. Department of Health and Human Services, National Institutes

of Health. https://nida.nih.gov/publications/drugfacts/mdma-ecstasymolly

National Institute on Drug Abuse. (2022b). *What is the scope of cocaine use in the United States?* U.S. Department of Health and Human Services, National Institutes of Health. https://nida.nih.gov/publications/research-reports/cocaine/what-scope-cocaine-use-in-united-states

National Institute on Drug Abuse. (2022c). *What is the scope of heroin use in the United States?* U.S. Department of Health and Human Services, National Institutes of Health. https://nida.nih.gov/publications/research-reports/heroin/scope-heroin-use-in-united-states

National Poison Control Center. (2024). *Is the one chip challenge dangerous?* https://www.poison.org/articles/is-the-one-chip-challenge-dangerous

Odgers, C. L., & Jensen, M. R. (2020). Annual research review: Adolescent mental health in the digital age: Facts, fears, and future directions. *Journal of Child Psychology and Psychiatry, 61*(3), 336–348. https://doi.org/10.1111/jcpp.13190

Palamar, J.J., Rutherford, C., & Keyes, K.M. (2019). "Flakka" use among high school seniors in the United States. *Drug and Alcohol Dependence, 196*, 86-90. https://doi.org/10.1016/j.drugalcdep.2018.12.014

Park, J. H., Moon, J. H., Kim, H. J., Kong, M. H., & Oh, Y. H. (2020). Sedentary lifestyle: Overview of updated evidence of potential health risks. *Korean Journal of Family Medicine, 41*(6), 365. https://doi.org/10.4082/kjfm.20.0165

Passos, P. F., Pintor, A. V. B., Marañón-Vásquez, G. A., Campos, T., Abrahão, A. C., Ferreira, D. M. T., … & Visconti, M. A. (2022). Oral manifestations arising from oral piercings: A systematic review and meta-analyses. *Oral Surgery, Oral Medicine, Oral Pathology and Oral Radiology, 134*(3), 327–341. https://doi.org/10.1016/j.oooo.2022.04.051

Patterson, K., Brady, J., & Olympia, R. P. (2017). School nurses on the front lines of medicine: Uppers and downers: The approach to the student with altered mental status. *NASN School Nurse, 32*(6), 350–355. https://doi.org/10.1177/1942602X17706380

Price, S. N., Studts, J. L., & Hamann, H. A. (2019). Tobacco use assessment and treatment in cancer patients: A scoping review of oncology care clinician adherence to clinical practice guidelines in the US. *The Oncologist, 24*(2), 229–238. https://doi.org/10.1634/theoncologist.2018-0246

Proebstl, L., Kamp, F., Koller, G., & Soyka, M. (2018). Cognitive deficits in methamphetamine users: How strong is the evidence? *Pharmacopsychiatry, 51*(6), 243–250. https://doi.org/10.1055/s-0043-123471

Rau, W., & Lytle, M. (2020). The role of the school nurse in increasing instructional time using multi-tiered systems of support for behavior (MTSS-B): A quality improvement project. *NASN School Nurse, 35*(5), 276–283. https://doi.org/10.1177/1942602X20942492

Ryan, J. E., McCabe, S. E., & Boyd, C. G. (2021). Medicinal cannabis: Policy, patients, and providers. *Policy, Politics, and Nursing Practice, 22*(2), 126–133. https://doi.org/10.1177/1527154421989609

Sajwani, H. S. (2023). The dilemma of new psychoactive substances: A growing threat. *Saudi Pharmaceutical Journal, 31*(3), 348–350. https://doi.org/10.1016/j.jsps.2023.01.002

Samoggia, A., & Rezzaghi, T. (2021). The consumption of caffeine-containing products to enhance sports performance: An application of an extended model of the theory of planned behavior. *Nutrients, 13*(2), 1–18. https://doi.org/10.3390/nu13020344

Sawyer, S. M., Azzopardi, P. S., Wickremarathne, D., & Patton, G. C. (2018). The age of adolescence. *The Lancet Child & Adolescent Health, 2*(3), 223–228. https://doi.org/10.1016/S2352-4642(18)30022-1

Selekman, J. (2019). Vaping: It's all a smokescreen. *Pediatric Nursing, 45*(1), 12–15.

Shenoi, R. P., Spirito, A., Linakis, J. G., Bromberg, J. R., Mello, M. J., Chun, T. H., Charles Casper, T., & Richards, R. (2019). Predictive validity of the CRAFFT for substance use disorder. *Pediatrics, 144*(2), 1–12. https://doi.org/10.1542/peds.2018-3415

Siegmund, L. A. (2022). Appearance and performance enhancing drugs and substances: The role of the school nurse. *NASN School Nurse, 37*(5), 263–269. https://doi.org/10.1177/1942602X221093938

Soós, R., Gyebrovszki, Á., Tóth, Á., Jeges, S., & Wilhelm, M. (2021). Effects of caffeine and caffeinated beverages in children, adolescents and young adults: Short review. *International Journal of Environmental Research and Public Health, 18*(23), 1–20. https://doi.org/10.3390/ijerph182312389

Stanescu, D. F., & Romascanu, M. C. (2020). Are tattooing indicators of dark personalities? An analysis of body modification within the framework of dark triad of personality. *Journal of Social and Development Sciences, 11*(4), 7–14. https://doi.org/10.3390/ijerph182312389

Stewart, T. (2023, April). *Overview of motor vehicle traffic crashes in 2021.* National Highway Traffic Safety Administration. https://crashstats.nhtsa.dot.gov/Api/Public/ViewPublication/813435

Stockdale, L., & Coyne, S. M. (2018). Video game addiction in emerging adulthood: Cross-sectional evidence of pathology in video game addicts as compared to matched healthy controls. *Journal of Affective Disorders, 225*, 265–272. https://doi.org/10.1016/j.jad.2017.08.045

Strasburger, V. C., Zimmerman, H., Temple, J. R., & Madigan, S. (2019). Teenagers, sexting, and the law. *Pediatrics, 143*(5). https://doi.org/10.1542/peds.2018-3183

Substance Abuse and Mental Health Services Administration. (2020). *Focus on prevention*. https://store.samhsa.gov/product/Focus-on-Prevention/SMA10-4120

Substance Abuse and Mental Health Services Administration. (2021a). *Facts of underage drinking*. https://store.samhsa.gov/sites/default/files/pep21-03-10-008.pdf

Substance Abuse and Mental Health Services Administration. (2021b). *Underage drinking*. https://www.samhsa.gov/underage-drinking-topic

Substance Abuse and Mental Health Services Administration. (2022a). *Drug testing resources*. https://www.samhsa.gov/workplace/drug-testing-resources

Substance Abuse and Mental Health Services Administration. (2022b). *Parent & caregiver resources*. https://www.samhsa.gov/talk-they-hear-you/parent-resources

Substance Abuse and Mental Health Services Administration. (2022c). *Risk and protective factors*. https://www.samhsa.gov/sites/default/files/20190718-samhsa-risk-protective-factors.pdf

Substance Abuse and Mental Health Services Administration. (2022d). *SBIRT: screening, brief intervention, and referral to treatment*. https://www.samhsa.gov/sbirt

Substance Abuse and Mental Health Services Administration. (2023). *Types of commonly misused or abused drugs*. https://www.samhsa.gov/prescription-drug-misuse-abuse/types

Suppiah, H. T., Swinbourne, R., Wee, J., Tay, V., & Gastin, P. (2021). Sleep characteristics of elite youth athletes: A clustering approach to optimize sleep support strategies. *International Journal of Sports Physiology & Performance, 16*(9), 1225–1233. https://doi.org/10.1123/ijspp.2020-0675

Tabuchi, T. (2021). *Science and practice for heated tobacco products*. Springer.

Tanz, L. J., Dinwiddie, A. T., Mattson, C. L., O'Donnell, J., & Davis, N. L. (2022). Drug overdose deaths among persons aged 10–19 years—United States, July 2019–December 2021. *Morbidity and Mortal Weekly Report, 71*, 1576–1582. http://dx.doi.org/10.15585/mmwr.mm7150a2

Tariq, N., & Gupta, V. (2022, July 11). *High risk behaviors*. StatPearls. https://www.ncbi.nlm.nih.gov/books/NBK560756/

Temple, J. L. (2019). Review: Trends, safety, and recommendations for caffeine use in children and adolescents. *Journal of the American Academy of Child & Adolescent Psychiatry, 58*(1), 36–45. https://doi.org/10.1016/j.jaac.2018.06.030

Thompson, K. M. (2021). Beyond roofies: Drug- and alcohol-facilitated sexual assault. *Journal of the American Academy of Physician Assistants, 34*(1), 45–49. https://doi.org/10.1097/01.JAA.0000723940.92815.0b

U.S. Department of Health and Human Services & U.S. Department of Education. (2019). *Joint guidance on the application of the Family Educational Rights and Privacy Act (FERPA) and the Health Insurance Portability and Accountability Act of 1996 (HIPAA) to student records.* https://rems.ed.gov/docs/2019%20HIPAA%20FERPA%20Joint%20Guidance.pdf

U.S. Drug Enforcement Administration. (n.d.). *Drug scheduling.* U.S. Department of Justice. https://www.dea.gov/drug-scheduling

U.S. Drug Enforcement Administration. (2018a). *Designer drugs.* U.S. Department of Justice. https://www.dea.gov/taxonomy/term/341

U.S. Drug Enforcement Administration. (2018b). *Prescription for disaster: How teens abuse medicine.* U.S. Department of Justice. https://www.dea.gov/sites/default/files/2018-11/DEA_PrescriptionForDisaster-2018ed_508.pdf

U.S. Drug Enforcement Administration. (2020a). *Drug fact sheet: Amphetamines.* U.S. Department of Justice. https://www.dea.gov/sites/default/files/2020-06/Amphetamines-2020_0.pdf

U.S. Drug Enforcement Administration. (2020b). *Drug fact sheet: Marijuana/cannabis* U.S. Department of Justice. https://www.dea.gov/sites/default/files/2020-06/Marijuana-Cannabis-2020_0.pdf

U.S. Drug Enforcement Administration. (2022a). *Drug fact sheet: Fentanyl.* U.S. Department of Justice. https://www.dea.gov/sites/default/files/2023-06/Fentanyl%202022%20Drug%20Fact%20Sheet-update.pdf

U.S. Drug Enforcement Administration. (2022b). *Drug fact sheet: Methamphetamines.* U.S. Department of Justice. https://www.dea.gov/sites/default/files/2020-06/Methamphetamine-2020_0.pdf

U.S. Food and Drug Administration. (2016). *Deadly synthetic drugs: The need to stay ahead of the poison peddlers.* https://www.fda.gov/news-events/congressional-testimony/deadly-synthetic-drugs-need-stay-ahead-poison-peddlers

U.S. Food and Drug Administration. (2017a). *Think before you ink: Are tattoos safe?* https://www.fda.gov/consumers/consumer-updates/think-you-ink-are-tattoos-safe

U.S. Food and Drug Administration. (2017b). *Tobacco control act.* https://www.fda.gov/tobaccoproducts/labeling/rulesregulationsguidance/ucm246129.htm

U.S. Food and Drug Administration. (2018). *Spilling the beans: How much caffeine is too much?* https://www.fda.gov/consumers/consumer-updates/spilling-beans-how-much-caffeine-too-much

U.S. Food and Drug Administration. (2020a, January 2). *FDA finalizes enforcement policy on unauthorized flavored cartridge-based e-cigarettes that appeal to children, including fruit and mint.* https://www.fda.gov/news-events/press-announcements/fda-finalizes-enforcement-policy-unauthorized-flavored-cartridge-based-e-cigarettes-appeal-children

U.S. Food and Drug Administration. (2020b). *FDA's youth tobacco prevention plan.* https://www.fda.gov/tobacco-products/youth-and-tobacco/fdas-youth-tobacco-prevention-plan#:~:text=Preventing%20youth%20access%20to%20tobacco,key%20role%20in%20protecting%20youth

U.S. Food and Drug Administration. (2023, March 29). *FDA approves first over-the-counter naloxone nasal spray.* https://www.fda.gov/news-events/press-announcements/fda-approves-first-over-counter-naloxone-nasal-spray

Waldman, E. G. (2023). *Just extracurriculars?* Minnesota Law Review, Forthcoming. https://ssrn.com/abstract=4378879

Wellershoff, G. (2018). Severe accidental intoxication by caffeine anhydrous. *Notarzt, 34*(2), 85–89. https://doi.org/10.1055/s-0044-100718

White, M., Brennan, E., Ren, K. Y. M., Shi, M., & Thakrar, A. (2018). Anabolic androgenic steroid use as a cause of fulminant heart failure. *Canadian Journal of Cardiology, 34*(10), 1369. https://doi.org/10.1016/j.cjca.2018.06.008

Whitten, P., Stoner, J., Aulakh, B. S., Verma, K., & Copelen, K. (2020). *#BeTheFirst Tobacco-Free Generation.* [Conference session]. American Thoracic Society Conference. https://doi.org/10.1164/ajrccm-conference.2020.201.1_MeetingAbstracts.A1078

Williams, J. F., & Lundahl, L. H. (2019). Focus on adolescent use of club drugs and "other" substances. *The Pediatric Clinics of North America, 66*(6), 1121–1134. https://doi.org/10.1016/j.pcl.2019.08.013

Wright, P. J., Herbenick, D., & Paul, B. (2019). Adolescent condom use, parent-adolescent sexual health communication, and pornography: Findings from a U.S. probability sample. *Health Communication, 35*(13), 1576–1582. https://doi.org/10.1080/10410236.2019.1652392

World Health Organization. (2017). *Health topics: Adolescent health.* http://www.who.int/topics/adolescent_health/en/

Yu, L., Mei, H., Shi, D., Wang, X., Cheng, M., Fan, L., Xiao, Y., Liang, R., Wang, B., Yang, M., & Chen, W. (2022). Association of caffeine and caffeine metabolites with obesity among children and adolescents: National Health and Nutrition Examination Survey (NHANES) 2009–2014. *Environmental Science and Pollution Research International, 29*(38), 57618–57628. https://doi.org/10.1007/s11356-022-19836-1

Zuckerman, M. (2007). The Sensation Seeking Scale V (SSS-V): Still reliable and valid. *Personality and Individual Differences, 43*(5), 1303–1305. https://doi.org/10.1016/j.paid.2007.03.021

part VII

School Health Services Leadership

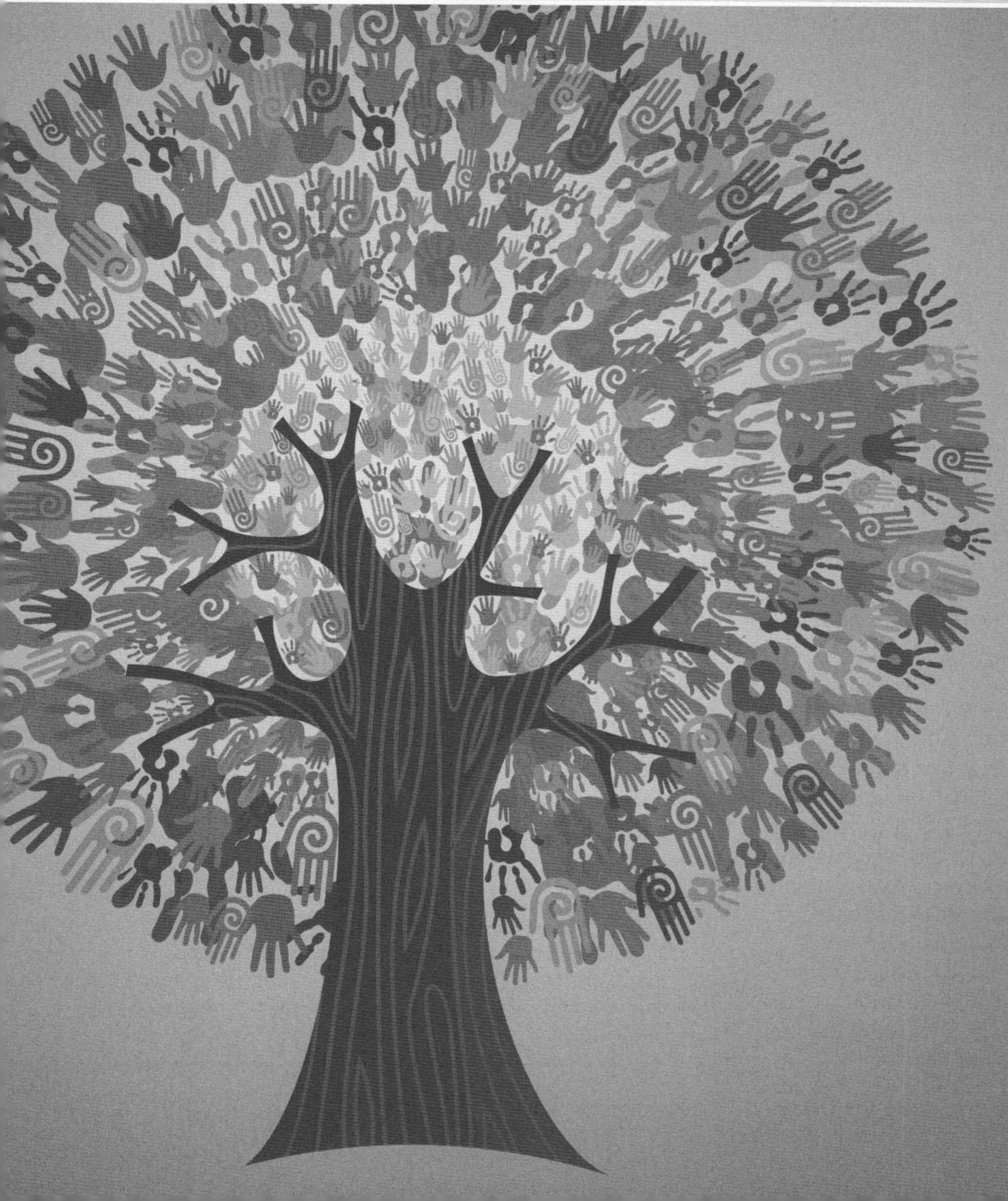

Chapter 30

Managing the School Health Office

Rachel McClanahan ▪ Cynthia Hiltz

CHAPTER OUTLINE

The school health office serves as the headquarters for the school nurse to carry out the activities outlined in the National Association of School Nurses' (NASN's) *School Nursing Practice Framework:* standards of practice, care coordination, leadership, quality improvement, and community and public health (NASN, 2024). The presence of a school nurse in a well-functioning health office on campus is crucial to advancing wellness and managing complex healthcare needs in the school population. Students and staff need to understand that the school health office is a safe and welcoming place where they will be cared for and respected by the school nurse.

Factors that affect the needs of a school health office include the number of students and others who access services; the health status of students and staff; the predominant social, economic, and health concerns of the community; school and district policies and procedures; and municipal, state, and federal laws. An assessment of the school health data can identify tertiary prevention issues such as students with special health needs and those who require ongoing nursing assessments and interventions in the school health office. An assessment of the school community can reveal health concerns and populations of students at risk where the school nurse can focus primary and secondary prevention efforts to improve health.

There is tremendous variability in school health offices and school health programs across the nation. NASN's *School Nursing: Scope and Standards of Practice* (2022b) provides a framework for evaluating school nursing practice according to national standards (see Chapter 3). The goal of this chapter is to assist the school nurse in establishing a safe environment and effective processes to

> **Focus on the Framework**
> **Leadership**
>
> **School Health Advisory Committee**
>
> The school nurse should provide leadership in identifying stakeholders and consultation for developing and directing a *School Health Advisory Committee.*
>
> - A multidisciplinary School Health Advisory Committee can be an important resource in planning effective school health services.
> - Members knowledgeable in health, child development, area health systems, and community resources can recognize the school's and community's needs and assets.

deliver efficient school health services in the health office to improve the health and education of children.

THE SCHOOL HEALTH OFFICE

The school nurse should be actively involved when health offices are being constructed, redesigned, or renovated to ensure that the space allows for safe and effective care delivery. One of the first considerations in setting up a school health office is the term that will be used to name the space. Many schools call this area the *nurse's office* or *school nurse's office.* It is important to be mindful of what the name suggests. Is there a nurse present in the office full time? Or does an unlicensed assistive personnel (UAP), such as a health clerk or aide, staff the office in addition to or in the absence of a nurse? There are important differences between a school nurse and a nurse in a school. Some models of school health service delivery employ registered nurses (RNs) or licensed practical/vocational nurses (LPNs/LVNs) whose role is limited to caring for school health office visitors and who do not assume the specialty role of the school nurse. Unless a full-time school nurse is consistently present, referring to the space as the *school health office* or *school health room* avoids indicating the full-time presence of a professional school nurse.

Some districts refer to the school health office as a *clinic,* which may cause confusion. Clinics typically are healthcare facilities that deliver primary or ambulatory care. Using the term *clinic* may create misperceptions that students can receive diagnostic and prescriptive services, such as in a primary care clinic, federally qualified health center, or school-based health center. Understanding the distinction between the care students receive from school health services and *school-based health centers* is essential since both focus on student health and well-being.

School health services provide triage, assessment, intervention, and referral for students with chronic conditions, illnesses, and injuries, as well as health promotion and prevention activities during the school day, at no cost to the student. Where allowed by state nurse practice acts, some of these services may be delegated by the school nurse to UAP.

In contrast, *school-based health centers* partner with school districts but are independent entities that deliver fee-for-service primary care services to individual children whose families pay out of pocket or who are covered as patients through their private or public health insurance, such as Medicaid. Typically located at or near middle or high schools, school-based health centers provide preventive and primary care services, such as well-child care (physicals and immunizations), urgent care, case management, counseling for mental and behavioral health problems and substance use, and oral health (NASN & School-Based Health Alliance, 2021) (see Online Materials OM30-1). School nurses with school-based health centers in their districts should partner with them closely so that students can access the quality health care they need. See Chapter 3 for more information on school-based health centers.

It is important that students, families, and the school staff clearly understand the roles and educational preparation of the school health office staff. The school nurse's name and credentials should be clearly posted outside and inside the school health office. The names, credentials, and titles of other health office staff should also be posted. Professional RN or LPN/LVN licenses should be displayed. NASN (2021a) recommends that the minimum educational level for entry into school nursing practice is a bachelor of science in nursing (BSN). Therefore framed copies of diplomas from accredited colleges of nursing highlight the BSN school nurse's level of expertise. RN or LPN/LVN badges can be clipped onto the school employee identification badge. Additionally, the school nurse's schedule should be posted to notify students, teachers, and families of the times the school nurse can be expected to be present. It is equally important that school health staff identify themselves and their position when greeting health office visitors or answering the phone. For example, parents/guardians may assume they are talking to the school nurse if a UAP answers the phone by saying, "School Nurse's Office. How may I help you?" To avoid confusion, persons answering the phone should clarify the name of the office and the title of who is answering, for example, "Hello, this is *Name,* the School Nurse. How may I help you?"; or "Good afternoon, school health office; this is *Name,* the health aide. How may I help you?"

Practice Connection

The American Academy of Pediatrics (AAP) offers two important programs to improve school health services toward the better health of the school community.

1. Enhancing school health services through *Training, Education, Assistance, Mentorship, and Support* (*TEAMS*; AAP, 2022b): A three-person team consisting of a district health services representative, a health department partner, and a physician partner can register and build skills to
   - Engage stakeholders and foster partnerships to support improvements in school health services.
   - Assess their current school health services policies, practices, and infrastructure.
   - Identify and prioritize key areas for improvement and develop a strategic action plan.
   - Implement and evaluate changes.
2. The *Health Services Assessment Tool for Schools* (*HATS*; AAP, 2022a) helps school nurses determine the strengths and weaknesses, infrastructure, policies, and procedures to support a high-quality health services program. This tool helps school nurses understand what works well and where improvements are needed to determine priorities and focus resources.

Location and Design

Many factors need to be considered when choosing an optimal location for the school health office, principally that the area should be used solely for school health services and allow for student and staff privacy. The office should be located on the ground floor in a readily available area to students, families, and staff. It should meet all Americans With Disabilities Act (ADA) accessibility and design standards requirements (U.S. Department of Justice [USDOJ], 2010). Attention should be given to the most current version of the law that stipulates specific requirements regarding minimizing architectural barriers, ramps, door width, shelves, and accessibility of computers and furniture. Bathrooms must meet specific requirements, including size; grab bars in stalls; raised toilet seats; sinks; soap and towel dispensers at an unobstructed and accessible height; and mirrors must be situated with the bottom edge 35 to 40 inches from the ground (USDOJ, 2010).

Ideally, the health office should be situated in a quieter area of the school, away from playgrounds, music rooms, gymnasiums, or noisy machinery, to promote a calm environment and optimize careful physical assessment. Locating the health office near student support personnel and administrators (e.g., principal, counselors, psychologists, social workers, etc.) allows collaboration with other school support professionals to meet student needs.

Space allocation for school health services varies widely from school to school. There must be enough room to carry out the essential functions of the health office. General requirements necessary to perform the functions of the school health office include the following:

- Private space where the nurse, student, teachers, parent, or others can confidentially discuss specific health issues and concerns
- Private examination area where the school nurse can conduct physical assessments of students, administer treatments or procedures, or where ill students can rest
- Isolated area for students suspected of having a communicable condition
- Adequate space for mandated health screenings (e.g., vision, hearing)
- Clean sink area for hand washing (not in a bathroom)
- Secure, readily accessible area for student emergency medications, a school emergency box, and a go kit
- Desk area with computer and phone for health office staff and the school nurse
- Storage area for health supplies, equipment, and health education materials
- Secured area with locked storage for paper records
- Secured area with locked storage for medications that meet state requirements for safeguarding controlled substances
- ADA-accessible bathroom with adequate ventilation, a toilet, and a sink with running water
- Cots separated by curtains hung from ceiling tracks for privacy

Basic space must be considered when designing a school health office. Some states have developed *adequacy standards* for schools that include the square footage allowed (both maximum and minimum) for a school health office, medication storage, security, and the number of bathrooms. The square footage recommendations for the school health office increase with the size of the school population. As was learned from the COVID-19 pandemic, it is essential to have a dedicated space where students suspected of contagious illness can be isolated. Figure 30-1 shows a sample school health office design.

Healthy Environment

Understanding a healthy environment's impact on student health is fundamental to school nursing practice (NASN, 2021b). The ventilation, temperature, and lighting of the health office environment will influence students' comfort and stress levels. Indoor air and water quality, building materials, and exposure to chemicals, waste, and mold are important considerations whether building or remodeling an old school. The school administrator and building engineers must ensure that the facility meets current building codes.

Other environmental considerations in the school health office include the availability of functioning

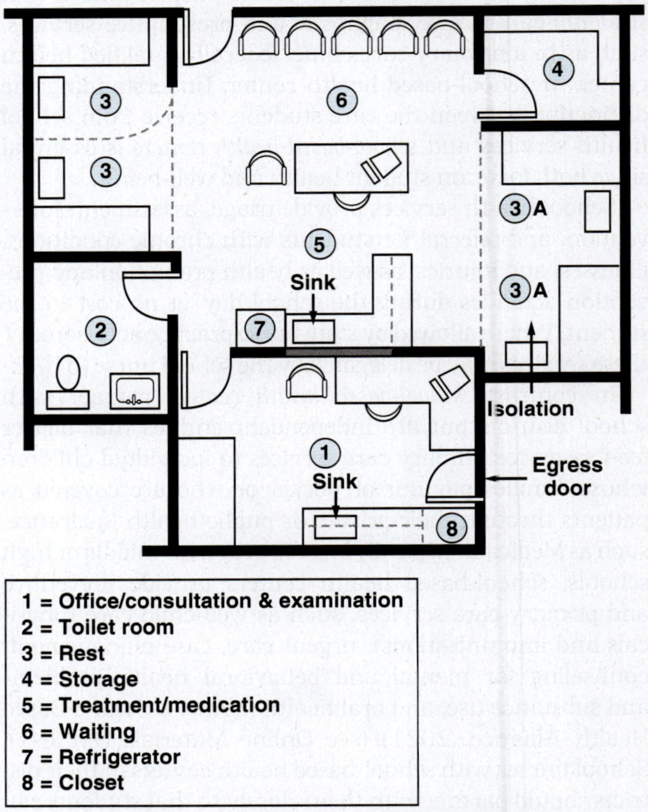

FIGURE 30-1. Sample school health office design.

windows to provide fresh air, ventilation, and natural light. Refer to local school district policy regarding whether windows can be opened. Assessment, treatment, storage areas, and bathrooms must be adequately lit. Dimmable lighting in at least one area is preferable when performing ophthalmological assessments and helpful when students are ill or resting. It is recommended that health offices be carpet-free because carpet is difficult to clean, can harbor moisture and mold, and may contain latex to which some students and staff may be allergic. Walls, flooring, and furniture should be sturdy and easy to clean and disinfect if soiled. Surfaces that are visibly soiled need to be cleaned and disinfected immediately. Bathrooms, desks, countertops, doorknobs, faucets, and phones should be routinely cleaned to prevent the spread of infection (see Chapter 13). The health office should be clean, neat, sanitary, and free of clutter to create an aesthetically pleasing, calming, and restful atmosphere.

The health office bathroom should only be used by students and staff requiring school health services. School staff who use the health office bathroom for convenience risk spreading the bacteria and viruses of sick children to themselves and others at school. The health office should have an additional "clean" sink outside the bathroom for hand hygiene before and after performing first aid or administering medications and procedures. Soap and paper towels and hand sanitizer should be easily accessible and located in the bathroom and near the office sink.

Safety and Hazard Reduction

Student and staff safety is a priority when designing the school health office. Visual supervision is critical in providing a safe and secure environment. The physical layout should allow the school nurse and health office staff to face the main door and visually supervise all health room areas while providing students privacy. Ideally there is a second egress door in case of emergency. The health office should have a well-marked, unobstructed, wheelchair-accessible entry. Hallway and exterior office windows should have blinds, shades, or curtains for privacy or safety in the event of a lockdown. Doors should have working locks with keys for the nurse and health office staff. Floors should be kept clean, dry, and uncluttered to prevent falls.

Connection to backup generator power in case of electrical interruption is an important safety consideration for students who require electric/electronic technology or whose medications require refrigeration. Battery-powered lighting and flashlights with extra batteries should be on hand in case of power outages.

Installation of a "panic button" may be prudent for help in case of an aggressive visitor, especially for school health offices that are distant or isolated from administrative offices. School- or district-provided radios or cellphones assist communications when phone lines are busy or down, when an emergency arises, or when the nurse needs to leave the health office. See Chapter 15 for information about emergency and disaster preparedness in schools.

Chemical products create hazards in schools. School nurses need to be aware of what chemicals are in the school and what hazards they present in the event of exposure, spills, or ingestion. This information is contained on *Safety Data Sheets* that must be relayed to poison control, medical providers, or emergency medical services. Schools may have a risk manager or health and safety officer who is in charge of hazardous materials management (U.S. Department of Labor & Occupational Safety and Health Administration [OSHA], 2015).

Cleaning, disinfecting, and sanitizing agents must effectively eliminate microorganisms. However, certain cleaning agents can aggravate pulmonary conditions and cause mucosal irritation, especially in students with allergies or asthma. Schools should use products that meet *Environmental Protection Agency Safer Product Standards* (U.S. Environmental Protection Agency, 2017). School nurses should follow the school's procedures for cleaning and verify that best cleaning practices are consistently practiced by custodial staff.

Standard precautions must be strictly followed to minimize the risk of bloodborne pathogen exposure to students and staff. Personal protective equipment (e.g., gloves, masks, eye protection, gowns) must be readily accessible. Needles should be disposed of in an approved sharps container with a biohazard label. The school nurse is responsible for ensuring that sharps containers are disposed of according to federal and state guidelines. OSHA has *Bloodborne Pathogen and Hazard Communications Standards* to protect employees in the workplace, including schools (U.S. Department of Labor & OSHA, 2003). See Chapter 13 for more information on pathogens, and cleaning, sanitizing, and disinfecting.

SCHOOL HEALTH OFFICE EQUIPMENT AND SUPPLIES

Each school district will have established protocols to follow when ordering equipment. The school nurse should advocate for adequate health office budgeting to secure the requisite health office supplies for student health and safety (see Budgetary Considerations in Chapter 32).

Storage

Adequate storage space is necessary for medical supplies, medications, and records. Locked cabinets for medications and hard-copy health records are required. All nonemergency medication should be in locked storage. Emergency medications should be kept in a *secure unlocked* and clearly labeled location to be easily accessible in an urgent situation. All medication should be secured after school hours. Controlled substances should be in a double-locked storage area (NASN, 2021c).

A refrigerator with a separate freezer compartment is essential for storing medications and cold packs; an icemaker is an added convenience. Storage of food items in refrigerators with medications should be avoided (i.e., snacks, supplies for students with diabetes, staff lunches, etc.). Refrigerators should be able to lock so that medications inside are secure (NASN, 2021c). Refrigerator temperature should be monitored regularly to ensure specifications for the medications.

School nurses are very creative in storing individual students' medication and supplies. Storage methods include small plastic containers with lids that can be stacked, a lockable storage cart with multiple drawers, sealable plastic bags, or pencil boxes labeled for each student. Containers can include copies of medical orders or emergency action plans. With parental/guardian consent, the student's picture can be included as an extra identifier to reduce the risk of medication error, especially during an emergency.

Equipment

The school nurse maintains an inventory of health office equipment that includes recording the purchase dates, purchase order number, and inventory control number for efficient tracking. The population of students and grade levels will dictate what equipment is needed. Students with special healthcare needs may require specific equipment at school that is written into their individualized educational program (IEP) or Section 504 plan. The party responsible for supplying the equipment (district or parent/guardian) may also be stipulated in the appropriate plan. A storage area in or near the health office to house larger equipment such as a wheelchair, stretcher, crutches, and other bulky items is necessary. Automated external defibrillators should be mounted at easily accessible locations and where most likely to be needed such as near the health office, in a central hallway, the cafeteria, and the gymnasium and playing fields. Schools with extended emergency medical service response times may have additional emergency equipment and medication stored in the health office. Box 30-1 shows a sample school health office equipment inventory.

Supplies

As with equipment, the school nurse maintains an inventory of health office supplies that varies depending on the population and needs of each school. Supplies may be recommended by a medical advisor or school nurse administrator, or supply inventory may be or determined by state/local protocols, annual budget constraints, needs assessment results, and staff input. An ongoing supply list overseen by the school nurse provides a record of supplies currently in the health office and those used during the school year. Box 30-2 shows a list of routine health office supplies.

Health offices should also have an emergency "Go Bag" or box that can be quickly retrieved and taken to the site of an emergency. See Chapter 15 for a sample school nurse emergency Go Bag content checklist.

The school nurse must understand the resources available to support school health services as each state and school district allocates funds differently. The general school budget typically funds school health services, equipment, and supplies. Therefore it is prudent for the school nurse to interact regularly with the principal or health services director to communicate the supply needs of the health office and understand the budget and ordering procedures. In large school districts, supplies may be bought in bulk as a cost-savings measure and stored in a central location. Needs must be prioritized, and resources used effectively and efficiently. Partnerships and sharing within districts can be leveraged to ensure that equipment is available to the school nurse when needed. For instance, screening dates can be staggered so that vision and hearing screening equipment can be shared to minimize overhead costs for purchasing and maintaining machines.

Funding sources may be pieced together from noneducational state funds, nonprofits, and other agencies. Medicaid, private insurance, state and federal grants, and foundation monies may cover specific equipment and supplies to provide school health services. The school nurse should work with the district finance department when considering grants, community partnerships, and local public health dollar applications and use to make sure documentation of funds used is adequate to meet the demands of the offer. Seeking new funding sources relieves some of the school's financial burden and engages new collaborative partners. Community connections and partnerships can be established to help fund specific supplies and equipment.

Accessing leaders and stakeholders in civic organizations, local hospitals, community centers, primary care providers, religious organizations, and business organizations may provide avenues of support for needed supplies. Nonprofit organizations related to specific health conditions can be strong partners. See Chapter 32 for more information on funding and budgeting school health services.

DOCUMENTATION AND RECORD-KEEPING

Whether paper or electronic, student health records are a critical component of safe, effective health care. Student health records include information related to demographics, immunizations, screening assessments, school physicals, and referrals. Student health records may contain a record of health office visits, treatment and medication orders from healthcare providers, and parent/guardian authorization for treatment and sharing of information. Student health records may also contain treatment and medication logs; medical reports; correspondence; incident or injury reports; information related to the delegation of care to unlicensed personnel (if state nurse practice acts allow); records of consultations with the student,

BOX 30-1
Health Office Equipment Inventory

Books:
Communicable Diseases Manual ________
Drug Manual ________
IHP Book ________
Pediatric Textbook ________
Physical Assessment Book ________
School Health Policy and Procedure Manual ________
School Nursing: A Comprehensive Text (4th edition) ________
School Health Legal Resource ________
Albuterol (if allowed by state law)
Automated external defibrillator with adult and child pads: Model ________ Serial # ________
Audiometer: Model ________ Serial # ________
Biohazard disposal box (sharps container)
Computer: Model ________ Serial #________
Cots/beds (sheets, blankets, and pillows)
CPR masks: adult # ________ and child # ________
Manual resuscitator (Ambu) bag masks: adult # ________ child # ________
Emesis basins, wash basins
Epinephrine (stock, if allowed by state law)
Eye charts (Sloan, LEA, HOTV)
Examining lamps, flashlights and batteries, penlight and batteries
Two first-aid kits: one emergency "go box" (bag), one disaster box
Narcan (stock, if allowed by state law)
Ophthalmoscope and otoscope: extra batteries and bulbs
Oxygen: capacity ________ Expiration date: ________
Peak flow meter: disposable mouthpieces #________ ________ ________
Personal protective equipment (gloves, masks, eye protectors, gowns)
Printer/fax/scanner ________
Pulse oximeter: Model ________ Serial #________
Refrigerator with separate freezer compartment
Scale
Stadiometer
Sphygmomanometer and three cuffs (child, adult, and extra-large adult cuffs)
Three stethoscopes: office, emergency, go bag
Suction unit
Thermometers: oral, tympanic temporal, extras for emergency go bag and disaster bag
Tympanometer: Model ________ Serial #________
Vision screening equipment: Model: ________ Serial # ________
Wheelchair, stretcher, crutches

BOX 30-2

Health Office Supply List*

DESCRIPTION

Automated external defibrillator (AED) replacement pads (adult and pediatric)
Alcohol (rubbing)
Alcohol swabs
Alcohol-acetone pads
Ammonia inhalants capsules
Applicator cotton-tipped 6-inch
Bags: brown paper, reclosable plastic bags (assorted sizes)
Bandages and dressing supplies (assorted sizes): adhesive (elastic) strip bandages, butterfly bandages, stretch gauze rolls, nonadherent pads, gauze sponges, transparent film dressing (4 × 4 inch), cloth tape rolls
Batteries (replacement for all equipment types)
Biohazard sharps container
Blanket
Bleach
Bleeding control kit with tourniquet
Cotton balls
Dental floss, waxed
Equipment calibration schedule
Disinfectant spray
Disposable eye cups
Disposable drinking cups—paper, 3- and 5-ounce
Epinephrine pen (0.15 mg, 0.3 mg) as allowed by law
Eyeglass repair kit and extra eyeglass screws
Eye wash bottle
Eye pads
Flashlight or penlight with batteries
Forceps: mosquito straight stainless, 5-inch; splinter stainless, 4-½-inch
Gauze sponges—2 × 2 inch, 4 × 4 inch
Gloves—vinyl, powder free—L, M, S
Hand sanitizer
Ice packs (may be purchased or made with ice in plastic resealable bags)
Liquid soap (hand and dish)
Medicine cups, 1 oz.
Nail clipper and nail brush
Normal saline for irrigation
Otoscope covers (disposable)
Orthodontic wax
Oxygen refill (or condenser)
Paper roll smooth, 18-inch
Peak flow monitor with disposable mouthpieces
Pillow (poly filled) with zippered cover
Pocket mask with one-way valve and case
Safety pins (small, medium, large)
Salt, noniodized
Skin lotion or cream (unscented)
Scissors: bandage, cuticle
Scissor-cuticle—3-¼ inch
Slings (or triangular cloth bandage with pins)
Splints (assorted sizes)
Surface disinfectant
Thermometer (probe covers)
Tissues
Tongue depressors
Tooth holders
White petroleum jelly
Additional items needed: ______________________

____

*Excel spreadsheets can be configured to track *Quantity on Hand*, *Quantity Needed*, and *Expiration Dates* as indicated.

parents, healthcare providers, and other support staff; and emergency action plans (EAPs), emergency evacuation plans, and individualized healthcare plans (IHPs), when indicated. Individualized education programs (IEPs) and Section 504 plans are considered educational records though they may contain health information.

Student health office visits should always be documented, including time of entry and exit, chief complaint, history of the problem, vital signs if appropriate, assessment, treatment or course of action, medication administration, referral, follow-up if needed, and disposition of the student. Staff health visits should also be recorded following the same criteria used for student data entry.

Health information on either paper or electronic forms must be confidential, secure, and accessible only by authorized staff with legitimate educational interests and protected from loss or destruction. Practices for maintaining the confidentiality of student health records must adhere to guidelines mandated by both the *Family Educational Rights and Privacy Act* (FERPA) and the *Health Insurance Portability and Accountability Act* (HIPAA; U.S. Department of Health and Human Services [USDHHS] & U.S. Department of Education, 2008). See Chapter 6 for more information about the legal confidentiality, privacy, and security mandates regarding protected health information in schools under HIPAA and FERPA.

Procedures for safe storage, limited access, retrieval of files, and access to technology that can transmit and receive electronic information securely should be developed and followed. Hard copy and written student records should be kept in locked cabinets and accessed only by authorized personnel with a legitimate educational interest. A log should be kept to record each time a record is accessed by someone with *legitimate educational interest* and by whom. The school nurse is considered the “keeper” of the health record and does not need to sign the log when accessing written health records. Procedures should be developed concerning who maintains student records, how they are managed, who is responsible for releasing records when a student withdraws from school or transfers to another school, who receives records when a student transfers into the school, how to transmit electronic records, and notification when records will be destroyed. The school nurse should collaborate with the district information system administrator to ensure adequate policies and procedures are in place.

School nurses are often asked by teachers, school staff, or administrators to provide a list of names of students with health conditions for safety purposes. Additionally, a common practice for convenience is to keep a running health office sign-in log on the same sheet or electronic tablet screen that records multiple students' names and the reason for their health office visit. However, compiling the health information of more than one student on a page is problematic and should be avoided. Such lists or logs are *not* FERPA-compliant and should not be used, because they contain the protected health information of more than one individual, which might be seen by other students, staff, and even visitors without consent or a legitimate educational interest in that information (Moss, 2023; Roberts & Zittoun, 2017). Importantly, such health office visit logs cannot be easily divided into discrete records for an individual student if requested by parents or subpoenaed for legal purposes.

School nurses should also avoid the use of "personal notes" that contain sensitive or protected information about a student or their family or that include a nurse's personal recollections or perspectives about a situation. Personal notes, or writing used to refresh one's memory, may be discoverable or subpoenaed in the event of a legal proceeding (Committee on the Judiciary, House of Representatives, 116th Congress, 2019). Best practice is to document objectively and in detail in the official health record (Moss, 2023).

Electronic Health Records

Most school nurses use *electronic health records* (EHRs). EHRs are made up of data entry fields that comprise a series of databases. These essential data collection tools allow school nurses to efficiently track and monitor the health status of individual students and school populations over time. The school nurse needs an up-to-date computer, printer, copier, scanner, and shredder in the school health office to manage health records effectively. NASN holds that all school nurses should have access to a software platform for student EHRs that "complies with standards of confidentiality, security, and privacy" (NASN, 2019). EHRs promote the meaningful use of school health data. According to NASN, "EHRs facilitate improved quality, safety and efficiency of care; lower the costs of healthcare; improve the privacy of health information; and allow greater patient access to their own health records" (2019, para. 3). EHRs must be password protected with role-designated log-in privileges to limit access by unauthorized personnel (Johnson, 2024). For instance, a health aide should only have access to specific fields such as routine health office visits or immunization data entry.

School nurses can use EHRs to create data-rich reports necessary to improve the quality of care and provide key data points for NASN's *National School Health Data Set* (see Chapter 5). The effective use of EHR reports allows school nurses to do the following:

- Describe health service activities: understand where and how much time is spent on activities.
- Develop evidence for practice: create and/or participate in quality improvement projects using existing data.
- Describe nurse-sensitive student outcomes: better understand the connection between nursing activities and student health outcomes.
- Analyze population health: create an accurate portrait of the population's health to prioritize activities.
- Evaluate the effectiveness of care delivery: examine outcomes and trends.
- Manage appropriate resource allocation: determine where resources should be used for best outcomes.

School and district-level electronic data can inform decision and policy making, budgets and resource allocation, and staffing needs. De-identified student data can be collected and aggregated in school health/nursing research (see Chapter 5). In some regions of the country, school nurses have access to hospital and clinic health records for students with special healthcare needs through shared electronic interfaces with healthcare systems. School nurses should work with district and health system administrators to develop relationships that improve the sharing of health information, which can lead to more comprehensive and coordinated care.

School nurses must be integrally involved in district decisions regarding purchasing and implementing EHRs. When choosing a quality system from a large field of competing EHR products, many factors must be considered. The functionality of EHRs depends on the quality of Internet connections, computer hardware and software, and operating systems. The level of customer support and the capacity to customize data entry and reporting functions are vital considerations when choosing an EHR platform.

EHR systems should have structured and unstructured methods of data entry. Structured methods facilitate data analysis and reporting by entering facts or figures that can be encoded in a standardized way, such as checklists, checkoffs, or dropdown menus. Ideally, structured data entry incorporates standardized nursing terminology, supporting the nursing process as integral to clinical decision making in school nursing practice. Standardized nursing language terminology also supports communication or *interoperability* between EHR programs for school nursing research. EHRs should facilitate unstructured data entry, such as notes or narrative text, to record nursing assessments, interventions, and evaluations (Johnson, 2024).

Some EHRs also include templates for IHPs, parent notifications, forms, and communications, as well as the capacity to upload related documents, such as records from healthcare providers' offices.

A growing number of "free" EHR products are emerging. The pros and cons of free cloud-based systems must be carefully evaluated (Wilburn, 2017). Such products are attractive to cash-strapped school districts for economic reasons. However, it is important for school districts and parents to understand that they may be required to authorize the sale of de-identified student data in exchange for the free service, the ramifications of which may or may not be fully understood by the consenting parties. These companies profit by selling the de-identified student data to other businesses, such as pharmaceutical companies, health products, or service providers. The ethical and legal considerations relating to questions such as who owns the data once exchanged, how the data are used, and how privacy, security, and confidentiality are maintained are complicated. Unforeseen technological advances or threats against cloud-based data are also factors. School districts should seek advice from informatics experts, district legal counsel, and state school nurse consultants before entering such agreements (Wilburn, 2017).

Ideally, EHRs are integrated with student educational records whereby the school nurse can enter generic health alerts visible to teachers when they access their students' individual records. Such alerts, often in the form of a symbol such as a medical cross or caduceus, should prompt teachers to seek relevant information from the school nurse and serve as a regular reminder that a student has a safety concern or chronic condition. Interoperability between school EHRs and the EHRs of hospitals and specialty and primary care providers improves care coordination and provider communication, with the recognition that the school nurse is an integral member of the student's healthcare team (Johnson, 2024).

School nurses can support confidentiality by providing universal training for teachers, school staff, or administrators on the most common student health conditions. School personnel should learn how to respond to any student who may present with a significant condition, such as students with diabetes, seizures, asthma, or anaphylaxis.

Faxes, E-mails, Texting, and Social Media Messaging

All forms of communication involve some level of risk. Student health information must be protected when sending or receiving faxed, e-mailed, or texted information between the school nurse, primary care providers, or parents. The school health office should have a fax machine and private fax number so that the school nurse can send or receive health information privately without it being viewed by other school staff. If a private fax for the school nurse is not feasible, there should be a plan with the main office to keep faxes with protected health information confidential.

Best practices regarding faxes and e-mail transmission include the following:

- Always use fax cover sheets and instruct senders of the requested information to do the same.
- Ensure the correct fax number or recipient address is entered on the fax so that information is not sent to an unknown location or person.
- Verify transmission on the fax machine.
- Keep a copy of the fax transmission receipts in a secure location or separate electronic or paper file folder; faxed health records should then be kept in the student's locked file.
- Personal student health information should not be sent via e-mail unless the system is encrypted or within the district-secured servers.
- Include a request for a "read receipt" for all e-mail communications that contain protected information. Similar precautions apply to scanned documents in e-mail. Questions should be referred to the district technology department.

Texting and social media offer numerous advantages for school nursing practice. It is often the fastest and most efficient way of communicating and sending information. Texting for professional communications at work should only be conducted on district-issued devices and should follow district policy. Protected health information should never be sent, received, or stored on a personal smart phone or tablet. Text messages may reside on

Practice Connection

E-mail and fax messages should include a formal signature from the school nurse, including full name, credentials, certifications, and contact information. Signatures should also contain a confidentiality statement as part of the signature. Here is a sample professional school nurse e-mail signature:

Your Name, BSN, RN, NCSN
School Nurse
School Name, District Name
Address
E-mail
Phone
Fax
Web site URL

CONFIDENTIALITY NOTICE: This e-mail, including attachments, is confidential and privileged information intended solely for the use of the designated addressee(s) and may be legally privileged communication. If you are not the intended recipient, you are hereby notified that any disclosure, copying, dissemination, or distribution of this communication, or taking any action in reliance on its contents is strictly prohibited by law. If you have received this communication by mistake, please notify [school nurse name] immediately and destroy all copies of this e-mail and attachments.

a mobile device or a server indefinitely, putting the information exchanged at risk for access by unauthorized third parties due to theft, loss, or recycling of the device. Special considerations are necessary before texting on social media platforms and should adhere to district policies. Without adequate safeguards, anyone with access to the device may have access to text messages. School nurses must address any privacy and security risks texting poses and consult with information technology specialists for guidance. School nurses should limit texting to general use to avoid sharing patient health information with students, parents, and school staff. Remember that documentation and correspondence by the school nurse is discoverable: the "e" in *electronic* also stands for ***e**vidence!*

When copiers, scanners, computers, cellphones, printers, and fax machines with memory are to be discarded, their memory must be deleted and destroyed before removing the device from the school health office.

Emergency Cards

Many school nurses keep separate emergency cards containing demographic information and emergency phone numbers, including home phone numbers, parent/guardian work numbers, and the phone numbers of individuals authorized to retrieve students from school if the parent/guardian cannot be reached. These cards often contain protected health information, such as allergies or chronic conditions, and phone numbers of primary care providers, dentists, or other healthcare professionals for each student in the school. The confidentiality and security of these cards should be maintained in the same manner as other health records. Although these cards are part of the student health record, many school nurses keep them in a separate folder or binder for easy access in an emergency.

Record Retention

School nurses should know the federal and state laws, regulations, and guidelines about school health record maintenance, storage, disclosure, and destruction. School nurses must adhere to state and district policies regarding the retention and destruction of records. School nurses should be familiar with what records are considered temporary and permanent and manage those records accordingly. Many states and school districts require a records manager or officer who oversees these complex processes and can serve as a resource to school staff, including the school nurse. State School Nurse Consultants are another good resource to help the school nurse determine the state requirements around student health records.

MEDICATION ADMINISTRATION

Many children require medication during the school day for chronic, acute, or episodic conditions or life-threatening emergencies. One of the primary responsibilities of school nursing practice is to ensure the proper and safe management and administration of medications to students. The most common conditions for which students take prescription medication at school align with the prevalence of those conditions in childhood—attention deficit-hyperactivity disorder, asthma, diabetes, mental health conditions, allergies, seizures, and bowel or bladder management issues (Maughan et al., 2017). School nurses should utilize NASN's (2021c) *School Nursing Evidence-Based Clinical Practice Guideline: Medication Administration in Schools* as a decision-making tool for developing and updating policies and procedures for medication management and administration. This clinical practice guideline provides detailed guidance in the following domains:

- Medication policies
- Delegation
- Training
- Security
- Medication administration
- As needed (prn) and over-the-counter (OTC) medications
- Emergency medications
- Alternative, off-label, and experimental medications
- Field trips and off-campus events
- Quality improvement
- Medication disposal
- Self-carry and self-administration
- Medication reconciliation
- Verbal orders

The *rights of medication administration* must be upheld in the school setting.

- Right student
- Right medication
- Right dose
- Right time
- Right route
- Right documentation

The school nurse is also responsible for conducting the *right* assessment and the *right* evaluation of the student's response to the medication related to efficacy and potential adverse effects. The school nurse provides the *right* health teaching to students and families about their medications. Furthermore, the school nurse has the right to refuse to give medications when sound nursing judgment demands.

Policies and Protocols

School districts need to have policies and procedures to ensure safe student medication management and administration based on established state regulations, state nurse practice acts, school policies, and evidence-based guidelines (AAP, 2009; NASN, 2021c). As the professionals responsible for medication management and administration, school nurses should lead these policy and procedure development decisions. Best practices for school medication management and administration include the following (not a comprehensive list). School nurses are encouraged to utilize NASN's (2021c) *School Nursing Evidence-Based Clinical Practice Guideline: Medication Administration in Schools* to develop a comprehensive best practice protocol.

- A written order from the licensed prescriber (e.g., physician, nurse practitioner) is required. Orders should contain all the information required for all prescriptions: student name, medication, indication, dose, route, and time. Prescriber name and contact information, pharmacy name and contact information, and medication expiration date should also be included.
- The school nurse should include additional information for safe administration, such as adverse reactions and student disposition following administration (especially for prn medications). School nurses should contact the provider immediately if clarification is needed or as changes in the student's status warrant. HIPAA allows school nurses to seek clarification about an ordered medication or treatment from the licensed prescriber without parental permission (USDHHS, 2013).
- Signed parent/guardian authorization for the medication administration includes HIPAA-compliant release of information language.
- Medication orders should be provided to the school nurse at least each school year or as changes in the student's status warrant.
- Stock medications (if allowed), including OTC and emergency medications, require standing licensed prescriber orders and parent/guardian permission. Parents should be notified when a stock medication is administered. Follow local or state regulations to ensure legal compliance.
- Changes in medication orders must be written and signed by the licensed prescriber. When allowed by school board policy, state law, and the state's nurse practice act, verbal orders may be taken by the school nurse and signed by the provider within district or state legal parameters.
- Medication should be delivered to school by the parent in the original container labeled with the student's name, name of the drug, drug dosage, route of administration, directions or interval for the drug to be given, name of the licensed prescriber, expiration date, and pharmacy contact information.
- Only medications that must be given during school hours should be administered. For example, antibiotics prescribed three times a day may be given at home before school, after school, and at bedtime depending on the student's school schedule. If medication compliance at home is inconsistent, administration at school may be warranted.
- Medication orders should be reviewed before each administration to ensure the *rights of medication administration*.
- Medication should not be prepoured or prepared early for later administration by another nurse or UAP.
- Medication administration should be completed on time and promptly documented. Medication may be administered 30 minutes before or after the scheduled time if ordered every 4 hours or more often (NASN, 2021c).
- Students should not receive the initial dose of a newly prescribed medication at school.
- Students receiving medication in a particular manner (e.g., via g-tube, crushed in food, etc.) require detailed instructions and training for the UAP, if delegated.
- All student medications, except emergency rescue medications, should be in a locked cabinet or drawer, and access should be restricted to specific school personnel. Medication cabinets should be securely mounted to a solid surface with solid doors (without glass/plastic windows) to prevent breaking and ensure privacy. Emergency rescue medications should be well labeled and readily accessible during school hours.
- The temperature of refrigerators used to store medications should be monitored. Like all medication storage, medication refrigerators should be locked. Medicines should not be stored with food.
- An inventory system of counting and tracking medications should be followed. Liquid medications can be tracked by documenting the original volume and subtracting the volume of each dose. All medications should be counted upon receipt, and the count should be documented. Controlled substances should be counted each time administered. Use a two-person counting method for controlled substances at least once a week. Controlled substances should be double-locked to ensure security (NASN, 2021c).
- A system to prevent, minimize, and remediate medication errors should be in place to promote a culture of safety. All medication errors should be reported and documented (AAP, 2009; NASN, 2021c).

See Figure 30-2 for a sample medication or special procedure order form. A downloadable and fillable version of this form is available in Online Materials OM30-2.

Delegation

The school nurse works closely with the educational team, student, family, and provider to ensure that students receive the medication or treatments they need to be in school learning. Unlicensed assistive personnel can play essential roles in assisting school nurses in meeting students' health needs, including administering medications in states where the practice is allowed. When school nurses delegate the responsibility for completing a task to a UAP, they maintain responsibility for outcomes. Whether or not to delegate is a nursing judgment that occurs only

Your School District
Licensed Prescriber and Parent/Guardian Request for Administration of Medicine or Special Procedure by School Personnel

Medications and special healthcare procedures may be administered at school when necessary for school attendance and cannot otherwise be accomplished. Prescribed medication may be administered by a nurse or by a non-health professional designee of the principal and delegatee of the school nurse. The medication should be brought to the school in a properly labeled container from a pharmacy (parents/guardians may request the pharmacist to dispense two labeled bottles, one for home and one for school). Submit this completed form and the medication or special equipment to the school nurse.*

Medical Order

1. Student ________________ Birth date ________________
2. Address ________________ School ________________
3. Condition for which the treatment is required ________________
4. Medication or procedure ________________

   Dosage, route, time, protocol, or special instructions ________________
5. Precautions, potential side effects, unfavorable reactions ________________
6. Disposition of student following medication or procedure administration (return to class, rest, home, 911, seek medical attention, contact prescriber) ________________
7. If applicable, indicate if the student has been instructed and is competent to self-carry those medications allowed by District Medication Policy (asthma inhalers, epinephrine pens) ________________
8. Request date ________________ Stop date ________________
9. Prescriber name (print) ________________ Signature ________________

   Address ________________ Phone ________________

Parent Authorization of Administration

I (we), the undersigned, parent/guardian of (student's name) ________________ request the administration of the above medication or procedure at school and consent to confidential communications between the licensed prescriber and the school nurse regarding treatment.

Name (print) ________________

Signature ________________ Relationship ________________

Phone #1 ________________ Phone #2 ________________

Email ________________

Filed in the Health Office by (print) ________________ **Initials** ________________

Title ________________ **Date** ________________

*As allowed by state nurse practice act delegation rules.

FIGURE 30-2. Sample school medication order form.

after a comprehensive assessment that carefully considers the benefits and risks to students. The *National Guidelines for Nursing Delegation* from the National Council of State Boards of Nursing (NCSBN) and the American Nurses Association (ANA) provides guidance on delegation best practices (2019). The school nurse should consider the *five rights of delegation* when deciding whether an activity is appropriate to delegate. The five rights of delegation outline the considerations for the transfer of accountability for tasks: (1) right task, (2) right circumstances, (3) right person, (4) right directions and communication, and (5) right supervision and evaluation (NCSBN & ANA, 2019). The school nurse is best positioned to understand and assess the student's condition and needs, what can or should be delegated, and to whom in specific situations.

When a decision is made to delegate to a UAP, the school nurse provides training, observes the UAP demonstrate competence, and monitors the UAP's performance on an ongoing basis (AAP, 2009; NASN, 2021c). NASN's (2021a) *School Nursing Evidence-Based Clinical Practice Guideline: Medication Administration in Schools* provides detailed guidance on training. LPNs or LVNs working in schools administer medication under their own license. Licensed practical and vocational nurses should have initial and annual training on medication administration in schools, including information about the scope of practice and clear direction on how to proceed if there are questions about the medication. See Chapters 6 and 31 for more detailed discussion about delegation.

Over-the-Counter Medications

OTC medications may provide symptomatic relief of a minor complaint, allowing a student to return to class and preventing a parent from missing work to come to administer the medication or take the student home. However, OTC medications are not without side effects and can pose a risk of harm to students and potential liability to school districts (AAP, 2009). OTC medications can mask signs of more serious health conditions or contagious diseases that require medical attention or exclusion from school.

School districts need clear policy and procedures on OTC medications that align with state rules and regulations. The policies and procedures applied to prescribed medications also pertain to OTC medications, namely that nurses do not administer medications without a licensed prescriber order (NASN, 2021c). Many districts partner with a school physician or cooperating primary care provider to write standing orders and protocols for stock OTC medications, particularly in upper grade centers like middle or high schools where students have more independence. Although this removes the need to get a separate medical order for each student, parent/guardian authorization for the administration of stock OTC medications should be required and must be renewed at least annually. The school nurse uses their professional judgment on whether to notify parents when their child receives an OTC at school (NASN, 2021c). Parental direction on notification can be sought when the OTC is ordered.

Medications Not Approved by the U.S. Food and Drug Administration

Medications that are not approved by the U.S. Food and Drug Administration (USFDA) include alternative, off-label, and experimental medications (USDHHS & NIH, 2021). School districts need clear policies regarding administering substances not tested for safety and effectiveness by the USFDA and not approved for use in children.

Often prescribed by homeopathic or naturopathic practitioners, **complementary and alternative treatments** include herbs, homeopathic medicines, traditional or cultural treatments, essential oils, salves, and dietary supplements (i.e., nutraceuticals). Claims of the benefits of complementary and alternative therapies abound in lay literature, on the Internet, and in advertisements. Scientific research has validated the effectiveness of very few of these products: some have been found *not* to be safe, and more rigorous research is lacking for many if not most products. Some parents assume that such products are inherently safe because they are labeled "natural." Many parents/guardians might be surprised to learn that the USFDA does not regulate alternative substances and products. Therefore in many instances the active ingredients and their strength, proper dosing, efficacy, and side effects may be unpredictable or unknown.

School nurses need to know whether they can accept medical orders from the prescribers of complementary or alternative treatments under the regulations of their state nurse practice acts. Even so, under an RN's scope of practice, the school nurse is responsible for knowing the active ingredients, proper dose ranges, actions, therapeutic value, and side-effect profile of medications administered. Because safety and efficacy cannot be determined for alternative and homeopathic medications, those substances should not be administered in schools (NASN, 2022a).

Districts should develop sound policies on **medicinal marijuana and cannabidiol** (CBD) products derived from the cannabis plants at school. Marijuana contains the psychoactive ingredient, tetrahydrocannabinol (THC). Marijuana remains federally prohibited and is considered by the U.S. Drug Enforcement Administration (USDEA) as

Did You Know?

The National Institutes of Health (NIH) Center for Complementary and Integrative Health describes the difference between complementary and alternative medicine as follows: "If a non-mainstream practice is **together with** conventional medicine, *'complementary.'* If a non-mainstream practice is used **in place of** conventional medicine, *'alternative'* (USDHHS & NIH, 2021, para. 3).

a Schedule I drug, which means that it has "no currently accepted medical use and a high potential for abuse." (n.d., para. 3). The American Nurses Association (2021) has a position statement to support changing the classification to a Schedule II controlled substance to allow research. However, as of 2023, 15 states permit legal use of medical marijuana, and 24 states permit legal use of both medical and recreational marijuana for adults only (Brittanica ProCon.org, 2023). Research has shown that school nurses from states that have legal marijuana laws have less concerns about medical marijuana administration at school than their peers from states where marijuana is not legal (Jochen & Holben, 2022).

Medical cannabis is sometimes considered to treat refractory seizures, irritability in children with autism spectrum disorder, Tourette syndrome, and spasticity, though such treatments remain controversial. Some states allow parents/guardians to take the child off school property and administer the medical cannabis, then bring the child back to the school. Some states allow the parent to administer medical marijuana at school, but not the nurse, because state nurse practice acts prohibit the administration of illegal substances. There is general agreement that medical marijuana should not be smoked on school grounds or in the building, but oral administration may be allowed in specific circumstances. Standards must be developed for prescribing, indications for use, dose, route, expected effect, possible side effects, and indications for stopping the medication. There also must be protection from criminal penalties for the school nurse and the student before the school nurse is allowed to administer marijuana.

Cannabidiol (CBD) products are derived from cannabis plants but do not contain THC, which produces the "high," and are not widely regulated. CBD may help relieve certain symptoms, such as pain in adults, though evidence of efficacy and safety in children is lacking. In 2018, the USFDA approved a pure plant-derived CBD compound, cannabidiol (Epidiolex), for treatment of medically refractory seizures in children with Dravet and Lennox-Gestaut syndromes, two severe forms of epilepsy in children (Abu-Sawwa & Stehling, 2020).

Though not universally embraced, the use of medical marijuana or CBD for children with certain health conditions is increasingly accepted and appears to benefit some children. More research is needed to establish safe use. Some states have legislation that permits students with certain conditions, such as intractable seizures, to receive medical marijuana at school. Medical marijuana is available in many delivery routes. Due to the frequency of changes to state laws, school nurses should check for current legislation and state nurse practice act stipulations on this issue. See Chapter 29 for more information on marijuana.

School nurses may occasionally be asked to administer **off-label or experimental medications.** *Off-label* is when a provider prescribes a drug that the USFDA has approved to treat a different condition or approved for a different age group or dose range. According to the American Academy of Pediatrics (2014, para. 1) "the term 'off-label' does not imply an improper, illegal, contraindicated, or investigational use." Off-label prescribing is legal and common: approximately 20% of prescriptions are written for off-label use (Agency for Healthcare Quality and Research, 2015). School nurses require accurate drug information that supports sound clinical decision making regarding the appropriateness and safety of carrying out medical orders for off-label medications at school. Again, clear policies and procedures for schools are needed for the administration of medication prescribed for off-label use.

Experimental medications are drugs used in clinical trials. Clinical trials in children require special human subject protections (National Institutes of Health, 2019). School nurses must communicate closely with families, investigators, and school administrators regarding the information needed by the school nurse and the best way to support students in clinical trials in adherence with school board policy.

School nurses can decline to carry out medical orders to administer non–USFDA-approved, off-label, or experimental medications, dosages that exceed manufacturer recommendations, and nutritional supplements (AAP, 2009; NASN, 2021c). The school nurse is obligated to record such requests and work with parents and providers to achieve an acceptable resolution of the conflicts. School nurses may face ethical dilemmas when prescribed drugs are not USFDA approved but no other effective treatment options are available for disabling conditions in children. NASN (2022a) holds that school nurses should advocate for evidence-based interventions. Additionally:

> *When deciding whether or not to incorporate the use of non-FDA approved therapies or dietary supplements into school nurse practice, it is important that the school nurse first determine what is known about the product, such as ingredients, precautions, recommended dose, and any potential adverse effects. Secondly, determine whether administration is allowable under federal and state law, including applicable state nurse practice acts, and district policy. Additionally, complementary and integrative therapies in the school setting should not disrupt the educational process. (NASN, 2022a, para. 4)*

As indicated, school districts are advised to seek the counsel of state school nurse consultants, school physicians, district attorneys, and even medical ethicists when developing policies on administering non–USFDA-approved substances at school.

Emergency Medications

Some students require medication that must be given immediately in a life-threatening situation at school. During the event, a school nurse may not be available to respond immediately and/or emergency medical services might have prolonged response times. Therefore the school nurse develops an emergency action plan (EAP) for students with known life-threatening conditions and trains the delegated school staff to act according to the plan, including medication administration under very specific parameters. Emergency medication administration policy and procedures should adhere to state and local laws and the nurse practice act. Examples of rescue medications ordered specifically for individual students include insulin, glucagon, epinephrine, naloxone, bronchodilators, diazepam, and oxygen. Schools must ensure that the student's parents/guardians provide an adequate supply of emergency medication. Emergency medications should be stored securely and clearly labeled but need to be immediately accessible (AAP, 2009).

Increasingly, schools have standing medical orders for undesignated or *stock* emergency medications for students with known life-threatening conditions who do not have medication at school or for students who may experience an unanticipated life-threatening event at school. Many families cannot afford the cost of providing expensive rescue medications for school. Additionally, approximately 20% to 25% of students who experience anaphylaxis at school have no documented history of severe allergy (McCaughey et al., 2020). School districts need to collaborate with a medical advisor to provide standing orders when undesignated emergency or rescue medication use is allowed by state law and/or school board policy. Since the medical orders are not for specific individual students, these medications are "stocked" for use on any students who require the rescue medication in an emergency. Epinephrine, followed by albuterol inhalers and glucagon, are the most commonly stocked emergency medications for undesignated use (McCaughey et al., 2020). Undesignated nasal naloxone is increasingly stocked, as are glucagon and oxygen.

School districts must ensure compliance with the state rules and regulations surrounding the acquisition, storage, record-keeping, and disposal of stock rescue medications, as well as requirements for reporting to local or state authorities after an administration. In states that lack regulations on stock rescue medication in schools, school nurses work with legislators to advocate for allowing this life-saving practice (Yonkaitis & Jacobs, 2022).

The school district needs to ensure that policies and protocols are in place to direct the proper use of undesignated rescue medications, including when to use them and who may administer them. Standardized training for UAP designated to administer an emergency medication must be in place, including symptom recognition and proper medication administration. Competency in skills demonstration by UAP should be documented. An additional consideration is whether stock rescue medications are available during after-school activities.

Self-Administration of Medications

State regulations and/or district policies and guidelines often govern the right of students to carry and self-administer medications. Districts should follow state laws regarding student self-carry and self-administration of medications and develop policies to ensure safety. Students who demonstrate the ability to safely carry and self-administer medications, especially emergency medications, should be allowed to do so. Following district procedures, the school nurse is responsible for assessing the student's abilities and risks to self-carry and for teaching the necessary self-care skills. The student must be developmentally able to accept responsibility, understand when the medication is indicated, demonstrate proper medication administration techniques, and know when to seek further help. The school nurse should provide periodic monitoring and education to ensure these skills are maintained. School nurses should consider obtaining an extra dose of the self-carry, self-administered medication for the health office. Students should not be allowed to carry controlled substances. Self-carry medications should always be with the student and not left unattended (NASN, 2021c). Schools may require a contract between the student and the school before allowing a student to self-carry medications. Figure 30-3 shows a sample student self-carry contract.

Field Trips

Some students may need medication or special procedure administration during field trips. Because field trips are part of the school day, it is the school's legal responsibility to ensure that students receive their medications on field trips. All established district policies and procedures related to medication administration also apply during field trips (NASN, 2021c). Students should be allowed to self-carry and self-administer if all established requirements have been met. The nurse should ensure that the UAP assigned to administer medications has the appropriate training and skills to give the medication safely and document administration. Medication should be in an original container (NASN, 2021c). Additionally, there should be mechanisms for safe storage of the medication and any associated supplies. If nursing judgment is needed to administer the medication or procedure, a nurse or a substitute nurse should attend the field trip. Based on the healthcare demands or potential risks of the student population, school nurses should make prudent decisions about whether they can personally go on the field trip and leave the building unattended or whether they need to hire another nurse. Parents/guardians may attend the field trip to administer medications if they wish but must adhere to school policy regarding field trips; family members or caregivers cannot be required to attend field trips to administer medications. If proper field trip accommodations cannot be made and the student cannot participate, the fieldtrip should be canceled—holding the student back at school and providing alternative activities is considered a denial of their right to a free and appropriate public education (FAPE) and is therefore unacceptable.

Medication Errors

NASN's *School Nursing Evidence-Based Clinical Practice Guideline: Medication Administration in Schools* (2021c) is a standardized and evidence-based process for medication

Your School District
Student Contract to Self-Carry and Self-Administer Medication

Student ______________________________ Date __________

School ______________ Grade ________ Teacher/Homeroom __________

Health issue: ______________________________

Symptoms requiring medication: ______________________________

Medication ______________________________

Emergency medication may be self-carried and self-administered if the following conditions are met:

Yes	No	Condition for Permission to Self-Carry and Administer Medication
		Complete and current *Physician/Parent Request for Administration of Medicine or Special Procedure by School Personnel* form on file
		Student verbalizes adequate understanding of health condition requiring medication self-administration
		Student verbalizes triggers, exposure, or predisposing factors that precede symptoms
		Student states symptoms that require self-administration of medication
		Student states proper dosing and prescribed timing of medication
		Student demonstrates proper technique/skills for medication administration
		Student agrees to carry medication in appropriate manner and not to share medication with other students
		Student agrees to seek immediate adult help or go directly to the health office as indicated if no relief of symptoms following self-administration of medication
		Student acknowledges that failure to demonstrate the above responsibilities may result in losing medication self-carry and administration privileges

Student Signature ______________________________ Date: __________

School Nurse (print) ______________ Signature ______________ Date: __________

See Parent and MD signatures on Medication Authorization form.

FIGURE 30-3. Sample student medication self-carry contract.

administration that can help to decrease medication errors. According to these guidelines, "A medication error is any preventable event that may cause or lead to inappropriate medication use or patient harm while the medication is in the control of the healthcare professional, patient, or consumer" (NASN, 2021c, p. 8). Medication errors in school include missed doses, wrong time, wrong dose, wrong medication, wrong student, spilled or dropped doses, administration without appropriate authorization, incorrect or missing documentation, and improper storage of temperature-controlled medications. *Whether or not a medication error causes an adverse outcome for the student, all medication errors should be documented and evaluated.* School districts should use a standardized error reporting system to identify contributing factors, risk-reduction strategies, and corrective actions (NASN, 2021c). A *culture of safety* that includes a nonpunitive reporting system focused on decreasing the stigma surrounding reporting medication errors should be established. A culture of safety in an institution is focused on increased vigilance for medication errors and establishing a just culture through training and continuous quality improvement activities (NASN, 2021c). Support for the licensed provider or UAP who experiences a medication error should also be provided.

When students forget, neglect, or refuse to come to the health office for medication, every effort should be made to find the student and administer the medication in a timely fashion. Failure to give a medication may adversely affect the student's health, affect the student's learning, and put the school at risk for litigation. The school nurse should work with the student on strategies to remember to come to the health office and coordinate with teachers and other school personnel to remind the student to go to the health office or locate the student to give the medication. If cellphone use is allowed, a student can easily set a reminder alarm.

Medication administration records should be systematically reviewed to identify incidents and issues. EHRs can be programmed to notify the school nurse of pending scheduled medications and alert the nurse to missed doses. EHRs can also recognize errors that might not otherwise be reported. School nurses must carefully look at medication error reports to identify human and system factors that need improvement. Figure 30-4 shows a sample medication error reporting form. See Chapter 31 for more information on medication errors.

Unused Medications

Schools must make every effort to return medications to the parents/guardians at the end of the school year, when the child transfers to another school, or if the medication is discontinued or expired. Nurses should try various methods of informing parents/guardians of the date medications must

Your School District
Medication/Procedure Incident Report

A medication error is defined as failure to administer the prescribed medication or procedure according to medical orders and in accordance with accepted practice. *Use reverse side if necessary.*

Name of Student		Grade	Date
Teacher/Homeroom		School	
Home Address Street, City, State, Zip			
Medication	Dose	Route	Scheduled Time
Name of Licensed Prescriber		Reason Medication was Prescribed	
Date/Time of Incident		Person Administering Medication	
Describe the incident and how it occurred:			
Immediate Action Taken:			
Describe the Outcome:			
Licensed Prescriber		Notified ☐ Yes ☐ No Date/Time	By whom:
Parent/Guardian		Notified ☐ Yes ☐ No Date/Time	By whom:
Supervising School Nurse		Notified ☐ Yes ☐ No Date/Time	By whom:
Other Persons Notified		Date/Time	By whom:
Name (Print)		Signature	Date
Supervising School Nurse follow-up:			
Name (Print)		Signature	Date

FIGURE 30-4. Sample medication/procedure incident report form.

be claimed or they will be destroyed, such as newsletters, announcements, notes sent home, phone calls, or e-mails. Ideally, parents/guardians should pick medication up from the health office. School nurses should document on the medication record or medication return form the receiving parent/guardian or designee's name, the name of the school personnel dispersing the medication, and the date and time. Both parties should sign the form. Sometimes it is not practical for parents/guardians to pick up medication. If medications are sent home with a student, a secure process should be followed and documented including permission from the parent/guardian, secure packaging, and counts of the amount sent. Controlled medications should not be sent home with minor students.

The medication must be properly disposed of if medications expire or remain unclaimed after the specified pick-up date. School districts can partner with USDEA-authorized collectors such as retail pharmacies, hospital or clinic pharmacies, or local law enforcement agencies who have community-based drug "take-back" programs to collect and destroy medications (U.S. Food and Drug Administration [USFDA], 2020). If no local take-back program is available, unclaimed medication can be thrown in the trash if the following steps are taken:

1. Count and record the number or volume of unclaimed drugs.
2. Destroy the medication.
   a. Remove medication from the original container.
   b. Place medication into a sturdy sealable container.
   c. Medication destruction products can be purchased or mix the medication with coffee grounds or cat litter and add water to the mix.
3. Seal the container tightly.
4. Dispose of the container in the regular trash.
5. Remove or scratch out the label from the student's empty medication bottle and discard it.
6. Document in the student record that the medication was discarded (USFDA, 2020).

School nurses should document the disposal of medication, including controlled substances, noting the amount of medication disposed of, using a two-person method including signatures.

CONCLUSION

School nurses provide vital services that promote optimal student health and learning. The school health office is the headquarters for these activities. Students, families, and staff benefit when school health offices are well-designed, clean, welcoming, and safe spaces. To fulfill their professional responsibilities, school nurses need adequate space, staffing, resources, and supplies. School nurses engage in continuous quality improvement by having school health office policies, processes, and procedures that follow legal regulations and nursing best practices. A well-managed school health office supports student health, safety, privacy, dignity, wellness, and well-being. The school nurse is recognized as the health expert in the school community when quality nursing services are delivered from an exemplary school health office.

The Editors gratefully acknowledge the work of the 3rd edition chapter authors, Rachel McClanahan, Robin Adair Shannon, and Pamela Kahn.

References

Abu-Sawwa, R., & Stehling, C. (2020). Epidiolex (cannabidiol) primer: Frequently asked questions for patients and caregivers. *The Journal of Pediatric Pharmacology and Therapeutics, 25*(1), 75–77. https://doi.org/10.5863/1551-6776-25.1.75

Agency for Healthcare Quality and Research. (2015). *Off label drugs: What you need to know.* https://www.ahrq.gov/patients-consumers/patient-involvement/off-label-drug-usage.html

American Academy of Pediatrics. (2009). Policy statement: Guidance for the administration of medication in school. *Pediatrics, 124*(4), 1244–1251. http://publications.aap.org/pediatrics/article-pdf/124/4/1244/1012175/zpe01009001244.pdf

American Academy of Pediatrics. (2014). Off-label use of drugs in children (Policy Statement). *Pediatrics, 133*(3), 563–567. https://publications.aap.org/pediatrics/article-pdf/133/3/563/1100558/peds_2013-4060.pdf

American Academy of Pediatrics. (2022a). *Health services Assessment Tool for Schools (HATS).* https://www.aap.org/en/patient-care/school-health/teams-enhancing-school-health-services/health-services-assessment-tool-for-schools-hats/

American Academy of Pediatrics. (2022b). *Training, Education, Assistance, Mentorship and Support (TEAMS) to enhance school health services.* https://www.aap.org/en/patient-care/school-health/teams-enhancing-school-health-services/

American Nurses Association. (2021). *Therapeutic use of marijuana and related cannabinoids.* https://ojin.nursingworld.org/table-of-contents/volume-27-2022/number-1-january-2022/therapeutic-use-of-marijuana/

Britannica ProCon.org. (2023, June 5). *State-by state medical marijuana laws.* https://medicalmarijuana.procon.org/legal-medical-marijuana-states-and-dc/

Committee on the Judiciary, House of Representatives, 116th Congress. (2019, December). *Federal rules of evidence.* U.S. Government Publishing Office. https://www.uscourts.gov/sites/default/files/federal_rules_of_evidence_-_dec_1_2019_0.pdf

Jochen, A., & Holben, D. (2022). School nurse perspectives of medical cannabis policy in K-12 schools: An exploratory descriptive study. *Journal of School Nursing.* https://doi.org/10.1177/10598405221136

Johnson, K. H. (2024). School health records. In C. A. Resha & V. L. Taliaferro (Eds.), *Legal resource for school health services* (pp. 123–150). SchoolNurse.com

Maughan, E., McCarthy, A. M., Hein, M., Perkhounkova, Y., & Kelly, M. W. (2017). Medication management in schools: 2015 survey results. *Journal of School Nursing, 34*(6), 468–479. https://doi.org/10.1177/1059840517729739

McCaughey, R. A., McCarthy, A. M., Maughan, E., Hein, M., Perkhoundkova, Y., & Kelly, M. W. (2020). Emergency medication access and administration in schools: A focus on epinephrine, albuterol inhalers, and glucagon. *Journal of School Nursing, 38*(4), 326–335. https://doi.org/10.1177/1059840520934185

Moss, E. (2023). Legal issues 101: Documentation and school records. *NASN School Nurse, 39*(2), 84-87 . https://doi.org/10.1177/1942602X231186095

National Association of School Nurses. (2019). *Electronic health records: An essential tool for school nurses to keep students healthy. Journal of School Nursing, 40*(3), 352-354, https://doi.org/10.1177/10598405241241804

National Association of School Nurses. (2021a). *Education, licensure, and certification of school nurses* (Position Statement). Author.

National Association of School Nurses. (2021b). *Environmental health* (Position Statement). Author.

National Association of School Nurses. (2021c). *School nursing evidence-based clinical practice guideline: Medication administration in schools.* Author. https://cdn.fs.pathlms.com/eMfakewQq20XiLuoim9w

National Association of School Nurses. (2022a). *Complementary and integrative therapies* (Position Statement). Author.

National Association of School Nurses. (2022b). *School nursing: Scope and standards of practice* (4th ed.). Author.

National Association of School Nurses. (2024). A contemporary framework update for today's school nursing landscape: Introducing the School Nursing Practice Framework. *NASN School Nurse, 39*(3), 140-147. https://www.doi.org/10.1177/1942602X241241092

National Association of School Nurses & School-Based Health Alliance. (2021, May). *Joint statement: School nursing & school-based health centers. Working together for student success.* https://www.nasn.org/nasn-resources/professional-practice-documents/joint-endorsed-statementshttp://www.sbh4all.org/school-health-care/aboutsbhcs/

National Council of State Boards of Nursing & American Nurses Association. (2019). *National guidelines for nursing delegation.* https://www.ncsbn.org/NGND-PosPaper_06.pdf

National Institutes of Health. (2019). *Vulnerable and other populations requiring additional protections.* https://grants.nih.gov/policy/humansubjects/policies-and-regulations/vulnerable-populations.htm

Roberts, W. J., & Zittoun, G. J. (2017). Family Educational Rights and Privacy Act ("FERPA")/Health Insurance Portability and Accountability Act ("HIPAA"). In C. A. Resha & V. L. Taliaferro (Eds.), *Legal resource for school health services* (pp. 125–135). SchoolNurse.com

U.S. Department of Health and Human Services. (2013). *HIPAA administrative simplification: Regulation text, 45 CFR, Parts 160, 162 and 164.* https://www.hhs.gov/sites/default/files/hipaa-simplification-201303.pdf

U.S. Department of Health and Human Services & National Institutes of Health, National Center for Complementary and Integrative Health. (2021). *Complementary, alternative, and integrative health: What's in a name.* https://www.nccih.nih.gov/health/complementary-alternative-or-integrative-health-whats-in-a-name

U.S. Department of Health and Human Services & U.S. Department of Education. (2008). *Joint guidance on the application of the Family Educational Rights and Privacy Act (FERPA) and the Health Insurance Portability and Accountability Act of 1996 (HIPAA) to student health records.* https://www2.ed.gov/policy/gen/guid/fpco/doc/ferpa-hipaa-guidance.pdf

U.S. Department of Justice, Civil Rights Division, Disability Rights Section. (2010). *2010 ADA standards for accessible design.* https://www.ada.gov/law-and-regs/design-standards/2010-stds/

U.S. Department of Labor & Occupational Safety and Health Administration. (2003). *Model plans and programs for the OSHA Bloodborne Pathogens and Hazard Communications Standards.* Retrieved from https://www.osha.gov/Publications/osha3186.pdf

U.S. Department of Labor & Occupational Safety and Health Administration. (2015). *OSHA quick card: Hazard communication safety data sheets.* https://www.osha.gov/Publications/HazComm_QuickCard_SafetyData.html

U.S. Drug Enforcement Administration. (n.d.). *Drug scheduling.* https://www.dea.gov/drug-information/drug-scheduling

U.S. Environmental Protection Agency. (2017). *Healthy schools, healthy kids.* https://www.epa.gov/schools

U.S. Food and Drug Administration. (2020). *Disposal of unused medicines: What you should know.* https://www.fda.gov/drugs/safe-disposal-medicines/disposal-unused-medicines-what-you-should-know

Wilburn, A. (2017). Nursing informatics: Ethical considerations for adopting electronic records. *NASN School Nurse, 33*(3), 1–4. https://doi.org/10.1177/1942602X17712020

Yonkaitis, C. F., & Jacobs, J. (2022). Undesignated glucagon in Illinois: An issue of access and equity. *NASN School Nurse, 37*(6), 331–336. https://doi.org/10.1177/1942602X221120

Chapter 31

Supervising School Health Services

Yvonne Clarke ▪ Laurie G. Combe

CHAPTER OUTLINE

Effective program management is essential to the productive functioning of all organizations, including schools. School health systems are affected by trends in local and national economic, cultural, legal, business, political, scientific, public health, and health systems. Consequently, policies and practices, service models, and job performance expectations require regular review. Administrators of school health services must function within the mission, vision, and core values of the organization. The role of school health leadership is to support student health and academic success and to provide high-quality, cost-effective, and ethical school health services.

Important factors that determine school health staffing patterns include budgets, student enrollment, health acuity of students, the number and skill of available staff, the number of schools, and the values of district administration. There are no national mandates for school nurse staffing, preparation, or credentials. One or more persons in a school district may perform the duties of a school health staff supervisor. School health staff may be directed and managed by various levels of school nurses or nonnurses with titles such as school health or school nursing administrator, director, supervisor, or manager. Therefore this chapter addresses multiple audiences and aims to provide guidance on the roles and responsibilities of being an effective school health services leader.

HEALTH SERVICES ROLES

School health services staffing varies by state, region, county, and school district. School nurse staff may be directly employed by schools, school systems, state agencies (Nelson, 2023), health departments, or hospital systems.

When school nurses are employees of agencies external to school systems, they must adhere to all programmatic and professional legal expectations of both agencies. Before initiating services, incongruent policies and practices must be negotiated with memoranda of agreement or memoranda of understanding. The school nurse must keep in mind the professional obligation to adhere to federal and state laws regarding school health.

There is a difference between a school nurse and a nurse in a school. A school nurse should be licensed as a registered nurse (RN). Licensed practical/vocational nurses (LPNs/LVNs) typically provide routine care to students under the supervision of an RN according to the stipulations of their state nurse practice act. Additionally, some jurisdictions require the school nurse to have a state specific or national school nurse certification in order to practice in this role. School nurse supervision also varies. Ideally, an RN with an advanced nursing degree functions in the school health services director or administrator role. The school health services supervisor may be a lead nurse who may also have a campus to manage. However, campus principals or individuals without nursing licensure are also identified as supervisors in some school districts. With the variety in health services supervisory staffing, this chapter aims to provide information and resources for a variety of circumstances.

Job Descriptions

Job descriptions detail the knowledge, skills, and abilities required of the person filling a position. The job description should provide the employee with information about the culture and vision of the organization, their direct report, compensation scale, and expectations of the role's work priorities, competencies, and duties. Accurate job descriptions provide a sound basis for performance evaluations. They should be clearly written using action verbs (i.e., assesses, provides, manages) that provide measurable descriptions of duties. Job descriptions are also important tools when disputes arise between the employer and the employee about the scope or quality of the work performed. Job descriptions may be used to support management decisions for increased school nurse responsibility, remediation, or removal of an employee from a position. Conversely, job descriptions can benefit employees should they be asked to perform duties they consider outside the parameters of their role. See Box 31-1 for a sample school nurse job description.

School nurse job descriptions will vary depending on the role, school district policies, supervisory department, and overall responsibilities. Factors influencing duties may include characteristics of the school population, enrollment, available school and community resources, and federal and state regulations. Nurses planning to practice in the school health field should recognize that health care is not the primary focus of the schools. Therefore the full scope of the school nurse role is difficult to appreciate from the nonnurse administrator perspective. Administrators with limited understanding of the role should not be responsible for creating the school nurse job description, organizational standards, and nurse evaluation (Reising & Cygan, 2022).

The National Association of School Nurses' (NASN's) *School Nursing Practice Framework* (2024), hereinafter referred to as the *Framework*, provides five tenets of school nurse practice: *Standards of Practice, Care Coordination, Community/Public Health, Leadership,* and *Quality Improvement* (see Chapter 3). When comparing school nurse job descriptions to this framework, care coordination was identified as the primary duty of the school nurse (57%), followed by community/public health (29%). However, leadership and quality improvement tenets were missing from or underrepresented in the school nurse job descriptions (Reising & Cygan, 2022). In order to appreciate the

BOX 31-1
Sample School Nurse Job Description

POSITION TITLE: School Nurse, District Health Services

POSITION FUNCTION/PURPOSE: Enhance the educational process by removing health barriers to learning through planning, implementing, coordinating, monitoring, and evaluating health services in a specific school(s) assignment. Promote the health of the student body, staff, and school community.

ACCOUNTABILITY: Reports dually to health services nursing supervisor and building principal 185 days/10 months.

QUALIFICATIONS: Current state licensure as a registered nurse. Current cardiopulmonary resuscitation (CPR)/automated external defibrillator (AED) certification. Graduate of an accredited school of nursing. A bachelor of science degree in nursing is required. Proficient computer skills: word processing, e-mail, and data entry into software platforms.

Minimum of 1 year of RN experience required.

MAJOR RESPONSIBILITIES: Duties include but are not limited to the following:

- Establish and maintain the school health office to deliver comprehensive school health services according to *School Nursing Standards of Practice*, the state nurse practice act, and departmental procedures and protocols.
- Provide episodic and emergency health care to ill or injured students, staff, and visitors.
- Coordinate care for individual students and student populations via family engagement, education,

BOX 31-1

Sample School Nurse Job Description—cont'd

collaboration with interprofessional stakeholders, address infrastructure needs and advocate for improvements. Collaborates with other school professionals, family, caregivers, community, and healthcare providers to maximize communication and deliver culturally sensitive care.

- Assist students, families, and employees to achieve optimal levels of wellness through health assessments, medical referrals, interpretation of medical data, health counseling, and social services to students.
- Provide case management of students with special healthcare needs, including administration of medications and special procedures according to medical orders. Develop and implement individualized healthcare plans. Develop and train need-to-know school staff on emergency action plans for students with potentially life-threatening conditions.
- Serve as a member of the interprofessional student support team: assess the impact of students' physical and mental health needs on learning and school participation; develop and implement individualized health goals and interventions for students receiving special education services or Section 504 plan accommodations.
- Maintain communicable disease prevention and control measures in accordance with state regulations, local health department protocols, and district policies and department protocol. Conduct communicable disease surveillance and reporting. Manage the student immunization compliance program on campus. In case of communicable disease outbreaks, assist the health department in a school level immunization campaign to protect students and others in the school community.
- Communicate with students and families in culturally sensitive exchanges. Provide health information and resources for students, families, and staff at appropriate health literacy and reading levels. Demonstrate professional conduct and effective written, verbal, and nonverbal communication. Remain calm in emergency situations.
- Document all student health information in the electronic health record according to department guidelines and procedures. Maintain student confidentiality and privacy according to HIPAA and FERPA.
- Conduct state-mandated health and developmental screening. Participate in Child Find.
- Serve as a member of the school emergency and disaster preparedness and response team.
- Serve as a member of the school wellness committee.
- Seek professional development to expand knowledge and skills. Assist with professional and paraprofessional educational growth activities in areas of nursing, health, and communication skills.
- Promote a safe and healthy school environment and climate of school connectedness.
- Promote health and wellness education by serving as a health information resource to students and teachers, provide classroom teaching activities as requested or approved by the principal, and conduct district- and state-mandated health training for school staff.
- Identify and clarify the role of the school nurse in community/public health and continuous quality improvement. Pursue professional development and communicate self-identified learning needs to nursing supervisor.
- Perform duties of child abuse and neglect mandated reporting.
- Perform other tasks and duties as assigned.

SUPERVISORY RESPONSIBILITIES:

- Supervise and monitor LPN/LVN assigned to campus according to the scope of licensure under the state nurse practice act. Delegate nursing duties to LVN/LPN as indicated and maintain clear lines of responsibility and communication. Participate in evaluation of LVNs/LPNs under assignment.
- Supervise and monitor clinic attendants. Delegate healthcare tasks that can be conducted by or delegated to unlicensed assistive personnel according to district policy and the state nurse practice act. Participate in formal and/or informal evaluation of paraprofessionals under assignment.
- Communicate and monitor agency nurses (RNs or LVNs/LPNs) contracted to care for individual students on campus.

PHYSICAL DEMANDS: *The physical demands described here are representative of those that must be met by an employee to successfully perform the essential functions of this job. Reasonable accommodations will be made if necessary.*

While performing the duties of this job, the employee is regularly required to sit; stand; walk, bend, climb stairs and move throughout the facility; communicate verbally and electronically; use hands to finger, handle, or feel objects, tools, or controls; and reach with hands and arms. May be required to drive between school buildings. Occasionally required to stoop, kneel, crouch, and/or crawl. While performing the duties of this job, the employee is regularly required to lift or exert force of up to 10 pounds and occasionally may be required to lift or exert force of up to 100 pounds. Specific vision abilities required by this job include close vision, distance vision, color vision, and the ability to adjust focus. May be exposed to bacteria and communicable diseases.

Adapted from Klein Independent School District. Klein, TX (2018). With permission.

full scope of the school nurse role, job descriptions should represent the five aforementioned tenets of the Framework. Therefore school nurses should review the Framework with their supervisor, discuss the extent of their role, and advocate for job description review by an experienced nurse supervisor (Davis et al., 2021). Job descriptions for all levels of licensed nurses should address and support the licensure scope and responsibilities outlined in the state's nurse practice act.

Registered Nurses

School districts may hire different levels of school nursing staff such as RNs with graduate, baccalaureate, or associate degrees. Due to the complexity and autonomy of school nursing practice, NASN (2021a, 2022) and the American Academy of Pediatrics Council on School Health (2016) recommend every school nurse be licensed by their state of residence as a registered nurse (RN) and have the minimum qualification of a bachelor of science in nursing degree (BSN). Because approximately 5% of school-age children are uninsured (Mykyta et al., 2022), the school nurse often serves as the primary interface that students and their families have with a healthcare provider. It is essential the licensure of the school nurse enables comprehensive assessment and care planning. Additionally, school nurses are charged with overseeing the health and safety of the whole school community. BSN programs have required course content in concepts of leadership and public/population health nursing, which are essential competencies for the full scope of school nursing practice (NASN, 2022). The NASN *School Nursing: Scope and Standards of Practice* (2022) states the following:

> *Educational preparation for school nurse varies, however, the broad scope of the specialty practice of school nursing, and the complexity of issues addressed within a school community setting by the school nurse require advanced skills. These include the ability to practice independently, supervise others, apply community health concepts, manage programs, and delegate care. Therefore, the NASN recommends, and the American Nurses Association (ANA) has consistently affirmed, that the minimal educational preparation for a school nurse be a Bachelor of Science degree in Nursing (BSN) from an accredited college or university. BSNs are significantly better prepared in 12 out of 16 practice areas related to quality and safety including evidence-based practice (EBP), data analysis, and project implementation; therefore, could improve and safeguard the quality of patient care. (p. 47)*

NASN (2022) additionally supports state certification or licensure where required. NASN promotes national certification of school nurses through the National Board for Certification of School Nurses (2025). A bachelor's degree or higher is required to earn the distinction of earning the Nationally Certified School Nurse (NCSN) credential.

Health services delivery models vary. A school may have one RN assigned as the campus-wide school nurse and another RN responsible for direct nursing care delivered in the health office or for students with special healthcare needs. In order to control personnel costs, school districts may employ one school nurse to provide services to multiple buildings or schools. Depending on resources or geography, the school nurse may have to travel around the school district in order to provide coverage.

Licensed Practical/Vocational Nurses

The expected roles and responsibilities of licensed practical/vocational nurses (LPNs/LVNs) should be expressly outlined in the employee's job description. LPNs/LVNs function in a variety of routine direct care roles within school health under the stipulations of the state's nurse practice act (NASN, 2020b). Staffing models include the LPN/LVN as the only nurse available to the campus, part of a nursing team, or providing direct services to individual students with special healthcare needs. It is important to note that in most states, LPNs/LVNs require supervision by an RN or other licensed healthcare provider. However, LPNs/LVNs practice within the scope of their own license. The direct supervision of the LPN/LVN may be the responsibility of the campus RN, a district RN, or nursing supervisor (or agency supervisor). See Online Materials OM31-1 for a sample LPN/LVN job description.

Some school district LPNs/LVNs are assigned to care for students with special medical needs in the classroom. In some instances, the LPN/LVN also serves a dual role as the student's educational paraprofessional. Alternatively, some school districts contract with private staffing agencies to hire LPNs/LVNs to provide personal nursing care to students whose healthcare needs exceed what can be provided by the building nurse. Such contracts should detail the responsibility of the LPN/LVN supervision, skill set, and communication with school district healthcare team members.

Unlicensed Health Services Staff

Where legally permitted by state regulations or school board policy, unlicensed assistive personnel (UAP) can assist school nurses with tasks not requiring professional nursing judgment. UAP are not licensed healthcare professionals; they are individuals hired by the school, school

Practice Connection

The Cost of Covering Multiple Schools

If a nurse is asked to cover multiple schools, it is prudent to calculate the amount of time it takes to travel between schools (from leaving one's office and arriving at another), including during high traffic periods or bad weather. Then calculate how much of the nurse's salary is spent during that time in the car providing service to *no* students. Add the cost of mileage reimbursement. Present the total cost of these inefficiencies to district administration to make the case for more school nurses.

district, public health department, or a private entity to provide very limited elements of care to students (NASN, 2020b). Some UAP may hold certification as a medical assistant or nursing assistant. UAP are trained by the supervising school nurse to provide care in conjunction with, or in the absence of, the school nurse only when nursing judgment is not required.

Appropriate titles for UAP include *health office attendant, health office assistant, health clerk, health aide,* or *health tech.* UAP should never refer to themselves or allow others to refer to them as the school nurse. Nor should they answer the phone with the salutation, "Nurse's Office," which may lead the caller to believe they are speaking to the school nurse. Similarly, if staffed by a nonnurse, the office space should be called the *health office* rather than the nurse's office. The staffing schedule, including job titles, should be clearly posted. Transparency about school health office staffing allows parents to make informed decisions regarding their child's health care during the school day. See Online Materials OM31-2 for a sample UAP job description.

In some school districts, the nonnurse administrator or principal is legally responsible for hiring or designating a lay staff person to help in the health office. The school nurse should be involved in interviews and hiring decisions; provide training, ongoing supervision, and performance evaluation; and retain the authority to delegate healthcare tasks. School nurse delegation of healthcare tasks to UAP is discussed later in this chapter.

ORIENTATION OF HEALTH SERVICES STAFF

School nursing is a specialty practice. However, many nursing schools offer limited to no clinical experience in school nursing for their students. Nurses accepting a school nurse position are often not aware of the autonomous role and unique responsibilities of nursing practice in the community setting of schools. As of 2021, 31 states had regulatory policies that required nurses employed in schools to have specific educational qualifications, such as a BSN, or certification or licensure (Steed et al., 2022). Additionally, there is often a perception that the school nurse role is not demanding or does not require a true skill set (Flippo & Helms, 2022). To eliminate this perception, a detailed review of the job description should be provided during the candidate interview phase. Explanation of the specialized role, available resources, and anticipated support could be viewed as the first step in the orientation process.

The Orientation Process

School nurse orientation should be based on the role, student population, and school community, as well as the size of the district and number of campuses the school nurse will cover. Instructors should consider adult learning theories when determining the content and setting to effectively teach orientees (Mukhalalati & Taylor, 2019). With school nursing being a specialized role, there is a considerable amount of educational content to review. To prevent overwhelming the newly hired nurse, it is recommended the instructor adopt a measured approach to orientation content delivery. Consider which items need to be delivered immediately to ensure student safety, and which can be presented later in the semester.

Transitioning from a graduate nurse to an experienced nurse encompasses Benner's (1982) framework of *Novice to Expert.* Candidates coming to school nursing with previous nursing experience may have already advanced to the proficient or expert practitioner level in another area. However, orienting to this new specialized role will return them to the Novice stage. Previous nursing experience provides the orientee with knowledge, skills, and critical thinking, which can be applied to this new role (Ozdemir, 2019). These established abilities will assist the orientee to transition from the Novice level faster than a graduate nurse. Therefore school nurse orientation programs should not be "one size fits all."

Orientation content should address the uniqueness of the school nurse's role and interprofessional relationships that are vital to delivering care in the educational system (Tsai & McClanahan, 2022). Effective school nurse orientation programs do the following:

- Foster an understanding of the organizational culture, values, mission, and goals.
- Help new employees understand the responsibilities of their role and fit within the organization, including development of strategic relationships.
- Clarify the evaluation process and its relation to the job description, policies, procedures, and the nurse practice act.
- Verify nurse competency in essential skills.

Orientation programs should employ a variety of teaching/learning modalities and strategies to reach diverse learners and maintain interest (Tsai & McClanahan, 2022). Examples of instructional methods include face-to-face classroom teaching (lectures, case studies, small group discussion), hybrid/blended instruction (synchronous or asynchronous sessions), skills labs with simulations, or team/group activities (games, role-playing, presentations). Providing a comprehensive orientation and mentorship to the new school nurse can improve their job satisfaction and retention (Tsai & McClanahan, 2022).

Substitute nurses also require orientation to the school nurse role. Licensed nurses need to be oriented to school procedures and school health room management, including retrieval and input of information into the electronic health record (EHR) using their own password. The substitute nurse orientation may not be as comprehensive as full-time employees but should ensure they can practice safely in the school environment. The orientation content may have to be adjusted if the substitute nurse will cover multiple schools versus a designated campus.

New Employee Support

Nurses require motivation and mentorship in order to succeed in their new role (Karam, 2022). New members to any group generally have some level of anxiety and uncertainty about expectations and processes. As school nurses are traditionally autonomous practitioners, they may lack an onsite peer for support. Partnering a new school nurse with a more experienced one is an effective way to reinforce the orientation concepts and provide ongoing support.

Development of peer relationships through social events, formal introductions, and assignment are strategies that support the orientation process (Tsai & McClanahan, 2022). The supervisor should make every effort to ensure the candidate is prepared for their new role, which in turn will support student safety.

Preceptors

Nurse preceptors are skilled experienced practitioners who assist nurses with orientation to a new practice area through skills training and clinical reasoning modeling. A preceptor is responsible for providing the orientation content as well as evaluating its translation into practice (Kennedy, 2019). The preceptor designation is different from an experienced peer discussed earlier; preceptors are a source of organizational knowledge, provide coaching, and may complete performance evaluations. Their selection should be based on professionalism, reliability, and communication style, as opposed to convenience or proximity to the new nurse (Tsai & McClanahan, 2022).

Preceptors typically have a dual role; in addition to supporting the orientee, they may also be responsible for managing their own caseload or school assignments. Therefore creating a schedule and expectations should provide a clear outline and a balanced program for both the preceptor and preceptee. Preceptors are the designated point of contact for support. Providing clear orientation program objectives and expectations in advance helps prevent the preceptee from receiving contradictory information from differing sources in the district (Tsai & McClanahan, 2022). To ensure preceptor retention and adequate preparation, it is important to provide them with support, education strategies, and a balanced workload (Kennedy, 2019).

Onboarding Unlicensed Assistive Personnel

Unlicensed assistive personnel (UAP) are not healthcare professionals. The UAP job description should detail the work's scope, responsibilities, and accountability, as well as who the UAP will be supervised by and report to. With student health conditions becoming more complex, the UAP will require training and supervision to understand their role in these situations. The UAP requires detailed training for interventions they can perform, including when they should alert a licensed nurse. Schools may utilize UAP to assist the school nurse with the daily management of students presenting with acute illnesses and injuries, maintenance of student's chronic health conditions, performance of health-related functions, and clerical assistance. As allowed by state law and school policy, UAP may also be asked to accomplish routine health tasks in the absence of a nurse, such as administration of oral medication or daily procedures.

Beyond the overall role review, a UAP orientation program should include the following items:

- Documentation expectations and tools, including mass and individual data entry methods
- Record retention policies and procedures
- Enrollment procedures and immunization record review
- Communicable illness management
- State required screenings such as vision and hearing
- Emergency response protocols
- Communication expectations and protocols
- Delegated procedures, if appropriate

Peer support is important for all job categories and the UAP should not be overlooked. Partnering the UAP with an experienced peer can assist in translating didactic orientation content into practice. The supervisor should take into consideration their learning style and ability to transfer new concepts into practice.

SCHOOL HEALTH SERVICES STAFFING

School Nurse Workload

Student success is supported by appropriate school nurse staffing (NASN, 2020a). School health service delivery models and staffing formulas vary within and across states, school districts, and schools. Currently, only Delaware and Vermont have a legal mandate for a bachelor's degree–prepared school nurse in every school (Steed et al., 2022). The *National School Nurse Workforce Study* 2.0 (Willgerodt et al., 2023) identified that approximately 70% of urban schools and only 56% of rural schools employ a full-time nurse, with regional differences ranging from 33.3% in the West to 88% in the Northeast. Factors that affect safe school nurse staffing include legal mandates; health acuity of students; social influences on health; nursing staff experience, training, and expertise; and school/community effects on students' health (Jameson et al., 2018; NASN, 2020a). Additionally, workload determinations must consider school nurse health promotion and disease prevention interventions geared to the student body at large (Jameson et al., 2022).

School nurse staffing should be based on workload rather than rigid, predetermined caseload ratios that are not evidence-based (Jameson et al., 2022; NASN, 2020a). For example, Washington state guidance calls for a ratio not to exceed 1:1,500; however, this ratio can be adjusted based on health acuity and social needs (Nelson, 2023). Ideally, each school health office should be staffed with a full-time BSN-RN supported by additional staff as determined by criteria previously described. School health managers have an ethical, legal, and professional responsibility to provide staffing that safeguards students' health (NASN, 2022) as well as the professional integrity of nurses they lead.

The 2020–2023 COVID-19 pandemic brought school nurse staffing concerns to the forefront of education, public health, and federal agencies. The pandemic highlighted the need for flexible emergency operation plans to address critical increases in health services staff and health services delivery models (Duff, 2020). During the pandemic, school nurse leaders collaborated to devise communication enhancements, remote support and connection for health services staff, and varied models of school nurse service delivery (Combe, 2020; Duff, 2020; Galemore et al., 2022).

Many state, regional, and/or local school boards of education require regular nursing and health program service reports. In addition to state reports, NASN's *Every Student Counts!* (2023a) (discussed later in this chapter) serves as a data collection template to track student health indicators that are sensitive to school nursing practice. Data reports can be pulled from the EHR that include student and staff visits within a specific period and the disposition of the student following the visit (i.e., return to class, sent home, referred for medical care, activated emergency medical services), the types of care required, health acuity levels of the student population, and other mandated activities performed by the school nurse. If the current staffing plan does not safely meet workload demands, the school nurse supervisor should present workload data and concerns to school district administrative staff and/or the district's school board to request more staff. School health supervisors also need to identify the maximum number of staff one can oversee safely based on the scope of their supervisory responsibilities.

Substitute or Alternative School Nurses

School campuses are often left without nursing coverage when nurses are assigned to multiple schools or when the nurse is absent. School systems vary in their procedures to provide students with seamless delivery of health care in the absence of the assigned school nurse. School nurses should advocate for a support system that includes float school nursing staff or a reliable pool of school nurse substitutes to care for the students in the absence of the assigned nurse. However, substitute school nurses are often in short supply due to low hourly wage, district budget constraints, lack of availability of qualified nurses, and general lack of knowledge of many nurses about the school nursing specialty. Many school districts contract with nursing staffing agencies to cover school nurse shifts. However, the cost of agency nurses is typically much higher than what a district might pay a substitute nurse.

Parents/guardians of students who require daily school nurse support must be informed of how their child's care will be delivered when the assigned nurse is not available. School administrators must understand that failure to provide students with needed health care at school may constitute a denial of a student's right to a free and appropriate public education (Individuals With Disabilities Education Improvement Act [IDEA], 2004) or accommodations necessary for the student to access educational content and other school activities (Section 504 of the Rehabilitation Act of 1973).

Ideally, alternative nurses are oriented to their responsibilities and the functions of the school health office in advance; yet this is not always the case. The school nurse should maintain a confidential "subfolder," binder, or electronic file in each health office that includes the information needed by the alternate school nurse to provide nursing services for students. Necessary information includes licensed prescriber orders for medications and procedures, individualized healthcare plans (IHPs), emergency action plans (EAPs), a map of the school, information about delegated care, who to call when nursing questions arise, and any special instructions or schedules. Alternate nurses should have access to all student health records (paper and electronic) to ensure care can be provided and properly documented in the absence of the assigned school nurse. Alternate nurses should use a designated login/password to access the EHR and never use the primary school nurse's login.

Optimally, substitute or alternate school nurse orientation includes time spent in the school health office with the assigned school nurse so to gain familiarity with students' needs; the heath office layout; and location of IHPs, EAPs, daily and emergency medications, and supplies, and how to document. Communication between the alternate school nurse and the assigned school nurse via documentation, written notes, and verbal conversation is important to ensure necessary information related to student health is communicated and continuity of care is maintained.

Volunteers in the School Health Office

Caution is warranted when using volunteers for the delivery of school health services or assistance with other tasks in the school health office. Volunteers may interact with the children of their neighbors and friends, creating a conflict of interest when gaining access to protected student health information. Regardless of a volunteer's relationship with students or their families, the mandates of the Family Educational Rights and Privacy Act (FERPA) and Health Insurance Portability and Accountability Act (HIPAA) must be considered when allowing such activity in the school health office. Consultation with the school's legal counsel is advisable before initiating new commitments with volunteers. Schools should develop policies for the use of volunteers that coincide with state legal requirements for school volunteers. Thorough background checks of volunteer prospects should be conducted. Volunteers require specific training on their roles and responsibilities, as well as the principles of privacy and confidentiality (HIPAA, FERPA). For each volunteer, the school district should obtain written acknowledgment of training and agreement to act accordingly. Volunteers, whether licensed or unlicensed, should only be used to assist the school nurse—not to act in the place of the school nurse.

All professionals providing school health services are obligated to provide the service within the relevant standard of care, including volunteers. Failure to do so may create malpractice exposure for the person and the school. Good Samaritan laws apply only during emergencies and only when the person rendering assistance does not have a duty or preexisting professional relationship with the client (Association of State and Territorial Health Officials, 2012). The school nurse must use volunteers in accordance with state nurse practice acts, must verify the competency of the volunteer in providing assigned tasks, and is accountable for training and supervising the volunteer.

DELEGATION

For the purposes of the following discussion, the term *assignment* is used to describe nurse and nonnurse administrators' general task transfer to school staff. The term *delegation* is used to describe RN transfer of nursing tasks to a UAP when it is appropriate to do so. It is never appropriate to delegate nursing judgment or any part of the nursing process. Therefore, the term *healthcare tasks* will be used in lieu of *nursing tasks.* The nurse who delegates is referred to as the *delegator;* the individual who accepts delegation is referred to as the *delegatee* (National Council of State Boards of Nursing [NCSBN] & American Nurses Association [ANA], 2019). Nonnurse school administrators, such as a principal, can identify and *designate* a staff member to be a *delegatee.* The delegatee must agree to accept the responsibility for the delegated task(s) and the school nurse delegator must assess and verify the competence of the delegatee to perform the task. It is important that school administrators understand that only the nursing profession, via state nurse practice acts, defines the scope of nursing practice and identifies who can delegate nursing tasks. Delegation requires nursing judgment on the part of the delegator, and therefore lay administrators who delegate nursing tasks to a UAP may be considered by courts and state boards of nursing to be practicing nursing without a license (*Mitts v. Hillsboro Union High School District,* 1987). Consequently, nonnurse administrators should restrict their assignments to those duties outside the realm of nursing practice.

Task Delegation by School Nurses

The rules and regulations of each state's nurse practice act define the guidelines and standards for delegation of nursing tasks. When making delegation decisions, school nurses must also be knowledgeable about federal law, their state nurse practice act, school policy, and guidance principles from nursing organizations such as the National Council of State Boards of Nursing (NCSBN) and ANA (2019), as well as NASN (2022). Some states and territories restrict the procedures that can be delegated; others do not allow delegation at all (see Chapter 6). Some states consider that RNs can delegate to LPNs/LVNs, whereas states recognize the licensed LPN/LVN as independently accountable for care assigned by the RN. It should be noted that there are some states that allow LPNs/LVNs to be the delegator (NCSBN & ANA, 2019).

School health services must be provided as a related service or as an accommodation for all eligible students with disabilities under the Americans With Disabilities Act, IDEA (2004), and Section 504 of the *Rehabilitation Act of 1973.* Where allowed by state nurse practice acts, school districts may meet this mandate, in part, through school nurse delegation of healthcare tasks to UAP. Schools may also use UAP to *assist* the school nurse with the daily management of students presenting with acute illnesses and injuries, maintenance of students' chronic health conditions, performance of health-related functions, and clerical assistance. As allowed by state law and school policy, UAP may also be asked to accomplish routine health tasks in the absence of a nurse, such as administration of oral medication or rescue medications and daily special procedures.

When making the decision to delegate, the school nurse retains authority, responsibility, and accountability for delegated nursing functions. The school nurse must follow the *Five Rights of Delegation* (NCSBN & ANA, 2019) and delegate healthcare tasks only when it is safe and appropriate to do so (Box 31-2). A thorough nursing assessment is critical to determine whether the student's health condition is *stable and predictable,* thus allowing delegation. The task must *not* require the UAP to use nursing judgment or critical decision making. The UAP must be willing and competent to complete the delegated task safely and be provided with student-specific training by the school nurse. The UAP may not transfer the responsibility for the delegated task to another individual, nor may the training be transferred to provision of care for another student. The UAP should be provided with written guidance and training for reporting changes in the student's health status (NCSBN & ANA, 2019).

Safe and proper delegation of healthcare tasks in the school setting requires collaboration between the district leadership, nursing staff, and the UAP delegatee (NCSBN & ANA, 2019). Central to this shared responsibility is public protection. Therefore the necessary protocols and procedures that prioritize the safety of the student should be in place. See Figure 31-1 for the NCSBN & ANA *Delegation Model.*

Nevertheless, delegation is not without risks. The school nurse should take every precaution to reduce those risks for the safety of the student. The school nurse provides and documents the correct task training via detailed

BOX 31-2
Five Rights of Delegation

Right task: The activity falls within the delegatee's job description or is included as part of the established written policies and procedures of the nursing practice setting. The facility needs to ensure the policies and procedures describe the expectations and limits of the activity and provide any necessary competency training.

Right circumstance: The health condition of the patient must be stable. If the patient's condition changes, the delegatee must communicate this to the licensed nurse, and the licensed nurse must reassess the situation and the appropriateness of the delegation.

Right person: The licensed nurse along with the employer and the delegatee is responsible for ensuring that the delegatee possesses the appropriate skills and knowledge to perform the activity.

Right directions and communication: Each delegation situation should be specific to the patient, the licensed nurse, and the delegatee. The licensed nurse is expected to communicate specific instructions for the delegated activity to the delegatee; the delegatee, as part of two-way communication, should ask any clarifying questions. This communication includes any data that need to be collected, the method for collecting the data, the time frame for reporting the results to the licensed nurse, and additional information pertinent to the situation. The delegatee must understand the terms of the delegation and must agree to accept the delegated activity. The licensed nurse should ensure that the delegatee understands that they cannot make any decisions or modifications in carrying out the activity without first consulting the licensed nurse.

Right supervision and evaluation: The licensed nurse is responsible for monitoring the delegated activity, following up with the delegatee at the completion of the activity, and evaluating patient outcomes. The delegatee is responsible for communicating patient information to the licensed nurse during the delegation situation. The licensed nurse should be ready and available to intervene as necessary. The licensed nurse should ensure appropriate documentation of the activity is completed.

NCSBN & ANA (2019). With permission.

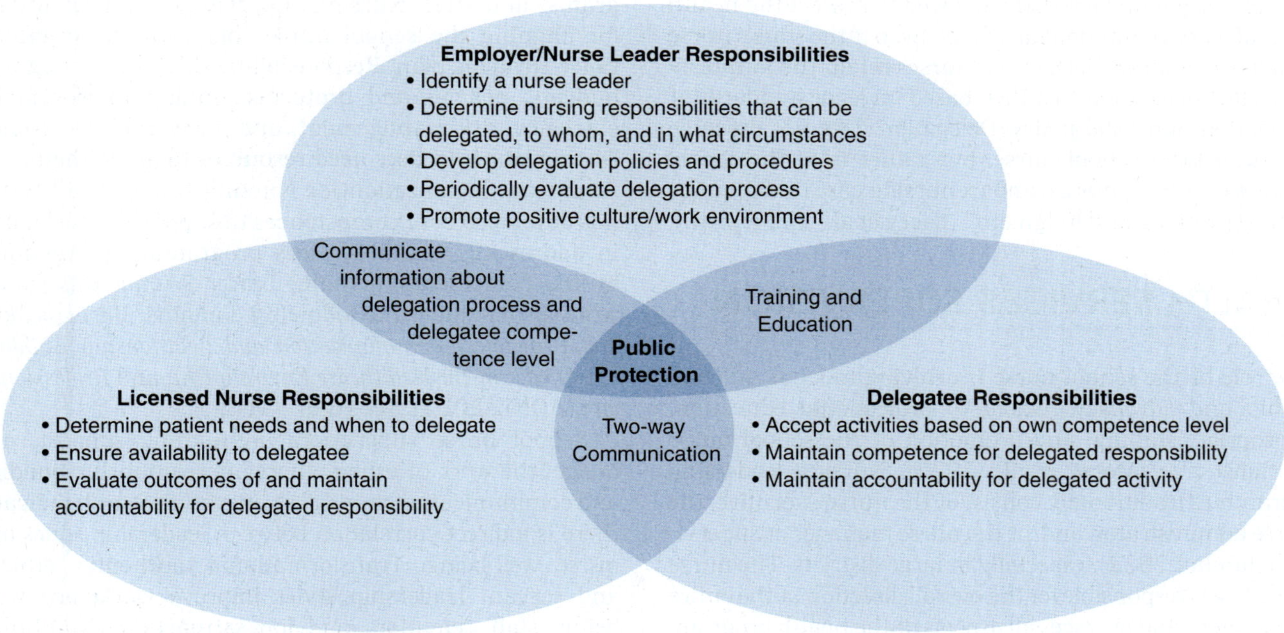
Employer/Nurse Leader Responsibilities
• Identify a nurse leader
• Determine nursing responsibilities that can be delegated, to whom, and in what circumstances
• Develop delegation policies and procedures
• Periodically evaluate delegation process
• Promote positive culture/work environment
Communicate information about delegation process and delegatee competence level
Training and Education
Public Protection
Licensed Nurse Responsibilities
• Determine patient needs and when to delegate
• Ensure availability to delegatee
• Evaluate outcomes of and maintain accountability for delegated responsibility
Two-way Communication
Delegatee Responsibilities
• Accept activities based on own competence level
• Maintain competence for delegated responsibility
• Maintain accountability for delegated activity

FIGURE 31-1. NCSBN & ANA Delegation Model. *(NCSBN & ANA [2019]. With permission.)*

skills checklists, including demonstration, return demonstration, and scheduled monitoring to ensure safe delivery of care (Shannon & Kubelka, 2013a, 2013b). See Online Materials OM31-3 for a sample *UAP Delegation Skills Checklist.*

The school nurse delegator must be available to the UAP delegatee for consultation either in person, by close proximity, or via telephone. Periodic supervision of the delegated task is a necessity, with higher frequency at the onset of delegation and decreasing frequency as

> **Focus on the Framework**
> **Leadership**
>
> School nurse delegation can be more complex than nurse delegation in other settings. At the behest of Texas school nurses, the Texas Board of Nursing (BON) convened a work group, including school nurses, charged with development of algorithms to guide school nurses' delegation decision making (Texas Board of Nursing & Texas Department of State Health Services, n.d.). Do the school nurses in your community need to approach your BON for additional delegation guidance?

competent skill in delivery of the task is observed and documented. As the skill of the UAP increases, the frequency of supervision may decrease; however, regular supervision must continue throughout the entire period of delegation. The school nurse should promptly retrain the UAP if any issues or complications arise.

The school nurse decides when delegation is not safe. School staff and parents may require education about the legal parameters surrounding nursing delegation in the school setting and how that differs from care provided in a student's home. The school nurse advocates that the principles of delegation be strictly followed to protect the health and safety of the student at school. Even if the state's nurse practice act allows delegation, nurses retain the authority to decline delegation to a UAP based on legal standards of delegation and local policy. Delegation does not preclude the need for a school nurse, but rather frees the school nurse to "provide more complex nursing care that requires critical thinking and judgment" (Lacey et al., 2024, p. 48).

HEALTH SERVICES SUPERVISION

The role of the school nurse is evolving to focus on leadership and advocacy related to professional education, appropriate staffing, and promotion of the school nurse specialist role (Morse et al., 2022). Nursing leadership hierarchies traditionally consist of the nurse executive, the nurse administrator, and/or the nurse manager or supervisor (Hamlin, 2022), especially in large districts. The nurse executive is responsible for the overall direction of the entire department and oversees all aspects of the health program. The nurse administrator monitors policy, procedure, and staffing, while the nurse supervisor has administrative and clinical duties (Hamlin, 2022).

However, in medium-sized districts, the nursing leader may serve all three of these roles, in effect. Many smaller districts lack a formal nursing leadership structure where the school nurses have coordinated but parallel positions on the district organizational chart. In some small districts, there may be only one school nurse who covers all responsibilities. It is still common in many districts for the leader of school health services to be a nonnurse.

School Nurse Leadership

The responsibilities of the school health director or coordinator position include oversight, coordination, and provision of supervision for the school health services program. Ideally, school nurse leaders have advanced degrees, such as a master of science in nursing (MSN) or doctor of nursing practice (DNP), that prepare them for their roles as systems leaders. The nurse supervisor should act as liaison and spokesperson to improve communication within, about, and for school nursing practice. School nurse leaders can further distinguish themselves as experts in the specialty practice by earning National Certification in School Nursing (National Board for Certification of School Nurses, 2023).

School nurse leaders should engage in practices that

- Challenge the status quo
- Help others work toward collective goals that improve circumstances for school nurses
- Enable care delivery that has a positive impact on the health and safety of students and staff

Leadership plays a vital role in the supervision and management of effective school health services, programs, and staff. Nursing supervisors are accountable for aligning the school nurse role with the organization's strategic plan. Responsibilities include oversight of budgets, policies and protocols, quality improvement, efficiency, risk management, and measurable outcomes. District nurse leaders need resources to guide them. The American Organization for Nursing Leadership (AONL) has developed core competences to support nurse leaders in addressing health services programming. Anchored by the competency domain, *Leader Within*, this framework also includes the following domains: *Business Skills and Principles*, *Communication and Relationship Building*, *Knowledge of the Healthcare Environment*, and *Professionalism* (AONL, 2022). See Figure 31-2.

School nurse supervisors orchestrate, support, and budget the work of others; therefore relationship building and communication are vital strengths. Research indicates there is a direct correlation between leadership styles and nurse well-being. Transformational, authentic, ethical, and servant leadership styles improve workplace well-being, staff retention, and job satisfaction (Niinihuhta & Häggman-Laitila, 2022). Utilization of education, self-assessments, and resources from leadership organizations can assist the new, emerging, or experienced leader learn about their personal leadership style. School nurse supervisors require advanced preparation on topics such as leadership, budget control, influence without authority, conflict management, and emotional intelligence. Therefore they should search out resources beyond the typical

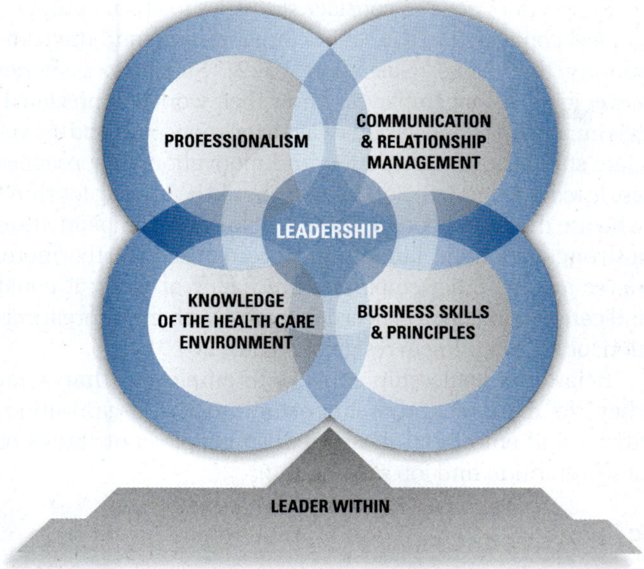

FIGURE 31-2. Nurse Leader Core Competencies Model. *(American Organization for Nursing Leadership [2022]. With Permission.)*

school nurse systems to organizations such as the AONL (2022).

According to *Nursing Administration: Scope and Standards of Practice* (ANA, 2016, pp. 8–18), core elements of the nursing staff manager's role include the following:

- Safety, quality, and risk management: Create environments that take into account nursing ethics as well as the goals and legal obligations of the organization, while providing processes that drive quality nursing practice.
- Patient and population health advocacy: Focus on client-centered policy development, nursing care delivery, and decision making in addressing the needs of individual patients and/or communities.
- Clinical care delivery and optimal patient outcomes: Establish policies and procedures that drive the provision of quality clinical services, hold nursing staff accountable to the scope and standards of nursing practice, and promote nursing professionalism.
- Healthy work environment: Emphasize diversity and inclusion; a healthy physical, emotional, and interpersonal work environment; safe staffing; and appropriate recognition.
- Strategic, financial, and human resources management: Participate in strategic planning to identify the organization's mission and vision. Translate the strategic focus into patient care activities, recruitment and retention of quality staff, and efficient financial resource management.
- Legal and regulatory compliance: Administer nursing services within the legal mandates of local, state, and federal statutes that regulate client confidentiality, employee rights, nursing practices, financial practices, service reimbursement, and other institutional standards.
- Networking, collaborating, and partnering: Network both within and outside of healthcare organizations to enhance understanding of nursing roles and objectives. Cultivate partnerships that facilitate patient services and transitions. Collaborate to advance health outcomes.

Clinical supervision and evaluation of school nurses should be based on school systems' job descriptions, *School Nursing: Scope and Standards of Practice* (NASN, 2022), and the *School Nursing Practice Framework* (NASN, 2024). It is best practice that school nurses should be supervised by school nurses.

> *It is the position of the National Association of School Nurses (NASN) that the clinical practice of the registered professional school nurse (hereinafter referred to as the school nurse) be supervised and evaluated by a registered nurse knowledgeable about school nurse practice in accordance with School Nursing: Scope and Standards of Practice (NASN, 2022) and the Framework for 21st Century School Nursing Practice™ (NASN, 2016, 2020a). Nursing supervision and evaluation of school nursing foster professionalism, competency, and quality standards of school nursing clinical care necessary to equitably promote the health, safety, and learning of all students and the school community (Campbell & Minor, 2017). (NASN, 2023b, para. 1)*

Nonnurse Supervisor

In reality, because the school nurse may be the only healthcare professional in a school or district, they may be supervised by a professional other than a nurse. In the absence of a nurse supervisor, the responsibility of hiring, supervising, and evaluating the school nurse typically falls on the district superintendent, building principal, or nonnurse health services/related services director or coordinator. Customarily, individuals in these positions are responsible for all staff and students assigned to that building. This level of responsibility is typically assigned to a leader who has demonstrated mastery of school district policy, procedure, communication, and other predetermined measures. It is typical for the nonnurse supervisor to have been a teacher that advanced through the ranks in various educational facilities.

The fundamental role of the school nurse and principal is to have students in class and able to learn. School nurses should keep this shared responsibility as a focus for discussions regarding duties and expectations. The school may surmise that a change in the school culture is needed when administrators and educational staff have limited awareness of the complexity and significance of the role of the school nurse. School nurses need to educate administrators and school staff about the value of school nurse to the students' education and advocate the right quality, quantity, and accessibility of supplies, equipment, space, and tools. Without appropriate nursing supervision or unclear expectations of practices, new school nurses can quickly become demotivated.

Promoting Employee Motivation

Job satisfaction and work-related burnout have a direct impact on staff retention. Nurses are accustomed to handling stressful clinical situations, but burnout happens when that stress is prolonged, interpersonal, and emotional. Burnout may be attributed to high workload demands, inability to complete tasks, lack of supervisor support, and role conflict (Jameson & Bowen, 2020). Decreased job satisfaction is directly correlated to quality of care, increased patient dissatisfaction, and employee turnover (Buchan et al., 2022). The COVID-19 pandemic contributed to additional stressors and demands on nursing staff, which has resulted in higher rates of turnover and reduced feelings of job satisfaction (Buchan et al., 2022). When staff members leave, they take with them institutional knowledge and work experience, which takes time to replace while adding strain to the remaining staff. Recruitment and onboarding of professional staff is costly for districts. Therefore it is the role of the supervisor, on behalf of the organization, to provide and instill confidence, trust, and satisfaction in employees to increase their motivational drive and intent to stay.

Job satisfaction can come from both intrinsic and extrinsic sources. Intrinsic or internal motivators include satisfaction, which is self-initiated, such as a feeling of accomplishment or importance and pride in one's work. Studies have shown employees with higher levels of personal accomplishment have reduced levels of burnout (Jameson & Bowen, 2020). Extrinsic or external motivators are incentives, such as rewards, job benefits, promotions, and money, coming from outside the employee.

Supervisors need to consider strategies to ensure employees feel connected to the school, organization, and the community they serve (Galemore, 2022). Supervisors should never assume that employees know their work is appreciated. It is important to find various ways to acknowledge and appreciate staff's work. Celebration and motivational approaches are listed in Box 31-3. Supervisors should be looking for those who are the "silent good." These people never complain, have a strong work ethic, but are rarely recognized. Furthermore, never assume quiet employees are happy at work; it could indicate they do not feel heard, have lost faith in the organization, or are planning to resign (Thomas, 2019).

Relational leadership conveys to employees that what they do matters and is important to the organization. Social and emotional investment in people contributes to staff retention and job satisfaction.

Self-Advocacy

School nurses without a nursing supervisor must be their own advocate. Even when a school nurse lacks a school district nursing supervisor, the school nurse is professionally accountable for adherence to the standards of nursing practice and the quality of their practice. The boards of nursing expect the licensed nurse to be their own advocate and seek additional training when encountering unfamiliar practice situations (Ballard et al., 2016). Unknowingly, principals, teachers, and parents may expect the school nurse to perform duties or tasks that are beyond the scope of nursing licensure. Making an effort to understand the responsibilities, standards of practice, and the challenges faced by administrators can help the school nurse foster a collegial relationship with their campus and/or district administrators (Davis & Lynch, 2018). In order to understand and achieve their shared goal, the school nurse and the principal

BOX 31-3

Celebratory and Motivational Approaches for Staff Recognition

Empowerment	Give staff more responsibility and decision-making authority to encourage ownership in the work.
Interesting or creative work	Align assignments with natural interests and talents; encourage creativity, problem-solving, and change.
Personal development	Mindfulness and resilience training (Buchan et al., 2022)
Recognition	Recognize performance and celebrate accomplishments for nurses at all stages of their school nursing career (Galemore, 2022). Consider a recognition at a school board meeting or in newsletters, and sharing accomplishments when announcing staff promotions.
Quality work environment	Facilitate a safe and sanitary work environment.
Enhance trust and communication	Demonstrate reliability through actions consistent with organizational values. Consistently follow through with promises. Listen to what employees say, giving them full attention. Connect to and talk with employees.

Did You Know?

Self-Advocacy

The school nurse is professionally accountable for adherence to the standards of nursing practice, their state's nurse practice act, and the quality of their practice. Practicing without a nurse supervisor is not a valid reason for nonadherence to the nurse practice act.

should have regularly scheduled meeting times. It is recommended that both stakeholders review the following:

Job description
- Clearly listed duties and responsibilities
- Duties and responsibilities are within the nurse's scope of practice per the state nurse practice act
- Need for additional training or supervision in required skills

Expectations, timelines, and reporting responsibilities
- Duty hours and days
- Principal notification expectations
- Parent notification expectations
- Established procedures for this role
- Community stakeholder engagement guidelines

Legal constructs
- Applicable school district policies
- Health department requirements
- Nurse licensing authority requirements
- Professional nursing standards of practice
- Solutions for lack of nursing supervision (i.e., contract agency, public health department, neighboring school district, educational service center, or state school nurse consultant)

Additionally, membership enrollment in the National Association of School Nurses provides the school nurse with tiered membership in their state and regional organizations. Membership provides access to countless resources, including discussion boards where advice, support, and knowledge are shared among peers.

PERFORMANCE EVALUATION

Supervision of school nursing care based on performance review and evaluation is a quality management process that provides employees with recognition for good performance and identifies areas for growth or improvement. An effective performance review motivates, gives direction, and establishes expected contributions, as well as identifies professional development needs.

Evaluation Processes

Performance evaluation is a supervisory responsibility that should be conducted using established agency or school district policies and guidelines, state laws governing nursing practice, employee job descriptions, and preestablished performance goals. School nurse performance should be measured by competencies, standards, performance indicators, and outcome measures as determined by the school or hiring organization (NASN, 2022). NASN's *School Nursing: Scope and Standards of Practice* (2022) and *School Nursing Practice Framework* (2024) are guiding documents for evaluating the quality of school nursing practice.

Competence in nursing practice should be evaluated by the individual school nurse (self-assessment), nurse peers, and nurses in the roles of supervisor, coach, mentor, or preceptor. Competency assessment includes not only evaluating knowledge and skills, but also the impact, relevance, necessity, and appropriateness of the nurse's interventions in meeting the standard of care. Each school nurse is an individual practitioner whose previous experience, educational preparation, and school nurse tenure will affect how they meet assessment indicators. Other influencing factors may include the nurse's workload, geographical size of the assignment, number and sizes of schools covered, population demographics, community expectations, supervisory responsibilities, and other duties as assigned (Jameson et al., 2022). Just as school nurses may need to educate others about their job roles, they should also advocate for evaluation processes and tools that fairly assess and document the full scope of their role.

Evaluation Tools

A robust evaluation system allows the school nurse to demonstrate their practice, professional growth, and evidence of achievements (Wallin & Rothman, 2020). Employee performance review typically occurs on an annual basis, but regardless of tenure, employees should be afforded adequate time for a meaningful evaluation. As RNs, school nurses should be evaluated by nurses (NASN, 2023b). However, nonnurse administrators are an important part of the evaluation process because they provide input on nonclinical performance expected of all school professionals such as attendance, teamwork, communication skills, and cultural effectiveness (Wallin & Rothman, 2020).

Evaluation techniques and tools vary depending on the purpose of the evaluation, whether it is for routine quality evaluation or to address performance concerns. A variety of evaluation approaches may be used, such as one performance rater, multiple raters, peer evaluations, self-evaluation, and professional portfolios. Evaluation tools should be provided to the nurses in advance, so they are aware of the criteria on which they will be evaluated. A few exemplars of evaluation tools are provided here.

Evaluations should align with the school nurse job description, *School Nursing: Scope and Standards of Practice* (NASN, 2022), and the principles of the *School Nursing Practice Framework* (NASN, 2024). A comprehensive performance evaluation correlating to the Framework is the gold standard of evaluation, providing school nurses and school administrators with insight into the full scope of school nursing as a specialty practice (Wallin & Rothman, 2020). Parkway School District has created a tool based on the *Framework* principles as demonstrated by the competencies of the school nurse standards. The evaluation includes school nurse self-reflection, as well as school administrator and health services director input (Wallin & Rothman, 2020). This evaluation tool allows for demonstration of growth, goal setting, and quality improvement. See Figure 31-2a for a section of this tool and Online Materials OM31-4 for the complete tool.

The performance evaluation process must be fair and consistent from one employee to another. Therefore many school districts rely on skills-based evaluation tools related to specific tasks or behaviors and direct observations. These tools provide objective evidence of clinical task attainment such as medication administration, health record maintenance, or data submission. Tools that utilize a simple scoring system support the validity and reliability across evaluations by different evaluators (i.e., interrater reliability), which allows evaluations to be compared individually over time or collectively with other nursing staff.

Audits, data reports, and school nurse portfolios are important sources of performance information. A professional portfolio contains complied documentation of effective practice that demonstrates professional growth over time and provides opportunity for self-reflection, an essential component of the evaluation. Portfolios also provide the school nurse with an opportunity to showcase initiatives or innovations that may be outside the typical job expectations, such as population-focused interventions (e.g., teaching health lessons in the classroom or leading wellness programs for school staff). School nurse portfolios may also include qualitative data or commendations, such

Principle: Leadership School nurse completes all self-evaluation standards. School Administrator completes the unshaded evaluation standards. Director of Health Services completes all evaluation standards.	**School Nurse Self-Evaluation**				**Building Administrator**				**Director of Health Services**			
	Unsatisfactory	Emerging	Proficient	Exemplary	Unsatisfactory	Emerging	Proficient	Exemplary	Unsatisfactory	Emerging	Proficient	Exemplary
L1: The school nurse leads within the professional practice setting and the profession. (Standard 12-Leadership)												
L2: The school nurse seeks knowledge and competence that reflects current nursing practice and promotes innovative, anticipatory thinking. (Standard 13-Education).												
L3: The school nurse demonstrates advocacy in all roles and setting. (Standard 8 - Advocacy)												

School Nurse Comments:

Building Administrator's Comments:

Director of Health Services' Comments:

FIGURE 31-2A Parkway School District school nurse evaluation form: leadership section.
(Parkway School District. [2024]. School nurse evaluation form. *Acknowledgments to R. Wallin & S. Rothman. With permission.)*

as positive feedback from families and school staff, awards, news articles, or official social media posts.

The school nurse should employ the electronic health record (EHR) data to create reports that demonstrate the amount of effort the school nurse spends on caring for students. NASN's *Every Student Counts!* offers uniform data points to be included in standardized reporting, as well as utilized in health services program evaluation (discussed later) (NASN, 2023a; Stanislo, 2023a). The school nurse can analyze school health data in the context of school health data to tell a story of their contributions to the health of students and the school community. Through *data storytelling*, the school nurse can convey complex data in an impactful way to leadership and stakeholders (Stansilo, 2023b). See Chapter 5 for more information on Every Student Counts!

School nurse performance indicators and outcome measures may include the following:

- Number of health office student visits (EHR reports)
- Impact on student attendance or instructional time (number of students sent home or back to class, i.e., student disposition)
- Health and wellness initiatives conducted with outcomes
- Examples of individual healthcare plans and contributions to IEPs and Section 504 plans
- Provision of developmentally and culturally appropriate student health resources
- Monies reimbursed to the school district from Medicaid billing
- Decreased absenteeism due to school nurse interventions
- Improved academic performance because of school nurse interventions
- Professional development activities
- Membership on school-wide committees (wellness committee, emergency response team, school improvement committee)
- Parent letters praising expert school nurse care
- Community partnerships
- Quality improvement measures
- Cost efficiencies to budgets

Utilizing an evaluation tool that displays competencies over several levels can encourage the nurse to reach for the next level. Benner's *Novice to Expert Model* (1982) provides stages of competency along a continuum, which allows the nurse to evaluate their current practice and areas to grow. See Table 31-1 for an example of a self-evaluation rubric based on the Novice to Expert Model and the *School Nursing Scope and Standards of Practice: Standard 7, Ethics* (NASN, 2022). The nurse would provide the supervisor with samples/evidence to support their self-rating. This form of evaluation can be subjective but allows for discussion and opportunities to identify areas for professional growth.

Once evaluations are completed, the school nurse and supervisor meet to discuss the results and jointly develop a development plan to assist the school nurse to build on strengths and overcome identified obstacles or limitations. Employees should be informed in person and in writing about any concerns regarding their job performance in a timely manner following district protocols. Written documentation of all formal evaluations will be retained by the administrator within the personnel file and in accordance with agency or school policies on employee records. Such documentation supports the legal need for an organization to track employee performance and validate grounds for promotion or termination. The school nurse should retain a copy of their evaluation to use as a resource for reflection or

TABLE 31-1 Self-Evaluation Based on Standard 7 of School Nursing Scope and Standards of Practice: Ethics

Topic	**Standard of School Nursing Practice 7: Ethics**			
Level	***Beginner***	***Competent***	***Proficient***	***Expert***
Examples of competence	Provides compassionate care to staff and students.	Maintains professional relationships with staff, students, and peers.	Maintains a professional, respectful, caring relationship with the parent and student even when there is disagreement with their healthcare choices.	Consistent self-reflection to ensure hidden bias or personal choices do not influence interactions with parent/student.
	Collaborates with teachers, administration, and/or parents to ensure the safety and privacy of students' health needs in the school setting.	Seeks guidance from experienced peers or supervisor when faced with a difficult situation.	Participates in professional learning related to nursing ethics or participates on a nursing peer review committee.	Takes accountability for nursing actions and utilizes professional nursing judgment when making student healthcare assignments.

NASN (2022).

as part of their portfolio. Nurses who demonstrate an accurate and thorough understanding of the school nurse's role should be encouraged to further develop their competencies and leadership skills, and pursue advanced degrees in nursing that promote advancement and promotion.

SUPPORT FOR DIFFICULT SITUATIONS

Medication Errors

Administration of student medications is performed by school nurses and may be delegated by the school nurse to a variety of school employees as state nurse practice acts allow (Lowe et al., 2022). There is a risk of unsafe practice or medication errors when policies, procedures, and training methods are not followed. NASN's (2021b) *School Nursing Evidence-Based Clinical Practice Guideline: Medication Administration in Schools* provides structured processes for medication management for school nurses (DuChateau & Carr, 2022).

> *A medication error is any preventable event that may cause or lead to inappropriate medication use or patient harm while the medication is in the control of the healthcare professional, patient, or consumer. Such events may be related to professional practice, healthcare products, procedures, and systems including prescribing, order communication, product labeling, packaging, and nomenclature, compounding, dispensing, distribution, administration, education, monitoring, and use (National Coordinating Council for Medication Error Reporting and Prevention, 2021). Medication errors include incorrect person, incorrect medication, incorrect dose, incorrect time, incorrect route, incorrect or missing documentation, missing dose, and wrong weight. (NASN, 2021b, p. 8)*

Errors may be a result of unclear procedures, simple human error, straying from standard procedures, or even conscious and intentional errors. All medication errors should be documented, reported, and evaluated—whether or not there is an adverse outcome for students. However, nurses and UAP may fear they will get in trouble for reporting medication errors. Creating a *culture of safety* or a *fair and just culture* is "a shift from the culture of blaming individuals responsible for medical errors to one of vigilance that is fair and just" (NASN, 2021b). Standardized reporting procedures are recommended, as well as postevent coaching, and student safety measures (NASN, 2021b). Health services leaders should examine medication errors for contributing factors, trends, and protocol deficiencies. Leaders should make process improvements as indicated to help prevent future errors.

Following medication error reporting, health services leaders should consider their approach to nonpunitive remediation. Coaching allows the employee to share their experience with trusted colleagues, which is an important step in preventing *second victim phenomenon* (Stillwater, 2018). This phenomenon results when the practitioner experiences emotional trauma from the event, including guilt, shame, and feelings of inadequacy (Stillwater, 2018). Punitive reprimands following medication error reports may limit reporting and the ability to identify system-wide process defects. Yet obviously, negligence, willful misconduct, or diverting student medications for personal use should not be tolerated and should be reported to appropriate authorities. See Chapter 30 for more discussion on medication errors in the health office and a sample medication/procedure incident report form.

Board of Nursing Complaint

A complaint to the state board of nursing can be made by anyone when they judge a licensed nurse's practice to be unethical, unsafe, or not in compliance with regulations. Boards of nursing handle complaints or allegations that are within their jurisdiction and that warrant investigation. If a nurse receives a complaint from their board of nursing, it should be taken seriously and addressed immediately. Investigation by the board of nursing can be distressing for the nurse, even when they believe they did not commit a nurse practice act violation. If employers have questions regarding the nurse's ability to practice safely during the investigation period, they should seek guidance from the board of nursing. The National Council of State Boards of Nursing (NCSBN; n.d.a, n.d.b) has resources for patients, nurses, and nurse leaders in regard to scope of practice complaints. Nurse leaders can utilize the NCSBN *Adverse Event Decision Pathway* (2016) to assist in action steps for unprofessional conduct or practice errors (Russell & Radtke, 2014). The board of nursing and state nurse practice acts require licensed nurses to be knowledgeable of rules and regulations related to their licensure. It is recommended nurses visit their board of nursing Web site frequently to update their knowledge of the applicable rules for their licensure and role.

Employee Corrective Action

It is legally prudent to have school district policies that address performance concerns, the discipline process, and behaviors for which an employee could be immediately terminated. Some school districts require each employee to acknowledge in writing their understanding of personnel policies provided via print, online, or both on an annual basis. School nurse supervisors should work closely with the human resources and legal departments when employee corrective action or discipline is required. When unionized health services staff are recommended for corrective action, they are typically entitled to union representation. It is imperative to respect union guidelines for disciplinary action to avoid workplace disputes.

Conflict Management

Conflict management is a common challenge for managers and supervisors. Conflict is characteristic of human relationships influenced in the workplace by interpersonal relationships, subjective interpretation of events, and organizational behaviors (Ellis, 2021). Conflicts are often caused by communication failures, by either failing to listen or misinterpreting the intent of others. The need to be right is a strong drive in all humans and is a primary contributor to conflict. Many nurses prefer to avoid addressing conflict directly, but this can have a significant negative impact on the health and well-being of the employee. Additionally, conflict can affect the quality and timeliness of patient care, which can perpetuate a lack of trust and erosion of communication (Ellis, 2022a).

The *NASN Code of Ethics for School Nurses* (NASN, 2022) and the *Code of Ethics for Nurses With Interpretive Statements* (ANA, 2015) emphasize the responsibilities of nurses to collaborate with colleagues in ways that promote self-growth, positive work environments, and the provision of quality school nursing care. Examples of situations that create ethical conflicts for school nurses and other members of the educational team may involve the following:

- Unsafe school nurse–to–student workloads
- Accountability for care delegated to UAPs
- Documentation of expectations that do not align with the standards of nursing practice
- Assignment of nursing tasks to UAPs without the input of the school nurse
- Attempts by nonlicensed administrators to direct practice (NASN, 2022, p. 131)

Often conflict is perceived as a negative process to be avoided. On the other hand, conflict can ignite quality improvement, team communication, and change processes (Ellis, 2022b). School nurse supervisors may need to act as mediators, facilitators, or coaches in conflict resolution between employees. Barriers to conflict resolution may include workload demands, power imbalances, avoidance, and team culture (Ellis, 2021, 2022c). Effective supervisors investigate the source of conflict and encourage negotiation, compromise, and acceptance of accountability. The school nurse's strong sense of emotional intelligence is essential when negotiating with education team members regarding areas of conflict (Ellis, 2022b).

Formal employer conflict management may be facilitated by human resource processes and encompass a range of activities, including communication, problem-solving, managing emotions, and relationship building. Supervisors should monitor for changes in employees' behavior, including irritability, anxiety, absences, and hypervigilance (Ellis, 2022c).

Harassment

Employers, including schools, have an obligation to maintain a workplace free from harassment and adhere to written policies that address hostile work environments. School health administrators should ensure that all employees within their supervision have completed all required harassment and discrimination trainings. Unlawful "harassment is a form of discrimination that violates Title VII of the Civil Rights Act of 1964, the Age Discrimination in Employment Act of 1967, and the Americans with Disabilities Act of 1990" (U.S. Equal Employment Opportunity Commission [USEEOC], n.d., para. 1). Harassment can be "based on race, color, religion, sex (including sexual orientation, gender identity, or pregnancy), national origin, older age (beginning at age 40), disability, or genetic information (including family medical history)" (USEEOC, n.d., para. 1).

District-wide harassment policies should be written into the employee handbook, included in new employee orientation, and reviewed periodically. Such policies should include the following:

- Define *harassment* and *aggression.*
- Outline steps employees must take to report harassment.
- Protect complainants and reporters from retaliation.
- Ensure confidentiality when possible.
- Outline investigation protocols.
- Provide standards for corrective action when it is determined that harassment has occurred.

Additionally, *Title IX of the Education Amendments of 1972* requires schools to adopt and publish grievance procedures to investigate and resolve sex discrimination and sexual harassment complaints (U.S. Department of Education, 2021). Schools are liable for permitting harassment to continue once notice of the behavior is made. Therefore school nurse administrators must familiarize themselves with these legal statutes and associated school policies and take prompt action once a report of such behaviors is made.

Workplace Bullying

Workplace bullying is widely talked about in health care, but there is no universal definition (Hawkins et al., 2023). Unfortunately, workplace bullying is not addressed by any law unless it crosses over into the legally defined areas of harassment. Bullying presents as persistent and systematic attempts to humiliate. Incivility presents itself as rudeness, discourteous behavior, gossiping, spreading rumors, and refusal to assist in completion of work processes. Supervisors should be cognizant of risk factors for bullying in employees who are either bullies or who are susceptible to bullying (Hawkins et al., 2023). Supervisor intervention must occur to stop the negative behaviors and to foster safe work environments free of intimidation for students and staff.

School nurses themselves may be at risk of being bullied due to their status as autonomous healthcare practitioners in an educational setting where fellow workers may have limited awareness of the nurse's role complexity (Peters et al., 2021). School nurse supervisors must provide leadership in instances of incivility, bullying, and harassment of nursing staff from administrators, educational staff, student family members, and sometimes even students. An interprofessional and unified approach from all school administrators is needed to address unacceptable or threatening behavior at school, no matter the source. At any time that the school environment is not safe, school security personnel and law enforcement involvement is warranted.

HEALTH SERVICES PROGRAM MANAGEMENT AND EVALUATION

Professional accountability for program management is infused throughout *School Nursing: Scope and Standards of Practice* (2022), calling for the school nurse to

- Participate in initiatives that improve the health of the school community.
- Engage diverse stakeholders in partnerships.
- Collaborate to develop health policies and programming.
- Pursue health services funding.
- Integrate telehealth services to improve student access to care (NASN, 2022).

Attention to high-quality, evidence-based practice in the delivery of health care to students is paramount—whether it is the individual school nurse delivering health services and health programming within one school or the school health supervisor who is responsible for managing the overall school health program in a district or state.

Total Quality Management

The NASN *Framework for School Nursing Practice* (2024) principle, *Quality Improvement*, leads to enhanced school nursing outcomes through systematic processes across the other principles: *Standards of Practice, Care Coordination, Leadership,* and *Community/Public Health*. Quality of practice is a professional standard for all levels of professional school nursing practice (ANA, 2016; NASN, 2022).

Quality does not just happen; it must be intentional and managed. The terms *total quality management* (TQM), *quality improvement*, and *continuous quality improvement* (CQI) are used to identify this activity and connote that quality is a continuous journey rather than an attained event. Quality improvement is a systematic process to analyze and improve practice. TQM supports an organizational culture of service via focus on the customer and organizational performance (Aggarwal et al., 2019). Health quality domains include the following:

- Effectiveness
- Efficiency
- Equity
- Patient-centeredness
- Safety
- Timeliness (Agency for Healthcare Research and Quality [AHRQ], 2020)

Measuring Quality

According to the AHRQ (2020), "a quality measure is a mechanism to assign a quantity to quality of care by comparison with a criterion. Healthcare quality measurement for children is described as the process of using scientifically sound tools to assess the extent to which children are receiving quality healthcare" (Section 5). AHRQ prescribes rigorous and systematic processes to attain quantifiable data using measurement tools that are reliable (obtain the same reading by all persons doing the measurement), valid (measures what it is intended to measure), and standardized (definitions of the data and processes are readily understood and applied in the same way, regardless of who uses them).

Quality measurement can demonstrate the contributions of school nurses and school health programs to the academic success of students. School nurses have many opportunities to demonstrate effectiveness in managing several quality indicators for the student population, such as educational outcomes, health outcomes, and economic savings (Roesler et al., 2022; Wang et al., 2014; Wolfe et al., 2019).

Standardized data are necessary to drive informed decision making for practice and policy development. School health program outcomes include standard data point measurements of school demographics, school health staffing, student chronic conditions, health office visits, and the related disposition of students (Stanislo, 2023b). School nurse care of students with acute, episodic, or chronic conditions; injuries; medications; or special procedures should be documented, as well as parent or teacher consultations/meetings, special education meetings, and home visits. Community agency partnerships and preventive services, such as dental, vision, or mental health services, have important data points. Also consider data from obesity prevention, sexual health, and parenting programs, as well as enrollment in federal/state insurance programs, to demonstrate the value of the school health program.

Evidence-Based Practice

Evidence-based practice (EBP) is a "problem-solving approach to health care using healthcare provider expertise, the best scientific evidence, and the consumer's values and preference to determine and guide the plan of care" (NASN, 2022, p. 101). Attention to quality evidence-based delivery of health care to students is paramount. School nurse administrators must recognize when evidence indicates a need for change in practice and when steps should be taken to better align policy or protocol with the evidence. When embarking upon quality improvement projects, school nurses should design interventions based on evidence. The *Plan, Do, Study, Act Cycle* guides establishment of a goal, design and deployment of an intervention, observation of outcomes, and a decision to abandon or expand the intervention (Bergren &

Maughan, 2019, p. 98; Institute for Healthcare Improvement, 2017). This process should occur within the constraints of nursing's scope of practice and in consultation with school administration and legal counsel. See Chapter 5 for more detailed information regarding quality improvement, evidence-based practice, and school nursing research.

Evaluation of School Health Services

Evaluation of school health services programs is an essential standard of practice for school nurse administrators that provides a systematic, outcomes-based assessment of progress toward program goals (ANA, 2016, 2022; NASN, 2022). Program evaluation must include pertinent stakeholders, including school nurses, school nurse administrators, nonnurse administrators, UAP, teachers, parents, and community members (ANA, 2016, 2022; NASN, 2022). As the primary consumers of school health services, student input should also be incorporated in evaluation strategies as appropriate. The evaluation should be designed to measure desired outcomes.

The design of evaluation models should align with a theoretical and conceptual framework such as the *School Nursing Practice Framework* (NASN, 2016) or the Centers for Disease Control and Prevention's (CDC's) *Whole School, Whole Community, Whole Child* model (2018a). The CDC Program Performance and Evaluation Office provides a *Framework for Program Evaluation* (2017) that is useful for public health settings. This framework includes standards of evaluation, stakeholder engagement, description of the program, evaluation design, evidence gathering, conclusion, and sharing of lessons learned.

The *School Health Index* is a program evaluation tool used by many schools to assess a broad range of school health indices (CDC, 2018b). The School Health Index includes questionnaires, surveys, interviews, documentation review, observation, focus groups, and case studies. School health services stakeholders must be involved in selection of program evaluation methods to ensure buy-in to effectively respond to evaluation results. Accurate and thorough recording of the School Health Index data analysis can drive process improvements in the school health program in support of student success.

In addition to reasons discussed earlier in this chapter, school nurse leaders can use NASN's *National School Health Data Set: Every Student Counts!* (2023a) to supplement evaluation of school health services. School health data sets are useful in the organization, analysis, and reporting of "school demographics and workforce capacity, school health program staffing, student health chronicity, and health office disposition by staff job description" (Stanislo, 2023a, p. 27). Reporting Every Student Counts! data locally to school administrators provides crucial information about service delivery, student needs, and school nurse impact on student access to learning. These data are critical to school administrators' understanding of student health and school health services. Through yearly contribution of these data to NASN's Every Student Counts! initiative, school nurses can inform policy, best practices, and an appreciation of student health status and needs over time (NASN, 2023a).

Some school districts are under the misperception that school nurses are an unwarranted expense and that a nonnurse can accomplish their work. Therefore it is imperative to show that quality school nursing services can have a cost benefit to school districts and to the wider community (Cowell, 2018; Wang et al., 2014). The school nurse should shift the evaluation of their practice beyond task examination and competencies to evaluating their impact on student health and educational outcomes. The *3S Model: Student–School Nurse–School Community* (Fig. 31-3A and Fig. 31-3B) utilizes available data and helps determine what further data can demonstrate school nurse intervention results (Wolfe et al., 2018). In fact, evidence and examples of school nurse impact abound throughout this textbook.

Examples of school nurse outcomes that may influence student health and education outcomes include the following:

- The full-time presence of a school nurse at one school decreased the rate of students being sent home ill by 75% compared with having an aide or secretary handle these cases.
- A school nurse–led an initiative to increase student awareness of *Myplate* portion sizes improved student self-report of dietary intake and estimated calories in seventh-grade students.
- Four families were connected to social services to ensure sufficient food and clothing in the home so their children could come to school ready to learn.
- A school nurse–initiated antismoking program resulted in a 50% decrease in the number of students who reported that they had smoked a cigarette in the past 30 days.
- The school nurse accessed the services of a speaker on cyberbullying free of charge to the school, at a savings to the school of $1,000.
- One child was referred for symptoms of diabetes and one for symptoms of hypertension; both received early diagnosis and early intervention, thus preventing long-term sequelae.
- Safety recommendations by the school nurse regarding playground ground cover resulted in a 25% decrease in playground injuries over 1 academic year.
- An employee stress management program initiated by the school nurse resulted in significant decreases in staff absences, saving the district thousands of dollars in substitute pay.

The usefulness of outcome measures is multidimensional. Administrators and school nurses themselves need to know that school nursing care makes a difference;

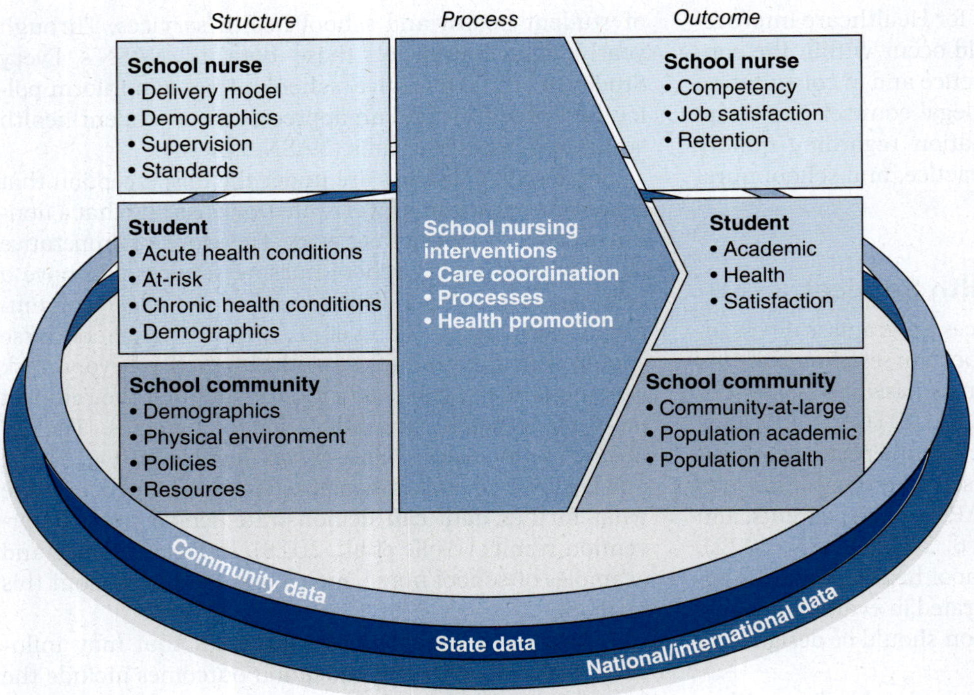

FIGURE 31-3A. The 3S Model: Students–School Nurse–School Community, example 1.

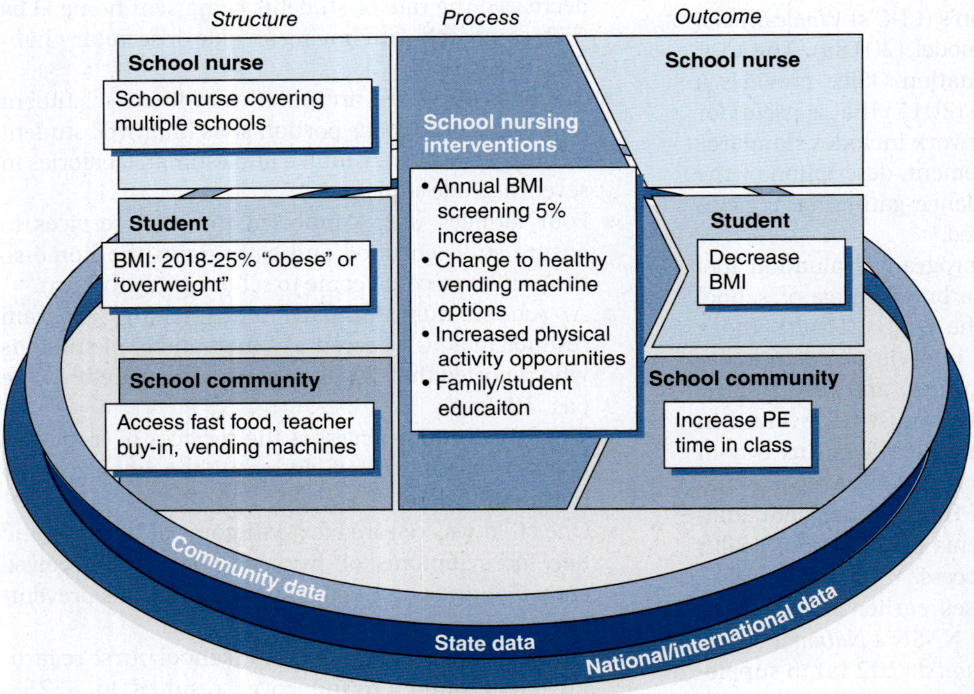

FIGURE 31-3B. The 3S Model: Students–School Nurse–School Cmmunity, example 2. *(Wolfe et al. [2018]. With permission.)*

school boards want to benchmark performance; and taxpayers want to know what they are getting for their money. It is up to school nurse leaders to determine what measures best reflect the efficacy of school nursing practice and demonstrate the impact of school nursing interventions on individual students and the larger school community.

CONCLUSION

Every employee is entitled to competent supervision. School health supervisors and lead school nursing staff must be continuous learners who are able to accept and implement change through proper use, teaching, and mentorship of the future workforce. Each staff member wants a feeling of connection and respect for and from their administration. Therefore the school health supervisor's responsibilities include representing the needs, interests, and well-being of their staff. Being effective in a supervisory role is critical to individual employee and organizational successes.

Effective school nursing management includes the ability to recruit, evaluate, supervise, mentor, and motivate. It requires communication and conflict management skills, as well as knowledge of legal statutes, rules, and regulations affecting practice. The school nurse and the school nurse supervisor have important roles in the development of school health policy based on scientific evidence, as well as in evaluation of one's own practice, evaluation of the healthcare program within one's school, and evaluation of the healthcare program and policies within a district or state.

School nurses must systematically measure and evaluate the outcomes of their care. Not only does measurement demonstrate accountability—it also demonstrates cost-effectiveness and the ability to assist the school in its mission to have students in their seats at optimal levels of health and learning. Policy and program decisions are based on need and what best serves the entire organization. Effective school nurse leadership contributes to improved quality of school nursing care, enhances the health and education that all students deserve, and demonstrates why every child deserves access to a school nurse all day, every day.

References

Agency for Healthcare Research and Quality. (2020). *Understanding quality measurement.* https://www.ahrq.gov/patient-safety/quality-resources/tools/chtoolbx/understand/index.html

Aggarwal, A., Aeran, H., & Rathee, M. (2019). *Quality management in healthcare: The pivotal desideratum. Journal of Oral Biology and Craniofacial Research, 9*(2), 80–182. https://doi.org/10.1016/j.jobcr.2018.06.006

American Academy of Pediatrics Council on School Health. (2016). Policy statement—Role of the school nurse in providing school health services. *Pediatrics, 137*(6). http://pediatrics.aappublications.org/content/137/6/e20160852

American Nurses Association. (2015). *Code of ethics for nurses with interpretive statements.* Author.

American Nurses Association. (2016). *Nursing administration: Scope and standards of practice* (2nd ed.). Author.

American Nurses Association. (2022). *Public health nursing: Scope and standards of practice* (3rd ed.). Author.

American Organization for Nursing Leadership. (2022). *AONL nurse leader core competencies.* https://www.aonl.org/resources/nurse-leader-competencies

Association of State and Territorial Health Officials. (2012). *Emergency volunteer toolkit: Volunteer protection acts and Good Samaritan laws.* https://legacy.astho.org/Programs/Preparedness/Public-Health-Emergency-Law/Emergency-Volunteer-Toolkit/Volunteer-Protection-Acts/

Ballard, K., Haagenson, D., Christiansen, L., Damgaard, G., Halstead, J. A., Jason, R. R., Joyner, J. C., O'Sullivan, A. M., Silvestre, J., Cahill, M., Radtke, B., & Alexander, M. (2016). Scope of nursing practice decision-making framework. *Journal of Nursing Regulation, 7*(3), 19–21.

Benner, P. (1982). From novice to expert. *The American Journal of Nursing, 82*(3), 402–407. https://doi.org/10.2307/3462928

Bergren, M., & Maughan, E. (2019). The school nurse's role in evidence-based practice, quality improvement, and research. In J. Selekman, R. A. Adair, & C. F. Yonkaitis (Eds.), *School nursing: A comprehensive text* (pp. 96–115). F.A. Davis.

Buchan, J., Catton, H., & Shaffer, F. A. (2022). *The global nursing workforce and the COVID-19 pandemic.* International Centre on Nurse Migration. https://www.intlnursemigration.org/2022/01/24/new-report-calls-for-global-action-plan-to-address-nursing-workforce-crisis-and-prevent-an-avoidable-healthcare-disaster/

Campbell, T., & Minor, L. (2017). Supervision of school nurses. In C. Resha & V. Taliaferro (Eds.), *Legal resource for school health services* (pp. 49–54). Schoolnurse.com

Centers for Disease Control and Prevention. (2017). *A framework for program evaluation.* https://www.cdc.gov/evaluation/framework/index.htm

Centers for Disease Control and Prevention. (2018a). *Whole school, whole child, whole community.* https://www.cdc.gov/healthyyouth/wscc/model.htm/

Centers for Disease Control and Prevention. (2018b). *School Health Index.* https://www.cdc.gov/healthyschools/shi/

Combe L. G. (2020). School nurses: Living the framework during COVID-19. *NASN School Nurse, 35*(4), 183–187. https://doi.org/10.1177/1942602X20929533

Cowell, J. M. (2018). Population health: School health services and school nursing. *The Journal of School Nursing, 34*(1), 10. https://doi:10.1177/1059840517748720

Davis, C. R., & Lynch, E. J. (2018). Administrator leadership styles and their impact on school nursing part II. A high-performance school nurse-building administrator relationship model. *NASN School Nurse, 33*(5), 311–316. https://doi.org/10.1177/1942602X18774534

Davis, D., Maughan, E. D., White, K. A., & Slota, M. (2021). School nursing for the 21st century: Assessing scope of practice in the current workforce. *The Journal of School Nursing, 37*(5), 374–386. https://doi.org/10.1177/1059840519880605

DuChateau, T., & Carr, B. (2022). Introducing NASN's medication administration in schools implementation toolkit. *NASN School Nurse, 37*(4), 179–181. https://doi.org/10.1177/1942602X221091845

Duff, C. L. (2020). School nursing—always student-centered: Leading and innovating on the frontlines of the pandemic. *American Nurse Journal, 15*(10), 48. https://link.gale.com/apps/doc/A640512927/HRCA?u=anon~2815424e&sid=googleScholar&xid=974818db

Ellis, P. (2021). Conflict management (art 1). *Wounds UK, 17*(4), 91–93. https://www.wounds-uk.com/journals/issue/653/article-details/conflict-management-part-1

Ellis, P. (2022a). Conflict management (part 2). *Wounds UK, 18*(1), 72–74. https://www.wounds-uk.com/journals/issue/657/article-details/conflict-management-part-2

Ellis, P. (2022b). Conflict management (part 3). *Wounds UK, 18*(2), 67–69. https://www.wounds-uk.com/journals/issue/660/article-details/conflict-management-part-3-dealing-conflict

Ellis, P. (2022c). Dealing with the effects of conflict. *Wounds UK, 18*(3), 67–69. https://www.wounds-uk.com/journals/issue/664/article-details/dealing-effects-conflict

Family Educational Rights and Privacy Act of 1974 (FERPA) (20 U.S.C. § 1232g; 34 CFR Part 99). https://www.law.cornell.edu/uscode/text/20/1232g

Flippo, R. & Helms, C.A. (2022). Case study in academic and school nursing partnerships. *NASN School Nurse, 37*(2), 96–102. https://doi.org/10.1177/1942602X211039884

Galemore, C. A. (2022). Sustaining and retaining school nurses using fish! *NASN School Nurse, 37*(5), 238–239. https://doi.org/10.1177/1942602X221115226

Galemore, C. A., Marion, S., Moran Fossile, K., O'Toole, S., Ragan, K., & Robertson, B. (2022). Leading during a pandemic: A school nurse administrator roundtable. *NASN School Nurse, 37*(3), 155–164. https://doi.org/10.1177/1942602X221084069

Hamlin, K. (2022). Nurse leadership roles: The differences among nurse executives, administrators, and managers. *Nurse Journal.* https://nursejournal.org/resources/nurse-exec-vs-admin-vs-manager/

#:~:text=Nurse%20executives%20are%20the%20top,day%20 activities%20of%20the%20 staff

Hawkins, N., Jeong, S. Y. S., Smith, T., Sim, J., & Clapham, M. (2023). Creating respectful workplaces for nurses in regional acute care settings: A quasi-experimental design. *Nursing Open, 10*(1), 78–89. https://doi.org/10.1002/nop2.1280

Health Insurance Portability and Accountability Act of 1996 (HIPAA) (Pub. L. No. 104–191, 110 Stat. 1936). https://www.gpo.gov/fdsys/pkg/PLAW-104publ191/html/PLAW-104publ191.htm

Individuals With Disabilities Education Improvement Act. (2004), 20 U.S.C. §1400 et seq.

Institute for Healthcare Improvement. (2017). *Tools: Plan-Do-Study-Act (PDSA) Worksheet.* https://www.ihi.org/resources/Pages/Tools/PlanDoStudyActWorksheet.aspx

Jameson, B. E., Anderson, L. S., & Endsley, P. (2022). Identification of workload measurement indicators for school nursing practice. *The Journal of School Nursing, 38*(3), 287–298. https://doi:10.1177/1059840520946833

Jameson, B. E., & Bowen, F. (2020). Use of the worklife and levels of burnout surveys to assess the school nurse work environment. *Journal of School Nursing, 36*(4), 272–282. https://doi.org/10.1177/1059840518813697

Jameson, B. E., Engelke, M. K., Anderson, L. S., Endsley, & P. Maughan, E. D. (2018). Factors related to school nurse workload. *Journal of School Nursing, 34*(3), 211–221. https://doi.org/10.1177/1059840517718063

Karam, S. (2022). Train and retain from orientation to leadership, here are the strategies that experienced staff developers use. *ONS Voice.* https://voice.ons.org/news-and-views/train-and-retain-from-orientation-to-leadership-here-are-the-strategies-that

Kennedy, A. (2019). Nurse preceptors and preceptor education: Implications for preceptor programs, retention strategies, and managerial support. *MEDSURG Nursing, 28*(2), 107–113.

Klein Independent School District. (2018). Sample school nurse job description.

Lacey, K., Prendergast, K., & Resha, C. (2024). In C.A. Resha & V.L. Taliaferro (Eds.). *Legal resource for school health services* (2nd ed., pp. 37–51). schoolNurse.com.

Lowe, A. A., Gerald, J. K., Clemens, C., Gaither, C., & Gerald, L. B. (2022). Medication administration practices in United States' schools: A systematic review and meta-synthesis. *The Journal of School Nursing, 38*(1), 21–34. https://doi.org/10.1177/10598405211026300

Mitts, Carol v. Hillsboro Union High School district 3-8 Jt et al., Washington County Circuit Court Case 87-1142C (1987)

Morse, B. L., Anderson, L., Combe, L. G., Delack, S., Ondeck, L., & Homme, C. (2022). U.S. school nursing job analysis. *The Journal of School Nursing, 38*(2), 126–137. https://doi:10.1177/1059840520930075

Mukhalalati, B. A., & Taylor, A. (2019). Adult learning theories in context: A quick guide for healthcare professional educators. *Journal of Medical Education and Curricular Development, 6*, 1–10. https://doi.org/10.1177/2382120519840332

Mykyta, L., Keisler-Starkey, K., & Bunch, L. (2022 Sept 13). *More children were covered by Medicaid and CHIP in 2021.* United States Census Bureau. https://www.census.gov/library/stories/2022/09/uninsured-rate-of-children-declines.html

National Association of School Nurses. (2016). Framework for 21st century school nursing practice. *NASN School Nurse, 31*(1), 45–53. https://doi.org/10.1177/1942602X15618644

National Association of School Nurses. (2020a). *School nurse workload: Staffing for safe care* (Position Statement). https://www.nasn.org/nasn-resources/professional-practice-documents/position-statements/ps-workload

National Association of School Nurses. (2020b). *The school health services team: Supporting student outcomes* (Position Statement). https://www.nasn.org/nasn-resources/professional-practice-documents/position-statements/ps-team

National Association of School Nurses. (2021a). *Education, licensure, and certification of school nurses* (Position Statement). https://www.nasn.org/nasn-resources/professional-practice-documents/position-statements/ps-education

National Association of School Nurses. (2021b). *School nursing evidence-based clinical practice guideline: Medication administration in schools.* https://cdn.fs.pathlms.com/eMfakewQq20XiLuoim9w?cache=true&_ga=2.251096518.1544331792.16

National Association of School Nurses. (2022). *School nursing: Scope and standards of practice* (4th ed.). Author.

National Association of School Nurses. (2023a). *The National School Health Data Set: Every Student Counts!* https://www.nasn.org/research/everystudentcounts/uniform-data-points

National Association of School Nurses. (2023b). *Supervision and evaluation of the school nurse* (Position Statement). https://www.nasn.org/nasn-resources/professional-practice-documents/position-statements/ps-supervision

National Association of School Nurses. (2024). A contemporary framework update for today's school nursing landscape: Introducing the School Nursing Practice Framework. *NASN School Nurse, 39*(3), 140-147. https://www.doi.org/10.1177/1942602X241241092

National Board for Certification of School Nurses. (2023). *Certification: Eligibility and readiness.* https://www.nbcsn.org/eligibility-readiness/

National Certification for School Nurses. (2025). *Certification.* https://nbcsn.org/

National Coordinating Council for Medication Error Reporting and Prevention. (2021). *About medication errors: What is a medication error?* https://www.nccmerp.org/about-medication-errors

National Council of State Boards of Nursing. (n.d.a). *About U.S. nursing regulatory bodies.* https://www.ncsbn.org/nursing-regulation/about-nursing-regulatory-bodies.page

National Council of State Boards of Nursing. (n.d.b). *Discipline.* https://www.ncsbn.org/nursing-regulation/discipline.page

National Council of State Boards of Nursing. (2016). *Adverse events decision pathway for nurse leaders/administrators.* https://www.ncsbn.org/public-files/21_AEDP_Updated.pdf

National Council of State Boards of Nursing & American Nurses Association. (2019). *National guidelines for nursing delegation.* https://www.ncsbn.org/public-files/NGND-PosPaper_06.pdf

Nelson, L. (2023, February 8). *School nurse staffing in Washington State.* Personal phone and email communication.

Niinihuhta, M. & Häggman-Laitila, A. (2022). A systematic review of the relationships between nurse leaders' leadership styles and nurses' work-related well-being. *International Journal of Nursing Practice.* https://doi.org/10.1111/ijn.13040

Ozdemir, N. G. (2019). The development of nurses' individualized care perceptions and practices: Benner's novice to expert model perspective. *International Journal of Caring Sciences, 12*(2). https://internationaljournalofcaringsciences.org/docs/81_ozdemir_special_12_2.pdf

Parkway School District. (2024). *School nurse evaluation form: Leadership section.* Parkway School District.

Peters, A., El-Ghaziri, M., Quinn, B., Simons, S., & Taylor, R. (2021). An exploratory study of bullying exposure among school nurses: Prevalence and impact. *The Journal of School Nursing, 37*(6), 449–459. https://doi.org/10.1177/1059840519897308

Reising, V., & Cygan, H. (2022). School nurse job descriptions in urban districts: Alignment with the Framework for 21st-Century School Nursing Practice. *The Journal of School Nursing, 38*(4) 410–417. https://doi:10.1177/1059840520963621

Roesler, M., Fato, P., & Obst, B. (2022). Long COVID—The new "invisible" illness: How school nurses can support the nursing and educational teams for student success. *NASN School Nurse, 37*(2), 90–95. https://doi.org/10.1177/1942602X211059427

Russell, K. A., & Radtke, B. K. (2014). An evidence-based tool for regulatory decision making: The regulatory decision pathway. *Journal of Nursing Regulation, 5*(2), 5–9. https://www.ncsbn.org/public-files/21_AEDP_Updated.pdf

Shannon, R. A., & Kubelka, S. (2013a). Reducing the risks of delegation: Use of procedure skills checklists for unlicensed assistive personnel in schools, Part 1. *NASN School Nurse, 28*(4), 178-181. doi:10.1177/1942602X13489886

Shannon, R. A., & Kubelka, S. (2013b). Reducing the risks of delegation: Use of procedure skills checklists for unlicensed assistive personnel in schools, Part 2. *NASN School Nurse, 28*(5), 222-226. doi:10.1177/1942602X13490030

Stanislo, K. J. (2023a). Revisiting the National School Health Data Set: Every Student Counts! *NASN School Nurse, 38*(1), 26–30. https://doi.org/10.1177/1942602X221137519

Stanislo, K. J. (2023b, November 23). Data sharing: HOW to tell your story. *NASN School Nurse,* OnlineFirst. https://doi.org/10.1177/1942602X2312142

Steed, H., O'Toole, D., Lao, K., Nunez, B., Surani, K., & Stuart-Cassel, V. (2022, August 8). State laws on school nursing outline copious responsibilities for nurses. *Child Trends.* https://www.childtrends.org/publications/state-laws-on-school-nursing-outline-copious-responsibilities-for-nurses

Stillwater, A. R. (2018). Medication errors: The school nurse as second victim. *NASN School Nurse, 33*(3), 163–166. https://doi.org/10.1177/1942602X17747294

Texas Board of Nursing & Texas Department of State Health Services. (n.d.). *Algorithms for determining the school RN's role in delegating tasks to unlicensed persons (UP) and supervising tasks delegated or assigned by others.* https://www.bon.texas.gov/pdfs/delegation_pdfs/School%20Nurse%20Delegation%20Decision%20Trees.pdf

Thomas, G. (2019, November 21). *When your most passionate employees become quiet.* Leadershipfirst.net. https://www.leadershipfirst.net/post/when-your-most-passionate-employees-become-quiet

Tsai, S., & McClanahan, R. (2022). Smoothing the way into school nursing practice. *NASN School Nurse, 37*(4), 199–205. https://doi.org/10.1177/1942602X221077236

U.S. Department of Education. (2021). Title IX and sex discrimination. https://www.ed.gov/laws-and-policy/civil-rights-laws/sex-discrimination/Title-IX-and-Sex-Discrimination

U.S. Equal Employment Opportunity Commission. (n.d.). *Overview.* https://www.eeoc.gov/overview

Wallin, R. L., & Rothman, S. (2020). A new framework for school nurse self-reflection and evaluation. *NASN School Nurse, 35*(1), 35–42. https://doi:10.1177/1942602X19852295

Wang, L. Y., Vernon-smiley, M., Gapinksi, M. A., Desisto, M., Maughan, E., & Sheetz, A. (2014). Cost-benefit study of school nursing services. *JAMA Pediatrics, 168*(7), 642–648. https://doi.org/10.1001/jamapediatrics.2013.5441

Willgerodt, M. A., Brock, D., & Tanner, A. (2023). National School Nurse Workforce Study 2.0. Manuscript in preparation. https://www.nasn.org/research/school-nurse-workforce

Wolfe, L. C., Maughan, E. D., & Bergren, M. D. (2018). Introducing the 3S (Student–School Nurse–School Community) model. *NASN School Nurse, 34*(1), 30–34. https://doi.org/10.1177/1942602X18814233

Chapter 32

Funding and Budgeting for School Health Services

Elizabeth Clark

CHAPTER OUTLINE

School nursing is guided by the National Association of School Nurse's (NASN's) *School Nursing Practice Framework* (2024) and *School Nursing: Scope and Standards of Practice* (4th ed.) (NASN, 2022b). The *Leadership* principle of the *School Nursing Practice Framework* includes directing health services, which entails stewardship of program budgets, funding, and reimbursement. Standard 17 of the *Scope and Standards of Practice* is *Resource Stewardship,* which states "that the school nurse utilizes appropriate resources to plan, provide, and sustain evidence-based nursing services that are safe, effective, financially responsible, and used judiciously" (2022b, p. 94). School nurse leaders strive to acquire healthcare funding to support cost-effective, evidence-based school health services that reduce barriers to learning and promote the health of the nation's youth.

National momentum is gaining for the need for reliable financial resources for school health services. The *Future of Nursing Report 2030: Charting a Path to Achieve Health Equity* substantiates funding school health (National Academies of Sciences, Engineering, and Medicine, 2021). Recommendation 5 advises sustainable payment structures, from federal to local, including private and public options directed at supporting school nurses in the provision of school health services. The NASN Position Statement, *Equitable Reimbursement for School Nursing Services* (NASN, 2023), holds that nursing services that are similarly reimbursed in other healthcare delivery systems can also be reimbursed in schools. The National Healthy Schools Collaborative (NHSC) released the *Ten-Year Roadmap for Healthy Schools* in 2022. Priority 2 emphasized the importance of building and maintaining healthy schools through the establishment of sufficient and unbiased funding standards at the federal, state, and local levels.

While school nursing services may appear expensive on district or school budget sheets, these services are an investment with many rewards. The connection between health and learning is well understood (Robert Wood Johnson Foundation, 2019). School nurses have a powerful and positive impact on improving student health and attendance. School nursing/school health services may also be a potential source of reimbursement for school districts. Importantly, investments in essential school health services save society millions of dollars annually in healthcare costs, in addition to reducing costs related to lost parent and teacher productivity (Wang et al., 2014). This chapter reviews potential funding models and cost recovery sources. Proposal writing and marketing skills that promote school health services are discussed. Basic budgeting considerations are outlined, such as managing the essential costs of school health offices and health services staff.

GENERAL SCHOOL FUNDING

Public education in the United States costs billions of dollars each year. During the 2020–2021 academic year alone, $927 billion was spent on primary and secondary schools (National Center for Education Statistics [NCES], 2024). The cost of instruction is expensive in terms of human resources: employee salaries and benefits for teachers, instructional support staff, professional student support services, and administration make up 80% of these expenditures.

Education funding and expenses varied widely among states and within states themselves. In 2020–2021, per-pupil annual spending allocations ranged from lowest in Idaho ($11,700) and Utah ($12,301) to highest in New York ($32,200) and the District of Columbia ($37,800) (NCES, 2024). Public schools attempt to balance budgets calculating incoming revenues with outgoing expenses. In most states, federal funds are passed through state departments of education or state departments of health and are added to state tax dollars made available to pay for public education. The formulas that determine the amount of revenue generated from the federal, state, and local taxes are complex and often politically contentious. Counties, townships, cities, and towns levy their own taxes that contribute to education revenue, typically in the form of real estate taxes. State and local revenues combined constitute most of the school funding that covers the costs of public education in the United States (NCES, 2024).

States use a variety of funding models based on attendance rates, including single count, multiple counts, enrollment period, attendance average, and membership average (Syverson & Duncombe, 2022). The number of students eligible to be included in the attendance count determines the annual allocation of state funds the district received.

The federal government historically provides about 8% of public-school funding, some of which is allotted to school health services. Some funds derive from safety net programs such as Medicare, Medicaid, and Social Security (NCES, 2021). Other funds must be periodically reauthorized, whereby Congress recommends changes, additions, and deletions to specific funding initiatives.

Local and state budget constrictions can result in an imbalanced school health funding equation, especially in states where school nursing services are not legislatively mandated. Consequently, school budgets are at risk for underfunding through traditional school funding sources and are increasingly dependent on a variety of funding streams to support student health services.

School nursing services are traditionally covered under school support services budgets, which constitute approximately 4% of education spending nationally (NCES, 2021). There are multiple and mixed sources of funding for public school nurses. See Figure 32-1. However, over half of school nurses report that they are not aware of how their positions are funded (Willgerodt et al., 2023).

Schools may also receive additional funding in response to national emergencies. In response to the COVID-19 pandemic, the federal government provided several unprecedented and temporary funding streams to K-12 schools. The American Rescue Plan (ARP), Elementary and Secondary School Emergency Relief (ESSER), and Coronavirus Response and Relief Supplemental Appropriations (CRRSA) provided $122 billion in federal funding to safely reopen K-12 schools. This funding was authorized to support student health and well-being by hiring school staff, including school nurses (U.S. Department of Education [USDOE], 2021a, 2021b). Additionally, the Centers for Disease Control and Prevention allocated $10 billion to states for school-based COVID-19 screening testing for students, teachers, and staff in K-12 (USDOE, 2021a). School districts had a spending deadline of September 2024 for ESSER monies, unless an extension was granted until January 2025 (Jordan, 2023).

EVERY STUDENT SUCCEEDS ACT

Federal education dollars were reauthorized in 2015 under the Elementary and Secondary Education Act, called the *Every Student Succeeds Act* (ESSA; 2015). Beginning in the 2018–2019 school year, full implementation of ESSA was mandated to support education system reform, including removal of obstacles that impede students' academic success, such as poor health. ESSA has shifted the locus of control from the federal government to the states, allowing for innovation in addressing the population-focused needs of students. Unfortunately, federal funding allocations are variable and often fall short (Blackborrow et al., 2018).

Through their NASN state affiliates, many school nurses contributed through active voice in advocating for school health services during the ESSA (2015) planning process. ESSA emphasizes the imperative to address the whole child to provide a well-rounded education. Absenteeism, student engagement, and student safety were included among the indicators of success.

Funding for Public School Nurses

NASN
National Association of School Nurses

While bridging health and education, school nursing can sometimes feel like it doesn't fit solidly in either. Funding for school nursing comes from a variety of sources, with 56.0% of public school nurses (RN/LVN/LPN) surveyed reporting that they weren't sure where the funding for their role came from. Of those that responded, the majority were funded by the education sector. Other funding for school nurses include the health department, local organizations, federal and state organizations.

Medicaid Funding in the Education Sector

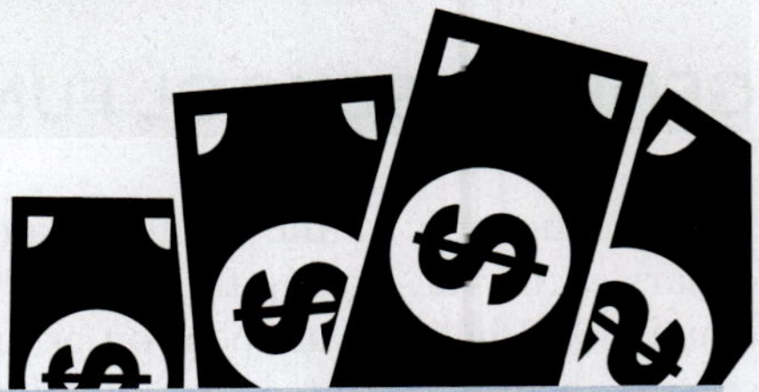

42.3%

of respondents reported their buildings billed for Medicaid.

Medicaid offers a potential sustainable revenue stream to pay for school nurses as schools may bill for certain services performed by school nurses for Medicaid-eligible students (requirements and reimbursable services vary by state).

Sources of Funding for Public School Nurses:

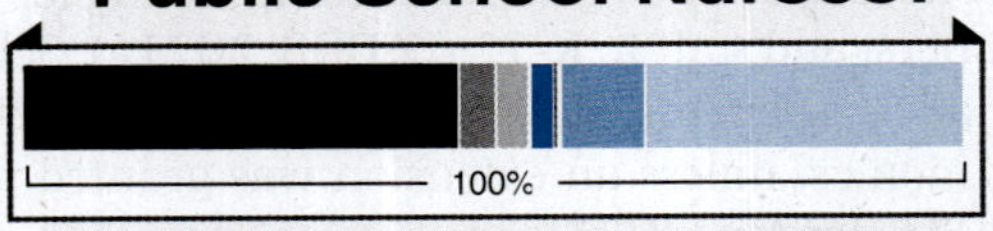

- Department of Education Only: 41.9%
- Health Department Only: 5.3%
- Grants Only: 3.5%
- Special Education funds only: 2.8%
- Medicaid Only: 0.2%
- Other: 14.8%
- Multiple Sources: 31.4%

[NOTE: numbers below show percentages of various entities within multiple sources]

- Department of Education: 63.6%
- Medicaid: 11.5%
- Special education funds: 13.9%
- Health Department: 11.5%
- Grants: 18.5%
- Other: 30.7%

Funding for school nurses is often blended through several sources. Respondents were allowed to select multiple responses; therefore, summed percentages are greater than 100%.

The percentage of schools that bill for Medicaid reimbursements differ by urbanicity and region of the country.

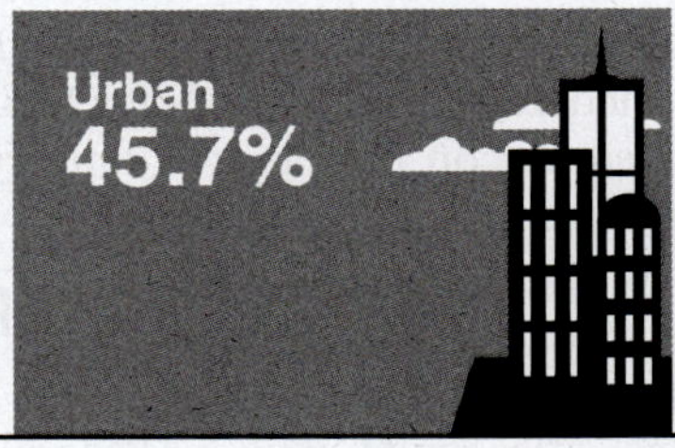

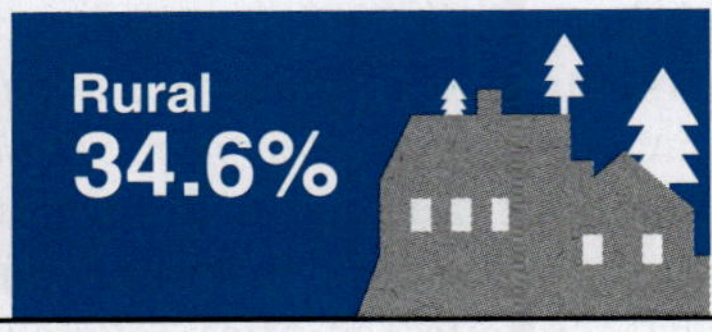

Billing for Medicaid by Region

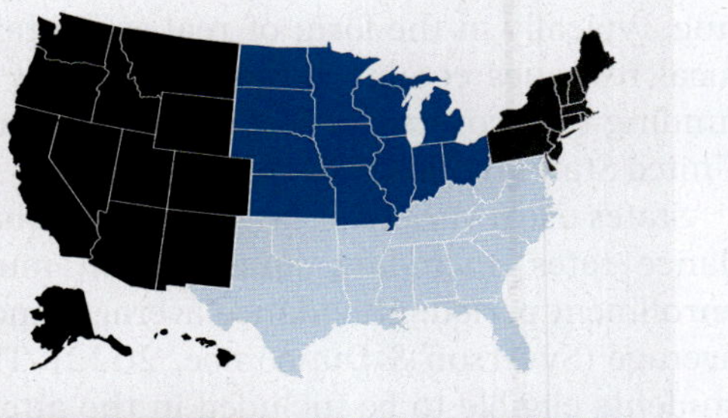

West: 47.3%

Midwest: 45.4%

Northeast: 31.8%

South: 43.2%

These results were obtained during a 2021 study. With a 36.8% survey response rate and variable response rate per survey question, 2,568 respondents reported to be a public school nurse. Of these respondents, 2,392 provided information regarding licensure, with 2,141 reporting as RN and 251 reporting as LPN/LVN.

nasn.org

FIGURE 32-1. Funding for public school nurses. *(Willgerodt, M. A., Brock, D., & Tanner, A. [2023]. National School Nurse Workforce Study 2.0. Used with NASN permission.)*

Did You Know?

ESSA consists of nine sections, called *Titles*, three of which have health-related benefits for students:

- *Title I* funds are intended to provide opportunities for all children to meet the state's student academic achievement standards and are particularly intended to address the needs of disadvantaged children. Such opportunities include necessary health and social services not funded by other sources. Schools can use this funding to develop school-wide health programs, such as hiring a school nurse or counselor, implementing nutrition and physical activity programs, or offering positive behavior and social-emotional support strategies. A community needs assessment must be completed by schools to receive ESSA funding over $30,000. School nurses can contribute valuable school health data to this needs assessment.
- *Title II* provides funds for training, recruiting, and retaining teachers, principals, and specialized instructional support personnel. School nurses are identified in ESSA as specialized instructional support personnel. Title II funds may be used to support effective instruction and improve school climate and safety. School nurses can use Title II training funds to provide training for school staff, to receive training, or to support student behavioral health needs.
- *Title IV,* Part A, is a grant program that combines 49 programs focused on providing a well-rounded education, supporting safe and healthy students, and supporting effective use of technology. The allocation can be used for school-based initiatives directed toward behavioral health prevention programs, such as suicide, drug, violence, bullying, and harassment prevention. Title IV(A) supports school programs that "(ii) support a healthy, active lifestyle, including nutritional education and regular, structured physical education activities and programs that may address chronic disease management with instruction led by school nurses, nurse practitioners, or other appropriate specialists or professionals to help maintain the wellbeing of students" (ESSA, 2015). School nurses are essential to achieving the health and educational outcomes under ESSA (Blackborrow et al., 2018).

MEDICAID FUNDING

According to the U.S. Department of Health and Human Services (USDHHS; 2021), *Medicaid* and the *Children's Health Insurance Program* (CHIP) provide coverage for episodic and long-term health services to millions of eligible low-income and disabled individuals, including approximately 38 million children. Medicaid is a federal financial participation program available to school districts through the Centers for Medicare and Medicaid Services (CMS), the national public healthcare financing program (CMS, 2009a) authorized by *Title XIX of the Social Security Act* (Social Security Administration, n.d.). Every U.S. state participates in Medicaid, even though it is not federally mandated (Bundy & Gormley, 2023).

Medicaid is funded by both the federal government and individual states. Participating states are guaranteed federal matching funds based on state expenditures for Medicaid and the income level of state residents, called the *Federal Medicaid Assistance Percentage.* The state portion for Medicaid funding is typically provided from the state general fund budget (Medicaid and CHIP Payment and Access Commission, 2017).

Although the federal government determines specific guidelines for the administration of Medicaid, it is administered by the states. Thus each state has some flexibility in the creation of its *State Plan Amendments,* which is the Medicaid contract between the federal government and the state. Changes to state plans require federal approval and changes in state laws and regulations. The policies and programs by which individual states administer Medicaid vary widely and are extremely complex, affecting what is funded at the school level (CMS, n.d.). School nurses can educate themselves on their state's administration of Medicaid and actively support enrollment for eligible students and families.

Early and Periodic Screening, Diagnostic, and Treatment

Title XIX of the Social Security Act, also called *Early and Periodic Screening, Diagnostic, and Treatment* (EPSDT), is Medicaid's comprehensive and preventive child health program for low-income children and adolescents (CMS, 2014a). EPSDT is a required service under Medicaid for categorically needy children and youth from birth through age 21 years; children whose families have poverty-level income receive Supplemental Security Income or receive federal foster care or adoption assistance.

EPSDT was created to provide comprehensive healthcare services to ensure that health problems are identified and treated in a timely manner, before becoming more serious and expensive to treat. EPSDT examinations may be performed by or under the supervision of a certified Medicaid provider such as a physician, dentist, nurse practitioner, physician assistant, or other qualified providers under state law to provide primary healthcare services (CMS, 2014a).

EPSDT billing is based on a fee-for-service system, and providers are obligated by Medicaid to bill third-party liable resources. If the state is *not* in a managed care program, a school district may bill Medicaid under the EPSDT program if the district is a qualified provider of covered services for children and if permitted under the state plan. In states with managed care plans, districts may not bill for EPSDT services for students who are enrolled in managed care plans unless otherwise contracted. The goals of the EPSDT program are to ensure the availability and accessibility of required healthcare resources and to help Medicaid recipients and their families effectively use these resources (CMS, 2014a).

School Medicaid

Schools can seek Medicaid reimbursement for the services that school healthcare professionals provide, including school nurses, to increase funding for school health services in schools and access to needed health services for students (Berhmann & Mazyck, 2022). In 1997, CMS published *Medicaid and School Health: A Technical Assistance Guide.* In 2003, CMS developed the *Medicaid School-Based Administrative Claiming Guide* to provide guidance on expenditures for administrative activities that support school-based services and the reimbursement process for these claims. In 2023, CMS in consultation with the U.S. Department of Education released new guidance, *Delivering Service in School-Based Settings: A Comprehensive Guide to Medicaid Services and Administrative Claiming* (CMS, 2023).

The goal of the new guidance is to reduce the administrative burden for local education agencies (LEAs) and school-based providers and expand opportunities for school participation in the delivery of Medicaid services for students (CMS, 2023). Additionally, the *Bipartisan Safer Communities Act* directed CMS to establish a technical assistance center (TAC) and create $50 million in grants for schools to implement or expand medical services in schools through school Medicaid or CHIP (USDHHS & CMS, 2022).

Almost all states reimburse school Medicaid dollars for nursing services. However, unless legislated, school districts have discretion on how these monies are spent. This means that school Medicaid reimbursement dollars may or may not be allocated by the district to help fund school health services (Bundy & Gormley, 2023). For individual schools or school providers to seek reimbursement through Medicaid, the school's LEA must be enrolled as a provider, and the services must be (1) covered under Medicaid, (2) medically necessary, and (3) furnished by a qualified practitioner (CMS, 2023). Federal Medicaid regulations dictate certain Medicaid provider qualifications, whereas other provider qualifications are enacted by the state. When a school or school district offers a variety of Medicaid-covered services, the school must meet all federal and state provider qualifications related to each provided service. In instances where states have enacted provider qualifications, the state standards must be applied universally to all applicants. The health services provided must be among those identified in the Medicaid law and included in the state's Medicaid plan, or be offered through EPSDT (CMS, 2023).

School districts that seek to receive Medicaid reimbursement must have provider agreements in place with the state Medicaid agency. School districts may furnish services directly by qualified school-based providers or through contracts with independent service providers (CMS, 2023).

LEAs must also keep detailed and confidential records of services to students and maintain the records for specified periods in the event of an audit. Historically, many school districts found the issue of *third-party liability* particularly problematic. In the new CMS guidance, school districts may suspend or terminate the process to seek reimbursement from a third party if it is not cost effective to do so (CMS, 2023). Medicaid is traditionally the payer of last resort; however, under the 2023 CMS guidance, Medicaid is the payer of first resort for medical services required in the individualized education program (IEP), individualized family service plan (IFSP), and Section 504 plan services included in the IEP. Due to the complexity of Medicaid billing, many LEAs hire vendors to assist with the billing activities. Although the vendors can provide guidance through the billing process, school districts can also avail themselves of the free technical assistance and information offered by the federal government's TAC and their state Medicaid and education agencies (CMS, 2023).

The Individuals With Disabilities Education Improvement Act

The *Individuals With Disabilities Education Improvement Act* (IDEA, 2004) is a federal civil rights law that mandates partial funding for students with disabilities who receive special education, including nursing/health service minutes (see Chapter 7). When an IEP for students actively enrolled in Medicaid includes school nursing or other health services, the school district can seek reimbursement from Medicaid *if* the related service is specifically outlined in the plan. Likewise, if the IEP indicates, an LEA can submit Medicaid claims for specific transportation services the student needs (e.g., special equipment, shortened route, bus attendant) due to a medical condition on the day that a medically necessary service is provided at school (CMS, 2023).

Free Care

Free Care is described as health services that are provided to all students at school without charge. In 2014, CMS provided clarification to State Medicaid Directors regarding Medicaid payment for services provided without charge. Theoretically, this clarification removed administrative barriers related to Medicaid claiming and provided school districts the opportunity to submit claims for general education students with Medicaid *without* IEPs (CMS, 2014b). As mentioned previously, in 2022 USDHHS and CMS issued an informational bulletin promoting school Medicaid expansion to increase health equity through the delivery of physical and mental health services that are needed (USDHHS & CMS, 2022).

However, practical barriers to implementing the "Free Care Rule" remain due to the complexity of each state's Medicaid plan, as well as how and when states adjust their plans to allow for billing under Free Care. School districts can advocate for the timely and effective implementation of Free Care and seek advice from state Medicaid agencies on how to include Free Care into school claiming activities. Twenty-five states have expanded their state plans through an amendment and serve as models for other states (Healthy Schools Campaign, 2021).

Practice Connection

Important information about school Medicaid resources can be found at the following Web sites:

- Centers for Medicare and Medicaid Services (n.d.). Resources for states. Medicaid technical assistance. Medicaid school-based services.
- National Alliance for Medicaid in Education (NAME; 2022). NAME provides advocacy for the Medicaid in Schools Program.
- Healthy Schools Campaign, Healthy Schools, Promising Futures (2021).

Medicaid Administrative Claiming

Medicaid reimburses LEAs under *Medicaid Administrative Claiming* for activities required for the efficient and appropriate management of Medicaid programs. For administrative services to be reimbursable under Medicaid, the provider furnishing the services must participate in the Medicaid program and participate in a randomized time study (CMS, 2023). LEAs are reimbursed for health-related administrative duties and training, including the following:

- Providing outreach to families, such as assisting families to enroll their children in the state's Children's Health Insurance Program (CHIP) and Medicaid programs
- Referring, coordinating, and monitoring covered services
- Transportation-related activities for Medicaid/CHIP services
- Providing translations related to Medicaid services
- Promoting interagency coordination
- Medicaid and CHIP training
- Developing related policies and programs
- Referral, coordination, and monitoring of Medicaid services (CMS, 2023)

Delivering Service in School-Based Settings: A Comprehensive Guide to Medicaid Services and Administrative Claiming (CMS, 2023) provides guidance to determine whether an activity qualifies for reimbursement. Even if performed in the best interest of the student and their family, activities unrelated to the Medicaid program are generally not reimbursable (e.g., assistance finding suitable housing or community food resources). The activity must be in the approved Medicaid state plan for its related administrative costs to be eligible for reimbursement under the Medicaid program (CMS, 2023). Depending on the size of the school district and whether the district has elected to participate in the federal Medicaid reimbursement programs, school nurses need specifics on how these programs work so they can effectively support their district's participation.

Participation in school programs for Medicaid reimbursement is complicated and time-consuming. The mandated process to obtain parent/guardian permission to submit Medicaid claims for reimbursement is a serious barrier for school systems. The School Superintendent Association (AASA), the National Alliance for Medicaid in Education (NAME), and the Association of Education Service Agencies (AESA) surveyed school districts and school Medicaid leaders to obtain data on the challenges related to the parent consent process. The findings verified that 70% of parents conveyed hesitation in signing a Medicaid consent form, 66% of school staff expressed serious liability with the time commitment for tracking and reaching out to caregivers for unsigned forms, and 56% of survey participants reported that obtaining consent is more challenging today than it was 5 years ago (AASA et al., 2023). Small or underresourced LEAs may find that Medicaid reimbursement for health services and administrative claiming requires more personnel and technical assets than are available to invest in the process. Note that Medicaid compensation covers a portion of the cost; it does not cover the full cost of providing services. However, school Medicaid programming is a valuable source of added revenue for student health services in districts with sizable numbers of Medicaid-eligible students with health-care needs.

Section 1115 of the Social Security Act

The purpose of *Section 1115 of the Social Security Act* is to give the U.S. Secretary of Health and Human Services authority to approve experimental, pilot, or demonstration projects that show promise in advancing Medicaid objectives (CMS, 2005). Section 1115 waivers allow for the provision of health services that would otherwise not be eligible for federal matching funds. Waivers can expand eligibility for individuals who without the waiver would not

Did You Know?

The following is an example of a Section 1115 waiver: Effective July 1, 2001, the Maryland State Department of Education began administering the *Autism Waiver*, targeted to children ages 1 through the end of the semester that the child turns 21. In determining eligibility, a child must be diagnosed with autism spectrum disorder, meet an *Intermediate Care Facility for the Intellectually Disabled* level of care, not be enrolled in any other waiver, have an IEP or IFSP, and receive at least 15 hours of special education and related services per week. The services provided under the Autism Waiver are respite care, family training, environmental accessibility adaptations, family consultation, residential habilitation, intensive individual support services, therapeutic integration, and adult life planning (Maryland Department of Education, 2022).

be eligible for Medicaid. For instance, the savings achieved from the induction of Medicaid-eligible individuals into managed care programs can be used to finance coverage for people previously ineligible for Medicaid. A key factor in the federal decision to accept or decline a waiver is that the pilot cannot be anticipated to cost more than it would have cost without the waiver (CMS, 2005). School nurse leaders are wise to be aware of the status of their state's Section 1115 waivers and educate school administrators of this potential source of financial support for school-based health programs.

Case Management

Defined by Sections 1905(a)(19) and 1915(g)(2) of the Social Security Act, *case management* includes those activities that help eligible individuals under a state's Medicaid plan gain access to necessary medical, social, educational, and other services. It also involves coordinating services to prevent duplication while maximizing the individual's access to those services. A school district's opportunity for reimbursement for case management activities is dependent on the individual state's Medicaid plan and outlined in *Delivering Service in School-Based Settings: A Comprehensive Guide to Medicaid Services and Administrative Claiming* (CMS, 2023).

States have the flexibility to seek approval from Medicaid for reimbursement of several different forms of case management:

- Schools may provide case management as a medical service, such as the coordination of care for specific medical needs identified in EPSDT activities.
- Schools may provide case management under Medicaid waivers, such as when school-related health services are exempted from a state's managed care waiver.
- Schools may provide targeted case management, such as managing services provided to a targeted group of individuals (e.g., students with disabilities who are served under an IEP) (CMS, 2023).

School nurses can play major roles in case management by identifying students' health problems and facilitating contacts among the families, health services, and social services. Case management activities can assist families in identifying, choosing, and maintaining contact with healthcare providers, making appointments, finding transportation, maintaining records, and providing follow-up to ensure that students receive needed services.

ADDITIONAL FUNDING SOURCES

Children's Health Insurance Program

Health insurance coverage is a key factor in determining children's access to and use of health care. In 2021, about 5% (more than 4 million) children younger than 19 years in the United States were uninsured (Kaiser Family Foundation, 2021). This number is unacceptably high. Uninsured children are more likely to go without necessary medical care and more likely to get their health care in emergency departments. The school nurse is often the main provider of healthcare services for many of these children.

As a complement to Medicaid, the State Children's Health Insurance Program (SCHIP) was established as part of *Title XXI of the Social Security Act* (P.L. 105–33 of the Balanced Budget Act of 1997). The goal was to provide coverage to low-income uninsured children who were not eligible for Medicaid. This piece of legislation was the largest expansion of children's healthcare coverage since the inception of Medicaid more than 40 years earlier; it has since been amended in 2022. In 2009, the *Children's Health Insurance Program Reauthorization Act* (CHIPRA) (P.L. 111–3) was established to extend and expand SCHIP, now known simply as the *Children's Health Insurance Program* (CHIP). Note: The similar acronyms can be confusing. CHIPRA refers to the children's health insurance *legislation;* CHIP refers to the children's health insurance *program.*

The Children's Health Insurance Program Reauthorization Act of 2009 (CHIPRA) does not mandate universal insurance coverage for every child, but the Children's Health Insurance Program (CHIP) is designed to provide coverage to eligible uninsured children through age 18 (CMS, 2009b). The purpose is to provide health insurance to children whose families make too much money to qualify for Medicaid, but too little money to purchase private health insurance, such as parents who do not receive or are unable to afford employee-related healthcare benefits. As such, CHIP extends health insurance coverage to millions of children of working families.

Like Medicaid, CHIP is jointly funded by the federal and state governments. Using broad federal guidelines, each state designs its own CHIP by determining eligibility groups and benefits packages, establishing payment levels for coverage, and developing and implementing administrative and operating procedures. As with Medicaid, federal funds are used to match state allocations for CHIP, but at an enhanced rate compared with the rate available to states for Medicaid. However, each state receives a capped allotment of federal CHIP dollars based on the state's actual and projected expenditures, as well as inflation and child population growth factors (CMS, 2009b).

States may be eligible for performance bonuses that encourage the enrollment of eligible uninsured children. CHIPRA requires state CHIP plans to include dental coverage. It also requires mental health parity for states that include mental health or substance abuse services in their state plan. CHIPRA also permits a supplemental dental-only coverage for qualified children who already have other health insurance but no dental benefits. Although CHIPRA excludes adult coverage, the law establishes a statutory option permitting states to use CHIP funds to cover women who are pregnant. States may provide CHIP-covered services through school-based health centers (CMS, 2009b).

The impact of the uninsured population on schools is a significant issue for education. It is the school nurse's responsibility to be aware of potentially reimbursable school nursing services under CHIP and increase access to care by providing information to families about enrollment. CHIP is reauthorized regularly and therefore is subject to political deal-making between and among state and federal policymakers and legislators. Healthcare reform agendas affect CHIP and other federal funding programs for children's health initiatives. School nurses are well positioned to support parents/guardians to enroll their children in CHIP and Medicaid to improve students' access to health care, thereby supporting successful learners (USDHHS & CMS, 2022).

Private Insurance Reimbursement

Some school districts have successfully received reimbursement from private insurance companies for school nursing/health services, even though these monies represent small sources of revenue, and most private insurance carriers do not reimburse for health services provided at school. However, in a changing healthcare landscape, school districts are wise to investigate service agreements with private insurance companies, health maintenance organizations (HMOs), and managed care plans. Telehealth services for physical and behavioral health services is an expanded opportunity for partnership with local hospital systems or community health organizations that are equipped to seek reimbursement from private insurance companies.

Managed Care Reimbursement

Managed care plans administered by managed care organizations combine the delivery and financing of healthcare services into one system to offer their members a broad spectrum of medical services and specialties. According to Medicaid.gov (n.d.),

> *Managed care is a health care delivery system organized to manage cost, utilization, and quality. Medicaid managed care provides for the delivery of Medicaid health benefits and additional services through contracted arrangements between state Medicaid agencies and managed care organizations (MCOs) that accept a set per member per month (capitation) payment for these services. (para. 1)*

Managed care plans profit by keeping their members healthy through increased access to preventive and primary care. Each member is assigned to a primary healthcare provider, often referred to as the *medical home,* who is responsible for coordinating the member's care within the system (CMS, 2023). Managed care has the potential to increase healthcare access, reduce unnecessary care, improve the quality of care, and contain related costs. Managed care plans typically reimburse healthcare providers at a capitated, prepaid premium for providing a set package of health services. In exchange for the premium, the managed care plan accepts the financial liability for provision of the health services package. The managed care plan pays healthcare providers, develops a provider network, and informs providers and plan members about covered services (CMS, 2023).

Approximately 69% of Medicaid beneficiaries are enrolled in managed care (Hinton & Stolyar, 2022). The growth of managed care plans has created complications for LEAs pursuing Medicaid reimbursement for school health services. School providers who operate under the Medicaid fee-for-service practice may find the system very different when a state decides to move its Medicaid beneficiaries into a managed care program (CMS, 1997). When a state is mandated to move Medicaid beneficiaries into managed care, it does so under a waiver. Efforts by states to enroll Medicaid-eligible individuals in managed care programs have increased as states have faced budget reductions and increased healthcare costs.

There are no specific statutory requirements for states to establish relationships between school-based providers and managed care entities. As states apply for waivers related to managed care, CMS encourages collaboration between school districts and managed care plans to establish relationships when waivers are being developed. In many states, *carved-out* direct services do not require a referral by a managed care provider, such as for immunizations, sexual health services, tuberculosis and lead services, and dental and vision care. However, many providers are not aware of such provisions.

Although managed care providers understand primary care delivery, they are not usually well acquainted with school health programs. Therefore school nurses can work with their state Medicaid agency to create a role for themselves in managed care when 1915(b) and 1115 waivers are developed and implemented. Agreements or contracts can be established with managed care organizations that describe each organization's responsibility regarding the provision of health services and the receipt of reimbursements. The details of these agreements need to be locally determined because they will depend on the types of local services that are available from both the LEA and the local managed care providers (CMS, 2023).

School nurses are the ideal healthcare professionals to act as liaisons between their schools and the managed care community because they have the skills and knowledge to effectively communicate with both to ensure that students receive the services they need.

Public and Private Grants

There are numerous sources of outside public and private funds for school-related programs and projects. Many of these resources are narrow categories typically funded for a prescribed amount of time. Grants are usually offered competitively to forward an objective of interest to the funders. Rarely are grants geared toward providing resources for school health services for the general population of students. Consequently, although these funds allow for creativity, the result is a piecemeal approach to short-term, problem- or population-specific funding that is frequently given only once. Even so, school nurses can consider and not overlook these sources of dollars to fill school health budget gaps.

Public grantors and private foundations operate somewhat differently from each other. Public grants may be provided directly to a school district or partner organization. Public grants tend to require more detail, including evidence of need, collaboration with community stakeholders, and an evaluation component. Funding is often more generous and spread over a longer time frame than private grants.

Private foundations tend to supply smaller amounts of funding and applications may be more informal. Grants may be available from the local, state, and national organizations that offer funding for a variety of health initiatives such as behavioral health, oral health, physical activity, or nutrition. Nurses can search the Internet for grant opportunities based on their passion to improve identified health concerns for students. School nurses benefit by developing relationships with local community funders and signing up for e-mail notifications for upcoming grant opportunities.

Small grants are available from nursing organizations, especially for research on the efficacy of school nursing practice. NASN and its state chapter affiliates, the Society of Pediatric Nurses, and local chapters of Sigma Theta Tau International Honor Society of Nursing are excellent beginning sources for research grant money. Dissertation research and doctorate of nursing practice scholarly projects can be supported by grant money from government or other national or organizational funding groups. When a school nurse is involved in research, some portion of the nurse's salary may be paid by the grant.

Local Resources

A variety of local resources may be available to help fund school health programs. Some cities have implemented community-wide children's services initiatives addressing children's needs. Funds to support school programs may be available from local service clubs (e.g., Elks Kiwanis, Lions, Rotary, Shriners, and Soroptimists) and local chapters of professional associations (e.g., American Lung Association, American Heart Association, American Diabetes Association, and American Dental Association). Schools can also partner with regional volunteer organizations such as the American Red Cross.

According to the American Hospital Association (2022), over half of hospitals in the United States operate as nonprofit organizations with tax exempt status. Under the *Patient Protection and Affordable Care Act* (i.e., the ACA) (2010), nonprofit hospitals must meet a *community benefit* requirement to maintain their tax exemption (Rozier et al., 2019). The community benefit requirement stipulates that hospitals provide some level of charity care and support community health improvement based on a community needs assessment. Hospitals have room for flexibility and creativity in how they meet the identified community needs. School nurses can partner with local nonprofit hospitals to meet health needs of their students or support school health programs. For example, providers could develop an initiative to lower emergency department visits of pediatric populations for nonemergency reasons.

Local corporations (e.g., biotechnology companies and pharmaceutical firms) are other sources of funds for schools because these entities have a vested interest in health, particularly in the health of their employees and their families (as well as potential tax benefits). In addition to monetary assistance, some organizations participate in adopt-a-school programs that could offer resources for school health programs.

> **Practice Connection**
>
> The Colorado Department of Education (CDOE) initiated a *School Health Professional Grant Program* funded by marijuana tax revenue in 2015 after recreational marijuana was legalized in the state. The School Health Professional Grant Program was developed to provide funds to school districts to increase school health professionals to address substance use in elementary and secondary schools, including school nurses, school psychologists, school social workers, and school counselors (CDOE, 2022a). The grant funds vary annually based on legislative priorities: $2.5 million dollars were available in 2015, over $12 million in 2017, and slightly over $6 million in 2021 (CDOE, 2022b).

Grant Proposal Writing

A large amount of information on grant writing is available on the Internet, in libraries, at local universities, and through nonprofit organizations and for-profit companies. According to Clark and Carter (2019), successful grant writing entails following the "four *F*'s":

- *Fit:* The goals for the proposal need to align with the funding organization's application request.
- *Fabulous narrative:* A well-written description for the project plan including details for implementation is essential.
- *Follow-through:* Meeting the deadlines for the application and providing additional clarification requested by the funder.
- *Finish-line details:* Active communication with the funder to clear up any questions regarding the approval or rejection of the request.

Important components of the grant writing phase of a project include attention to the specific information required by the funder; use of clear, concise, and persuasive language; and a realistic project budget. Budgets are essential components of grants. Each granting agency will have stipulations on what can and cannot be included in a budget.

It is essential to know these parameters before the grant is written. If the grant is to support a school nurse position, the team writing the grant needs to know how much of the salary can be included and if benefits can be included as well. School system human resources and finance departments are resources for personnel cost information. Depending on the nature of the grant, the grant writing team can inquire about what specific project costs can be funded, such as durable equipment (e.g., computers, supplies, and equipment for the health office) or travel or professional development costs (e.g., meetings or conferences).

In some cases, the school or LEA may be asked to match the funds requested. This requires communication with administration to garner support. Some grants allow matching funds to be in the form of *in-kind* funds, such as release time for the school nurse to engage in the program planning and activities or for a nurse administrator's time to oversee the project.

Some grantors do not allow indirect costs or overhead to be charged. These are resources that will be consumed by implementing the grant, but are not specific just to the project, such as costs to operate a facility or salaries of staff members assigned to coordinate the grant. However, overhead can be accounted for. For example, if the nurse uses grant money to attend a school nurse conference, overhead fees may allow the district to pay a substitute nurse in their absence.

It is imperative to adhere to the technical specifications in grant proposal guidelines. The directions for submission must be followed exactly or the application might be excluded. For instance, many grant proposals will not be considered if the strict page limit is exceeded.

Although larger LEAs may have grant writers, smaller school districts usually rely on professional staff to write grants, in addition to their other duties. Collaboration with larger organizations or university partners (schools/colleges of nursing) can open opportunities for grant-writing support to increase the success of funding. Regardless of whether the proposal is accepted for funding, follow-up with the funder will provide valuable information about the proposal's strengths and weaknesses. This information will be of assistance in preparing future proposals.

In-Kind Funds

Although dollars are essential to keep school health programs and school nurses funded, *in-kind* funds can also be considered as sources of funding. These include programs that support and enhance the mission of the school, as well as donated services and equipment that would otherwise be paid for by the school or district. School systems typically have policies regarding donations. The school nurse should keep a list of donated equipment, supplies, and services and their value. Examples include vision screening equipment donated by the Lions Club or toothbrushes from a local dentist. Parent/guardian–teacher organizations may be reliable resources for in-kind health supplies, such as digital thermometers or blood pressure cuffs. A *wish list* can be prominently displayed in the health office and shared with parent/guardian–teacher organizations or community partners. School nurses should speak with administration before accepting donations and be careful about accepting equipment that may have associated costs (e.g., calibration, warranties, batteries, or expensive replacement parts).

Health System Partnerships

School health services may be paid for by a variety of funding models and sources but are predominantly covered by school districts (Willgerodt et al., 2023). See Figure 32.3. Increasingly, districts are partnering with healthcare systems to manage and fund school nursing services. For example, school nurses in the Austin Independent School District (AISD) are employees of Dell Children's Medical Center and Seton Family of Hospitals (AISD, 2022). The Colorado Children's Hospital provides registered nurses to several Denver metro school districts through contracted services (Colorado Children's Hospital, 2022).

PROGRAM MARKETING TO ENSURE FUNDING

Marketing and public relations are key components for successfully supporting and funding school health services and programs. NASN advocacy tools (2022a) are an excellent resource to market school nursing services. It is essential that school boards appreciate what school nurses do to further the district's mission, vision, and value statements. When budget allocations for health services are being considered, school nurses can communicate with leadership the fact that school nurses provide financial benefits to the school and community and support student well-being and readiness to learn (NASN, 2022a). School nurses can document and report data on standardized school health data sets to administration and stakeholders that demonstrate the value of comprehensive school nursing services (see Chapter 5).

As mentioned previously, most states use complex state school funding formulas tied to some degree of student attendance; schools with higher attendance measures receive more state education funding, and schools with lower attendance measures receive less funding (Syverson & Duncombe, 2022). School nurses can make dedicated efforts to decrease student absenteeism and report their successes to school leadership to demonstrate a positive impact on school funding. Additionally, data can be presented to the school board regarding total dollars recouped in Medicaid reimbursement for school nursing services. School nurses need to convey the message loud and clear: "I make a difference and you need me."

Education policymaking in the United States tends to be based on local priorities and opinions. Decision makers may be more likely to value a school health program that has strong public support from community stakeholders, including parents/guardians, parent/guardian–teacher associations, youth-serving community organizations, civic agencies, respected business leaders, and key private-sector employees. Religious leaders and congregations are often strong allies. A well-organized public relations campaign may help increase school and community awareness of the value of school health programs. An important aspect of marketing is deciding which of the markets is the most important and narrowing the focus based on those determinations. Presenting the school health message in a public forum is a skill every school nurse can develop. Support will follow a school nurse who is competent, knowledgeable, and professional. See Box 32-1 for suggestions on increasing school nurse visibility to stakeholders. Box 32-2 highlights the value of school nursing services.

BOX 32-2

Cost-Benefit Study of School Nursing Services

Results from a *Cost-Benefit Study of School Nursing Services* in Massachusetts validated that quality school nursing services pay for themselves and more. School nursing services in 78 Massachusetts districts prevented an estimated

- $20.0 million in healthcare use costs
- $28.1 million in parents' productivity costs
- $129.1 million in teachers' productivity costs

In total, school health services in these districts were estimated to have contributed a net benefit of $98.2 million. The return on investment was approximated to be $2.20 for every dollar spent (Wang et al., 2014). The authors developed a spreadsheet-based Excel model and data collection instruments to support school nurses to collect data and perform cost-benefit analyses of their own programs. The materials can be found on the NASN Web site by searching *cost-benefit analysis*.

SCHOOL HEALTH SERVICES BUDGET CONSIDERATIONS

LEAs commonly set aside a portion of their annual budgets to address student healthcare needs. Annual state budgets for school health services vary by state. In states where there are no state mandates for school health services, the annual budget can vary greatly from district to district. Budgets also may vary from school to school in districts with decentralized budgets where building level administrators control nursing positions. School nurses and health services administrators have a duty to be involved in the budget process. Decision makers must have a clear picture of core health services that every school can provide, funding streams, and the costs associated with those essential services.

BOX 32-1

Suggestions for Increasing School Nurse Visibility

- *Complete a needs assessment* of the school and community to identify the priority health needs.
- *Be visible.* Speak at school meetings and events. Be present at "Meet the Teacher Night" and encourage families to meet the nurse. Speak to community groups to share what is happening at the school related to health promotion and disease prevention. Get the word out to the local newspaper. Create a school nurse Web site for your school or district. Be active on social media.
- *Participate in ESSA implementation.*
- *Collect data* on predetermined activities to demonstrate the efficacy of your interventions and promote the results in school newsletters and memos to administrators. Examples are return-to-class rates, decreasing exacerbations for asthma, or decreasing body mass index for a grade level.
- *Work with teachers* to identify their classroom needs and develop ways to assist them in the content they need to teach or the issues they must address.
- *Keep the administrator informed* of your ideas and plans. Administrators want to know about policy and program initiatives being planned, especially if the matter might be addressed to the school board.
- *Collaborate with fellow school nurses* in other schools in the district or state to develop a combined campaign to promote the role of, and the need for, school nurses.

School health managers can develop budget proposals in consideration of federal, state, and local mandates; mandated or recommended nurse staffing levels; and screening and EPSDT services. Additional considerations for health services budgets include equipment to support nursing assessment and treatment. Computer technology, including an electronic health record platform, is essential to collect and track data and support continuous quality improvement. Nondesignated discretionary funds are also essential to support unplanned needs that arise during the school year.

In 2020, the Washington State Nursing Care Quality Assurance Commission and the Washington State Office of Superintendent of Public Instruction developed a staff model for school health services. It is divided into two parts. *Part 1: Levels of Nursing Care for Student Diseases and Conditions: Severity Coding* includes a nursing assessment to obtain levels of nursing services essential for individual students in a school setting. *Part 2: School District Model for the Delivery of Health Services* has nursing staffing guidance for the school unit.

Salaries may be covered under the school health services budget or may be under the instructional or support services personnel budget. The recommended minimal preparation for school nurses is a bachelor's degree in nursing (NASN, 2021). Professional school nurses should be paid according to the same salary scale and receive the same benefits as other qualified school professionals in the district. In unionized LEAs, school nurse salaries may be protected by a union contract. Some states require licensure or certification for school nurses, which supports pay parity with certified teaching staff. Costs for school nurses' educational preparation and professional development should be considered.

School health services are provided in a designated health office that has appropriate physical facilities, equipment, and supplies for meeting the health needs of the school community. A budget for supplies can be established. Disposable supplies must be replaced. Durable goods need to be maintained, calibrated, repaired, and replaced as needed. The school nurse can keep an accurate record of the number of supplies used each month to estimate the school's future budget needs. See Chapter 30 for discussion of health office supplies and equipment. See Table 32-1 and Table 32-2 for considerations for school health service budgets.

TABLE 32-1 **Budget Considerations for School Nurse/School Nurse Administrators**

Title	Description	Annual Budget
Nursing Services Personnel	Registered nurse (RN) positions and full-time equivalents (FTEs)	Based on the salaries of the nurses or other professionals in the school, or school district
	RNs or Certified School Nurses	
	Licensed practical nurse/licensed vocational nurse if authorized in state	
	Substitutes for school nurses	
	Nurse administrator(s)	Based on the salaries of administrators in the school district
	Lead nurse(s)	Based on lead teacher or other professional lead position salaries
	Health paraprofessionals/unlicensed assistive health personnel may be included with health services, or in building level budgets	Based on the salaries of paraprofessionals/unlicensed assistive personnel (UAP) in the school district
	Administrative assistant staff	Based on the salaries of administrative assistants in the school district
FTEs to support the department		
	Health screeners	May be employed by the school district or may be contracted services
	Cardiopulmonary resuscitation (CPR) instructors	
Benefits	Health, life, dental, Medicare, pension plans	According to the National Labor Statistics, benefits average 31% (https://www.bls.gov/news.release/pdf/ecec.pdf)
Contracts	Medical advisory	Nurse practitioner or physician
Nonsalary expenses	Cellphone stipends	District pays a monthly rate for the phone plans
	Purchased professional educational services	Funds speakers to provide professional development
	Repairs and maintenance	Funds to repair or calibrate equipment in health rooms
	Mileage reimbursement	Funds for travel between schools and to meetings
	In-service travel	Conference fees, hotel costs (for professional development)
	General supplies	Funds to support new and ongoing health supplies for health room
	Food	Funds to provide food and beverages for staff meetings and trainings sponsored by health services staff
	Technology, computer software, and supplies	Funds software and supplies to support school nurse role

Continued

TABLE 32-1 Budget Considerations for School Nurse/School Nurse Administrators—cont'd

Title	Description	Annual Budget
	Telephone/fax	Costs for phone/fax replacement
	Noncapital equipment	Funds equipment less than $5,000 for school nurses
	Other miscellaneous	Funds unexpected needs that arise during the year
	Copy and printing, mailing, and postage	Funds handouts for required training certificates, letters to families, etc.
	Furniture and fixtures	Desks, chairs, lights, etc.
	Dues and fees	Funds may be used to support professional membership dues

TABLE 32-2 Budget Considerations for the School Health Office

Title	Description	Annual Budget
Health Supplies	Disposable supplies that need regular replacement: first aid supplies, cups, thermometer covers, cot paper, ice packs, gloves, masks, etc.	Often this can be determined based on the number of students attending the school, such as $5 per pupil × 300 students = $1,500 for supplies for the school year.
Health Equipment	Thermometers, otoscopes, blood pressure cuffs, stethoscopes, scales to measure height and weight, etc.	Determine costs of maintenance and replacement of durable medical equipment.
Repair and Maintenance	Audiometers and scales require regular calibration. Vision screening light boxes may need repair.	Determine the cost of calibration and estimate repair costs.
Copy and Print Costs	Printing health education plans and materials for students and parents, such as hand washing, head lice, and head injury sheets.	Determine cost based on average from last year's budget.
Professional Development (PD)	PD for the school nurse and a health office unlicensed assistive personnel (UAP) may be funded by the school budget, rather than the local educational agency budget.	Based on comparable costs of PD for other professional staff in the school: teachers, counselors, and therapists. PD for health office UAP would be comparable to the other professional office staff.
Furniture and Fixtures	Health room desks, tables, chairs, cots, and privacy screens or curtains	Determine cycle of replacement due to the frequent use.
Electronic Health Records (EHRs)	Funds for purchasing, maintaining, and upgrading EHRs	Consider programs that work with school district student data system, state immunization information systems, special education software, and ability to create Medicaid claims.
Dues and Fees	Funds for professional dues, such as NASN membership	Encourage schools to fund NASN membership to obtain vision service plan vouchers to subsidize glasses for students.
Other Miscellaneous	Funds for unexpected items for the health office	Funds for unplanned expenses

CONCLUSION

School nursing services affect academic success and positive health outcomes for students. School nurses serve as a main point of healthcare intervention for students with barriers to accessing health care. Professional school nurses realize the importance of legislation on school funding and advocate for the needs of the students and school community. As experts on school healthcare delivery, it is essential that school nurses understand the issues involved in educational and health funding and spending. School nurses are decision makers that promote funding for school nurse positions and school health resources. It is imperative that school nurses vocally and visibly market the value and benefits of school health programs to gain funder and stakeholder support. School nursing services have proven to benefit the fiscal bottom line; but more important, school nursing benefits the health, well-being, and safety of students, school communities, and society at large.

References

AASA (School Superintendent Association), National Alliance for Medicaid in Education, & Association of Education Service Agencies. (2023). *Obtaining parental consent to bill Medicaid: An unnecessary, time consuming, and emotionally fraught process for districts and parents.* https://www.aasa.org/uploadedFiles/Policy_and_Advocacy/Resources/Medicaid_Parental_Consent_2023.pdf

American Hospital Association. (2022). *Fast facts on hospitals, 2022.* https://www.aha.org/statistics/fast-facts-us-hospitals

Austin Independent School District. (2022). *AISD student health services.* https://www.dellchildrens.net/services-and-programs/aisd-student-health-services/

Berhmann, E., & Mazyck, D. (2022, December 3). Expanding Medicaid services in neighborhood schools makes healthcare more equitable and accessible. *Mathematica.* https://mathematica.org/blogs/expanding-medicaid-services-in-neighborhood-schools-makes-health-care-more-accessible-and-equitable

Blackborrow, M., Clark, E., Combe, L., Morgitan, J., & Tupe, A. (2018). There's a new alphabet in town: ESSA and its implications for students, schools, and school nurses. *NASN School Nurse, 33*(2), 116–122. https://doi.org/10.1177/1942602X17747207

Bundy, B., & Gormley, J. M. (2023). Introduction to school Medicaid for school nurses. *NASN School Nurse, 39*(3), 148-155. https://doi.org/10.1177/1942602X231213604

Centers for Medicare and Medicaid Services. (n.d.). *State Medicaid and CHIP profiles.* https://www.medicaid.gov/medicaid/by-state/by-state.html

Centers for Medicare and Medicaid Services. (1997). *Medicaid and school health: A technical assistance guide.* https://www.medicaid.gov/medicaid/financing-and-reimbursement/downloads/school_based_user_guide.pdf

Centers for Medicare and Medicaid Services. (2003). *Medicaid school-based administrative claiming guide.* https://www.cms.gov/research-statistics-data-and-systems/computer-data-and-systems/medicaidbudgetexpendsystem/downloads/schoolhealthsvcs.pdf

Centers for Medicare and Medicaid Services. (2005). *Section 1115 demonstrations.* https://www.medicaid.gov/medicaid/section-1115-demo/index.html

Centers for Medicare and Medicaid Services. (2009a). *Brief summaries of Medicare & Medicaid.* https://www.cms.gov/Research-Statistics-Data-and-Systems/Statistics-Trends-and-Reports/MedicareProgramRatesStats/downloads/MedicareMedicaidSummaries2009.pdf

Centers for Medicare and Medicaid Services. (2009b). *Children's Health Insurance Program (CHIP).* https://www.medicaid.gov/chip/index.html

Centers for Medicare and Medicaid Services. (2014a). *EPSDT—A guide for states.* https://www.medicaid.gov/medicaid/benefits/downloads/epsdt_coverage_guide.pdf

Centers for Medicare and Medicaid Services. (2014b). *SMD #14-006, Re: Medicaid payment for services provided without charge (free care).* https://www.medicaid.gov/federal-policy-guidance/downloads/smd-medicaid-payment-for-services-provided-without-charge-free-care.pdf

Centers for Medicare and Medicaid Services. (2023). *Delivering service in school-based settings: A comprehensive guide to Medicaid services and administrative claiming.* https://www.medicaid.gov/sites/default/files/2023-07/sbs-guide-medicaid-services-administrative-claiming-ud.pdf

Children's Health Insurance Program Reauthorization Act of 2009 (CHIPRA). (2009). Public Law 111–3. 123 Stat. 8. 42 U.S.C. 1305 (H.R. 2). https://www.medicaid.gov/chip/chipra/index.html

Clark, R. C., & Carter, K. F. (2019). Successful grant applications: Follow the 4 F's. *Nursing, 49*(2), 55–58, https://doi.org/10.1097/01.NURSE.0000552701.73372.b4

Colorado Children's Hospital. (2022). *School nurse program delivers localized care to kids* https://www.childrenscolorado.org/community/community-health/school-health/

Colorado Department of Education. (2022a, November). *School health professional grant program.* https://www.cde.state.co.us/healthandwellness/shpg

Colorado Department of Education. (2022b, July). *2020–2021 school health professional grant legislative report.* https://www.cde.state.co.us/healthandwellness/schoolhealthprofessionalgrantprogram

Every Student Succeeds Act of 2015, Pub. L. No. 114-95 § 114 Stat. (2015). https://www.gpo.gov/fdsys/pkg/BILLS-114s1177enr/pdf/BILLS-114s1177enr.pdf

Healthy Schools Campaign. (2021). *Healthy students promising futures: State data on Medicaid eligible school health services and providers.* https://healthystudentspromisingfutures.org/map-school-medicaid-programs/

Hinton, E., & Stolyar, L. (2022). *10 things to know about Medicaid managed care. Issue Brief.* Kaiser Family Foundation. https://www.kff.org/medicaid/issue-brief/10-things-to-know-about-medicaid-managed-care/

Individuals With Disabilities Education Improvement Act of 2004 (Pub. L. 108-446). https://www.gpo.gov/fdsys/pkg/PLAW-108publ446/content-detail.html

Jordan, P. W. (2023, May 11). *What congressional funding means for K-12 schools.* FutureEd. https://www.future-ed.org/what-congressional-covid-funding-means-for-k-12-schools/

Kaiser Family Foundation. (2021). *Health insurance coverage of children 0-18.* https://www.kff.org/other/state-indicator/children-0-18/

Maryland Department of Education. (2022). *Maryland Medicaid home and community-based services waiver for children with autism spectrum disorder (Autism Waiver).* https://www.marylandpublicschools.org/programs/Pages/Special-Education/autismfactsheet.aspx

Medicaid.gov. (n.d.). *Managed care.* https://www.medicaid.gov/medicaid/managed-care/index.html

Medicaid and CHIP Payment and Access Commission. (2017). *March 2017 report to Congress on Medicaid and CHIP.* https://www.macpac.gov/wp-content/uploads/2017/03/March-2017-Report-to-Congress-on-Medicaid-and-CHIP.pdf

National Alliance for Medicaid in Education. (2022). *About Us.* https://www.medicaidforeducation.org/about

National Academies of Sciences, Engineering, and Medicine. (2021). *The future of nursing 2020–2030: Charting a path to achieve health equity.* Washington. DC: The National Academies Press. https://doi.org/10.17226/25982

National Association of School Nurses. (2021). *Education, licensure, and certification of school nurses* (Position Statement). https://www.nasn.org/nasn-resources/professional-practice-documents/position-statements/ps-education

National Association of School Nurses. (2022a). *Advocacy tools.* https://www.nasn.org/nasn-resources/advocacy-tools

National Association of School Nurses. (2022b). *School nursing: Scope and standards of practice* (4th ed.). Author.

National Association of School Nurses. (2023). *Equitable reimbursement for school nursing services* (Position Statement). https://www.nasn.org/nasn-resources/professional-practice-documents/position-statements/ps-reimbursement

National Association of School Nurses. (2024). A contemporary framework update for today's school nursing landscape: Introducing the School Nursing Practice Framework. *NASN School Nurse, 39*(3), 140–147. https://www.doi.org/10.1177/1942602X241241092

National Center for Education Statistics. (2021). *Revenues and expenditures for public and elementary education: School year 2018–2019 (fiscal year 2019).* U.S. Department of Education. https://nces.ed.gov/pubs2021/2021302.pdf

National Center for Education Statistics. (2024). Public school expenditures. *Condition of education.* U.S. Department of Education, Institute of Education Sciences. https://nces.ed.gov/programs/coe/indicator/cmb

National Healthy Schools Collaborative. (2022). *Healthy schools ten-year road map*. https://www.healthyschoolsroadmap.org/

Patient Protection and Affordable Care Act, 42 U.S.C, § 18031. (2010). https://www.hhs.gov/sites/default/files/ppacacon.pdf

Robert Wood Johnson Foundation. (2019). *Healthy schools research findings from surveys of parents, teachers, and administrators*. https://www.rwjf.org/en/insights/our-research/2019/09/healthy-schools-research-phase—ii.html

Rozier, M., Goold, S., & Singh, S. (2019). How should non-profit hospitals' community benefit be more responsive to health disparities? *American Medical Association Journal of Ethics, 21*(30), 273–280. https://journalofethics.ama-assn.org/article/how-should-nonprofit-hospitals-community-benefit-be-more-responsive-health-disparities/2019-03

Social Security Administration. (n.d.). *Compilation of the Social Security laws: Title XIX—Grants to states for medical assistance programs*. https://www.ssa.gov/OP_Home/ssact/title19/1900.htm#act-1900

Syverson, E., & Duncombe, C. (2022). *Student counts in K-12 funding models*. Education Commission. (Policy Brief). https://files.eric.ed.gov/fulltext/ED617186.pdf

Title XXI—State Children's Health Insurance Program. (P.L. 117-328). (2022, December 29). https://www.govinfo.gov/content/pkg/COMPS-8770/pdf/COMPS-8770.pdf

U.S. Department of Education. (2021a). *Department of education announces American rescue plan funds for all 50 states, Puerto Rico, and the District of Columbia to help schools reopen*. https://www.ed.gov/news/press-releases/department-education-announces-american-rescue-plan-funds-all-50-states-puerto-rico-and-district-columbia-help-schools-reopen

U.S. Department of Education. (2021b). *U.S. Department of Education fact sheet: American rescue act of 2021, elementary and secondary school relief fund (ARP ESSR)*. https://oese.ed.gov/files/2021/03/FINAL_ARP-ESSER-FACT-SHEET.pdf

U.S. Department of Health and Human Services. (2021). *New Medicaid and CHIP enrollment snapshot shows almost 10 million Americans enrolled in coverage during the COVID-19 public health emergency*. https://www.hhs.gov/about/news/2021/06/21/new-medicaid-and-chip-enrollment-snapshot-shows-almost-10-million-americans-enrolled.html#:~:text=In%20the%2050%20states%20that%20reported%20total%20Medicaid,50%25%20of%20the%20total%20Medicaid%20and%20CHIP%20enrollment

U.S. Department of Health and Human Services & Centers for Medicare and Medicaid Services. (2022). *CMCS informational bulletin—Information on school-based services in Medicaid: Funding, documentation and expanding services*. https://www.medicaid.gov/federal-policy-guidance/downloads/sbscib081820222.pdf

Wang, L. Y., Vernon-Smiley, M., Gapinski, M. A., Desisto, M., Maughan, E., & Sheets, A. (2014). Cost-benefit study of school nursing services. *JAMA Pediatrics, 168*(7), 642–648. https://doi.org/10.1001/jamapediatrics.2013.5441

Washington State Nursing Care Quality Assurance Commission & Washington State Office of Superintendent of Public Instruction. (2020, April). *Staff model for the delivery of school health services*. https://doh.wa.gov/sites/default/files/legacy/Documents/6000/StaffModel.pdf

Willgerodt, M. A., Brock, D., & Tanner, A. (2023). *National school nurse workforce study 2.0*. National Association of School Nurses. https://higherlogicdownload.s3.amazonaws.com/NASN/8575d1b7-94ad-45ab-808e-d45019cc5c08/UploadedImages/PDFs/Advocacy/2023-08-28-FundingforPublicSchoolNurses-Final.pdf

Chapter 33

Promoting School Staff Wellness

Eileen Moss ▪ Robin Adair Shannon

CHAPTER OUTLINE

Workplace health programs are widely recommended as evidenced by the *Healthy People 2030* goal to "strengthen the workforce by promoting health and well-being" (Office of Disease Prevention and Health Promotion, para. 1, n.d.). The Centers for Disease Control and Prevention's (CDC's) *Workplace Health Model* provides employers with resources and guidance on the development of health protection, promotion, and disease prevention programs (CDC, 2016). See Figure 33-1. Additionally, one of the 10 central tenets of the CDC's (2018b) *Whole School, Whole Child, Whole Community Model* is Employee Wellness. A comprehensive school employee wellness approach is described by the CDC as "a coordinated set of programs, policies, benefits, and environmental supports designed to address multiple risk factors (e.g., lack of physical activity, tobacco use) and health conditions (e.g., diabetes, depression) to meet the health and safety needs of all employees" (CDC, 2018b, para. 15).

Despite the movement to support workplace health, the policy database of the National Association of School Boards of Education demonstrates that there are vast differences in state policies and protocols that promote the health of school employees (Faggert, 2019). School districts are not alone in the lack of structured programming for employee health. The *Workplace Health Survey in America* demonstrated that in 2017 the prevalence of workplace health programs had increased between 2004 and 2017 but remained low; few worksites have comprehensive health programs (Linan et al., 2019).

Workplace health and wellness programs benefit employees and the employer. Programs can help employees modify their lifestyles to adopt habits to prevent the development of disease, reduce the risk of chronic disease, and manage stress. Additional benefits include improvements in employee emotional, social, spiritual, and financial health (National Association of Chronic Disease Directors [NACDD], 2018). Enhancing the well-being of staff can improve employee retention, resulting in cost savings (Wisconsin Department of Health Services [WDHS] et al., 2018). Employers in general may see a reduction in health care costs and worker's compensation claims, as well as improved employee morale and retention (CDC, 2016).

School nurses support the health and safety of the whole school community, including educational staff. As health professionals in the school environment, school nurses are in a unique position to promote health and initiate change among the health of school staff. The purpose of this chapter is to discuss the school nurse's leadership

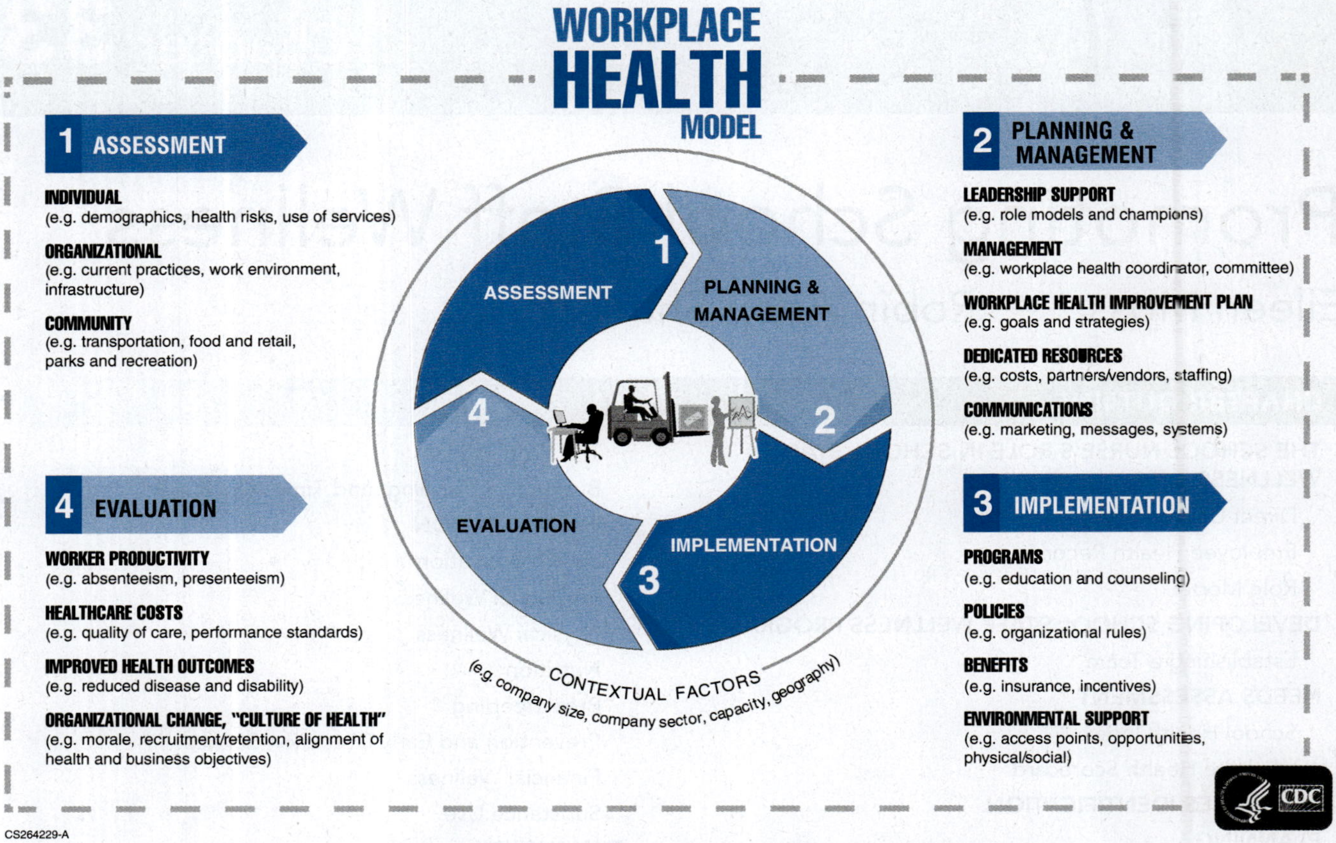

FIGURE 33-1. Workplace Health Model. *(CDC, 2016)*

role in the development and implementation of a school staff wellness program to promote the physical and emotional health of the school community.

THE SCHOOL NURSE'S ROLE IN SCHOOL STAFF WELLNESS

Direct Care of Staff

Typically, school staff wellness programs are population-focused, addressing the health needs of the whole school staff. Additionally, the school nurse can assist in supporting the health of individual staff members who come to school with a wide variety of acute, subacute, and chronic health conditions or who become ill or injured at work. The school nurse acts as first responder in all cases of emergency illness or injury at school and often provides basic first aid for staff. Employee health conditions may require either direct care or monitoring, and some may require accommodations for the individual to be successful on the job.

The extent of direct care that school nurses provide to individual staff members is dependent on state and local laws, as well as school board policy, job descriptions, and local school resources (Morse, 2023). The school nurse should collaborate with school officials to establish the scope of services provided to staff, as well as adequate staffing resources and professional liability coverage. The school nurse's primary responsibility, however, is to provide services to students. Serving in the role of occupational health nurse presents challenges and questions regarding responsibilities, capacity, and liability unless reasonable parameters are set. Responsibilities for staff health should be delineated in the professional school nurse's job description (Morse, 2023).

The practice of schools supplying over-the-counter (OTC) medications for school staff is accepted practice in some schools. However, such practices are not without risk. Policies should be developed regarding the school nurse's role in giving medication advice or dispensing OTC medications to staff members. As in all areas of practice, school nurses should follow the stipulations of their state's nurse practice act regarding medication administration. If the school administration is willing to accept liability for providing OTC medications to staff, a policy should be developed based on legal statutes. Standing orders from a licensed prescriber may be needed. The school nurse should accept medical orders for employees who need rescue medications at school, such as glucagon or epinephrine.

Employee Health Records

School staff employment records are typically maintained by the school or district human resources department. Such records may include each employee's complete physical form, the school district's reasonable accommodation for an employee's disability, workers' compensation claims, accident/incident reports, bloodborne pathogen exposure reports, immunization records, sick or long-term disability records, emergency contact information, and family or medical leave requests. Mental health and substance use assessments may also be required if there is concern about the employee's ability to function in the school setting.

Employee medical records are maintained as a confidential component of the employee's personnel file protected under the Health Insurance Portability and Accountability Act (HIPAA) (U.S. Department of Health and Human Services [USDHHS], 2021b) and regulated by federal laws, specifically the Americans With Disabilities Amendment Act (ADA) (ADA, 2008). Employee health information is not covered under the Family Education Rights and Privacy Act (FERPA), which pertains to student records (U.S. Department of Education, 2021).

In addition to human resource medical records, any medical information that the school employee elects to share with the school nurse is also protected health information under HIPAA. The confidential notes regarding an employee's health created by the school nurse should be kept in a locked file separate from student health records in the health office or in a password-protected electronic health record. An employee's medical information cannot be obtained or shared without a HIPAA-compliant release of information consent form signed by the employee. The school nurse must work with district human resources and records management staff to determine how and where staff health records should be stored. Pertinent protected information about an employee's health condition may need to be shared with administrators, emergency medical services, and police or safety officers when there is a risk of harm to self or others or when the health condition may require emergency treatment (ADA, 2008).

On rare occasions, an employee with a life-limiting health condition may provide the school nurse with a *Do Not Attempt Resuscitation* (DNAR) or *Physician Orders for Life-Sustaining Treatment* (POLST) advance directive. When respecting DNAR requests, careful consideration, planning, and coordination are needed among administrators, the employee, and their family. The district's legal counsel should also be consulted to make sure that the proper policies and procedures are in place to support the employee's wishes in the unlikely event that they should die at school. Many of the factors considered for students with end-of-life orders also apply to employees. See Chapter 20 for more information on DNAR orders in schools.

Role Model

School nurses are systems-level leaders who provide community/public health interventions to improve the health of the whole school community. The *Scope and Standards of Professional School Nursing Practice* (NASN, 2022) states that school nurses, in collaboration with school personnel, are responsible for the health and well-being of the broader school community.

As all nurses know, knowledge about healthy behaviors does not necessarily translate into behavior change in individuals, including themselves. Nurses are more likely to be overweight, get less sleep, and have more stress than the average American adult (ANA Enterprise, 2022). In 2017, the ANA launched the *Healthy Nurse Healthy Nation*™ campaign to improve the health of the nation's 43 million nurses. Healthy Nurse Healthy Nation is a free wellness program that encourages nurses, nursing students, employers of nurses, nursing organizations, schools of nursing, and other stakeholders to take action within the domains of physical activity, rest, nutrition, quality of life, safety, and mental health (ANA Enterprise, 2021). A school nurse who cares for their personal health and well-being serves as a role model to students and staff.

DEVELOPING SCHOOL STAFF WELLNESS PROGRAMS

The number of hours that employees spend at work provides employers with the opportunity to enhance the health and well-being of employees with staff wellness programs. The district should focus on creating an employee-centered wellness culture that includes health protection, health promotion, and disease prevention (CDC, 2016). The school nurse has the knowledge and skills to be an advocate, leader, and provider for school staff wellness programs. The school nurse can advocate for the need for an employee wellness program by providing general data on the benefits of programs. The program should align with the district's mission and vision, strategic plans, and other school health initiatives (NACDD, 2018). Initiatives should use evidence-based resources and available data from the district, and local

Focus on the Framework

The role of the school nurse in promoting employee health is supported by the National Association of School Nurses' *School Nursing Practice Framework* (2024) principle of **Community/Public Health.** The school nurse supports the health of the school community, including the employees. As the professional health expert in the school setting, it is vital that the school nurse is a member of the team that develops the Employee Wellness Program (NASN, 2024).

and state health departments. Employee physical and mental health priorities must be considered.

Establishing a Team

The first step in developing a wellness program is to build a team to approach the initiative. Most of the control of employee health promotion programming lies with the school administration. Therefore it is important to gain the support of someone in a senior leadership position who can assure that the program will have financial and organizational support (Kaiser Permanente, 2021). The responsibilities of the identified key administrator could include the following:

- Approving wellness program plans
- Communicating with the employees about the program and its importance
- Identifying resources such as time, space, and funding
- Facilitating changes to policy and practice
- Ensuring that employee wellness is part of strategic planning and district improvement plans (NACDD, 2018)

Organizational support from teacher and labor unions who represent the best interests of the employees could help support program initiation. Be sure to notify district leadership before engaging union leaders (CDC, 2016; NACDD, 2018).

The next step is to assemble a team or committee to share the responsibilities of creating a program. Include individuals with experience working on other initiatives. Employees with relevant knowledge in health, such as school nurses, school counselors, social workers, athletic staff members, and physical education and health teachers can serve as content experts in program development. Ensure diversity by including individuals from different departments and various levels of the organizational chart. Consider recruiting a representative from the school board and employees from human resources, maintenance, food service, and transportation to provide a comprehensive understanding of employee needs. The size of the committee should be commensurate with the number of employees. See Table 33-1.

The wellness committee work can be facilitated by a nonadministrative leader who has a passion for wellness.

TABLE 33-1 Recommended Size of Wellness Committee

Number of Employees	Number of Committee Members
Less than 300	3–8
300–999	8–12
1,000 or more	12+

Kaiser Permanente (2021).

The magnitude of the responsibilities would warrant a stipend or compensation of time. Responsibilities of the leader would include the following:

- Lead efforts to implement the school district's vision for employee health education, prevention, and wellness.
- Serve as the liaison to district administration, wellness committee, or school board.
- Develop relationships with external partners and serve as the point person for communication.
- Oversee the program and regularly convene the committee.
- Prepare the annual budget and manage purchases and billing for the purpose of ensuring the fiscal stability of the program.
- Monitor outcomes of implemented programs for the purpose of measuring the effectiveness of the wellness initiative (CDC, 2016; NACDD, 2018).

Schools can seem like silos in a large school district. Leadership within each building is necessary to communicate and lead wellness initiatives. A *wellness champion* can serve this role and the individual must be a passionate, enthusiastic leader who is in close proximity to the participants and has the skills to motivate others. The wellness champion can be a volunteer or be assigned to the role. The responsibilities of the wellness champion are to disseminate information about the program, promote activities and programs, generate enthusiasm, provide feedback to the committee, and to assist with on-site wellness activities (NACDD, 2018; WDHS et al., 2018; Wood et al., 2019).

School nurses will recognize that the steps to systematically creating a workplace health promotion program mirror the nursing process. See Figure 33-2.

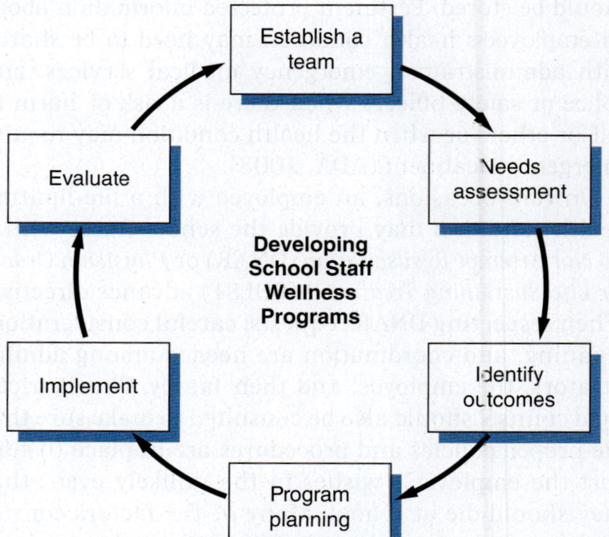

FIGURE 33-2. Developing school staff wellness programs.

NEEDS ASSESSMENT

Gathering information about employee needs and interests, employee health status, existing programs and supports, and district and community resources is instrumental in building a results-oriented wellness program (NACDD, 2018). An assessment of employee wellness can include demographic data, employee attendance records, workers' compensation claims, and data from health insurance carrier claims. Job satisfaction surveys are also a key source of data to elucidate opportunities to improve employee mental well-being and workplace policies (CDC, 2016).

Interest surveys can assess employee behaviors, enthusiasm, and readiness to change to inform the wellness team's planning. An employee wellness program interest survey creates a sense of ownership by allowing school staff to express what health issues are important to them and what activities they would like implemented. The surveys let staff express their opinions confidentially and know their suggestions are valued by the school administration. Box 33-1 provides an example of a school employee wellness program interest survey.

Did You Know?

There are many factors to assess that influence health in the workplace and can be affected by supportive changes within the following levels of influence:

- Individual—elements of an employee's health, such as their health behaviors, health risk factors such as high blood pressure, and current health status
- Interpersonal—elements of an employee's social network, including relationships with managers, coworkers, and family that provide support, mentoring, or role models
- Organizational—elements of the workplace structure, culture, practices, and policies such as benefits, health promotion programs, work organization, and leadership, as well as management support for workplace health and safety initiatives
- Environmental—elements of the physical workplace such as facilities and settings where employees work, as well as access and opportunities for health promotion provided by the surrounding community where employees live (CDC, 2016)

BOX 33-1

Sample Employee Interest Survey for Initiation of a Staff Wellness Program

Our school is planning a wellness program for our employees. Please help us learn more about your health needs and interests by completing this anonymous and confidential interest survey.

A committee of volunteers has reviewed the survey and noted that it took approximately 5 minutes to complete. A summary of the survey results will be communicated in the near future. We sincerely appreciate your help with this important activity. Your participation will help ensure that our health promotion programming meets the unique needs and interests of our employees.

1. What health topics would you like to learn more about? Put an "X" next to your top 5 picks.

_____ Weight loss
_____ Healthy eating
_____ Financial education
_____ Exercise routines
_____ Coping with stress
_____ Smoking cessation
_____ Depression/anxiety
_____ Understanding health insurance
_____ High blood pressure
_____ Cholesterol
_____ Other _______________

2. If the following opportunities were offered through work, mark the ones that interest you with an "X."

_____ Fitness competitions
_____ Nutrition webinars/classes
_____ Money management webinars/classes
_____ Exercise classes
_____ Stress management classes
_____ Smoking cessation resources
_____ Blood pressure testing
_____ Blood tests to rule out diabetes, high cholesterol, etc.
_____ Vaccine clinics—flu, shingles, routine boosters
_____ Discounted gym memberships

3. What do you think is the best way for the school to promote healthy eating?

_____ Have vending machines at work
_____ Provide food in the lunchroom
_____ Provide healthy snacks at meetings
Other: _______________

4. Where are you most likely to exercise?

_____ At home
_____ At a local fitness center
_____ At a workplace
Other _______________

5. If an opportunity to exercise at work were offered, when would you prefer to attend?

_____ Before work
_____ After work

6. Other program considerations—indicate yes or no

_____ I would need childcare to be able to participate in programs.
_____ I have family members who would be interested in participating in programs.
_____ I would be willing to share the cost of certain programs/screenings.

Maine Center for Disease Control and Prevention (n.d.).

Another strategy is to collect individual health information via employee health risk appraisals (CDC, 2016). Health risk appraisals are electronic or hard-copy questionnaires used to gather information about employee health behaviors and health risk factors (e.g., exercise, tobacco, and alcohol use) or biometric health information (e.g., blood pressure, cholesterol levels, and blood glucose). This approach requires occupational health and administrative resources using expertise and experience in storing and analyzing employee confidential protected health information. The employee wellness team may find the de-identified (i.e., anonymous) aggregate data useful in creating wellness programs that target population-focused interventions, rather than focusing on the individual. Therefore the collection of specific individual employee health data must be considered carefully and may be beyond the scope and capacity of the employee wellness team. School districts may face an ethical dilemma and be put at risk for liability if an employee identifies a significant physical or mental health issue and no action is taken to help. Reassure staff that their survey answers and assessment data will be kept confidential and will in no way affect their employment status or eligibility for health benefits (CDC, 2016).

School Health Index

The CDC's (2017) *School Health Index* (SHI) is a downloadable or online health and safety assessment and planning tool for schools. The SHI comes in one version for elementary schools and another for middle and high schools. Each is designed to (1) identify the strengths and weaknesses of a school's health promotion policies and programs; (2) help develop a plan for improving student, staff, and school health and safety; and (3) engage teachers, students, parents, and the school community in health promotion activities. The Employee Wellness and Health Promotion module within the SHI is valuable in assessing the availability, cost, and accessibility of programs to ensure equitable access to all employees (CDC, 2017). The school nurse can be a leader in the interdisciplinary team approach to the comprehensive collection of data of health promotion needs and opportunities. See Chapter 3 for more information on the SHI.

Worksite Health Scorecard

The *CDC Worksite Health Scorecard* (2019) is a free online assessment tool that asks 154 questions to help employers evaluate the effectiveness of their health promotion strategies. Though not specifically designed for schools, this workplace survey assists employers to identify gaps and track improvements in their programs over time. The Worksite Health Scorecard can be used to set priorities for program development based on strengths and weaknesses identified in the following areas:

- Organizational supports (8 questions)
- Tobacco use (8 questions)
- High blood pressure (6 questions)
- High cholesterol (5 questions)
- Physical activity (10 questions)
- Weight management (4 questions)
- Nutrition (14 questions)
- Heart attack and stroke (12 questions)
- Prediabetes and diabetes (6 questions)
- Depression (7 questions)
- Stress management (7 questions)
- Alcohol and other substance use (6 questions)
- Sleep and fatigue (6 questions)
- Musculoskeletal disorders (7 questions)
- Occupational health and safety (9 questions)
- Vaccine-preventable diseases (7 questions)
- Maternal health and lactation (7 questions)
- Cancer (8 questions)

OUTCOMES IDENTIFICATION

It may take months or years to accurately measure the outcomes of the school staff wellness program and determine whether the program has positively affected employee well-being (Marken & Agrawal, 2022). The interventions are designed to enhance career, social, and physical well-being. Career well-being describes an educator's perceived level of support on the job, which can be affected by policy changes. Programs that address emotional support can have a positive impact on employee social well-being. Improvement of physical health and well-being is the goal of exercise and nutrition initiatives. In supporting all areas of well-being, the employer may see outcomes in the form of educator retention and decreased healthcare costs.

PLANNING

Now that the assessment has provided data to direct program development, decisions must be made to fit the needs of the school community. It is not realistic to address all the health needs of the school staff. Rather, priority goals should target the most common and modifiable health issues identified from the needs assessment. The School Health Index suggests that health promotion activities be prioritized by rating their importance, cost, time that it would take to implement the activity, the level of enthusiasm that the activity might generate, and the ease at which the activity could be implemented (CDC, 2017). Consult with the district school improvement team, safety personnel, and committees or groups that make decisions for employee insurance coverage for comprehensive input (NACDD, 2018).

Legal Regulations and Wellness Programs

As the planning phase begins, caution must be used to comply with federal laws. Wellness programs must comply with Title I of the American With Disabilities Act (ADA),

Title II of the Genetic Information Nondiscrimination Act, the Health Insurance and Portability and Accountability Act, and the Affordable Care Act (Federal Register, 2016). These laws prohibit denying access to wellness programs based on disability, provide guidance on conducting medical examinations, set requirements for the collecting and safeguarding of health information, require reasonable alternatives to and limits on incentives, and require that wellness programs be voluntary (NACDD, 2018). Employers must be sensitive to the needs of employees with disabilities and make accommodations as necessary.

Policy Changes

The staff wellness strategies should support as well as guide changes to school and district policies. The health of the entire school community is affected by local policies and the overall school climate. Policies can facilitate access or create barriers to health programs and services. The school physical structure and emotional climate have a direct impact on the daily health and well-being of students and staff. The school nurse can be instrumental in assessing these components and facilitating an organizational response to ensure a healthy and safe work environment. Allowing staff to leave work immediately after student dismissal to attend a wellness class is an example of a supportive school environment specific to worksite wellness. Policies regarding nutritious items in vending machines and food items sold for fundraising activities or at school-sponsored events are examples of wellness policies that have a positive impact on both students and staff.

Wellness Promotion Resources

Schools may already have many resources that can be used to initiate and implement a wellness program, such as physical space and equipment. Most school buildings have a gym or other large room that would facilitate exercise classes. High schools likely have weight rooms, and some schools house indoor swimming pools. Outdoor resources such as playing fields, tracks, and walking paths provide additional possibilities. If school space is not available, community partners such as local health departments, hospitals and health systems, parent organizations, voluntary health organizations, fitness clubs, and civic organizations may have resources, staff, or existing programs that could promote school staff health. Local businesses may be able to donate money, goods, and services. Social media can provide public service announcements or publicity for school-sponsored health events.

The Written Plan

It is essential to put the school staff wellness promotion plan in writing. Establishing a comprehensive plan takes time and energy. Creating an operating plan provides a map of the program's direction and content. The plan should clearly designate what the program intends to accomplish, the methods of accomplishment, and a timeline. Effective plans include the following:

- A wellness mission statement
- Measurable program goals
- SMART (specific, measurable, achievable, relevant, and time-based) objectives (CDC, 2018a)
- A timeline for accomplishments
- Plans of action
- A detailed budget
- An evaluation strategy (CDC, 2018a; WDHS et al., 2018)

Budgeting, Funding, and Time Allocation

Once the desired program elements have been identified, a budget can be finalized. Creating an itemized budget is important regardless of the amount of money available. Examples of budget items include the costs for

Practice Connection

The following initiatives are examples of school staff wellness program offerings that might be outlined in the written plan:

- Preventive services—vaccines, health assessments, and screenings for physical and emotional needs
- Chronic disease management classes or support groups
- Safety and injury prevention within the school setting
- Classes for first aid and cardiopulmonary resuscitation (CPR)
- Physical activity—opportunities to be active in the school environment, such as a walking club or yoga classes
- Nutrition—healthy foods on site, farmers' markets, cooking classes, recipe sharing, and school gardens
- Substance use—education, support groups, and employee assistance programs
- Social-emotional health and stress—implement policies and culture that support work-life balance, professional development, and mental health support classes
- Conflict resolution—policies and workshops
- Sleep—increase natural light in workspaces and offer sleep hygiene classes
- Breastfeeding—provide resources and develop policies that support employees
- Emergency preparedness—emergency response team, staff training, and ensure availability of emergency supplies
- Benefits—health literacy and employee benefit classes
- Financial wellness—financial literacy and retirement planning workshops

CDC (2017); NACDD (2018).

the space, printing, incentives, instructors, speakers, equipment, and staff time. Opportunities for external funding should be explored, such as gifts or grants from nonprofit organizations, corporate sponsorships, philanthropic contributions, fundraisers, incentives from health insurers, and hospital community benefit dollars. Educational resources can be obtained by chronic disease organizations, such as the American Heart Association, American Cancer Society, and American Diabetes Association.

When using the resources on site such as gymnasiums, weight rooms, and outdoor tracks to accommodate physical fitness programs, a school district's building rental policy and schedule need to be consulted before proceeding with planned usage of facilities or equipment. Identify extra costs such as paying for custodial expenses after regular working hours.

One of the biggest challenge in offering educational wellness classes is identifying a convenient time that employees can attend and convincing them of the value in attending. Stipend pay or staff development points incentivizes participation in activities outside of employee contract time. Programs may be offered for employees during duty-free lunch periods, on professional development days, or in combination with faculty meetings. Offering various days and times and online options encourages greater participation in health education programs.

Rewards and Incentives

Health behaviors are controlled by intrinsic and extrinsic motivation. Extrinsic motivations such as weight loss, money, prizes, medals, and praise are generally effective for short-term goals. Longer-term change comes from intrinsic motivation and is obtained by valuing health, finding joy or social connection with exercise, or helping others become healthy (WDHS et al., 2018). The use of rewards and incentives in worksite wellness programs can provide encouragement when tailored to the school culture by helping employees remain committed to the program. Incentives can be monetary such as cash and gift cards, or nonmonetary in the form of recognition with the use of social media, social events, or special recognition or honors. School districts must keep abreast of laws that limit the monetary amount of tax-free gifts (including wellness prizes) that each employee may earn per year. The district's insurance carrier may be another way to supply prizes or rewards. It is recommended that districts provide incentives for participation as well as for achievements to make the program equitable (NACDD, 2018). Ultimately, the goal of worksite health promotion is the establishment of intrinsic rewards that result in feeling better through an improved lifestyle, and not relying on incentives alone.

Program Promotion

Developing appropriate communication strategies to share wellness program planning and progress is critical for the success of the initiative. Communication messages to staff with a focus on what they can gain as opposed to the negative impact of poor health will be more attractive. Multiple modes of communication are necessary to disseminate this information. Simple methods of communication such as social media, e-mails, announcements, bulletin boards, and presentations are effective, but personal outreach by wellness leaders may have the most impact (NACDD, 2018).

IMPLEMENTATION

Interventions are chosen to meet the stated program objectives and focus on the identified employee health risks, needs, and interests. Themed messaging or classes could coincide with national health observances of the month or health awareness weeks/days. Examples of the National Health Observances Calendar include the following:

- January: *Glaucoma and cervical cancer*
- February: *American Heart*
- March: *Colorectal cancer, kidney disease, and nutrition*
- April: *Minority health and STD awareness*
- May: *Physical fitness, women's health, and mental health* (USDHHS, 2023)

See Table 33-2 for a sample calendar of employee health promotion activities.

Health Education

Adults commonly turn to the Internet for health information, which is a rich resource for both valid and spurious information. School staff have varying levels of health literacy and may not always understand what scientifically sound health information is and is not. The realities of the Internet and social media era are that health misinformation and disinformation are rampant across a variety of electronic platforms. According to the American Psychological Association (2024, para. 1), "*Misinformation* is false or inaccurate information—getting the facts wrong. *Disinformation* is false information which is deliberately intended to mislead—intentionally misstating the facts." Therefore an important objective of employee health promotion education is to teach what comprises a reputable source of online health information and how to search and access them. To improve employee self-care, the school nurse can compile a resource list of reputable evidence-based Web sites, such the CDC, MedlinePlus, WebMD, American Heart Association, American Diabetes Association, or health system Web sites. Search and navigation skills should be included in teaching. Health education can also be disseminated through health promotion literature, newsletters, educational sessions, and classes. Any of the following topics would be appropriate for health education initiatives.

TABLE 33-2 Sample School Year Employee Wellness Programming Timeline

Month	Program	Description and Incentive
August	Nutrition classes	Plan topics and schedule dates for fall semester.
	First-quarter fitness classes	Plan and implement a variety of fitness classes held at least one time per week.
	Wellness Champion or building rep meeting	Plan and schedule meeting to update Wellness Champions on upcoming events and programming.
September	Health screening, health risk appraisal, health coaching	Schedule to precede benefit enrollment timeline if participation linked to premium discount.
October	Vaccination campaign	Provide convenient time and location (multiple sites or at each building) for staff, spouses, and children.
November	Healthy Thanksgiving cooking class	Offer after school and have potluck lunch of prepared recipes the next day for lunch.
December	Enjoying a mindful and peaceful winter break.	Offer class on stress reduction techniques for the holidays.
	Second-quarter fitness classes	Modify from first quarter as needed; enroll participants.
January	Nutrition book study	1 week/chapter, self-study with e-mail prompts.
	Begin health tracker step contest	Staff resource to record individual health information.
	Third-quarter fitness classes	Modify from second quarter as needed; enroll participants.
February	Nutrition classes	Plan topics and schedule dates for spring semester.
March	Fourth-quarter fitness classes	Modify from third quarter as needed; enroll participants.
April/May	Jointly with human resources and teacher bargaining unit, begin announcements and promotion for fall semester's health screenings	Allows staff time over summer break to schedule examination with personal physician if desired.
	Compile annual evaluation data	
	Fitness classes	Summer fitness classes; enroll participants.
June/July	Planning for following school year	Seasonal engagement programs to be offered, bulletin board topics, monthly or quarterly newsletter topics

Emotional Wellness

Emotional health and physical health are interconnected, and it is imperative to address both areas in employee health initiatives. Staff well-being is necessary to enhance the education of students (Gray et al., 2017). Interventions that address maintaining a positive organizational culture as well as strengthening personal emotional stability should be included in program planning. To assist teachers and support staff with job-related stress, districts can offer various programs, such as after-school peer support groups, fitness activities, journaling, music therapy, mindfulness training, and Eastern arts (e.g., yoga, tai chi, meditation). Emotional health can affect sleep and teaching methods of sleep hygiene may benefit employees.

School nurses serve as a trusted source to employees in crisis and need to have resources available for prompt referral. It is important to note the difference between school staff wellness programs and *employee assistance programs* that provide confidential individualized counseling to help employees take charge of their health, work, and life. Employee assistance services typically include assistance with workplace conflict, marriage and family concerns, financial issues, stress management, alcohol and drug addiction, and legal consultation. Many employee assistance programs also offer online resources and services, as well as group presentations on various topics (USDHHS, 2022).

Physical Wellness

Physical wellness is one of the most common components of employee wellness programs. The level of physical activity for many Americans is not sufficient to prevent and manage chronic health conditions. Physical activity is one of the most important measures that can be taken to improve health by controlling weight, reducing the risks of cardiovascular disease, diabetes, metabolic syndrome, and some types of cancers. Regular exercise improves bone strength, balance, cognition, and emotional health, as well as increasing the chances of living longer (USDHHS, 2018).

Group workout sessions offer motivation and a sense of community support. Taking the activity to the employee is one strategy to increase physical activity among school personnel. Fitness classes could be offered in an onsite district facility or in various district buildings at a convenient time. Ideally, fitness classes would be offered for a nominal fee and provide a relaxed and comfortable environment

Did You Know?

Adults need at least:

- 2 hours and 30 minutes (150 minutes) of moderate intensity aerobic activity (i.e., brisk walking, ballroom dancing, water aerobics, bicycling slower than 10 miles per hour) every week AND *muscle-strengthening activities* on 2 or more days a week that work all major muscle groups (legs, hips, back, abdomen, chest, shoulders, and arms).

OR

- 1 hour and 15 minutes (75 minutes) of vigorous intensity aerobic activity (i.e., race walking, running, aerobic dancing, swimming laps, bicycling at least 10 miles per hour) every week AND *muscle-strengthening activities* on 2 or more days a week that work all major muscle groups (legs, hips, back, abdomen, chest, shoulders, and arms).

OR

- An equivalent mix of moderate- and vigorous-intensity *aerobic activity* AND *muscle-strengthening activities* on 2 or more days a week that work all major muscle groups (legs, hips, back, abdomen, chest, shoulders, and arms) (USDHHS, 2018).

for the novice and the experienced exerciser. Offering childcare will improve participation among staff who are working parents. Identifying instructors for fitness classes requires networking. There may be district employees certified and willing to teach classes for a stipend or community members in fitness professions. For the safety of employees, it is crucial to use fitness instructors with a degree in an exercise-related field or a certification from a reputable organization. Having each participant sign a waiver releasing the district from any liability is essential.

It is important to consider the various ages and physical abilities among staff when choosing the types of classes to offer. Accommodations must be made for employees with disabilities. Ideas for classes to offer include yoga, Pilates, aquatic exercise, ballroom dancing, classes for toning, and cardiovascular exercises. Some programs, such as weight loss and daily steps challenges, do not require instruction and may be effective for those who are motivated by competition. Fitness tracking devices and mobile applications are effective at helping individuals track their own activity and the activity of competitors. Tracking can increase team encouragement and accountability, thereby heightening the excitement of the challenge (Townsley et al., 2021). Employer health insurance carriers may offer a discount on fitness tracking devices for employees.

Nutrition

A healthy dietary intake is instrumental in overall physical and emotional wellness. The promotion of nutrition in the school environment benefits staff and students. Educators can serve as role models to students by modeling the intake of healthy food choices while at work. Policy changes surrounding food at staff meetings and the provision of water sources in place of soft drinks on school campuses promote staff wellness (NACDD, 2018). Healthy potluck lunches allow staff to try new foods and model healthy habits to the students. Wellness teams should consider displaying nutrition information in the form of posters and bulletin boards as visual reminders of healthy choices. Educational opportunities in the form of classes on reading food labels, food preparation, healthy meal planning, and cooking classes can be led by staff who are passionate about healthy eating. Creative ways to promote nutrition include a school garden and a periodic on-site farmers' market (WDHS et al., 2018).

Breastfeeding

Federal law requires employers who employ more than 50 individuals to provide lactation support in the form of allowing break time and providing a place for employees to express milk during work hours (U.S. Department of Labor, 2022). Breastfeeding is known to enhance the health of infants and therefore has the potential to reduce absences of employees. Part of a wellness program is ensuring that policies are in place to support the health of breastfeeding employees with the accommodations provided by law. Wellness program initiatives are an ideal time to ensure the presence of a policy and to assess how well the district is supporting breastfeeding employees.

Prevention and Early Detection Services

School nurses can facilitate disease prevention and early detection services through a workplace wellness program. A common workplace wellness intervention is providing influenza vaccinations to employees. Flu viruses are detected year-round but typically increase in October and can continue to be present through the end of the school year (CDC, 2022b). Flu viruses can have a significant impact on student and staff attendance at school. The COVID-19 experience immersed schools in disease prevention in ways never before experienced. Although not new, school-located vaccine events (SLVEs) were very important in providing COVID-19 vaccines for staff and the school community (Park et al., 2021). SLVEs are in alignment with goal 4 of the Department of Health and Human Services' *Vaccines National Strategic Plan 2021–2025* to "increase access to and use of all routinely recommended vaccines" (USDHHS, 2021a).

Resources for hosting an SLVE are available on the NASN Web site. Steps in the process of organizing an SLVE include the following (NASN & Association of Immunization Managers, n.d.):

- Obtain district leadership support.
- Identify community partners such as local health department, local hospital, pharmacy, or mobile clinics.

- Collaborate with community partners to develop orders for vaccines, obtain supplies, develop emergency response procedures, obtain liability insurance coverage, create a memorandum of agreement, and outline the billing process, consent process, and privacy procedures.
- Identify location, timing, and target population.
- Create a communication plan to promote the event.
- Collaborate with employee insurance provider to identify potential sources of funding.

See Online Materials (OM33-1) for a *School-Located Vaccination School Nurse Planning Checklist* (NASN & Association of Immunization Managers, n.d.).

In addition to influenza and COVID-19 vaccines, schools may consider offering routine adult vaccinations and boosters. For example, hepatitis A and B, herpes zoster (shingles), tetanus, diphtheria, and pertussis (Tdap), meningococcal, and pneumococcal may be incorporated into the initiative (CDC, 2022a). Bringing vaccines to the staff may increase participation in the prevention campaign because of convenience.

Health screenings are an important component of wellness that are often overlooked by busy adults. The school nurse and wellness team can be instrumental in coordinating on-site health assessments or motivating employees to obtain screenings through their healthcare provider. Blood pressure readings, cholesterol, and diabetes are appropriate for on-site initiatives. Mobile mammography may be considered in a wellness initiative, because it can lead to early detection in asymptomatic individuals (NACDD, 2018; Spak et al., 2022). A referral source for mental health screenings is also important to include in the wellness plan if not provided by the school's employee assistance program.

Financial Wellness

Many college graduates, including educators, enter the workforce with significant student loans. Educators are underpaid compared with other college graduates and teacher pay has been relatively flat for 25 years (National Education Association, 2022). Financial stress can affect job performance and sometimes causes educators to leave the profession. A comprehensive wellness program includes resources for employees to seek assistance in finance management. Classes on financial literacy, credit counseling, retirement planning, and financial planning for life events provide the opportunity for employees to reduce stress related to financial issues (NACDD, 2018). Participants can take advantage of free resources for financial wellness through the federal government (Financial Literacy and Education Commission, 2022; Office of the Comptroller of the Currency, n.d.).

Substance Use

Substance use and abuse can affect job performance and safety and is known to have a negative impact on the health of the employee. Common workplace wellness initiatives geared to reduce the risks of substance use among staff include running a tobacco cessation campaign, running a substance use awareness campaign, and providing substance use resources and information (NACDD, 2018). Employee assistance programs are designed to help employees with personal problems that affect their work performance, including supports for staff who struggle with substance abuse (USDHHS, 2022). An initiative to increase awareness of available services from the employee assistance program is a good way to support employees in need (CDC, 2018b).

EVALUATION

A thorough evaluation of the employee wellness promotion should be conducted to guide future programming. It is important to gather data from the wellness team and the program participants. The program can be evaluated by looking at the process and outcome measures to provide a snapshot of the effectiveness of the interventions (NACDD, 2018). Process measures assess whether the program initiatives were implemented as intended and assess the quality of the interventions. Examples of process measures assessments include examining participation data, evaluating the use of resources, obtaining satisfaction surveys from participants, and making improvements in policies (WDHS, 2018).

Outcome measures assess the health impact on the participants but are difficult to assess until the interventions have been in place for a long period of time. Weight loss, exercise program attendance, and nutrition challenges are examples of initiatives that can be measured by outcomes. Assessment tools such as pre- and post-surveys, focus groups, and feedback from wellness champions can be used to understand employee perceptions of the impact of the program on employee morale, health, and quality of life. Data from the school staff wellness needs assessment can be benchmarked at regular intervals as the health promotion activities are implemented.

School administrators are interested in return on investment calculations. Several strategies may be useful. Tracking the district's employee absenteeism and presenteeism is one measure to evaluate cost savings associated with school staff wellness programs. A sophisticated approach entails collaboration between the human resources department and employer insurance providers to analyze data for associations between wellness program participation and employee healthcare utilization costs. Last, evaluation of programs should include stories of success by participating staff members both during and after the activity. Companies, including schools, need to consider more than numbers; numbers represent people, but it is their stories that educate and motivate others.

Although it may take at least three years to actualize the benefits of an employee wellness program, annual assessments of outcomes are necessary to track progress and to make necessary modifications to interventions and incentives. The expertise of the school nurse is integral to interpreting evaluation results and advocating for effective and timely improvements in health promotion initiatives. Results of the evaluation should be communicated to the school administration, board members, community stakeholders, and participants. And of course—successes should be celebrated! The school nurse's health bulletin board and school Web site are excellent venues to spread the word about the fun and benefits of participating in the school employee wellness program.

CONCLUSION

Through implementation of evidence-based models and team collaboration, employee wellness programs can be developed to enhance the school staff's overall physical and mental health and personal job satisfaction. Employee wellness programs show promise in reducing not only healthcare costs, but employer costs associated with disease and functional disability. Healthy educational staff serve as role models for student health and are more likely to incorporate health into teaching.

The role of the school nurse in promoting employee health is supported by the CDC's *Whole School, Whole Child, Whole Community Model* (2018b); NASN's *School Nursing Practice Framework* (2024); and the *School Nursing: Scope and Standards of Practice* (NASN, 2022). The school nurse provides health expertise and program leadership on the staff wellness committee to deliver health promotion activities that are evidence-based, effective, and fun for school employees.

References

American Psychological Association. (2024). *Misinformation and disinformation.* https://www.apa.org/topics/journalism-facts/misinformation-disinformation#:~:text=Misinformation%20is%20false%20or%20inaccurate,mislead%E2%80%94intentionally%20misstating%20the%20facts

Americans With Disabilities Amendment Act of 2008. 42 U.S.C. § 12101-12102. https://www.ada.gov/regs2016/adaaa.html

ANA Enterprise. (2021, October). Healthy nurse healthy nation year four highlights 2020-2021. *American Nurse Journal.* https://www.healthynursehealthynation.org/~4a9f4b/globalassets/hnhn-assets/all-images-view-with-media/about/hnhn-oct21-issue-921.pdf?__hstc=53609399.e87691f6d18b2f7cb2921739b7ffb d1d.1671805869277.1671820538445.1672497452563.3 &__hssc=53609399.3.1672497452563&__hsfp=626429062

ANA Enterprise. (2022). *Healthy nurse healthy nation.* https://www.healthynursehealthynation.org/?__hstc=53609399.e87691f6d18b2f7cb2921739b7ffb d1d.1671805869277.1671820538445.1672497452563.3 &__hssc=53609399.2.1672497452563&__hsfp=626429062

Centers for Disease Control and Prevention. (2016, May 13). *Workplace health model.* https://www.cdc.gov/workplacehealthpromotion/model/index.html

Centers for Disease Control and Prevention. (2017). *School Health Index: A self-assessment and planning guide.* https://www.cdc.gov/healthyschools/shi/pdf/Elementary-Total-2017.pdf

Centers for Disease Control and Prevention. (2018a). *Evaluation brief: Writing SMART objectives.* https://www.cdc.gov/healthyyouth/evaluation/pdf/brief3b.pdf

Centers for Disease Control and Prevention. (2018b). *Whole School, Whole Child, Whole Community.* https://www.cdc.gov/healthyyouth/wscc/

Centers for Disease Control and Prevention. (2019). *CDC worksite health scorecard: An assessment tool to promote employee health and well-being.* https://www.cdc.gov/workplacehealthpromotion/initiatives/healthscorecard/pdf/CDC-Worksite-Health-ScoreCard-Manual-Updated-Jan-2019-FINAL-508.pdf

Centers for Disease Control and Prevention. (2022a). *Adult immunization schedule.* https://www.cdc.gov/vaccines/schedules/hcp/imz/adult.html?CDC_AA_refVal=https%3A%2F%2Fwww.cdc.gov%2Fvaccines%2Fschedules%2Fhcp%2Fadult.html

Centers for Disease Control and Prevention. (2022b). *Flu season.* https://www.cdc.gov/flu/about/season/flu-season.htm

Faggert, M. (2019, September). Supporting educators through employee wellness initiatives. *Policy update: National Association of State Boards of Education, 26,* 4. https://files.eric.ed.gov/fulltext/ED601007.pdf

Federal Register, The Daily Journal of the United States Government. (2016). *Regulations under the Americans with Disabilities Act.* https://www.federalregister.gov/documents/2016/05/17/2016-11558/regulations-under-the-americans-with-disabilities-act

Financial Literacy and Education Commission. (2022). *Life events.* https://www.mymoney.gov/lifeevents

Gray, C., Wilcox, G., & Nordstokke, D. (2017). Teacher mental health, school climate, inclusive education, and student learning: A review. *Canadian Psychology, 58*(3), 203–210. https://doi.org/10.1037/cap0000117

Kaiser Permanente (2021). *Wellness committee toolkit.* https://docs.google.com/viewerng/viewer?url=http://business.kaiserpermanente.org/wp-content/uploads/2021/03/Kaiser-Permanente-Wellness-Committee-Toolkit.pdf&hl=en_US

Linan, L., Cluff, L., Lang, J., Penne, M., & Leff, M. (2019). Results of the workplace health survey in America. *American Journal of Health Promotion, 33*(5), 652–665. https://doi.org/10.1177/0890117119842047

Maine Center for Disease Control and Prevention. (n.d.). *Good work! Linking health to the bottom line: Cost effective strategies for a healthier workplace.* https://www.maine.gov/dhhs/mecdc/nav-tabs/business-work.shtml#healthwellness

Marken, S., & Agrawal, S. (2022). *Gallup Panel Workforce study: K-12 workers have highest burnout rate in U.S.* Gallup.com. https://news.gallup.com/poll/393500/workers-highest-burnout-rate.aspx

Morse, B. L. (2023). School staff: Provision of health services. In C. A. Resha & V. L. Taliaferro (Eds.), *Legal resource for school health services* (2nd ed., pp. 687–693). SchoolNurse.com

National Association of Chronic Disease Directors. (2018). *Healthy school, healthy staff, healthy students.* https://chronicdisease.org/resource/resmgr/school_health/school_employee_wellness/nacdd_schoolemployeewellness.pdf

National Association of School Nurses. (2022). *School nursing: Scope and standards of practice* (4th ed.). Author.

National Association of School Nurses. (2024). A contemporary framework update for today's school nursing landscape: Introducing the School Nursing Practice Framework. *NASN School Nurse, 39*(3), 140–147. https://www.doi.org/10.1177/1942602X241241092

National Association of School Nurses & Association of Immunization Managers. (n.d.). *School-located vaccination school nurse planning checklist.* https://higherlogicdownload.s3.amazonaws.com/NASN/fb30a5b7-1233-4956-af59-ac9059f01034/UploadedImages/NASN_AIM_School_Located_Vaccination_School_Nurse_Planning_Checklist.pdf

National Education Association. (2022). *Educator pay and student spending: How does your state rank?* https://www.nea.org/resource-library/educator-pay-and-student-spending-how-does-your-state-rank

Office of Disease Prevention and Health Promotion. (n.d.). *Workforce. Healthy People 2030.* U.S. Department of Health and Human Services. https://health.gov/healthypeople/objectives-and-data/browse-objectives/workforce

Office of the Comptroller of the Currency. (n.d.). *Financial literacy resource directory*. https://www.occ.gov/topics/consumers-and-communities/community-affairs/resource-directories/financial-literacy/index-financial-literacy-resource-directory.html

Park, K., Cartmill, R., & Wallin, R. (2021). Preparing for a school-located COVID-19 vaccination clinic. *NASN School Nurse, 36*(3), 156–163. https://doi.org/10.1177/1942602X21991643

Spak, D., Foxhall, L., Rieber, A., Hess, K., Helvie, M., & Whitman, G. (2022). Retrospective review of a mobile mammography screening program in an underserved population within a large metropolitan area. *Academic Radiology, 29*(1). https://doi.org/10.1016/j.acra.2020.07.012

Townsley, M., Waldron, J., Alborn-Yilek, S., Schares, D., Huckstadt, K., McNamara, S., & Gute, D. (2021). School administrators' experiences in a 6-month health and wellness community of practice. *Journal of School Health, 91*(10), 857–866. https://doi-org.proxy.cc.uic.edu/10.1111/josh.13073

U.S. Department of Education. (2021). *Laws and guidance: Family educational rights and privacy act (FERPA)*. https://www2.ed.gov/policy/gen/guid/fpco/ferpa/index.html

U.S. Department of Health and Human Services. (2018). *Physical activity guidelines for Americans* (2nd ed.). https://health.gov/sites/default/files/2019-09/Physical_Activity_Guidelines_2nd_edition.pdf

U.S. Department of Health and Human Services. (2021a). *Vaccines national strategic plan 2021–2025*. https://www.hhs.gov/vaccines/vaccines-national-strategic-plan/vision-and-goals/index.html

U.S. Department of Health and Human Services. (2021b). *HIPAA for professionals.* https://www.hhs.gov/hipaa/for-professionals/index.html

U.S. Department of Health and Human Services. (2022). *Provide support*. Substance Abuse and Mental Health Services Administration. https://www.samhsa.gov/workplace/employer-resources/provide-support

U.S. Department of Health and Human Services. (2023). *National health observances.* https://healthfinder.gov/NHO/nhoyear.aspx?year=2018

U.S. Department of Labor. (2022). *Section 7(r) of the fair labor standards act—Break time for nursing mothers provision*. https://www.dol.gov/agencies/whd/nursing-mothers/law

Wisconsin Department of Health Services, Division of Public Health, Chronic Disease Program, Wisconsin Partnership for Activity and Nutrition. (2018). *Wisconsin worksite resource kit to prevent obesity and related chronic diseases.* https://www.dhs.wisconsin.gov/publications/p4/p40135.pdf

Wood, J., Huggins, A., Clausen, L., & Lailari, S. (2019). Finding fit: School nurses lead the way in the development of employee wellness program. *NASN School Nurse, 34*(4), 205–209. https://doi.org/10.1177/1942602X18811550

INDEX

Note: The italicized *f, t,* and *b* following page numbers refer to figures, tables, and boxes respectively.

B

C

D

E

H

I

J

K

L

M

N

O

P

Q

R

S

U

V

W

Y

Z